High-Yield Q & A Review for USMLE Step 1:

Biochemistry and Genetics

High-Yield Q & A Review for USMLE Step 1:

Biochemistry and Genetics

Michael W. King, PhD

Peggy L. Sankey Professor of Medical Education
Professor of Biochemistry and Molecular Biology
Indiana University School of Medicine
Terre Haute, Indiana

Mc
Graw
Hill

High-Yield Q & A Review for USMLE Step 1: Biochemistry and Genetics

ISBN 978-1-265-55084-4
MHID 1-265-55084-0

This book was set in Adobe Garamond Pro by KnowledgeWorks Global Ltd.
The editor was Michael Weitz.
The production supervisor was Catherine H. Saggese.
Project management was provided by Abhishek Singh, KnowledgeWorks Global Ltd.

Contents

Preface

This High-Yield Q&A review text has been designed with the intention of preparing individuals, including current medical students as well as medical graduates, for the Biochemistry and Medical Genetics questions in the USMLE Step 1 exam. To accomplish this goal, there are 35 chapters that briefly review the high-yield concepts of Metabolic Biochemistry, Cellular and Molecular Biology, and Medical Genetics. Each chapter emphasizes the integration of these concepts to physiology, pharmacology, and pathology and to important diseases associated with defects in these processes. In this update, several topics have been added such as lipoprotein lipase synthesis and functions in Chapter 16, apoptosis in Chapter 34, and uniparental disomy (UPD) in Chapter 35. In addition, several new Clinical Boxes have been added including Cori disease in Chapter 7, Fabry disease in Chapter 12, Familial chylomicronemia syndrome (FCS) in Chapter 16, and cystic fibrosis in Chapter 25.

To aid in the preparation for the USMLE Step 1 exam, the text now includes **1038** multiple choice questions, throughout each of the chapters. This is an increase of 150 questions from the initial printing, which includes 32 new questions in the Medical Genetics section. These questions are formatted in the current NBME Item format or the USMLE Step 1 format. Nearly all 1038 questions are written as clinical or laboratory vignettes.

Many questions in this text utilize the double- and triple-jump format of NBME questions. This refers to a style of question where the student is required to recognize one or two related concepts (eg, pathophysiology and pharmacology) and then use that knowledge to conclude the most correct option to the question that may be biochemistry (or some other subject) related. As such, these questions require a knowledge base that exceeds the primary topics of Biochemistry and Genetics that are reviewed in this text, similar to what is required to successfully answer USMLE Step 1 questions.

In keeping with the focus of the Step 1 exam being about process, there are numerous questions with similar question stems but that ask distinctly different questions. In addition, many questions have more than one correct answer but only one of which is the most correct. The purpose of including similar, yet distinct questions, as well as questions with more than one possible correct answer, is to ensure that students obtain a clear idea of the different ways the NBME prepares questions for its assessments that cover the same concept yet asks the student to utilize their knowledge base and their problem-solving skills to determine the single best answer.

This review book is divided into five broad sections. The first section, Foundational Biochemistry, covers the basics of the major building blocks of all cells and tissues, protein structure-function relationships, and the role of vitamins and minerals in metabolic processes including enzymes. The second section, Metabolic Biochemistry, and by far the major bulk of any Medical Biochemistry text, covers metabolic biochemistry with a strong emphasis on clinical correlations and clinical disorders related to these all-important pathways. The third section, Cellular and Molecular Biology, reviews the concepts of DNA, RNA, and protein metabolism, cellular structures and the components of these structures, signal transduction processes, and the molecular tools utilized in the diagnosis and treatment of disease. The fourth section, Integrative Biochemistry, reviews the concepts of digestive processes, insulin and diabetes, hormones, blood coagulation, and cancer. The fifth section, Medical Genetics, reviews the high-yield concepts of medical genetics including single-gene inheritance, population genetics, cytogenetics, and linkage.

Every chapter begins with a list of high-yield terms related to the included content. Each chapter includes numerous explanatory figures and tables aimed at allowing increased understanding and focus on the critical high-yield content. Most chapters include detailed Clinical Boxes that describe and discuss the high-yield information concerning diseases and disorders related to defects in the processes being reviewed. Although every chapter does not warrant one or more Clinical Boxes, there are over 95 such high-yield topics throughout the book. Each chapter content section is followed by a series of multiple-choice questions. Following the questions, there are detailed explanations as to why the correct choice is the most correct, as well as explanations as to why the other options do not represent the most correct choice. Finally, at the end of each section or chapter is a Checklist designed to refocus the reader to the most important and high-yield concepts covered by each chapter. If a student finds concepts and/or content confusing or unclear when completing any chapter, it is highly recommended that for further detailed information they go to http://themedicalbiochemistrypage.org. This is the most complete resource for a more comprehensive study of the material reviewed in this book, excluding the Medical Genetics content.

Acknowledgments

I would like to acknowledge the invaluable contributions provided by the McGraw Hill editorial team of Michael Weitz and Catherine Saggese and Abhishek Singh from KnowledgeWorks Global for helping make this review text successful. I am grateful to the Peggy L Sankey family for their kind and generous support of my endeavors to provide the best possible medical education to students around the globe. Finally, I would like to thank my wife Kara Wright for her incredible support and encouragement throughout the process of completing the updating of this text.

PART I FOUNDATIONAL BIOCHEMISTRY

CHAPTER 1

Biological Building Blocks

High-Yield Terms	Ionic Equilibrium
pH	Defined as the negative logarithm of the hydrogen ion (H^+) concentration of any given solution
pK_a	Represents a relationship between pH and the equilibrium constant (K_a) for the dissociation of weak acids and bases in a solution. The value of pK_a is the negative logarithm of K_a
Isoelectric point	Defines the pH at which a molecule or substance carries no net electric charge
Henderson-Hasselbalch equation	Defines the relationship between pH and pK_a for any dissociation reaction of a weak acid or base such that when the concentration of any conjugate base (A^-) and its acid (HA) is equal, the pK_a for that dissociation is equivalent to the pH of the solution
Buffering	Relates to the property that when the pH of a solution is close to the pK_a of a weak acid or base, the addition of more acid or base will not result in appreciable change in the pH

High-Yield Terms	Amino Acids
α-Amino group	The $-NH_2$ (primary amine) group attached to the tetrahedral α-carbon
α-Carboxylate group	The –COOH group attached to the tetrahedral α-carbon
R-group	Constitutes the side chain that is unique to each amino acid

High-Yield Terms	Carbohydrates
Carbohydrate	Any organic molecule composed exclusively of carbon, hydrogen, and oxygen where the hydrogen to oxygen ratio is usually 2:1; biological synonym is saccharide, commonly called sugar
Saccharide	Synonym for carbohydrate in biological systems; lay terminology is sugar
Aldose	A monosaccharide that contains only one aldehyde (–CH=O) group per molecule
Ketose	A monosaccharide that contains only one ketone (–C=O) group per molecule
Glycosidic bond	Any of the type of covalent bond that joins a carbohydrate molecule to another group

High-Yield Terms	Lipids
Essential fatty acid	Fatty acid required in the diet due to the inability of human cells to synthesize
Omega fatty acid	Refers to the location of sites of unsaturation relative to the omega end (farthest from the carboxylic acid) of a fatty acid
Monounsaturated fatty acid	A fatty acid with a single site of unsaturation; oleic acid is the most common monounsaturated fatty acid
Polyunsaturated fatty acid (PUFA)	Any fatty acid with multiple sites of unsaturation; omega-3 and omega-6 PUFA are the most significant clinically
Plasmalogen	Any of a group of ether phospholipids
Sphingosine	An amino alcohol that serves as the backbone for the sphingolipid class of lipid which includes the sphingomyelins and the glycosphingolipids
Ceramide	Sphingosine containing a fatty *N*-acylation, serves as the backbone for the glycosphingolipids
Glycosphingolipid	Any ceramide to which a carbohydrate or carbohydrates have been added constitutes the cerebrosides, globosides, sulfatides, and gangliosides

High-Yield Terms	Nucleic Acids
Nucleoside	Refers to the complex of non-phosphorylate ribose sugar and a nucleobase such as purine or pyrimidine
Nucleotide	Refers to the complex of phosphorylated ribose sugar and a nucleobase such as purine or pyrimidine
Phosphodiester bond	The bond formed when the phosphate of one nucleotide is esterified to the hydroxyls of two ribose sugars typical in polynucleotides
Phosphoanhydride bond	An anhydride is a bond formed between two acids; a phosphoanhydride is the bond formed from two phosphoric acids such as with the β-and γ-phosphates of di- and triphosphate nucleosides, respectively

AMINO ACIDS

There are 20 α-amino acids that are relevant to mammalian proteins (Table 1–1). Several other amino acids (eg, ornithine and citrulline; see Chapter 17) and amino acid derivatives (eg, serotonin and epinephrine; see Chapter 19) perform critical functions not related to protein synthesis. The α-amino acids in peptides and proteins consist of a carboxylic acid (–COOH) and primary amine (–NH_2) attached to the same tetrahedral carbon (α-carbon) atom. Distinct functional moieties (R-groups) that distinguish one amino acid from another also are attached to the α-carbon, except in the case of glycine where the R-group is hydrogen. The fourth substitution on the tetrahedral α-carbon of amino acids is hydrogen. Proline is the exception to this structure in that it is composed of a secondary amine (imine) and is, thus, an imino acid.

Each of the 20 α-amino acids found in proteins can be distinguished by the R-group substitution on the α-carbon atom (Table 1–1). There are two broad classes of amino acids based on whether the R-group is hydrophobic or hydrophilic.

The hydrophobic amino acids tend to repel the aqueous environment and, therefore, reside predominantly in the interior of proteins. The hydrophilic amino acids tend to interact with the aqueous environment, are often involved in the formation of hydrogen bonds, and are predominantly found on the exterior of proteins or in the reactive centers of enzymes.

The α-COOH and α-NH_2 groups can donate or accept protons as well as the acidic and basic R-groups of the amino acids. For the α-COOH and α-NH_2 groups of the amino acids, the equilibrium reactions are designated as follows:

$$\text{R-COOH} \leftrightarrow \text{R-COO}^- + \text{H}^+$$
$$\text{R-NH}_3^+ \leftrightarrow \text{R-NH}_2 + \text{H}^+$$

At physiologic pH (around 7.4), the carboxyl group will be unprotonated and the amino group will be protonated.

HIGH-YIELD CONCEPT

At physiologic pH, an amino acid with no ionizable R-group would be electrically neutral since the carboxylic acid would be negatively charged and the amino group would be positively charged. This state is referred to as a **zwitterion.** The term zwitterion defines an electrically neutral molecule with one positive and one negative charge at different sites within that molecule.

TABLE 1–1 L-α-amino acids present in proteins.

Name	Symbol	Structural Formula	pK_1	pK_2	pK_3
With Aliphatic Side Chains			α-COOH	α-NH_3^+	R Group
Glycine	Gly [G]	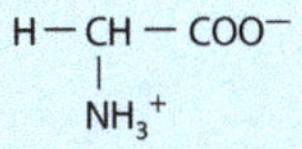	2.4	9.8	
Alanine	Ala [A]	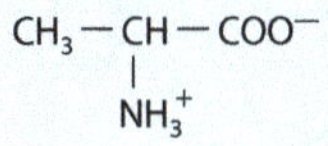	2.4	9.9	
Valine	Val [V]	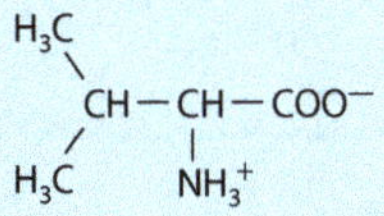	2.2	9.7	
Leucine	Leu [L]	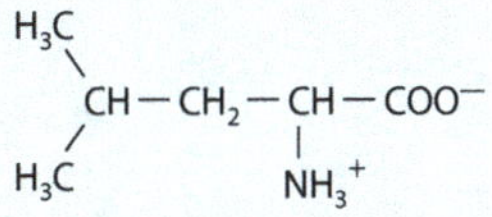	2.3	9.7	
Isoleucine	Ile [I]	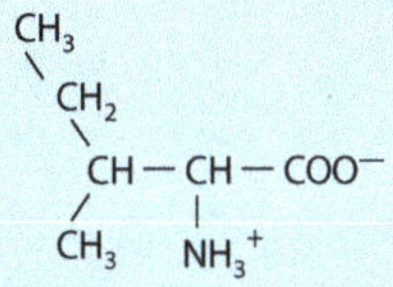	2.3	9.8	
With Side Chains Containing Hydroxylic [OH] Groups					
Serine	Ser [S]	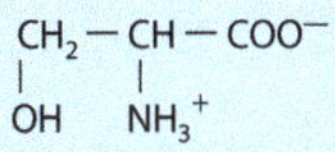	2.2	9.2	About 13
Threonine	Thr [T]	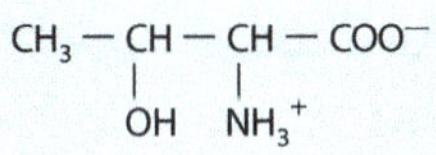	2.1	9.1	About 13
Tyrosine	Tyr [Y]	See below			
With Side Chains Containing Sulfur Atoms			α-COOH	α-NH_2^+	R Group
Cysteine	Cys [C]	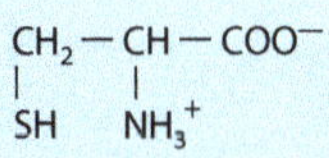	1.9	10.8	8.3
Methionine	Met [M]	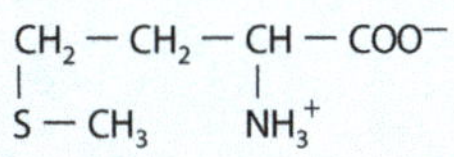	2.1	9.3	
With Side Chains Containing Acidic Groups or Their Amides					
Aspartic acid	Asp [D]	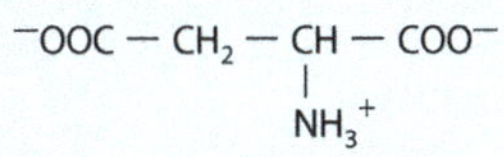	2.1	9.9	3.9
Asparagine	Asn [N]	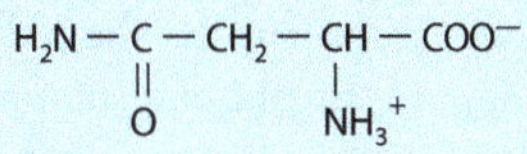	2.1	8.8	

(Continued)

TABLE 1–1 L-α-amino acids present in proteins. (*Continued*)

Name	Symbol	Structural Formula	pK_1	pK_2	pK_3
Glutamic acid	Glu [E]	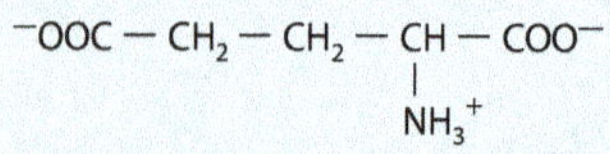	2.1	9.5	4.1
Glutamine	Gln [Q]	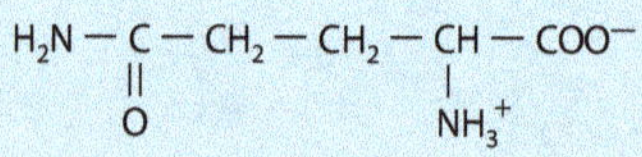	2.2	9.1	
With Side Chains Containing Basic Groups					
Arginine	Arg [R]	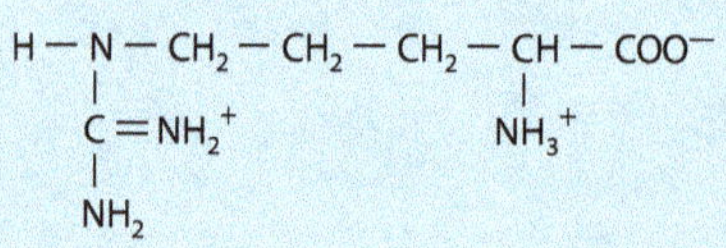	1.8	9.0	12.5
Lysine	Lys [K]	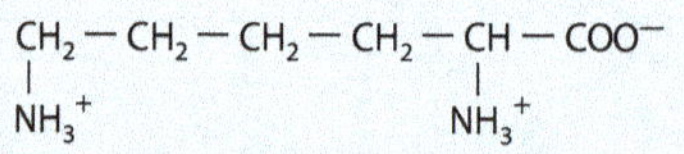	2.2	9.2	10.8
Histidine	His [H]	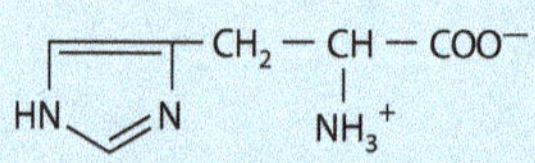	1.8	9.3	6.0
Containing Aromatic Rings					
Histidine	His [H]	See above			
Phenylalanine	Phe [F]	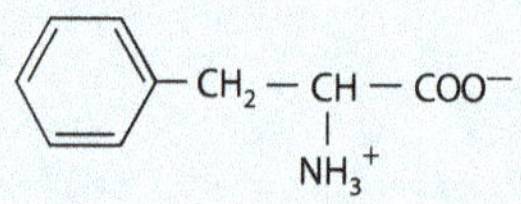	2.2	9.2	
Tyrosine	Tyr [Y]	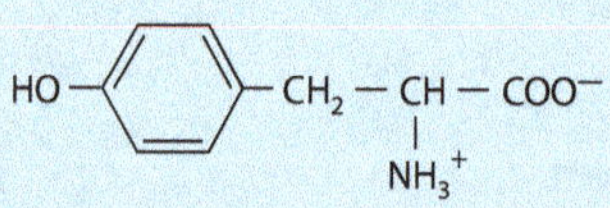	2.2	9.1	10.1
Tryplophan	Trp [W]	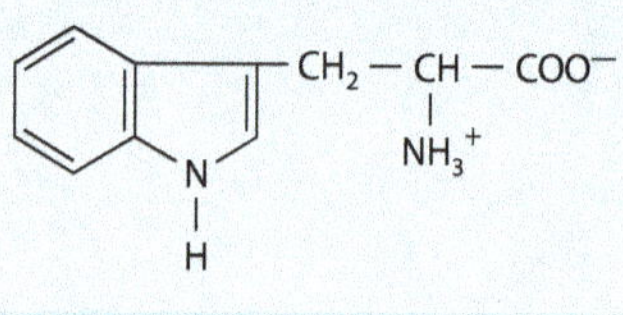	2.4	9.4	
Imino Acid					
Proline	Pro [P]	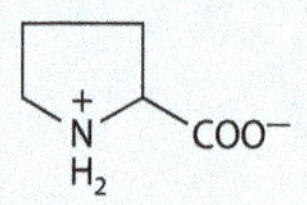	2.0	10.6	

Reproduced with permission from Rodwell VW, Bender DA, Botham KM, et al: *Harper's Illustrated Biochemistry*, 31st ed. New York, NY: McGraw Hill; 2018.

The acidic strength of the carboxyl, amino, and ionizable R-groups in amino acids can be defined by the equilibrium constant (K_a) or, more commonly, the negative logarithm of K_a ($-\log K_a$), the pK_a. This value is determined for any given acid or base from the Henderson-Hasselbalch equation:

$$pH = pK_a + \log\frac{[A^-]}{[HA]}$$

The net charge of any amino acid, peptide, or protein will depend on the pH of the surrounding aqueous environment. As the pH of a solution of an amino acid or protein changes, so too does the net charge. This phenomenon can be observed during the titration of any amino acid (Figure 1–1) or protein. When the net charge of an amino acid or protein is zero, the pH will be equivalent to the isoelectric point, pI.

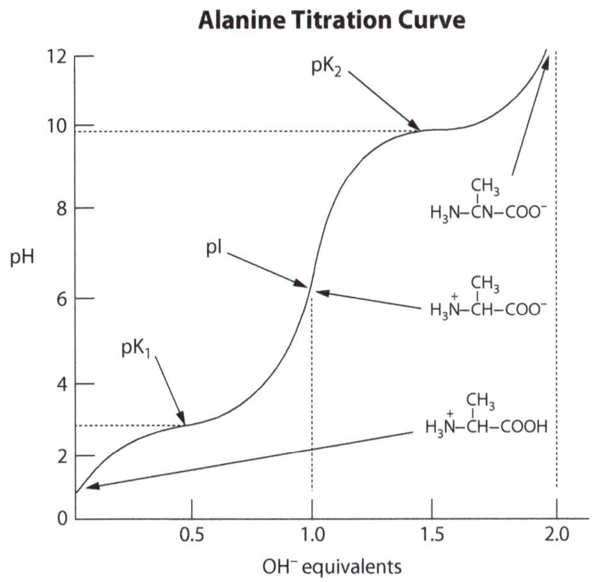

FIGURE 1–1 Titration of alanine. (Reproduced with permission from themedicalbiochemistrypage, LLC.)

Functional Significance of Amino Acid R-Groups

It is the nature of interaction of the amino acid R-groups that dictate structure-function relationships of peptides and proteins in a solution (see Chapter 2). For example, the imidazole ring of histidine allows it to act as either a proton donor or acceptor at physiologic pH. Hence, it is frequently found in the reactive center of enzymes. Equally important is the ability of histidine in hemoglobin to buffer the protons (H^+ ions) from carbonic acid ionization in red blood cells. This property of hemoglobin allows it to exchange O_2 and CO_2 at the tissues or lungs, respectively (see Chapter 2).

The Peptide Bond

A peptide bond is the covalent interaction of α-NH_2 group of one amino acid with the α-COOH group of another amino acid. The presence of the carbonyl group in a peptide bond allows electron resonance stabilization to occur such that the peptide bond exhibits rigidity not unlike the typical –C=C– double bond. The peptide bond is, therefore, said to have partial double-bond character (Figure 1–2).

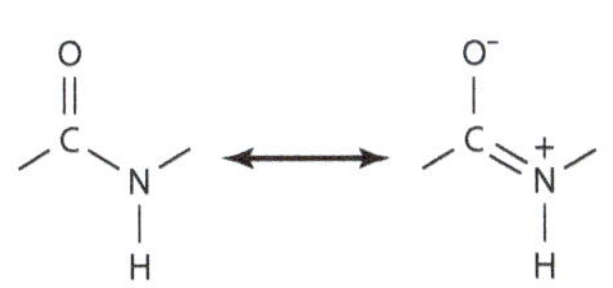

FIGURE 1–2 Resonance stabilization forms of the peptide bond. (Reproduced with permission from Rodwell VW, Bender DA, Botham KM, et al: *Harper's Illustrated Biochemistry*, 31st ed. New York, NY: McGraw Hill; 2018.)

CHECKLIST

- ☑ All amino acids found in human proteins exist as L-α-amino acids, although D-amino acids are found in nature.
- ☑ All amino acids contain at least two weakly acidic groups, the α-NH_2 and the α-COOH groups. Many amino acids also contain weakly acidic function groups designated as the R-group.
- ☑ The R-groups of the amino acids determines their classification, for example, acidic or basic.
- ☑ The association constant, pK_a, can be determined for H^+ dissociation from any of the ionizable groups of each amino acid.
- ☑ As with all acids and bases, when titrating amino acids the pH at which the net charge on the molecule is neutral is referred to as the isoelectric point, pI.
- ☑ Amino acids form peptide bonds creating polymers called peptides and proteins. Due to resonance stabilization of electrons about the peptide bond, there is limited mobility leading to restricted protein conformations.

CARBOHYDRATES

Carbohydrates are biological compounds composed solely of carbon, oxygen, and hydrogen that generally contain hydroxyl groups (–OH). The presence of the hydroxyl groups allows carbohydrates to interact with the aqueous environment and to participate in hydrogen bonding.

In biochemistry carbohydrate is synonymous with saccharide and the more common term, sugar. The simplest carbohydrates also contain either an aldehyde moiety and are termed aldoses (Figure 1–3), or a ketone moiety and are termed ketoses (Figure 1–4). The predominant carbohydrates encountered in the body are structurally related to the aldose glyceraldehyde and the ketose dihydroxyacetone. The numbering of the carbons in carbohydrates proceeds from the carbonyl carbon, for aldoses, or the carbon nearest the carbonyl, for ketoses.

All carbohydrates can be classified as either **monosaccharides**, **oligosaccharides**, or **polysaccharides**. Anywhere from 2 to 10 monosaccharide units, linked by glycosidic bonds, make up an oligosaccharide. Polysaccharides are much larger, generally containing hundreds of monosaccharide units. Derivatives of the carbohydrates can contain nitrogen, phosphate, and/or sulfur compounds. Carbohydrates also can combine with lipid to form glycolipids (see Chapter 12) or with protein to form glycoproteins (see Chapter 24).

Carbohydrate Structure and Nomenclature

All carbohydrates contain at least one asymmetrical (chiral) carbon and are, therefore, optically active. In addition, carbohydrates can

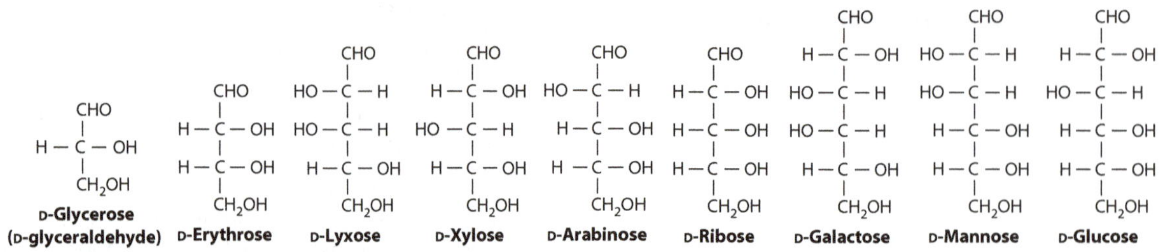

FIGURE 1–3 Examples of aldoses of physiologic significance. (Reproduced with permission from Rodwell VW, Bender DA, Botham KM, et al: *Harper's Illustrated Biochemistry*, 31st ed. New York, NY: McGraw Hill; 2018.)

exist in either of two conformations, as determined by the orientation of the hydroxyl group about the asymmetric carbon farthest from the carbonyl. With a few exceptions, those carbohydrates that are of physiologic significance exist in the D-conformation. The mirror-image conformations, called **enantiomers**, are in the L-conformation.

Monosaccharides of five or six carbon atoms exist in solution in an equilibrium between linear and ring forms (Figure 1–5). The ring structures form from a carbonyl group and a relatively distant hydroxyl group. Glucose, for example, forms a six-membered ring. The ring structures of the carbohydrates can be depicted by either **Fischer** or **Haworth** (also called the chair form) style diagrams (Figure 1–5).

The rings can open and re-close, allowing rotation to occur about the carbon bearing the reactive carbonyl yielding two distinct configurations, α and β. The carbon about which this rotation occurs is the **anomeric carbon**, and the two forms are termed anomers. Carbohydrates can change spontaneously between the α and β configurations, a process known as **mutarotation**. When drawn in the Fischer projection, the α configuration places the hydroxyl attached to the anomeric carbon to the right, toward the ring. When drawn in the Haworth projection, the α configuration places the hydroxyl downward. Constituents of the ring that project above or below the plane of the ring are axial and those that project parallel to the plane are equatorial. In the chair conformation, the orientation of the hydroxyl group about the anomeric carbon of α-D-glucose is axial and equatorial in β-D-glucose.

Monosaccharides

The monosaccharides commonly found in humans are classified according to the number of carbons they contain in their backbone structures. The major monosaccharides in humans contain three to six carbon atoms. The 5-carbon sugars (the pentoses; Table 1–2) and the 6-carbon sugars (the hexoses; Table 1–3) represent the largest groups of physiologically important carbohydrates in human metabolism.

The amino sugars are another class of biologically significant monosaccharides that contain nitrogen. These include *N*-acetylglucosamine (GlcNAc; Figure 1–6), *N*-acetylgalactosamine (GalNAc), and *N*-acetylneuraminic acid (NANA; also known as sialic acid, Sia).

Disaccharides

Covalent bonds between the anomeric hydroxyl of one carbohydrate and the hydroxyl of a second carbohydrate (or another alcohol containing compound) are termed **glycosidic bonds**, and the resultant molecules are **glycosides**. The linkage of two monosaccharides to form disaccharides involves a glycosidic bond (Figure 1–7).

Sucrose is the dominant carbohydrate in sugarcane and sugar beets and is composed of glucose and fructose linked via an α-(1,2)-β-glycosidic bond. Lactose is found exclusively in the milk of mammals and consists of galactose and glucose linked via a β-(1,4) glycosidic bond. Maltose is the major degradation product of starch, and it is composed of two glucose monomers linked via an α-(1,4) glycosidic bond.

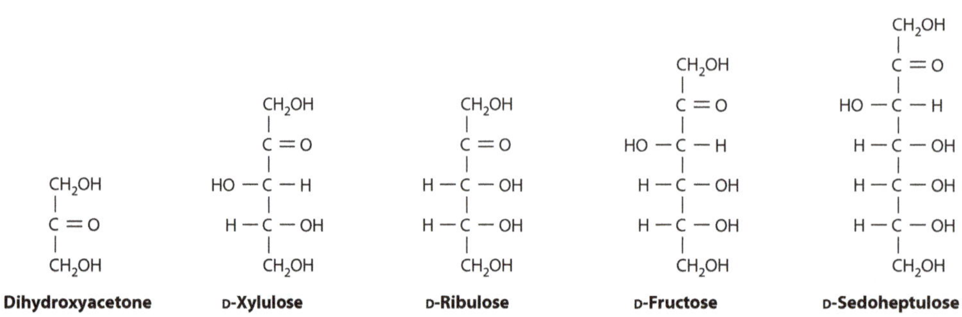

FIGURE 1–4 Examples of ketoses of physiologic significance. (Reproduced with permission from Rodwell VW, Bender DA, Botham KM, et al: *Harper's Illustrated Biochemistry*, 31st ed. New York, NY: McGraw Hill; 2018.)

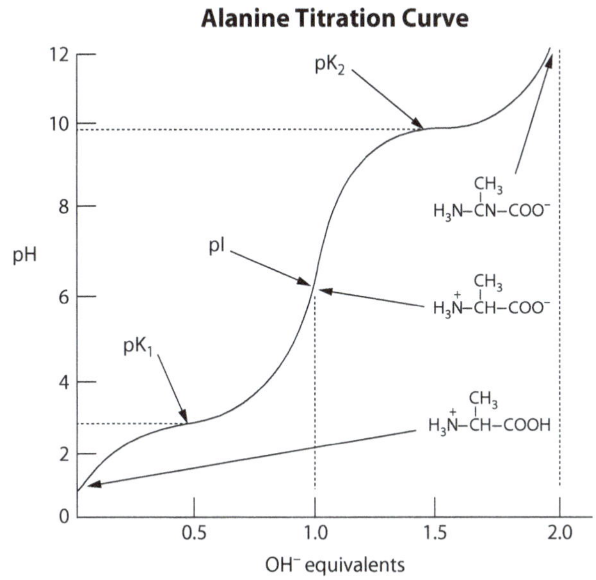

FIGURE 1–1 Titration of alanine. (Reproduced with permission from themedicalbiochemistrypage, LLC.)

CHECKLIST

- ☑ All amino acids found in human proteins exist as L-α-amino acids, although D-amino acids are found in nature.
- ☑ All amino acids contain at least two weakly acidic groups, the α-NH_2 and the α-COOH groups. Many amino acids also contain weakly acidic function groups designated as the R-group.
- ☑ The R-groups of the amino acids determines their classification, for example, acidic or basic.
- ☑ The association constant, pK_a, can be determined for H^+ dissociation from any of the ionizable groups of each amino acid.
- ☑ As with all acids and bases, when titrating amino acids the pH at which the net charge on the molecule is neutral is referred to as the isoelectric point, pI.
- ☑ Amino acids form peptide bonds creating polymers called peptides and proteins. Due to resonance stabilization of electrons about the peptide bond, there is limited mobility leading to restricted protein conformations.

Functional Significance of Amino Acid R-Groups

It is the nature of interaction of the amino acid R-groups that dictate structure-function relationships of peptides and proteins in a solution (see Chapter 2). For example, the imidazole ring of histidine allows it to act as either a proton donor or acceptor at physiologic pH. Hence, it is frequently found in the reactive center of enzymes. Equally important is the ability of histidine in hemoglobin to buffer the protons (H^+ ions) from carbonic acid ionization in red blood cells. This property of hemoglobin allows it to exchange O_2 and CO_2 at the tissues or lungs, respectively (see Chapter 2).

The Peptide Bond

A peptide bond is the covalent interaction of α-NH_2 group of one amino acid with the α-COOH group of another amino acid. The presence of the carbonyl group in a peptide bond allows electron resonance stabilization to occur such that the peptide bond exhibits rigidity not unlike the typical –C=C– double bond. The peptide bond is, therefore, said to have partial double-bond character (Figure 1–2).

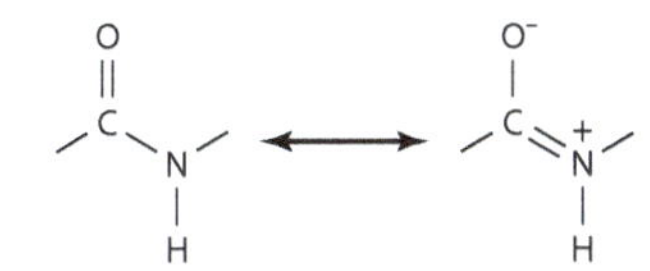

FIGURE 1–2 Resonance stabilization forms of the peptide bond. (Reproduced with permission from Rodwell VW, Bender DA, Botham KM, et al: *Harper's Illustrated Biochemistry*, 31st ed. New York, NY: McGraw Hill; 2018.)

CARBOHYDRATES

Carbohydrates are biological compounds composed solely of carbon, oxygen, and hydrogen that generally contain hydroxyl groups (–OH). The presence of the hydroxyl groups allows carbohydrates to interact with the aqueous environment and to participate in hydrogen bonding.

In biochemistry carbohydrate is synonymous with saccharide and the more common term, sugar. The simplest carbohydrates also contain either an aldehyde moiety and are termed aldoses (Figure 1–3), or a ketone moiety and are termed ketoses (Figure 1–4). The predominant carbohydrates encountered in the body are structurally related to the aldose glyceraldehyde and the ketose dihydroxyacetone. The numbering of the carbons in carbohydrates proceeds from the carbonyl carbon, for aldoses, or the carbon nearest the carbonyl, for ketoses.

All carbohydrates can be classified as either **monosaccharides**, **oligosaccharides**, or **polysaccharides**. Anywhere from 2 to 10 monosaccharide units, linked by glycosidic bonds, make up an oligosaccharide. Polysaccharides are much larger, generally containing hundreds of monosaccharide units. Derivatives of the carbohydrates can contain nitrogen, phosphate, and/or sulfur compounds. Carbohydrates also can combine with lipid to form glycolipids (see Chapter 12) or with protein to form glycoproteins (see Chapter 24).

Carbohydrate Structure and Nomenclature

All carbohydrates contain at least one asymmetrical (chiral) carbon and are, therefore, optically active. In addition, carbohydrates can

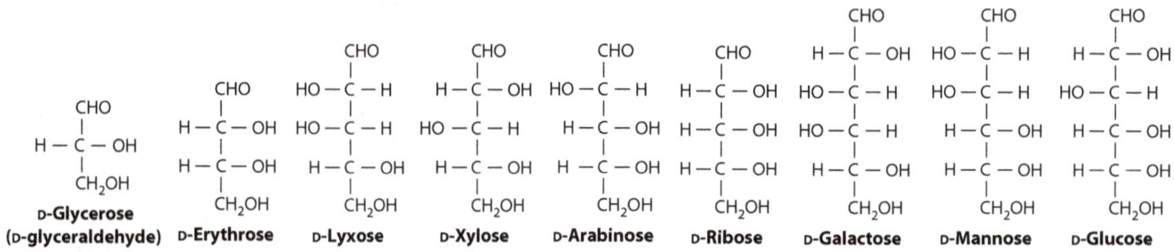

FIGURE 1–3 Examples of aldoses of physiologic significance. (Reproduced with permission from Rodwell VW, Bender DA, Botham KM, et al: *Harper's Illustrated Biochemistry*, 31st ed. New York, NY: McGraw Hill; 2018.)

exist in either of two conformations, as determined by the orientation of the hydroxyl group about the asymmetric carbon farthest from the carbonyl. With a few exceptions, those carbohydrates that are of physiologic significance exist in the D-conformation. The mirror-image conformations, called **enantiomers**, are in the L-conformation.

Monosaccharides of five or six carbon atoms exist in solution in an equilibrium between linear and ring forms (Figure 1–5). The ring structures form from a carbonyl group and a relatively distant hydroxyl group. Glucose, for example, forms a six-membered ring. The ring structures of the carbohydrates can be depicted by either **Fischer** or **Haworth** (also called the chair form) style diagrams (Figure 1–5).

The rings can open and re-close, allowing rotation to occur about the carbon bearing the reactive carbonyl yielding two distinct configurations, α and β. The carbon about which this rotation occurs is the **anomeric carbon**, and the two forms are termed anomers. Carbohydrates can change spontaneously between the α and β configurations, a process known as **mutarotation.** When drawn in the Fischer projection, the α configuration places the hydroxyl attached to the anomeric carbon to the right, toward the ring. When drawn in the Haworth projection, the α configuration places the hydroxyl downward. Constituents of the ring that project above or below the plane of the ring are axial and those that project parallel to the plane are equatorial. In the chair conformation, the orientation of the hydroxyl group about the anomeric carbon of α-D-glucose is axial and equatorial in β-D-glucose.

Monosaccharides

The monosaccharides commonly found in humans are classified according to the number of carbons they contain in their backbone structures. The major monosaccharides in humans contain three to six carbon atoms. The 5-carbon sugars (the pentoses; Table 1–2) and the 6-carbon sugars (the hexoses; Table 1–3) represent the largest groups of physiologically important carbohydrates in human metabolism.

The amino sugars are another class of biologically significant monosaccharides that contain nitrogen. These include *N*-acetylglucosamine (GlcNAc; Figure 1–6), *N*-acetylgalactosamine (GalNAc), and *N*-acetylneuraminic acid (NANA; also known as sialic acid, Sia).

Disaccharides

Covalent bonds between the anomeric hydroxyl of one carbohydrate and the hydroxyl of a second carbohydrate (or another alcohol containing compound) are termed **glycosidic bonds**, and the resultant molecules are **glycosides**. The linkage of two monosaccharides to form disaccharides involves a glycosidic bond (Figure 1–7).

Sucrose is the dominant carbohydrate in sugarcane and sugar beets and is composed of glucose and fructose linked via an α-(1,2)-β-glycosidic bond. Lactose is found exclusively in the milk of mammals and consists of galactose and glucose linked via a β-(1,4) glycosidic bond. Maltose is the major degradation product of starch, and it is composed of two glucose monomers linked via an α-(1,4) glycosidic bond.

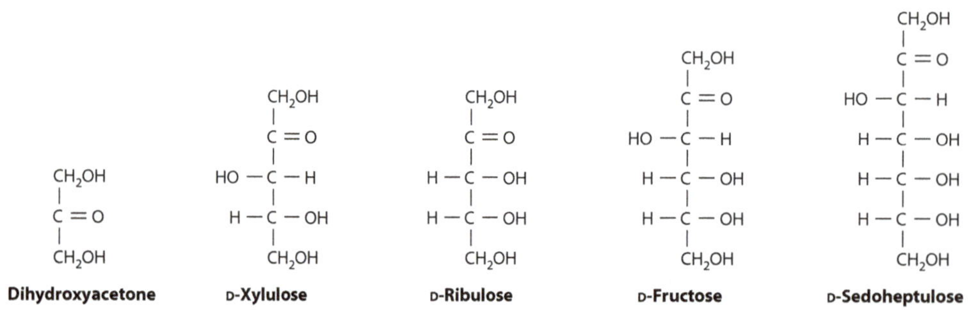

FIGURE 1–4 Examples of ketoses of physiologic significance. (Reproduced with permission from Rodwell VW, Bender DA, Botham KM, et al: *Harper's Illustrated Biochemistry*, 31st ed. New York, NY: McGraw Hill; 2018.)

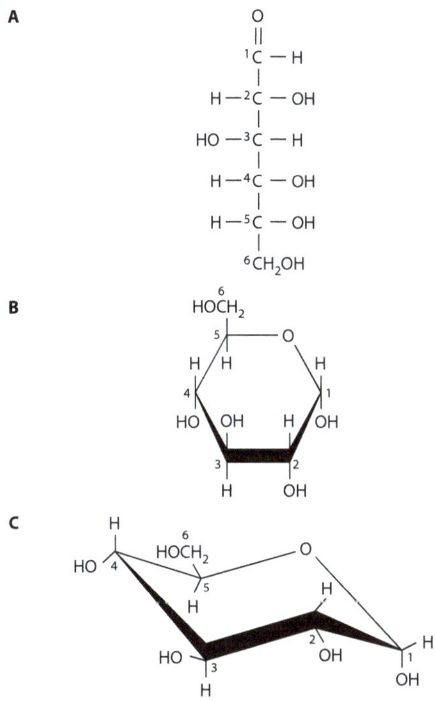

FIGURE 1–5 D-Glucose. (A) Straight-chain form. (B) α-D-glucose; Haworth projection. (C) α-D-glucose; chair form. (Reproduced with permission from Rodwell VW, Bender DA, Botham KM, et al: *Harper's Illustrated Biochemistry*, 31st ed. New York, NY: McGraw Hill; 2018.)

Polysaccharides: Glycogen

Most of the carbohydrates found in nature occur in the form of high-molecular-weight polymers called **polysaccharides**. Glycogen, the major form of stored carbohydrate in animals, is a polysaccharide composed solely of glucose (Figure 1–8). The majority of the glucose monomers in glycogen are linked together via α-(1,4) glycosidic bonds. Glycogen is also highly branched where each branch is generated via an α-(1,6) glycosidic bond. Glycogen is a very compact structure that results from the coiling of the polymer chains. This compactness allows large amounts of carbon energy to be stored in a small volume, with little effect on cellular osmolarity.

TABLE 1–2 Pentoses of physiologic importance.

Sugar	Source	Biochemical and Clinical Importance
D-Ribose	Nucleic acids and metabolic intermediate	Structural component of nucleic acids and coenzymes, including ATP, NAD(P), and flavin coenzymes
D-Ribulose	Metabolic intermediate	Intermediate in the pentose phosphate pathway
D-Arabinose	Plant gums	Constituent of glycoproteins
D-Xylose	Plant gums, proteoglycans, glycosaminoglycans	Constituent of glycoproteins
L-Xylulose	Metabolic intermediate	Excreted in the urine in essential pentosuria

Reproduced with permission from Rodwell VW, Bender DA, Botham KM, et al: *Harper's Illustrated Biochemistry*, 31st ed. New York, NY: McGraw Hill; 2018.

TABLE 1–3 Hexoses of physiologic importance.

Sugar	Source	Biochemical Importance	Clinical Significance
D-Glucose	Fruit juices, hydrolysis of starch, cane or beet sugar, maltose, and lactose	The main metabolic fuel for tissues; "blood sugar"	Excreted in the urine (glucosuria) in poorly controlled diabetes mellitus as a result of hyperglycemia
D-Fructose	Fruit juices, honey, hydrolysis of cane or beet sugar and inulin, enzymic isomerization of glucose syrups for food manufacture	Readily metabolized either via glucose or directly	Hereditary fructose intolerance leads to fructose accumulation and hypoglycemia
D-Galactose	Hydrolysis of lactose	Readily metabolized to glucose; synthesized in the mammary gland for synthesis of lactose in milk. A constituent of glycolipids and glycoproteins	Hereditary galactosemia as a result of failure to metabolize galactose leads to cataracts
D-Mannose	Hydrolysis of plant mannan gums	Constituent of glycoproteins	

Reproduced with permission from Rodwell VW, Bender DA, Botham KM, et al: *Harper's Illustrated Biochemistry*, 31st ed. New York, NY: McGraw Hill; 2018.

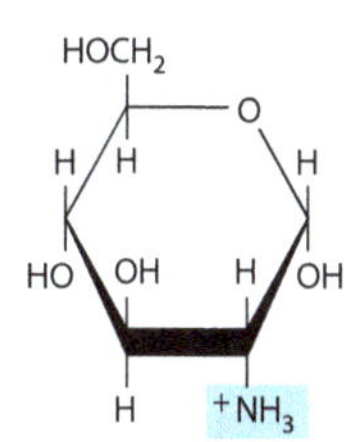

FIGURE 1–6 Glucosamine (2-amino-D-glucopyranose) (α form). Galactosamine is 2-amino-D-galactopyranose. Both glucosamine and galactosamine occur as *N*-acetyl derivatives in more complex carbohydrates, for example, glycoproteins. (Reproduced with permission from Murray RK, Bender DA, Botham KM, et al: *Harper's Illustrated Biochemistry*, 29th ed. New York, NY: McGraw Hill; 2012.)

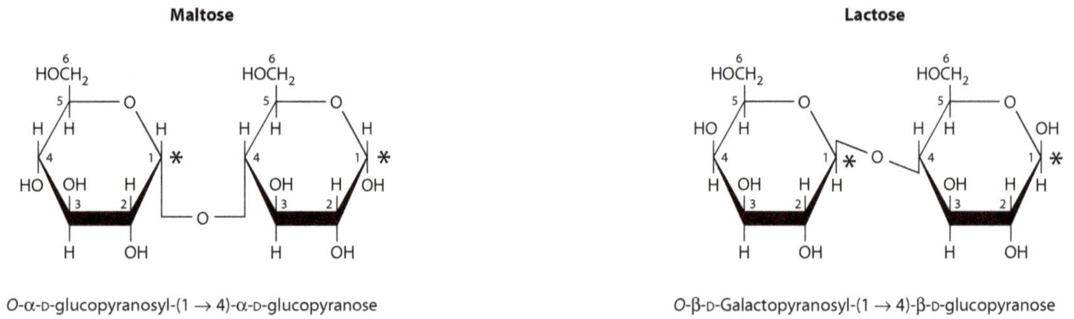

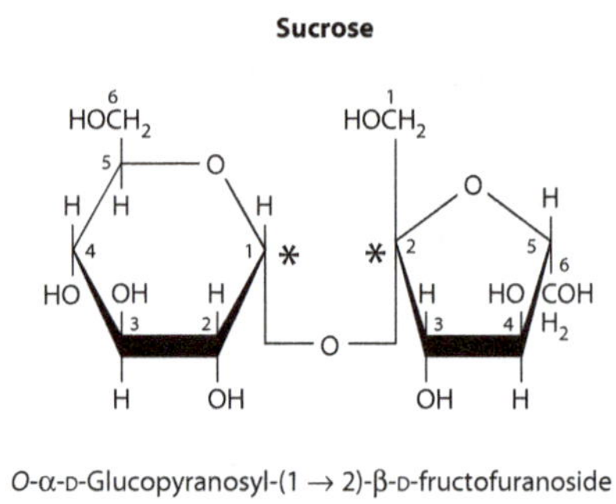

FIGURE 1–7 Structures of important disaccharides. α and β refer to the configuration at the anomeric carbon atom (*). When the anomeric carbon of the second residue takes part in the formation of the glycosidic bond, as in sucrose, the residue becomes a glycoside known as a furanoside or a pyranoside. As the disaccharide no longer has an anomeric carbon with a free potential aldehyde or ketone group, it no longer exhibits reducing properties. (Reproduced with permission from Murray RK, Bender DA, Botham KM, et al: *Harper's Illustrated Biochemistry*, 29th ed. New York, NY: McGraw Hill; 2012.)

Starch is another polysaccharide that constitutes the major form of stored carbohydrate in plant cells. Its structure is identical to glycogen, except for a much lower degree of branching (about every 20–30 residues). Unbranched starch is called **amylose**; branched starch is called **amylopectin**.

Complex Carbohydrates Structures

A variety of complex carbohydrate-containing compounds exist that are important both structurally and functionally. The major classes of these molecules are the glycoproteins (see Chapter 24),

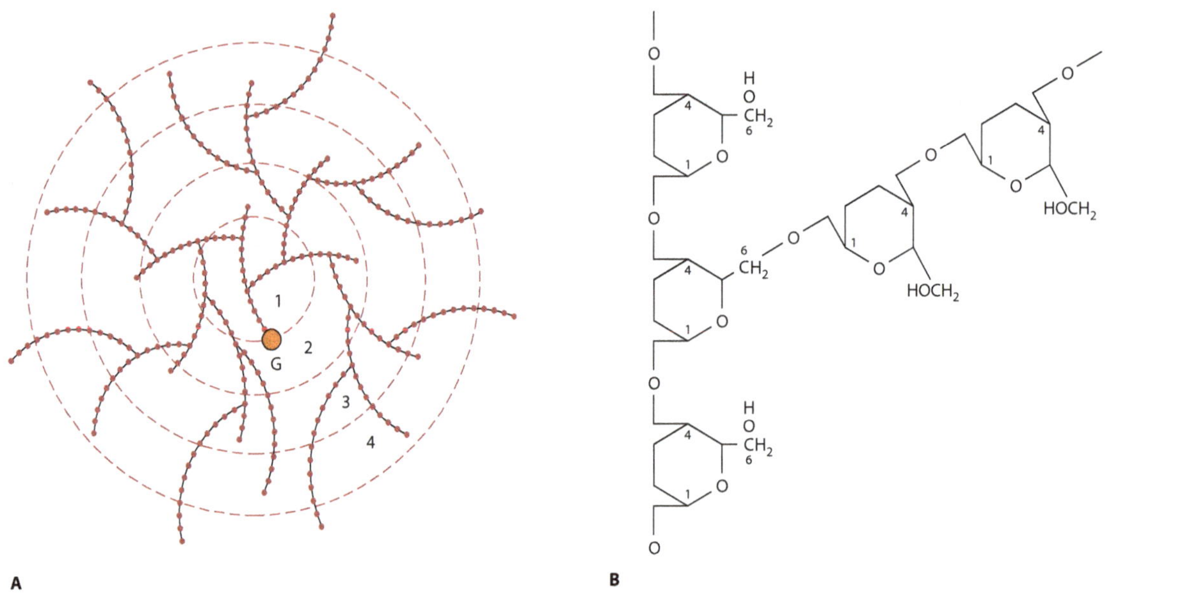

FIGURE 1–8 The glycogen molecule. (A) General structure. (B) Enlargement of structure at a branch point. The molecule is a sphere ~21 nm in diameter that can be seen in electron micrographs. It has a molecular mass of ~10^7 Da and consists of polysaccharide chains, each containing about 13 glucose residues. The chains are either branched or unbranched and are arranged in 12 concentric layers (only four are shown in the figure). The branched chains (each has two branches) are found in the inner layers and the unbranched chains in the outer layer. (G, glycogenin, the primer molecule for glycogen synthesis.) (Reproduced with permission from Murray RK, Bender DA, Botham KM, et al: *Harper's Illustrated Biochemistry*, 29th ed. New York, NY: McGraw Hill; 2012.)

glycolipids (see Chapter 12), and glycosaminoglycans and proteoglycans (see Chapter 25). The physiologic significance of protein glycosylation can be emphasized by the fact that approximately 50% of all proteins are known to be glycosylated, and at least 1% of the human genome is represented by glycan biosynthesis genes.

CHECKLIST

- ☑ Carbohydrates (saccharides) are major sources of energy for human tissues, and they also represent major storage forms of energy in both plants and animals. Biologically significant carbohydrates contain different amounts of carbon (generally from 3 to 6 atoms) and can be found as monosaccharides, disaccharides, or polysaccharides.
- ☑ Glucose is the most important monosaccharide in humans. It is the storage form of carbohydrate, can be readily catabolized to generate energy, even in the absence of oxygen, and most all other carbohydrates can be converted into glucose.
- ☑ Ribose is another physiologically significant monosaccharide as it serves as a constituent of the nucleotides.
- ☑ Carbohydrates exist in different configurations and conformations in solution due to the presence of several asymmetric carbon atoms.
- ☑ The most significant disaccharides are sucrose (glucose and fructose) which is a major sweetener and dietary carbohydrate, maltose (2 glucose) which is an intermediate in the digestion of starch from plants, and lactose (glucose and galactose) which is the major carbohydrate of milk.
- ☑ Polymers of glucose found in plants are called starch and those in animals are called glycogen. Starch is a major source of dietary energy, whereas glycogen is a major form of intracellular stored energy.
- ☑ Complex carbohydrates are formed to serve both structural and functional roles in cells and tissues. These complex carbohydrates include the amino sugars, uronic acids, and sialic acids. Proteoglycans, glycosaminoglycans, glycoproteins, and glycolipids represent the major classes of complex carbohydrates in human tissues.

LIPIDS

Fatty Acids

Fatty acids are long-chain hydrocarbon molecules containing a carboxylic acid group at one end. The numbering of carbons in fatty acids begins with the carbon of the carboxylate group. At physiologic pH, the carboxylic acid group will be ionized, rendering a negative charge onto fatty acids in bodily fluids.

Fatty acids perform the following three major roles in the body:

1. They serve as components of more complex membrane lipids (see Chapter 25).
2. They are the major components of stored energy in the form of triglycerides (see Chapter 11).
3. They serve as the precursors for the synthesis of the numerous types of bioactive lipids (see Chapter 12).

Fatty acids that contain no carbon-carbon double bonds are termed saturated fatty acids; those that contain carbon-carbon double bonds are unsaturated fatty acids. Fatty acids with multiple sites of unsaturation are termed polyunsaturated fatty acids (PUFA). The numeric designations used for fatty acids come from the number of carbon atoms, followed by the number of sites of unsaturation (eg, palmitic acid is a 16-carbon fatty acid with no unsaturation and is designated by 16:0; Table 1–4). The site of unsaturation in a fatty acid is indicated by the symbol Δ, and the number of the first carbon of the double bond where the carboxylic acid group carbon is designated carbon #1. For example, palmitoleic acid is a 16-carbon fatty acid with one site of unsaturation between carbons 9 and 10 and its designation is $16{:}1^{\Delta 9}$.

HIGH-YIELD CONCEPT

The melting point of fatty acids increases as the number of carbon atoms increases. In addition, the introduction of sites of unsaturation results in lower melting points when comparing a saturated and an unsaturated fatty acid of the same number of carbons. Saturated fatty acids of less than eight carbon atoms are liquid at physiologic temperature, whereas those containing more than 10 are solid.

The steric geometry of unsaturated fatty acids can vary such that the acyl groups can be oriented on the same side or on opposite sides of the double bond. When the acyl groups are both on the same side of the double bond it is referred to as a *cis* bond, such as is the case for oleic acid (18:1). When the acyl groups are on opposite sides the bond is termed *trans* such as in elaidic acid, the *trans* isomer of oleic acid (Figure 1–9).

The majority of naturally occurring unsaturated fatty acids exist in the *cis*-conformation.

HIGH-YIELD CONCEPT

The *cis*-conformation predominates in naturally occurring fats. *Trans* fatty acid content increases as a result of the process of hydrogenating unsaturated fatty acids to make them solids at room temperature, such as in partially hydrogenated vegetable oils. Diets high in *trans* fatty acids have been associated with an increased risk of cardiovascular disease and development of the metabolic syndrome.

TABLE 1–4 Physiologically relevant fatty acids.

Numerical Symbol	Common Name and Structure	Comments
14:0	Myristic acid 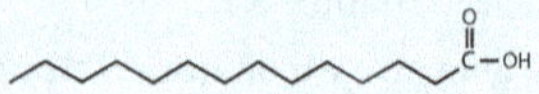	Often found attached to the *N*-terminus of plasma membrane–associated cytoplasmic proteins
16:0	Palmitic acid 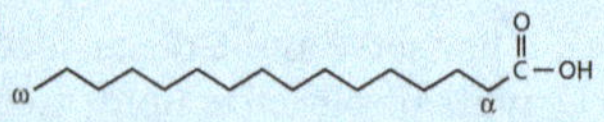	End-product of mammalian fatty acid synthesis
$16{:}1^{\Delta 9}$	Palmitoleic acid 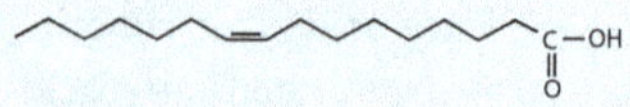	Major monounsaturated fatty acid (MUFA) in humans; omega-7 fatty acid
18:0	Stearic acid 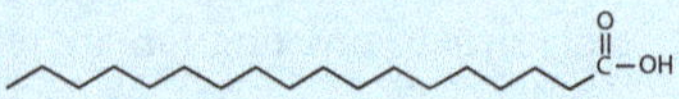	
$18{:}1^{\Delta 9}$	Oleic acid 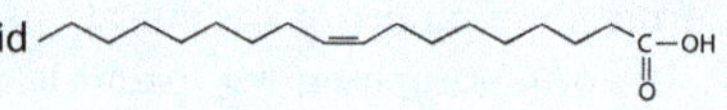	Physiologically most important omega-9 monounsaturated fatty acid (MUFA)
$18{:}2^{\Delta 9,12}$	Linoleic acid 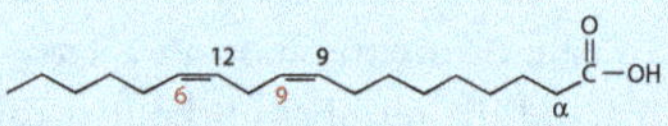	Essential fatty acid, an omega-6 PUFA
$18{:}3^{\Delta 9,12,15}$	α-Linolenic acid (ALA) 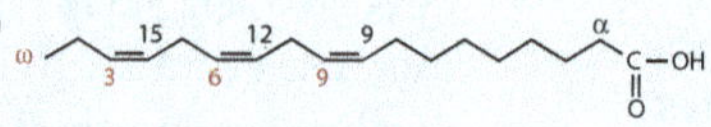	Essential fatty acid, an omega-3 PUFA; can exist in two configurations, of which the α-configuration is shown; is the substrate for the synthesis of eicosapentaenoic acid (EPA) and docosahexaenoic acid (DHA)
$20{:}4^{\Delta 5,8,11,14}$	Arachidonic acid 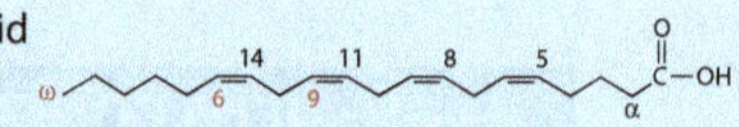	An omega-6 PUFA, precursor for eicosanoid synthesis; systematic nomenclature is all-cis-5,8,11,14-eicosatetraenoic acid (ETAn-6); also exists in an omega-3 configuration identified as ETAn-3
$20{:}5^{\Delta 5,8,11,14,17}$	Eicosapentaenoic acid (EPA) 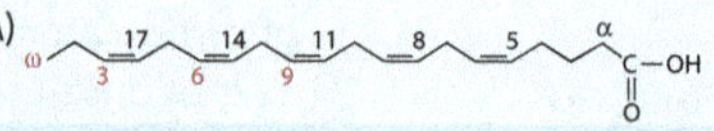	An omega-3 PUFA, enriched in krill and fish oils
$22{:}6^{\Delta 4,7,10,13,16,19}$	Docosahexaenoic acid (DHA) 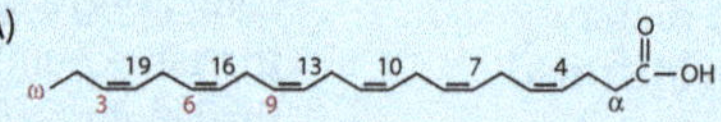	An omega-3 PUFA, enriched in krill and fish oils

Reproduced with permission from King MW: *Integrative Medical Biochemistry Examination and Board Review*. New York, NY: McGraw Hill; 2014.

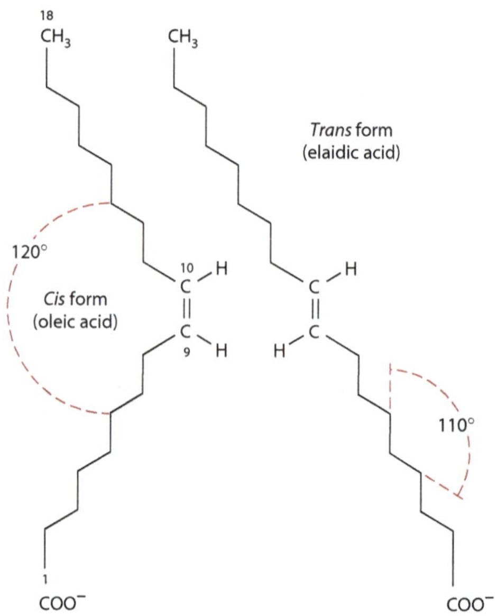

FIGURE 1–9 Geometric isomerism of Δ^9, 18:1 fatty acids (oleic and elaidic acids). (Reproduced with permission from Rodwell VW, Bender DA, Botham KM, et al: *Harper's Illustrated Biochemistry*, 31st ed. New York, NY: McGraw Hill; 2018.)

The lipid biosynthetic capacity of the body can generate nearly all the various fatty acid structures needed. Two key exceptions to this are the PUFA, linoleic acid and α-linolenic acid (ALA). These two fatty acids cannot be synthesized from precursors in the body and are therefore, essential fatty acids. These two essential fatty acids are members of a family of fatty acids referred to as omega fatty acids.

Omega-3 and -6 Polyunsaturated Fatty Acids

The term omega, as it relates to fatty acids, refers to the terminal carbon atom farthest from the carboxylic acid group (–COOH). The designation of a polyunsaturated fatty acid (PUFA) as an omega-3 fatty acid, for example, defines the position of the first site of unsaturation relative to the omega end of that fatty acid. Thus, an omega-3 fatty acid like α-linolenic acid (ALA; Table 1–4), which harbors three sites of unsaturation (carbon-carbon double bonds), has a site of unsaturation between the third and fourth carbons from the omega end.

There are three major omega-3 fatty acids that are ingested in foods and used by the body—ALA, eicosapentaenoic acid (EPA), and docosahexaenoic acid (DHA). Once consumed, the body converts ALA to EPA and DHA. Both EPA and DHA serve as important precursors for lipid-derived modulators of cell signaling, gene expression, and inflammatory processes. The primary dietary omega-6 PUFA is the essential fatty acid, linoleic acid. Linoleic acid is ultimately converted to arachidonic acid (see Chapter 12).

Triglycerides

Triglycerides (also termed triacylglycerols) are composed of a glycerol backbone to which three fatty acids are esterified. Triglycerides represent the storage form of fatty acids in all cells but synthesis predominates in adipose tissue (see Chapter 11).

Phospholipids

The basic structure of phospholipids is very similar to that of the triglycerides except that carbon 3 (*sn*3) of the glycerol backbone is esterified to phosphoric acid. Phospholipids constitute major components of biological membranes. The different forms of phospholipids result from the esterification of various polar substituents to the phosphate of phosphatidic acid (Figure 1–10). These substitutions include ethanolamine (phosphatidylethanolamine: PE), choline (phosphatidylcholine: PC, also called lecithins), serine (phosphatidylserine: PS), glycerol (phosphatidylglycerol: PG), *myo*-inositol (phosphatidylinositol: PI), and phosphatidylglycerol (diphosphatidylglycerol more commonly known as cardiolipins). Phosphotidylinositols most often have one to several of the inositol hydroxyls esterified to phosphate generating polyphosphatidylinositols.

Plasmalogens

Plasmalogens (Figure 1–11) are complex membrane lipids that resemble phospholipids except that the fatty acid at carbon 1 (*sn*1) of glycerol contains either an *O*-alkyl (–O–CH_2–) or *O*-alkenyl ether (–O–CH=CH–) species.

Sphingolipids

Sphingolipids are composed of a backbone of sphingosine which is derived from glycerol and palmitic acid (Figure 1–12). Sphingosine is *N*-acetylated by a variety of fatty acids generating a family of molecules referred to as ceramides (see Chapter 12). Sphingolipids predominate in the myelin sheath of nerve fibers.

Sphingomyelin is an abundant sphingolipid generated by the transfer of phosphocholine of phosphatidylcholine to a ceramide. Thus sphingomyelin is a unique form of a phospholipid. The other major class of sphingolipids is the glycosphingolipids generated by substitution of carbohydrates to a ceramide. There are four major classes of glycosphingolipids:

Cerebrosides: Contain a single carbohydrate, principally galactose
Sulfatides: Sulfuric acid esters of galactocerebrosides
Globosides: Contain two or more carbohydrates
Gangliosides: Similar to globosides except they also contain sialic acid (*N*-acetylneuraminic acid, NANA).

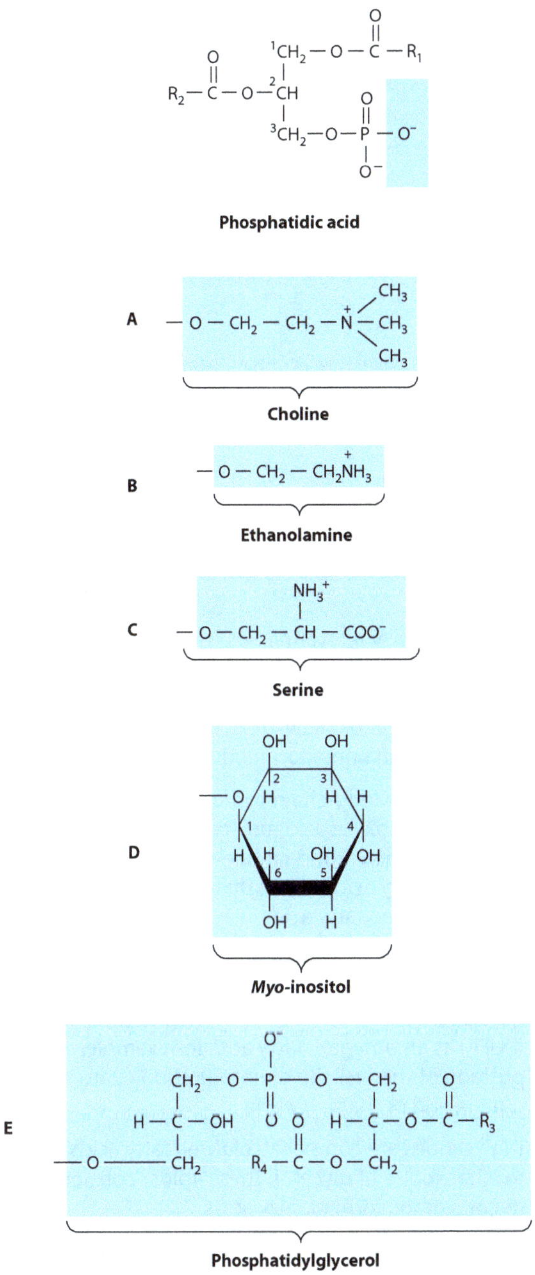

FIGURE 1–10 Phosphatidic acid and its derivatives. The O— shown shaded in phosphatidic acid is substituted by the substituents shown to form in (A) 3-phosphatidylcholine, (B) 3-phosphatidylethanolamine, (C) 3-phosphatidylserine, (D) 3-phosphatidylinositol, and (E) cardiolipin (diphosphatidylglycerol). (Reproduced with permission from Rodwell VW, Bender DA, Botham KM, et al: *Harper's Illustrated Biochemistry,* 31st ed. New York, NY: McGraw Hill; 2018.)

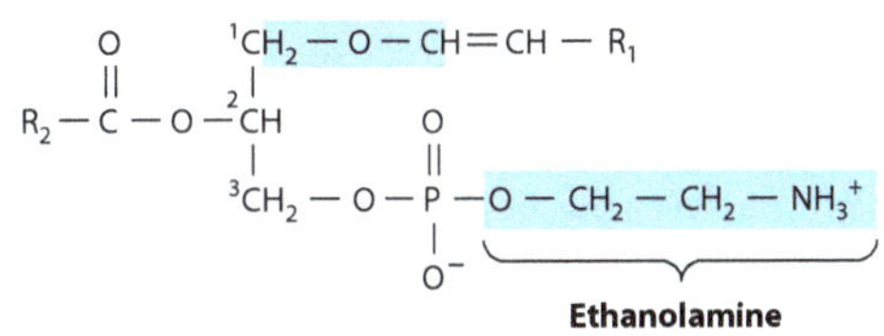

FIGURE 1–11 Plasmalogen. (Reproduced with permission from Rodwell VW, Bender DA, Botham KM, et al: *Harper's Illustrated Biochemistry*, 31st ed. New York, NY: McGraw Hill; 2018.)

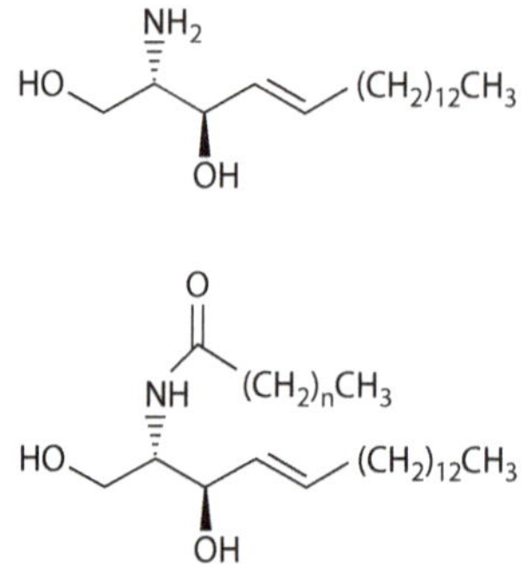

FIGURE 1–12 Structure of sphingosine and a basic ceramide. (Reproduced with permission from King MW: *Integrative Medical Biochemistry Examination and Board Review*. New York, NY: McGraw Hill; 2014.)

CHECKLIST

- ☑ The biologically relevant lipids consist of the fatty acids, triglycerides, phospholipids, sphingolipids, ceramides, cholesterol, bile acids, eicosanoids, omega fatty acid derivatives, and bioactive lipid derivatives which also include the inflammation-modulating lipid derivatives.
- ☑ Fatty acids are long-chain hydrocarbon molecules containing a carboxylic acid moiety at one end. Fatty acids that contain no carbon-carbon double bonds are termed saturated fatty acids; those that contain double bonds are unsaturated fatty acids.
- ☑ The term omega, as it relates to fatty acids, refers to the terminal carbon atom farthest from the carboxylic acid group. The designation of a polyunsaturated fatty acid (PUFA) as an omega-3 fatty acid, for example, defines the position of the first site of unsaturation relative to the omega end of that fatty acid.
- ☑ Triglycerides are composed of three fatty acids esterified to a backbone of glycerol. These lipids represent the major storage form of fatty acids.
- ☑ Phospholipids have a structure similar to that of the triglycerides except that C-3 (*sn*3) of the glycerol backbone is esterified to phosphoric acid.
- ☑ The sphingolipids represent a complex class of lipid composed of a sphingosine backbone with the majority also containing carbohydrate forming the glycosphingolipids.

NUCLEIC ACIDS

Nucleotides are found primarily as the monomeric units comprising the major nucleic acids of the cell, RNA and DNA. However, they also are required for numerous other important functions within the cell.

The nucleotides found in cells are derivatives of the heterocyclic, highly basic compounds, purine and pyrimidine (Figure 1–13).

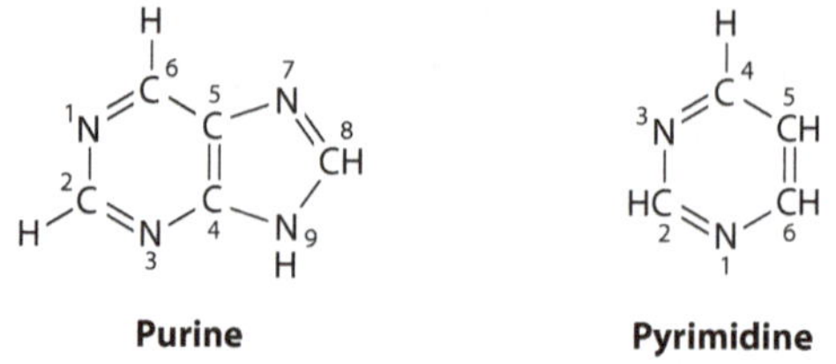

FIGURE 1–13 Purine and pyrimidine. The atoms are numbered according to the international system. (Reproduced with permission from Rodwell VW, Bender DA, Botham KM, et al: *Harper's Illustrated Biochemistry*, 31st ed. New York, NY: McGraw Hill; 2018.)

HIGH-YIELD CONCEPT

Chemically the nucleotides are basic compounds, which is the reason for the common term "bases" in the context of DNA and RNA. There are five major bases found in cells. The derivatives of purine are called adenine and guanine, and the derivatives of pyrimidine are called thymine, cytosine, and uracil. The common abbreviations used for these five bases are, A, G, T, C, and U, respectively.

The purine and pyrimidine bases in cells are linked to ribose-5-phosphate and in this form are termed, nucleosides (Table 1–5). The carbon atoms of the ribose present in nucleotides are designated with a prime (′) mark to distinguish them from the backbone numbering in the bases. Nucleosides normally exist in cells in the mono-, di-, or tri-phosphorylated state (eg, AMP, ADP, or ATP).

The ribose of nucleotides can be D-ribose such as the nucleotides of RNA, or 2′-deoxy-D-ribose as in the nucleotides of DNA (Figure 1–14). The deoxynucleotides are designated with a lowercase "d" as in dAMP.

The nucleotide uridine is never found naturally in DNA and thymine is almost exclusively found in DNA. The primary modified base in DNA is 5-methylcytosine (see Chapter 22). A variety of modified bases appear in the tRNAs (see Chapter 23). Many modified nucleotides are encountered outside of the context of DNA and RNA that serve important biological functions.

Nucleotide Derivatives

The most common adenosine derivative is the cyclic form, 3′-5′-cyclic adenosine monophosphate, cAMP. Formation of cAMP is catalyzed by adenylate cyclase, itself activated by cell surface receptors of the G protein-coupled receptor (GPCR) family (see Chapter 26). Cyclic AMP serves as the "second messenger" of the signal transduction process where the primary signal is the hormone or growth factor that binds to a particular GPCR. A cyclic form of GMP (cGMP) is also produced in cells and also acts as a second messenger molecule, such as in the visual process (see Chapter 3).

Another important adenosine derivative is S-adenosylmethionine (see Chapter 18), which is a form of activated methionine serving as a methyl donor in methylation reactions and as a source of propylamine in the synthesis of polyamines.

TABLE 1–5 Purine bases, ribonucleosides, and ribonucleotides.

Purine or Pyrimidine	X = H	X = Ribose	X = Ribose Phosphate
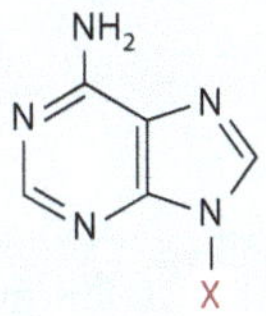	Adenine	Adenosine	Adenosine monophosphate (AMP)
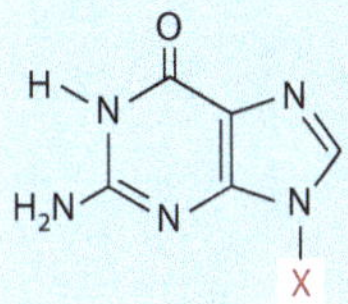	Guanine	Guanosine	Guanosine monophosphate (GMP)
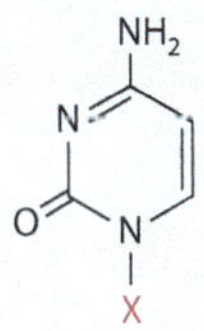	Cytosine	Cytidine	Cytidine monophosphate (CMP)
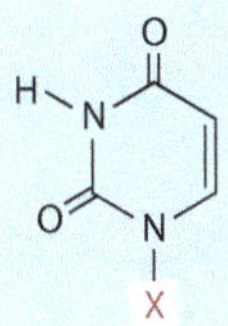	Uracil	Uridine	Uridine monophosphate (UMP)
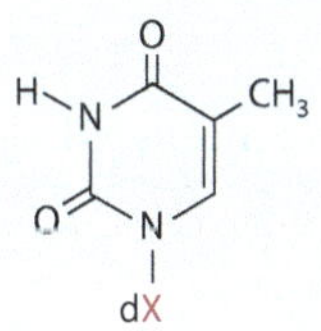	Thymine	Thymidine	Thymidine monophosphate (TMP)

Reproduced with permission from Rodwell VW, Bender DA, Botham KM, et al: *Harper's Illustrated Biochemistry*, 31st ed. New York, NY: McGraw Hill; 2018.

Polynucleotides

Polynucleotides are formed by the condensation of two or more nucleotides. The condensation most commonly occurs between the alcohol of a 5′-phosphate of one nucleotide and the 3′-hydroxyl of a second forming a phosphodiester bond. The primary structure of DNA and RNA (the linear arrangement of the nucleotides) proceeds in the 5′→3′ direction, written for example, 5′-GATC-3′.

CHECKLIST

- ☑ The nucleotides found in cells are derivatives of the heterocyclic, highly basic compounds, purine and pyrimidine.
- ☑ Nucleosides are composed of a nucleobase (purine or pyrimidine) attached to ribose but containing no phosphate. Nucleotides are the result of phosphate addition to nucleosides and they can be either mono-, di-, or tri-phosphate modified.
- ☑ The triphosphate and diphosphate groups of nucleotides are phosphanhydride bonds imparting high transfer energy for participation in covalent bond synthesis, such as in the case of ATP.
- ☑ The nomenclature for the atoms in nucleosides and nucleotides includes a prime (′) designation to distinguish the atoms in the sugar from those in the base.
- ☑ Polynucleotides are composed of two or more nucleotides linked together via a phosphodiester bond between the 5′ phosphate of the sugar in one nucleotide and the 3′ hydroxyl of the sugar in another nucleotide. The common left-to-right nomenclature for polynucleotides is 5′ → 3′ for example, 5′-pApGpCpT-3′ or just 5′-AGCT-3′.
- ☑ Cyclic adenosine and guanine nucleotides act as second messengers in signal transduction events.
- ☑ Nucleotide analogs are used as antimicrobial and anti-cancer agents via their ability to interfere with nucleotide biosynthesis or DNA replication.

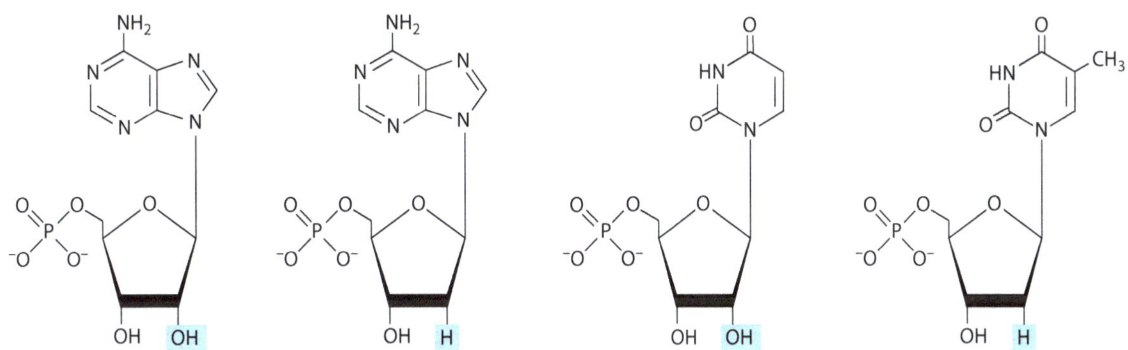

AMP **dAMP** **UMP** **TMP**

FIGURE 1–14 Structures of AMP, dAMP, UMP, and TMP. (Reproduced with permission from Rodwell VW, Bender DA, Botham KM, et al: *Harper's Illustrated Biochemistry*, 31st ed. New York, NY: McGraw Hill; 2018.)

REVIEW QUESTIONS

1. Acids in solution, such as amino acids, exhibit an equilibrium between the acid and conjugate base forms. Which of the following most correctly defines the value associated with this equilibrium?
   (A) It is the ion constant of water
   (B) It is the negative log of the concentration of H^+
   (C) It is the pH at which a molecule is neutrally charged
   (D) It is the pH at which an equivalent distribution of acid and conjugate base exists in solution
   (E) It is the value of the dissociation of HA to A^- and H^+

2. Which of the following most correctly defines the isoelectric point (pI) of an amino acid?
   (A) It is the ion constant of water
   (B) It is the negative log of the concentration of H^+
   (C) It is the pH at which a molecule is neutrally charged
   (D) It is the pH at which an equivalent distribution of acid and conjugate base exists in solution
   (E) It is the value of the dissociation of HA to A^- and H^+

3. Amino acids are characterized by the presence or absence of charge, affinity for water, or repulsion of water. Which one of the following amino acids is most likely to repel water at physiologic pH?
   (A) Arginine
   (B) Aspartic acid
   (C) Glycine
   (D) Isoleucine
   (E) Threonine

4. Various amino acids interact with the aqueous environment by being able to buffer protons (H^+). Which of the following has the greatest capacity to buffer at physiologic pH 6?
   (A) Alanine
   (B) Cysteine
   (C) Glutamate
   (D) Histidine
   (E) Tyrosine

5. The formation of a disaccharide is most likely going to involve which of the following types of chemical bond?
   (A) Carbonyl
   (B) Double
   (C) Glycosidic
   (D) Hydrogen
   (E) Phosphodiester

6. The measurement of the levels of HbA_{1c} is diagnostic for the chronic state of hyperglycemia in patients with type 2 diabetes. Which of the following is the most likely mechanism for the formation of this form of hemoglobin?
   (A) GlcNAcylation
   (B) Glycation
   (C) *N*-glycosylation
   (D) *O*-glycosylation
   (E) Phosphorylation

7. Which of the following carbohydrates most likely belongs to the ketose family?
   (A) Fructose
   (B) Galactose
   (C) Glucose
   (D) Lactose
   (E) Maltose

8. Patients with Gaucher disease accumulate lipid compounds in cells of the monocyte lineage. Which of the following most closely represents the class of accumulating lipid in this disease?
   (A) Fatty acid
   (B) Glycosphingolipid
   (C) Phospholipid
   (D) Sphingomyelin
   (E) Triglyceride

9. A cell that lacked expression of the glycerol kinase gene would most likely be incapable of synthesizing which of the following lipid classes?
   (A) Cholesterol
   (B) Fatty acids
   (C) Phospholipids
   (D) Sphingolipids
   (E) Triglycerides

10. Which of the following lipids is most likely to have the highest melting point?
    (A) Arachidonic acid
    (B) Linoleic acid
    (C) Oleic acid
    (D) Palmitic acid
    (E) Palmitoleic acid

11. The formation of polymers of nucleic acids is most likely going to involve which of the following types of chemical bond?
    (A) Carbonyl
    (B) Double
    (C) Glycosidic
    (D) Hydrogen
    (E) Phosphodiester

12. Males with Lesch-Nyhan syndrome cannot properly salvage nucleotides and as a result are most likely to excrete large quantities of which of the following?
    (A) Adenosine
    (B) Hypoxanthine
    (C) Thymidine
    (D) Uracil
    (E) Uric acid
    (F) Xanthine

13. Which of the following is most likely to be found only in transfer RNA molecules?
    (A) cAMP
    (B) Cytidine
    (C) cGMP
    (D) Dihydrouridine
    (E) Thymidine

ANSWERS

1. Correct answer is **E.** The dissociation constant of an acid or a base, defined as K_a, is the product of the concentrations of the conjugate acid (eg, A^-) and conjugate base (eg, H^+) divided by the concentration of acid (eg, HA). The ion constant for water, K_w (choice A), is the product of the concentration of protons (H^+) and hydroxyl ions (OH^-). The value of pH is defined as the negative log of the hydrogen ion (H^+) concentration (choice B). The isoelectric point (pI) is defined by

the pH at which a molecule is electrically neutral (choice C). The value of pK_a (choice D) is defined as the pH at which an equivalent distribution of acid and conjugate base exists in a solution.

2. Correct answer is **C.** The isoelectric point is that pH at which a substance exhibits no net charge. In other words, all the negative and positive charges, say for instance in a protein, are equal in number such that the molecule is electrically neutral. The ion constant for water, K_w (choice A), is the product of the concentration of protons (H^+) and hydroxyl ions (OH^-). The value of pH is defined as the negative log of the hydrogen ion (H^+) concentration (choice B). The value of pK_a (choice D) is defined as the pH at which an equivalent distribution of acid and conjugate base exists in a solution. The dissociation constant of an acid or base (choice E), defined as K_a, is the product of the concentrations of the conjugate acid (eg, A^-) and conjugate base (eg, H^+) divided by the concentration of the acid (eg, HA).

3. Correct answer is **D.** Hydrophobic amino acids, like isoleucine, are those with side chains that do not like to reside in an aqueous environment. For this reason, these amino acids are more often found buried within the hydrophobic core of a protein, or within the lipid portion of a membrane. All of the other amino acids (choices A, B, C, and E) are composed of R-groups that can ionize in an aqueous environment and, therefore, are hydrophilic and as such interact with water at physiologic pH.

4. Correct answer is **D.** Histidine contains an imidazole ring as its R-group. The nitrogen in this ring possesses a pK_a around 6.0; thus it is able to accept or donate a proton at physiologic pH. This fact makes the amino acid an ideal buffering component of a protein containing several histidine residues. In addition, histidine is often found in the reactive centers of enzymes where it participates in H^+ interactions. Alanine (choice A) is hydrophobic and possesses an R-group that does not ionize. Cysteine (choice B), glutamate (choice C), and tyrosine (choice E) all contain ionizable R-groups but the pKa values of these R-groups are outside the range of physiologic pH and as such are less capable of buffering protons at this pH.

5. Correct answer is **C.** The formation of disaccharides, as well as polysaccharides, involves the covalent attachment of monosaccharide units via glycosidic bonds. Carbonyl bonds (choice A) are composed of oxygen atoms double bonded to carbon atoms. Double bonds (choice B) are any covalent bonds that are formed between two atoms (eg, carbon and carbon or carbon and oxygen) that involves four bonding electrons. Hydrogen bonds (choice D) are noncovalent bonds that result from an electrostatic attraction between a proton in one molecule and an electronegative atom (such as oxygen) in the other. Phosphodiester bonds (choice E) result when a phosphoric acid group in a nucleotide forms covalent bonds with the hydroxyl groups in the ribose sugar of two different nucleotides forming a polynucleotide.

6. Correct answer is **B.** Glycation is the nonenzymatic covalent attachment of a carbohydrate, most often glucose, to protein or lipid. The formation of HbA_{1c} results from the glycation of amino groups in the protein subunits of the major form of hemoglobin (HbA_1). Hemoglobin glycation is often incorrectly identified as nonenzymatic glycosylation. GlcNAcylation (choice A) refers to the attachment of *O*-GlcNAc to serine or threonine residues in cytosolic and nuclear proteins via the action of the enzyme, *O*-GlcNAc transferase, OGT. *N*-glycosylation (choice C) and *O*-glycosylation (choice D) are the enzymatic attachment of carbohydrate to asparagine or serine residues, respectively, in protein. Phosphorylation (choice E) is the covalent attachment of phosphate to serine, threonine, or tyrosine residues in protein.

7. Correct answer is **A.** Ketoses are monosaccharides that contain one ketone (−C=O) in the acyclic form of the molecule. In addition to fructose, several other important ketoses in humans are dihydroxyacetone, ribulose, xylulose, and sedoheptulose. All of the other carbohydrates are monosaccharides that are aldoses (choices B and C) or disaccharides composed of monosaccharides that are aldoses (choices D and E).

8. Correct answer is **B.** Gaucher disease is a lysosomal storage disease that results from mutations in the gene (GBA) encoding the lysosomal hydrolase, glucosylceramidase beta, also called acid β-glucosidase or glucocerebrosidase. As a result of the enzyme defect the glycosphingolipid, glucosylceramide (glucocerebroside) accumulates in lysosomes. None of the other options (choices A, C, D, and E) represent the class of molecule accumulating in Gaucher disease.

9. Correct answer is **E.** Triglycerides are composed of a backbone of glycerol to which three fatty acids are esterified. One of the pathways to triglyceride synthesis in hepatocytes is initiated by the phosphorylation of glycerol via the action of glycerol kinase. Therefore, a defect in glycerol kinase activity in these cells would result in reduced capacity to synthesize triglycerides. Adipocytes of adipose tissue do not express the glycerol kinase gene and, therefore, required the glycolytic intermediate, dihydroxyacetone phosphate, as the intermediate in triglyceride synthesis. Synthesis of the other lipids (choices A, B, C, and D) does not involve the use of glycerol kinase.

10. Correct answer is **D.** The melting point of palmitic acid is 63°C. The important consideration is not the absolute melting points of various fatty acids, but the factors that contribute to fatty acid melting points. The melting point of fatty acids increases as the number of carbon atoms increases. In addition, the introduction of sites of unsaturation results in lower melting points when comparing a saturated and an unsaturated fatty acid of the same number of carbon atoms. Saturated fatty acids of less than eight carbon atoms are liquid at physiologic temperature, whereas those containing more than 10 carbon atoms are solid. The melting point of arachidonic acid (choice A) is -50°C, linoleic (choice B) is -5°C, oleic (choice C) is 16°C, and palmitoleic (choice E) is 0.5°C.

11. Correct answer is **E.** The formation of polynucleotides (RNA and DNA) involves the formation of a phosphodiester bond between two nucleotides. Phosphodiester bonds result when a phosphoric acid group in a nucleotide forms covalent bonds with the hydroxyl groups in the ribose sugar of two different nucleotides during the formation of a polynucleotide. Carbonyl bonds (choice A) are composed of oxygen atoms double bonded to carbon atoms. Double bonds (choice B) are any covalent bonds that are formed between two atoms (eg, carbon and carbon or carbon and oxygen) that involves four bonding electrons. A glycosidic bond (choice C) is formed between the hemiacetal or hemiketal group of a saccharide and the hydroxyl group of some other compound

such as another saccharide or any other compound such as an alcohol. Hydrogen bonds (choice D) are noncovalent bonds that result from an electrostatic attraction between a proton in one molecule and an electronegative atom (such as oxygen) in the other.

12. Correct answer is **E.** Lesch-Nyhan syndrome results from deficiencies in hypoxanthine-guanine phosphoribosyltransferase (HGPRT). HGPRT is a purine nucleotide salvage enzyme that converts guanine to GMP and hypoxanthine to inosine monophosphate (IMP). Loss of this salvage enzyme results in decreased levels of AMP, GMP, and IMP, all of which normally feedback inhibit the rate-limiting enzyme of purine nucleotide biosynthesis, 5-phosphoribosyl-1-pyrophosphate (PRPP) amidotransferase. The loss of feedback inhibition results in excess synthesis of purines with the consequences being increased rates of purine nucleotide catabolism whose end product is uric acid. Although the consequences of defective HGPRT are increased purine synthesis leading to increased adenosine (choice A) followed by increased catabolism to hypoxanthine (choice B) and xanthine (choice F), these do not accumulate due to their complete catabolism to uric acid. Thymidine (choice C) and uracil (choice D) are pyrimidine nucleotides, and their synthesis and metabolism are not affected in Lesch-Nyhan syndrome.

13. Correct answer is **D.** Modified nucleotides are found in all three classes of RNA: tRNA, rRNA, and mRNA. As many as 25% of the nucleotides found in tRNAs are modified post-transcriptionally. At least 80 different modified nucleotides have been identified at more than 60 different positions in various tRNAs. The two most commonly occurring modified nucleotides in tRNA are dihydrouridine (abbreviated D) and pseudouridine (designated with the Greek capital Psi: Ψ), each of which is found in a characteristic loop structure in tRNAs. Pseudouridine is the 5-ribosyl isomer of uridine that is generated a 180-degree rotation of the uridine base such that the base is attached to the 1′ carbon of the ribose via a carbon-carbon glycosidic bond instead of the normal nitrogen-carbon glycosidic bond. Dihydrouridine is found in the D-loop (hence the name of the loop) and pseudouridine is found in the TΨC loop (hence the name of the loop). Both cAMP (choice A) and cGMP (choice C) are modified nucleotides, but they are not found in RNA but rather serve as second messengers in numerous cell signaling pathways. Cytidine (choice B) is present in all three classes of RNA as well as DNA. Thymidine (choice E), specifically thymidine attached to deoxyribose, is found only in DNA. However, the thymidine nucleobase attached ribose (ribothymidine) is found in tRNAs and is the T found in the TΨC loop.

CHAPTER

2

Protein Structure: Hemoglobin and Myoglobin

High-Yield Terms

Fibrous protein	Any protein that is generally insoluble in water and exists in an elongated and rigid conformation; most structural proteins are fibrous
Globular protein	Any protein that is generally soluble in water and exists in more compact spherical conformation; most functional proteins are globular
Methemoglobin	The form of the hemoglobin protein that contains ferric iron (Fe^{3+}) in the heme prosthetic groups due to oxidation
Hemoglobinopathy	Any disease resulting from either (or both) quantitative or qualitative defects in α-globin or β-globin proteins
Thalassemia	Specifically refers to quantitative hemoglobinopathies due to either α-globin or β-globin protein defects
Sickle cell anemia	Most commonly occurring qualitative hemoglobinopathy, results from a single amino acid substitution in the adult β-globin gene
Cooley anemia	Is thalassemia major which is either β^0- and β^+-thalassemia

FORCES CONTROLLING PROTEIN STRUCTURE

The interaction of different domains is governed by several forces. These include hydrogen bonding, hydrophobic interactions, electrostatic interactions, and van der Waals forces.

Hydrogen Bonding

Polypeptides contain numerous proton donors and acceptors both in their backbone and in the R-groups of the amino acids. The environment in which proteins are found also contains the ample H-bond donors and acceptors of the water molecule. H-bonding, therefore, occurs not only within and between polypeptide chains but with the surrounding aqueous medium.

Hydrophobic Forces

Proteins are composed of amino acids that contain either hydrophilic or hydrophobic R-groups. It is the nature of the interaction of the different R-groups with the aqueous environment that plays the major role in shaping protein structure. The spontaneous folded state of globular proteins is a reflection of a balance between the opposing energetics of H-bonding between hydrophilic R-groups and the aqueous environment and the repulsion from the aqueous environment by the hydrophobic R-groups. The hydrophobicity of certain amino acid R-groups tends to drive them away from the exterior of proteins and into the interior. This driving force restricts the available conformations into which a protein may fold.

Electrostatic Forces

Electrostatic forces are mainly of three types; charge-charge, charge-dipole, and dipole-dipole. Typical charge-charge interactions that favor protein folding are those between oppositely charged R-groups such as K or R and D or E. A substantial component of the energy involved in protein folding is charge-dipole interactions. This refers to the interaction of ionized R-groups of amino acids with the dipole of the water molecule.

van der Waals Forces

There are both attractive and repulsive van der Waals forces that control protein folding. Attractive van der Waals forces involve the interactions among induced dipoles that arise from fluctuations in the charge densities that occur between adjacent uncharged nonbonded atoms. Repulsive van der Waals forces involve the interactions that occur when uncharged nonbonded atoms come very close together but do not induce dipoles. The repulsion is the result of the electron-electron repulsion that occurs as two clouds of electrons begin to overlap.

PRIMARY STRUCTURE IN PROTEINS

The primary structure of proteins refers to the linear order of the amino acids present. The convention for the designation of the order of amino acids is that the N-terminal end (ie, the end bearing the residue with the free α-amino group) is to the left (and the number 1 amino acid) and the C-terminal end (ie, the end with the residue containing a free α-carboxyl group) is to the right, for example, NH_2-Asp-Glu-Tyr-Ala-COOH.

SECONDARY STRUCTURE IN PROTEINS

The ordered array of amino acids in a protein confers regular conformational forms on that protein. These conformations constitute the secondary structures of a protein. The primary secondary structures are formed through hydrogen bonding (H-bonding) between atoms in the peptide bond. In general, proteins fold into two broad classes of structure termed globular proteins or fibrous proteins. Globular proteins are compactly folded and coiled. Fibrous proteins are filamentous or elongated.

The α-Helix

The formation of the α-helix (Figure 2–1) is spontaneous and is generated through H-bonding between an amide nitrogen and a carbonyl oxygen of peptide bonds spaced four residues apart. This orientation of H-bonding produces a helical coiling of the peptide backbone such that the R-groups lie on the exterior of the helix and perpendicular to its axis.

Not all amino acids favor the formation of the α-helix due to steric constraints of the R-groups. This is particularly true for P since it is an imino acid whose structure significantly restricts movement about the peptide bond in which it is present, thereby, interfering with extension of the helix.

β-Sheets

Like the α-helix, β-sheets (Figure 2–2) are formed from H-bonding of the atoms in peptide bonds. In β-sheets, the H-bonding adjacently opposed stretches of the polypeptide backbone consisting of at least 5–10 amino acids. Beta-sheets are either parallel or antiparallel. In parallel sheets, adjacent

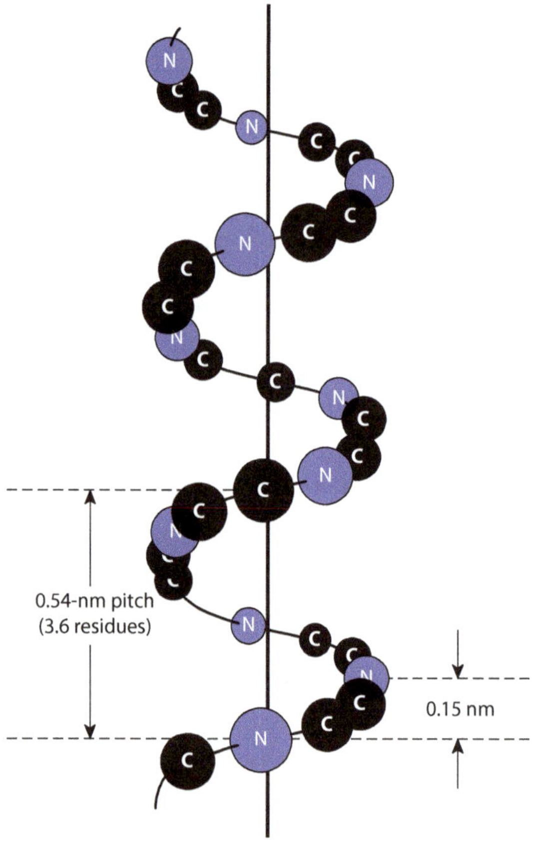

FIGURE 2–1 Orientation of the main chain atoms of a peptide about the axis of an α-helix. (Reproduced with permission from Rodwell VW, Bender DA, Botham KM, et al: *Harper's Illustrated Biochemistry*, 31st ed. New York, NY: McGraw Hill; 2018.)

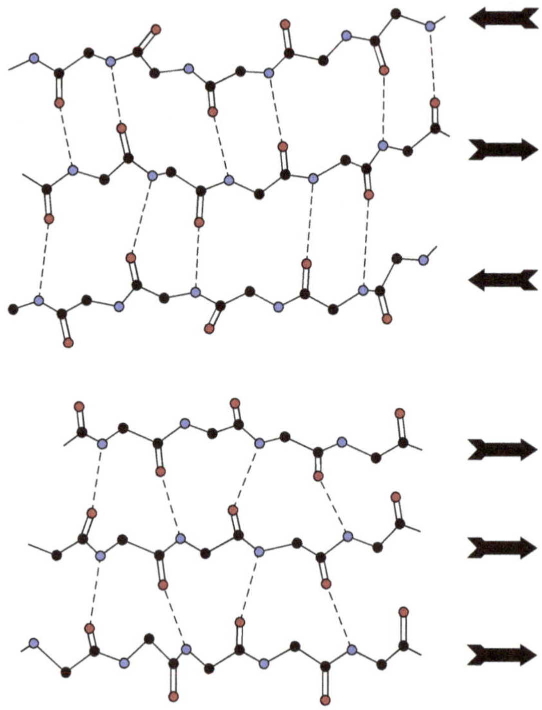

FIGURE 2–2 Spacing and bond angles of the hydrogen bonds of antiparallel and parallel pleated β-sheets. Arrows indicate the direction of each strand. Hydrogen bonds are indicated by dotted lines with the participating α-nitrogen atoms (hydrogen donors) and oxygen atoms (hydrogen acceptors) shown in blue and red, respectively. Backbone carbon atoms are shown in black. For clarity in presentation, R groups and hydrogen atoms are omitted. Top: Antiparallel β-sheet. Pairs of hydrogen bonds alternate between being close together and wide apart and are oriented approximately perpendicular to the polypeptide backbone. Bottom: Parallel β-sheet. The hydrogen bonds are evenly spaced but slant in alternate directions. (Reproduced with permission from Rodwell VW, Bender DA, Botham KM, et al: *Harper's Illustrated Biochemistry*, 31st ed. New York, NY: McGraw Hill; 2018.)

peptide chains proceed in the same direction (ie, the direction of N-terminal to C-terminal ends is the same), whereas in antiparallel sheets adjacent chains are aligned in opposite directions. Beta-sheets can be depicted in ball and stick format or as ribbons in certain protein formats.

SUPER-SECONDARY STRUCTURE

Some proteins contain an ordered organization of secondary structures, termed super-secondary structures. These structures form distinct functional domains in proteins. Examples include the helix-loop-helix and zinc finger domains of eukaryotic transcriptional regulators or the leucine zipper domain that promotes protein-protein interactions. These domains are termed super-secondary structures.

TERTIARY STRUCTURE OF PROTEINS

Tertiary structure refers to the complete three-dimensional structure that a given protein occupies. Included in this description is the spatial relationship of different secondary structures to one another within a protein and how these secondary structures themselves fold into the three-dimensional form of the protein.

QUATERNARY STRUCTURE

Proteins with multiple polypeptide chains are oligomeric proteins. The overall structure formed by the interaction of at least two protein subunits in an oligomeric protein is known as quaternary structure. One of the best models for quaternary structure and function is hemoglobin.

HEMOGLOBIN: MODEL OF QUATERNARY STRUCTURE & FUNCTION

Hemoglobin and the related protein, myoglobin, are heme-containing proteins whose physiologic importance is related to their ability to bind molecular oxygen. Hemoglobin is a heterotetrameric oxygen transport protein found in red blood cells (erythrocytes). Adult hemoglobin is a heterotetrameric protein composed of two α-globin proteins and two β-globin proteins (Figure 2–3). Myoglobin is a monomeric protein found mainly in muscle tissue where it serves as an intracellular storage site for oxygen. The oxygen carried by hemoglobin and myoglobin is bound directly to the ferrous iron (Fe^{2+}) atom of the heme prosthetic group. The oxidation state of iron dramatically alters the binding of oxygen to hemoglobin. (see Clinical Box 2–1).

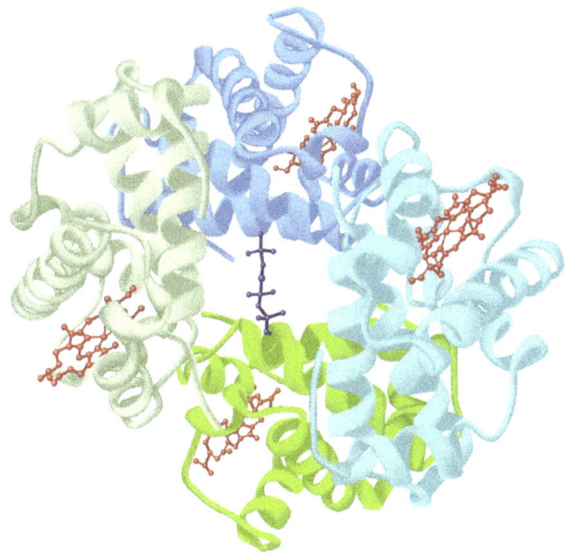

FIGURE 2–3 Hemoglobin. Shown is the three-dimensional structure of deoxyhemoglobin with a molecule of 2,3-bisphosphoglycerate (dark blue) bound. The two α-subunits are colored in the darker shades of green and blue, the two β-subunits in the lighter shades of green and blue, and the heme prosthetic groups in red. (Modified with permission from Protein Data Bank ID no. 1b86.)

CLINICAL BOX 2–1 EFFECT OF IRON OXIDATION ON OXYGEN BINDING TO HEMOGLOBIN

Oxidation of the ferrous (Fe^{2+}) iron to the ferric (Fe^{3+}) oxidation state renders a globin monomer incapable of normal oxygen binding. When one or more of the heme iron molecules exists in the ferric state, the hemoglobin is termed methemoglobin. Formation of the reactive oxygen species (ROS), superoxide anion, can occur in erythrocytes as a result of O_2 oxidation of ferrous iron to ferric iron in hemoglobin. The consequence of the latter reaction is the generation of methemoglobin. Since hemoglobin is a heterotetramer, and each subunit contains Fe^{2+} iron in its heme there is the potential for multiple Fe^{3+} irons to be present in methemoglobin. The Fe^{3+} form of iron does not bind O_2; however, the presence of at least one Fe^{3+} in the hemoglobin tetramer results in enhanced binding of the O_2 to the remaining Fe^{2+} irons causing reduced delivery of the O_2 to the tissues with potential for cyanosis. Normal daily levels of methemoglobin range from 0.5 to 3%. The ferric iron in methemoglobin is reduced to ferrous via the action of the NADH-requiring enzyme, methemoglobin reductase (cytochrome b_5 reductase 3: CYB5R3). The NADPH produced in the pentose phosphate pathway (see Chapter 8) and the antioxidant glutathione (GSH; see Chapter 19) are both necessary for the continual removal of ROS from within the erythrocyte to help prevent accumulation of methemoglobin.

OXYGEN-BINDING CHARACTERISTICS

Oxygen binding to hemoglobin is a cooperative process that can be evidenced in the sigmoidal characteristics in a saturation binding curve (Figure 2–4). The cooperative binding is the consequence of the quaternary structure of hemoglobin. In contrast, the monomeric myoglobin protein exhibits linear oxygen saturation kinetics.

When oxygen binds to the first subunit of deoxyhemoglobin it increases the affinity of the remaining subunits for oxygen. As additional oxygen is bound to the second and third subunits, oxygen-binding affinity is increased even further. At the oxygen pressure in lung alveoli hemoglobin is easily fully saturated with oxygen.

CLINICAL BOX 2-2 EFFECT OF CARBON MONOXIDE ON THE FUNCTION OF HEMOGLOBIN

Carbon monoxide (CO) also binds coordinately to heme iron atoms in the ferrous state (Fe^{2+}) in hemoglobin in a manner similar to that of oxygen. However, the binding of CO to heme iron is much stronger (>200-fold) than that of O_2. When CO is bound to hemoglobin, the resulting protein is referred to as carboxyhemoglobin (HbCO). In addition to a higher affinity of CO over that of O_2 for ferrous iron in hemoglobin, the result of CO binding to at least one globin monomer causes a higher affinity of the remaining subunits for O_2. This effect contributes to reduced O_2 release in the tissues. These combined effects of the preferential binding of CO to heme iron is largely responsible for the lethality that results from carbon monoxide poisoning.

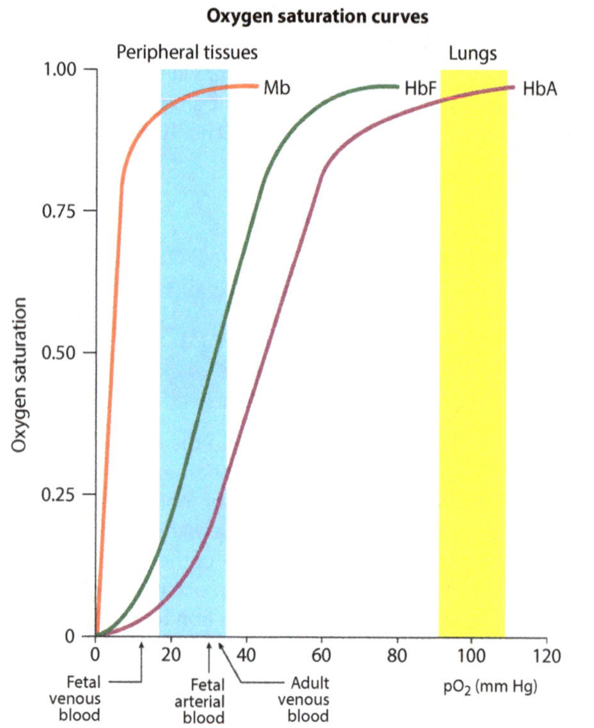

FIGURE 2–4 Oxygen saturation curves for myoglobin and hemoglobin. The saturation curve for myoglobin shows the typical rapid oxygen concentration–dependent saturation of this monomeric oxygen-binding protein. The other two curves show the typical sigmoidal saturation curves for cooperative oxygen binding exhibited by fetal hemoglobin (HbF) and adult hemoglobin (HbA). Also indicated in the diagram are the typical oxygen concentrations in peripheral tissues and the lungs. Note that whereas myoglobin can be fully oxygen saturated in the tissues, hemoglobin requires much higher oxygen tension to become fully saturated, which only occurs in the lungs. The position of HbF saturation to the left of HbA (ie, at lower oxygen tension) reflects the fact that fetal hemoglobin binds oxygen with higher affinity than adult hemoglobin and this is so that the fetus can acquire oxygen from the maternal circulation. (Reproduced with permission from themedicalbiochemistrypage, LLC.)

The cooperative oxygen-binding properties of hemoglobin arise directly from the interaction of oxygen with the iron atom of the heme prosthetic groups and the resultant effects of these interactions on the quaternary structure of the protein. The low affinity state of deoxygenated hemoglobin (Hb) is known as the T (tense) state. Conversely, the high affinity state of hemoglobin (HbO_2) is known as the R (relaxed) state.

Carbon monoxide will also bind the heme prosthetic group of hemoglobin but does so with an affinity on the order of 200 times higher than that of oxygen. The effect of CO binding to hemoglobin is significantly reduced oxygen delivery to the tissues (see Clinical Box 2–2).

The primary regulator of the transition between the T and R states is 2,3-bisphosphoglycerate (2,3-BPG or also just BPG). Additional regulators of hemoglobin affinity for oxygen are CO_2, hydrogen ion (H^+: proton), and chloride ion (Cl^-). Although all four regulators can influence O_2 binding independent of each other, CO_2, H^+, and Cl^- primarily function collectively on the affinity of hemoglobin for O_2.

In the high O_2 environment (high pO_2) of the lungs, there is sufficient O_2 to overcome the inhibitory nature of the T state of hemoglobin. During the O_2 binding-induced alteration from the T state to the R state, several amino acid side groups on the surface of hemoglobin subunits will dissociate protons (H^+) as depicted in the following equation.

$$4O_2 + Hb \leftrightarrow nH^+ + Hb(O_2)_4$$

Proton dissociation from hemoglobin in the lungs plays an important role in the expiration of the CO_2 that arrives from the tissues. Although protons exert a negative influence on oxygen binding to hemoglobin, the pH of the blood in the lungs (≈7.4–7.5) is not sufficiently low enough to exert this negative influence. In addition, the high pO_2 of the lungs can overcome the effect of any protons released from hemoglobin. Conversely, when the oxyhemoglobin reaches the tissues the pO_2 is sufficiently low and the pH (≈7.2) is such that the T state is favored and the O_2 released.

Catabolic reactions in tissues produce CO_2 which diffuses into the blood and enters the circulating erythrocytes. Within erythrocytes the CO_2 is rapidly converted to carbonic acid through the action of carbonic anhydrase. The carbonic acid then rapidly ionizes leading to increased production of H^+.

$$CO_2 + H_2O \leftrightarrow H_2CO_3 \leftrightarrow H^+ + HCO_3^-$$

The H^+ released from carbonic acid influences an R to T state transition in hemoglobin leading to release of O_2. The effect of this H^+ on hemoglobin is referred to as the Bohr effect (Figure 2–5).

The bicarbonate ion is transported out of the erythrocyte and is carried in the blood to the lungs. Coupled with bicarbonate transport out of the erythrocyte is transport of Cl^- into the cell. The antiporter that carries out this transport is the anion exchanger 1 (AE1) encoded by the SLC4A1 gene. Approximately 80% of the CO_2 produced in metabolizing cells is transported to the lungs as bicarbonate ion. A small percentage of CO_2 is transported in the blood as a dissolved gas.

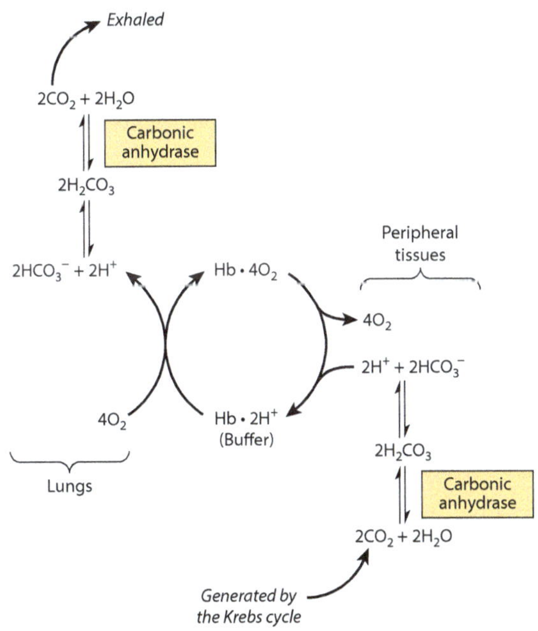

FIGURE 2–5 The Bohr effect. Carbon dioxide generated in peripheral tissues combines with water to form carbonic acid, which dissociates into protons and bicarbonate ions. Deoxyhemoglobin acts as a buffer by binding protons and delivering them to the lungs. In the lungs, the uptake of oxygen by hemoglobin releases protons that combine with bicarbonate ion, forming carbonic acid, which when dehydrated by carbonic anhydrase becomes carbon dioxide, which then is exhaled. (Reproduced with permission from Rodwell VW, Bender DA, Botham KM, et al: *Harper's Illustrated Biochemistry,* 31st ed. New York, NY: McGraw Hill; 2018.)

HIGH-YIELD CONCEPT

The reactions forming bicarbonate ion and proton (H^+) are essentially freely reversible. Indeed, during periods of metabolic acidosis, the increased levels of H^+ in the blood trigger the activation of chemoreceptors (proton-sensitive receptors; primarily G-protein coupled receptor 4 [GPR4]) in neurons of the retrotrapezoid nucleus (RTN) in the brainstem. Activation of these chemoreceptors triggers an increase in respiration rate leading to increased expiration of CO_2, which in turn drives the reaction in the leftward direction resulting in a reduction in H^+ levels in the blood and thus, decreased acidity (increased pH).

HIGH-YIELD CONCEPT

As much as 15% of CO_2 is transported to the lungs bound to N-terminal amino groups of the T form of hemoglobin. This reaction forms what is called carbamino-hemoglobin.

$$CO_2 + \text{Hb-NH}_2 \leftrightarrow H^+ + \text{Hb-NH-COO}^-$$

The formation of H^+ via this reaction enhances the release of the bound O_2 to the surrounding tissues. Within the lungs, the high O_2 content results in O_2 binding to hemoglobin with the concomitant release of H^+. The released protons then promote the dissociation of the carbamino to form CO_2 which is then released with expiration.

ROLE OF 2,3-BISPHOSPHOGLYCERATE (2,3-BPG)

The compound 2,3-bisphosphoglycerate (2,3-BPG), derived from the glycolytic intermediate 1,3-bisphosphoglycerate, is a potent allosteric effector on the oxygen-binding properties of hemoglobin.

HIGH-YIELD CONCEPT

Since 2,3-BPG decreases the affinity of hemoglobin for O_2, it is beneficial at high altitude and other low oxygen conditions (hypoxia), to increase the amount associated with hemoglobin to facilitate the release of as much O_2 as possible under limiting conditions. The processes of erythrocyte metabolic reprogramming at high altitude and other hypoxic conditions involve sphingosine-1-phosphate (S1P: see Chapter 12) mediated release of several glycolytic enzymes from membrane association with anion exchanger 1 (AE1; originally identified as band 3). The release of glycolytic enzymes results in an increase in the rate of glycolysis and increased 2,3-BPG synthesis. An additional change that occurs in red blood cells under hypoxic conditions is activation of AMP-activated kinase (AMPK), which phosphorylates and enhances the activity of the bifunctional enzyme, 2,3-bisphosphoglycerate mutase (BPGM) of the Rapoport–Luebering shunt, further enhancing 2,3-BPG synthesis.

The pathway of red blood cell 2,3-BPG synthesis is referred to as the Rapoport–Luebering shunt. The interaction of 2,3-BPG with hemoglobin occurs via the β-globin subunits.

Hemoglobin molecules differing in subunit composition have different 2,3-BPG binding. For example, fetal hemoglobin (HbF) poorly binds 2,3-BPG with the result that HbF binds oxygen with greater affinity than the mother's adult hemoglobin (HbA). This effect results in the fetus acquiring oxygen carried by the mother's circulatory system.

THE HEMOGLOBIN GENES

The α- and β-globin proteins contained in functional hemoglobin tetramers are derived from gene clusters. Both gene clusters contain not only the major adult genes, α and β, but other expressed sequences that are utilized at different stages of development (Figure 2–6).

Hemoglobin synthesis begins in the first few weeks of embryonic development. The major hemoglobin at this stage of development is a tetramer composed of two zeta (ζ) chains encoded within the α cluster and two epsilon (ε) chains from the β cluster. By 6–8 weeks of gestation, the embryonic genes are turned off in both clusters. At this time, expression from the α cluster consists of identical proteins from the α1 and α2 genes and two genes are expressed throughout life. During fetal development, the genes of the β-globin cluster that are expressed are the gamma (γ) genes. The gamma proteins are called Gγ and Aγ, the derivation of which stems from the single amino acid difference between the two fetal genes: glycine in Gγ and alanine in Aγ at position 136. Fetal hemoglobin is designated HbFA.

Shortly before birth γ-globin genes expression ceases and adult β-globin gene expression ensues. The major adult hemoglobin is designated HbA_1. A minor adult hemoglobin, identified as HbA_2, is a tetramer of two α chains and two delta (δ) chains. Expression from the δ globin gene is low due to poor efficiency of the promoter region. The overall hemoglobin composition in a normal adult is approximately 97.5% HbA_1, 2% HbA_2, and 0.5% HbF (Figure 2–6).

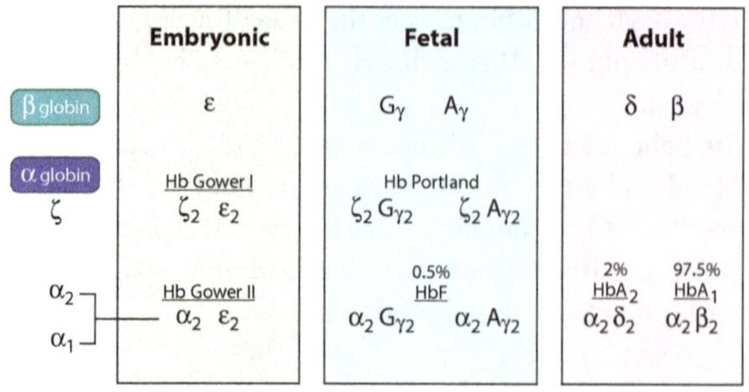

FIGURE 2–6 Major types of hemoglobin proteins found during embryonic, fetal, and adult life. (Reproduced with permission from themedicalbiochemistrypage, LLC.)

THE HEMOGLOBINOPATHIES

The term hemoglobinopathy refers to a family of disorders resulting from the synthesis of abnormal or reduced levels of one of the globin chains of the hemoglobin molecule. Hemoglobinopathies are classified dependent on whether the defect results in reduced (quantitative) or altered (qualitative) hemoglobin. More commonly the term hemoglobinopathy is used to imply structural abnormalities in the globin proteins themselves. In contrast, the term thalassemia is used to define hemoglobinopathies that are due to underproduction of normal globin proteins (see Clinical Boxes 2–3, 2–4, and 2–5).

CLINICAL BOX 2–3 ABNORMAL HEMOGLOBINS

Hemoglobin C: Hemoglobin C results from a relatively common mutation at codon 6, the same codon harboring the mutation in sickle cell anemia. In the case of HbC, the mutation converts the Glu codon to a Lys codon (AAG). Like sickle cell anemia, HbC disease is inherited as an autosomal recessive condition. Homozygous HbC/HbC individuals manifest a relatively benign disease consisting of mild hemolytic anemia, mild splenomegaly, and blood smears that show the presence of codocytes (target cells). HbC homozygous individuals may appear to have a very mild form of sickle cell anemia. However, in compound heterozygotes expressing an HbS and an HbC allele (SC disease) there is a much more significant pathology.

Hemoglobin E: Hemoglobin E is a form of hemoglobin resulting from mutation at amino acid 26 in the β-globin gene. This mutation changes the normal Glu (GAG) residue to a Lys (AAG). In addition to the change in amino acid sequence resulting in a qualitative hemoglobinopathy, the HbE mutation results in the generation of a cryptic splice site at codons 25–27 that results in 40% of β-globin mRNA being shorter than normal by 16 nucleotides. This shortened β-globin mRNA does not give rise to detectable β-globin protein, typical of quantitative β-thalassemias. The HbE form of hemoglobin is quite common in individuals of Southeast Asian descent. Hemoglobin E disease is inherited as an autosomal recessive disease where homozygous individuals (HbE/HbE) experience a mild form of β-thalassemia in the postnatal period. Heterozygotes (HbA/HbE) do not show any symptoms. Homozygotes for the HbE allele do not exhibit symptoms at birth because of the presence of normal fetal hemoglobin (HbF). Symptoms will begin to appear after the expression of the γ-globin gene ceases and the adult

CLINICAL BOX 2–3 (CONTINUED)

β-globin gene is activated. The typical symptoms are mild hemolytic anemia and mild splenomegaly. Serious pathology is present in individuals who are compound heterozygotes harboring one HbE allele and one β-thalassemia allele (HbE/β-thal). These individuals experience growth retardation, hepatosplenomegaly, hyperbilirubinemia (presenting as jaundice), bone abnormalities, and cardiovascular issues.

Hemoglobin M: Hemoglobin M (HbM) refers to group of autosomal dominant methemoglobinemias that are caused by heterozygous mutations in either the α- or β-globin genes. These mutations result in the production of what is referred to as M hemoglobin (HbM) which is a form of hemoglobin that stabilizes the heme iron in the ferric (Fe^{3+}) state and which is not amenable to reduction. The designation HbM also can refer to a form of hemoglobin that exhibits an unusual susceptibility to oxidizing agents. At least five different forms of hemoglobin M have been characterized. Four of these, HbM (Boston), HbM (Hyde Park), HbM (Iwate), and HbM (Saskatoon), are due to mutations that alter the critical His residues to Tyr in the heme binding pocket of either α-globin or β-globin proteins. The fifth form of HbM (Milwaukee-1) results from a Glu for Val substitution at a position four amino acid residues from the distal His of the heme binding pocket. These mutations all stabilize the heme iron in the ferric (oxidized) state. The primary pathology in patients harboring HbM mutations is cyanosis, but otherwise they are asymptomatic. If the HbM mutation is in the α-globin gene, the cyanosis is apparent at birth. If the HbM mutation is in the β-globin gene, then cyanosis appears later or intensifies when β-subunit production increases. Neonates that harbor mutations in the γ-globin gene will exhibit cyanosis at birth but it will disappear when the complete γ-globin to β-globin gene expression switch occurs.

CLINICAL BOX 2–4 SICKLE CELL ANEMIA

Sickle cell anemia is an autosomal recessive disorder affecting the function of hemoglobin. In order for full disease symptoms to manifest in an individual, they must carry two copies (homozygous genotype = SS) of the HbS gene. However, individuals who are heterozygous (genotype = AS) have what is referred to as sickle cell trait, a phenotypically dominant trait. Although AS individuals are clinically normal, their red blood cells can sickle under very low oxygen pressure, for example, when at high altitudes or in airplanes with reduced cabin pressure. Because of this phenomenon, AS individuals exhibit phenotypic dominance yet are genotypically recessive. The mutation causing sickle cell anemia is a single nucleotide substitution (A to T) in the codon for amino acid 6. The change converts a Glu codon (GAG) to a Val codon (GTG). The form of hemoglobin in persons with sickle cell anemia is referred to as HbS. The underlying problem in sickle cell anemia is that the valine for glutamic acid substitution results in hemoglobin tetramers that aggregate into arrays on deoxygenation in the tissues. This aggregation leads to deformation of the red blood cell into a sickle-like shape making it relatively inflexible and unable to traverse the capillary beds. This structural alteration in the red blood cell can easily be seen under light microscopy and is the source of the name of this disease. Repeated cycles of oxygenation and deoxygenation lead to irreversible sickling. Sickle cell anemia is characterized by persistent episodes of hemolytic anemia and the occurrence of acute episodes referred to as sickling crises. The sickling red cells result in clogging of the fine capillary beds. In addition, due to these recurrent vasculo-occlusive episodes there are a series of complications. Because bones are particularly affected by the reduced blood flow, frequent and severe bone pain results. This is the typical symptom during a sickle cell crisis. In long term, the recurrent clogging of the capillary beds leads to damage to the internal organs, in particular the kidneys, heart, and lungs. The continual destruction of the sickled red blood cells leads to chronic anemia and episodes of hyperbilirubinemia. Sickle cell anemia usually presents in infancy although milder cases will only manifest later in life. The hallmark presentations are failure to thrive and repeated infections and repeated attacks of painful hand-foot syndrome, termed dactylitis. This symptom is characterized by sudden onset of a painful swelling of the back (dorsum) of the hands and feet. Presenting infants will be pale with slight jaundice (icterus) visible in the sclera of the eyes and the spleen will be palpable. The clinical course of sickle cell anemia is variable even within the afflicted individuals of the same sibship. Children with sickle cell anemia have an increased susceptibility to infections due to *Streptococcus pneumonia*, *Salmonella*, and *Hemophilus influenza*. The increased propensity to infection results in impaired splenic function that resembles infections in children who have had their spleens removed for other reasons. Pneumococcal pneumonia and septicemia are the most devastating consequences of sickle cell anemia. Septicemia and shock is a common cause of death particularly in infants and during childhood.

CLINICAL BOX 2–5 THE THALASSEMIAS

The thalassemias are quantitative hemoglobinopathies that result from abnormalities in hemoglobin synthesis and affect both α-globin and β-globin gene clusters. Deficiencies in β-globin synthesis result in the β-thalassemias and deficiencies in α-globin synthesis result in the α-thalassemias. The term thalassemia is derived from the Greek word thalassa meaning "sea" and was applied to these disorders because of the high frequency of their occurrence in individuals living around the Mediterranean Sea. In normal individuals an equal amount of both α- and β-globin proteins are made allowing them to combine stoichiometrically to form the correct hemoglobin tetramers. In the α-thalassemias normal amounts of β-globin are made but not the α-globin proteins. The β-globin proteins are capable of forming homotetramers (β4) and these tetramers are called hemoglobin H, (HbH). An excess of HbH in red blood cells leads to the formation of inclusion bodies commonly seen in patients with α-thalassemia. In addition, the HbH tetramers have a markedly reduced oxygen carrying capacity. In β-thalassemia, where the β-globins are deficient, the α-globins are in excess and will form α-globin homotetramers. The α-globin homotetramers are extremely insoluble which leads to premature red cell destruction in the bone marrow and spleen. With the α-thalassemias the level of α-globin production can range from none to very nearly normal levels. This is due in part to the fact that there are two identical α-globin genes on chromosome 16. Thus, the α-thalassemias involve inactivation of one to all four α-globin genes. If three of the four α-globin genes are functional, individuals are completely asymptomatic. This situation is identified as the "silent carrier" state or sometimes as α-thalassemia 2. Genotypically this situation is designated αα/α– (where the dash indicates a nonfunctional gene) or α–/αα. If two of the four genes are inactivated, individuals are designated as α-thalassemia trait or as α-thalassemia 1. Genotypically this situation is designated αα/– –. In individuals of African descent with α-thalassemia 1, the disorder usually results from the inactivation of one α-globin gene on each chromosome and is designated α–/α–. This means that these individuals are homozygous for the α-thalassemia 2 chromosome. The phenotype of α-thalassemia 1 is relatively benign. The mean red cell volume (designated MCV in clinical tests) is reduced in α-thalassemia 1, but individuals are generally asymptomatic. The clinical situation becomes more severe if only one of the four α-globin genes is functional. Because of the dramatic reduction in α-globin chain production in this latter situation, a high level of β4 tetramer is present. Clinically this is referred to as hemoglobin H (HbH) disease. Afflicted individuals have moderate to marked anemia and their MCV is quite low, but the disease is not fatal. The most severe situation results when no α-globin chains are made (genotypically designated – –/– –). This leads to prenatal lethality or early neonatal death. The predominant fetal hemoglobin in afflicted individuals is a tetramer of γ-chains and is referred to as hemoglobin Barts. This hemoglobin has very high affinity for oxygen resulting in poor oxygen release and thus, oxygen starvation in the fetal tissues. Heart failure results as the heart tries to pump more oxygenated blood to oxygen starved tissues leading to marked edema. This latter situation is called hydrops fetalis. A large number of mutations have been identified leading to decreased or absent production of β-globin chains resulting in the β-thalassemias. In the most severe situation mutations in both the maternal and paternal β-globin genes lead to loss of normal amounts of β-globin protein. A complete lack of HbA is denoted as β^0 thalassemia. If one or the other mutations allows production of a small amount of functional β-globin then the disorder is denoted as β^+ thalassemia. Both β^0 and β^+ thalassemias are referred to as thalassemia major, also called Cooley anemia after Dr. Thomas Cooley who first described the disorder. Afflicted individuals suffer from severe anemia beginning in the first year of life leading to the need for blood transfusions. As a consequence of the anemia the bone marrow dramatically increases its effort at blood production. The cortex of the bone becomes thinned leading to pathologic fracturing and distortion of the bones in the face and skull. In addition, there is marked hepatosplenomegaly as the liver and spleen act as additional sites of blood production. Without intervention these individuals will die within the decade of life. As indicated, β-thalassemia major patients require blood transfusions, however, in the long term these transfusions lead to the accumulation of iron in the organs, particularly the heart, liver, and pancreas. Organ failure ensues with death in the teens to early twenties. Iron chelation therapies appear to improve the outlook for β-thalassemia major patients, but this requires continuous infusion of the chelating agent. Individuals heterozygous for β-thalassemia have what is termed thalassemia minor. Afflicted individuals harbor one normal β-globin gene and one that harbors a mutation leading to production of reduced or no β-globin. Individuals that do not make any functional β-globin protein from one gene are termed β^0 heterozygotes. If β-globin production is reduced at one locus, the individuals are termed β^+ heterozygotes. Thalassemia minor individuals are generally asymptomatic. The term thalassemia intermedia is used to designate individuals with significant anemia and who are symptomatic but unlike thalassemia major do not require transfusions. This syndrome results in individuals where both β-globin genes express reduced amounts of protein or where one gene makes none and the other makes a mildly reduced amount. A person who is a compound heterozygote with α-thalassemia and β^+ thalassemia will also manifest as thalassemia intermedia. The primary cause of α-thalassemias is deletion, whereas for β-thalassemias the mutations are more subtle. In β-thalassemias, point mutations in the promoter, mutations in the translational initiation codon, a point mutation in the polyadenylation signal, and an array of mutations leading to splicing abnormalities have been characterized.

CHECKLIST

- ☑ Proteins are classified based on numerous factors such as solubility, hydrophobicity, conformation, function, or the presence of specific types of prosthetic groups or cofactors.
- ☑ Proteins structure and function are dictated, in part, by a combination of primary amino acid sequence and the forces that control the overall three-dimensional conformation.
- ☑ Overall protein structure is a combination of primary, secondary, and tertiary structures. Quaternary structure represents an additional level of complexity imparted by multiple subunit proteins.
- ☑ Defects in protein structure, due primarily to mutations in the encoding gene, can have profound effects on function resulting in potentially debilitating disorders.
- ☑ Myoglobin and hemoglobin are the oxygen carrying proteins of the body. Myoglobin is monomeric protein and hemoglobin is a heterotetrameric protein.
- ☑ Both myoglobin and hemoglobin contain the prosthetic group, heme, required for oxygen binding.
- ☑ Myoglobin binds oxygen with hyperbolic kinetics, whereas, hemoglobin binds oxygen cooperatively and thus, demonstrates sigmoidal binding characteristics.
- ☑ Hemoglobin binds oxygen with reduced affinity in the low oxygen environment of the tissues but with high affinity in the high oxygen pressures of the lungs.
- ☑ The affinity of hemoglobin for oxygen is controlled by several factors including hydrogen ion concentration, the partial pressure of CO_2, the level of chloride ion, and the concentration of bound 2,3-bisphosphoglycerate.
- ☑ Mutations in the genes encoding both the α-globin and β-globin proteins have been identified and these mutations are classified as to whether they result in decreased function (qualitative) or decreased amounts (quantitative) of hemoglobin tetramers.
- ☑ The most common qualitative hemoglobinopathy is sickle cell anemia, resulting from a single mutation in the adult β-globin gene.
- ☑ Quantitative hemoglobinopathies are referred to as the thalassemias and reflect defects in either the α-globin (α-thalassemias) or β-globin (β-thalassemias) genes.

REVIEW QUESTIONS

1. A 68-year-old man was rushed to the Emergency Department after being found unconscious by his wife in his running car inside the garage. In the ambulance he regains consciousness but is confused, nauseated, lethargic, and unaware of time or place. When the wife is asked about any past medical history, she indicates that her husband has high blood pressure but that he does not smoke cigarettes. Upon arrival at the Emergency Department, his temperature is 38.7°C (101.6°F), his respiration rate is 18 breaths per minute, his pulse is 115 beats per minute, and his blood pressure is 143/97. Laboratory studies find the following:

	Patient value	Normal value
HCO_3^-	18 mEq/L	22–30 mml/L
Venous pH	7.25	7.35–7.45
PaO_2	84 mm Hg	75–100 mm Hg
$PaCO_2$	33 mm Hg	35–45 mm Hg

An increase in which of the following in the patient's red blood cells is the most likely underlying cause of the laboratory findings?
(A) Carbaminohemoglobin
(B) Carboxyhemoglobin
(C) Glycated hemoglobin
(D) Oxyhemoglobin
(E) Methemoglobin

2. Numerous missense mutations have been identified in the pyruvate kinase gene that result in erythrocyte pyruvate kinase deficiency. One identified mutation causes an arginine (Arg) residue to be changed to a tryptophan (Trp). This mutation is associated with reduced stability of the enzyme. Another mutation changes the same arginine to a glutamine (Gln), but this form of the enzyme exhibits normal stability. Which of the following, with respect to the R-group of tryptophan, is the most likely explanation for the reduced stability of the Arg to Trp mutation versus the Arg to Gln mutation?
(A) It cannot form hydrogen bonds
(B) It creates an enlarged active site which destabilizes the protein
(C) It disrupts the required alpha helix of the active site
(D) It is hydrophilic and destabilizes the active site of the protein
(E) It repels negatively charged carbonyl groups of adjacent peptide bonds

3. Numerous missense mutations have been identified in the gene encoding the enzyme that catalyzes the conversion of phenylalanine to tyrosine. One mutation affects a specific arginine residue near the catalytic domain. Mutation of this site to which of the following would most likely be the least disruptive to the structure of this enzyme?
(A) Glutamate
(B) Glycine
(C) Leucine
(D) Lysine
(E) Phenylalanine

4. A 12-year-old boy has suffered from chronic sinopulmonary disease including persistent infection of the airway with *Pseudomonas aeruginosa*. He has constant and chronic sputum production as a result of the airway infection. Additionally, he suffers from gastrointestinal and nutritional abnormalities that include biliary cirrhosis, meconium ileus, and pancreatic insufficiency. The symptoms are most likely associated with a defect in which of the following proteins?
(A) Cystic fibrosis transmembrane conductance regulator
(B) Ferritin
(C) Ferrochelatase
(D) Hepcidin
(E) Intrinsic factor

5. A 4-year-old boy brought to the physician because his mother says that he has been very tired and has soreness in his joints. Physical examination shows marked yellowing of the sclera. Laboratory studies show a mean corpuscular volume (MCV) of 62 fL. An analysis of his blood by nondenaturing electrophoresis shows the following composition of hemoglobin isoforms: HbF = 75%, HbA_1 = 23%, HbA_2 = 2%, HbS = 0%. This patient is most likely homozygous for which of the following?
(A) Complete deletion of the α-globin locus
(B) Complete deletion of the β-globin locus
(C) Mutation in the promoter of one of the α-globin genes
(D) Mutation in the promoter of the β-globin gene
(E) Nonsense mutation in one of the α-globin genes
(F) Nonsense mutation in the β-globin gene

6. In healthy 2- to 3-month-old infants, there will be a measurable increase in the level of oxygen delivery to the tissues. This is, in part, due to the removal of red blood cells containing HbF with new cells containing predominantly HbA_1. Which of the following changes is most likely contributing to the observed increases in oxygen delivery in these infants?
(A) Decreased production of 2,3-bisphosphoglycerate
(B) Decreased production of HbA_2
(C) Decreased production of transferrin
(D) Increased production of 2,3-bisphosphoglycerate
(E) Increased production of HbA2
(F) Increased production of transferrin

7. Numerous missense mutations have been identified in the gene encoding the enzyme that catalyzes the conversion of phenylalanine to tyrosine. One mutation affects a specific glutamate residue within the catalytic domain. Mutation of this site to which of the following would most likely be the least disruptive to the function of this enzyme?
(A) Arginine
(B) Aspartate
(C) Lysine
(D) Serine
(E) Tyrosine

8. A 37-year-old woman of eastern Mediterranean descent is being examined by her physician with a primary complaint of increasing fatigue and mild shortness of breath. Results of blood work find the following: hemoglobin of 10.4 g/dL, (N = 12–15 g/dL), MCV (mean corpuscular volume) of 76 fL (N = 82–98 fL), MCHC (mean corpuscular hemoglobin concentration) of 29 g/dL (N = 31–38 g/dL), and TIBC (total iron binding capacity) of 420 μg/dL (N = 250–370 μg/dL). Other blood values find that white blood cell (WBC) and platelet counts are within normal ranges. Which of the following is the most likely reason for this patient's pathology?
(A) Anemia of chronic disease
(B) Aplastic anemia
(C) Iron deficiency anemia
(D) Pernicious anemia
(E) Sideroblastic anemia
(F) β-Thalassemia

9. Numerous missense mutations have been identified in the gene encoding the monomeric G-protein RAS. The normal subcellular location of this protein is association with lipids in the plasma membrane. One mutation affects this normal localization property, and the mutant protein is found in the cytosol. This mutation is most likely to have introduced which of the following amino acid into the protein?
(A) Aspartate
(B) Isoleucine
(C) Leucine
(D) Methionine
(E) Valine

10. In one form of β-thalassemia, patients have significantly reduced levels of β-globin transcripts. Notably these β-globin transcripts are less than half the length of the normal β-globin mRNA. These patients exhibit elevated levels of HbF and no detectable HbA_1. Which of the following best explains the molecular reason for these observations?
(A) Addition of 7-methylguanosine to the β-globin mRNA
(B) Covalent modification of the β-globin protein
(C) Improper folding of the β-globin protein
(D) Promoter mutations in the β-globin gene
(E) Splicing alteration of the β-globin mRNA

11. A 2-year-old girl with a history of microcytic anemia is being examined by her pediatrician during a routine follow-up. Laboratory studies show the presence of inclusion bodies in erythrocytes. Electrophoresis of erythrocyte protein extracts shows a large excess of β-globin protein and a near complete lack of α-globin protein. Which of the following is the most likely diagnosis in this patient?
(A) Hemoglobin Bart's
(B) Hemoglobin H disease
(C) Hereditary persistence of fetal hemoglobin
(D) Hydrops fetalis
(E) Sickle cell anemia
(F) β-Thalassemia major

12. Experiments are being conducted on the oxygen-binding characteristics of a synthetic oxygen transport compound. The design of the compound must be such that it most closely mimics the oxygen affinity of native hemoglobin protein. If these studies successfully identify this type of synthetic transport compound, addition of which of the following to a test solution would have the greatest negative effect on the ability of the compound to bind oxygen?
(A) Bicarbonate ion
(B) 2,3-Bisphosphoglycerate
(C) Carbonic acid
(D) Chloride ion
(E) Carbamino-hemoglobin
(F) Thiosulfate

13. A 27-year-old apparently healthy African-American woman who is applying for life insurance comes to the physician for a physical examination. Laboratory studies show a hematocrit of 35%, a mean corpuscular volume (MCV) of 83 fL (N = 82–98 fL), and a mean corpuscular hemoglobin concentration (MCHC) of 32% (N = 31–38%). Hemoglobin electrophoresis shows: HbA_1, 62%; HbS, 35%; HbF, 1%; HbA_2, 1% with no detection of variant C, D, G, or H bands. Which of the following is the most likely diagnosis in this patient?
(A) Sickle cell disease
(B) Sickle thalassemia minor
(C) Sickle trait
(D) Thalassemia intermedia
(E) Thalassemia major
(F) Thalassemia minor

14. Experiments are being carried out to compare the localization and function of a protein found to be encoded by a mutant gene in melanoma. In wild-type skin fibroblasts the protein is found anchored to the inner leaflet of the plasma membrane. The protein isolated from the melanoma cells is found within the cytoplasm. Which of the following properties of the wild-type protein is most likely defective in the mutant protein, accounting for its altered localization?
(A) Disulfide bond formation to its phosphatidylinositol anchor
(B) Disulfide bond formation to its sphingomyelin anchor
(C) Hydrogen bonding of amino acid side chains to membrane phospholipid tails
(D) Hydrophobic interactions between the amino acid side chains and membrane phospholipid tails
(E) Formation of ionic bonds between the amino acid side chains and membrane phospholipids
(F) Formation of β-pleated sheet structures that interact with membrane phospholipids

15. Experiments are being conducted on the toxin produced by the lysogenic bacteriophage of *Vibrio cholerae*. The toxin exerts its effects only after its two polypeptide subunits dissociate from each other when exposed to an environment of reduced pH. Which of the following is the most likely subcellular location where the toxin subunits dissociate from each other?
(A) Cytosol
(B) Endoplasmic reticulum
(C) Endosome
(D) Mitochondrial matrix
(E) Nucleus
(F) Peroxisome

16. Experiments are being conducted on the structure-function relationships of pyruvate kinase. These experiments focus on the thermodynamic properties relating to formation of a critical α-helical domain in the enzyme. This domain forms with a lower energy requirement in an alcohol-based medium than in an aqueous medium. Which of the following is the best explanation for this difference?
(A) Competition for hydrogen bonding is lower for ethanol than for water
(B) Ethanol forms covalent interactions with amino acids in the domain
(C) Hydrophobic forces are greater in ethanol than in water
(D) The peptide aggregates in water but not in ethanol
(E) van der Waals interactions are lower in ethanol than in water

17. A 2-year-old boy has sustained several fractures over the course of the past 8 months. His pediatrician is concerned there is a molecular cause and orders DNA testing. Results of the test find a missense mutation in the COL1A1 gene. Which of the following substitutions is most likely to be associated with the symptoms in this child?
(A) Glu to Asp
(B) Glu to Gln
(C) Gly to Leu
(D) Leu to Gly
(E) Lys to Pro

18. A 23-year-old man sees his physician on a regular basis because he has suffered from bronchiectasis, chronic sinusitis, rhinitis, and secretory otitis media since childhood. He is currently being evaluated for infertility because he and his wife have been unable to conceive. His wife has been evaluated, and no abnormalities were found. The volume of his ejaculate and his sperm count are within reference ranges. Molecular studies find that the patient harbors a nonsense mutation in a gene encoding a member of the dynein family. Given his history and current findings, his infertility could best be explained by a deficiency in the functions of which of the following?
(A) Dystrophin glycoprotein complex
(B) Integrins
(C) Intermediate filaments
(D) Microtubules
(E) Proteoglycans

19. Experiments are being carried out on cultures of dopaminergic neurons isolated from the substantia nigra. These experiments involve the use of the microtubule inhibitor, colchicine. Which of the following will be the most likely result in these cells in response to the addition of the drug to the culture medium?
(A) Induction of dendrites
(B) Induction of dopamine secretion
(C) Inhibition of dopamine secretion
(D) Inhibition of dopamine synthesis
(E) Stimulation of Ca^{2+} transporter activity
(F) Stimulation of Na^+-K^+ ATPase activity

20. A 7-month-old infant is being examined by his pediatrician due to concerns of his parents that he has had a persistent fever and appears pale. Physical examination finds that the infants' hands and feet are swollen and painful to manipulation, he has icteric sclera, and his temperature is 38.2°C. Blood cells sickle in the presence of sodium metabisulphite. Given the signs and symptoms in this patient, which of the following is most likely to be elevated?
(A) HbA_{1c}
(B) HbA_2
(C) HbC
(D) HbF
(E) HbH

21. A 47-year-old woman was rushed to the Emergency Department after being found by her husband unconscious in her running car inside the garage. In the ambulance the patient is administered 100% oxygen and she regains consciousness but is confused, unaware of time and place, and complains of a severe headache. When venous blood is drawn for laboratory studies it is noted to be quite red in color. Which of the

following is the most likely underlying cause of the observations in this patient?
(A) Accumulation of CO_2 in the blood
(B) Competitive inhibition of O_2 binding sites in hemoglobin
(C) Increased levels of oxalic acid in the blood
(D) Lactic acidosis
(E) Methemoglobinemia

22. A 9-year-old African-American girl is being examined in the Emergency Department to ascertain the cause of the painful swelling of her hands and feet. Her parents indicate that the swelling began the following evening and that this is an issue that has plagued their daughter several times over the past 18 months. The patient has had no other significant medical history. Family history reveals that a maternal aunt and a paternal uncle experienced similar issues, with the maternal aunt losing her life to a severe bacterial infection at the age of 17 years. Physical examination shows dactylitis and scleral icterus. Which of the following molecular alterations is most likely to account for the patient's presentation?
(A) Deletion within the delta globin gene
(B) Gamma globin gene promoter mutation
(C) Glutamate to lysine substitution
(D) Glutamate to valine substitution
(E) Histidine to tyrosine substitution

23. A 9-year-old African-American boy is being examined in the Emergency Department to ascertain the cause of the painful swelling of his hands and feet. His parents indicate that the swelling began the following evening and that this is an issue that has plagued their son several times over the past 18 months. The patient has had no other significant medical history. Family history reveals that a maternal aunt and a paternal uncle experienced similar issues, with the maternal aunt losing her life to bacteremia at the age of 17 years. Physical examination shows dactylitis and scleral icterus. The attending physician orders blood tests, which reveal a hematocrit of 28% (N = 35–45%) and a reticulocyte count of 8.5% (N = 0.98–1.94%). Given the most likely diagnosis in this patient, which of the following represents the most clinically significant future complication?
(A) Hemochromatosis
(B) Hepatic cancer
(C) Macrocytic anemia
(D) Methemoglobinemia
(E) Streptococcal pneumonia

24. A 9-year-old African-American boy is being examined in the Emergency Department to ascertain the cause of the painful swelling of his hands and feet. His parents indicate that the swelling began the following evening and that this is an issue that has plagued their son several times over the past 18 months. The attending physician orders blood tests which reveal hemoglobin of 10.4 g/dL (N = 11.5–15.5 g/dL), hematocrit of 28% (N = 35–45%), and a reticulocyte count of 8.5% (N = 0.98–1.94%). A peripheral blood smear shows the presence of Howell-Jolly bodies. The attending recommends the patient be prescribed once-daily hydroxy urea therapy. Which of the following best explains the clinical benefits of the prescribed therapy?
(A) Decreases α-globin synthesis
(B) Decreases the concentration of hemoglobin A_2
(C) Increases erythropoiesis
(D) Increases the concentration of hemoglobin F
(E) Induces a rightward shift in the oxygen dissociation curve

25. Within the periphery, the CO_2 generated via the normal processes of metabolism is taken up by red blood cells and converted to carbonic acid through the actions of carbonic anhydrase. Carbonic acid ionizes and the bicarbonate ions leave the red blood cells, but the hydrogen ions remain. Which of the following best explains the mechanism by which red blood cells maintain electrical neutrality under these circumstances?
(A) Bicarbonate exchange for chloride ions
(B) Bicarbonate exchange for potassium ions
(C) Buffering of the protons (H^+) by chloride ions
(D) Buffering of the protons (H^+) by hemoglobin
(E) Transport of potassium ions out of the red blood cell
(F) Transport of sodium ions out of the red blood cell

ANSWERS

1. Correct answer is **B.** Despite the reasons that may be behind the patient being unconscious in a running car in an enclosed space, such as the garage, the continuous inhalation of the exhaust from the car will lead to a significant increase in the intake of carbon monoxide (CO). CO also binds coordinately to heme iron atoms in the ferrous state (Fe^{2+}) in hemoglobin in a manner similar to that of oxygen (O_2). However, the binding of CO to heme iron is much stronger (>200 fold) than that of O_2. When CO is bound to hemoglobin, the resulting protein is referred to as carboxyhemoglobin (HbCO). In addition to a higher affinity of CO over that of O_2 for ferrous iron in hemoglobin, the result of CO binding to at least one globin monomer causes a higher affinity of the remaining subunits for O_2. This effect contributes to reduced O_2 release in the tissues. These combined effects of the preferential binding of CO to heme iron is largely responsible for the asphyxiation that results from carbon monoxide poisoning. Carbaminohemoglobin (choice A) is the form of hemoglobin with CO_2 covalently bound to N-terminal amino groups of the T form of hemoglobin. Around 15% of the CO_2 generated by metabolic processes is transported from the tissues to the lungs in carbaminohemoglobin form. Glycated hemoglobin (choice C) is the form of hemoglobin with covalently attached glucose molecules. This form of hemoglobin is clinically referred to as HbA_{1c} (or simply as A1c). Oxyhemoglobin (choice D) is the normal form of hemoglobin with O_2 bound to the ferrous iron in each heme moiety. Methemoglobin (choice E) is the form of hemoglobin where some, or all, of the ferrous (Fe^{2+}) iron has been oxidized to the ferric (Fe^{3+}) state. The Fe^{3+} form of iron does not bind O_2, however, the presence of at least one Fe^{3+} in the hemoglobin tetramer results in enhanced binding of the O_2 to the remaining Fe^{2+} irons causing reduced delivery of the O_2 to the tissues with potential for cyanosis.

2. Correct answer is **A.** Tryptophan has a large bulky hydrophobic R-group that does not ionize and thus has no hydrogen bonding potential which most likely would contribute to the lower stability of the enzyme. Tryptophan, being a nonpolar amino acid would most likely be found on the outside of a protein, and therefore, if the Arg was originally in the active site of the enzyme the substitution for Trp would distort the active site, it would not enlarge the active site (choice B). Alpha helices are formed by hydrogen bonding between the carbonyl oxygens and amide nitrogens attached to the α-carbon of amino acids and do not involve the R-groups (choice C). The R-group of Trp is aliphatic and nonpolar, not hydrophilic (choice D). There is no net charge to the R-group of Trp and thus, it would not repel the charge of carbonyl oxygens (choice E).

3. Correct answer is **D.** Arginine exhibits a net positive charge at physiologic pH. Lysine possesses an R-group that is closest in size and charge to arginine; therefore, it could participate in the same hydrogen bonding as arginine resulting in the least disruption to the structure and function of the enzyme. Glutamate (choice A) possesses an R-group that would be negatively charged at physiologic pH and, although it could participate in hydrogen bonding the difference in charge may disrupt the catalytic function. The other amino acid side chains (choices B, C, and E) are nonpolar and/or have no hydrogen bonding potential, therefore they would not contribute to normal function of the active site of the enzyme.

4. Correct answer is **A.** The boy has the hallmark symptoms of cystic fibrosis. Cystic fibrosis (see Chapter 25) results from mutations in the gene encoding the cystic fibrosis transmembrane conductance regulator (CFTR). The disease is characterized by abnormal transport of chloride and sodium across an epithelium, leading to thick, viscous mucus secretions. This mucus builds up in the breathing passages of the lungs, as well as in the pancreas and intestines. Difficulty breathing is the most serious symptom and results from frequent lung infections, particularly with *Pseudomonas aeruginosa*. The secretions in the pancreas block the exocrine movement of the digestive enzymes into the duodenum and result in irreversible damage to the pancreas. The lack of digestive enzymes leads to difficulty absorbing nutrients with their subsequent excretion in the feces resulting in a malabsorption disorder. Defects in ferritin (choice B) would result in the inability of intracellular iron storage and manifests as an iron deficient anemia. Ferrochelatase deficiency (choice C) results in erythropoietic protoporphyria, EPP. Defects in hepcidin (choice D) result in a form of iron overload (hemochromatosis) called juvenile hemochromatosis type 2B. Deficiency in intrinsic factor (choice E) most often results from autoimmune destruction of intrinsic factor secreting parietal cells of the stomach resulting in a lack of vitamin B12 absorption from the distal ileum which leads to a form of macrocytic anemia termed pernicious anemia.

5. Correct answer is **D.** A mutation in the promoter region of the β-globin genes would result in reduced expression. This is evidenced by the lower-than-normal amount of HbA_1 in this child. Under these circumstances the body will tend to compensate by continuing to express the fetal hemoglobin genes at higher-than-normal levels resulting in potentially dramatic increases in measured HbF. Normal levels of HbF in a 4-year-old child would be around 0–2%, whereas this child shows significant increase in HbF of 75%. Complete deletion of the α-globin genes (choice A) results in prenatal lethality or early neonatal death. The predominant fetal hemoglobin in afflicted individuals is a tetramer of γ-chains and is referred to as hemoglobin Bart's. Complete deletion of the β-globin locus (choice B) would result in the form of thalassemia termed β^0-thalassemia and there would be no detectable HbA_1. A promoter mutation in one of the two α-globin genes (choice C) would result in what is termed α-thalassemia trait which is associated with relatively normal levels of HbA_1 and HbF. Nonsense mutations in one of the α-globin genes (choice E) would also most likely result in α-thalassemia trait, depending upon where the nonsense mutation occurred in the coding region. Nonsense mutation in the β-globin gene (choice F) would result in no HbA_1 and increased levels of HbA_2 from the δ-globin gene, depending upon where in the coding region the nonsense mutation occurred.

6. Correct answer is **D.** Following birth, the increased production of red blood cells expressing the adult β-globin gene coincides with increased production of 2,3-bisphosphoglycerate (2,3-BPG). In addition to producing more 2,3-BPG, the affinity of adult β-globin for 2,3-BPG, relative to fetal β-globin (Gγ or Aγ) is much higher promoting oxygen release in the tissues. Synthesis of 2,3-BPG increases not decreases (choice A) following birth. The level of HbA2 will increase (choice E) not decrease (choice B) following birth but the level of HbA2 does not contribute to increased oxygen delivery. Changes in the levels of transferrin (choices C and F) can affect the level of iron available for production of normal hemoglobin but would not affect the delivery of oxygen to the same extent as that contributed to by 2,3-BPG levels.

7. Correct answer is **B.** Since glutamic acid is a negatively charged amino acid at physiologic pH, any other negatively charged amino acid, such as aspartic acid, could potentially be substituted without significant loss of enzyme activity. Although arginine (choice A) and lysine (choice C) will be charged at physiologic pH, their negative charge may prevent normal charge-charge interaction required for normal enzyme function. The pK_a values of the hydroxyl groups of serine (choice D) and tyrosine (choice E) are such that they would not be charged at physiologic pH, and if they did ionize, they would be negatively charged and as such could not contribute to the required charge interactions that would be a likely function of the arginine.

8. Correct answer is **C.** Laboratory findings of a hypochromic anemia with a decrease in MCV and MCHC and a decreased reticulocyte count suggest a hypoproliferative anemia. The various microcytic, hypochromic anemias belong to this category and a partial differential diagnosis for these includes iron deficiency anemia, anemia of chronic disease (ACD), thalassemias, and sideroblastic anemias. Serum iron and ferritin levels are low and total iron binding capacity (TIBC) is elevated in iron deficiency anemia. Anemia of chronic disease (choice A) can be distinguished from iron deficiency anemia by the additional iron studies that were performed in this case. While serum iron and ferritin levels are low and TIBC is elevated in iron deficiency anemia, in anemia of chronic disease ferritin is typically normal or elevated, iron and TIBC is low. Aplastic anemia (choice B) is most often diagnosed by a low reticulocyte count and through a bone marrow biopsy that shows reduced levels of all blood cells. Pernicious anemia (choice D) is a form of macrocytic anemia and as such the MCV value would be found to be greater than 98 fL. Although sideroblastic anemias (choice E) are forms of microcytic, hypochromic anemias, the MCV value is found to be normal or slightly elevated in these types of anemias. A person with a β-thalassemia (choice F) would present with symptoms long before the age of 37 unless it is a thalassemia minor which generally remains asymptomatic.

9. Correct answer is **A.** Lipids would most likely interact with equally hydrophobic substances. Aspartic acid is an acidic amino acid and as such would be more likely to interact with an aqueous environment than a hydrophobic lipid one. Isoleucine (choice B), leucine (choice C), methionine (choice D), and valine (choice E) are all hydrophobic nonpolar amino

acids that would likely interact with the hydrophobic lipid environment of the membrane.

10. Correct answer is **E.** Numerous β-thalassemias result from mutations in the sequences that control proper splicing of the β-globin transcript. These mutations lead to β-globin mRNAs that are shorter or longer than the normal β-globin mRNA. The cap structure found on most mRNAs, including β-globin mRNAs, is composed of a 7-methylguanosine residue (choice A) so this would not affect the mRNA or protein. The β-globin proteins are not normally subjected to post-translational modifications (choice B). Glycation, due to high levels of plasma glucose in diabetes, is an observable covalent modification of the β-globin protein. Mutations that result in abnormally structured β-globin proteins (choice C) could lead to degradation, and thus reduced levels of HbA_1; however, most of these types of mutations do not result in mRNAs that are less than half the normal length. Although mutations in the promoter region (choice D) of the β-globin gene will lead to reduced levels of expression, and thus, to reduced levels of β-globin mRNA, they generally do not result in mRNAs nor proteins that are shorter than normal.

11. Correct answer is **B.** The α-thalassemias result when there is reduced or no expression at one or both of the α-globin genes. When only one of the four α-globin genes is functional the dramatic reduction in α-globin chain production results in a high level of β4 tetramers. Clinically this is referred to as hemoglobin H disease, HbH. When no α-globin protein is made it leads to prenatal lethality, or early neonatal lethality. The predominant fetal hemoglobin in afflicted individuals is a tetramer of γ-chains and is referred to as hemoglobin Bart's (choice A). Hereditary persistence of fetal hemoglobin, HPFH (choice C) is usually not associated with hypochromia and microcytosis in heterozygotes. Because the HPFH syndrome is benign most individuals do not even know they carry a hemoglobin abnormality. Many HPFH individuals harbor deletions in the δ-globin and/or β-globin gene coding regions of within the β-globin gene cluster. In the circumstance where hemoglobin Bart's is produced, this tetrameric form of hemoglobin has very high affinity for oxygen resulting in poor oxygen release and thus, oxygen starvation in the fetal tissues. Heart failure results as the heart tries to pump more oxygenated blood to oxygen starved tissues leading to marked edema. This latter situation is called hydrops fetalis (choice D). Sickle cell anemia (choice E) results from a single nucleotide mutation in the β-globin gene and is not associated with altered levels of expression from the α-globin genes nor with altered levels of α-globin protein. Beta-thalassemia major (choice F) is one of three major forms of β-thalassemia. At the level of the β-globin proteins the β-thalassemias are characterized by whether or not there is partial or complete defect in protein production. A complete lack of protein is denoted as β^0-thalassemia (beta-zero-thalassemia). If mutation(s) allows production of a small amount of functional β-globin, then the disorder is denoted as β^+-thalassemia (beta-plus-thalassemia). Thalassemia major is often referred to as Cooley anemia.

12. Correct answer is **C.** Addition of carbonic acid (H_2CO_3) to the solution would result in its ionization to bicarbonate (HCO_3^-) and proton (H^+). The increase in H^+ would, therefore, be expected to exert a large negative effect on oxygen binding by the synthetic hemoglobin construct just as is the case for the negative effect of increasing H^+ on the affinity of natural hemoglobin for oxygen. Bicarbonate ion (choice A), although being derived from carbonic acid, does not have any impact itself on the binding of oxygen to hemoglobin. The ability of 2,3-BPG (choice B) to reduce the affinity of hemoglobin for oxygen is dependent on the binding of 2,3-BPG to the β-globin proteins of hemoglobin. Since the hypothetical oxygen carrying compound would not likely be composed of β-globin protein there would be no interaction with 2,3BPG. The role of chloride ion (choice D) relates to ensuring that when red blood cells generate bicarbonate and hydrogen ions and the negatively charged bicarbonate ion is transported out of the cell chloride is transported in to ensure electrical neutrality. Chloride ion itself has no effect on oxygen binding to hemoglobin. Carbamino-hemoglobin (choice E) is the form of hemoglobin to which carbon dioxide is covalently bound and as such plays no role in oxygen binding. Thiosulfate (choice F) is produced from the amino acid cysteine as a natural cyanide detoxifier and is unrelated to hemoglobin binding oxygen.

13. Correct answer is **C.** Individuals who are heterozygous (genotype = AS) for the sickle cell allele have what is referred to as sickle cell trait. Although AS individuals are clinically normal their red blood cells can sickle under very low oxygen pressure, for example, when at high altitudes in airplanes with reduced cabin pressure. Individuals with sickle trait are healthy and not anemic. Hemoglobin electrophoresis of individuals with sickle trait demonstrates a minor proportion of HbS and a major proportion of HbA_1. Fetal hemoglobin (HbF) and HbA_2 are usually normal. Sickle trait confers the benefit of protecting erythrocytes from some forms of malarial infection. About 9% of African Americans in the United States have sickle trait. Conversely, in sickle cell disease (choice A) almost all hemoglobin is HbS, no HbA_1 is detected, and patients have a clinical history of severe anemia. Sickle thalassemia minor (choice B) presents as a chronic microcytic anemia with a major HbS component and elevated HbA_2. The three forms of thalassemia (choices D, E, and F) would not present with detectable HbS.

14. Correct answer is **D.** Membranes are predominantly lipid and thus, most likely to interact with hydrophobic amino acids. The interaction between the hydrophobic R-groups of amino acids and the hydrophobic lipid tails of membrane phospholipids anchors integral membrane proteins to the membrane. Disulfide bonds (choices A and B) are not shown to exist between membrane lipids and proteins due to the lack of –SH groups in the membrane constituents. Membrane phospholipid tails are hydrophobic and lack the ability to form hydrogen bonds (choice C) of to form ionic bonds (choice E) with proteins. Although hydrophobic R-groups or amino acids in β-pleated sheet structures (choice F) could participate in interactions with lipids in membranes, specific structures such as these are not required for the interaction.

15. Correct answer is **C.** Endosomes are membrane-bound compartments inside cells. They are compartments of the endocytic membrane transport pathway from the plasma membrane to the lysosome. For example, when LDL binds the LDL receptor the complex is internalized and fused to the endosomal membranes. Because of the slightly acidic environment of the endosome, ligands, such as LDL, dissociate. None of the other compartments (choices A, B, D, E, and F) are involved with the dissociation of cholera toxin subunits.

16. Correct answer is **A.** The α-helix results from the formation of hydrogen bonds between the carbonyl oxygens and amide hydrogens of nearby amino acids in the protein. Because these same atoms in the amino acids can form hydrogen bonds with water there can be competition for the formation of the bonds required for the α-helix. In the presence of ethanol there would be less competition from the water molecules thus, explaining the increased rate of α-helix formation in this medium. Ethanol does not form covalent bonds with amino acids (choice B). Due to the chemical nature of ethanol, there will be less hydrophobic forces in this medium than in water (choice C). Depending on composition a peptide might aggregate more in water than in ethanol (choice D), but this would not directly influence the formation of domains such as an α-helix. Overall van der Waals interaction (choice E) would be similar in a protein in water and ethanol.

17. Correct answer is **C.** The triple-helical structure of collagen arises from an unusual abundance of three amino acids: glycine, proline, and hydroxyproline. These amino acids make up the characteristic repeating motif Gly-Pro-X, where X can be any amino acid. The side chain of glycine, an H atom, is the only one that can fit into the crowded center of a three-stranded helix. Hydrogen bonds linking the peptide bond nitrogen of a glycine residue with a peptide carbonyl group in an adjacent polypeptide help hold the three chains together. It is because of this role of glycine in collagen that it is indispensable for normal collagen structure and function. Therefore, a mutation causing a substitution of glycine for leucine would result in the production of defective collagen. A Glu to Asp substitution (choice A) represents an identical charge and would not exert much, if any, effect on collagen structure. Although Glu and Gln are oppositely charged (choice B), they are both charged and thus, the substitution would have limited effect on collage structure. Leu and Gly (choice D) are both nonpolar and so this substitution would exert minimal effect on collagen structure. Substituting Lys for Pro (choice E) could alter collagen structure since proline does not participate in the formation of α-helical structures, but it is not likely to be as disruptive as losing a Gly residue.

18. Correct answer is **D.** The patient has Kartagener syndrome, also known as primary ciliary dyskinesia. Kartagener syndrome can result from mutations in several different genes, all of which are important to the structure and function of cilia which require microtubule dynamics to function properly. Microtubules are filamentous intracellular structures that are responsible for various kinds of movements in all eukaryotic cells. Microtubules are involved in nuclear and cell division, organization of intracellular structures, and intracellular transport, as well as ciliary motility. The symptoms observed in this individual, bronchiectasis, sinusitis, rhinitis, and secretory otitis media are all the result of defective ciliary function. Deficiency in the function of the dystrophin glycoprotein complex (choice A) can occur by mutations in any of the multiple genes encoding components of the complex, such as α-dystroglycan or dystrophin, resulting in a family of disorders termed the muscular dystrophy-dystroglycanopathies (MDDG). The integrins (choice B) and proteoglycans (choice E) are primarily components of the extracellular matrix and although many different disorders are known to result from the many genes encoding these cellular components, they do not manifest with the constellation of symptom in this patient. Intermediate filaments (choice C) interact with components of the microtubule machinery but are not directly involved in their organization and function.

19. Correct answer is **C.** Colchicine is an inhibitor of microtubule function. Secretion of hormone requires migration and fusion of secretory vesicles with the plasma membrane. The migration of secretory vesicles is mediated via their interactions with the microtubule network inside the cell. The addition of colchicine would inhibit, not induce dendrite formation (choice A), would inhibit not induce dopamine secretion (choice B), would not inhibit dopamine synthesis (choice D), and would more likely inhibit, as opposed to stimulate transporter activity (choices E and F).

20. Correct answer is **D.** The infant most likely has sickle cell anemia. The presence of the HbS hemoglobin in the erythrocytes of sickle cell patients leads to reduced overall oxygen carrying capacity. This results in a compensatory increase in the expression of fetal hemoglobin (HbF) in an attempt to increase oxygen delivery to the tissues. HbA_{1c} (choice A) is the glycated form of HbA_1 found in red blood cells of individuals with chronic hyperglycemia such as type 2 diabetics. The level of HbA_2 (choice B) may increase slightly in sickle cell anemia patients but not significantly or to the extent of increased HbF. HbC (choice C) is the form of hemoglobin that results from a different mutation in the same codon 6 of the β-globin gene. This form of hemoglobin would not be increased in a sickle cell anemia patient. HbH (choice E) results in individuals with only one of the four α-globin genes producing function protein.

21. Correct answer is **B.** The continuous inhalation of the exhaust from a running car in an enclosed space, such as a garage, will lead to a significant increase in the intake of carbon monoxide (CO). CO also binds coordinately to heme iron atoms in the ferrous state (Fe^{2+}) in hemoglobin and as such will compete with O_2 for binding to heme in hemoglobin. The binding of CO to heme iron is much stronger (>200 fold) than that of O_2. When CO is bound to hemoglobin the resulting protein is referred to as carboxyhemoglobin (HbCO). When CO binds to heme in hemoglobin it alters the chromophoric character such that venous blood appears bright red instead of the normal bluish-red color imparted by deoxyhemoglobin. In addition to a higher affinity of CO over that of O_2 for ferrous iron in hemoglobin, the result of CO binding to at least one globin monomer causes a higher affinity of the remaining subunits for O_2. This effect contributes to reduced O_2 release in the tissues. These combined effects of the preferential binding of CO to heme iron is largely responsible for the asphyxiation that results from carbon monoxide poisoning. Under conditions of CO poisoning, the level of CO_2 in the blood (choice A) will not change significantly. Oxalate (choice C) is present in many foods and is also derived from the metabolism of ascorbic acid, and the amino acids glycine, serine, and 4-hydroxyproline. Whereas CO can indirectly affect the metabolism of oxalate, there is no direct relationship, and thus, oxalate levels would not likely be elevated in this patient. Increased CO bound to hemoglobin impairs both the binding of O_2 and the release of any O_2 that is bound within the tissues, resulting in tissue hypoxia. This hypoxic state will lead to increased levels of lactate (choice D), a state of metabolic acidosis, but does not correlate to the original unconscious state of the patient, the confusion, nor the red venous blood. Methemoglobinemia (choice E) results from the oxidation of the ferrous (Fe^{2+}) iron in the heme moieties of hemoglobin to ferric (Fe^{3+}) iron. The spontaneous formation of superoxide anion in red blood cells is the predominant cause of iron oxidation. Carbon monoxide does not significantly, if at all, increase the levels of methemoglobin in the blood.

22. Correct answer is **D.** The patient is most likely exhibiting complications associated with sickle cell anemia. Sickle cell anemia is caused by a single nucleotide substitution in the sixth codon of the *HBB* gene which encodes the adult β-globin protein. This mutation changes the normal glutamate residue to a valine which results in hemoglobin tetramers that aggregate into arrays upon deoxygenation in the tissues. This aggregation leads to deformation of the red blood cell, making it relatively inflexible and unable to traverse the capillary beds. Repeated cycles of oxygenation and deoxygenation lead to irreversible sickling. The result is clogging of the fine capillaries. Because bones are particularly affected by the reduced blood flow, frequent and severe bone pain results. This is the typical symptom during a sickle cell "crisis". In long term, the recurrent clogging of the capillary beds leads to damage to the internal organs, in particular the kidneys, heart, and lungs. Deletion within the delta globin gene (choice A) results in a condition referred to as delta-beta thalassemia which is a mild form of thalassemia similar to thalassemia minor. Gamma globin gene promoter mutation (choice B) is associated with a disorder referred to as hereditary persistence of fetal hemoglobin (HPFH) which is most often a benign disorder associated with expression fetal hemoglobin (HbF) into adulthood. Glutamate to lysine substitution (choice C) is seen in hemoglobin E (HbE) at amino acid 26. This mutation results in the activation of a cryptic splice site such that 40% of the β-globin mRNA produced is shorter than normal by 16 nucleotides. Histidine to tyrosine substitution (choice E) in the heme binding pocket of either the α-globin or the β-globin protein results in the formation of hemoglobin M, which refers to a group of autosomal dominant methemoglobinemias.

23. Correct answer is **E.** The patient is most likely exhibiting complications associated with sickle cell anemia. Sickle cell anemia is caused by a single nucleotide substitution in the sixth codon of the *HBB* gene which encodes the adult β-globin protein. This mutation changes the normal glutamate residue to a valine which results in hemoglobin tetramers that aggregate into arrays upon deoxygenation in the tissues. This aggregation leads to deformation of the red blood cell making it relatively inflexible and unable to traverse the capillary beds. Repeated cycles of oxygenation and deoxygenation lead to irreversible sickling. The result is clogging of the fine capillaries. Because bones are particularly affected by the reduced blood flow, frequent and severe bone pain results. This is the typical symptom during a sickle cell "crisis". In long term, the recurrent clogging of the capillary beds leads to damage to the internal organs, in particular the kidneys, heart, and lungs. Capillary bed clogging contributes to dactylitis which refers to a condition of diffuse swelling of one or more fingers or toes, often associated with pain. The continual destruction of the sickled red blood cells leads to chronic anemia and episodes of hyperbilirubinemia which leads to jaundice as evidenced by scleral icterus. Due to the effects in the lungs, sickle cell anemia patients are highly susceptible to chronic lung disease referred to as acute chest syndrome (ACS). ACS is most commonly caused by repeated pulmonary infestation with *Streptoccocus pneumoniae.* Although sickle cell disease is associated with numerous complications, these do not include the iron overload disorder, hemochromatosis (choice A) or hepatic cancer (choice B). Macrocytic anemia (choice C) can be found in sickle cell disease patients but usually only in conjunction with folate or vitamin B12 deficiency or with the use of hydroxyurea. Methemoglobinemia (choice D) can occur in patients with sickle cell disease due to the fact that HbS is more susceptible to oxidation, but this condition is not as clinically significant as chronic lung infections and the development of ACS.

24. Correct answer is **D.** The patient is most likely exhibiting complications associated with sickle cell anemia. Treatment of sickle cell anemia patients is aimed at relieving symptoms and preventing complications. Most common treatments include blood transfusions and medications. The commonly used medications for treating the complications of sickle cell anemia include pain-relieving medications and medications to prevent infections. Hydroxyurea has been used in the treatment of sickle cell disease for several decades and functions primarily via inducing increases in the concentration of fetal hemoglobin, HbF. The increase in HbF reduces the acute clinical complications of sickle cell disease such as painful vaso-occlusive events and acute chest syndrome (ACS), as well as the need for blood transfusions. Hydroxyurea does not decrease α-globin synthesis (choice A) or the concentration of HbA_2 (choice B), nor does it affect the binding characteristics of hemoglobin for oxygen (choice E). Hydroxyurea inhibits ribonucleotide reductase which leads to a reduction in erythropoiesis as opposed to an increase (choice C).

25. Correct answer is **A.** Within red blood cells (RBC), the CO_2 generated by metabolism is rapidly converted to carbonic acid through the action of carbonic anhydrase as shown in the equation below:

$$CO_2 + H_2O \leftrightarrow H_2CO_3 \leftrightarrow HCO_3^- + H^+$$

The bicarbonate ion produced in this dissociation reaction diffuses out of the RBC and is carried in the blood to the lungs. Approximately 80% of the CO_2 produced in metabolizing cells is transported to the lungs in this way. Coupled to the diffusion of bicarbonate out of RBCs in the tissues, there must be ion movement into the RBCs to maintain electrical neutrality. This is the role of chloride ions (Cl^-) and is referred to as the "chloride shift" (see following figure). In this way, Cl^- plays an important role in bicarbonate production and diffusion and thus also negatively influences O_2 binding to hemoglobin.

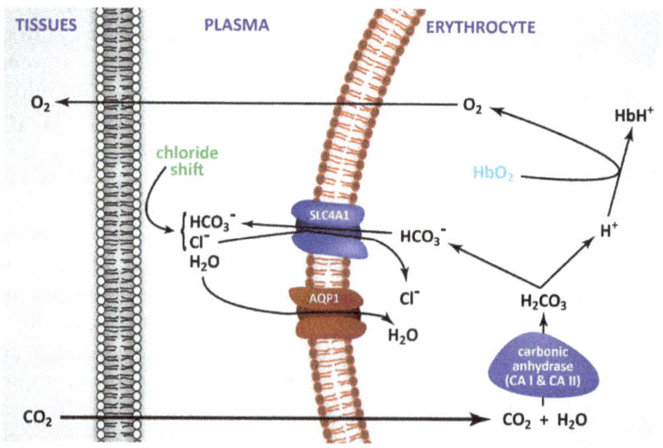

CHAPTER

3

Vitamins and Minerals

High-Yield Terms

Beriberi	Result of a diet that is carbohydrate rich and thiamine deficient; characterized by difficulty walking, loss of sensation in hands and feet, loss of muscle function of the lower legs, mental confusion/speech difficulties, nystagmus
Wernicke encephalopathy	Manifests with symptoms similar to those of beriberi but not associated with carbohydrate-rich diet
Wernicke-Korsakoff syndrome	Extreme consequence of chronic thiamine deficiency, resulting in loss of short-term memory and mild to severe psychosis
Pellagra	Classically described by the 3 D's: diarrhea, dermatitis, and dementia, caused by a chronic lack of niacin
Pernicious anemia	One of many types of megaloblastic anemias; caused by loss of secretion of intrinsic factor which is necessary for intestinal absorption of vitamin B_{12}
Megaloblastic anemia	A macrocytic anemia resulting from inhibition of DNA synthesis during erythrocyte progenitor proliferation
Xeropthalmia	Pathologic dryness of the conjunctiva and cornea due to progressive keratinization of the cornea
Rickets	Characterized by improper mineralization during the development of the bones resulting in soft bones
Osteomalacia	Characterized by demineralization of previously formed bone leading to increased softness and susceptibility to fracture
Ferrous iron	Iron with an oxidation state of +2 [Fe^{2+} or Fe(II)]
Ferric iron	Iron with an oxidation state of +3 [Fe^{3+} of Fe(III)]
Cuprous copper	Copper with an oxidation state of +1 [Cu^{1+} or Cu(I)]
Cupric copper	Copper with an oxidation state of +2 [Cu^{2+} or Cu(II)]
Ferroxidase	Any of a class of enzyme that oxidizes ferrous (Fe^{2+}) iron to ferric (Fe^{3+}) iron
Ferrireductase	Any of a class of enzyme that reduces ferric (Fe^{3+}) iron to ferrous (Fe^{2+}) iron
Reticuloendothelial cells	Comprise phagocytic cells located in different organs of the body; responsible for engulfing bacteria, viruses, other foreign substances, and abnormal body cells
Hemosiderin	An intracellular complex of iron, ferritin, denatured ferritin, and other material; most commonly found in macrophages; accumulates in conditions of hemorrhage and iron excess
Ceruloplasmin	Major ferroxidase in the blood
Metallothioneins	A family of cysteine-rich proteins that bind a variety of metals and are thought to provide protection against metal toxicities

WATER-SOLUBLE VITAMINS

Thiamine: Vitamin B_1

Thiamine (also written thiamin) is also known as vitamin B_1. Thiamine is rapidly converted to its active form, thiamine pyrophosphate (TPP), in the brain and liver by the enzyme thiamine diphosphotransferase (Figure 3–1).

TPP is necessary as a cofactor for a number of dehydrogenases including the pyruvate dehydrogenase complex (PDHc), the 2-oxoglutarate dehydrogenase complex (OGDH; commonly called α-ketoglutarate dehydrogenase), and the branched-chain α-keto acid dehydrogenase complex (BCKD). The PDHc and OGDH are critical to the function of the TCA cycle (see Chapter 9) and the BCKD is required for the oxidation of the branched-chain amino acids (see Chapter 18).

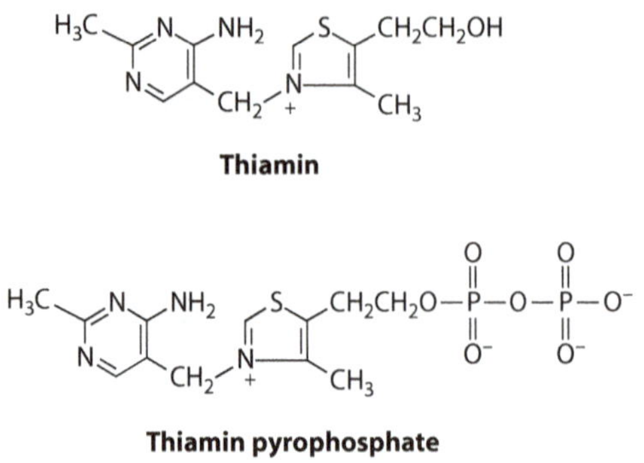

FIGURE 3–1 Structures of thiamin and thiamin pyrophosphate. (Reproduced with permission from themedicalbiochemistrypage, LLC.)

HIGH-YIELD CONCEPT

As is evident from these enzymes, thiamine plays a critical role in overall energy homeostasis and thus, a deficiency in this vitamin will lead to a severely reduced capacity of cells to generate energy (see Clinical Box 3–1).

CLINICAL BOX 3-1 THIAMINE DEFICIENCY

The earliest symptoms of thiamine deficiency include constipation, appetite suppression, nausea as well as mental depression, peripheral neuropathy, and fatigue. Chronic thiamine deficiency leads to more severe neurologic symptoms including ataxia, mental confusion, and loss of eye coordination resulting in nystagmus. Other clinical symptoms of prolonged thiamine deficiency are related to cardiovascular and musculature defects.

The severe thiamine deficiency disease known as Beriberi is the result of a diet that is carbohydrate rich and thiamine deficient. An additional thiamine deficiency-related disease is known as Wernicke encephalopathy. This disease is commonly found in chronic alcoholics due to their poor diet and has symptoms similar to those of beriberi. Wernicke-Korsakoff syndrome is an extreme manifestation of chronic deficiency of thiamine. It is characterized by acute encephalopathy followed by chronic impairment of short-term memory and mild to severe psychosis.

Riboflavin: Vitamin B_2

Riboflavin is also known as vitamin B_2. Riboflavin is the precursor for the coenzymes, flavin mononucleotide (FMN; Figure 3–2), and flavin adenine dinucleotide (FAD; Figure 3–2). The enzymes that require FMN or FAD as cofactors are termed flavoproteins, and they are involved in a wide range of reduction and oxidation (redox) reactions as well as in the process of electron transport and oxidative phosphorylation (see Chapter 10).

The enzymes that require FMN or FAD as cofactors are termed flavoproteins. Several flavoproteins also contain metal ions and are termed metalloflavoproteins. Both classes of enzyme are involved in a wide range of redox reactions, for example, succinate dehydrogenase (of the TCA cycle, see Chapter 9) and xanthine oxidase (of purine nucleotide catabolism, see Chapter 20). The roles of FMN and FAD in a wide array of different reactions underscore the consequences of deficiency in riboflavin (see Clinical Box 3–2).

Nicotinic Acid (Niacin): Vitamin B_3

Nicotinic acid (commonly referred to as niacin) and nicotinamide are also known as vitamin B_3. Both nicotinic acid and nicotinamide can serve as the dietary source of vitamin B_3. Niacin is required for the synthesis of the active forms of vitamin B_3, nicotinamide adenine dinucleotide (NAD^+), and nicotinamide adenine dinucleotide phosphate ($NADP^+$; Figure 3–3). Both NAD^+ and $NADP^+$ function as cofactors for several hundred different redox enzymes. The roles of NAD^+ and $NADP^+$ in a wide array

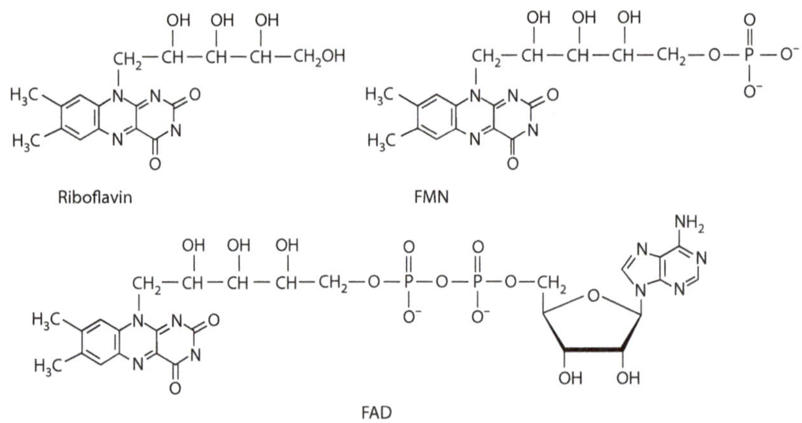

FIGURE 3–2 Riboflavin and the coenzymes flavin mononucleotide (FMN) and flavin adenine dinucleotide (FAD). (Reproduced with permission from Murray RK, Bender DA, Botham KM, et al: *Harper's Illustrated Biochemistry*, 29th ed. New York, NY: McGraw Hill; 2012.)

CLINICAL BOX 3–2 RIBOFLAVIN DEFICIENCY

Riboflavin deficiencies are rare in the United States due to the presence of adequate amounts of the vitamin in eggs, milk, meat, and fortified cereals. Riboflavin deficiency is often seen in chronic alcoholics due to their poor dietary habits. Symptoms associated with riboflavin deficiency include itching and burning eyes, angular stomatitis and cheilosis (cracks and sores in the mouth and lips), bloodshot eyes, glossitis (inflammation of the tongue leading to purplish discoloration), seborrhea (dandruff, flaking skin on scalp and face), trembling, sluggishness, and photophobia (excessive light sensitivity). Riboflavin decomposes when exposed to visible light. This characteristic can lead to riboflavin deficiencies in newborns treated for hyperbilirubinemia by phototherapy.

of different reactions underscore the consequences of deficiency in nicotinic acid (see Clinical Box 3–3).

Outside the context of metabolic pathways that utilize NAD^+ or $NADP^+$ in redox reactions, NAD^+ is required for a wide array of biological processes. There are two major cell signaling pathways that utilize NAD^+ as a cosubstrate. The sirtuin proteins and the poly-ADP-ribose polymerases (PARP) are all NAD^+-dependent enzymes that function in processes that include mitochondrial metabolism, inflammation, meiosis, autophagy, apoptosis, transcriptional regulation, RNA biogenesis and processing, DNA damage repair, chromatin remodeling, the unfolded protein response (UPR), and circadian rhythms.

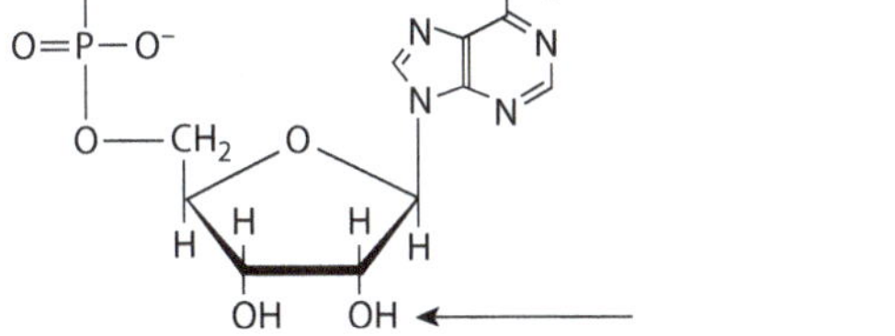

FIGURE 3–3 Structure of NAD^+. Inset box shows structure of the nicotinamide where the –R represents the adenine dinucleotide of NAD^+ or $NADP^+$. The arrow designates the location of the phosphate in $NADP^+$. The red H represents the hydrogen that is added during reduction of NAD^+ or $NADP^+$ to NADH or nicotinamide adenine dinucleotide phosphate (NADPH). (Reproduced with permission from themedicalbiochemistrypage, LLC.)

HIGH-YIELD CONCEPT

Niacin is not a true vitamin in the strictest definition since it can be derived from the amino acid tryptophan (see Chapter 18). However, the ability to utilize tryptophan for niacin synthesis is inefficient (60 mg of tryptophan are required to synthesize 1 mg of niacin) to satisfy all of the daily requirements.

HIGH-YIELD CONCEPT

Nicotinic acid (but not nicotinamide), when administered in pharmacologic doses of 2–4 g/day, lowers plasma cholesterol levels and has been shown to be a useful therapeutic for hypercholesterolemia (see Chapter 15).

CLINICAL BOX 3–3 NICOTINIC ACID DEFICIENCY

A diet deficient in niacin (as well as tryptophan) leads to glossitis of the tongue (inflammation of the tongue leading to purplish discoloration), dermatitis, weight loss, diarrhea, depression, and dementia. The severe symptoms, depression, dermatitis, and diarrhea (referred to as the three D's), are associated with the condition termed pellagra. Chronic loss of niacin in the diet can result in death and as such the symptoms of deficiency are often referred to as the four D's. Several physiologic conditions such as Hartnup disorder (see Clinical Box 18–1) or malignant carcinoid syndrome, as well as certain drug therapies (eg, isoniazid) can lead to niacin deficiency. In Hartnup disorder, tryptophan uptake from the gut and reabsorption from the glomerular filtrate in the kidneys is impaired. Malignant carcinoid syndrome is associated with altered tryptophan metabolism resulting in excess serotonin synthesis. Isoniazid (the hydrazide derivative of isonicotinic acid) was, at one time, a primary drug for chemotherapeutic treatment of tuberculosis. Although still used, the chemotherapeutic control of tuberculosis involves isoniazid in combination with three other drugs, rifampicin, pyrazinamide, and ethambutol. This therapy is often referred to by the acronym "RIPE" therapy.

Pantothenic Acid: Vitamin B_5

Pantothenic acid is also known as vitamin B_5 (Figure 3–4). Pantothenate is required for the synthesis of coenzyme A (CoA) and is a component of the acyl carrier protein (ACP) domain of fatty acid synthase (FAS). Pantothenate is required for the metabolism of carbohydrate via the TCA cycle and all fats and proteins. At least 70 enzymes have been identified as requiring CoA or ACP derivatives for their function.

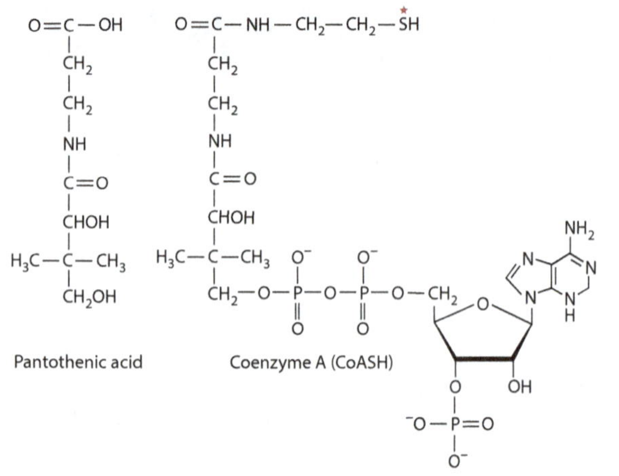

FIGURE 3–4 Pantothenic acid and coenzyme A. Asterisk shows site of acylation by fatty acids. (Reproduced with permission from Rodwell VW, Bender DA, Botham KM, et al: *Harper's Illustrated Biochemistry*, 31st ed. New York, NY: McGraw Hill; 2018.)

Vitamin B_6

Pyridoxal, pyridoxamine, and pyridoxine are collectively known as vitamin B_6. All three compounds are efficiently converted to the biologically active form of vitamin B_6, pyridoxal phosphate (PLP). This conversion is catalyzed by the ATP requiring enzyme, pyridoxal kinase (Figure 3–5). Pyridoxal kinase requires zinc for full activity, thus making it a metalloenzyme.

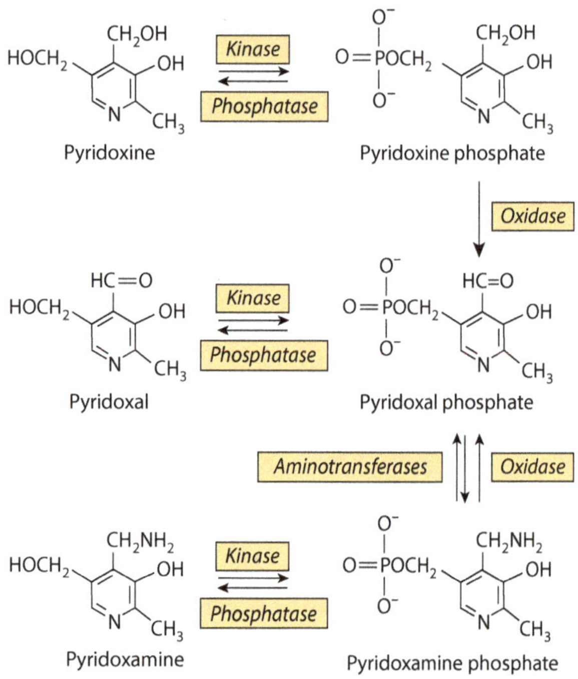

FIGURE 3–5 Interconversion of the vitamin B_6 vitamers. (Reproduced with permission from Rodwell VW, Bender DA, Botham KM, et al: *Harper's Illustrated Biochemistry*, 31st ed. New York, NY: McGraw Hill; 2018.)

PLP functions as a cofactor in enzymes involved in transamination reactions required for the synthesis and catabolism of the amino acids, is a critical cofactor for the heme biosynthetic enzyme (see Chapter 21) δ-aminolevulinic acid synthase (ALAS), the methionine metabolizing enzymes (see Chapter 18) cystathionine β-synthase (CBS) and cystathionase (cystathionine γ-lyase), as well as in glycogenolysis (see Chapter 7) as a cofactor for glycogen phosphorylase and as a cofactor for the synthesis of the inhibitory neurotransmitter γ-aminobutyric acid (GABA; see Chapter 19). Given the critical role of PLP in the synthesis of heme, deficiency of vitamin B_6 is associated with anemia (see Clinical Box 3–4).

Biotin

Biotin (Figure 3–6; also known as vitamin B_7 or vitamin H) is the cofactor required of enzymes that are involved in carboxylation reactions such as acetyl-CoA carboxylase (see Chapter 11) and pyruvate carboxylase (see Chapter 6). Biotin is found in numerous foods and also is synthesized by intestinal bacteria, and as

CLINICAL BOX 3–4 VITAMIN B_6 DEFICIENCY AND MICROCYTIC ANEMIA

Deficiencies of vitamin B_6 are rare and usually related to an overall deficiency of all the B-complex vitamins. Isoniazid (see Clinical Box 3–3) and penicillamine (used to treat rheumatoid arthritis and cystinurias) are two drugs that complex with pyridoxal and PLP resulting in a deficiency in this vitamin. The most severe symptoms of vitamin B_6 deficiency are related to the role of pyridoxal phosphate (PLP) in the synthesis of heme (see Chapter 21). PLP is required for the rate-limiting enzyme in heme biosynthesis, δ-aminolevulinic acid synthase (ALAS). Therefore, a deficiency in vitamin B_6 will result in loss of protoporphyrin IX synthesis and consequently the production of heme. As a result of this, role of vitamin B_6 a deficiency in the vitamin can be evidenced by a significant reduction in measurable ALAS product (δ-aminolevulinic acid, δ-ALA) and protoporphyrin. In erythroid progenitor cell heme regulates protein synthesis; thus the loss of heme production in vitamin B_6 deficiency results in poor protein synthesis and low heme levels in these cells leading to hypochromic microcytic anemia. The lack of protoporphyrin IX synthesis leads to iron deposits on mitochondria in bone marrow erythroblasts resulting in the formation of what are histopathologically referred to as ringed sideroblasts. The loss of iron incorporation into protoporphyrin IX leads to increased serum and intracellular iron concentration, the latter resulting in increased translation of ferritin as a means to prevent iron toxicity. Thus, vitamin B6 deficiency is associated with increased levels of serum ferritin. Deficiencies in pyridoxal kinase result in reduced synthesis of PLP and are associated with seizure disorders related to a reduction in the synthesis of GABA. Other symptoms that may appear with deficiency in vitamin B_6 include nervousness, insomnia, skin eruptions, loss of muscular control, anemia, mouth disorders, muscular weakness, dermatitis, arm and leg cramps, loss of hair, slow learning, and water retention.

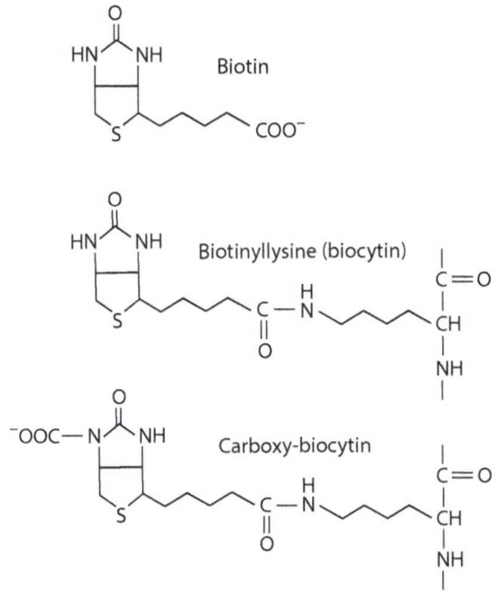

FIGURE 3–6 Biotin, biocytin, and carboxy-biocytin. (Reproduced with permission from Rodwell VW, Bender DA, Botham KM, et al: *Harper's Illustrated Biochemistry*, 31st ed. New York, NY: McGraw Hill; 2018.)

such deficiencies of the vitamin are rare. Deficiencies are generally seen only after long antibiotic therapies which deplete the intestinal microbiota or following excessive consumption of raw eggs. The latter is due to the affinity of the egg white protein, avidin, for biotin preventing intestinal absorption of the vitamin. Symptoms that may appear if biotin is deficient are extreme exhaustion, drowsiness, muscle pain, loss of appetite, depression, and grayish skin color.

Cobalamin: Vitamin B_{12}

Cobalamin is more commonly known as vitamin B_{12}. Vitamin B_{12} (as the hydroxocobalamin form) is synthesized exclusively by microorganisms and is stored in the liver of animals, including humans, bound to protein. The active forms of vitamin B_{12} in humans are methylcobalamin and 5′-deoxyadenosylcobalamin (Figure 3–7).

Cobalamin must be hydrolyzed from protein in order to be active and this occurs in the stomach via the activity of the gastric protease, pepsin. After being released, cobalamin is bound to the protein haptocorrin (also known as transcobalamin I) in the lumen of the stomach. Haptocorrin is a glycoprotein that is produced by oral salivary glands in response to intake of food. Within the small intestine pancreatic trypsin hydrolyzes the haptocorrin-cobalamin complexes allowing binding of cobalamin to another protein called intrinsic factor, IF. Intrinsic factor is also called gastric intrinsic factor. Intrinsic factor binds cobalamin only within the alkaline pH of the intestines. Cobalamin, bound to intrinsic factor, can then bind to a receptor complex called cubilin present on the apical membranes of intestinal enterocytes in the distal ileum. After transport to the blood, cobalamin is bound to transcobalamin II, a plasma globulin that is the primary transport protein for vitamin B_{12} in the blood.

HIGH-YIELD CONCEPT

There are only two clinically significant reactions in the body that require vitamin B_{12} as a cofactor, methylmalonyl-CoA mutase and methionine synthase (Clinical Box 3–5 and Clinical Box 3–6).

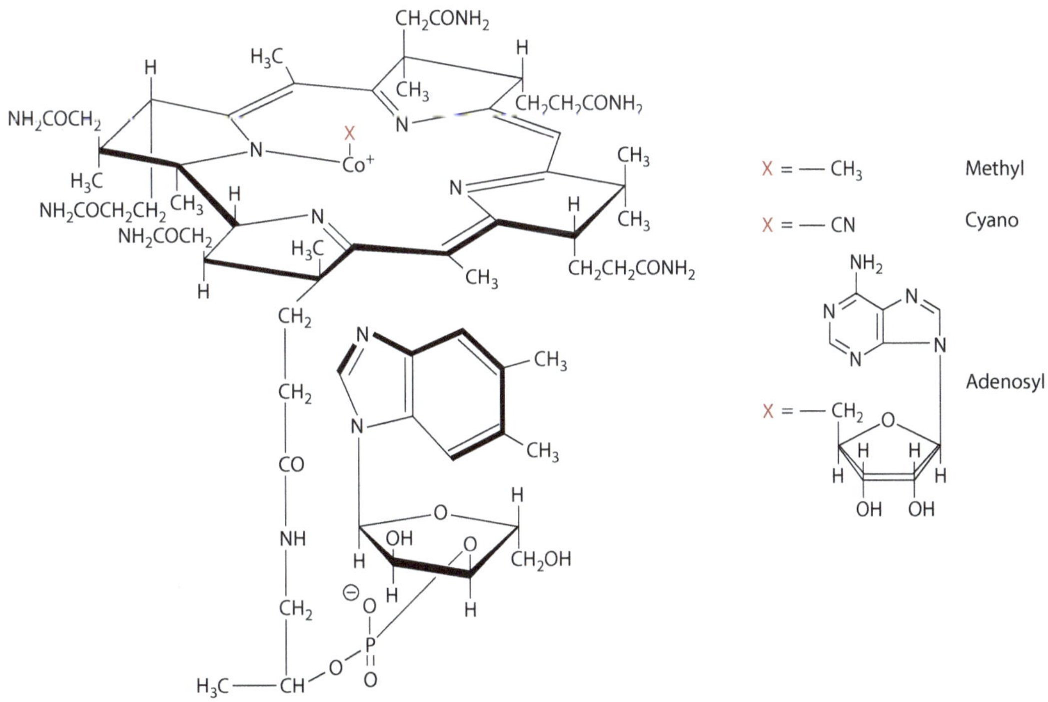

FIGURE 3–7 Structure of cobalamin. The red X indicates the position of the major substituents, methyl, cyano, or adenosyl, found in mammalian forms of vitamin B_{12}. (Reproduced with permission from themedicalbiochemistrypage, LLC.)

CLINICAL BOX 3–5 VITAMIN B_{12} DEFICIENCY AND MACROCYTIC ANEMIA

Given the ability of the liver to store vitamin B_{12}, deficiencies in this vitamin are rare and symptoms of deficiency do not appear rapidly. Pernicious anemia is a specific type of megaloblastic (macrocytic) anemia resulting from vitamin B_{12} deficiency. The loss of intrinsic factor production and release from stomach parietal cells leads to subsequent malabsorption of the vitamin from the distal ileum. The major cause of the loss of intrinsic factor is an autoimmune destruction of the parietal cells that secrete the factor. Surgical removal of a part of the stomach can also result in loss of intrinsic factor resulting in pernicious anemia. In rare cases, individuals inherit mutations in the *GIF* gene that encodes intrinsic factor resulting in pernicious anemia. The pernicious anemias result from impaired DNA synthesis due to a block in purine and thymidine biosynthesis. The block in nucleotide biosynthesis is a consequence of the effect of vitamin B_{12} on folate metabolism. When vitamin B_{12} is deficient essentially all of the folate becomes trapped as the N^5-methyltetrahydrofolate (5-methylTHF; or simply methylTHF) derivative as a result of the loss of functional methionine synthase (also called homocysteine methyltransferase). This trapping prevents the synthesis of other THF derivatives required for the purine and thymidine nucleotide biosynthesis pathways (see Chapter 20). The megaloblastic anemia is the consequence of the block to DNA synthesis such that erythroid progenitor cells, that enlarged during the G_1 phase of the cell cycle, are found in the blood along with hypersegmented neutrophils. Neurologic complications also are associated with vitamin B_{12} deficiency and result from a progressive demyelination of nerve cells. The demyelination results from the increase in methylmalonyl-CoA that results from vitamin B_{12} deficiency that is associated with loss of methylmalonyl-CoA mutase activity. The loss of methylmalonyl-CoA mutase activity with deficiencies in B_{12} results in an accompanying methylmalonic acidemia. Methylmalonyl-CoA is a competitive inhibitor of malonyl-CoA in fatty acid biosynthesis as well as being able to substitute for malonyl-CoA in any fatty acid biosynthesis that may occur. Since the myelin sheath that protects nerve cells is in continual flux the methylmalonyl-CoA-induced inhibition of fatty acid synthesis results in the eventual destruction of the sheath. The incorporation of methylmalonyl-CoA into fatty acid biosynthesis results in branched-chain fatty acids being produced that may severely alter the architecture of the normal membrane structure of nerve cells. Contributing to the neural degeneration seen in vitamin B_{12} deficiency is the reduced synthesis of *S*-adenosylmethione (SAM; also abbreviated AdoMet) due to loss of the methionine synthase catalyzed reaction. The conversion of phosphatidylethanolamine (PE) to phosphatidylcholine (PC) requires the enzyme phosphatidylethanolamine *N*-methyltransferase (encoded by the *PEMT* gene) which carries out three successive SAM-dependent methylation reactions. This reaction is a critically important reaction of membrane lipid homeostasis. Therefore, the reduced capacity to carry out the methionine synthase reaction, due to nutritional or disease-mediated deficiency of vitamin B_{12}, results in reduced SAM production and as a consequence contributes to the neural degeneration (ie, depression, peripheral neuropathy) seen in chronic B_{12} deficiency. Deficiencies in B_{12} can also lead to elevations in the level of circulating homocysteine and elevated excretion of the oxidized dimer of homocysteine called homocystine. Elevated levels of homocysteine are known to lead to cardiovascular dysfunction. Due to its high reactivity to proteins, homocysteine is almost always bound to proteins, thus thiolating them leading to their degradation. Homocysteine also binds to albumin and hemoglobin in the blood. Some of the detrimental effects of homocysteine are due to its binding to lysyl oxidase, an enzyme responsible for proper maturation of the extracellular matrix proteins collagen and elastin. Production of defective collagen and elastin has a negative impact on arteries, bone, and skin, and the effects on arteries are believed to be contributory to the cardiac dysfunction associated with elevated serum homocysteine. In individuals with homocysteine levels above $\approx 12 \mu M$, there is an increased risk of thrombosis and cardiovascular disease. The increased risk for thrombotic episodes, such as deep vein thrombosis (DVT), associated with homocysteinemia is due to homocysteine serving as a contact activation nucleus for activation of the intrinsic coagulation cascade (see Chapter 33).

During the catabolism of fatty acids with an odd number of carbon atoms and the amino acids methionine, valine, isoleucine, and threonine the resultant propionyl-CoA is converted to succinyl-CoA for oxidation in the TCA cycle. One of the enzymes in this pathway, methylmalonyl-CoA mutase, requires vitamin B_{12} as a cofactor in the conversion of methylmalonyl-CoA to succinyl-CoA. The 5′-deoxyadenosine derivative of cobalamin is required for this reaction. The combined pathway of metabolism of these different compounds is often referred to by the mnemonic "VOMIT pathway" where V is valine, O is fatty acids with an odd number of carbon atoms, M is methionine, I is isoleucine, and T is threonine.

The second reaction requiring vitamin B_{12} catalyzes the conversion of homocysteine to methionine and is catalyzed by methionine synthase (also called homocysteine methyltransferase). This reaction results in the transfer of the methyl group from N^5-methyltetrahydrofolate (methyl-THF) to hydroxycobalamin generating tetrahydrofolate (THF) and methylcobalamin (Figure 3–8).

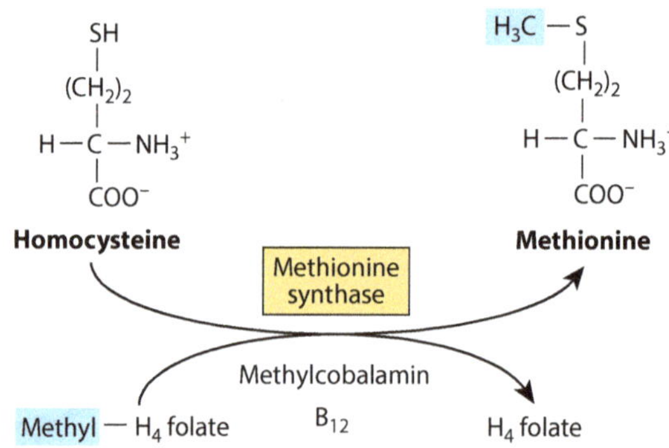

FIGURE 3–8 Homocysteine and the "folate trap." Vitamin B_{12} deficiency leads to impairment of methionine synthase, resulting in accumulation of homocysteine and trapping folate as methyltetrahydrofolate. (Reproduced with permission from Rodwell VW, Bender DA, Botham KM, et al: *Harper's Illustrated Biochemistry*, 31st ed. New York, NY: McGraw Hill; 2018.)

CLINICAL BOX 3–6 VITAMIN B_{12} DEFICIENCY AND METHYLMALONIC ACIDEMIA/ACIDURIA

The methylmalonic acidemias represent a family of disorders that have in common the elevation of methylmalonic acid in the blood and urine. Some of the methylmalonic acidemias also include the presence of homocystinuria and are referred to as combined methylmalonic acidemia and homocystinuria. Methylmalonic acid (as methylmalonyl-CoA) is an intermediate in the metabolism of four amino acids, methionine, isoleucine, valine, and threonine (see Chapter 18), as well as the metabolism of fatty acids that contain an odd number of carbon atoms (see Chapter 13). The catabolism of all five substrates yields propionyl-CoA which is converted to the TCA cycle intermediate, succinyl-CoA, by a series of three reactions catalyzed by, in order, propionyl-CoA carboxylase, methylmalonyl-CoA epimerase, and methylmalonyl-CoA mutase.

Inherited forms of the methylmalonic acidemias result from a number of different gene defects that occur either in the methylmalonyl-CoA mutase gene (*MMUT*) or genes responsible for the conversion of vitamin B_{12} to its active forms, adenosylcobalamin (AdoCbl) and methylcobalamin (MeCbl). In addition, dietary deficiency of vitamin B_{12} results in megaloblastic anemia accompanied by methylmalonic acidemia. Although there are numerous genes that, when defective, lead to methylmalonic acidemia, over 60% of identified cases are the result of mutations in the *MMUT* gene that encodes methylmalonyl-CoA mutase.

Within the family of methylmalonic acidemias, there are two subfamilies: those where symptoms are associated only with elevated levels of methylmalonic acid in the blood and urine and those where the symptoms are associated with increased methylmalonic acid and increased homocystine in the blood (homocystinemia) and urine (homocystinuria). Homocystine is the disulfide bonded molecule derived from oxidation of two homocysteine molecules.

The clinical spectrum of the methylmalonic acidemias is wide and can range from a benign condition to a fatal neonatal disease. The major primary symptoms include metabolic acidosis, ketosis, hyperammonemia, hypoglycemia or hyperglycemia, and neutropenia. The major secondary complications of the methylmalonic acidemias include variable developmental delay, tubulointerstitial nephritis with progressive renal failure, acute and chronic basal ganglia involvement, disabling movement disorder with choreoathetosis, dystonia, and para- or quadriparesis, pancreatitis, growth failure, functional immune impairment, and optic nerve atrophy. Infants with isolated methylmalonic acidemia commonly present with lethargy, failure to thrive, recurrent vomiting, dehydration, respiratory distress, and muscular hypotonia. Approximately 80% of infants that are null for the *MMUT* gene present during the first week of life and 90% before the end of the first month of life. The most characteristic extrapyramidal sign seen in methylmalonic acidemia infants is choreoathetosis (involuntary movements in a combination of chorea [irregular migrating contractions] and athetosis [twisting and writhing]). Clinical manifestations associated with methylmalonic acidemias with homocystinurias can be quite variable as well due to the various causes. In some cases, there is intrauterine growth retardation and, therefore, the clinical signs are evident at birth and include microcephaly. In infants, the symptoms include failure to thrive, delayed development, difficulty feeding, pallor (abnormally pale appearance), and intellectual disability. Neurological symptoms also manifest in patients with methylmalonic acidemia with homocystinuria. These symptoms include hypotonia and seizures. The signs and symptoms of methylmalonic acidemia with homocystinuria worsen over time and can result in life-threatening complications if not properly treated.

The accumulation of methylmalonic acid is associated with metabolism to 2-methylcitrate, propionate, and 3-hydroxypropionate, all of which either directly or indirectly inhibit complex II (succinate dehydrogenase) of the TCA cycle and the oxidative phosphorylation pathway. The inhibition of these processes results in the neuropathogenesis typical of the methylmalonic acidemias.

Due to the associated hyperammonemia with the methylmalonic acidemias, therapeutic intervention cannot be delayed. The initial medical treatment should include limitations in protein intake along with intravenous glucose. Treatment with drugs that include L-carnitine, hydroxocobalamin, biotin, sodium phenylbutyrate (nitrogen scavenger to reduce serum ammonia levels), L-arginine, and N-carbamylglutamate should be instituted. Long-term therapy for methylmalonic acidemia patients includes L-carnitine, vitamin B_{12} in responsive patients, antibiotics to reduce intestinal nitrogen producing bacteria, low protein diets, isoleucine and valine supplementation, and vitamin and mineral supplementation. Trimethylglycine (betaine) supplementation has some utility at lowering serum levels of homocysteine in methylmalonic acidemia patients. The drug Cystadane® (betaine anhydrous) has been approved as an adjunctive treatment of homocystinurias, including CBS deficiency, MTHFR deficiency, and diseases of cobalamin cofactor metabolism. The utility of oral betaine is that it activates betaine-homocysteine methyltransferase which converts homocysteine to methionine but bypasses the cobalamin-dependent methionine synthase reaction. Trimethylglycine and cystadane are used in combinations with vitamin B_6, vitamin B_{12}, folic acid, and in some forms of methylmalonic acidemias, a low methionine diet.

Folic Acid

Folic acid (folate) is sometimes referred to as vitamin B_9. Folate itself is not biologically active but in derivatives of the THF form it participates in a number of one-carbon transfer reactions (Figure 3–9). Dietary folates are predominately the N^5-methyl-THF form (methyl-THF). Dietary folate is converted first to dihydrofolate (DHF) and then to THF through the action of the enzyme, dihydrofolate reductase (DHFR).

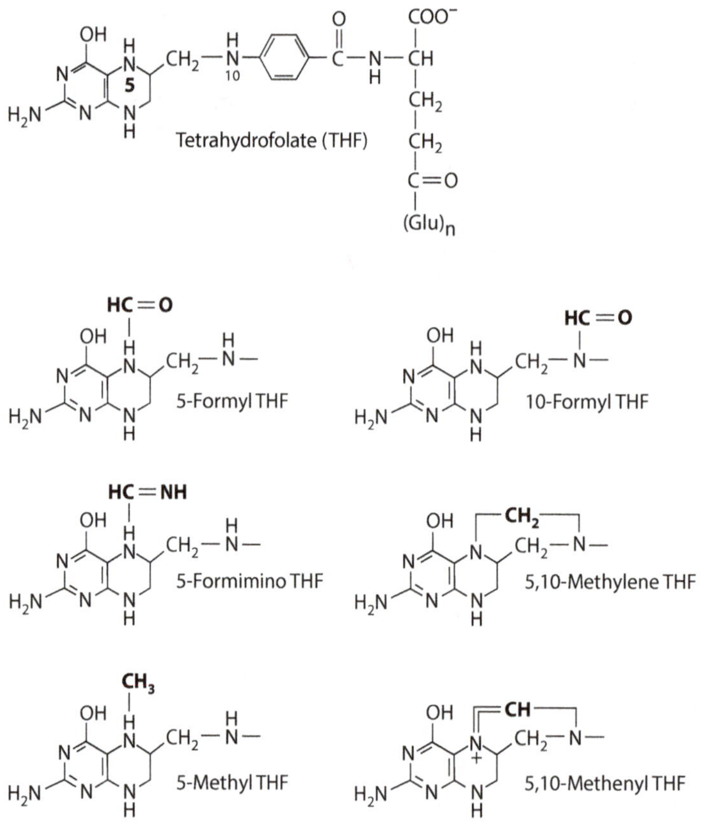

FIGURE 3–9 Tetrahydrofolic acid and the one-carbon substituted folates. (Reproduced with permission from Rodwell VW, Bender DA, Botham KM, et al: *Harper's Illustrated Biochemistry*, 31st ed. New York, NY: McGraw Hill; 2018.)

The function of THF derivatives is to carry and transfer various forms of one-carbon units during biosynthetic reactions. The one-carbon units are methyl, methylene, methenyl, formyl, and formimino groups. These one-carbon transfer reactions are required in the biosynthesis of amino acids and nucleotides (Figure 3–10).

The ability to acquire choline and amino acids from the diet and to salvage the purine nucleotides makes the role of N^5,N^{10}-methylene-THF in dTMP synthesis the most metabolically significant function for this vitamin (see Clinical Box 3–7). The role of vitamin B_{12} and N^5-methyl-THF in the conversion of

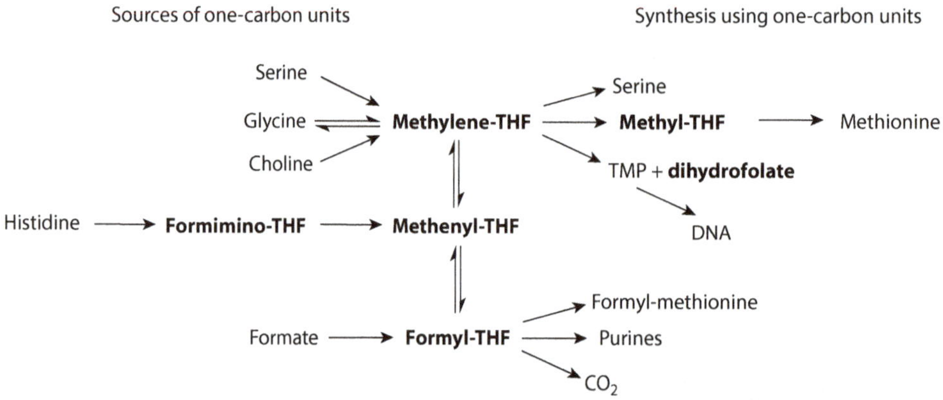

FIGURE 3–10 Sources and utilization of one-carbon substituted folates. (Reproduced with permission from Rodwell VW, Bender DA, Botham KM, et al: *Harper's Illustrated Biochemistry*, 31st ed. New York, NY: McGraw Hill; 2018.)

CLINICAL BOX 3–7 FOLATE DEFICIENCY AND MACROCYTIC ANEMIA

Folate deficiency results in complications nearly identical to those described for vitamin B_{12} deficiency. The most pronounced effect of folate deficiency on cellular processes is on DNA synthesis. This is due to an impairment in dTMP synthesis which leads to cell cycle arrest in S-phase of rapidly proliferating cells, in particular hematopoietic cells. The result is megaloblastic anemia as for vitamin B_{12} deficiency. The inability to synthesize DNA during erythroid progenitor cell proliferation leads to abnormally large erythrocytes and hypersegmented neutrophils being found in the blood, typical of megaloblastic (macrocytic) anemia. Since both folate and vitamin B_{12} deficiencies result in megaloblastic anemias, it is necessary to be able to clinically distinguish the cause as it relates to vitamin deficiency. Since B_{12} is required for both the methionine synthase reaction and the methylmalonyl-CoA mutase reaction, a megaloblastic anemia resulting from B_{12} deficiency is also associated with an accompanying methylmalonic acidemia, whereas megaloblastic anemias caused by folate deficiency are not. An additional critical diagnostic is related to the onset of symptoms. Because human cells cannot store any significant amount of folate but the liver can store B_{12}, folate deficient megaloblastic anemias manifest very quickly, whereas B_{12} deficient anemias take considerably longer to manifest. Folate deficiencies are rare due to the adequate presence of folate in food. Poor dietary habits, such as those of chronic alcoholics, can lead to folate deficiency. The predominant causes of folate deficiency in nonalcoholics are impaired absorption or metabolism or an increased demand for the vitamin. The predominant condition requiring an increase in the daily intake of folate is pregnancy. This is due to an increased number of rapidly proliferating cells present in the blood. The need for folate will nearly double by the third trimester of pregnancy. Certain drugs such as anticonvulsants and oral contraceptives can impair the absorption of folate. Anticonvulsants also increase the rate of folate metabolism.

Mutations in the methylene THF reductase gene (MTHFR) are associated with a disorder that was originally referred to as hyperhomocysteinemia. Characteristic features of this inherited disorder are a high plasma homocysteine level and an associated early onset of coronary artery disease (CAD). Additional symptoms of hyperhomocysteinemia include mild cognitive impairment and the potential for dementia. Indeed, there is evidence that links elevated serum homocysteine levels with Alzheimer disease. The most common mutation in the MTHFR gene resulting in this disorder is a C to T change at nucleotide position 677 (C677T).

homocysteine to methionine also can have a significant impact on the ability of cells to regenerate needed THF.

Ascorbic Acid: Vitamin C

Ascorbic acid (ascorbate) is more commonly known as vitamin C (Figure 3–11). The active form of vitamin C is ascorbate itself. The main function of ascorbate is to serve as a reducing agent in a number of different reactions. Ascorbate is the cofactor for Cu^{+}-dependent monooxygenases and Fe^{2+}-dependent dioxygenases. Several critical enzymes that require ascorbate as a cofactor include the collagen processing enzymes, the lysyl hydroxylases and the prolyl hydroxylases as well as the catecholamine synthesis enzyme dopamine β-hydroxylase. Many of the symptoms of vitamin C deficiency are the result of the loss of proper collagen processing (see Clinical Box 3–8).

Dietary ascorbate is also involved in nonheme iron absorption in the small intestine and in the overall regulation of iron homeostasis.

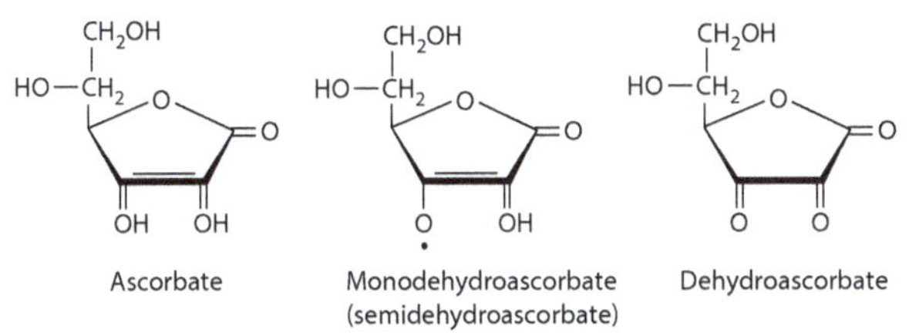

FIGURE 3–11 Vitamin C. (Reproduced with permission from Rodwell VW, Bender DA, Botham KM, et al: *Harper's Illustrated Biochemistry*, 31st ed. New York, NY: McGraw Hill; 2018.)

HIGH-YIELD CONCEPT

The most important reactions requiring ascorbate are those involved in the processing of the various collagens.

CLINICAL BOX 3–8 SCURVY

Deficiency in vitamin C leads to the disease scurvy due to the role of the vitamin in the posttranslational modification of collagens. Scurvy is characterized by easily bruised skin, muscle fatigue, soft swollen gums, decreased wound healing and hemorrhaging, osteoporosis, and anemia. Due to its role in collagen processing, the bleeding dysfunction associated with vitamin C deficiency is characterized by the lack of effect on prothrombin time (PT) but with a prolonged bleeding time. The latter effect is the result of the reduced ability for platelets to adhere to exposed subendothelial extracellular matrix collagen which is required for their activation. Vitamin C is readily absorbed and so the primary cause of vitamin C deficiency is poor diet and/or an increased requirement. The primary physiologic state leading to an increased requirement for vitamin C is severe stress (or trauma). This is due to a rapid depletion in the adrenal stores of the vitamin. The reason for the decrease in adrenal vitamin C levels is unclear but may be due either to redistribution of the vitamin to areas that need it or an overall increased utilization. Inefficient intake of vitamin C has also been associated with a number of conditions, such as high blood pressure, gallbladder disease, stroke, some cancers, and atherosclerosis.

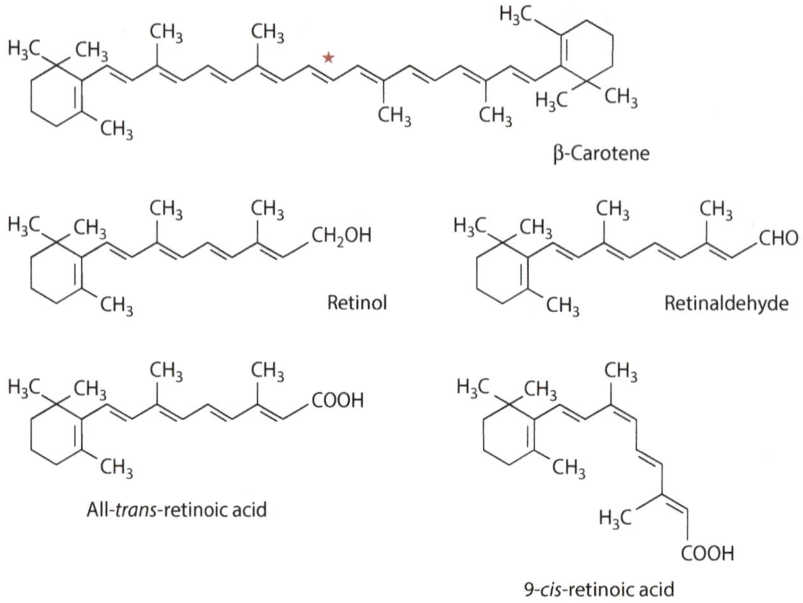

FIGURE 3–12 α-Carotene and the major vitamin A vitamers. Asterisk shows the site of cleavage of β-carotene by carotene dioxygenase, to yield retinaldehyde. (Reproduced with permission from Rodwell VW, Bender DA, Botham KM, et al: *Harper's Illustrated Biochemistry*, 31st ed. New York, NY: McGraw Hill; 2018.)

FAT-SOLUBLE VITAMINS

Vitamin A

Vitamin A consists of three biologically active retinoids: retinol, retinaldehyde (commonly called retinal), and retinoic acid. Each of these vitamin A compounds is derived from the plant precursor molecule, β-carotene (a member of a family of molecules known as carotenoids). Beta-carotene, which consists of two molecules of retinal linked at their aldehyde ends, is also referred to as the provitamin form of vitamin A (Figure 3–12). Additional provitamin A carotenoids are α-carotene and β-cryptoxanthin.

Ingested β-carotene is cleaved in the lumen of the intestine by β-carotene dioxygenases to yield free retinaldehyde. Retinaldehyde is reduced to retinol within intestinal enterocytes by one of a family of enzymes called retinol dehydrogenases. Retinol is esterified to palmitic acid and delivered to the blood via chylomicrons. The uptake of chylomicron remnants by the liver results in delivery of retinol to this organ for storage.

Role of Vitamin A in the Visual Process

Photoreception in the eye is the function of two specialized cell types located in the retina; the rod and cone cells. Both rod and cone cells contain a photoreceptor pigment in their membranes. The photosensitive compound of most mammalian eyes is a protein called opsin to which retinaldehyde is covalently coupled. The opsin of rod cells is called scotopsin. The photoreceptor of rod cells is specifically called rhodopsin or visual purple. This compound is a complex between scotopsin and the 11-*cis*-retinaldehyde form of vitamin A. Rhodopsin is member of the large superfamily of G-protein coupled receptors (GPCR: see Chapter 26). The G-protein to which rhodopsin is coupled is called transducing (G_t). Rhodopsin is present in the disc membranes inside rod cells (Figure 3–13). The earliest symptoms of deficiency in vitamin A are related to the role of this vitamin in the visual process (see Clinical Box 3–9).

When rhodopsin is exposed to a photon of light the associated 11-*cis*-retinaldehyde is converted to all-trans-retinaldehyde, a process referred to as photobleaching. The conformational change in retinaldehyde converts rhodopsin to metarhodopsin II. This conformational change activates the associated G-protein, transducin. Activated transducin, specifically the α-subunit, activates an associated cGMP phosphodiesterase (PDE) resulting in hydrolysis of cGMP to GMP. cGMP is required to maintain a cGMP-gated channel, present in the plasma membrane of rod cells, in the open state. These cyclic nucleotide-gated (CNG) channels transport both Na^+ and Ca^{2+} into the rod cell. The influx of these ions depolarizes the rod cell triggering the release of the neurotransmitter, glutamate. Glutamate binds to receptors on closely associated bipolar cells activating these cells to release the inhibitory neurotransmitter GABA. The release of GABA, from bipolar cells, inhibits neurotransmission along the optic nerve. The drop in cGMP concentration results in closure of the CNG channels leading to hyperpolarization of the rod cell and loss of glutamate release and cessation of bipolar cell stimulation. The net effect is that the optic nerve is no longer inhibited by GABA allowing propagation of nerve impulses to the visual center in the brain.

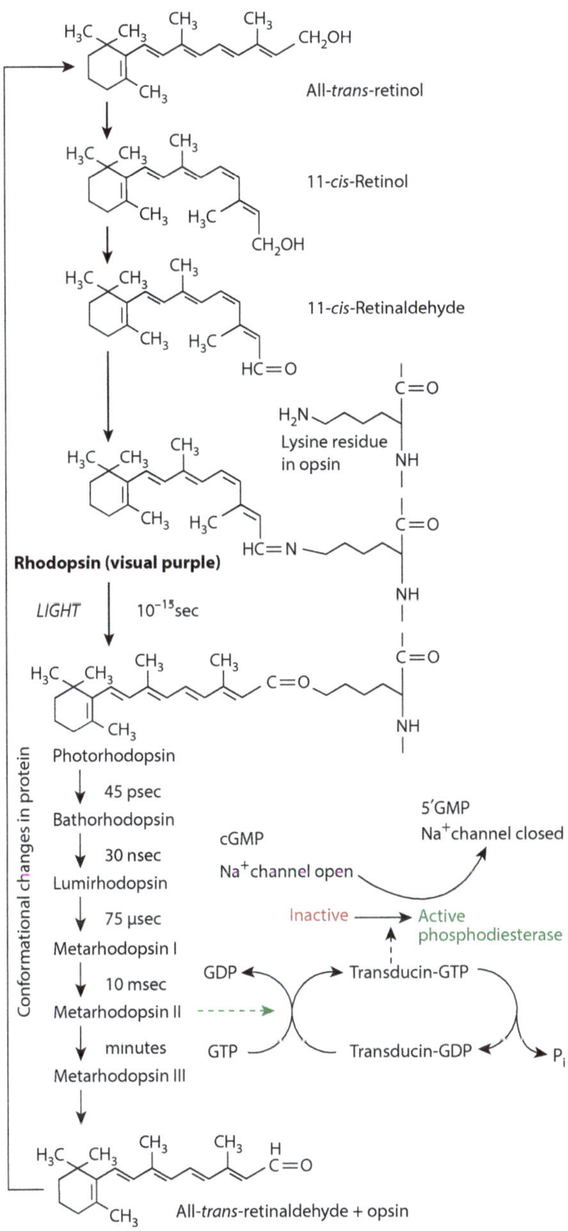

FIGURE 3–13 The role of retinaldehyde in the visual cycle. (Reproduced with permission from Rodwell VW, Bender DA, Botham KM, et al: *Harper's Illustrated Biochemistry*, 31st ed. New York, NY: McGraw Hill; 2018.)

Retinoic Acid: A Member of the Nuclear Hormone Receptor-Activating Hormones

Within cells retinoic acid (as well as the related compound 9-*cis*-retinoic acid) bind to specific receptors termed the retinoic acid receptors (RAR). A related family of receptors is the retinoid X receptors (RXR). The RAR and RXR are members of the steroid and thyroid hormone superfamily of nuclear receptors.

In the absence of hormone RAR and RXR are bound to target DNA sequences in conjunction with transcriptional repressor complexes. Following binding of hormone, the receptor-retinoic acid complex displaces the repressor complexes allowing for interaction with transcriptional activator complexes resulting in the activation of target gene expression.

CLINICAL BOX 3–9 VITAMIN A DEFICIENCY AND BLINDNESS

Vitamin A is stored in the liver and deficiency of the vitamin occurs only after prolonged lack of dietary intake. Any lipid malabsorption disorder can be associated with deficiency in vitamin A, as well as all the fat-soluble vitamins. Patients with cystic fibrosis are particularly prone to deficiencies in the fat-soluble vitamins due to defective pancreatic enzyme secretion and function. The earliest symptoms of vitamin A deficiency are night blindness. Additional early symptoms include follicular hyperkeratinosis, increased susceptibility to infection and cancer and anemia equivalent to iron-deficient anemia. Prolonged lack of vitamin A leads to deterioration of the eye tissue through progressive keratinization of the conjunctiva of the eye which results in abnormal dryness of the conjunctiva and the cornea and the lack of ability to produce tears, a condition known as xerophthalmia. The hyperkeratinization of the conjunctiva can be seen on examination of the eye, and the characteristic feature is referred to as Bitot spots after the French physician Pierre Bitot who first described this pathology in 1863.

The increased risk of cancer in vitamin A deficiency is thought to be the result of a depletion in β-carotene. Beta-carotene is a very effective antioxidant and is suspected to reduce the risk of cancers known to be initiated by the production of free radicals. Of particular interest is the potential benefit of increased β-carotene intake to reduce the risk of lung cancer in smokers. However, caution needs to be taken when increasing the intake of any of the lipid soluble vitamins. Excess accumulation of vitamin A in the liver can lead to toxicity which manifests as bone pain, hepatosplenomegaly, nausea, and diarrhea.

Vitamin D

The biologically active form of vitamin D is a steroid hormone that functions to regulate specific gene expression following interaction with its intracellular receptor, a member of the steroid and thyroid hormone receptor superfamily. The biologically active form of the hormone is 1,25-dihydroxy vitamin D_3 (1,25-$(OH)_2D_3$), which is commonly termed calcitriol. Calcitriol functions primarily to regulate calcium and phosphorous homeostasis by acting in the intestines, bone, and the kidney.

Active calcitriol is derived from ergosterol (produced in plants) and from 7-dehydrocholesterol, an intermediate in the synthesis of cholesterol (see Chapter 15). On exposure to ultraviolet (UV) wavelength light 7-dehydrocholesterol is nonenzymatically (thermal isomerization) converted to vitamin D_3 (cholecalciferol; Figure 3–14). Ergocalciferol (vitamin D_2) is formed by UV irradiation of ergosterol. Both vitamin D_2 and D_3 enter the bloodstream

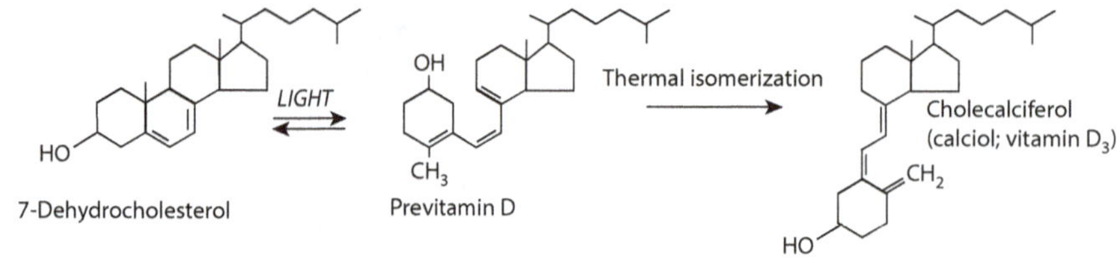

FIGURE 3–14 The synthesis of vitamin D in the skin. (Reproduced with permission from Rodwell VW, Bender DA, Botham KM, et al: *Harper's Illustrated Biochemistry*, 31st ed. New York, NY: McGraw Hill; 2018.)

and are taken up by the liver. Within the liver, vitamins D_2 and D_3 undergo the first of two activating hydroxylation reactions.

Dietary forms of vitamin D are absorbed from the intestine, packaged into chylomicrons, and delivered to the blood where they are transported to the liver. In the liver, cholecalciferol is hydroxylated at the 25 position by a specific 25-hydroxylase generating 25-hydroxy-D_3 (calcidiol) which is the major circulating form of vitamin D (Figure 3–15). Conversion of calcidiol to calcitriol occurs through the activity of a specific 25-hydroxyvitamin D_3 1-α-hydroxylase (1-hydroxylase) present in the proximal convoluted tubules of the kidneys, in bone, and in the placenta. The level of active 1-hydroxylase is controlled via the peptide hormone, parathyroid hormone (PTH; see Chapter 31).

Calcitriol functions as a steroid hormone, inducing the expression of calcium-binding proteins called calbindins that facilitate calcium transport within cells, particularly within the intestines and the kidneys. Calcitriol also enhances the expression of several intestinal calcium transporter genes. The steroid hormone action of vitamin D occurs via the action of calcitriol binding to a specific intracellular receptor that is a member of the nuclear receptor family of hormone receptors called the vitamin D receptor (VDR).

HIGH-YIELD CONCEPT

Calcitriol functions in concert with parathyroid hormone (PTH) to regulate serum calcium and phosphorous levels. Deficiency of vitamin D is principally associated with disturbances in calcium homeostasis (see Clinical Box 3–10) and is also true under conditions of supraphysiologic dosing of vitamin D supplements (see Clinical Box 3–11).

Vitamin E

Vitamin E is a mixture of several related compounds known as tocopherols and tocotrienols (Figure 3–16). The tocopherols are the major sources of vitamin E in the US diet. All tocopherols are able to act as free radical scavengers thus, they all have potent antioxidant properties, particularly against the formation of lipid hydroperoxides. Vitamin E is absorbed from the intestines packaged in chylomicrons. It is delivered to the tissues via chylomicron transport and then to the liver through chylomicron remnant uptake. The major site of vitamin E storage is in adipose tissue.

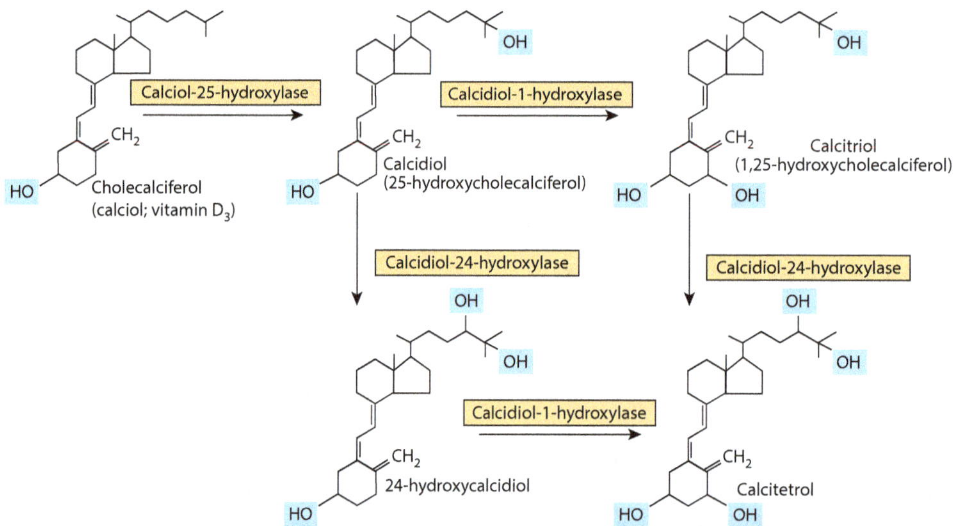

FIGURE 3–15 Metabolism of vitamin D. (Reproduced with permission from Rodwell VW, Bender DA, Botham KM, et al: *Harper's Illustrated Biochemistry*, 31st ed. New York, NY: McGraw Hill; 2018.)

CLINICAL BOX 3–10 VITAMIN D DEFICIENCY

As a result of the addition of vitamin D to milk, deficiencies in this vitamin are rare in most developed countries. As a fat-soluble vitamin, any lipid absorption disorder can be associated with deficiency in the vitamin. Patients with cystic fibrosis are particularly prone to deficiencies in the fat-soluble vitamins due to defective pancreatic enzyme secretion and function. The main symptom of vitamin D deficiency in children is rickets and in adults is osteomalacia. Rickets is characterized by improper mineralization during the development of the bones resulting in soft bones. Osteomalacia is defined as the softening of the bones caused by defective bone mineralization secondary to deficiency in available levels of phosphorous and calcium, or because of overactive resorption of calcium from the bone. Osteomalacia and osteoporosis do not describe the same bone defect. In osteoporosis, bone mineral density is reduced and the amount and variety of proteins in the bone are altered. Muscle weakness and achy bone pain are the major symptoms associated with osteomalacia. Treatment for osteomalacia involves replenishing low levels of vitamin D and calcium and treating any underlying disorders that may be causing the deficiencies. The resultant decrease in Ca^{2+} uptake due to vitamin D deficiency leads to hypocalcemia leading to excess parathyroid hormone release (referred to as secondary hyperparathyroidism) as a compensatory mechanism. The excess release of parathyroid hormone (PTH) can lead to over resorption of renal calcium leading to hypercalcemia. This hypercalcemia can cause calcification in soft tissues and peritrabecular fibrosis in bones. The peritrabecular fibrosis, associated with hyperparathyroidism, is quite distinct and is clinically called osteitis fibrosa cystica (OFC). OFC is also called von Recklinghausen disease of bone. This latter name is distinct from von Recklinghausen disease which is neurofibromatosis type 1.

CLINICAL BOX 3–11 VITAMIN D TOXICITY

Vitamin D toxicity is associated with supraphysiological dosing of vitamin D, considered to be any dose above 50,000 IU (2500 μg) per day for a duration of at least 1 month where the normal adult RDA for vitmain D is 600 IU/day. Whereas vitamin D toxicity is rare, it is a valid consideration in the context of the diagnosis of the causes of hypercalcemia. Both vitamin D_2 and D_3 (the cholecalciferols) are lipophilic and are rapidly taken up into skeletal muscle and adipose tissue where they can remain for several months. Given that the cholecalciferols are converted to calcidiol in the liver based solely on substrate availability, calcidiol will also accumulate under conditions of excess vitamin D intake. Calcidiol is also lipophilic and can be stored within adipose tissue for several months. Due to the storage of cholecalciferols and calcidiol in adipose tissue, vitamin D intoxication can take several weeks to resolve. In the event of excessive vitamin D intake there is a very characteristic toxicity profile. The excess vitamin results in an associated hypercalcemia. The hypercalcemia caused by vitamin D toxicity is primarily due to the significant increases in circulating levels of calcidiol, which when it enters cells, can bind to and activate the vitamin D receptor (VDR). In addition, at high concentrations calcidiol can displace calcitriol from vitamin D-binding protein resulting in increased free calcitriol that can then activate the VDR. Both of these pathophysiological phenomena result in increased intestinal calcium absorption and increased bone calcium resorption. The resultant hypercalcemia can lead to pathologies that are similar to those caused by the hypercalcemia that results from the secondary hyperparathyroidism in the context of vitamin D deficiency. One of the earliest tissues affected by the onset of the soft tissue calcification with vitamin D toxicity is the kidney. The symptoms that result from the damage to the renal tissue include polydipsia and polyuria. Additional symptoms of vitamin D toxicity include fatique, nausea, vomiting, and diminished mental capacity. Chronic vitamin D toxicity can lead to calcification of numerous soft tissues and may ultimately result in permanent renal failure.

HIGH-YIELD CONCEPT

The major function of vitamin E is to act as a natural antioxidant by scavenging free radicals and molecular oxygen, thereby preventing peroxidation of membrane-localized polyunsaturated fatty acids (PUFA).

No major disease states have been found to be associated with vitamin E deficiency due to adequate levels in the average American diet. The major symptom of vitamin E deficiency in humans is an increase in red blood cell fragility. Since vitamin E is absorbed from the intestines in chylomicrons, any disease associated with fat malabsorption can lead to deficiencies in vitamin E intake. Neurologic dysfunction has been correlated to vitamin E deficiencies associated with fat malabsorptive disorders. Increased intake of vitamin E is recommended in premature infants fed formulas that are low in the vitamin as well as in persons consuming

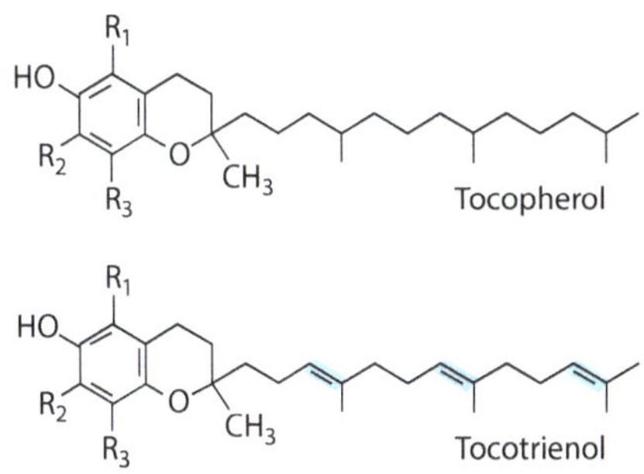

FIGURE 3–16 Vitamin E vitamers. In α-tocopherol and tocotrienol R1, R2, and R3 are all —CH3 groups. In the β-vitamers R2 is H, in the γ-vitamers R1 is H, and in the δ-vitamers R1 and R2 are both H. (Reproduced with permission from Rodwell VW, Bender DA, Botham KM, et al: *Harper's Illustrated Biochemistry*, 31st ed. New York, NY: McGraw Hill; 2018.)

a diet high in polyunsaturated fatty acids. Polyunsaturated fatty acids tend to form free radicals on exposure to oxygen and this may lead to an increased risk of certain cancers.

Vitamin K

The K vitamins exist naturally as K_1 (phylloquinone) in green vegetables and K_2 (menaquinone) produced by intestinal bacteria, and K_3 is synthetic menadione. When administered, vitamin K_3 is alkylated to one of the vitamin K_2 forms of menaquinone (Figure 3–17). Like all the fat-soluble vitamins, vitamin K is delivered from the diet to the blood via chylomicrons.

HIGH-YIELD CONCEPT

The major function of the K vitamins is the maintenance of normal levels of the γ-carboxylated blood clotting proteins, prothrombin, factors VII, IX and X, and protein C and protein S, which are all synthesized in the liver as inactive precursor enzymes (zymogens). In addition, several proteins involved in bone homeostasis are also subjected to vitamin K-dependent γ-carboxylation, which indicates this vitamin is also critically important for overall bone health.

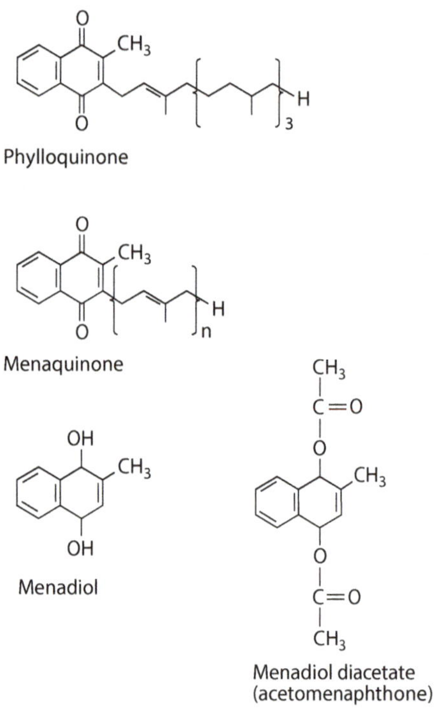

FIGURE 3–17 The vitamin K vitamers. Menadiol (or menadione) and menadiol diacetate are synthetic compounds that are converted to menaquinone in the liver. (Reproduced with permission from Rodwell VW, Bender DA, Botham KM, et al: *Harper's Illustrated Biochemistry*, 31st ed. New York, NY: McGraw Hill; 2018.)

Conversion from inactive to active clotting factor requires posttranslational carboxylation of specific glutamate (E) residues (Figure 3–18). This modification is a carboxylation that is catalyzed by the vitamin K-dependent enzyme, γ-glutamyl carboxylase. The resultant modified E residues are γ-carboxyglutamate (*gla*). The *gla* residues are responsible for calcium (Ca^{2+}) binding, a process required for factor association with phospholipids following which they are proteolyzed by the appropriate upstream activation factor. For example, prothrombin (factor II) is proteolyzed to active thrombin via the action of activated factor X (Xa).

HIGH-YIELD CONCEPT

The role of vitamin K in the function of γ-glutamyl carboxylase is the target of the anticoagulant drugs of the coumarin family (eg, Warfarin). Coumarins inhibit the enzyme that is required to maintain vitamin K in the hydroxyquinone state required by γ-glutamyl carboxylase. Because protein C, an anticoagulant factor, is the least stable of the *gla* residue factors, the use of coumarin drugs can result in a potentially lethal hypercoagulopathy if patients are not given the rapid-acting anticoagulant, heparin.

HIGH-YIELD CONCEPT

The intestine of newborn infants is sterile; therefore, vitamin K deficiency in infants is highly possible in breastfed infants. As a result, newborn infants are prone to a condition referred to as vitamin K deficiency-related bleeding (VKDB). Neonatal VKDB is defined as a bleeding disorder in which the coagulation deficit is rapidly corrected by vitamin K supplementation. Although the vast majority of neonates do not experience coagulation deficit, it is now generally considered routine to administer a prophylactic dose of vitamin K at birth in order to prevent classical and late VKDB.

MINERALS

The functions of the "minerals" are numerous and either quite broad or highly specific. The minerals that are needed for normal cellular functioning can be divided into two broad categories termed macrominerals and trace minerals.

Macrominerals

A. Calcium

Calcium ion (Ca^{2+}) is an extremely critical mineral required for numerous biochemical processes such as neural signaling, cell proliferation, bone mineralization, cardiac function, muscle contraction, digestive system function, and secretory processes. In the context of Ca^{2+} in secretion, the ion is required for neurotransmitter release and hormone release from a number of different tissues.

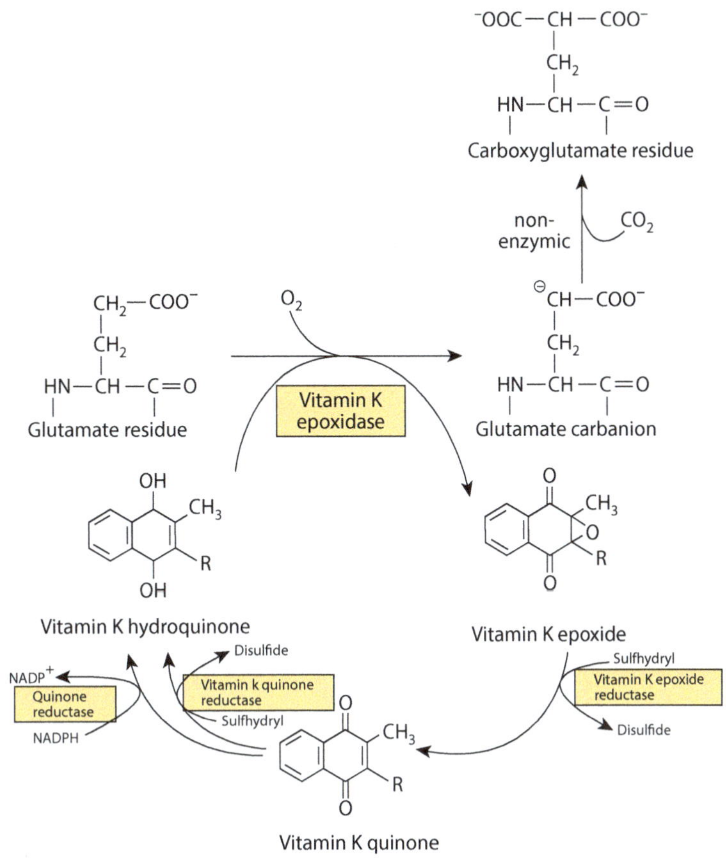

FIGURE 3–18 The role of vitamin K in the synthesis of γ-carboxyglutamate. (Reproduced with permission from Rodwell VW, Bender DA, Botham KM, et al: *Harper's Illustrated Biochemistry*, 31st ed. New York, NY: McGraw Hill; 2018.)

In addition, calcium is necessary for proper activity of a number of proteins involved in blood coagulation. Calcium concentrations in the blood are very tightly regulated within a narrow range. Within the blood over half of the Ca^{2+} is free while the rest is bound to albumin or complexed with other ions such as bicarbonate and phosphate.

Calcium functions both intracellularly and extracellularly. As an intracellular ion, Ca^{2+} serves the role of a second messenger. The difference between the Ca^{2+} concentration outside the cell, within the interstitial fluids, is on the order of 12,000 times that of the free intracellular concentration. This difference creates an inwardly directed electrical gradient as well as allowing for dramatic influxes of the ion in response to a variety of cellular stimuli.

Within the cell, most calcium is not free in the cytosol but is stored within the endoplasmic reticulum (ER) and other microsomal (membrane) compartments. This stored calcium is able to be rapidly mobilized to the cytosol via the activation of a family of ligand-gated calcium channels whose ligands are the lipid, inositol-1,4,5-trisphosphate ($IP_{3;\ Ins\text{-}1,4,5\text{-}P3}$). The activation of GPCR that are coupled to G_q-type G-proteins results in the activation of phospholipase Cβ (PLCβ). Active PLCβ, in turn, hydrolyzes membrane phosphatidylinositol-4,5-bisphosphate ($PIP_{2;\ PtdIns\text{-}4,5\text{-}P2}$) into diacylglycerol (DAG) and IP_3, the latter then activating the ligand-gated calcium channels.

Calcium exerts many of its biochemical effects by binding to Ca^{2+}-binding proteins. The vast majority of proteins, whose activities are controlled by Ca^{2+} binding, contain a structural motif referred to as the EF-hand. The EF-hand domain consists of two regions of α-helix linked by a short (usually 12 amino acids) loop region.

Several important examples of intracellular Ca^{2+}-binding proteins include the calmodulins, calcineurins, calbindins, and troponins, whereas important extracellular Ca^{2+}-binding proteins include the coagulation factors, prothrombin (factor II), VII, IX, X, protein C, and protein S, and the cell-cell communication/adhesion proteins of the cadherin family.

B. Chlorine

Chlorine (as chloride ion: Cl^-) is a major ion necessary for digestive processes as it is required for the formation of gastric acid (HCl) within the lumen of the stomach. The majority of the chloride ion in the body is found in the extracellular fluid compartment. Chloride ion represents approximately 3% of the total electrolyte composition of the human body. Chloride ion functions along with sodium ion (Na^+) and potassium ion (K^+) in the maintenance of electrolyte balance. Chloride ion is required for the function of several ligand-gated ion channels. Of particular importance is the role of Cl^- in the function of the inhibitory neurotransmitter,

GABA (γ-aminobutyric acid). The GABA-A receptor is a Cl^- channel that, in response to GABA binding, induces an inward flux of Cl^- into the neuron.

C. Magnesium

Magnesium ion (Mg^{2+}) is an activator for more than 300 enzymes. All enzymes that utilize ATP as a substrate or as an allosteric regulator require Mg^{2+} ion for activity. Magnesium is a highly critical ion in the nucleus where it interacts with DNA, an interaction necessary for stabilization of DNA structure.

With respect to the requirement for Mg^{2+} in ATP functions, essentially all of the ATP in the cell has Mg^{2+} bound to the phosphates. This Mg^{2+}:ATP complex allows ATP to more readily release the terminal phosphate (the γ-phosphate) when doing so to provide energy for cellular metabolism.

Magnesium is a required component of numerous signal transduction pathways as a result of its role as a substrate (activator) of adenylate cyclase leading to the production of cAMP which in turn activates the serine/threonine kinase, PKA. Magnesium is also important in the processes of electrolyte transport across membranes which facilitates, among numerous metabolic processes, glucose uptake and metabolism, ATP production via mitochondrial oxidative phosphorylation, and the functioning of nerve transmission via stabilization of ATP in Na^+/K^+-ATPases.

D. Phosphorous

Phosphorous is the most important systemic electrolyte acting as a significant buffer in the blood in the form of phosphate ion: PO_4^{3-} as well as the monobasic (HPO_4^{2-}) and dibasic ($H_2PO_4^-$) forms. In the context of biological systems, phosphate ion is commonly referred to as inorganic phosphate and written as P_i which is used to designate all phosphate ion forms.

In addition to its role as a critical blood buffer, phosphate is required in the biosynthesis of cellular components, such as ATP, nucleic acids, phospholipids, and proteins, and is involved in many metabolic pathways, including energy transfer, protein activation, and amino acid metabolism. Phosphate is also required for bone mineralization, and is necessary for energy utilization. One of the most important metabolic reactions that requires P_i is the phosphorolytic cleavage of glucose from glycogen by the enzyme glycogen phosphorylase.

Hormonal control of phosphate levels is exerted primarily via the actions of vitamin D and parathyroid hormone within the proximal tubules of the kidneys.

E. Potassium

Potassium ion is a key circulating electrolyte as well as being involved in the regulation of ATP-dependent channels along with sodium ion. These channels are referred to as Na^+/K^+-ATPases, and they regulate electrochemical gradients between the inside of cells and the interstitial spaces. The functions of the Na^+/K^+-ATPases in the body are numerous with primary roles being in the processes of nerve transmission in the central and peripheral nervous systems, in the functioning of muscle cells, in particular cardiac muscle function, and in the regulation of fluid and ionic balance via the kidneys. Numerous other forms of potassium channels utilize this ion to regulate action potential propagation in the context of the transmission of nerve impulses in the brain and in the control of cardiac muscle and skeletal muscle activity.

Potassium ions represent approximately 5% of the total electrolyte pool in the human body. The majority of potassium ion in the body is found intracellularly. The average intracellular potassium concentration in around 150 mM, whereas the concentration of potassium in the blood is only around 3.5 mM–5 mM.

F. Sodium

Sodium ion is a key circulating electrolyte and also functions in the regulation of Na^+/K^+-ATPases with potassium ion. Sodium ions represent approximately 2% of the total electrolyte composition in the human body. Along with chloride ion (Cl^-) and potassium ion (K^+), sodium ion is required for normal cellular osmolarity, maintenance of normal water distribution and water balance in the body, and maintenance of normal acid-base balance. Sodium ions are also critical to the initiation of action potentials in the context of nerve transmission, cardiac muscle, and skeletal muscle activity. The majority of sodium ion is found in the extracellular fluids. The intracellular Na^+ concentration is around 10 mM while the concentration in the blood is around 135 mM–145 mM.

G. Sulfur

Sulfur has a primary function in amino acid metabolism (methionine and cysteine) but is also necessary for the modification of complex carbohydrates present in proteins (glycoproteins) and lipids (glycolipids) where the sulfur is donated from the amino acid methionine.

TRACE MINERALS

Iron

Iron is the most abundant trace metal in the human body. Iron exists in the ferrous (Fe^{2+}) and ferric states (Fe^{3+}). Under conditions of neutral or alkaline pH, iron is found in the Fe^{3+} state and at acidic pH the Fe^{2+} state is favored. When in the Fe^{3+} state, iron will form large complexes with anions, water, and peroxides. These large complexes have poor solubility and on their aggregation lead to pathologic consequences.

Ferrous ion is a critical micronutrient with a major role in the transport of oxygen where it coordinates the oxygen molecule into heme of hemoglobin. Aside from its role in oxygen transport, iron is critical to the overall process of oxidative phosphorylation where it is also found in the heme of cytochromes and in the Fe-S (iron-sulfur) centers of the various complex of oxidative phosphorylation.

Iron is the only metal in the human body that is toxic if allowed to remain free in the plasma or the fluid compartments of cells. The toxicity of free iron is related to the ability of the ferrous (Fe^{2+}) ion to rapidly generate the highly toxic hydroxyl free radical ($^{\bullet}HO$) via the Fenton reaction.

Iron, consumed in the diet, is either ferric ion or heme iron. Ferric ion in the intestines is reduced to the ferrous state through the concerted actions of the duodenal ferrireductase (DCYTB) and ascorbate (vitamin C). Indeed, ascorbate is critical to overall iron homeostasis through its role in regulating the ferrous and ferric states of iron for cellular uptake. The dietary ferrous iron is then transported into the cells through the action of the divalent metal transporter, DMT1. Intestinal uptake of heme iron occurs through the interaction of dietary heme with the heme carrier protein (HCP1). The iron in the heme is then released within the enterocytes via the action the heme catabolizing enzyme heme oxygenase (see Figure 21–3).

Dietary iron (as well as peripheral tissue iron) is transported across the basolateral membranes, into the circulation, through the action of the transport protein called ferroportin 1. Associated with ferroportin 1 in intestinal enterocytes (but not other tissues) is the copper-containing ferroxidase, hephaestin. Hephaestin is related to the plasma copper-dependent ferroxidase, ceruloplasmin. Simultaneous with intestinal ferroportin 1 transport of ferrous iron it is oxidized to the ferric state.

Once in the circulation, ferric iron is bound to transferrin and passes through the portal circulation of the liver. The liver is the major storage site for iron. The major site of iron utilization is the bone marrow where it is used in heme synthesis (see Chapter 21). Transferrin, made in the liver, is the serum protein responsible for the transport of iron. Although several metals can bind to transferrin, the highest affinity is for the ferric iron. The ferrous form of iron does not bind to transferrin. Transferrin can bind two moles of ferric iron. Cells take up the transported iron through interaction of transferrin with cell-surface receptors. Internalization of the iron-transferrin-receptor complexes is initiated following receptor phosphorylation by PKC. Following internalization, the iron is released due to the acidic nature of the endosomes. The transferrin receptor is then recycled back to the cell surface.

Ferritin is the major protein used for intracellular storage of iron. Ferritin without bound iron is referred to as apo-ferritin. Apo-ferritin is a large polymer of 24 polypeptide subunits. This multimeric structure of apo-ferritin is able to bind up to 2000 iron atoms in the form of a complex ferric-phosphate. If the storage capacity of the ferritin is exceeded, iron will deposit adjacent to the ferritin-iron complexes in the cell. Histologically, these amorphous iron deposits are referred to as hemosiderin. Hemosiderin is composed of ferritin, denatured ferritin, and other materials and its molecular structure is poorly defined. Hemosiderin is found most frequently in macrophages and is most abundant following hemorrhagic events. The consequences of excess iron intake and storage can have profound consequences, the most significant of which is hemochromatosis (Clinical Box 3–12).

CLINICAL BOX 3–12 HEMOCHROMATOSIS

Hemochromatosis is defined as a disorder in iron metabolism that is characterized by excess iron absorption, saturation of iron-binding proteins, and deposition of hemosiderin in the tissues. The primary affected tissues are the liver, pancreas, and skin. Iron deposition in the liver leads to cirrhosis and in the pancreas causes diabetes. The excess iron deposition leads to bronze pigmentation of the organs and skin. The bronze skin pigmentation seen in hemochromatosis, coupled with the resultant diabetes, lead to the designation of this condition as bronze diabetes. Primary hemochromatosis is an autosomal recessive disorder that is referred to as type 1 hemochromatosis. The defective protein causing type 1 hemochromatosis has been designated the homeostatic iron regulator (HFE). The HFE protein is encoded by a major histocompatibility complex (MHC) class-1 gene. Hemochromatosis, that is associated with the HFE locus, is one of the most common inherited genetic defects. Manifestation of the symptoms of the disease is modified by several environmental influences. Dietary iron intake and alcohol consumption are especially significant to hemochromatosis. Menstruation and pregnancy can also influence symptoms. Hemochromatosis occurs about 5–10 times more frequently in men than in women. Symptoms usually appear between the ages of 40 and 60 in about 70% of individuals. The *HFE1* gene encodes an α-chain protein with three immunoglobulin-like domains. This α-chain protein associates with β_2-microglobulin, typical of MHC class 1 encoded proteins. Normal HFE has been shown to form a complex with the transferrin receptor, thus regulating the rate of iron transfer into cells. A mutation in HFE will therefore lead to increased iron uptake and storage. The majority of hereditary hemochromatosis patients have inherited a mutation in HFE that results in the substitution of Cys 282 for a Tyr (C282Y). Another mutation found in certain forms of hereditary hemochromatosis also affects the *HFE* gene and causes a change of His 63 to Asp (H63D). This latter mutation is found along with the more common C282Y mutation resulting in a compound heterozygosity. As a result of the C282Y mutation, the HFE protein remains trapped in the intracellular compartment. Because it cannot associate with the transferrin receptor there is a reduced uptake of iron by intestinal crypt cells. It is thought that this defect in intestinal iron-uptake results in an increase in the expression of the divalent metal transporter (DMT-1) on the brush border of the intestinal villus cells. Excess DMT-1 expression leads to an inappropriate increase in intestinal iron absorption. In hemochromatosis the liver is usually the first organ to be affected. Hepatomegaly will be present in more than 95% of patients manifesting symptoms. Initial symptoms include weakness, abdominal pain, change in skin color, and the onset of symptoms of diabetes mellitus. In advanced cases of hemochromatosis there will likely be cardiac arrhythmias, congestive heart failure, testicular atrophy, jaundice, increased pigmentation, spider angiomas, and splenomegaly. Diagnosis of the disease is usually suggested when there is the presence of hepatomegaly, skin pigmentation, diabetes mellitus, heart disease, arthritis, and hypogonadism. Treatment of hemochromatosis before there is permanent organ damage can restore life

CLINICAL BOX 3–12 (CONTINUED)

expectancy to normal. Treatment involves removal of the excess body iron. This is accomplished by twice-weekly phlebotomy at the beginning of treatment. Alcohol consumption should be curtailed and preferably eliminated in hemochromatosis patients. Iron chelating agents, such as deferoxamine, can be used to remove around 10–20 mg of iron per day. However, phlebotomy is more convenient and safer for most patients.

NON-HFE HEMOCHROMATOSIS: There are several additional causes of hemochromatosis, although none are as common as classic hemochromatosis. There are at least four additional genetic loci, that when defective lead to hemochromatosis. Two of which are juvenile forms identified as type 2A and 2B and two additional forms identified type 3 and type 4.

Juvenile hemochromatosis (JH) type 2A (sometimes called HFE2A) is the result of defects in the gene encoding hemojuvelin (HJV). The function of hemojuvelin is to regulate the expression of the hepcidin gene (HAMP). As suggested by the juvenile nomenclature, this disorder manifests in patients under the age of 30. Cardiomyopathy and hypogonadism are prevalent symptoms with type 2A hemochromatosis. Type 2A hemochromatosis is inherited as an autosomal recessive disorder.

JH type 2B (sometimes called HFE2B) results from defects in the gene encoding hepcidin (HAMP). As with type 2A disease, symptoms of type 2B disease appear in patients under 30 years of age and include cardiomyopathy and hypogonadism. Type 2B hemochromatosis is inherited as an autosomal recessive disorder.

Type 3 hemochromatosis (sometimes called HFE3) is caused by mutations in the transferrin receptor-2 gene (TFR2). TFR2 is a homolog of the classic transferrin receptor (identified as TFR1). Unlike the ubiquitous expression of TFR1, TFR2 expression is almost exclusively found in the liver. The function of TFR2 in the liver is not to act in the uptake of transferrin-bound iron but to sense iron levels and to act as a regulator of hepcidin function. The clinical features of type 3 hemochromatosis are similar to those of classic type 1 disease. Type 3 hemochromatosis is inherited as an autosomal recessive disorder.

Type 4 hemochromatosis (sometimes called HFE4) is also called ferroportin disease because it is caused by mutations in the ferroportin gene. Ferroportin is highly expressed in the liver, duodenum, and reticuloendothelial cells. The major function of ferroportin is to transport dietary iron across the basolateral membranes of intestinal enterocytes into the blood and to recycle iron via the reticuloendothelial system. Symptoms of type 4 hemochromatosis are similar to those of classic type 1 disease but are generally milder. The unique aspect of type 4 hemochromatosis is that it is inherited as an autosomal dominant disease.

Regulation of iron absorption, recycling, and release from intracellular stores is controlled through the actions of the hepatic iron regulatory protein, hepcidin. Hepcidin functions by inhibiting the presentation of ferroportin in intestinal enterocyte basolateral membranes and reticuloendothelial macrophages. With a diet high in iron the level of hepcidin mRNA increases and conversely its levels decrease when dietary iron is low.

HIGH-YIELD CONCEPT

Hepcidin is encoded by the *HAMP* (hepcidin antimicrobial protein) gene. Inflammation activates expression of the *HAMP* gene through the action of the proinflammatory cytokine, IL-6. IL-6 induces the phosphorylation of the transcription factor, signal transducer, and activator of transcription 3 (STAT3), which leads to its translocation to the nucleus and subsequent *HAMP* gene activation. The inflammation-mediated increase in hepcidin plays a critical role in the development of iron deficiency in chronic infections. This syndrome is commonly, although erroneously, referred to as **anemia of chronic disease.** It is more correctly an **anemia of chronic infection or inflammation.**

Dietary deficiency of iron, or excess loss of body iron results in the disorder aptly referred to as iron-deficiency anemia (see Clinical Box 3–13). This anemia is characterized by microcytic (small) and hypochromic (low pigment) erythrocytes. Iron-deficiency anemia is the most common form of anemia worldwide. Clinical determination of iron status can be made through a number of different blood tests (Table 3–1).

Copper

Like iron, copper exists in two oxidation states, cuprous (Cu^{1+} or Cu^{+}) and cupric (Cu^{2+}). Copper is involved in the formation of red bloods cells, the synthesis of hemoglobin, and the formation of bone. Additional functions of copper are energy production, wound healing, taste sensation, and skin and hair color. Copper is critical to the functions of cytochrome oxidase of the electron transport chain and copper-zinc-superoxide dismutase (SOD1) involved in the detoxification of the reactive oxygen species, superoxide. Copper is also involved in the proper processing of collagen and elastin via the action of the extracellular matrix-associated enzyme, lysyl oxidase. Thus, copper is critical to the proper production of connective tissue.

Dietary copper is taken up by intestinal enterocytes via the action of a specific transport protein, copper transporter 1 (CTR1) as well as by the divalent metal transporter 1 (DMT1). Uptake by other tissues (primarily the liver and kidneys) also involves CTR1. Once copper is transported into cells by CTR1 it is transferred directly to the intracellular chaperone identified as antioxidant 1 copper chaperone (ATOX1). The role of ATOX1 is to transport copper from the apical membrane to either intracellular vesicles or to the copper transporting ATPase (Cu-ATPase), ATP7A, within the trans-Golgi network (TGN) for ultimate export from intestinal enterocytes to the blood. The significance of ATP7A function to overall copper homeostasis is evidenced by

CLINICAL BOX 3–13 IRON DEFICIENCY ANEMIA

Iron deficiency is the leading cause of anemia, specifically microcytic anemia. Because iron incorporation into protoporphyrin IX is required to form functional heme, iron deficiency results in reduced heme production. Heme levels in erythroid progenitor cells control protein synthesis (see Figure 24–9) and low heme results in impaired protein synthesis. The reduced level of protein synthesis results in small (microcytic) erythrocytes. In addition, the reduced heme levels result in reduced erythrocyte color such that the anemia is a hypochromic microcytic anemia. The lack of heme production with iron deficiency results in loss of feedback inhibition of the rate-limiting enzyme of heme synthesis, δ-aminolevulinic acid synthase, (ALAS), therefore these patients will have an associated increase in measurable protoporphyrin IX. The loss of iron intake means reduced iron in the serum and reduced intracellular iron. When intracellular iron levels fall, there will be reduced ferritin translation and thus, reduced ferritin in the blood as well as increased translation of the transferrin receptor leading to increased levels of measurable transferrin receptor protein. The lack of iron for incorporation into protoporphyrin IX results in spontaneous, nonenzymatic incorporation of Zn^{2+} forming Zn-protoporphyrin (ZPP). ZPP causes erythrocytes to fluoresce under the appropriate wavelength illumination and is the basis of the ZPP test for iron deficiency or lead poisoning.

the fact that loss of its function results in the lethal disorder identified as Menkes disease (Clinical Box 3–14).

Within the liver and other nonintestinal cells ATOX1 can transfer copper to the primary copper-transporting ATPase (Cu-ATPase) of the secretory pathway. This ATPase is identified as ATP7B. The significance of ATP7B function to overall copper homeostasis is evidenced by the fact that loss of its function due to inherited mutations in the ATP7B gene result in the disorder identified as Wilson disease (Clinical Box 3–15).

Once in the blood, copper is transported throughout the body bound primarily to albumin and to a much lesser extent by α_2-macroglobulin. Although up to 95% of copper in the blood is associated with the ferroxidase called ceruloplasmin, ceruloplasmin copper is not part of the exchangeable plasma copper pool. Indeed, ceruloplasmin does not directly bind nor take up copper ions. Copper is incorporated into soluble ceruloplasmin only during the synthesis of the protein.

While stored inside the cell, copper is primarily localized to lysosome-like compartments stored bound to copper-binding proteins, with the major class of proteins being the metallothioneins.

Iodine

Iodine is required for the synthesis of the thyroid hormones and thus plays an important role in the regulation of energy metabolism via thyroid hormone functions.

Manganese

Manganese is involved in reactions of protein and fat metabolism, promotes a healthy nervous system, and is necessary for digestive function, bone growth, and immune function. Maintenance of blood glucose levels is controlled in large part via the ability of the liver to produce glucose from precursor carbon atoms in the pathway of gluconeogenesis (see Chapter 6). Two of the enzymes of gluconeogenesis, pyruvate carboxylase (PC) and phosphoenolpyruvate carboxykinase (PEPCK) require manganese for their activity.

Within the liver, kidneys, and brain manganese is critical in the regulation of ammonium ion (NH_4^+) levels via its role activating glutamine synthetase. Within the liver, manganese plays an additional role in the regulation of NH_4^+ levels in the body via its activation of the urea cycle enzyme arginase. Manganese also

TABLE 3–1 Changes in various laboratory tests used to assess iron-deficiency anemia.

Parameter	Normal	Negative Iron Balance	Iron-Deficient Erythropoiesis	Iron-Deficiency Anemia
Serum ferritin (μg/dL)	50–200	Decreased <20	Decreased <15	Decreased <15
Total iron-binding capacity (TIBC) (μg/dL)	300–360	Slightly increased >360	Increased >380	Increased>400
Serum iron (μg/dL)	50–150	Normal	Decreased <50	Decreased <30
Transferrin saturation (%)	30–50	Normal	Decreased <20	Decreased <10
RBC protoporphyrin (μg/dL)	30–50	Normal	Increased	Increased
Soluble transferrin receptor (μg/L)	4–9	Increased	Increased	Increased
RBC morphology	Normal	Normal	Normal	Microcytic Hypochromic

Data from Hillman RS, Finch CA: *Red Cell Manual*, 7th ed. Philadelphia, PA: FA Davis; 1966.

CLINICAL BOX 3–14 MENKES DISEASE

Menkes disease is inherited as an X-linked disorder of copper homeostasis. The disorder is associated with an inability to absorb copper from the gastrointestinal tract. As a consequence of the reduced delivery of copper to the brain, Menkes patients exhibit severe mental and developmental impairment. In addition, because there is a need for copper as a cofactor in numerous enzymes (eg, lysyl oxidases), Menkes patients also exhibit connective tissue abnormalities and twisting of blood vessels where there are normally supposed to be turns. The vessel twisting can lead to blockages if it is severe. Menkes disease is so named because it was originally described in 1962 by Dr. John H. Menkes. The incidence of Menkes disease ranges from 1:40,000 to 1:360,000 live births. Menkes disease is the result of defects in the P-type ATPase protein that is responsible for the translocation of copper across the intestinal basal-lateral membrane into the blood, thus allowing for uptake of dietary copper. This protein is encoded by the ATPase, Cu^{2+}-transporting, alpha polypeptide (ATP7A) gene. The structure of the ATP7A gene is highly similar to that of the ATP7B gene which is disrupted in another copper-transport defect disease called Wilson disease (Clinical Box 3–13). ATP7A has two important activities related to copper homeostasis. It delivers copper to several copper-requiring enzymes and is required for the ATP-driven efflux of copper from cells. ATP7A is expressed in numerous tissues except the liver. Copper homeostasis effected by the liver is the function of the ATP7B protein. When carrying out its function to supply copper-dependent enzymes with copper, the ATP7A protein is localized to the *trans*-Golgi network where it transports copper into the lumen of the Golgi. When copper levels rise, ATP7A is translocated to vesicular compartments closely associated with the plasma membrane where it can transport copper into these compartments. The copper in these vesicles can then be released by exocytosis. Numerous mutations have been identified in the ATP7A gene resulting in Menkes disease. To date at least 357 different mutations have been characterized. The most frequently occurring mutations, accounting for 22% of all cases, are insertion or deletion of a few base pairs. Additional alterations include missense mutations, partial gene deletions, splice site mutations, and mutations leading to premature termination of translation. The clinical spectrum associated with Menkes disease includes progressive neurodegeneration, connective tissue abnormalities, and wiry brittle hair. The distinctive clinical features of Menkes disease are usually present by 3 months of age. Infants will lose, or fail to demonstrate, specific developmental milestones and failure to thrive. Most patients with Menkes disease do not survive beyond early childhood, however there is phenotypic variability and some mildly affected patients have been reported to survive for longer periods. Because of the phenotypic variations Menkes disease has been divided into three classifications. Classic Menkes disease which results in early death, mild Menkes disease with longer survival times (accounting for 6% of all patients), and occipital horn syndrome, OHS (accounting for 3% of all patients). OHS was previously called X-linked cutis laxa, or Ehlers-Danlos syndrome type IX. In the classic form of Menkes disease infants have cherubic faces, sagging jowls, and no or scant eyebrows. Their hair is gray or white due to the lack of tyrosinase activity and has the appearance of feel of steel wool. The deficiency in lysyl oxidase activity accounts for most of the skeletal abnormalities present in Menkes infants. These anomalies include osteoporosis, metaphyseal dysplasia, wormian skull bones, and rib fractures. Progressive cerebral degeneration occurs primarily due to loss of cytochrome c oxidase, peptidyl α-amidating monooxygenase, and dopamine β-hydroxylase in the central nervous system. Unfortunately, there is no effective treatment for Menkes disease, and severely afflicted infants will not survive more than a few months after birth. In mildly afflicted patients there is some benefit to parenteral administration of various forms of copper such as copper histidine, copper chloride, and copper sulfate. Although this treatment can correct the hepatic copper deficiency, normalize serum copper, and ceruloplasmin levels it has not been shown to ameliorate the progressive neurologic deterioration.

CLINICAL BOX 3–15 WILSON DISEASE

Wilson disease (WD) is inherited as an autosomal recessive disorder of copper homeostasis. The disease is characterized by excessive copper deposition primarily in the liver and brain. These sites of copper deposition are reflective of the major manifestations of Wilson disease. Wilson disease is named after Dr. Samuel Alexander Kinnier Wilson who first described the disorder in 1912. The frequency of Wilson disease ranges from 1:5,000 to 1:30,000 live births. Wilson disease is the result of defects in the P-type ATPase protein that is primarily responsible for copper homeostasis effected by the liver. This protein is encoded by the ATPase, Cu^{2+}-transporting, beta polypeptide (*ATP7B*) gene. The *ATP7B* gene is expressed predominantly in the liver, but also in the kidney and placenta. Lower levels of expression are also detectable in the brain, heart, and lungs. The structure of the *ATP7B* gene is highly similar to that of the *ATP7A* gene which is disrupted in another copper-transport defect disease called Menkes disease (Clinical Box 3–12). The ATP7B protein is localized to the *trans*-Golgi network where it transports copper into the lumen of the Golgi. When copper levels rise, ATP7B is translocated to vesicular compartments closely associated with the plasma membrane where it can transport copper into these compartments. The copper in these vesicles can then be released by exocytosis. When copper is transferred from intestinal enterocytes to the plasma, through the action of the ATP7A protein, it is bound to albumin and delivered to the liver. In the liver the copper is transferred to intracellular storage sites by the chaperone ATOX1.

CLINICAL BOX 3–15 (CONTINUED)

Copper is stored intracellularly bound to the protein metallothionein. Any copper in excess of the binding capacity of metallothionein is excreted into the biliary canaliculi through the transport action of ATP7B. ATP7B also facilitates the transfer of copper to the major plasma copper transport protein, ceruloplasmin. Ceruloplasmin that does not have bound copper is referred to as apoceruloplasmin. Ceruloplasmin is then released in the blood. Greater than 90% of the copper in the blood is bound to ceruloplasmin and this functions in the transport of copper to peripheral organs such as the brain and kidneys. Deficiencies in ATP7B result in increased levels of apoceruloplasmin and a toxic build-up of copper in hepatocytes due to defective transfer to the biliary canaliculi. Numerous mutations have been identified in the *ATP7B* gene resulting in Wilson disease. The majority of these mutations are clustered in the transmembrane domains of the encoded protein. In Europeans and North Americans two mutations account for 38% of the observed mutations in this disease. These two mutations are a substitution of glutamine for histidine at amino acid 1069 (H1069Q) and arginine for glycine at amino acid 1267 (G1267R). The molecular basis for the observed phenotypic variations in Wilson disease are complex and involve both environmental influences and the effects of modifier genes such as *COMMD1* (copper metabolism MURR1 domain-containing protein 1). The MURR1 domain was first identified in a murine protein and refers to: **m**ouse **U**2af1-**r**s1 **r**egion. An additional ATP7B modifier protein is the chaperone protein ATOX1 (antioxidant protein 1). An additional locus affecting the phenotype of Wilson disease is apolipoprotein E ε3/3. Individuals harboring this particular apoE allele have a delayed onset in the presentation of Wilson disease symptoms. The majority of patients with Wilson disease present with hepatic or neuropsychiatric symptoms. All other patients, representing about 20% of all Wilson disease cases, manifest with symptoms that are attributable to involvement of other organs. Hepatic presentation in Wilson disease occurs in late childhood or adolescence. The symptoms in these patients include hepatic failure, acute hepatitis, or progressive chronic liver disease. Patients that manifest neurologic symptoms of Wilson disease present in the second to third decade of life. In these patients there will be extrapyramidal, cerebellar, and cerebral-related symptoms such as Parkinsonian tremors, diminished facial expressions and movement, dystonia, and choreoathetosis. About 30% of Wilson disease patients will exhibit psychiatric disturbances that include changes in behavior, personality changes, depression, attention deficit hyperactivity disorder, paranoid psychosis, suicidal tendencies, and impulsivity. As the disease progresses, copper deposition leads to vacuolar degeneration in the proximal tubular cells of the kidneys which causes a Fanconi syndrome (substances that are normally absorbed by the kidney are excreted in the urine). Acute release of copper into the circulation results in damage to red blood cells resulting in hemolysis. The most significant sign in the diagnosis of Wilson disease results from the deposition of copper in Descemet's membrane of the cornea. These golden-brown deposits can be seen with a slit-lamp and are called Kayser-Fleischer rings. Treatment of Wilson disease is aimed at reducing the toxic concentration of copper. This can be accomplished with copper chelating agents such as trientine and D-penicillamine. Once the copper levels have been reduced the chelating agents can be reduced or eliminated and zinc salt used to prevent systemic absorption of copper. Patients with progressive liver failure will require liver transplantation. Liver transplantation is also required in patients that do not respond to copper chelation therapy.

serves as an important antioxidant mineral since it is necessary for the proper function of mitochondrial superoxide dismutase (SOD2) which catalyzes the same reaction as that catalyzed by the cytosolic enzyme, SOD1.

Molybdenum

Molybdenum is primarily involved as a cofactor in oxidase enzymes such as xanthine dehydrogenase/oxidase necessary for purine nucleotide catabolism (see Chapter 20). Molybdenum is also a necessary cofactor in the detoxification reactions catalyzed by sulfite oxidase. Sulfite oxidase is the terminal enzyme in the pathways of the metabolism of sulfur-containing compounds such as the amino acid cysteine. The product of the sulfite oxidase reaction, sulfate, is then excreted.

Selenium

Selenium serves as a modifier of the activity of several enzymes through its incorporation into protein in the form of selenocysteine. The mechanism for selenocysteine incorporation during protein synthesis requires a special translation complex (see Chapter 24).

Two critical redox enzyme families that require selenocysteine residues are the glutathione peroxidase and thioredoxin reductase families. Glutathione peroxidases are critical enzymes involved in the protection of red blood cells from reactive oxygen species (ROS). Thioredoxin reductases are involved in the reduction of thioredoxin which itself is principally involved in the reduction of oxidized disulfide bonds in proteins. The enzymes of the deiodinase family are also important selenocysteine-containing enzymes. Clinically relevant enzymes in this family are the thyroid deiodinases that are critical for the maturation and catabolism of the thyroid hormones.

There is a very narrow clinically safe range for selenium intake; too little and there are serious clinical consequences, too much and some overlapping as well as a different set of serious clinical complications occur. Chronic selenium deficiency is associated with lethargy, dizziness, motor weakness and paresthesias, and an excess risk of amyotrophic lateral sclerosis. Selenium toxicity due to excess intake manifests most significantly with neurologic impairment evidenced by ataxia, hypotonia, hyperreflexia, dyasthesia, and paralysis. Lethargy and dizziness are also common with selenium intoxication as for selenium deficiency. Additional CNS effects of selenium intoxication include localized or generalized tremors and convulsions. Many individuals suffering from selenium intoxication experience behavioral disturbances that can lead to suicidal ideation. One characteristic feature associated with selenium intoxication is a garlic odor to the expired breath. This is similar to the consequences of arsenic poisoning, therefore, in and of itself a garlic odor to the breath is not exclusively diagnostic for selenium intoxication.

Zinc

After iron, zinc is the second most abundant trace metal in the human body. Zinc ion (Zn^{2+}) is found as a cofactor in more than 300 different enzymes and thus, is involved in a wide variety of biochemical processes. Zinc interacts with the hormone insulin to ensure proper function; thus, zinc participates in the regulation of blood glucose levels via insulin action. Zinc is necessary for the activity of a number of transcription factors such as those of the nuclear receptor (steroid and thyroid hormone receptor superfamily) family through its role in the formation of the structurally critical zinc finger domain that binds to DNA. Zinc also promotes wound healing, regulates immune function, serves as a cofactor for numerous antioxidant enzymes, and is necessary for protein synthesis and the processing of collagen.

CHECKLIST

- ☑ Vitamins are organic nutrients that are generally required in the diet since they cannot be synthesized by human tissues.
- ☑ Vitamin derivatives play essential roles as cofactors for enzyme-catalyzed reactions critical to overall metabolic homeostasis.
- ☑ The B vitamins are water-soluble vitamins involved in important roles in cellular metabolism. These consist of thiamine (B_1), riboflavin (B_2), niacin (B_3), pantothenate (B_5), pryidoxal (B_6), and cobalamin (B_{12}). Biotin and folic acid are sometimes also considered in the B vitamin class as B_7 and B_9, respectively.
- ☑ Vitamin C is a water-soluble antioxidant that is also critical as a cofactor for the modification of components of the extracellular matrix.
- ☑ Vitamin A is critical in the normal function of the visual processes, in the form of retinoic acid. Vitamin A plays an essential role in the control of genes involved in embryonic patterning.
- ☑ Vitamin D is a prohormone that when converted to active calcitriol functions as a steroid hormone in the regulation of calcium and phosphorous homeostasis.
- ☑ Vitamin E is a potent antioxidant and as such serves as the most important lipid-derived antioxidant.
- ☑ Vitamin K functions as a cofactor in the enzymatic modification of numerous enzymes involved in the process of blood coagulation.
- ☑ The minerals are inorganic micronutrients that are necessary for the functions of numerous processes involved in whole body homeostasis.
- ☑ Iron serves numerous important functions in the body. These include its role in heme binding of oxygen in hemoglobin and as a significant functional part of heme and iron-sulfur centers in numerous other proteins.
- ☑ Iron will form large complexes with anions, water, and peroxides. These large complexes have poor solubility and on their aggregation lead to pathologic consequences. In addition, iron can bind to and interfere with the structure and function of various macromolecules necessitating the need for tight regulation of iron homeostasis.
- ☑ Iron consumed in the diet is either free iron or heme iron. Free iron in the intestines is reduced from the ferric (Fe^{3+}) to the ferrous (Fe^{2+}) state on the luminal surface of intestinal enterocytes and transported into the cells through the action of the divalent metal transporter, DMT1. Intestinal uptake of heme iron occurs through the interaction of dietary heme with the heme carrier protein (HCP1).
- ☑ Iron is transported out of intestinal enterocytes into the circulation, through the action of the transport protein ferroportin (also called IREG1=iron-regulated gene 1). Associated with ferroportin is the enzyme hephaestin (a copper-containing ferroxidase with homology to ceruloplasmin) which oxidizes the ferrous form back to the ferric form
- ☑ Within the circulation the ferric form of iron is bound to transferrin and passes through the portal circulation of the liver. Cells take up iron through interaction of iron-transferrin complexes with the transferrin receptor. The iron-transferrin-receptor complexes are internalized, the iron is released due to the acidic nature of the endosomes and the transferrin receptor is returned to the cell surface.
- ☑ Iron can be stored within cells bound to ferritin in the ferrous state.
- ☑ If the storage capacity of the ferritin is exceeded, iron will deposit adjacent to the ferritin-iron complexes in the cell in amorphous iron deposits called hemosiderin.

- ☑ Regulation of iron absorption, recycling and release from intracellular stores occurs through the actions of the hepatic iron regulatory protein hepcidin. Hepcidin functions by inhibiting the presentation of one or more of the iron transporters (eg, DMT1 and ferroportin) in intestinal membranes.
- ☑ Defects in iron homeostasis can result from impaired intestinal absorption, excess loss of heme iron due to bleeding as well as to mutations in the iron response elements of iron-regulated mRNAs resulting in iron overload. Hemochromatosis is defined as a disorder in iron metabolism that is characterized by excess iron absorption, saturation of iron-binding proteins, and deposition of hemosiderin in the tissues. The primary affected tissues are the liver pancreas and skin.
- ☑ Copper is an essential trace element which plays a pivotal role in cell physiology as it constitutes a core part of copper-containing enzymes termed cuproenzymes. Copper exists in two oxidation states, cuprous (Cu^{1+} or Cu^{+}) and cupric (Cu^{2+}).
- ☑ Copper can be toxic when present in excessive amounts as it binds with high affinity to histidine, cysteine, and methionine residues of proteins which can result in their inactivation, and it also readily interacts with oxygen leading to the production of hydroxyl radical.
- ☑ Dietary copper is found primarily in the cupric state (Cu^{2+}) and is reduced to cuprous (Cu^{+}) prior to uptake which is effected by copper transport protein 1, CTR1.
- ☑ In cells, CTR1 is found at the plasma membrane and in intracellular vesicles. When CTR1 binds copper it is internalized and moves to endocytic vesicles. Copper-transporting P-type ATPases (Cu-ATPases) maintain intracellular copper levels.
- ☑ Two critical Cu ATPases are ATP7A and ATP7B. ATP7A is required for cuproenzyme biosynthesis, and in intestinal enterocytes it is required for copper efflux to the portal circulation. ATP7B is mainly expressed in the liver where it is required for copper incorporation into ceruloplasmin and for excretion of copper into the biliary circulation
- ☑ Mutations in ATP7A result in Menkes disease and mutations in ATP7B are the cause of Wilson disease

REVIEW QUESTIONS

1. A 14-month-old girl is brought to her physician because she seems to be in pain when she tries to move. Physical examination shows the infant exhibits a reluctance to move her arms and legs. She has bowing of her legs, a depression of the sternum with outward projection of the ends of the ribs, numerous bruises on her legs, and gingival hemorrhages. Which of the following vitamin deficiencies is most likely in this patient?

(A) Ascorbate
(B) Riboflavin
(C) Thiamine
(D) Vitamin A
(E) Vitamin B_{12}
(F) Vitamin D
(G) Vitamin K

2. A 16-month-old boy is brought to his physician because he seems to be in pain when he tries to move. Physical examination finds that the child is reluctant to move his arms and legs. He has numerous bruises on his legs and gingival hemorrhages. Blood work finds a mild microcytic hypochromic anemia. The signs and symptoms in this patient are most likely the result of a nutritional deficiency affecting which of the following processes?

(A) Amino acid metabolism
(B) Bone mineralization
(C) Extracellular matrix synthesis
(D) Heme biosynthesis
(E) Nucleotide biosynthesis

3. A 9-month-old male infant is brought to his pediatrician by his parents because they are concerned that their child has frequent diarrhea and occasional jerky movements of his arms and legs. Physical examination finds the infant is at the 15th percentile for both weight and length. When asked, the parents indicate that they are feeding their son via bottle using a nutritionally fortified formula. Physical examination shows several patches of dry scaly skin on the patient's arms, hands, and face. Given the most likely cause of this patient's symptoms, levels of which of the following enzyme cofactors is most likely to be negatively impacted?

(A) Flavin adenine dinucleotide
(B) Nicotinamide adenine dinucleotide
(C) Tetrahydrobiopterin
(D) Tetrahydrofolate
(E) Thiamine pyrophosphate

4. An emergency room physician is tending to a 59-year-old female patient who has a broken left fibula. Physical examination of the patient finds that she has multiple bruises on her arms, legs, and upper torso. The patient also complains of significant bleeding whenever she brushes her teeth. The patient indicates that her diet consists of bouillon soup, tea, plain pasta, and dinner rolls. Blood work demonstrates a mild microcytic anemia. Given these signs and symptoms this patient most likely is suffering from the effects of a deficiency in the activity of which of the following enzymes?

(A) Cystathionine β-synthase
(B) Lysyl hydroxylase
(C) Methionine synthase
(D) Methylmalonyl-CoA mutase
(E) Transketolase

5. A 3-month-old infant exhibiting failure to thrive is being examined by a pediatrician. Physical examination shows the infant has sagging jowls, brittle greyish hair, and no eyebrows. The infant exhibits a clear neurodegenerative deficit. This constellation of symptoms is most likely to be associated defect in which of the following processes?

(A) Copper oxidation
(B) Efflux of cellular copper
(C) Efflux of cellular iron
(D) Intestinal copper uptake
(E) Intestinal iron uptake
(F) Iron oxidation

6. A 27-year-old male is being examined for complaints of dry eyes and vision difficulties. Physical examination finds foamy appearing lesions on the temporal conjunctiva. This patient is most likely to be deficient in which of the following?
(A) Ascorbate
(B) Cobalamin
(C) Thiamine
(D) Vitamin A
(E) Vitamin D
(F) Vitamin K

7. During an examination of a 24-month-old infant the pediatrician finds the child has a slight bowing of the legs, a slightly misshapen skull, and a curvature to the spine. All of these symptoms are most likely the result of a deficiency in which of the following?
(A) Ascorbate
(B) Cobalamin
(C) Thiamine
(D) Vitamin A
(E) Vitamin D
(F) Vitamin K

8. A 62-year-old man, found unconscious in an alley, is brought to the Emergency Department by ambulance. The man is disheveled and reeking of alcohol, but does not present with any signs of physical trauma. Blood work finds the patient's blood alcohol level is 0.13 and his blood glucose is 47 mg/dL (normal non-fasting = 70–100 mg/dL). The patient is given an injection of naloxone and an intravenous infusion of D5W. The patient regains consciousness and tells the attending physician that he is homeless and an alcoholic, but that he does not use illicit drugs. Physical examination finds that his arms and legs are thin, and he has decreased sensation in both his hands and feet. When tested, his grip strength is 3/5 bilaterally. Examination of the patient's eyes finds horizontal nystagmus. Which of the following additional tests would be most useful in the diagnosis of the cause of the patient's underlying condition?
(A) Erythrocyte transketolase activity
(B) Peripheral blood smear
(C) Schilling test
(D) Serum methylmalonic acid levels
(E) Urine β-hydroxybutyrate levels

9. A patient, who has been bruising easily over the past 6 months, is being assessed for the cause of his condition. Results of a blood test find that her international normalized ratio (INR) value is 1.7 (N = 0.8–1.2). A deficiency in which of the following is most likely to be contributory to these findings?
(A) Ascorbic acid
(B) Biotin
(C) Cobalamin
(D) Vitamin D
(E) Vitamin A
(F) Vitamin K

10. A 45-year-old male, a known alcoholic for at least the past 10 years, is being examined by his physician. His chief complaints are burning eyes, a sore tongue, reduced appetite, and mild abdominal discomfort. Physical examination reveals cheilosis, glossitis, dull hair, seborrhea, and split nails. These signs and symptoms are most likely the result of a deficiency in which of the following?
(A) Biotin
(B) Niacin
(C) Riboflavin
(D) Thiamine
(E) Vitamin E
(F) Vitamin K

11. A 17-year-old male patient presents with hypogonadism and cardiomyopathy. Additional testing has confirmed that the patient is suffering from an atypical form of hemochromatosis. A mutation is identified in this patient in the gene encoding the hemojuvelin protein. Expression of which of the following proteins is most likely to be unregulated in this patient as a result of the identified mutation?
(A) Ceruloplasmin
(B) Ferroportin
(C) Hephaestin
(D) Hepcidin
(E) Transferrin
(F) Transferrin receptor

12. At autopsy, a sagittal section through the brain shows severe pigmentation of the mammillary bodies due to apparent hemorrhage. A deficiency in which of the following would most likely have contributed to the observed brain pathology?
(A) Ascorbate
(B) Folate
(C) Riboflavin
(D) Thiamine
(E) Vitamin D
(F) Vitamin K

13. A 27-year-old female is being examined for complaints of difficulty speaking, clumsiness while walking, uncontrolled twitching in her arms, fatigue, and depression. Physical examination shows distinct jaundice in skin and the eyes as well as a discoloration in the periphery of the cornea. These signs and symptoms are most likely indicative of which of the following disorders?
(A) Acute intermittent porphyria (AIP)
(B) Hemochromatosis type 1
(C) Menkes disease
(D) Porphyria cutanea tarda (PCT)
(E) Wilson disease

14. A deficiency in which of the following vitamins would most likely be responsible for the result of the blood smear shown in the accompanying image?

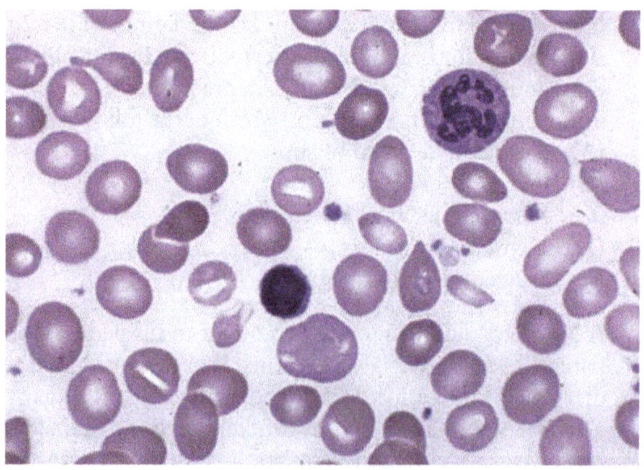

Reproduced with permission from Lichtman MS, Shafer MS, Felgar RE, et al: Lichtman's Atlas of Hematology 2016. New York, NY: McGraw Hill; 2017

(A) Ascorbate
(B) Cobalamin
(C) Pyridoxamine
(D) Thiamine
(E) Vitamin K

15. A patient presents with pale skin, sunken eyes, sore gums, muscle pain, loose teeth, and corkscrew shaped hair. Which of the following processes is most likely to be affected as a result of the nutritional deficiency causing the observed symptoms?
(A) Cholesterol synthesis
(B) Collagen processing
(C) Fatty acid synthesis
(D) Glycosaminoglycan synthesis
(E) *N*-linked glycoprotein processing

16. A deficiency in which of the following vitamins is most likely to be associated with a decrease in the metabolic process referred to as the methionine cycle?
(A) Biotin
(B) Folic acid
(C) Thiamine
(D) Vitamin A
(E) Vitamin D

17. A 38-year-old female is being examined by her physician with complaints of fatigue and depression. Physical examination finds the patient has patches of dry scaly skin, dry and splitting hair, a dry mouth, and dry eyes. The physician also finds petechia on several area on the patient's arms and legs. These signs and symptoms are most likely the result of a deficiency in which of the following?
(A) Ascorbate
(B) Cobalamin
(C) Thiamine
(D) Vitamin A
(E) Vitamin D

18. A 67-year-old male is being examined in the emergency department following a fainting spell. Physical examination shows pallor and signs of heart palpitations. The patient states that he has been very tired and light-headed for several weeks and that his fingers are numb and tingling. Blood work shows an MCV (mean corpuscular volume) value of 112 fL (N = 80–95 fL) and a hemoglobin value of 11.7 g/dL (N = 13.5–17.5 g/dL). The vitamin that is most likely deficient in this patient is involved in which of the following?
(A) As a cofactor in the biosynthesis of purine nucleotides required for the synthesis of DNA
(B) As a cofactor in the biosynthesis of thymidine nucleotides
(C) The absorption of folic acid from the gut
(D) The conversion of cystathionine to cysteine
(E) The conversion of N^5-methyl-tetrahydrofolate (THF) to THF

19. A 57-year-old male is being examined for symptoms that includes slurred speech, memory impairment, ataxia, and jaundice. The examining physician suspects the patient is suffering from iron overload. However, genetic analysis indicates the patient harbors the wild-type version of the gene encoding the primary protein normally found mutated in patients with iron overload. History reveals that no other family members, including the patient's parents and his children, have ever exhibited similar symptoms. Given these findings and test results which of the following proteins is most likely defective in this patient that would explain the observed symptoms?
(A) Ceruloplasmin
(B) Ferritin
(C) Ferroportin
(D) Hephaestin
(E) Transferrin

20. Fruits and cruciferous vegetables are sources of an important vitamin that is most likely to be involved in which of the following processes?
(A) Blood coagulation
(B) Cholesterol biosynthesis
(C) Connective tissue production
(D) Gluconeogenesis
(E) Glycogen breakdown

21. A patient with renal insufficiency is likely to experience a deficiency in production of a vitamin-derived factor. The lack of this factor is most likely to be associated with which of the following?
(A) Megaloblastic anemia
(B) Microcytic anemia
(C) Osteomalacia
(D) Peripheral neuropathy
(E) Xerophthalmia

22. The ability of rod cells in the eye to respond to light and transmit that response to the optic nerve requires the involvement of a vitamin-derived intermediate. This intermediate most likely exerts its effect through interaction with which of the following?
(A) cGMP phosphodiesterase
(B) Nuclear receptor
(C) Rod cell membrane localized GPCR
(D) Sodium channel
(E) Transducin

23. A 1-week-old infant is being examined for persistent bleeding from the umbilicus and the site of circumcision. The attending physician orders a series of blood tests with the results of the prothrombin time (PT) being 48 seconds (N = 11–15 seconds). These findings are indicative of a deficiency in a substance that is most likely to be involved in which of the following types of amino acid modification?
(A) Aspartate to β-carboxyaspartate
(B) Glutamate to γ-carboxyglutamate
(C) Lysine to hydroxylysine
(D) Lysine to β-methyllysine
(E) Proline to hydroxyproline

24. The inability to rapidly synthesize DNA during the process of erythrocyte maturation can result from a vitamin deficiency. Which of the following is the most likely vitamin involved?
(A) Ascorbate
(B) Biotin
(C) Folic acid
(D) Nicotinic acid
(E) Thiamine

25. Oxidation of fatty acids with odd numbers of carbon atoms involves a pathway to convert one of the products into a TCA cycle intermediate. The final step in this process is dependent upon adequate nutritional intake. Which of the following is the most likely vitamin required for the final step of this conversion?
(A) Ascorbate
(B) Cobalamin
(C) Riboflavin
(D) Thiamine
(E) Vitamin D

26. A 53-year-old woman diagnosed with Crohn disease has her terminal ileum resected. Five years later, she comes to the physician because of weakness and fatigue. Physical examination shows skin pallor. Laboratory studies show a hemoglobin concentration of 9 g/dL (N = 12–15 g/L), a MCV (mean corpuscular volume) value of 110 fL (N = 80–95 fL), and a hematocrit of 33% (N = 36–44%). Which of the following vitamin deficiencies is most likely in this patient?
(A) Ascorbate
(B) Cobalamin
(C) Riboflavin
(D) Thiamine
(E) Vitamin A
(F) Vitamin K

27. The terminal ileum was removed from a 50-year-old woman during excision of a tumor. About 3 years later, the patient was admitted to the hospital. She is very weak and pale. Hemoglobin is 9 g/dL (N = 12–15), MCV (mean corpuscular volume) is 110 fL (N = 80–95 fL). Measurement of which of the following would be useful in confirmation of a diagnosis in this patient?
(A) Bleeding time
(B) Ketones
(C) Lactic acid
(D) Methylmalonic acid
(E) Prothrombin time

28. The blood work from a 43-year-old male patient finds a hemoglobin level of 12.2 g/dL (N = 13.5–16.5 g/dL) and the MCV (mean corpuscular volume) value of 70 fL (N = 80–95 fL). A deficiency in which of the following is most likely to account for the findings in this patient?
(A) Acute bleeding
(B) Folate deficiency
(C) Iron deficiency
(D) Vitamin B_{12} deficiency
(E) Vitamin K deficiency

29. A 22-year-old primigravid woman comes to her physician for her first prenatal examination. She is currently taking phenytoin to control her seizures. The physician recommends that she switch to lamotrigine. If the patient fails to comply with this recommendation, which of the following process will most likely be deficient in her newborn?
(A) Blood coagulation
(B) Collagen processing
(C) Gluconeogenesis
(D) Heme biosynthesis
(E) Synthesis of GABA

30. A 38-year-old female is being examined by her physician with complaints of fatigue and depression. Physical examination finds the patient has patches of dry scaly skin, dry and splitting hair, a dry mouth, and dry eyes. The physician also finds petechia on several area on the patient's arms and legs. These signs and symptoms are most likely the result of a defect in which of the following processes?
(A) Bone marrow hematopoiesis
(B) Glycosaminoglycan synthesis
(C) Production of extracellular matrix
(D) Production of proteoglycans
(E) Synthesis of cholesterol

31. A physician is tending to a patient in the emergency department who presents in a confused state, is disheveled, and is smelling of alcohol and vomit. Physical examination identifies nystagmus and ataxia. Which of the following processes is most likely to be impaired contributing to the symptoms observed in this patient?
(A) Blood coagulation
(B) Cholesterol synthesis
(C) Night vision
(D) Peroxisomal fat oxidation
(E) Pyruvate oxidation

32. The parents of a 4-month-old infant bring their child to his pediatrician because they are concerned about his difficulty in feeding, irritability, and his overall floppiness. The pediatrician notes that the infant has pudgy, rosy cheeks and brittle, easily broken hair. The doctor suspects the child is suffering from Menkes disease. Given that the physician is correct in her diagnosis, the lack of which of the following processes of copper homeostasis would most likely be found in this patient?
(A) Incorporation into ceruloplasmin
(B) Storage in hepatocytes
(C) Transfer into the biliary circulation
(D) Transport from within intestinal enterocytes into the portal circulation
(E) Uptake by intestinal enterocytes

33. Which of the following symptoms are most likely to be found in a patient manifesting the hallmarks of Wernicke encephalopathy?
(A) Diarrhea, skin rash, confusion
(B) Megaloblastic anemia
(C) Nausea, peripheral neuropathy, mental depression, ophthalmoplegia
(D) Numbness, tingling, weakness, sore smooth tongue, diarrhea
(E) Seizures

34. A 32-year-old male is being seen by his physician with complaints of severe muscle pain. History reveals that he has been consuming large quantities of raw egg whites as part of his current body-building routine. Physical examination finds areas of scaly rash around his nose and mouth. His arms and legs have very sparse amounts of hair. The physician suspects a nutritional deficiency is causing the symptoms in his patient. Which of the following processes would most likely be impaired as a result of this deficiency?
(A) Fatty acid oxidation
(B) Fatty acid synthesis
(C) Glycogen breakdown
(D) Glycogen synthesis
(E) Glycolysis

35. A deficiency in either folate or vitamin B_{12} is most likely going to impact the circulating levels of which of the following?
(A) Homocysteine
(B) Lactate
(C) Norepinephrine
(D) Serotonin
(E) Thrombin

36. The attending physician in the emergency department is examining a 53-year-old man brought in by his wife because of a recent change in his mental status. Physical examination finds vertical nystagmus, bilateral facial nerve palsy, and truncal ataxia. These findings are indicative of a deficiency in a vitamin that is most likely to be involved in which of the following processes?
(A) Amino acid metabolism
(B) Gluconeogenesis
(C) Heme biosynthesis
(D) Posttranslational modification of collagen
(E) Posttranslational modification of prothrombin
(F) Thymidine nucleotide biosynthesis

37. A 29-year-old male is being examined by his physician with complaints of pain on inspiration and a persistent cough which frequently produces a bloody phlegm. History reveals that the patient has been losing weight due to a loss of appetite, experiences night sweats, chills, and extreme fatigue. Rales are detected via auscultation of the posterior and anterior chest walls. The physician makes a diagnosis, and he prescribes a medication that the patient will need to take for 9 months. Given the most likely therapeutic intervention in this patient which of the following processes is most likely to exhibit some level of impairment?
(A) Collagen processing
(B) Gluconeogenesis
(C) Heme biosynthesis
(D) Pyruvate oxidation
(E) Thymidine biosynthesis

38. Assessment of the activity of which of the following is most useful for the diagnosis of a deficiency of thiamine?
(A) Delta-aminolevulinic acid synthase
(B) Glycogen synthase
(C) Pyruvate carboxylase
(D) Pyruvate dehydrogenase
(E) Transketolase

39. A 37-year-old female is being examined by her physician for complaints of fatigue, memory loss, and confusion. Physical examination finds she has an unsteady gait and nystagmus. The physician believes that her patient is suffering from a nutritional deficiency. An increase in which of the following would be most useful to confirm the physician's diagnosis?
(A) Erythrocyte transketolase activity
(B) Leukocyte α-ketoglutarate dehydrogenase activity
(C) Plasma concentration of ferritin
(D) Plasma concentration of glucose
(E) Plasma concentrations of pyruvate and lactate

40. A clinic physician sees many transient workers. The physician finds that almost 30% of the patients are deficient in thiamine and their erythrocytes are markedly deficient in transketolase activity. Examination of liver function in these individuals would most likely show deficiency in which of the following metabolic processes?
(A) Biosynthesis of fatty acids from acetyl-CoA
(B) Biosynthesis of ketone bodies
(C) Conversion of glycerol to glucose during fasting
(D) Conversion of pyruvate to acetyl-CoA
(E) Incorporation of dietary glucose into hepatic glycogen

41. An emergency department physician is examining a 67-year-old woman. She was brought to the hospital by her neighbor because he found her passed out in the front yard. History reveals that she lives by herself and consumes a diet which consists primarily of lettuce and rice. She has not consumed any meat products for over 5 years and does not supplement her diet with vitamins. She reports that she is frequently quite tired. Blood work finds her MCV (mean corpuscular volume) is 118 fL (N = 80–95 fL) and MCH (mean corpuscular hemoglobin) is 38 pg (N = 26–34 pg). Which of the following reaction pathways is most likely impaired in this patient?
(A) Branched-chain amino acid degradation
(B) Glucose-6-phosphate being converted to ribulose-5-phosphate
(C) Gluconeogenesis
(D) Heme synthesis
(E) Thymidine nucleotide biosynthesis

42. A 27-year-old pregnant woman, who is at 32 week's gestation, is being examined by her physician with complaints of lethargy, weakness, and chronic fatigue. Blood work indicates the woman is suffering from a macrocytic anemia. Her diet consists mainly of starchy foods with little meat or green vegetables. Which of the following vitamins is most likely deficient in this woman?
(A) Folate
(B) Niacin
(C) Pyridoxine
(D) Riboflavin
(E) Thiamine
(F) Vitamin C
(G) Vitamin K

43. A 32-year-old female is undergoing a routine annual physical examination. History reveals that she has been on a strict vegan diet for the past 5 years. An analysis of her urine finds an elevated level of methylmalonic acid. The urine results are most likely indicative of which of the following?
(A) Deficiency of ascorbate
(B) Deficiency of cobalamin
(C) Deficiency in linolenic acid
(D) Excessive intake of protein
(E) Excessive intake of vitamin D
(F) Excess methylmalonate in the diet

44. Autoimmune destruction of specialized parietal cells in the stomach is most likely to result in an inability to metabolize which of the following compounds?
(A) Acetate
(B) Lactate
(C) Methionine
(D) Methylmalonate
(E) Propionate

45. A 62-year-old man has gone to his physician for an examination to determine why his teeth feel loose and that his gums bleed easily when he eats. History reveals that his diet is restricted and includes no fresh citrus fruits or leafy green vegetable. Which of the following vitamins is most likely to be deficient in this patient?

(A) Riboflavin
(B) Thiamine
(C) Vitamin A
(D) Vitamin C
(E) Vitamin K

46. Findings in a 52-year-old homeless man includes bleeding gums and numerous petechiae. These signs are most likely the result of a lack of a vitamin cofactor involved in which of the following processes?
(A) Cross-linking lysine and hydroxylysine residues
(B) Glycosylation of hydroxylysine residues
(C) Hydroxylation of proline residues
(D) Signal peptide removal from preprocollagen
(E) Translocation of collagen peptides into the endoplasmic reticulum

47. A defect in which of the following tissues is most likely to result in a reduced capacity to produce the hormonally active form of vitamin D?
(A) Bone
(B) Intestine
(C) Kidney
(D) Liver
(E) Spleen

48. A 57-year-old woman was diagnosed 2 years ago with primary biliary cirrhosis. Given her diagnosis, which of the following would be most likely to be detectable in her vasculature?
(A) Decreased ceruloplasmin
(B) Decreased cholesterol
(C) Decreased hematocrit
(D) Increased hemoglobin A_{1c}
(E) Increased lactate
(F) Increased oxidized LDL

49. An 11-year-old boy with cystic fibrosis is brought to the physician because his mother has noticed that it seems to take him significantly longer to stop bleeding when he has a cut. He had previously been prescribed pancreatic digestive enzyme supplements because of his stools were bulky, large, and malodorous. His mother admits that he does not take his supplements regularly. Physical examination shows several bruises on his skin. This patient is most likely deficient in which of the following?
(A) Ascorbic acid
(B) Calcium
(C) Essential fatty acids
(D) Folate
(E) Iron
(F) Methionine
(G) Vitamin K

50. A 29-year-old male is being examined by his physician with complaints of pain on inspiration and a persistent cough which frequently produces a bloody phlegm. History reveals that the patient has been losing weight due to a loss of appetite, experiences night sweats, chills, and extreme fatigue. Rales are detected via auscultation of the posterior and anterior chest walls. The physician makes a diagnosis, and he prescribes a medication that the patient will need to take for 9 months. Given the most likely therapeutic intervention in this patient which of the following is most likely to become deficient in this patient?
(A) Biotin
(B) Calcium
(C) Iron
(D) Pyridoxine
(E) Thiamine
(F) Vitamin B_{12}

51. A 53-year-old woman is being examined by her physician due to complaints of frequent oily bowel movements. History reveals that she bruises easily, suffers from chronic pancreatitis, and consumes numerous alcoholic drinks on a daily basis. Which of the following laboratory findings would be most revealing for a diagnosis in this woman?
(A) Comprehensive metabolic panel
(B) Erythrocyte count
(C) Fasting plasma glucose
(D) Mean corpuscular volume (MCV)
(E) Prothrombin time

52. A 61-year-old man is brought to the physician because of confusion and difficulty walking. His daughter says that he has been a heavy drinker for 35 years but does not believe that he has had alcohol recently. Physical examination shows ataxia and a sluggish pupillary light reflex. One week later, he returns to the physician for a follow-up examination. Physical examination shows a normal gait and pupillary light reflex. Neuropsychologic testing shows severe short-term memory impairment and frank confabulation. The vitamin deficiency most likely associated with his condition may also lead to which of the following conditions?
(A) Dermatitis
(B) Hypertrophic cardiomyopathy
(C) Megaloblastic anemia
(D) Night blindness
(E) Peripheral neuropathy

53. A 33-year-old woman comes to the physician for her first routine prenatal examination. The woman reports that she has recently noticed excessively dry and ulcerated skin over her knees and elbows. In addition, she states that she seems to have a difficult time seeing clearly at night. Ophthalmic examination shows gray plaques on the conjunctiva. Which of the following is the most likely cause of this patient's current condition?
(A) Ascorbic acid deficiency
(B) Excessive vitamin D intake
(C) Excessive vitamin E intake
(D) Excessive folate intake
(E) Thiamine deficiency
(F) Vitamin A deficiency

54. A 50-year-old woman comes to the emergency department because of insomnia, recurrent diarrhea, and gastric discomfort. She has smoked two packs of cigarettes daily for 25 years and has previously been diagnosed with moderate alcohol use disorder. Physical examination shows stomatitis, glossitis, and esophagitis. Exfoliative dermatitis with some vesicles on erythematous bases is seen on sunlight exposed areas of the skin. Neurologic examination shows confusion and memory loss. This patient most likely has a deficiency of which of the following vitamins?
(A) Biotin
(B) Niacin
(C) Riboflavin
(D) Thiamine
(E) Vitamin B_{12}
(F) Vitamin C
(G) Vitamin K

55. A 60-year-old chronic smoker and alcoholic man suffering from insomnia, intestinal discomfort, and recurrent diarrhea presented to the outpatient department of his local hospital. Clinical examination revealed memory disorientation, stomatitis, glossitis, and exfoliative dermatitis on sunlight exposed sites such as his hands, nose, and cheeks. Given the observed signs and symptoms in this patient, which of the following metabolic pathways would most likely be impaired?
(A) Catecholamine metabolism
(B) Fatty acid synthesis
(C) Gluconeogenesis
(D) Heme metabolism
(E) Thymidine nucleotide synthesis

56. A 3-month-old infant who otherwise appeared normal during the first 2 months of life except for a bout of hyperbilirubinemia is now clearly exhibiting developmental delay. In addition, the infant's hair has become grayish and dull and there is a stubble of broken hair over the occiput and temporal regions. The facial appearance has also changed such that the infant has very pudgy cheeks, abnormal eyebrows, and sagging jowls. The occurrence of frequent convulsions was the stimulus for the parents to bring their child to the emergency room. These rapidly deteriorating symptoms are most likely indicative of which of the following disorders?
(A) Crigler-Najjar syndrome type 2
(B) Gilbert syndrome
(C) Hemochromatosis
(D) Menkes disease
(E) Refsum disease

57. A 30-year-old patient is being treated for acute hepatitis and progressive chronic liver disease. The patient also shows Parkinsonian tremors, diminished facial muscle movement, and choreoathetosis. History reveals that the patient has become progressively more depressed and paranoid. Which of the following disorders most likely explains the signs and symptoms observed in this patient?
(A) Aceruloplasminemia
(B) GRACILE syndrome
(C) Hemochromatosis
(D) Menkes disease
(E) Wilson disease

58. A defect in which of the following proteins is most likely to interfere with the ability of dietary iron to be transported to the circulation?
(A) Ceruloplasmin
(B) Divalent metal transporter 1 (DMT1)
(C) Ferroportin
(D) Heme oxygenase
(E) Hephaestin

59. A 57-year-old male is being examined for symptoms that includes slurred speech, memory impairment, ataxia, and jaundice. Which of the following proteins is most likely absent or defective in this patient that would explain the observed symptoms?
(A) Divalent metal transporter-1 (DMT1)
(B) HLA complex iron protein (HFE)
(C) Ferritin
(D) Ferroportin
(E) Transferrin

60. The liver plays a critical role in overall iron homeostasis through the regulated expression of a liver-specific gene encoding a protein critical to this role. Loss of the hepatic protein can lead to severe iron overload with symptoms resembling those of classic hemochromatosis. Which of the following most closely describes the function of this important hepatic protein?
(A) Activates the expression of the iron-response element binding protein that regulates transferring receptor and ferritin mRNA translation
(B) Decreases the level of intestinal membrane iron transporters, resulting in reduced iron uptake
(C) Facilitation of the interaction of transferrin with the transferrin receptor
(D) Forms a complex with ferritin allowing for higher intracellular storage
(E) Promotes the formation of hemosiderin, thus detoxifying iron

61. Which of the following most likely represents the mechanism by which iron regulates the levels of ferritin inside cells?
(A) Binding of iron to ferritin leads to secretion of the complex from cells and subsequent excretion in the urine.
(B) Ferritin exists as a tetramer and when iron binds, the affinity for additional iron atoms increases.
(C) Iron binds an additional protein that acts as a regulator of ferritin mRNA translation; high iron leads to increased translation and thus increased iron-binding capacity
(D) When excess iron binds to ferritin it decreases the half-life of the protein allowing the iron to be released to the plasma and excreted

62. A 29-year-old male is being examined by his physician to determine the cause of his progressing tremors. His physician notes that the man has a diminished capacity to move his facial muscles and that the tremors in his arms are indicative of choreoathetosis. Serum analysis shows significantly elevated AST and ALT. Ophthalmic examination finds an orangish discoloration in the Descemet membranes of both eyes. The lack of which of the following processes related to copper homeostasis would most likely be found in this patient?
(A) Incorporation into ceruloplasmin
(B) Storage in renal tubule cells
(C) Transfer into the brain
(D) Transport from within intestinal enterocytes into the portal circulation
(E) Uptake by intestinal enterocytes

63. A 40-year-old female patient is being examined with complaints of fatigue. Blood work indicates her hemoglobin level is 12.2 g/dL (mean value = 15.5 g/dL) and her MVC (mean corpuscular volume) value is 73 fL (N = 80–95 fL). Given these findings, which of the following would most likely be present in this patient?
(A) Acute bleeding
(B) Cobalamin deficiency
(C) Folate deficiency
(D) Iron deficiency
(E) Vitamin K deficiency

64. A breast-fed 4-month-old infant, who was born at 34 weeks' gestation, is undergoing testing. Blood work shows MCV (mean corpuscular volume) is 70 fL (N = 80–95 fL) and

MCH (mean corpuscular hemoglobin) is 28 pg (N = 26–34 pg). A peripheral blood smear shows the following result:

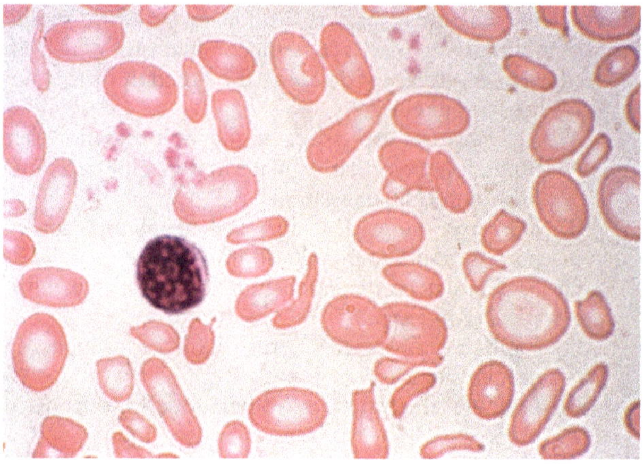

Given the signs in this infant which of the following is the most appropriate oral supplement?
(A) Copper
(B) Cobalamin
(C) Folate
(D) Iron
(E) Thiamine

65. A 28-year-old pregnant female has come to her personal physician with complaints of persistent, dry, ulcerated skin over her knees and elbows. Physical examination finds foamy grey patches on the conjunctiva of both of the patient's eyes. These signs and symptoms are most likely due to which of the following?
(A) Deficiency of ascorbate
(B) Deficiency in β-carotene
(C) Deficiency in thiamine
(D) Excessive cholecalciferol intake
(E) Excessive menadione intake
(F) Excessive α-tocopherol intake

66. A 55-year-old female presents with bleeding gums, loose teeth, and delayed wound healing. On questioning she admits that her food lacks fresh fruits and vegetables. Her symptoms are most likely caused by low activity of an enzyme found in which of the following compartments?
(A) Golgi apparatus
(B) Lysosomes
(C) Mitochondria
(D) Nucleus
(E) Rough endoplasmic reticulum

67. A 65-year-old male patient presents in the emergency department with a fractured arm that resulted from a fall. The patient has a history of precancerous skin lesions and has limited his sun exposure by avoiding outdoor activity and remaining fully covered when outside. The patient is otherwise healthy, and a physical examination is unremarkable with exception of the fractured arm. Serum measurements of calcidiol are below normal. Which of the following blood tests are expected to be above normal in this patient?
(A) Calcium
(B) Corticotropic-releasing hormone
(C) Growth hormone
(D) Parathyroid hormone
(E) Phosphate

68. A 57-year-old man has come to see his physician with complaints of feeling weak and off balance. The patient reports that there is a pounding sensation in his chest, his mouth is dry, his tongue feels numb, and his fingers and toes tingle all the time. History reveals that these symptoms have been apparent and progressive over the past year. Physical examination indicates that the patient has lost 20 pounds since his last visit 14 months ago. Given these signs and symptoms, which of the following is most likely deficient or defective in this patient?
(A) Ceruloplasmin
(B) Intrinsic factor
(C) Lysyl oxidase
(D) Pyridoxal kinase
(E) Thiamine pyrophosphokinase

69. A 39-year-old female is being examined by her physician with a primary complaint of excessive fatigue, weight loss, and vision problems over the past several months. The patient reports that she has strictly adhered to a vegan diet for the past 4 years. The patient's records indicate no significant past medical history. Physical examination finds that the patient has pale conjunctiva and glossitis. Her physician orders several tests with the following results:

	Patient Values	Normal Values
Hemoglobin	9.7 g/dL	12–16 g/dL
Hematocrit	31%	36–44%
MCV	111 fL	80–100 fL
MCHC	33 g/dL	32–36 g/dL

Histopathological analysis of a peripheral blood smear demonstrates hypersegmented neutrophils and poikilocytosis. Measuring serum levels of which of the following would be most useful for the determination of a correct diagnosis?
(A) δ-Aminolevulinic acid
(B) Anti-citrullinated peptide antibodies
(C) Ferritin
(D) Homocysteine
(E) Methylmalonic acid

70. An 18-month-old girl was brought to her pediatrician by her adoptive parents to have her examined for an unexplained rash. The infant's parents just recently adopted her following her being orphaned in Syria. The parents do not have information regarding the infant's medical history but state that the infant was definitely malnourished when they adopted her. Physical examination shows the child is in the 5th percentile for both weight and height, has conjunctival pallor, scaling and fissures at the corners of her mouth, inflamed lips, and a swollen tongue. There is also evidence of erythema on the face and the back of both thighs. The patient's signs and symptoms are most likely the result of a vitamin deficiency, the consequences of which are a defect in which of the following processes?
(A) DNA synthesis
(B) Heme synthesis
(C) Histone deacetylation
(D) Methionine synthesis
(E) Succinate oxidation

71. A 53-year-old woman is being examined by her physician because she has been experiencing increasing fatigue over the past 5 months. When asked if she has experienced any other significant changes, the patient notes that her stools have been much darker than what she considers normal, being almost tar-colored and that her hands and feet seem cold all the time. Physical examination of the patient's mouth shows mucosal pallor and glossitis, and examination of her hands shows koilonychia. The physician orders blood work which finds hemoglobin concentration is 8.2 g/dL (N = 12 – 15.5 g/dL), MCV is 73 fL (N = 80 – 95 fL), and MCHC is 27 g/dL (N = 32 – 36 g/dL). Given these signs and symptoms, which of the following changes in additional lab results are most likely to be found with this patient?

	Serum Iron	Serum Ferritin	TIBC	Transferrin Receptor
A.	↓	↓	↑	↑
B.	↓	↑	↓	↑
C.	↓	none	↑	↓
D.	↑	↑	↓	↑
E.	↑	none	↓	↑
F.	none	none	↑	↓

(A)
(B)
(C)
(D)
(E)
(F)

72. A 40-year-old woman is being examined by her physician because she has been experiencing increasing fatigue over the past 5 months that is even worse than the level of fatigue that led to her being diagnosed with systemic lupus erythematosus 2 years ago. In addition to the fatigue, the patient reports that she experiences a rapid onset of shortness of breath with mild exertion. Physical examination shows generalized pallor. The physician orders blood work which finds hemoglobin concentration is 7.4 g/dL (N = 12–15.5 g/dL), MCV is 74 fL (N = 80–95 fL), and MCHC is 28 g/dL (N = 32–36 g/dL). Increased expression of which of the following is the most likely contributing factor to this patient's signs and symptoms?
(A) Hepcidin
(B) Hephaestin
(C) Ferritin
(D) Ferroportin
(E) Transferrin

73. A 5-year-old girl, who was recently adopted from a refugee camp in Syria, is undergoing a first examination by a pediatrician with her new parents. They report that they are concerned about their child's vision, indicating that she frequently bumps into furniture, especially in the evening just prior to going to bed. Physical examination finds all vital signs to be within normal ranges but she is in the 10th percentile for weight and height and has a textured appearance to her skin which is also dry and flaky on her extremities as well as areas of her abdomen. Ophthalmoscopic examination shows she has a normal red reflex in both pupils with no apparent abnormalities on her retinas, but that her conjunctivae are dry and thickened. Given the most likely deficiency in this patient, which of the following processes is most likely to be impaired?
(A) Activation of a cGMP-specific phosphodiesterase
(B) Activation of coagulation factor X
(C) Catabolism of phytanic acid
(D) Expression of intestinal Na^+-Ca^{2+} exchanger, NCX1
(E) Protection of membrane lipids from peroxidation
(F) Synthesis of heme

74. A 14-year-old African-American female is being examined by the family physician with the primary complaint of easily becoming exhausted while playing soccer and a general feeling of constant fatigue. She reports that she has been experiencing these symptoms for the past several months. There is no prior significant medical history, and she does not take any medications. The patient tells the doctor that she has been adherent to a vegan diet for the past year. Family history is significant for a fraternal uncle and grandfather, both of whom have sickle cell anemia. Physical examination finds no palpable abdominal masses but does show conjunctival pallor. The physician orders blood tests and the results show the patient's hemoglobin is 9.2 g/dL (N = 12–15 g/dL), MCV is 57 fL (78–98 fL), and MCHC is 25 g/dL (32–36 g/dL). Which of the following is the most likely cause of the signs and symptoms in this patient?
(A) Erythrocyte pyruvate kinase deficiency
(B) Glucose-6-phosphate dehydrogenase deficiency
(C) Iron deficiency anemia
(D) Sickle cell anemia
(E) Vitamin B_{12} deficiency

75. A 49-year-old man is being examined by his physician to determine the cause of his progressively worsening fatigue and pain in most of his joints. He tells his physician that these symptoms have been plaguing him for over a year and adding to this discomfort is a significant drop in his sex drive. He claims that he does not drink alcohol or smoke cigarettes. History reveals that he is a type 2 diabetic and that he has been taking metformin for the past 3 years to help control his blood glucose levels. Family history is significant for the fact that his father died from liver failure at the age of 63 and his 61-year-old brother was recently diagnosed with cirrhosis. Physical examination finds palpable hepatomegaly and a bronze skin coloration. Which of the following is the most likely underlying cause of the signs and symptoms in this patient?
(A) Decreased hepatic excretion of iron
(B) Dubin-Johnson syndrome
(C) Fatty infiltration of hepatocytes
(D) Hepatocellular carcinoma
(E) Increased cellular uptake of iron
(F) Wilson disease

76. A 10-month-old female infant is being examined by her pediatrician because her mother is concerned about an apparent lack of growth compared to her best friend's daughter who is the same age. In addition, the mother reports that her daughter seems much more irritable than her friend's daughter. Physical examination shows that the patient is in the 25th percentile for weight and length. The mother indicates that her daughter is exclusively breast-fed. The mother reports that her mother died from skin cancer and so she is very afraid to take her daughter outside and ensures that she is completely covered when doing so. Physical examination shows that the infant's wrists and ankles are slightly wider than normal and that there is frontal bossing present on the infant's head. Given the signs and symptoms in this patient which of the following is most likely to be deficient?

(A) Ascorbate
(B) Folate
(C) Protein
(D) Total calories
(E) Vitamin D
(F) Vitamin K

77. A 43-year-old man is being examined by his physician due to night sweats, chills, fever, and a persistent cough with hemoptysis for the past 2 months. The patient states that he is easily fatigued, has no appetite, and has been losing weight during this same period. History reveals that the patient has worked as a volunteer in a homeless shelter for the past 2 years. Auscultation reveals bronchial breathing, wheezes, and crackles. The physician orders a chest X-ray, the results of which show enlarged lymph nodes and infiltrates. The physician makes a diagnosis and prescribes the most common prescription therapy for this diagnosis. Given the physician's diagnosis and prescribed treatment, which of the following is most likely to be a beneficial addition to the patient's treatment?
(A) Ascorbate
(B) Pyridoxine
(C) Thiamine
(D) Vitamin B_{12}
(E) Vitamin D

78. A 35-year-old man is being examined by his physician with complaints of chronic fatigue and numbness and tingling in his fingers and toes. History reveals that the patient has a history of hypertension and fatty liver due to chronic and excessive alcohol consumption. Physical examination shows no palpable abdominal masses nor evidence of jaundice, however, there is the presence of conjunctival pallor. The physician orders several blood tests, and these find the patient's hemoglobin concentration is 8.9 g/dL (N = 13.5–17.5 g/dL) and MCV is 74 fL (N = 80–100 fL). A peripheral blood smear shows clear evidence of hypochromic anemia. A deficiency in which of the following is most likely to be the underlying cause of the signs and symptoms in this patient?
(A) Folate
(B) Iron
(C) Pyridoxine
(D) Thiamine
(E) Vitamin B12

79. A 7-day-old female infant is rushed to the Emergency Department by her mother because she is bleeding from the nose and mouth. The infant was delivered via Caesarian section at 38 weeks gestation following an uncomplicated pregnancy. History reveals that the infant has not undergone any neonatal inborn disease testing due to opposition from the mother, is exclusively breast-fed, appears to be developing normally, and has gained weight since birth. Examination of the patient shows an otherwise healthy female infant with the only significant finding being multiple areas of bruising in the oral and nasal mucosa. All vital signs are stable and within normal limits. Blood tests find that the infant's bleeding time is normal but that her prothrombin time is significantly prolonged. Which of the following is the most likely cause of the abnormal bruising and bleeding observed in this infant?
(A) Factor VIII deficiency
(B) Folate deficiency
(C) Intestinal bacteria deficiency
(D) Metabolic enzyme deficiency
(E) Vitamin C deficiency

80. A 53-year-old woman is brought to the Emergency Department by her husband who is concerned about his wife's state of confusion and her complaining of intense abdominal pain. History reveals that the patient has no significant prior medical conditions and that she currently takes no prescription medications. She does inform the attending physician that she has been adherent to a vegan diet for the past 8 months and takes numerous nonprescription supplements. Physical examination finds the patient has a diffusely tender abdomen. The attending physician orders blood studies and an abdominal X-ray and CT scan. The results of the blood work show elevated serum calcium and phosphate. The result of the abdominal X-ray shows that the colon is full of stool throughout, and the CT scan finds nephrolithiasis in both the left and right renal pelvises. Given these findings, which of the following is the most likely underlying cause of the symptoms presenting in this patient?
(A) Addison disease
(B) Cushing syndrome
(C) Hyperthyroidism
(D) Hypothyroidism
(E) Vitamin D deficiency
(F) Vitamin D toxicity

ANSWERS

1. Correct answer is **A.** The patient is most likely exhibiting the signs and symptoms associated with a deficiency in vitamin C, ascorbic acid. The main function of ascorbate is as a reducing agent in a number of different reactions. Ascorbate is the cofactor for Cu^{+}-dependent monooxygenases and for several 2-oxoglutarate and Fe^{2+}-dependent dioxygenases (2OG-oxygenases). Several critical enzymes that require ascorbate as a cofactor include the collagen processing enzymes, the lysyl hydroxylases and the prolyl hydroxylases as well as the catecholamine synthesis enzyme dopamine β-hydroxylase. The most important reactions requiring ascorbate as a cofactor are the hydroxylation of lysine and proline residues in collagen. Vitamin C is, therefore, required for the maintenance of normal connective tissue as well as for wound healing since synthesis of connective tissue is the first event in wound tissue remodeling. Vitamin C also is necessary for bone remodeling due to the presence of collagen in the organic matrix of bones. Deficiency in vitamin C leads to the disease scurvy due to the role of the vitamin in the posttranslational modification of collagens. Scurvy is characterized by easily bruised skin, petechia, muscle fatigue, soft swollen gums, decreased wound healing, hemorrhaging, osteoporosis, and anemia. Ascorbate deficiency also leads to hemarthrosis (bleeding into joints) that makes movement very painful. Due to its role in collagen processing, the bleeding dysfunction associated with vitamin C deficiency is characterized by the lack of effect on prothrombin time (PT) but with a prolonged bleeding time. The latter effect is the result of the reduced ability for platelets to adhere to exposed sub-endothelial extracellular matrix collagen which is required for their activation. The major clinical symptoms of riboflavin deficiency (choice B) include itching and burning eyes, angular stomatitis, and cheilosis (cracks and sores in the mouth and lips), bloodshot eyes, glossitis (inflammation of the tongue leading to purplish discoloration), seborrhea (dandruff, flaking skin on scalp and face), trembling, sluggishness, and photophobia (excessive light sensitivity). The early symptoms of thiamine deficiency (choice C) include constipation, appetite suppression, and nausea. Progressive deficiency will lead to mental depression, peripheral neuropathy, and fatigue. Chronic thiamine deficiency leads to more severe neurologic symptoms including ataxia, mental confusion, and loss of eye coordination (nystagmus). A highly diagnostic physical test of thiamine deficiency is vertical nystagmus. Dietary thiamine deficiency is known as beriberi and is most often the result of a diet that is carbohydrate rich and thiamine deficient. An additional thiamine deficiency related syndrome is known as Wernicke syndrome which is most often associated with chronic alcohol consumption. The earliest symptoms of vitamin A deficiency (choice D) are night blindness. Additional early symptoms include follicular hyperkeratosis, increased susceptibility to infection and cancer, and anemia equivalent to iron-deficient anemia. Prolonged lack of vitamin A leads to deterioration of the eye tissue through progressive keratinization of the cornea which results in abnormal dryness of the conjunctiva and cornea and the lack of ability of produce tears, a condition known as xerophthalmia. The major clinical symptoms of vitamin B_{12} deficiency (choice E) is a megaloblastic anemia, referred to as pernicious anemia, resulting from the lack of intrinsic factor being released from stomach parietal cells leading to subsequent malabsorption of the vitamin. The major cause of the loss of intrinsic factor is an autoimmune destruction of the parietal cells that secrete it. Neurologic complications also are associated with vitamin B_{12} deficiency and result from a progressive demyelination of nerve cells. The demyelination is thought to result from the increase in methylmalonyl-CoA that results from vitamin B_{12} deficiency that is associated with loss of methylmalonyl-CoA mutase activity. The loss of methylmalonyl-CoA mutase activity with deficiencies in B_{12} results in an accompanying methylmalonic acidemia. Methylmalonyl-CoA is a competitive inhibitor of malonyl-CoA in fatty acid biosynthesis as well as being able to substitute for malonyl-CoA in any fatty acid biosynthesis that may occur. Since the myelin sheath that protects nerve cells is in continual flux the methylmalonyl-CoA-induced inhibition of fatty acid synthesis results in the eventual destruction of the sheath. Contributing to the neural degeneration seen in vitamin B_{12}, deficiency is the reduced synthesis of *S*-adenosylmethione (SAM; also abbreviated AdoMet) due to loss of the methionine synthase catalyzed reaction. The conversion of phosphatidylethanolamine (PE) to phosphatidylcholine (PC) requires the enzyme phosphatidylethanolamine *N*-methyltransferase (encoded by the PEMT gene) which carries out three successive SAM-dependent methylation reactions. This reaction is a critically important reaction of membrane lipid homeostasis. Therefore, the reduced capacity to carry out the methionine synthase reaction, due to nutritional or disease-mediated deficiency of vitamin B_{12}, results in reduced SAM production and as a consequence contributes to the neural degeneration (ie, depression, peripheral neuropathy) seen in chronic B_{12} deficiency. The major clinical symptom of vitamin D deficiency (choice F) in young children is the development of rickets and in adults is the development of osteomalacia. Rickets is characterized by improper mineralization during the development of the bones resulting in soft bones. Osteomalacia is characterized by demineralization of previously formed bone leading to increased softness and susceptibility to fracture. The major clinical symptom of vitamin K deficiency (choice G) is dysfunction in the processes of blood coagulation. Since the defect will be at the level of prothrombin, factors VII, IX, X, and protein C and protein S, the effects of vitamin K deficiency can be seen in the context of the prothrombin time (PT) assay. Whereas vitamin C deficiency is associated with bleeding dysfunction at the level of platelet adhesion to collagen and is, therefore, measurable with an associated increase in bleeding time, vitamin K deficiency has no effect on bleeding time.

2. Correct answer is **C.** The patient is most likely experiencing the symptoms of a deficiency in vitamin C, ascorbic acid. The main function of ascorbate is as a reducing agent in a number of different reactions. Ascorbate is the cofactor for Cu^+-dependent monooxygenases and for several 2-oxoglutarate and Fe^{2+}-dependent dioxygenases (2OG-oxygenases). Several critical enzymes that require ascorbate as a cofactor include the collagen processing enzymes, the lysyl hydroxylases and the prolyl hydroxylases as well as the catecholamine synthesis enzyme dopamine β-hydroxylase. The most important reactions requiring ascorbate as a cofactor are the hydroxylation of lysine and proline residues in collagen. Vitamin C is, therefore, required for the maintenance of normal connective tissue as well as for wound healing since synthesis of connective tissue is the first event in wound tissue remodeling. Vitamin C also is necessary for bone remodeling due to the presence of collagen in the organic matrix of bones. Deficiency in vitamin C leads to the disease scurvy due to the role of the vitamin in the posttranslational modification of collagens. Scurvy is characterized by easily bruised skin, petechia, muscle fatigue, soft swollen gums, decreased wound healing, hemorrhaging, osteoporosis, and anemia. Ascorbate deficiency also leads to hemarthrosis (bleeding into joints) that makes movement very painful. Due to its role in collagen processing, the bleeding dysfunction associated with vitamin C deficiency is characterized by the lack of effect on prothrombin time (PT) but with a prolonged bleeding time. The latter effect is the result of the reduced ability for platelets to adhere to exposed subendothelial extracellular matrix collagen which is required for their activation. Deficiencies in none of the other processes (choice A, B, D, and E) would result in the symptoms observed in this patient.

3. Correct answer is **B.** The infant is most likely suffering from the effects of Hartnup disease, a disease whose symptoms are very similar to those seen in patients with a deficiency in niacin (vitamin B_3). Since the infant is being fed a fortified formula it is not likely that the presenting symptoms are the result of a nutritional deficiency such as vitamin B_3. Hartnup disorder is caused by mutations in the intestinal neutral amino acid transporter encoded by the *SLC6A19* gene. SLC6A19 is also known as the system B(0) (also written as B^0) neutral amino acid transporter 1 [B(0)AT1 or B^0AT1]. The B refers to a broad specificity transporter, the 0 denotes the transporter as one for neutral amino acids, and the superscripting of the 0 denotes that the transporter is a Na^+-dependent transporter. The SLC6A19 transporter prefers large aliphatic neutral amino acids. Of significance to overall amino acid homeostasis is the fact that the SCL6A19 encoded transporter transports eight of the ten essential amino acids, namely leucine, isoleucine, valine, methionine, phenylalanine, tryptophan, threonine, and histidine. In the context of SLC6A19 deficiency, the lack of adequate tryptophan absorption from the intestines is the primary cause of the symptoms observed in Hartnup disease. Tryptophan is utilized to support the vital production of NAD^+ (see Figure 18-12), and lack of this contribution in Hartnup disease is the cause of the symptoms that are similar to those of dietary niacin deficiency. Vitamin B_2

(riboflavin) is the precursor for flavin adenine dinucleotide (choice A). Dietary riboflavin is absorbed from the small intestine through the action of the solute carrier family member transporter encoded by the *SLC52A3* gene. Cellular uptake of riboflavin occurs through the actions of the SLC transporters encoded by the *SLC52A1* and *SLC52A2* genes. Tetrahydrobiopterin (choice C) is synthesized from the nucleotide GTP. Tetrahydrofolate (choice D) is synthesized from dietary folic acid. Folates in the diet are predominantly the N^5-methyltetrahydrofolate (5-methyl-THF) form. Dietary folates are absorbed by jejunal enterocytes primarily via the SLC46A1 encoded transporter which is a proton (H^+)-coupled transporter more commonly referred to as the proton-coupled folate transporter, PCFT. Thiamine pyrophosphate (choice E) is derived from dietary thiamine (vitamin B_1). Thiamine uptake from the intestines is a function of the solute carrier transporter family member encoded by the *SLC19A2* gene. Uptake of thiamine into cells from the blood occurs primarily through the activity of the SLC19A3-encoded transporter.

4. Correct answer is **B.** The patient is most likely exhibiting the signs and symptoms of scurvy which results from a deficiency of vitamin C (ascorbate). The main function of ascorbate is as a reducing agent in a number of different reactions. Ascorbate is the cofactor for Cu^+-dependent monooxygenases and for several 2-oxoglutarate and Fe^{2+}-dependent dioxygenases (2OG-oxygenases). Several critical enzymes that require ascorbate as a cofactor include the collagen processing enzymes, the lysyl hydroxylases and the prolyl hydroxylases, as well as the catecholamine synthesis enzyme dopamine β-hydroxylase. The most important reactions requiring ascorbate as a cofactor are the hydroxylation of lysine and proline residues in collagen. Vitamin C is, therefore, required for the maintenance of normal connective tissue as well as for wound healing since synthesis of connective tissue is the first event in wound tissue remodeling. Vitamin C also is necessary for bone remodeling due to the presence of collagen in the organic matrix of bones. Dietary ascorbate is also involved in non-heme iron absorption in the small intestine and in the overall regulation of iron homeostasis. As a result of the role of ascorbate in iron absorption and homeostasis, vitamin C deficient patients often exhibit mild form of iron-deficiency anemia which is a microcytic hypochromic anemia. Cystathionine β-synthase (choice A) is a vitamin B_6-dependent enzyme. Methionine synthase (choice C) is a folate- and vitamin B_{12}-dependent enzyme. Methyl malonyl-CoA mutase (choice D) is a vitamin B_{12}-dependent enzyme. Transketolase (choice E) is a thiamine-dependent enzyme.

5. Correct answer is **D.** The patient is most likely manifesting the signs and symptoms of Menkes disease. Menkes disease is inherited as an X-linked recessive disorder of copper homeostasis. The disorder is associated with an inability to absorb copper from the gastrointestinal tract and an inability of tissues to absorb copper from the blood. Menkes disease is the result of defects in the P-type ATPase protein that is responsible for the translocation of copper across the intestinal basolateral membrane into the blood, thus allowing for uptake of dietary copper. This protein is encoded by the ATPase, Cu^{2+}-transporting, alpha polypeptide (*ATP7A*) gene. The loss of copper transport results in the reduced, or loss of, function of copper-dependent proteins. The clinical spectrum associated with Menkes disease is due in large part to the reduced activity of cytochrome c oxidase, dopamine β-hydroxylase, and ceruloplasmin, all of which are critical Cu^{2+}-dependent enzymes. The clinical spectrum of Menkes disease includes progressive neurodegeneration, connective tissue abnormalities, and wiry brittle hair. Progressive cerebral degeneration in Menkes disease occurs primarily due to loss of the Cu^{2+}-dependent enzymes, ceruloplasmin, cytochrome c oxidase, peptidylglycine α-amidating monooxygenase, and dopamine β-hydroxylase in the central nervous system and to the loss of iron homeostasis in the brain. The defective brain iron homeostasis is due to the loss of activity of the ferroxidase, ceruloplasmin. Within most tissues, ceruloplasmin is bound to the plasma membrane via a glycosylphosphatidylinositol (GPI) linkage and the function of GPI-ceruloplasmin is iron efflux from the tissues. Without adequate iron homeostasis, the brain accumulates iron resulting in the toxic effects of iron overload. The iron overload due to defective, or no, ceruloplasmin activity is a form of hemochromatosis termed hemosiderosis. The distinctive clinical features of Menkes disease are usually present by 3 months of age. Infants will lose, or fail to demonstrate, specific developmental milestones and failure to thrive. Most patients with Menkes disease do not survive beyond early childhood. Although the loss of copper uptake will lead to failure of functional ceruloplasmin and, therefore, reduced iron oxidation (choice F), this is secondary to the loss of copper absorption, the primary deficiency leading to Menkes disease. None of the other options (choices A, B, C, and E) correctly define the efficient process associated with the signs and symptoms in this patient.

6. Correct answer is **D.** The patient is most likely exhibiting the symptoms of a deficiency in vitamin A. The earliest symptom of vitamin A deficiency is night blindness. Additional early symptoms include follicular hyperkeratosis, increased susceptibility to infection and cancer, and anemia equivalent to iron deficient anemia. Prolonged lack of vitamin A leads to deterioration of the eye tissue through progressive keratinization of the cornea which results in abnormal dryness of the conjunctiva and cornea and the lack of ability to produce tears, a condition known as xerophthalmia. The progressive drying and keratinization of the conjunctiva, particularly on the nasal and temporal conjunctiva, results in the development of irregularly shaped spots termed Bitot ("bee toe") spots after the French physician, Pierre Bitot, who first described them. For the major symptoms of deficiencies in ascorbate (choice A), cobalamin, vitamin B_{12} (choice B), thiamine (choice C), vitamin D (choice E), and vitamin K (choice F) please read the answer descriptions in question 1.

7. Correct answer is **E.** The infant is most likely experiencing the symptoms of a deficiency in vitamin D. The hormonally active form of vitamin D is 1,25-dihydroxy vitamin D_3 (1,25-$(OH)_2D_3$, also called 1,25-dihydroxycholecalciferol or more commonly, calcitriol). Calcitriol functions primarily to regulate calcium and phosphorous homeostasis. The major clinical symptom of vitamin D deficiency in infants and young children is the development of rickets and in adults is the development of osteomalacia. Rickets is characterized by improper mineralization during the development of the bones resulting in soft bones. Osteomalacia is characterized by demineralization of previously formed bone leading to increased softness and susceptibility to fracture. In toddlers with rickets a common skeletal deformity is bowed legs. For the major symptoms of deficiencies in ascorbate (choice A), cobalamin, vitamin B_{12} (choice B), thiamine (choice C), vitamin A (choice D), and vitamin K (choice F) please read the answer descriptions in question 1.

8. Correct answer is **A.** The patient is most likely manifesting the signs and symptoms of thiamine deficiency. The earliest symptoms of thiamine deficiency include constipation, appetite suppression, and nausea. Progressive deficiency will lead to mental depression, peripheral neuropathy, and fatigue. Chronic thiamine deficiency leads to more severe neurologic symptoms, including ataxia, mental confusion, and loss of eye coordination (nystagmus). Prolonged thiamine deficiency is most commonly found in chronic alcoholics due to the fact that alcohol impairs thiamine uptake from the small intestine as well as the fact that these individuals generally have poor dietetic lifestyles. The major symptoms of chronic thiamine deficiency are due to the requirement for thiamine of the pyruvate dehydrogenase complex (PDHc). Confirmation of thiamine deficiency can be accomplished by measuring the level of activity of the pentose phosphate pathway enzyme, transketolase. This assay is relatively easy to perform, compared with assaying for PDHc activity, and the collection of samples is a simple matter of drawing blood from the patient. Peripheral blood smears (choice B) are useful for examining the morphology of blood cells to help diagnose various blood disorders. The Schilling test (choice C) is performed to ascertain whether a patient's vitamin B_{12} deficiency is due to the lack of absorption from the distal ileum. The measurement of serum methylmalonic acid levels (choice D) is performed to ascertain whether a patient with megaloblastic anemia has a deficiency in vitamin B_{12}. Measurement of urinary β-hydroxybutyrate levels is useful for the determination of excess ketone body production, particularly in the context of diabetic ketoacidosis, DKA.

9. Correct answer is **F.** The patient is most likely exhibiting a deficiency in the processes of blood coagulation. From a dietary perspective defective blood coagulation is the consequence of a vitamin K or a vitamin C (ascorbate) deficiency. Two types of assays can be used to assess blood coagulation, the bleeding time and the prothrombin time. The prothrombin time (PT) is an assay designed to screen for defects in fibrinogen, prothrombin, and factors V, VII, and X. Functional prothrombin, factor VII, and factor X require a vitamin K-dependent modification. When any of these factors is deficient, or defective, the PT is prolonged. A normal PT is 11.0–12.5 seconds. A PT greater than 20 seconds is indicative of coagulation deficit. The PT is measured using plasma after the blood cells are removed. A blood sample is collected in a tube containing citrate or EDTA to chelate any calcium and thus inhibit coagulation and then the cells are removed by centrifugation. After the cells are removed, excess calcium is added to the plasma to initiate coagulation. The most common measure of PT is to divide the time of coagulation of a patient's blood by that of a known standard and the resultant value is referred to as the international normalized ratio (INR). Normal INR values range from 0.8–1.2. PT is used to determine the correct dosage of the warfarin class of anticoagulation drugs (eg, Coumadin), for the presence of liver disease or damage, and to evaluate vitamin K status. In addition to prothrombin, factor VII, and factor X, vitamin K is required for the activation of factor IX, protein C, and protein S. Conversion from inactive to active clotting factor requires a posttranslational modification of specific glutamate (Glu) residues. This modification is a carboxylation and the enzyme responsible, γ-glutamyl carboxylase (GGCX), requires vitamin K as a cofactor. The resultant modified Glu residues are termed γ-carboxyglutamate (*gla*) residues. Thus, a deficiency in vitamin K will result in prolonged bleeding due to loss of clotting factor functions. Due to its role in collagen processing, the bleeding dysfunction associated with vitamin C deficiency (choice A) is characterized by the lack of effect on prothrombin time (PT) but with a prolonged bleeding time. The latter effect is the result of the reduced ability for platelets to adhere to exposed subendothelial extracellular matrix collagen which is required for their activation. Given that biotin (choice B) is synthesized by intestinal bacteria, deficiencies of the vitamin are rare. Deficiencies are generally seen only after long antibiotic therapies, which deplete the intestinal microbiota, or following excessive consumption of raw eggs. The latter is due to the affinity of the egg white protein, avidin, for biotin preventing intestinal absorption of the biotin. For the major symptoms of deficiencies in cobalamin, vitamin B_{12} (choice C), vitamin D (choice D), and vitamin A (choice E) please read the answer descriptions in question 1.

10. Correct answer is **C.** The patient is most likely exhibiting the symptoms associated with a deficiency in vitamin B_2, riboflavin. Symptoms associated with riboflavin deficiency include itching and burning eyes, angular stomatitis and cheilosis (cracks and sores on the mouth and lips), bloodshot eyes, glossitis (inflammation of the tongue leading to purplish discoloration), seborrhea (dandruff, flaking skin on scalp and face), trembling, sluggishness, and photophobia (excessive light sensitivity). Riboflavin decomposes when exposed to visible light. This characteristic can lead to riboflavin deficiencies in newborns treated for hyperbilirubinemia by phototherapy requiring dietary supplementation in these infants. Although thiamine deficiency (choice D) is common in chronic alcoholics, this patient does not exhibit the characteristic signs and symptoms of thiamine deficiency. Given that biotin (choice A) is synthesized by intestinal bacteria, deficiencies of the vitamin are rare. Deficiencies are generally seen only after long antibiotic therapies, which deplete the intestinal microbiota, or following excessive consumption of raw eggs. The latter is due to the affinity of the egg white protein, avidin, for biotin preventing intestinal absorption of the biotin. A diet deficient in niacin (choice B) leads to glossitis of the tongue (inflammation of the tongue leading to purplish discoloration), dermatitis, weight loss, diarrhea, depression, and dementia. The severe symptoms, depression, dermatitis, and diarrhea (referred to as the "3-D's"), are associated with the condition known as pellagra. Several physiologic conditions (eg, Hartnup disorder and malignant carcinoid syndrome) as well as certain drug therapies (eg, isoniazid) can lead to niacin deficiency. In Hartnup disorder, tryptophan absorption is impaired and in malignant carcinoid syndrome tryptophan metabolism is altered resulting in excess serotonin synthesis. Isoniazid was, at one time, a primary drug for chemotherapeutic treatment of tuberculosis. Conditions that result from vitamin E deficiency (choice E) are related to disturbances in nerve cell membrane lipid homeostasis. These conditions include cerebellar ataxias, myopathies, retinopathy, loss of deep tendon reflexes, and dysarthria (speech problem associated with difficulty articulating due to defects in the motor component of speech). Another major symptom of vitamin E deficiency in humans is an increase in red blood cell fragility due to the increased level of erythrocyte membrane lipid peroxidation in the absence of tocopherols. For the major symptoms of deficiencies in thiamine (choice D) and vitamin K (choice F) please read the answer descriptions in question 1.

11. Correct answer is **D.** The function of hemojuvelin is to regulate the expression of the gene (*HAMP*) encoding hepcidin via bone morphogenetic protein (BMP) signaling pathways, specifically BMP5, BMP6, and BMP7 proteins. The hemojuvelin protein is one of three members of a family of glycosylphosphatidylinositol (GPI)-linked cell membrane-associated proteins that were originally identified as repulsive guidance molecules, RGM. Hemojuvelin is also known as RGMc and is expressed predominantly in the liver and skeletal muscle. Mutations in the gene (*HJV*) encoding hemojuvelin are the cause of the form of hemochromatosis known as juvenile hemochromatosis (JH) type 2A. As suggested by the juvenile nomenclature, this disorder manifests in patients under the age of 30. The lack of hemojuvelin function results in impairment of the BMP signaling required to activate the expression of hepcidin. Hepcidin functions by binding to the basolateral membrane iron efflux transporter ferroportin 1 in intestinal enterocyte and reticuloendothelial macrophage membranes. On interaction with hepcidin, ferroportin 1 is internalized and degraded. An increased level of HAMP gene expression occurs as a consequence of iron status, erythropoiesis, inflammation, and hypoxia. When there is excess iron in the body, or under conditions of inflammation, the HAMP gene is turned on resulting in decreased iron absorption and decreased iron release from macrophages. The decreased release of iron from macrophages during infections is believed to result in iron deprivation from invading bacteria which require the metal for their growth. Conversely, when iron levels are deficient or during erythropoiesis or hypoxic events, expression of the HAMP gene decreases. When hepcidin expression is decreased there is increased iron absorption and increased iron release from macrophages. The function of none of the other proteins (choices A, B, C, E, and F) would be directly impacted by a loss of hemojuvelin.

12. Correct answer is **D.** The mammillary bodies are a pair of small round structures, located on the undersurface of the brain, that, as part of the diencephalon, form part of the limbic system. Damage to the mammillary bodies due to thiamine deficiency is implied in the pathogenesis of Wernicke-Korsakoff syndrome. Symptoms include impaired memory, also called anterograde amnesia, suggesting that the mammillary bodies may be important for memory. The early symptoms of thiamine deficiency include constipation, appetite suppression, and nausea. Progressive deficiency will lead to mental depression, peripheral neuropathy, and fatigue. Chronic thiamine deficiency leads to more severe neurologic symptoms including ataxia, mental confusion, and loss of eye coordination (nystagmus). A highly diagnostic physical test of thiamine deficiency is vertical nystagmus. Dietary thiamine deficiency is known as beriberi and is most often the result of a diet that is carbohydrate rich and thiamine deficient. Folate deficiency (choice B) results in complications nearly identical to those associated with vitamin B_{12} deficiency. The most pronounced effect of folate deficiency on cellular processes is on DNA synthesis. This is due to an impairment in dTMP synthesis which leads to cell cycle arrest, in S-phase, of rapidly proliferating cells, in particular hematopoietic cells. The result is megaloblastic anemia as for vitamin B_{12} deficiency. The inability to synthesize DNA during erythrocyte maturation leads to abnormally large erythrocytes termed macrocytic (megaloblastic) anemia. For the major symptoms of deficiencies in ascorbate (choice A), riboflavin (choice C), vitamin D (choice E), and vitamin K (choice F), please read the answer descriptions in question 1.

13. Correct answer is **E.** The patient is most likely experiencing the signs and symptoms of Wilson disease. Wilson disease is the result of defects in the P-type ATPase protein that is primarily responsible for copper homeostasis within the liver. This protein is encoded by the ATPase, Cu^{2+}-transporting, beta polypeptide (*ATP7B*) gene. The ATP7B protein is localized to the trans-Golgi network where it transports copper into the lumen of the Golgi. When copper levels rise, ATP7B is translocated to vesicular compartments closely associated with the plasma membrane where it can transport copper into these compartments. The copper in these vesicles can then be released by exocytosis. In the liver, copper is stored intracellularly bound to the protein metallothionein. Any copper in excess of the binding capacity of metallothionein is excreted into the biliary canaliculi through the transport action of ATP7B. ATP7B also facilitates the transfer of copper to the copper-dependent ferroxidase, ceruloplasmin. Copper-containing ceruloplasmin, produced in the liver, is then released to the blood. In all other tissues the form of ceruloplasmin is a plasma membrane GPI-linked form that is responsible for iron efflux from the cell. The majority of patients with Wilson disease present with hepatic or neuropsychiatric symptoms. The most significant sign in the diagnosis of Wilson disease results from the deposition of copper in the Descemet membrane of the cornea. These golden-brown deposits can be seen with a slit-lamp and are referred to as Kayser-Fleischer rings. Acute intermittent porphyria, AIP (choice A) is a disorder of heme biosynthesis. AIP is classified as an acute hepatic porphyria and results from defects in gene (HMBS) encoding the enzyme commonly called porphobilinogen deaminase (PBGD). PBGD is also known as hydroxymethylbilane synthase (HMBS). The clinical manifestations of AIP are related to the visceral, autonomic, peripheral, and central nervous system involvement of the disease. In fact, almost all of the symptoms of AIP result from neurologic dysfunction. Hemochromatosis, type 1, also known as primary hemochromatosis (choice B) is a disorder resulting from iron overload. Hemochromatosis is defined as a disorder in iron metabolism that is characterized by excess iron absorption, saturation of iron-binding proteins, and deposition of hemosiderin (amorphous iron deposits) in the tissues. The primary affected tissues are the liver, pancreas, and skin. In hemochromatosis the liver is usually the first organ to be affected. Hepatomegaly will be present in more than 95% of patients manifesting symptoms. Initial symptoms include weakness, abdominal pain, change in skin color and the onset of symptoms of diabetes mellitus. In advanced cases of hemochromatosis there will likely be cardiac arrhythmias, congestive heart failure, testicular atrophy, jaundice, increased pigmentation, spider angiomas, and splenomegaly. Diagnosis of the disease is usually suggested when there is the presence of hepatomegaly, skin pigmentation, diabetes mellitus, heart disease, arthritis, and hypogonadism. Menkes disease (choice C) is a disorder of copper homeostasis. The disorder is associated with an inability to absorb copper from the gastrointestinal tract and an inability of tissues to absorb copper from the blood. Menkes disease is the result of defects in the P-type ATPase protein that is responsible for the translocation of copper across the intestinal basolateral membrane into the blood, thus allowing for uptake of dietary copper. This protein is encoded by the ATPase, Cu^{2+}-transporting, alpha polypeptide (*ATP7A*) gene. The clinical spectrum of Menkes disease includes progressive neurodegeneration, connective tissue abnormalities, and wiry brittle hair. The distinctive clinical features of Menkes disease are usually present by 3 months of age. Infants will lose, or fail to demonstrate, specific developmental milestones and failure to thrive. Most patients with Menkes disease do not survive beyond early childhood. Porphyria cutanea tarda, PCT (choice D) is a disorder of heme biosynthesis. PCT is the result of deficiency in the activity of the heme biosynthetic enzyme, uroporphyrinogen decarboxylase. PCT is a late-onset disease with most affected individuals manifesting symptoms in the fifth to sixth decade of life. The symptoms of PCT are characterized by blistering skin lesions on sun-exposed areas of the skin. Because of this characteristic feature, PCT is strongly indicated in persons who develop skin lesions, particularly on the back of the hands and back of the neck, on exposure to sunlight. In addition to blistering skin lesions, the typical sign of PCT is dark red or purple coloration of the urine.

14. Correct answer is **B.** The image is a microscope field from a blood smear showing the characteristic features of a megaloblast typical of that seen in patients with various forms of megaloblastic anemia. Megaloblastic anemias are most often the result of deficiency of folate or vitamin B_{12} (cobalamin). Pernicious anemia is a megaloblastic anemia resulting from vitamin B_{12} deficiency that develops as a result of a lack of intrinsic factor in the stomach leading to malabsorption of the vitamin. The anemia results from impaired DNA synthesis due to a block in purine and thymidine nucleotide biosynthesis. The block in nucleotide biosynthesis is a consequence of the effect of vitamin B_{12} on folate metabolism. When vitamin B_{12} is deficient essentially all of the folate becomes trapped as the N^5-methyl-THF derivative as a result of the loss of functional methionine synthase. Methionine synthase is a folate and vitamin B_{12}-dependent enzyme. The trapping of folate prevents the synthesis of other THF derivatives required for the purine and thymidine nucleotide biosynthesis pathways. During G_1 phase of the cell cycle, erythroid progenitor cells are synthesizing protein and RNA in preparation for DNA synthesis in the S-phase. The lack of adequate nucleotide synthesis prevents erythroid progenitor cell progression beyond the G_1 phase, which results in their enlarged size and the presence of noncondensed chromatin. Deficiency of none of the other vitamins (choices A, C, D, and E) is associated with the development of megaloblastic anemia.

15. Correct answer is **B.** The patient is most likely exhibiting the signs and symptoms associated with a deficiency in vitamin C, ascorbic acid. The main function of ascorbate is as a reducing agent in a number of different reactions. Ascorbate is the cofactor for Cu^+-dependent monooxygenases and for several 2-oxoglutarate and Fe^{2+}-dependent dioxygenases (2OG-oxygenases). Several critical enzymes that require ascorbate as a cofactor include the collagen processing enzymes, the lysyl hydroxylases and the prolyl hydroxylases as well as the catecholamine synthesis enzyme dopamine β-hydroxylase. The most important reactions requiring ascorbate as a cofactor are the hydroxylation of lysine and proline residues in collagen. Vitamin C is, therefore, required for the maintenance of normal connective tissue as well as for wound healing since synthesis of connective tissue is the first event in wound tissue remodeling. Vitamin C also is necessary for bone remodeling due to the presence of collagen in the organic matrix of bones. Deficiency in vitamin C leads to the disease scurvy due to the role of the vitamin in the posttranslational modification of collagens. Scurvy is characterized by easily bruised skin, petechia, muscle fatigue, soft swollen gums, decreased wound healing, hemorrhaging, osteoporosis, and anemia. Ascorbate deficiency also leads to hemarthrosis (bleeding into joints) that makes movement very painful. Due to its role in collagen processing, the bleeding dysfunction associated with vitamin C deficiency is characterized by the lack of effect on prothrombin time (PT) but with a prolonged bleeding time. The latter effect is the result of the reduced ability for platelets to adhere to exposed subendothelial extracellular matrix collagen which is required for their activation. Nutritional deficiency of pantothenic acid and nicotinic acid could lead to impairment of cholesterol (choice A) and fatty acid (choice B) synthesis due to the role of pantothenic acid in CoA synthesis and nicotinic acid in NADPH synthesis. However, impairment in neither of these pathways would result in the signs and symptoms apparent in this patient. Impairment of glycosaminoglycan synthesis (choice D) or protein *N*-glycosylation (choice E) would not manifest with the signs and symptoms apparent in this patient.

16. Correct answer is **B.** Methionine can be recycled in the context of conversion to, and utilization of, *S*-adenosylmethionine (SAM). The enzymes and intermediates in the methionine recycling constitute what is referred to as the methionine cycle. There are four enzymes in the methionine cycle with one critical enzyme, methionine synthase (also called homocysteine methyltransferase), being dependent on folate and vitamin B_{12} for activity. None of the other vitamins (choices A, C, D, and E) are necessary as cofactors for enzymes of the methionine cycle.

17. Correct answer is **A.** The patient is most likely exhibiting the signs and symptoms associated with a deficiency in vitamin C, ascorbic acid. The main function of ascorbate is as a reducing agent in a number of different reactions. Ascorbate is the cofactor for Cu^+-dependent monooxygenases and for several 2-oxoglutarate and Fe^{2+}-dependent dioxygenases (2OG-oxygenases). Several critical enzymes that require ascorbate as a cofactor include the collagen processing enzymes, the lysyl hydroxylases and the prolyl hydroxylases as well as the catecholamine synthesis enzyme dopamine β-hydroxylase. The most important reactions requiring ascorbate as a cofactor are the hydroxylation of lysine and proline residues in collagen. Vitamin C is, therefore, required for the maintenance of normal connective tissue as well as for wound healing since synthesis of connective tissue is the first event in wound tissue remodeling. Vitamin C also is necessary for bone remodeling due to the presence of collagen in the organic matrix of bones. Deficiency in vitamin C leads to the disease scurvy due to the role of the vitamin in the posttranslational modification of collagens. Scurvy is characterized by easily bruised skin, petechia, muscle fatigue, soft swollen gums, decreased wound healing, hemorrhaging, osteoporosis, and anemia. Ascorbate deficiency also leads to hemarthrosis (bleeding into joints) that makes movement very painful. Due to its role in collagen processing, the bleeding dysfunction associated with vitamin C deficiency is characterized by the lack of effect on prothrombin time (PT) but with a prolonged bleeding time. The latter effect is the result of the reduced ability for platelets to adhere to exposed subendothelial extracellular matrix collagen which is required for their activation. For the major symptoms of deficiencies in cobalamin (choice B), thiamine (choice C), vitamin A (choice D), and vitamin D (choice E) please read the answer descriptions in question 1.

18. Correct answer is **E.** The patient is most likely experiencing the signs and symptoms of a megaloblastic anemia. Megaloblastic anemias are most often the result of deficiency of folate or vitamin B_{12} (cobalamin). Pernicious anemia is a megaloblastic anemia resulting from vitamin B_{12} deficiency that develops as a result of a lack of intrinsic factor in the stomach leading to malabsorption of the vitamin. The anemia results from impaired DNA synthesis due to a block in purine and thymidine nucleotide biosynthesis. The block in nucleotide biosynthesis is a consequence of the effect of vitamin B_{12} on folate metabolism. When vitamin B_{12} is deficient essentially all of the folate becomes trapped as the N^5-methyl-tetrahydrofolate (N^5-methylTHF) derivative as a result of the loss of functional methionine synthase. Methionine synthase is a folate and vitamin B_{12}-dependent enzyme that catalyzes the methylation of homocysteine generating methionine. The methyl group is donated from N^5-methylTHF and the THF is released for use in other THF derivative synthesis pathways. The distinguishing feature exerted by this patient that indicates the symptoms are the result of vitamin B_{12} deficiency and not folate deficiency is the peripheral neuropathy, the numbness and tingling the patient reports he is experiencing in his fingers. Folate derivatives are required for purine nucleotide synthesis (choice A) and thymidine nucleotide biosynthesis (choice B). Folate is absorbed from the gut (choice C) through the action of specific transporters that are not dependent on any other vitamin for activity. The conversion of cystathionine to cysteine (choice D) requires vitamin B_6. A deficiency in vitamin B_6 would lead to microcytic, not macrocytic anemia.

19. Correct answer is **A.** The patient is most likely experiencing the signs and symptoms of a form of aceruloplasminemia leading to iron overload of a form referred to as hemosiderosis. The most severe form of hemosiderosis is that associated with the lethal disorder, Menkes disease. Ceruloplasmin is the major copper-dependent ferroxidase in the blood. Ceruloplasmin binds 6–7 Cu^{2+} (cupric) ions which are required for its ferroxidase activity. Ceruloplasmin plays a major role in ensuring no free ferrous (Fe^{2+}) iron remains in the circulation and that Fe^{2+} iron can be exported from cells. Ceruloplasmin oxidizes Fe^{2+} to Fe^{3+} (ferric) iron which can then be bound to transferrin (choice E), the major iron transporting protein in the blood. Ceruloplasmin is often misrepresented as the major copper transporting protein of the blood due to the fact that up to 95% of copper in the blood is found in this enzyme, however, the major function of ceruloplasmin is as a ferroxidase not as a copper transporter. The primary copper transporting protein in the blood is albumin. There are two ceruloplasmin isoforms generated via alternative mRNA splicing, one form is secreted while the other is attached to the plasma membrane via a glycosylphosphatidylinositol (GPI) linkage. The secreted form of ceruloplasmin is synthesized exclusively by the liver. The GPI-linked isoform is expressed by numerous organs including the brain, liver, kidneys, and lungs. The GPI-linked ceruloplasmin is primarily responsible for iron efflux from tissues. Aceruloplasminemia, due to mutations in the gene encoding ceruloplasmin is not associated with abnormal copper homeostasis but manifests with iron overload of a form referred to as hemosiderosis. Aceruloplasminemia is a rare, recessively inherited neurodegenerative disorder characterized by a lack of ceruloplasmin in the circulation. The lack of ceruloplasmin results in abnormal iron use in the body and leads to iron deposits in various body tissues such as the brain, pancreas, and liver. The iron overload results in neurodegeneration, diabetes, and numerous other symptoms. Ferritin (choice B) is the major intracellular iron storage protein. Ferroportin (choice C) is the basal lateral membrane-associated iron transporter. Mutations in the gene *SLC4A1* that encoded ferroportin results in a form of hemochromatosis, hemochromatosis type 4. Symptoms of type 4 hemochromatosis are similar to those of classic type 1 disease but are generally milder. The unique aspect of type 4 hemochromatosis is that it is inherited as an autosomal dominant disease. Hephaestin (choice D) is the ferroxidase associated with the iron transporter, ferroportin, in hepatocyte and intestinal enterocyte basolateral membranes. Disorders of hephaestin have not been identified in humans, but when the gene (HEPH) encoding this protein is knocked-out in mice it results in iron deficiency and anemia. Transferrin (choice E) is the serum iron transport protein. Reduced levels of transferrin can be observed in patients with liver dysfunction or through excessive urinary excretion, or in certain cancers, or during an infection. Atransferrinemia, which is due to the absence of transferrin synthesis, results in a form of hemosiderosis affecting primarily the heart and liver, which can lead to heart and liver failure.

20. Correct answer is **C.** Fruits and cruciferous vegetables, especially the dark green cruciferous vegetable such as broccoli and kale, are rich sources of vitamin C (ascorbate). The main function of ascorbate is as a reducing agent in a number of different reactions. Ascorbate is the cofactor for Cu^+-dependent monooxygenases and for several 2-oxoglutarate and Fe^{2+}-dependent dioxygenases (2OG-oxygenases). Several critical enzymes that require ascorbate as a cofactor include the collagen processing enzymes, the lysyl hydroxylases and the prolyl hydroxylases as well as the catecholamine synthesis enzyme dopamine β-hydroxylase. The most important reactions requiring ascorbate as a cofactor are the hydroxylation of lysine and proline residues in collagen. Vitamin C is, therefore, required for the maintenance of normal connective tissue as well as for wound healing since synthesis of connective tissue is the first event in wound tissue remodeling. Deficiency in vitamin C leads to the disease scurvy due to the role of the vitamin in the posttranslational modification of collagens. Scurvy is characterized by easily bruised skin, petechia, muscle fatigue, soft swollen gums, decreased wound healing, hemorrhaging, osteoporosis, and anemia. Although fruits and cruciferous vegetables contain numerous vitamins that are important for many metabolic processes in the body, the other processes (choices A, B, D, and E) are not specifically dependent on ascorbate which is present at high levels in fruits and cruciferous vegetables.

21. Correct answer is **C.** The biologically active form of vitamin D, calcitriol, is synthesized in renal tubular epithelial cells. In the liver cholecalciferol (vitamin D_3) is hydroxylated at the 25 position by a specific vitamin D 25-hydroxylase generating 25-hydroxy-D3 [25-(OH)D_3: more commonly called calcidiol]. Conversion of calcidiol to its biologically active form, calcitriol, occurs through the activity of a specific 25-hydroxyvitamin D_3 1-α-hydroxylase (commonly just called 1-α-hydroxylase) present in the inner mitochondrial membrane of cells of the proximal convoluted tubules of the kidneys, and in several extrarenal sites such as in keratinocytes, macrophages, and placenta. Calcitriol functions primarily to regulate calcium and phosphorous homeostasis. The main symptom of vitamin D deficiency in children is rickets and in adults is osteomalacia. Osteomalacia is characterized by demineralization of previously formed bone leading to increased softness and susceptibility to fracture. None of the other pathologies (choices A, B, D, and E) would be directly attributable to renal failure and the loss of calcitriol synthesis.

22. Correct answer is **C.** Photoreception in the eye is the function of two specialized neuron types located in the retina; the rod and cone cells. Both rod and cone cells contain a photoreceptor pigment in their membranes. The photosensitive compound of most mammalian eyes is a protein called opsin to which is covalently coupled an aldehyde of vitamin A. The opsin of rod cells is called scotopsin. The photoreceptor of rod cells is specifically called rhodopsin or visual purple. This compound is a complex between scotopsin and the 11-cis-retinal (also called 11-cis-retinene) form of vitamin A. Rhodopsin is a G-protein coupled receptor (GPCR) embedded in the membrane of the discs inside the outer segment of rod cells. Coupling of 11-cis-retinal occurs at three of the transmembrane domains of rhodopsin. The rod cells are utilized only for seeing at night. During the day rod cells continuously release the excitatory neurotransmitter glutamate. The released glutamate binds to the synaptic membranes of specialized cells called bipolar cells. Activation of bipolar cells induces them to release the inhibitory neurotransmitter, GABA. Release of GABA thus leads to inhibition of the optic nerve. Intracellularly, rhodopsin is coupled to a specific heterotrimeric G-protein called transducing (choice E). The specific G_α-subunit of transduction is identified as $G_{\alpha t}$. The activation of transducin subsequently leads to activation of a cGMP-specific phosphodiesterase (choice A). This phosphodiesterase hydrolyzes the cGMP that is required to maintain a cyclic nucleotide-gated (CNG) ion channel in the open conformation. The CNG ion channel (choice D), when opened via cGMP interaction, transports both Na^+ and Ca^{2+} ions into the rod cell maintaining the cell in a state of depolarization. The loss of cGMP results in closure of the CNG channel resulting in hyperpolarization of the rod cell resulting in termination of glutamate release with disinhibition of the optic nerve being the ultimate role of vitamin A in the visual process. Vitamin A, specifically retinoic acid, functions as a growth factor through its ability to activate a receptor of the nuclear receptor (choice B) superfamily of ligand-activated transcription factors.

23. Correct answer is **B.** The infant is most likely exhibiting a deficiency in the processes of blood coagulation. Neonates are prone to vitamin K deficiency due to the limited levels in their bodies at birth and to limited intake. As a result, newborn infants are prone to a condition referred to as vitamin K deficiency-related bleeding (VKDB). Neonatal VDKB is defined as a bleeding disorder in which the coagulation deficit is rapidly corrected by vitamin K supplementation. The diagnosis of VDKB in an infant is indicated when the prothrombin time (PT) is found to be up to four times longer than the control value even though the infants platelet count and fibrinogen levels are normal. The prothrombin time (PT) is an assay designed to screen for defects in fibrinogen, prothrombin, and factors V, VII, and X. Functional prothrombin, factor VII, and factor X require a vitamin K-dependent modification. When any of these factors is deficient, or defective, the PT is prolonged. In addition to prothrombin, factor VII, and factor X, vitamin K is required for the activation of factor IX, protein C, and protein S. Conversion from inactive to active clotting factor requires a posttranslational modification of specific glutamate (Glu) residues. This modification is a carboxylation and the enzyme responsible, γ-glutamyl carboxylase (GGCX), requires vitamin K as a cofactor. The resultant modified Glu residues are termed γ-carboxyglutamate (*gla*) residues. Thus, a deficiency in vitamin K will result in prolonged bleeding due to loss of clotting factor functions. Modification of lysine (choices C) and proline (choice E) by hydroxylation is required for the normal processing of collagen. Abnormal collagen processing is associated with bleeding dysfunction that is indicative of a normal PT but a prolonged bleeding time. None of the other options (choices A and D) are associated with the processes of hemostasis, blood coagulation.

24. Correct answer is **C.** The ability to synthesize DNA requires a pool of deoxynucleotides, including thymidine nucleotides. The synthesis of the purine nucleotides and thymidine requires the folate derivatives, N^{10}-formyl tetrahydrofolate (N^{10}-formylTHF) and N^5,N^{10}-methyleneTHF, respectively. Although folate derivatives are required for multiple metabolic processes the most pronounced effect of folate deficiency on cellular processes is at the level of DNA synthesis. The reduced capacity to carry out DNA synthesis, as a result of folate deficiency, leads to cell cycle arrest in S-phase of rapidly proliferating cells, in particular hematopoietic cells such as erythroid progenitor cells. The result is a megaloblastic anemia. Although NAD^+, derived from nicotinic acid (choice D), is required for the synthesis of GMP and the synthesis of UMP, deficiency in this vitamin derived cofactor is not associated with the inability of erythroid progenitor cell DNA synthesis to the extent that is observed with a folate deficiency. None of the other vitamins (choices A, B, and E) are directly involved in nucleotide biosynthesis and as a consequence DNA synthesis.

25. Correct answer is **B.** The byproduct of the oxidation of fatty acids with an odd number of carbon atoms is propionyl-CoA. The conversion of propionyl-CoA to the TCA cycle intermediate, succinyl-CoA, occurs through a series of three reactions. The terminal reaction is catalyzed by methylmalonyl-CoA mutase which is dependent on vitamin B_{12} (cobalamin) as a cofactor. The first enzyme in this pathway, propionyl-CoA carboxylase, is a biotin-dependent enzyme. None of the other vitamins (choices A, C, D, and E) are involved in the metabolism of the end-product of oxidation of fatty acids with an odd number of carbon atoms.

26. Correct answer is **B.** The patient is most likely experiencing the signs and symptoms of a megaloblastic anemia apparent from the MCV value. Megaloblastic anemias are most often the result of deficiency of folate or vitamin B_{12} (cobalamin). Pernicious anemia is a megaloblastic anemia resulting from vitamin B_{12} deficiency that develops as a result of a lack of intrinsic factor in the stomach leading to malabsorption of the vitamin. The anemia results from impaired DNA synthesis due to a block in purine and thymidine nucleotide biosynthesis. The block in nucleotide biosynthesis is a consequence of the effect of vitamin B_{12} on folate metabolism. When vitamin B_{12} is deficient essentially all of the folate becomes trapped as the N^5-methyl-THF derivative as a result of the loss of functional methionine synthase. Methionine synthase is a folate and vitamin B_{12}-dependent enzyme. The trapping of folate prevents the synthesis of other THF derivatives required for the purine and thymidine nucleotide biosynthesis pathways. During G_1 phase of the cell cycle, erythroid progenitor cells are synthesizing protein and RNA in preparation for DNA synthesis in the S-phase. The lack of adequate nucleotide synthesis prevents erythroid progenitor cell progression beyond the G_1 phase, which results in their enlarged size and the presence of noncondensed chromatin. Deficiency of vitamin B_{12} results in hematologic, neurologic, and gastrointestinal effects. The hematologic symptoms include a low red blood cell count with large-sized macrocytic red blood cells as evidenced by the MCV value. Absorption of vitamin B_{12} is relatively complicated. The large and not very lipophilic molecule is released from food by the low pH of the stomach and pepsin digestion and binds to haptocorrin produced by salivary glands. Pancreatic proteases then digest the haptocorrin releasing cobalamin in the duodenum. Within the duodenum cobalamin (vitamin B_{12}) complexes with intrinsic factor which is produced by parietal cells of the stomach. Intrinsic factor-cobalamin complexes bind to a specific receptor in the apical membranes of enterocytes of the terminal ileum. Hence, vitamin B_{12} absorption will be low in this patient due to the surgical removal of this region of her small intestine. Liver storage is thought to be sufficient for 2–4 years so that the 3-year latency of the anemia further supports a vitamin B_{12} deficiency. For the major symptoms of deficiencies in ascorbate (choice A), riboflavin (choice C), thiamine (choice D), vitamin A (choice E), and vitamin K (choice F) please read the answer descriptions in question 1.

27. Correct answer is **D.** The patient is most likely experiencing the signs and symptoms of a megaloblastic anemia apparent from the MCV value. Megaloblastic anemias are most often the result of deficiency of folate or vitamin B_{12} (cobalamin). The megaloblastic anemia resulting from vitamin B_{12} deficiency is referred to as pernicious anemia. Pernicious anemia is primarily the result of the lack of intrinsic factor being released from stomach parietal cells leading to subsequent malabsorption of the vitamin. The major cause of the loss of intrinsic factor is an autoimmune destruction of the parietal cells that secrete it. The anemia results from impaired DNA synthesis due to a block in purine and thymidine nucleotide biosynthesis. The block in nucleotide biosynthesis is a consequence of the effect of vitamin B_{12} on folate metabolism. When vitamin B_{12} is deficient essentially all of the folate becomes trapped as the N^5-methyl-THF derivative as a result of the loss of functional methionine synthase. Methionine synthase is a folate and vitamin B_{12}-dependent enzyme. The trapping of folate prevents the synthesis of other THF derivatives required for the purine and thymidine nucleotide biosynthesis pathways. During G_1 phase of the cell cycle, erythroid progenitor cells are synthesizing protein and RNA in preparation for DNA synthesis in the S-phase. The lack of adequate nucleotide synthesis prevents erythroid progenitor cell progression beyond the G_1 phase, which results in their enlarged size and the presence of noncondensed chromatin. Deficiency of vitamin B_{12} results in hematologic, neurologic, and gastrointestinal effects. The hematologic symptoms include a low red blood cell count with large-sized macrocytic red blood cells as evidenced by the MCV value. Absorption of vitamin B_{12} is relatively complicated. The large and not very lipophilic molecule is released from food by the low pH of the stomach and pepsin digestion and binds to haptocorrin produced by salivary glands. Pancreatic proteases then digest the haptocorrin releasing cobalamin in the duodenum. Within the duodenum cobalamin (vitamin B_{12}) complexes with intrinsic factor which is produced by parietal cells of the stomach. Intrinsic factor-cobalamin complexes bind to a specific receptor in the apical membranes of enterocytes of the terminal ileum. Hence, vitamin B_{12} absorption will be low in this patient due to the surgical removal of this region of her small intestine. Liver storage is thought to be sufficient for 2–4 years so that the 3-year latency of the anemia further supports a vitamin B_{12} deficiency. A second B_{12}-dependent enzyme is methylmalonyl-CoA mutase which is involved in the metabolism of propionyl-CoA. The loss of methylmalonyl-CoA mutase activity with deficiencies in B_{12} results in an accompanying methylmalonic acidemia. Measurement for the presence or absence of methylmalonic acidemia is, in fact, diagnostic for the determination of a megaloblastic anemia being the result of vitamin B_{12} deficiency or folate deficiency, respectively. Measurement of none of the other substances (choices A, B, C, and E) would be useful in the diagnosis of the cause of the patient's megaloblastic anemia.

28. Correct answer is **C.** The blood work from of this patient is most likely indicative of a microcytic anemia. Microcytic anemia can often be associated with defective hemoglobin synthesis such as in the case of the β-thalassemias. Microcytic anemia can also result from nutritional deficiency of vitamin B_6 or iron and may also be the result of heavy metal intoxication such as in lead poisoning. Iron deficiency is the most common cause of anemia worldwide. In the absence of adequate iron, heme cannot be synthesized from protoporphyrin IX via the action of ferrochelatase. The lack of heme biosynthesis, in erythroid progenitor cells, results in a block to protein synthesis. Since protein synthesis is impaired in erythroid progenitor cells as a consequence of iron deficiency these cells do not grow during the G_1 phase of the cell cycle resulting in the typical microcytic anemia of iron deficiency. Anemia due to B_{12} or folate deficiency is macrocytic. A deficiency in folate (choice B) or vitamin B_{12} (choice D) would result in a macrocytic, not a microcytic anemia. Acute bleeding (choice A) or vitamin K deficiency (choice E) will not result in microcytic anemia.

29. Correct answer is **A.** Neonates are prone to vitamin K deficiency due to the limited levels in their bodies at birth and also to limited intake. As a result, newborn infants are prone to a condition referred to as vitamin K deficiency-related bleeding (VKDB). Neonatal VDKB is defined as a bleeding disorder in which the coagulation deficit is rapidly corrected by vitamin K supplementation. There are various forms of VKDB that are defined by the age of onset (early, classic, and late) and as either idiopathic or secondary. Early onset VKDB presents within 24 hours of birth and is almost exclusively seen in infants of mothers taking drugs which inhibit vitamin K. These drugs include anticonvulsants (eg, phenytoin, carbamazepine, or barbiturates), antituberculosis drugs (eg, rifampicin), certain antibiotics (eg, cephalosporins), and vitamin K antagonists (eg, warfarin). Loss of vitamin K, as a cofactor, leads to reduced hepatic γ-carboxylation of glutamate residues in several proteins of the coagulation cascade including prothrombin, factors VII, IX, X, and also protein C and protein S. The net effect is defective, potentially fatal, bleeding disorder in a neonate. Deficiency in none of the other processes (choices B, C, D, and E) would be apparent in a pregnant woman taking phenytoin.

30. Correct answer is **C.** The patient is most likely exhibiting the signs and symptoms associated with a deficiency in vitamin C, ascorbic acid. The main function of ascorbate is as a reducing agent in a number of different reactions. Ascorbate is the cofactor for Cu^{+}-dependent monooxygenases and for several 2-oxoglutarate and Fe^{2+}-dependent dioxygenases (2OG-oxygenases). Several critical enzymes that require ascorbate as a cofactor include the collagen processing enzymes, the lysyl hydroxylases and the prolyl hydroxylases as well as the catecholamine synthesis enzyme dopamine β-hydroxylase. The most important reactions requiring ascorbate as a cofactor are the hydroxylation of lysine and proline residues in collagen. Vitamin C is, therefore, required for the maintenance of normal connective tissue as well as for wound healing since synthesis of connective tissue is the first event in wound tissue remodeling. Deficiency in vitamin C leads to the disease scurvy due to the role of the vitamin in the posttranslational modification of collagens. Scurvy is characterized by easily bruised skin, petechia, muscle fatigue, soft swollen gums, decreased wound healing, hemorrhaging, osteoporosis, and anemia. A deficiency in none of the other processes (choices A, B, D, and E) would directly result from a deficiency in vitamin C.

31. Correct answer is **E.** The patient is most likely experiencing the signs and symptoms of Wernicke-Korsakoff syndrome that is caused, in large part, by deficiency of thiamine. The earliest symptoms of thiamine deficiency include constipation, appetite suppression, and nausea. Progressive deficiency will lead to mental depression, peripheral neuropathy, and fatigue. Chronic thiamine deficiency leads to more severe neurologic symptoms including ataxia, mental confusion, and loss of eye coordination (nystagmus). Wernicke-Korsakoff syndrome is most commonly found in chronic alcoholics due to the fact that alcohol impairs thiamine uptake from the small intestine as well as the fact that these individuals generally have poor dietetic lifestyles. Wernicke syndrome is also referred to as dry beriberi. Prolonged dietary deficiency in thiamine leads to wet beriberi. The wet form of the disease is the result of the cardiac involvement in the deficiency. At this stage in the deficiency all four chambers of the heart enlarge due to loss of energy generation and fluid retention resulting in what is called dilated cardiomyopathy. The result of the enlarged chambers is that they can't fill completely resulting in systolic failure. Systole relates to the force associated with cardiac contraction expelling blood to arteries. Blood pumped from the left ventricle enters the aorta and is delivered to the body, whereas blood pumped from the right ventricle is sent to the lungs. Thiamine is rapidly converted to its active form, thiamine pyrophosphate, TPP, by the enzyme thiamine pyrophosphokinase 1, TPK1. TPP is necessary as a cofactor for three critical dehydrogenases. These enzymes are the pyruvate dehydrogenase complex (PDHc) and α-ketoglutarate (2-oxoglutarate) dehydrogenase (OGDH), both of which are associated with the TCA cycle, and branched-chain keto acid dehydrogenase (BCKD) necessary for metabolism of the branched-chain amino acids, leucine, isoleucine, and valine. A deficiency in thiamine intake leads to a severely reduced capacity of cells to generate energy and to carry out reductive biosynthetic reactions as well as to synthesize nucleotides because of its role in the three critical dehydrogenase complexes. A deficiency in vitamin K would lead to deficiency of blood coagulation (choice A). Deficiency of vitamin A would lead to night blindness (choice C). Deficiency of nicotinic acid (niacin) would result in reduced capacity for cholesterol biosynthesis (choice B) and peroxisomal fat oxidation (choice D) as well as contributing to reduced function of the PDHc, OGDH, and BCKD.

32. Correct answer is **E.** Menkes disease is inherited as an X-linked recessive disorder of copper homeostasis. Menkes disease is the result of defects in the P-type ATPase protein that is responsible for the translocation of copper across the intestinal basolateral membrane into the blood, thus allowing for uptake of dietary copper as well as cellular uptake of copper from the blood. This protein is encoded by the ATPase, Cu^{2+}-transporting, alpha polypeptide (*ATP7A*) gene. The reduced uptake of copper results in decreased, or loss of, function of copper-dependent proteins. The clinical spectrum associated with Menkes disease is due in large part to the reduced activity of cytochrome c oxidase, dopamine β-hydroxylase, and ceruloplasmin, all of which are critical Cu^{2+}-dependent enzymes. The clinical spectrum of Menkes disease includes progressive neurodegeneration, connective tissue abnormalities, and wiry brittle hair. The distinctive clinical features of Menkes disease are usually present by 3 months of age. Infants will lose, or fail to demonstrate, specific developmental milestones and failure to thrive. Most patients with Menkes disease do not survive beyond early childhood. Incorporation of copper into copper-dependent proteins, such as ceruloplasmin (choice A), is apparent and contributes to the pathology of Menkes disease, however, this is secondary to the primary defect of impaired uptake of dietary copper. None of the other processes (choices B, C, and D) are directly related to the loss of dietary copper uptake and delivery to tissues.

33. Correct answer is **C.** The signs and symptoms of Wernicke encephalopathy (Wernicke-Korsakoff syndrome) are caused, in large part, by deficiency of thiamine. The earliest symptoms of thiamine deficiency include constipation, appetite suppression, and nausea. Progressive deficiency will lead to mental depression, peripheral neuropathy, and fatigue. Chronic thiamine deficiency leads to more severe neurologic symptoms including ataxia, mental confusion, loss of eye coordination (nystagmus), and paralysis of the extraocular muscles that control the movements of the eye (ophthalmoplegia). None of the other pathologies (choice A, B, D, and E) are found at any significant level in patients with Wernicke encephalopathy.

34. Correct answer is **B.** The patient is most likely experiencing the signs and symptoms of an isolated deficiency in biotin. Given that biotin is synthesized by intestinal bacteria deficiencies of the vitamin are rare. Deficiencies are generally seen only after long antibiotic therapies which deplete the intestinal microbiota or following excessive consumption of raw eggs. The latter is due to the affinity of the egg white protein, avidin, for biotin preventing intestinal absorption of the biotin. The symptoms of biotin deficiency typically appear gradually and can include thinning hair with progression to loss of all hair on the body, scaly, red rash around the eyes, nose, mouth, and perineum, conjunctivitis, seizures, brittle nails, and neurologic findings (eg, depression, lethargy, hallucinations, and paresthesia of the extremities) in adults. Metabolic abnormalities associated with biotin deficiency include lactic acidosis and aciduria. In humans, the biotin-requiring enzymes include acetyl-CoA carboxylase (ACC: humans express two distinct ACC genes), pyruvate carboxylase (PC), propionyl-CoA carboxylase (PCC), and 3-methylcrotonyl-CoA carboxylase (3MCC). The critically important biotin-requiring enzymes are ACC, PC, and PCC. Acetyl-CoA carboxylase is the rate-limiting and highly regulated enzyme required for initiation of fatty acid synthesis.

None of the other processes (choices A, C, D, and E) would be significantly impaired as a result of a deficiency in biotin.

35. Correct answer is **A.** The enzyme methionine synthase (also called homocysteine methyltransferase) requires both folate, in the form of N^5-methyltetrahydrofolate (methyl-THF), and vitamin B_{12} (cobalamin) for its activity. In the direction of methionine synthesis, the enzyme utilizes the methyl group from methyl-THF in the methylation of homocysteine. During this reaction the methyl-group is initially transferred to cobalamin generating methylcobalamin and tetrahydrofolate (THF). The methyl group is then transferred to homocysteine generating methionine and cobalamin. A deficiency in either folate or vitamin B_{12} will, therefore, result in the accumulation of homocysteine. Homocysteine can be oxidized to homocystine which is two homocysteines disulfide bonded together. The accumulating homocystine is excreted in the urine and is referred to as homocystinuria. None of the other substances (choices B, C, D, and E) would be increased or decreased as a result of a deficiency of either folate or vitamin B_{12}.

36. Correct answer is **A.** The patient is most likely experiencing the signs and symptoms of Wernicke-Korsakoff syndrome that is caused, in large part, by deficiency of thiamine. The earliest symptoms of thiamine deficiency include constipation, appetite suppression, and nausea. Progressive deficiency will lead to mental depression, peripheral neuropathy, and fatigue. Chronic thiamine deficiency leads to more severe neurologic symptoms including ataxia, mental confusion, and loss of eye coordination (nystagmus). Wernicke-Korsakoff syndrome is most commonly found in chronic alcoholics due to the fact that alcohol impairs thiamine uptake from the small intestine as well as the fact that these individuals generally have poor dietetic lifestyles. Wernicke syndrome is also referred to as dry beriberi. Prolonged dietary deficiency in thiamine leads to wet beriberi. The wet form of the disease is the result of the cardiac involvement in the deficiency. At this stage in the deficiency all four chambers of the heart enlarge due to loss of energy generation and fluid retention resulting in what is called dilated cardiomyopathy. The result of the enlarged chambers is that they cannot fill completely resulting in systolic failure. Systole relates to the force associated with cardiac contraction expelling blood to arteries. Blood pumped from the left ventricle enters the aorta and is delivered to the body, whereas blood pumped from the right ventricle is sent to the lungs. Thiamine is rapidly converted to its active form, thiamine pyrophosphate, TPP, by the enzyme thiamine pyrophosphokinase 1, TPK1. TPP is necessary as a cofactor for three critical dehydrogenases. These enzymes are branched-chain keto acid dehydrogenase (BCKD) which is necessary for metabolism of the branched-chain amino acids, leucine, isoleucine, and valine and the pyruvate dehydrogenase complex (PDHc) and α-ketoglutarate (2-oxoglutarate) dehydrogenase (OGDH) complex, both of which are associated with the TCA cycle. Deficiency of biotin, as well as nicotinic acid (niacin), would result in a reduced capacity for gluconeogenesis (choice B) leading to hypoglycemia and lactic acidemia. A deficiency in vitamin B_6 would lead to impaired synthesis of heme (choice C) leading to microcytic anemia. A deficiency in vitamin C would lead to impaired collagen processing (choice D) which is the cause of the symptoms of scurvy. A deficiency in vitamin K would lead to impaired posttranslational processing of prothrombin (choice E) leading to prolonged bleeding. A deficiency in folate would result in impaired synthesis of thymidine (choice F) and purine nucleotides leading to the development of a megaloblastic anemia.

37. Correct answer is **C.** The patient is most likely exhibiting the signs and symptoms of tuberculosis. The standard treatment for nondrug resistant tuberculosis is with the use of isoniazid, ethambutol, rifampin, and pyrazinamide. Long-term administration of isoniazid will lead to impaired conversion of pyridoxine (vitamin B_6) to pyridoxal phosphate, PLP. In addition, metabolites of isoniazid deactivate pyridoxine. Pyridoxal phosphate is required for numerous enzymes including all aminotransferases, glycogen phosphorylase, cystathionine β-synthase, and δ-aminolevulinic acid synthase, ALAS. ALAS is the first and rate-limiting enzyme of heme biosynthesis. One of the consequences of long-term isoniazid therapy, in the treatment of tuberculosis, is microcytic anemia due to the reduced activity of ALAS and the resultant decreased synthesis of heme. None of the other processes (choices A, B, D, and E) would be significantly affected by the effects of the drugs used to treat tuberculosis.

38. Correct answer is **E.** Thiamine is rapidly converted to its active form, thiamine pyrophosphate, TPP, by the enzyme thiamine pyrophosphokinase 1, TPK1. TPP is necessary as a cofactor for three critical dehydrogenases. These enzymes are the pyruvate dehydrogenase complex (PDHc) and α-ketoglutarate (2-oxoglutarate) dehydrogenase (OGDH), both of which are associated with the TCA cycle, and branched-chain ketoacid dehydrogenase (BCKD) necessary for metabolism of the branched-chain amino acids, leucine, isoleucine, and valine. These three dehydrogenases also require the cofactors derived from the vitamins lipoic acid, pantothenic acid (CoA), riboflavin, and niacin. For this reason, these three dehydrogenases are often referred to as the Tender (thiamine) Loving (lipoic acid) Care (CoA) For (flavin) Nancy (niacin) enzymes. In addition to these three dehydrogenases, TPP is a required cofactor for the transketolase catalyzed reactions of the pentose phosphate pathway, and it is required for the catabolism of the methyl-substituted fatty acid (phytanic acid) at the 2-hydroxyphytanoyl-CoA lyase reaction. The three dehydrogenases are localized to the mitochondria and the 2-hydroxyphytanoyl-CoA lyase enzyme is localized to the peroxisomes. These locations make it very difficult to easily and rapidly assess their activity in association with thiamine deficiency. The transketolase enzyme is expressed at high levels in red blood cells because of the need for the pentose phosphate pathway in the generation of NADPH needed to maintain the redox state of red blood cells. For this reason, assay of red blood cells for transketolase activity is the primary diagnostic tool to assess patient suspected of being deficient in thiamine. Delta-aminolevulinic acid synthase, ALAS (choice A) and glycogen synthase (choice B) both require vitamin B_6 as a cofactor. Pyruvate carboxylase (choice C) is a biotin-dependent enzyme. As indicated, pyruvate dehydrogenase (choice D) is localized to the mitochondria and would be difficult to assay for activity in a patient suspected of having thiamine deficiency.

39. Correct answer is **E.** The patient is most likely experiencing the signs and symptoms of a deficiency of thiamine. The earliest symptoms of thiamine deficiency include constipation, appetite suppression, and nausea. Progressive deficiency will lead to mental depression, peripheral neuropathy, and fatigue. Chronic thiamine deficiency leads to more severe neurologic symptoms including ataxia, mental confusion, and loss of eye coordination (nystagmus). Wernicke-Korsakoff syndrome is most commonly found in chronic alcoholics due to the fact that alcohol impairs thiamine uptake from the small intestine as well as the fact that these individuals generally have poor dietetic lifestyles. Thiamine is rapidly converted to its active form, thiamine pyrophosphate (TPP) by the enzyme thiamine pyrophosphokinase 1, TPK1. TPP is necessary as a cofactor for three critical dehydrogenases. These enzymes are branched-chain keto acid dehydrogenase (BCKD) which is necessary for metabolism of the branched-chain amino acids, leucine, isoleucine, and valine and the pyruvate dehydrogenase complex (PDHc) and α-ketoglutarate (2-oxoglutarate) dehydrogenase (OGDH) complex, both of which are associated with the TCA cycle. Since TPP is necessary as a cofactor for the pyruvate dehydrogenase complex (PDHc) a deficiency in thiamine would result in impaired oxidation of pyruvate. This will lead to increased plasma concentrations of pyruvate. When lactate from erythrocyte and skeletal muscle metabolism reaches the liver, it will not be readily converted to pyruvate due to the reduced pyruvate oxidative capacity leading to elevated plasma lactate. In addition, the excess pyruvate will be a substrate for lactate dehydrogenase resulting in additionally increased levels of pyruvate. Erythrocyte transketolase requires TPP for activity, thus, in thiamine deficiency transketolase activity would be reduced, not increased (choice A). The requirement for thiamine by the OGDH complex results in reduced, not increased activity of leukocyte OGDH activity (choice B). Iron deficiency would result in a decrease serum ferritin level, not an increase (choice C). Nutritional deficiency of B6 would impair glycogen phosphorylase activity which could lead to decreased plasma glucose concentration, not increased (choice D).

40. Correct answer is **D.** Thiamine is rapidly converted to its active form, thiamine pyrophosphate, TPP, by the enzyme thiamine pyrophosphokinase 1, TPK1. TPP is necessary as a cofactor for three critical dehydrogenases. These enzymes are branched-chain keto acid dehydrogenase (BCKD) which is necessary for metabolism of the branched-chain amino acids, leucine, isoleucine, and valine and the pyruvate dehydrogenase complex (PDHc) and α-ketoglutarate (2-oxoglutarate) dehydrogenase (OGDH) complex, both of which are associated with the TCA cycle. Since TPP is necessary as a cofactor for the pyruvate dehydrogenase complex (PDHc) a deficiency in thiamine would result in impaired oxidation of pyruvate to acetyl-CoA. The biosynthesis of fatty acids from acetyl-CoA (choice A), the synthesis of ketone bodies (choice B), and the conversion of glycerol to glucose (choice C) all require the nicotinic acid derived cofactors NAD^+, NADH, or NADPH. There is no direct involvement of vitamins in the storage of glucose in glycogen (choice E).

41. Correct answer is **E.** The patient is most likely experiencing the signs and symptoms of a megaloblastic anemia apparent from the MCV value. Megaloblastic anemias are most often the result of deficiency of folate or vitamin B_{12} (cobalamin). The megaloblastic anemia resulting from vitamin B_{12} deficiency is referred to as pernicious anemia. The anemia results from impaired DNA synthesis due to a block in purine and thymidine nucleotide biosynthesis. The block in nucleotide biosynthesis is a consequence of the effect of vitamin B_{12} on folate metabolism. When vitamin B_{12} is deficient essentially all of the folate becomes trapped as the N^5-methyl-THF derivative as a result of the loss of functional methionine synthase. Methionine synthase is a folate and vitamin B_{12}-dependent enzyme. The trapping of folate prevents the synthesis of other THF derivatives required for the purine and thymidine nucleotide biosynthesis pathways. Rice contains niacin, thiamine, vitamin B_6, and riboflavin among the many nutritional compounds. Branched-chain amino acid catabolism (choice A), the pentose phosphate pathway (choice B), and heme biosynthesis (choice D) require niacin and/or vitamin B_6 and as such would not be significantly affected in this patient. Gut microbiota synthesize biotin which is required by pyruvate carboxylase of the pathway of gluconeogenesis (choice C), therefore, this pathway would also be minimally affected by this patient's diet.

42. Correct answer is **A.** Macrocytic (megaloblastic) anemias are most often the result of deficiency of folate or vitamin B_{12} (cobalamin). The megaloblastic anemia resulting from vitamin B_{12} deficiency as a result of the loss of intrinsic factor is referred to as pernicious anemia. The megaloblastic anemia caused by vitamin B_{12} deficiency results from impaired DNA synthesis due to a block in purine and thymidine nucleotide biosynthesis exactly as is the case for deficiency of folate itself. The block in nucleotide biosynthesis is a consequence of the effect of vitamin B_{12} on folate metabolism. When vitamin B_{12} is deficient essentially all of the folate becomes trapped as the N^5-methyl-THF derivative as a result of the loss of functional methionine synthase. Methionine synthase is a folate and vitamin B_{12}-dependent enzyme. The trapping of folate prevents the synthesis of other THF derivatives required for the purine and thymidine nucleotide biosynthesis pathways. Pyridoxine, vitamin B_6 (choice C) is the precursor for pyridoxal phosphate which is required of many enzymes including δ-aminolevulinic acid synthase (ALAS) which is the initial and rate limiting enzyme of heme biosynthesis. Deficiencies of vitamin B_6 results in microcytic, not macrocytic anemias, due to reduced capacity to synthesize heme. Deficiency in none of the other vitamins (choices B, D, E, F, and G) would directly lead to the development of macrocytic anemia.

43. Correct answer is **B.** Strict vegan diets are frequently deficient in bioavailable vitamin B_{12}. Vitamin B_{12} is a critical coenzyme in the methionine synthase and methylmalonyl-CoA mutase catalyzed reactions. Therefore, a deficiency in vitamin B_{12} results in defective activity of these two enzymes. Methylmalonyl-CoA mutase is involved in the conversion of propionyl-CoA to the TCA cycle intermediate, succinyl-CoA, specifically the reaction whereby methylmalonyl-CoA is converted to succinyl-CoA. The inability to convert methylmalonyl-CoA to succinyl-CoA leads to excess excretion of methylmalonic acid in the urine as well as increased concentrations in the blood. Indeed, in patients with megaloblastic anemias measurement of urinary methylmalonic acid allows for discrimination between deficiency of vitamin B_{12} and deficiency in folate as the cause of the anemia. Elevated urinary methylmalonic acid is not indicative of any of the other abnormalities (choices A, C, D, E, and F).

44. Correct answer is **D.** Parietal cells of the stomach are responsible for the production of gastric acid via transporter mediated efflux of proton (H^+) and chloride ion (Cl^-). In addition, parietal cells produce intrinsic factor, a highly glycosylated protein required for absorption of dietary vitamin B_{12} in the distal ileum. Secretion of intrinsic factor occurs from parietal cells simultaneous with the stimulation to produce gastric acid. Autoimmune destruction of intrinsic factor producing parietal cells results in a particular form of megaloblastic anemia referred to as pernicious anemia. The enzyme cofactor forms of vitamin B_{12} are required by only two enzymes in humans, methionine synthase and methylmalonyl-CoA mutase. Methylmalonyl-CoA mutase is involved in the conversion of propionyl-CoA to the TCA cycle intermediate, succinyl-CoA, specifically the reaction whereby methylmalonyl-CoA is converted to succinyl-CoA. A deficiency in vitamin B_{12}, which impairs the activity of methylmalonyl-CoA mutase, will be associated with elevated levels of methylmalonic acid, thereby being detectable at elevated levels is both the blood and urine. The role of vitamin B_{12} in methionine synthase would lead to an inability to synthesize methionine but are not its metabolism (choice C). The conversion of propionyl-CoA to succinyl-CoA would be reduced, as a consequence of a deficiency in vitamin B_{12}, but the first two enzymes of this pathway would be unaffected such that propionate metabolism (choice E) would continue to methylmalonic acid. Metabolism of acetate (choice A) and lactate (choice B) would not be affected by deficiency in vitamin B_{12} that results from autoimmune destruction of gastric parietal cells.

45. Correct answer is **D.** The patient is most likely exhibiting the signs and symptoms associated with a deficiency in vitamin C, ascorbic acid. The main function of ascorbate is as a reducing agent in a number of different reactions. Ascorbate is the cofactor for Cu^+-dependent monooxygenases and for several 2-oxoglutarate and Fe^{2+}-dependent dioxygenases (2OG-oxygenases). Several critical enzymes that require ascorbate as a cofactor include the collagen processing enzymes, the lysyl hydroxylases and the prolyl hydroxylases as well as the catecholamine synthesis enzyme dopamine β-hydroxylase. The most important reactions requiring ascorbate as a cofactor are the hydroxylation of lysine and proline residues in collagen. Vitamin C is, therefore, required for the maintenance of normal connective tissue as well as for wound healing since synthesis of connective tissue is the first event in wound tissue remodeling. Deficiency in vitamin C leads to the disease scurvy due to the role of the vitamin in the posttranslational modification of collagens. Scurvy is characterized by easily bruised skin, petechia, muscle fatigue, soft swollen gums, decreased wound healing, hemorrhaging, osteoporosis, and anemia. For the major symptoms of deficiencies in riboflavin (choice A), thiamine (choice B), vitamin A (choice C), and vitamin K (choice E) please read the answer descriptions in question 1.

46. Correct answer is **C.** The findings of bleeding gums and petechiae in this patient is most likely indicative of a deficiency in vitamin C, ascorbic acid. The main function of ascorbate is as a reducing agent in a number of different reactions. Ascorbate is the cofactor for Cu^+-dependent monooxygenases and for several 2-oxoglutarate and Fe^{2+}-dependent dioxygenases (2OG-oxygenases). Several critical enzymes that require ascorbate as a cofactor include the collagen processing enzymes, the lysyl hydroxylases and the prolyl hydroxylases as well as the catecholamine synthesis enzyme dopamine β-hydroxylase. The most important reactions requiring ascorbate as a cofactor are the hydroxylation of lysine and proline residues in collagen. Vitamin C is, therefore, required for the maintenance of normal connective tissue as well as for wound healing since synthesis of connective tissue is the first event in wound tissue remodeling. Deficiency in vitamin C leads to the disease scurvy due to the role of the vitamin in the posttranslational modification of collagens. Scurvy is characterized by easily bruised skin, petechia, muscle fatigue, soft swollen gums, decreased wound healing, hemorrhaging, osteoporosis, and anemia. Vitamin C is not directly involved in any of the other processes (choices A, B, D, and E).

47. Correct answer is **C.** The biologically active form of vitamin D, calcitriol, is synthesized in renal tubular epithelial cells. In the liver cholecalciferol (vitamin D_3) is hydroxylated at the 25 position by a specific vitamin D 25-hydroxylase generating 25-hydroxy-D3 [25-(OH)D_3: more commonly called calcidiol]. Conversion of calcidiol to its biologically active form, calcitriol, occurs through the activity of a specific 25-hydroxyvitamin D_3 1-α-hydroxylase (commonly just called 1-α-hydroxylase) present in the inner mitochondrial membrane of cells of the proximal convoluted tubules of the kidneys, and in several extrarenal sites such as in keratinocytes, macrophages, and placenta. Although liver dysfunction (choice D) will lead to reduced calcidiol production, and consequently a reduced capacity for the kidney to produce calcitriol, this is not the organ responsible for making the hormonally active form of vitamin D. None of the other tissues (choices A, B, and E) contribute to calcitriol synthesis.

48. Correct answer is **F.** Due to the biliary obstruction the patient will have poor fat digestion and absorption and so will have reduced uptake of fat-soluble vitamins. In order for the fat-soluble vitamins to be absorbed from the intestines they must be emulsified along with all the other fatty molecules in the diet. The primary mechanism for fat emulsification is the release of bile salts from the gallbladder in response to food intake. The bile salts are synthesized from cholesterol within hepatocytes and then transported to the gallbladder via the bile canaliculi. Thus, cirrhosis of the biliary circulatory system will lead to impaired absorption of fats including fat-soluble vitamins such as vitamin E. The major function of vitamin E is to act as a natural antioxidant by scavenging free radicals and molecular oxygen. In particular, vitamin E is important for preventing peroxidation of polyunsaturated membrane fatty acids and the lipids in circulating lipoprotein particles such as LDL. Reduced uptake of vitamin E will, therefore, result in an increase in the level of oxidized LDL (oxLDL) in the circulation. None of the other options (choice A, B, C, D, and E) would be directly correlated to the reduced fat digestion and absorption typical in a patient with biliary obstruction.

49. Correct answer is **G.** Patients with cystic fibrosis exhibit abnormal transport of chloride and sodium across an epithelium, leading to thick, viscous secretions. In addition, there is a reduced or lack of pancreatic secretions into the gut leading to difficulty absorbing nutrients with their subsequent excretion in the feces. Individuals with cystic fibrosis also have difficulties digesting and absorbing the lipid components of their diet, including the fat-soluble vitamins. The major function of vitamin K is in the maintenance of normal levels of the blood clotting proteins, prothrombin, and factors VII, IX, X, and protein C and protein S, which are synthesized in the liver as inactive precursor proteins. Conversion from inactive to active clotting factor requires a posttranslational modification of specific glutamate (E) residues. This modification is a carboxylation and the enzyme responsible, γ-glutamyl carboxylase (GGCX), requires vitamin K as a cofactor. The vitamin K deficiency typical in patients with cystic fibrosis contributes to their bleeding dysfunction. Deficiency in none of the other components (choices A, B, C, D, E, and F) significantly contribute to the bleeding dysfunction in the cystic fibrosis patients.

50. Correct answer is **D.** The patient is most likely exhibiting the signs and symptoms of tuberculosis. The standard treatment for nondrug resistant tuberculosis is with the use of isoniazid, ethambutol, rifampin, and pyrazinamide. Long-term administration of isoniazid will lead to impaired conversion of pyridoxine (vitamin B_6) to pyridoxal phosphate, PLP. In addition, metabolites of isoniazid deactivate pyridoxine. Pyridoxal phosphate, is required for numerous enzymes including all aminotransferases, glycogen phosphorylase, cystathionine β-synthase, and δ-aminolevulinic acid synthase, ALAS. ALAS is the first and rate-limiting enzyme of heme biosynthesis. One of the consequences of long-term isoniazid therapy, in the treatment of tuberculosis, is microcytic anemia due to the reduced activity of ALAS and the resultant decreased synthesis of heme. None of the other substances (choices A, B, C, E, and F) would be significantly defective by the effects of the drugs used to treat tuberculosis.

51. Correct answer is **E.** The steatorrhea evident in this patient is most likely indicative of a fat malabsorptive syndrome. The inability to digest and absorb lipids is associated with deficiencies in the fat-soluble vitamins. The major function of vitamin K is in the maintenance of normal levels of the blood clotting proteins, prothrombin, and factors VII, IX, X, and protein C and protein S, which are synthesized in the liver as inactive precursor proteins. Conversion from inactive to active clotting factor requires a posttranslational modification of specific glutamate (E) residues. This modification is a carboxylation and the enzyme responsible, γ-glutamyl carboxylase (GGCX), requires vitamin K as a cofactor. The prothrombin time (PT) is an assay designed to screen for defects in fibrinogen, prothrombin, and factors V, VII, and X and thus measures activities of the extrinsic pathway of coagulation. When any of these factors is deficient then the PT is prolonged. The vitamin K deficiency that would most likely be apparent in this patient would, therefore, be associated with an abnormal prothrombin time. None of the other diagnostic assays (choices A, B, C, and D) would be as useful in an accurate diagnosis in this patient.

52. Correct answer is **E.** The patient is most likely experiencing the signs and symptoms of Wernicke-Korsakoff syndrome that is caused, in large part, by deficiency of thiamine. The earliest symptoms of thiamine deficiency include constipation, appetite suppression, and nausea. Progressive deficiency will lead to mental depression, peripheral neuropathy, and fatigue. Chronic thiamine deficiency leads to more severe neurologic symptoms including ataxia, mental confusion, and loss of eye coordination (nystagmus). Wernicke-Korsakoff syndrome is most commonly found in chronic alcoholics due to the fact that alcohol impairs thiamine uptake from the small intestine as well as the fact that these individuals generally have poor dietetic lifestyles. Wernicke syndrome is also referred to as dry beriberi. Prolonged dietary deficiency in thiamine leads to wet beriberi. The wet form of the disease is the result of the cardiac involvement in the deficiency. At this stage in the deficiency all four chambers of the heart enlarge due to loss of energy generation and fluid retention resulting in what is called dilated cardiomyopathy which is distinct in pathology from hypertrophic cardiomyopathy (choice B). Dermatitis (choice A) can result from numerous causes one of which is deficiency in niacin. Megaloblastic anemia (choice C) is most often the result of a deficiency in folate or vitamin B_{12}. Night blindness (choice D) is the earliest symptoms of a deficiency in vitamin A.

53. Correct answer is **F.** The patient is exhibiting the signs and symptoms of a deficiency in vitamin A. The earliest symptoms of vitamin A deficiency are night blindness. Additional early symptoms include follicular hyperkeratosis, increased susceptibility to infection and cancer and anemia equivalent to iron-deficient anemia. Prolonged lack of vitamin A leads to deterioration of the eye tissue through progressive keratinization of the cornea which results in abnormal dryness of the conjunctiva and cornea and the lack of ability to produce tears, a condition known as xerophthalmia. The progressive drying and keratinization of the conjunctiva, particularly on the nasal and temporal conjunctiva, results in the development of irregularly shaped spots termed Bitot ("bee toe") spots after the French physician, Pierre Bitot, who first described them. None of the other options (choices A, B, C, D, and E) are contributory to night blindness and the development of Bitot spots on the conjunctiva of the eyes.

54. Correct answer is **B.** The patient is most likely experiencing the classic symptoms of a deficiency in niacin. A diet deficient in niacin (as well as tryptophan) leads to glossitis of the tongue (inflammation of the tongue leading to purplish discoloration), dermatitis, weight loss, diarrhea, depression, and dementia. The severe symptoms, depression (or dementia), dermatitis, and diarrhea (referred to as the "3-D's" of niacin deficiency), are associated with the condition known as pellagra. The symptoms of biotin deficiency (choice A) typically appear gradually and can include thinning hair with progression to loss of all hair on the body, scaly, red rash around the eyes, nose, mouth, and perineum, conjunctivitis, seizures, brittle nails, and neurologic findings (eg, depression, lethargy, hallucinations, and paresthesia of the extremities) in adults. Deficiency in vitamin C (choice F) leads to the disease scurvy due to the role of the vitamin in the posttranslational modification of collagens. Scurvy is characterized by easily bruised skin, petechia, muscle fatigue, soft swollen gums, decreased wound healing, hemorrhaging, osteoporosis, and anemia. Ascorbate deficiency also leads to hemarthrosis (bleeding into joints) that makes movement very painful. For the major symptoms of deficiencies in riboflavin (choice C), thiamine (choice D), vitamin B_{12} (choice E), and vitamin K (choice G) please read the answer descriptions in question 1.

55. Correct answer is **B.** The patient is most likely experiencing the classic symptoms of a deficiency in niacin. A diet deficient in niacin (as well as tryptophan) leads to glossitis of the tongue (inflammation of the tongue leading to purplish discoloration), dermatitis, weight loss, diarrhea, depression, and dementia. The severe symptoms, depression (or dementia), dermatitis, and diarrhea (referred to as the "3-D's" of niacin deficiency), are associated with the condition known as pellagra. Niacin is the precursor for the vitamin cofactor, nicotinamide adenine dinucleotide (NAD^+ and $NADP^+$). Most reductive biosynthetic reactions, such as fatty acid synthesis, require the reduced electron carrier NADPH. During the synthesis of the catecholamines (choice A), the enzyme DOPA decarboxylase requires vitamin B_6 and the enzyme dopamine β-hydroxylase requires vitamin C. Although the hepatic enzyme glyceraldehyde-3-phosphate dehydrogenase requires NADH in the direction of gluconeogenesis (choice C), this pathway cannot begin without prior activation of the biotin-dependent enzyme, pyruvate carboxylase. Heme biosynthesis (choice D) is initiated, and regulated, by the vitamin B_6-dependent enzyme, δ-aminolevulinic acid synthase. Thymidine nucleotide biosynthesis (choice E) requires folate in the form of N^5,N^{10}-methylene tetrahydrofolate.

56. Correct answer is **D.** The patient is most likely manifesting the signs and symptoms of Menkes disease. Menkes disease is inherited as an X-linked recessive disorder of copper homeostasis. The disorder is associated with an inability to absorb copper from the gastrointestinal tract and an inability of tissues to absorb copper from the blood. Menkes disease is the result of defects in the P-type ATPase protein that is responsible for the translocation of copper across the intestinal basolateral membrane into the blood, thus allowing for uptake of dietary copper. This protein is encoded by the ATPase, Cu^{2+}-transporting, alpha polypeptide (*ATP7A*) gene. The loss of copper transport results in the reduced, or loss of, function of copper-dependent proteins. The clinical spectrum associated with Menkes disease is due in large part to the reduced activity of cytochrome c oxidase, dopamine β-hydroxylase, and ceruloplasmin, all of which are critical Cu^{2+}-dependent enzymes. The clinical spectrum of Menkes disease includes progressive neurodegeneration, connective tissue abnormalities, and wiry brittle hair. Progressive cerebral degeneration in Menkes disease occurs primarily due to loss of the Cu^{2+}-dependent enzymes, ceruloplasmin, cytochrome c oxidase, peptidylglycine α-amidating monooxygenase, and dopamine β-hydroxylase in the central nervous system and to the loss of iron homeostasis in the brain. The defective brain iron homeostasis is due to the loss of activity of the ferroxidase, ceruloplasmin. Within most tissues, ceruloplasmin is bound to the plasma membrane via a glycosylphosphatidylinositol (GPI) linkage and the function of GPI-ceruloplasmin is iron efflux from the tissues. Without adequate iron homeostasis, the brain accumulates iron resulting in the toxic effects of iron overload. The iron overload due to defective, or no, ceruloplasmin activity is a form of hemochromatosis termed hemosiderosis. The distinctive clinical features of Menkes disease are usually present by 3 months of age. Infants will lose, or fail to demonstrate, specific developmental milestones and failure to thrive. Most patients with Menkes disease do not survive beyond early childhood. The Crigler-Najjar syndromes (choice A) are of two forms, type 1 and type 2, both of which result as a consequence of defects in the metabolism and/or excretion of bilirubin. Crigler-Najjar syndrome, type 1 results from mutations in the bilirubin-UDP-glucuronosyltransferase gene that result in complete loss of enzyme activity, whereas type 2 is the result of mutations that cause reduced levels of enzyme activity. Gilbert (pronounced "zheel-bear") syndrome (choice B) belongs to the family of disorders that result as a consequence of defects in the metabolism and/or excretion of bilirubin. Gilbert syndrome is also referred to as constitutional hepatic dysfunction and familial nonhemolytic jaundice. The syndrome is characterized by mild chronic, unconjugated hyperbilirubinemia. Almost all afflicted individuals have a degree of icteric discoloration in the eyes typical of jaundice. Serum bilirubin levels in Gilbert syndrome patients is usually less than 3 mg/dL. Many patients manifest with fatigue and abdominal discomfort, symptoms that are ascribed to anxiety, but are not due to bilirubin metabolism. Hemochromatosis (choice C) is defined as a disorder in iron metabolism that is characterized by excess iron absorption, saturation of iron-binding proteins, and deposition of hemosiderin (amorphous iron deposits) in the tissues. The primary affected tissues are the liver, pancreas, and skin. Iron deposition in the liver leads to cirrhosis and in the pancreas causes diabetes. The excess iron deposition leads to bronze pigmentation of the organs and skin. In fact, the bronze skin pigmentation seen in hemochromatosis, coupled with the resultant diabetes, led to the designation of this condition as bronze diabetes. Refsum disease (choice E) is due to deficiencies in the peroxisomal enzyme responsible for one of the initial steps in the oxidation of phytanic acid, a 3-methyl substituted fatty acid derived from the chlorophyll, phytol. The cardinal clinical features of Refsum disease are retinitis pigmentosa, chronic polyneuropathy, cerebellar ataxia, and elevated protein levels in cerebrospinal fluid. Most Refsum patients have electrocardiographic changes, and some have sensorineural hearing loss and/or ichthyosis. Multiple epiphyseal dysplasia (skeletal malformations) is a conspicuous feature in some cases. Refsum disease is a slowly developing, progressive peripheral neuropathy.

57. Correct answer is **E.** The patient is experiencing the signs and symptoms of Wilson disease. Wilson disease (WD) is characterized by excessive copper deposition primarily in the liver and brain. These sites of copper deposition are reflective of the major manifestations of Wilson disease. Wilson disease is the result of defects in the P-type ATPase protein that is primarily responsible for copper homeostasis effected by the liver. This protein is encoded by the ATPase, Cu^{2+}-transporting, beta polypeptide (*ATP7B*) gene. The majority of patients with Wilson disease present with hepatic or neuropsychiatric symptoms. Hepatic presentation in Wilson disease occurs in late childhood or adolescence. The symptoms in these patients include hepatic failure, acute hepatitis, or progressive chronic liver disease. Patients that manifest neurologic symptoms of Wilson disease present in the second to third decade of life. In these patients, there will be extrapyramidal, cerebellar, and cerebral-related symptoms such as Parkinsonian tremors, diminished facial expressions and movement, dystonia, and choreoathetosis. About 30% of Wilson disease patients will exhibit psychiatric disturbances that include changes in behavior, personality changes, depression, attention-deficit hyperactivity disorder, paranoid psychosis, suicidal tendencies, and impulsivity. As the disease progresses copper deposition leads to vacuolar degeneration in the proximal tubular cells of the kidneys which causes a renal Fanconi syndrome (substances that are normally absorbed by the kidney are excreted in the urine). Acute release of copper into the circulation results in damage to red blood cells resulting in hemolysis. The most significant sign in the diagnosis of Wilson disease results from the deposition of copper in Descemet membrane of the cornea. These golden-brown deposits can be seen with a slit-lamp and are Kayser-Fleischer rings. Aceruloplasminemia (choice A), due to mutations in the gene encoding ceruloplasmin, manifests with iron overload of a form referred to as hemosiderosis. Aceruloplasminemia is a rare, recessively inherited neurodegenerative disorder characterized by a lack of ceruloplasmin in the circulation. The lack of ceruloplasmin results in abnormal iron use in the body and leads to iron deposits in various body tissues such as the brain, pancreas, and liver. The iron overload results in neurodegeneration, diabetes, and numerous other symptoms. GRACILE (GRACILE = growth retardation, aminoaciduria, cholestasis, iron overload, lactic acidosis, early death) syndrome (choice B) is a very rare neonatal lethal disorder caused by defects in the BCS1L that encodes a member of the AAA family of ATPases that is necessary for the assembly of complex III of oxidative phosphorylation. Hemochromatosis (choice C) is a disorder resulting from iron overload. Hemochromatosis is defined as a disorder in iron metabolism that is characterized by excess iron absorption, saturation of iron-binding proteins, and deposition of hemosiderin (amorphous iron deposits) in the tissues. The primary affected tissues are the liver, pancreas, and skin. Initial symptoms include weakness, abdominal pain, change in skin color and the onset of symptoms of diabetes mellitus. In advanced cases of hemochromatosis there will likely be cardiac arrhythmias, congestive heart failure, testicular atrophy, jaundice, increased pigmentation, spider angiomas, and splenomegaly. Diagnosis of the disease is usually suggested when there is the presence of hepatomegaly, skin pigmentation, diabetes mellitus, heart disease, arthritis, and hypogonadism. Menkes disease (choice D) is a disorder of copper homeostasis. The disorder is associated with an inability to absorb copper from the gastrointestinal tract and an inability of tissues to absorb copper from the blood. Menkes disease is the result of defects in the P-type ATPase protein that is responsible for the translocation of copper across the intestinal basolateral membrane into the blood, thus allowing for uptake of dietary copper. This protein is encoded by the ATPase, Cu^{2+}-transporting, alpha polypeptide (*ATP7A*) gene. The clinical spectrum of Menkes disease includes progressive neurodegeneration, connective tissue abnormalities, and wiry brittle hair. The distinctive clinical features of Menkes disease are usually present by 3 months of age. Infants will lose, or fail to demonstrate, specific developmental milestones and failure to thrive. Most patients with Menkes disease do not survive beyond early childhood

58. Correct answer is **E.** Iron consumed in the diet is either free iron or heme iron. Free iron in the intestines is reduced from the ferric (Fe^{3+}) to the ferrous (Fe^{2+}) state primarily on the luminal surface (apical membrane) of intestinal enterocytes and then transported into the cell. The reduction reaction is catalyzed by the transmembrane ferrireductase called duodenal cytochrome b (DCYTB) a reaction facilitated by intracellular ascorbate. Ferrous iron is then transported into the intestinal enterocyte via the action of the divalent metal transporter, DMT1 (choice B). The DMT1 transporter is a member of the SLC family of transporters and is encoded by the SLC11A2 gene. Dietary iron is either stored in intestinal enterocytes bound to ferritin or it can be transported across the basolateral membrane into the circulation. Transport of iron from intestinal enterocytes to the blood is the function of ferroportin 1 (choice C). Ferroportin 1 is a member of the SLC family of membrane transporters and as such is encoded by the SLC40A1 gene. Associated with ferroportin 1 is the intestine-specific enzyme hephaestin (a copper-containing ferroxidase with homology to ceruloplasmin) which oxidizes the ferrous iron back to the ferric state. The inability of intestinal enterocytes to oxidize ferrous iron while it is being transported to the blood prevents ferroportin from carrying out the transport function. Therefore, a defect in hephaestin is most likely to impair dietary iron transport to the circulation. Ceruloplasmin (choice A) is the plasma ferroxidase responsible for oxidizing ferrous iron released from the liver. Ceruloplasmin is also tethered to the plasma membrane of numerous tissues where it serves a function identical to that of intestinal hephaestin. Heme oxygenase (choice D) is the enzyme responsible for the initial reaction of heme catabolism.

59. Correct answer is **B.** The patient is most likely experiencing the signs and symptoms of hemochromatosis. Hemochromatosis is defined as a disorder in iron metabolism that is characterized by excess iron absorption, saturation of iron-binding proteins, and deposition of hemosiderin (amorphous iron deposits) in the tissues. The primary affected tissues are the liver, pancreas, and skin. Primary hemochromatosis is referred to as type 1 hemochromatosis and it is caused by the inheritance of an autosomal recessive allele. Primary hemochromatosis is an autosomal recessive disorder that is referred to as type 1 hemochromatosis. The locus causing type 1 hemochromatosis has been designated the HFE locus (homeostatic iron regulator) and is a major histocompatibility complex (MHC) class-1 gene (symbol: HFE). In hemochromatosis the liver is usually the first organ to be affected. Hepatomegaly will be present in more than 95% of patients manifesting symptoms. Initial symptoms include weakness, abdominal pain, change in skin color, and the onset of symptoms of diabetes mellitus. In advanced cases of hemochromatosis there will likely be cardiac arrhythmias, congestive heart failure, testicular atrophy, jaundice, increased pigmentation, spider angiomas and splenomegaly. Diagnosis of the disease is usually suggested when there is the presence of hepatomegaly, skin pigmentation, diabetes mellitus, heart disease, arthritis, and hypogonadism. Type 4 hemochromatosis, also called ferroportin disease, is caused by mutations in the gene (*SLC40A1*) that encodes ferroportin (choice D). Symptoms of type 4 hemochromatosis are much milder than type 1 hemochromatosis and this disorder is inherited as an autosomal dominant disease. A defect in none of the other proteins (choice A, C, and E) are associated with the signs and symptoms of iron overload typified by hemochromatosis.

60. Correct answer is **B.** In humans approximately 70% of total body iron is found in hemoglobin. Because of storage and recycling very little (1–2 mg) iron will need to be replaced from the diet on a daily basis. Any excess dietary iron is not absorbed or is stored in intestinal enterocytes bound in ferritin. Control over iron delivery to the blood from intestinal enterocytes is the function of the hepatic iron regulatory protein hepcidin. Hepcidin is encoded by the HAMP (hepcidin antimicrobial peptide) gene. Hepcidin functions by binding to the basolateral membrane iron efflux transporter, ferroportin 1, in intestinal enterocytes and reticuloendothelial macrophage membranes. On interaction with hepcidin, ferroportin 1 is internalized and degraded. An increased level of HAMP gene expression occurs as a consequence of iron status, erythropoiesis, inflammation, and hypoxia. When there is excess iron in the body, or under conditions of inflammation, the HAMP gene is turned on resulting in decreased iron absorption and decreased iron release from macrophages. Conversely, when iron levels are deficient or during erythropoiesis or hypoxic events, expression of the HAMP gene decreases. When hepcidin expression is decreased there is increased iron absorption and increased iron release from macrophages. None of the other options (choice A, C, D, and E) correctly define the role of the critical hepatic protein, hepcidin, in the regulation of iron homeostasis.

61. Correct answer is **C.** Regulation of the translation of certain mRNAs occurs through the action of specific RNA-binding proteins. Proteins of this class have been identified that bind to sequences in either the 5′-untranslated region (5′-UTR) or 3′-UTR of target mRNAs. Two particularly interesting and important regulatory schemes related to iron homeostasis encompass an RNA-binding protein that binds to either the 5′-UTR of the ferritin mRNA or to the 3′-UTR of the transferrin receptor mRNA. This RNA-binding protein is called iron response element binding protein (IRBP) and it binds to a specific iron response element (IRE) formed by the overall structure of its target mRNAs. This IRE forms a hair-pin loop structure that is recognized by IRBP. Ferritin is an iron-binding protein that prevents toxic levels of ferrous iron (Fe^{2+}) from building up in cells. When iron levels are high, IRBP cannot bind to the IRE in the 5′-UTR of the ferritin mRNA. This allows the ferritin mRNA to be translated. Conversely, when iron levels are low, the IRBP binds to the IRE in the ferritin mRNA preventing its translation. None of the other options (choices A, B, and D) correctly define the mechanism by which iron controls the levels of ferritin protein inside cells.

62. Correct answer is **A.** The patient is experiencing the signs and symptoms of Wilson disease. Wilson disease (WD) is characterized by excessive copper deposition primarily in the liver and brain. These sites of copper deposition are reflective of the major manifestations of Wilson disease. Wilson disease is the result of defects in the P-type ATPase protein that is primarily responsible for copper homeostasis effected by the liver. This protein is encoded by the ATPase, Cu^{2+}-transporting, beta polypeptide (*ATP7B*) gene. The ATP7B protein is localized to the trans-Golgi network where it transports copper into the lumen of the Golgi. When copper levels rise, ATP7B is translocated to vesicular compartments closely associated with the plasma membrane where it can transport copper into these compartments. The copper in these vesicles can then be released by exocytosis. When copper is transferred from intestinal enterocytes to the plasma, through the action of the ATP7A protein, it is bound to albumin and delivered to the liver. In the liver the copper is transferred to intracellular storage sites by the chaperone ATOX1. Copper is stored intracellularly bound to the protein metallothionein. ATP7B also facilitates the transfer of copper to the copper-dependent ferroxidase, ceruloplasmin. Copper-containing ceruloplasmin, produced in the liver, is then released to the blood. None of the other processes (choice B, C, D, and E) would be lacking in the overall process of copper homeostasis in a patient with Wilson disease.

63. Correct answer is **D.** The patient is most likely experiencing the signs and symptoms of anemia, specifically a microcytic anemia. Microcytic anemia can often be associated with defective hemoglobin synthesis such as in the case of the β-thalassemias. Microcytic anemia can also result from nutritional deficiency of vitamin B_6 or iron and may also be the result of heavy metal intoxication such as in lead poisoning. Iron deficiency is the most common cause of anemia worldwide. In the absence of adequate iron, heme cannot be synthesized from protoporphyrin IX via the action of ferrochelatase. The lack of heme biosynthesis, in erythroid progenitor cells, results in a block to protein synthesis. Since protein synthesis is impaired in erythroid progenitor cells, as a consequence of iron deficiency, these cells do not grow during the G_1 phase of the cell cycle resulting in the typical microcytic anemia of iron deficiency. Chronic bleeding, but not acute (choice A), most often due to gastrointestinal bleeding, can also result in microcytic anemia. Deficiency in cobalamin (vitamin B_{12}) (choice B) and folate (choice C) will result in megaloblastic (macrocytic) anemia. Vitamin K deficiency (choice E) will lead to excessive bleeding on injury but will not result in an anemia.

64. Correct answer is **D.** The blood work in this patient is most indicative of iron-deficiency anemia. Neonates who are not breast-fed and do not receive fortified formula but are, instead, fed cow's milk are the most likely to become iron deficient. This is due to the reduced levels of iron in cow's milk and the interference to iron absorption in the neonate caused by milk. Oral administration of ferrous sulfate (drops or pills) is commonly used to supplement iron loss causing the anemia. The child should also be put on a diet of formula and foods enriched in iron. A deficiency of cobalamin (vitamin B_{12}) (choice B) or folate (choice C) would result in a megaloblastic (macrocytic) anemia. Deficiency in copper (choice A) or thiamine (choice E) would not be associated with a microcytic anemia.

65. Correct answer is **B.** The patient is most likely exhibiting the symptoms of a deficiency in vitamin A. Bioactive vitamin A compounds are derived from the plant precursor molecule, β-carotene (a member of a family of molecules known as carotenoids). Beta-carotene, which consists of two molecules of retinal linked at their aldehyde ends, is also referred to as the provitamin form of vitamin A. Additional provitamin A carotenoids are α-carotene and β-cryptoxanthin. The earliest symptom of vitamin A deficiency is night blindness. Additional early symptoms include follicular hyperkeratosis, increased susceptibility to infection and cancer, and anemia equivalent to iron-deficient anemia. Prolonged lack of vitamin A leads to deterioration of the eye tissue through progressive keratinization of the cornea which results in abnormal dryness of the conjunctiva and cornea and the lack of ability of produce tears, a condition known as xerophthalmia. The progressive drying and keratinization of the conjunctiva, particularly on the nasal and temporal conjunctiva, results in the development of irregularly shaped spots termed Bitot ("bee toe") spots after the French physician, Pierre Bitot, who first described them. Ascorbic acid (vitamin C) deficiency (choice A) leads to scurvy, which is characterized by poor wound healing, poor bone formation, gingival changes, and petechiae. Vitamin C excess can lead to decreased absorption of vitamin B_{12}, increased estrogen levels in females on estrogen replacement therapy, uricosuria, and oxalate kidney stones. Interestingly, small doses of the vitamin (200 mg daily) may effectively treat leukocyte abnormalities associated with Chédiak-Higashi syndrome. Mild thiamine (vitamin B1) deficiency (choice C) leads to peripheral neuropathy (dry beriberi). More severe vitamin depletion leads to high-output cardiac failure (wet beriberi) and the dementia, ataxia, and ophthalmoplegia of the Wernicke-Korsakoff syndrome frequently seen in chronic alcoholics. Excessive cholecalciferol (vitamin D) intake (choice D) can lead to vitamin D excess, resulting in hypercalcemia and widespread calcification of soft tissues. A deficiency of vitamin D occurs with lack of sunshine or renal failure and leads to rickets in children and osteomalacia in adults. Excessive intake of menadione (choice E), a form of vitamin K, is associated with hyperbilirubinemia, hemolytic anemia, and swelling of the eyelids and lips. Rarer symptoms of vitamin K excess include irregular heartbeat, difficulty swallowing, and dry itchy skin. Excessive α-tocopherol (vitamin E) intake (choice F) can lead to vitamin E excess, which is characterized by malaise, headaches, gastro-intestinal complaints, and, sometimes, hypertension. Vitamin E deficiency is characterized by areflexia, decreased proprioception and vibratory sense, hemolysis, gait disturbances, and paresis of gaze.

66. Correct answer is **E.** The patient is most likely exhibiting the signs and symptoms associated with a deficiency in vitamin C, ascorbic acid. The most important reactions requiring ascorbate as a cofactor are the hydroxylation of lysine and proline residues in collagen. The hydroxylation of proline and lysine residues in collagen occurs as protein is being synthesized in the rough endoplasmic reticulum (ER). Vitamin C is, therefore, required for the maintenance of normal connective tissue as well as for wound healing since synthesis of connective tissue is the first event in wound tissue remodeling. Vitamin C also is necessary for bone remodeling due to the presence of collagen in the organic matrix of bones. Deficiency in vitamin C leads to the disease scurvy due to the role of the vitamin in the post-translational modification of collagens. Scurvy is characterized by easily bruised skin, petechia, muscle fatigue, soft swollen gums, decreased wound healing, hemorrhaging, osteoporosis, and anemia. Due to its role in collagen processing, the bleeding dysfunction associated with vitamin C deficiency is characterized by the lack of effect on prothrombin time (PT) but with a prolonged bleeding time. The role of ascorbate in the synthesis and processing of collagen does not involve any of the other subcellular compartments (choices A, B, C, and D).

67. Correct answer is **D.** The patient is most likely experiencing the consequences of deficiency in calcium absorption resulting from insufficient levels of hormonally active vitamin D. Calcium and phosphorous homeostasis in humans is regulated through the concerted actions of vitamin D and parathyroid hormone. The hormonally active form of vitamin D is 1,25-dihydroxy vitamin D_3 (1,25-$(OH)_2D_3$, also called 1,25-dihydroxycholecalciferol or more commonly calcitriol). Active calcitriol is derived from ergosterol (produced in plants) and from 7-dehydrocholesterol which is an intermediate in the synthesis of cholesterol that accumulates in the skin. On exposure to ultraviolet B wavelength light from the sun, 7-dehydrocholesterol is nonenzymatically (thermal isomerization) converted first to pre-vitamin D_3 and then to vitamin D_3. Within the liver vitamin D_3 undergoes the first of two activating hydroxylation reactions by a specific vitamin D 25-hydroxylase generating 25-hydroxy-D_3 [25-$(OH)D_3$: more commonly called calcidiol]. Conversion of vitamin D_3 to calcidiol is dependent solely on substrate availability as there is no regulatory mechanism to control the formation of calcidiol. Parathyroid hormone (PTH) is synthesized and secreted by chief cells of the parathyroid glands. Secretion of PTH from the parathyroid gland is controlled via the activity of the Ca^{2+}-sensing receptor (CaSR). The CaSR is expressed in the parathyroid glands, renal tubule cells, bone marrow, thyroid gland C-cells, and several other tissues. When calcium levels fall signaling from the CaSR is reduced which allows for enhanced secretion of PTH. The body response to PTH is complex but is aimed in all tissues at increasing Ca^{2+} levels in extracellular fluids. In the kidney, PTH reduces renal Ca^{2+} clearance by stimulating its reabsorption. At the same time, PTH reduces the reabsorption of phosphate and thereby increases its clearance resulting in reduced, not increased (choice E) serum levels. PTH acts on the kidney to stimulate the production of the hormonally active form of vitamin D, calcitriol. As a result of the lack of exposure to sunlight, this patient has a significantly reduced capacity to generate calcidiol as evidenced by the blood work showing its levels are below normal. Low calcidiol will, in turn, result in low calcitriol. Low calcitriol will impair intestinal uptake of calcium. The reduced calcium absorption will lead to decreased, not increased (choice A) serum calcium which will result in less Ca^{2+} bound to the CaSR and, subsequently increased release of PTH from the parathyroid gland. Calcidiol and PTH do not exert effects on the levels of corticotropin releasing hormone (choice B) nor growth hormone (choice C).

68. Correct answer is **B.** The patient is most likely experiencing the signs and symptoms of a megaloblastic anemia. Megaloblastic anemias are most often the result of deficiency of folate or vitamin B_{12} (cobalamin). Pernicious anemia is a megaloblastic anemia resulting from vitamin B_{12} deficiency that caused by the lack of intrinsic factor being released from stomach parietal cells leading to subsequent malabsorption of the vitamin. The major cause of the loss of intrinsic factor is an autoimmune destruction of the parietal cells that secrete it. The anemia results from impaired DNA synthesis due to a block in purine and thymidine nucleotide biosynthesis. The block in nucleotide biosynthesis is a consequence of the effect of vitamin B_{12} on folate metabolism. When vitamin B_{12} is deficient essentially all of the folate becomes trapped as the N^5-methyl-tetrahydrofolate (N^5-methylTHF) derivative as a result of the loss of functional methionine synthase. Methionine synthase is a folate and vitamin B_{12}-dependent enzyme that catalyzes the methylation of homocysteine generating methionine. The methyl group is donated by N^5-methylTHF and the THF is released for use in other THF derivative synthesis pathways. The distinguishing feature exerted by this patient that indicates the symptoms are the result of vitamin B_{12} deficiency and not folate deficiency is the peripheral neuropathy, the numbness and tingling he is experiencing in his fingers. Deficiency in ceruloplasmin (choice A) results in aceruloplasminemia. Aceruloplasminemia is a rare, recessively inherited neurodegenerative disorder characterized by a lack of ceruloplasmin in the circulation. The lack of ceruloplasmin results in abnormal iron use in the body and leads to iron deposits in various body tissues such as the brain, pancreas, and liver. The iron overload results in neurodegeneration, diabetes, and numerous other symptoms. Deficiency in lysyl oxidase (choice C) would prevent extracellular processing of collagen which would manifest with numerous connective tissue-related symptoms as well as bleeding dysfunction. Pyridoxal kinase (choice D) is required for the activation of vitamin B_6 to pyridoxal phosphate, PLP. PLP is a required cofactor for numerous enzymes including δ-aminolevulinic acid synthase, the initial and rate-limiting enzyme of heme biosynthesis. A deficiency in pyridoxal kinase would result in microcytic hypochromic anemia due to a lack of PLP. Thiamine pyrophosphokinase (choice E) is required for the activation of thiamine to thiamine pyrophosphate, TPP. A deficiency in thiamine pyrophosphokinase would manifest with symptoms identical to those associated with thiamine deficiency.

69. Correct answer is **E.** The patient is most likely exhibiting the signs and symptoms associated with a deficiency in vitamin B_{12} which can be a common occurrence in individuals adhering to a strictly vegan diet. Vitamin B_{12} supplementation and/or the consumption of vitamin B_{12} fortified vegan foods is critical for acquiring sufficient levels of bioactive methylcobalamin and adenosylcobalamin, the two cofactor forms of vitamin B_{12}. The cofactor forms of vitamin B_{12} are used in only two reactions in the body, the methionine synthase (also known as homocysteine methyltransferase) reaction, which converts homocysteine to methionine, and the methylmalonyl-CoA mutase reaction, which is the third enzyme in the pathway converting propionyl-CoA to succinyl-CoA. This propionyl-CoA conversion pathway is often remembered by the mnemonic as the VOMIT pathway, where V stands for valine, O for odd-chain fatty acids, M for methionine, I for isoleucine, and T for threonine. Deficiency in vitamin B_{12} leads to trapping of folate (5-methyltetrahydrofolate) at the methionine synthase reaction which in turn depletes the active folate pool required for nucleotide biosynthesis. The impairment in DNA synthesis results in erythroid progenitor cells being trapped at the G1 phase of the cell cycle, and since they can't divide, they are enlarged resulting in macrocytic anemia, which is evident from the MCV value in the patient being above 100 fL. Peripheral blood smears from patients with vitamin B_{12} deficiency show macrocytosis, poikilocytosis (abnormally shaped red blood cells), schistocytes (fragmented red blood cells), and hypersegmented neutrophils (abnormally lobed nuclei). The loss of function of the methylmalonyl-CoA mutase reaction with vitamin B_{12} deficiency results in increased levels of methylmalonic acid in blood and urine, which is diagnostic for vitamin B_{12} deficiency and not folate deficiency in patients with macrocytic anemia. Delta-aminolevulinic acid (choice A) levels are associated with inherited defects in heme biosynthesis which are not associated with the blood-related symptoms observed in this patient. Anti-citrullinated peptide antibodies (choice B) are predictive and diagnostic for rheumatoid arthritis, whose symptoms are not observed in this patient. Ferritin (choice C) levels rise in the blood in conditions of iron excess, symptoms of which are not seen in this patient. Although homocysteine (choice D) levels are elevated in patients with vitamin B_{12} deficiency, due to impaired activity of methionine synthase, measurement of levels of this metabolite are not as useful for a differential diagnosis of primary causes of macrocytic anemia as is the measurement of methylmalonic acid levels.

70. Correct answer is **E.** The patient is exhibiting the classic signs associated with deficiency of riboflavin (vitamin B_2) which include itching and burning eyes, angular stomatitis, and cheilosis (cracks and sores in the mouth and lips), bloodshot eyes, glossitis (inflammation of the tongue leading to purplish discoloration), seborrhea (dandruff, flaking skin on scalp and face), trembling, sluggishness, and photophobia (excessive light sensitivity). Riboflavin is the precursor for the coenzymes, flavin mononucleotide (FMN) and flavin adenine dinucleotide (FAD). FAD is a necessary cofactor for the function of succinate dehydrogenase which is involved in the TCA cycle and also represents complex II of the electron transport chain of oxidative phosphorylation, thus deficiency in riboflavin is associated with reduced oxidative phosphorylation capacity. Folate is required for the synthesis of the purine nucleotides and thymidine nucleotides and is, therefore, required for DNA synthesis (choice A). Pyridoxine (vitamin B_6) is converted to pyridoxal phosphate, which is required by several enzymes, one of which is the rate-limiting enzyme of heme biosynthesis (choice B), δ-aminolevulinic acid synthase. Niacin (vitamin B_3) is required by numerous dehydrogenases, such as the pyruvate dehydrogenase complex (PDHc), and enzymes of reductive biosynthesis, as well as a wide array of other biological processes. These other processes include the sirtuin proteins and the poly-ADP-ribose polymerases (PARP). The major function of the SIRT proteins is the NAD^+-dependent deacetylation of lysine residues in target proteins, particularly histone proteins (choice C). Vitamin B_{12}, as methylcobalamin, is a required cofactor for the enzyme, methionine synthase, which converts homocysteine to methionine (choice D).

71. Correct answer is **A.** The patient is most likely exhibiting the symptoms associated with iron deficiency anemia. Common symptoms associated with the anemia resulting from iron deficiency include fatigue, generalized weakness, pallor (pale skin), cold hands and feet, inflammation of the tongue (glossitis), and brittle spoon-shaped nails (koilonychia), as well as strange non-nutritive cravings (pica) such as for ice. Individuals with iron deficiency anemia often have gastrointestinal bleeding that results in dark, tar-colored feces. The loss of iron results in decreased levels of hemoglobin in the blood, a reduced red blood cell size (microcytic anemia) as measured by the mean corpuscular volume (MCV), and a reduced hemoglobin concentration in red blood cells as measured by the mean corpuscular hemoglobin concentration (MCHC). Additional laboratory findings will include changes to the typical measurements for iron status, which include serum iron (decreased), ferritin (decreased), and transferrin receptor (increased). The total iron-binding capacity (TIBC) is a measure of the ability of transferrin, the major serum iron transporting protein, to bind iron. As the level of serum iron goes down, the binding capacity goes up and the opposite is true under conditions of iron overload. The changes in serum levels of ferritin and the transferrin receptor result from the effect of iron on the stability and translatability of the mRNAs encoding these proteins (see Chapter 24, Figure 24–9). None of the other combinations of changes (choices B, C, D, E, and F) correctly depicts what would be expected for these serum parameters related to iron homeostasis in conditions of iron deficiency.

72. Correct answer is **A.** The patient is most likely exhibiting the symptoms of anemia of chronic inflammation, most often incorrectly identified as anemia of chronic disease, which is an anemia with symptoms very similar to those of iron deficiency anemia. The patient has a previous diagnosis of the autoimmune disorder, systemic lupus erythematosus (SLE), a disorder frequently associated with anemia of chronic inflammation. Conditions of inflammation lead to increased levels of pro-inflammatory cytokines such as IL-6. Within the liver, IL-6 induces the phosphorylation of the transcription factor, signal transducer, and activator of transcription 3 (STAT3), which leads to its translocation to the nucleus and subsequent activation of expression of the *HAMP* gene. The *HAMP* gene encodes the protein identified as hepcidin, which is responsible for regulating transport of dietary iron to the blood by stimulating the removal of ferroportin from the basolateral membranes of intestinal enterocytes. Hepcidin exerts the same effect on ferroportin in the membranes of reticuloendothelial macrophages. The effect of inflammation-mediated increased hepcidin levels is reduced dietary iron delivery, resulting in a form of iron deficiency anemia. Hephaestin (choice B) is the ferroxidase associated with the ferroportin transporter, and its expression is not affected by inflammation or iron deficiency. Under conditions of iron deficiency, the levels of ferritin (choice C) decrease due to decreased translation of the ferritin mRNA, not due to changes in the expression of the gene encoding ferritin. The levels of ferroportin are decreased, not increased (choice D), due to the effects of hepcidin. Under conditions of iron deficiency the levels of transferrin (choice E), which is the major plasma iron transporting protein, do increase but this is due to increased translation of the mRNA, not to increased expression of the gene encoding transferrin.

73. Correct answer is **A.** The patient is most likey exhibiting the signs and symptoms associated with a deficiency in vitamin A as a consequence of a likely poor diet while the patient was in the refugee camp. The earliest symptom of vitamin A deficiency is night blindness. Additional early symptoms include follicular hyperkeratosis, increased susceptibility to infection and anemia equivalent to iron deficient anemia. Prolonged lack of vitamin A leads to deterioration of the eye tissue through progressive keratinization of the cornea which results in abnormal dryness of the conjunctiva and cornea and the lack of ability to produce tears, a condition known as xerophthalmia. The vision issues, particularly night blindness, with vitamin A deficiency reflects the role of vitamin A, specifically 11-*cis*-retinal, in photoreception. When photons of light interact with 11-*cis*-retinal, which is associated with the G-protein coupled receptor called rhodopsin, the receptor is activated which in turn activates an associated G-protein. The G-protein is called transducing and when activated transducing activates a cGMP-specific phosphodiesterase (PDE6B) resulting in the degradation of cGMP inside the discs of retinal rod cells. The decrease in cGMP ultimately leads to disinhibition of the optic nerve allowing visual signals to be propagated along the optic nerve. Activation of coagulation factor X (choice B) requires vitamin K and there is no indication of bleeding dysfunction in this patient. Catabolism of phytanic acid (choice C), a methyl-substituted fatty acid found in tissues of ruminants, certain fishes, and in dairy products. The metabolism of phytanate involves a series of enzymes, one of which requires thiamine pyrophosphate but there are no signs of thiamine deficiency in this patient. Expression of the NCX1 transporter (choice D) is stimulated by the hormonal actions of vitamin D but there are no signs of vitamin D deficiency in this patient. Vitamin E is a critical antioxidant that protects membrane lipids from peroxidation (choice E), but there are no signs of vitamin E deficiency in this patient. Synthesis of heme (choice F) requires pyridoxal phosphate, the cofactor form of pyridoxine (vitamin B_6), but there are no signs of pyridoxine deficiency in this patient.

74. Correct answer is **C.** The patient is most likely exhibiting the signs and symptoms associated with iron deficiency anemia. The chronic fatigue and conjunctival pallor are typical symptoms associated with iron deficiency anemia. Although there is a history of sickle cell anemia (choice D) in the patient's family, it is unlikely that she has the disease given her anemia is demonstrably microcytic (MCV is 57 fL). Sickle cell anemia is more commonly associated with a normal, or slightly elevated, MCV. The clinical spectrum of erythrocyte pyruvate kinase deficiency (choice A) varies from mild and fully compensated hemolysis to severe cases that require transfusions for survival. In the most severe cases, an affected fetus will die *in utero*. Most PKLR deficient patients are diagnosed in infancy or early childhood. Glucose-6-phosphate dehydrogenase (G6PDH) deficiency (choice B) is not commonly associated with microcytic anemia, instead patients will have normal to slightly elevated MCV. The vast majority of individuals that harbor a mutant form of the *G6PD* gene go their entire lives without knowing they carry a mutation. Deficiency in vitamin B_{12} (choice E) is one of the two most common causes of macrocytic anemia, evidenced by MCV values greater than 100 fL.

75. Correct answer is **E.** The patient is most likely experiencing the symptoms associated with hemochromatosis, a disorder of iron overload. The most common form of hemochromatosis is caused by mutations in the *HFE* (homeostatic iron regulator) gene. The normal *HFE*-encoded protein has been shown to form a complex with the transferrin receptor and in so doing is thought to regulate the rate of iron transfer into cells. A mutation in HFE will therefore lead to increased iron uptake and storage. In hemochromatosis the liver is usually the first organ to be affected. Hepatomegaly will be present in >95% of patients manifesting symptoms. Initial symptoms include weakness, abdominal pain, change in skin color, and the onset of symptoms of diabetes mellitus. Diagnosis of the disease is usually suggested when there is the presence of hepatomegaly, skin pigmentation, diabetes mellitus, heart disease, arthritis, and hypogonadism. Although patients with hemochromatosis have excessive iron accumulation in tissues, particularly the liver given that this is the major tissue for iron storage, the excessive iron accumulation is not due to decreased hepatic iron excretion (choice A). Dubin-Johnson syndrome (choice B) is a disorder caused by defective hepatic transport of conjugated bilirubin into the bile canaliculi. Jaundice is usually the only physical symptom detected in patients with Dubin-Johnson syndrome. Most patients remain asymptomatic, although some complain of weakness and abdominal pains. Only occasionally do patients develop hepatosplenomegaly. Fatty infiltration of hepatocytes (choice C) is typical in the disorder termed the metabolic syndrome, and this can result in hepatomegaly but is not typically associated with joint pain and jaundice as seen in this patient. Hepatocellular carcinoma (choice D) is commonly associated with jaundice but is also associated with persistent itching, weight loss, loss of appetite, nausea, and vomiting, symptoms not seen in this patient. Wilson disease (choice F) is a disorder associated with excessive copper accumulation in tissues, particularly the liver since this is the major organ for copper storage. The majority of patients with Wilson disease present with hepatic or neuropsychiatric symptoms. The classic outward symptom of Wilson disease is due to the deposition of copper in Descemet's membrane of the cornea, resulting in what is referred to as Kayser-Fleischer rings.

76. Correct answer is **E.** The infant is most likely manifesting the symptoms of a deficiency in vitamin D. Since the child is exclusively breast-fed and is rarely exposed to sunlight, there is a significant likelihood of insufficient conversion of 7-dehydrocholesterol to cholecalciferol, the precursor of bioactive vitamin D, calcitriol. Typical symptoms of vitamin D deficiency in infancy are referred to as ricket and include delayed growth and reduced bone mineralization which in the skull leads to delayed closure of the fontanelle which can cause bulging of the forehead (frontal bossing). The lack of proper bone mineralization will result in the typical symptom of rickets which is bowing of the legs and enlargement of the ankles and wrists. Additionally, infants with vitamin D deficiency are irritable and exhibit increased sweating. Deficiency in none of the other substances (choices A, B, C, and D) will lead to the signs and symptoms seen in this infant.

77. Correct answer is **B.** The patient is most likely exhibiting the symptoms of tuberculosis (TB), which is commonly found in individuals who work in prisons or homeless shelters. Typical symptoms of TB include a cough lasting more than three weeks that can be associated with hemoptysis (bloody sputum). TB is also associated with night sweats, chills, fever, weight loss, and loss of appetite. The most common treatment for TB is a combination drug therapy referred to as RIPE for rifampin, isoniazid, pyrazinamide, and ethambutol. Treatment usually requires the drugs to be administered for more than 2 months which can lead to a deficiency in vitamin B_6 (pyridoxine). The vitamin B_6 deficiency results from the fact that isoniazid impairs conversion of pyridoxine to pyridoxal phosphate (PLP), the cofactor form of vitamin B_6. In addition, metabolites of isoniazid deactivate pyridoxine. Deficiencies in none of the other vitamins (choices A, C, D, and E) are typically associated with TB or the treatment of the disorder.

78. Correct answer is **C.** The patient is most likely exhibiting the signs and symptoms associated with a deficiency in vitamin B_6 (pyridoxine). Alcoholism is the leading cause of deficiency in vitamin B_6. Typical symptoms associated with deficiency of vitamin B_6 include nervousness, insomnia, skin eruptions, loss of muscular control, microcytic anemia, dry cracking skin around the mouth (cheilosis and stomatitis), muscular weakness, dermatitis, arm and leg cramps, hair loss, and water retention. The microcytic anemia in vitamin B_6 deficiency is due to the role of pyridoxal phosphate as a cofactor for the rate-limiting enzyme of heme biosynthesis, δ-aminolevulinic acid synthase. The lack of heme synthesis causes erythroid progenitor cell protein synthesis to be inhibited, so these cells stay small during bone marrow development. Although both iron deficiency (choice B) and vitamin B_6 deficiency cause microcytic and hypochromic anemias, the presence of peripheral neuropathy is unique to vitamin B6 deficiency anemia. Deficiency of folate (choice A) or vitamin B12 (choice E) is associated with macrocytic, not microcytic, anemia. Also, although peripheral neuropathy is associated with vitamin B_{12} deficiency, the presence of microcytic anemia in this patient means that he cannot be suffering from deficiency in vitamin B_{12}. Deficiency in thiamine (choice D) is associated with constipation, appetite suppression, and nausea. Chronic deficiency will lead to fatigue, mental depression and confusion, peripheral neuropathy, ataxia, and loss of eye coordination (nystagmus). A highly diagnostic physical test of thiamine deficiency is vertical nystagmus.

79. Correct answer is **C.** The infant is most likely experiencing what is defined as neonatal vitamin K-dependent bleeding (VKDB). Neonates are prone to vitamin K deficiency due to the limited levels in their bodies at birth and to limited intake, especially in breast-fed neonates delivered via C-section. Delivery via C-section bypasses the exposure to resident bacteria an infant would encouncter during a vaginal birth, bacteria that contribute to the production of bioavailable vitamin K. Neonatal VDKB is defined as a bleeding disorder in which the coagulation deficit is rapidly corrected by vitamin K supplementation. The diagnosis of VDKB in an infant is indicated when the prothrombin time (PT) is found to be at least four times longer than the control value, even though the infant's platelet count and fibrinogen levels are normal. Factor VIII (choice A) is encoded by the *F8* gene which resides on the X chromosome. Inheritance of mutations in the *F8* gene is the cause of hemophilia A, whose manifestation in females is only on the order of 1 in 50 million. Folate deficiency (choice B) is associated with macrocytic anemia but not bleeding dysfunction. Most metabolic enzyme deficiencies (choice D) are not associated with neonatal bleeding and bruising. Vitamin C deficiency (choice E) is associated with easy bruising and bleeding, but the symptoms are almost never observed in a neonate. In addition, vitamin C deficiency causes an increase in the bleeding time but has no effect on the prothrombin time.

80. Correct answer is **F.** The patient is most likely exhibiting the signs and symptoms associated with vitamin D toxicity. Supraphysiological dosing of vitamin D (considered to be any dose above 50,000 IU [2500 μg] per day for a duration of at least 1 month; normal adult RDA for vitmain D is 600 IU/day), and the associated toxicities are rare, it is a valid consideration in the context of the diagnosis of the causes of hypercalcemia. Excessive vitamin D intake results in an associated hypercalcemia. The hypercalcemia caused by vitamin D toxicity is primarily due to the significant increases in circulating levels of calcidiol which, when it enters cells, can bind to and activate the VDR. In addition, at high concentrations calcidiol can displace calcitriol from vitamin D binding protein resulting in increased free calcitriol that can then activate the VDR. Both of these pathophysiological phenomena result in increased intestinal calcium absorption and increased bone calcium resorption. The resultant hypercalcemia can lead to pathologies that are similar to those caused by the hypercalcemia that results from the secondary hyperparathyroidism in the context of vitamin D deficiency. One of the earliest tissues affected by the onset of the soft tissue calcification with vitamin D toxicity is the kidney. The symptoms that result from the damage to the renal tissue include polydipsia and polyuria. Additional symptoms of vitamin D toxicity include fatigue, nausea, vomiting, and diminished mental capacity. Addison disease (choice A) is the result of adrenal insufficiency. The characteristic clinical presentation of acute primary adrenal insufficiency includes an insidious onset of asthenia (fatigability and weakness), cutaneous and mucosal pigmentation, agitation, nausea, vomiting, anorexia, weight loss, orthostatic (postural) hypotension (drop in blood pressure upon standing), confusion, circulatory collapse, abdominal pain, and fever. Cushing syndrome (choice B) is the result of hypercortisolemia. Central obesity was and continues to be the most common finding in Cushing syndrome. This feature is apparent in approximately 95% of adult patients and in 100% of pediatric patients. In addition to truncal adiposity, Cushing syndrome patients exhibit unique fat accumulations over the face and neck giving the classical "moon" facies and "buffalo hump". In addition to the unique patterns of fat deposition, Cushing syndrome patients have thin extremities (spider appearance) that are due to the effects of cortisol on protein disposition in skeletal muscle. Hyperthyroidism (choice C) is typified by Graves disease, the classical symptoms of which are weight loss despite increased appetite, heat intolerance, irritability, insomnia, sweatiness, diarrhea, palpitations, muscular weakness, and menstrual irregularity. Hypothyroidism (choice D) is most commonly the result of iodine deficiency. The classic symptoms of hypothyroidism include fatigue, weight gain, intolerance to cold, dry skin and hair, constipation, joint and muscle pain, slow heart rate, depression, and memory problems. The main symptom of vitamin D deficiency (choice E) in adults is osteomalacia, which is characterized by demineralization of previously formed bone, leading to increased softness and susceptibility to fracture.

CHAPTER

4

Enzymes Kinetics

High-Yield Terms

Coenzymes	Nonprotein components of enzymes
Isozyme	Member of a set of enzymes sharing similar/same substrate specificity
Ribozymes	RNA molecules that exhibit catalytic activity in the absence of any protein component
Reaction rate	Described by the number of molecules of reactant(s) that are converted into product(s) in a specified time period
Chemical reaction order	Relates to the number of molecules in a reaction complex that can proceed to product
Equilibrium constant	Related to the ratio of product concentration to reactant concentration or rate constants for forward and reverse reactions
Michaelis-Menten constant (K_m)	Relates the maximum reaction velocity to substrate concentration such that K_m is the substrate concentration [S] at which a reaction has attained half the maximal velocity
Lineweaver-Burk plots	Linear double reciprocal plots of substrate concentration versus reaction velocity
Allosteric enzymes	Defined as any enzyme whose activity is altered by binding small molecule regulators referred to as effectors; plots of substrate concentration versus reaction velocity are sigmoidal instead of curvilinear

ENZYME CLASSIFICATIONS

Enzymes are biological catalysts that are broadly categorized based on the type of reaction they catalyze (Table 4–1). The macromolecular components of almost all enzymes are composed of protein, except for a class of RNA modifying catalysts known as ribozymes. Ribozymes are molecules of ribonucleic acid that catalyze reactions on the phosphodiester bond of other RNA.

ROLE OF COENZYMES

Many enzymes are functional solely as a protein or protein complex while others required cofactors, often called coenzymes. Typical coenzymes are derived from vitamins (see Chapter 3), or they can be other small organic molecules or metal ions.

Coenzymes function as transporters of chemical groups from one reactant to another. The chemical groups carried can be as simple as the hydride ion ($H^+ + 2e^-$) carried by NAD^+ or the mole of hydrogen carried by FAD, or they can be more complex such as the amine ($-NH_2$) carried by pyridoxal phosphate. Since coenzymes are chemically changed as a consequence of enzyme action, it is often useful to consider coenzymes to be a special class of substrates, or second substrates.

ENZYMES & THEIR SUBSTRATES

Although enzymes are highly specific for the kind of reaction they catalyze, the same is not always true of substrates on which they act. For example, succinate dehydrogenase (SDH) always catalyzes an oxidation-reduction reaction and its substrate is succinic acid, whereas alcohol dehydrogenase (ADH) always catalyzes oxidation-reduction reactions but can act on a number of different alcohols.

As enzymes have a more or less broad range of substrate specificity, it follows that a given substrate may be acted on by a number of different enzymes, each of which uses the same substrate(s) and produces the same product(s). The individual members of a set of enzymes sharing such characteristics are known as isozymes. For example, there is a liver isozyme of glycogen phosphorylase and there is a distinct skeletal muscle isozyme, yet both enzymes catalyze the phosphorolysis of glucose from glycogen (see Chapter 7).

TABLE 4–1 International Union of Biochemistry (IUB) classification of enzymes.

Number	Classification	Biochemical Properties
1	Oxidoreductases	Act on many chemical groupings to add or remove hydrogen atoms
2	Transferases	Transfer functional groups between donor and acceptor molecules. Kinases are specialized transferases that regulate metabolism by transferring phosphate from ATP to other molecules
3	Hydrolases	Add water across a bond, hydrolyzing it
4	Lyases	Add water, ammonia, or carbon dioxide across double bonds, or remove these elements to produce double bonds
5	Isomerases	Carry out many kinds of isomerization: L to D isomerizations, mutase reactions (shifts of chemical groups), and others
6	Ligases	Catalyze reactions in which two chemical groups are joined (or ligated) with the use of energy from ATP

Reproduced with permission from King MW: *Integrative Medical Biochemistry Examination and Board Review*. New York, NY: McGraw Hill; 2014.

Many enzymes have clinical significance in addition to their primary biochemical function. The measurement of the level of a particular enzyme in the blood can provide utility in the diagnosis and treatment of disease (see Clinical Box 4–1).

CHEMICAL REACTIONS & RATES

The rate of a chemical reaction is described by the number of molecules of reactant(s) that are converted into product(s) in a

CLINICAL BOX 4–1 ENZYMES IN THE DIAGNOSIS OF PATHOLOGY

The measurement of the serum levels of numerous enzymes has been shown to be of diagnostic significance.

Transaminases: Commonly assayed enzymes in the blood useful in the assessment of liver pathology are alanine transaminase (ALT) and aspartate transaminase (AST). When assaying for both ALT and AST, the ratio of the level of these two enzymes can also be diagnostic. Normally in liver disease or damage that is not of viral origin the ratio of ALT/AST is less than 1. However, with viral hepatitis the ALT/AST ratio will be greater than 1. Measurement of AST is useful not only for liver involvement but also for heart disease or damage. The level of AST elevation in the serum is directly proportional to the number of cells involved as well as on the time following injury that the AST assay was performed. Following injury, levels of AST rise within 8 hours and peak 24–36 hours later. Within 3–7 days, the level of AST should return to preinjury levels, provided a continuous insult is not present or further injury occurs.

Cardiac Troponins: Cardiac troponins found in the serum, specifically troponin I and T, are excellent markers for myocardial infarction as well as for any other type of heart muscle damage. The measurement of plasma troponin I levels are highly diagnostic of necrosis of cardiac muscle. Serum levels of troponin I rise within 4–8 hours after the onset of chest pains caused by myocardial infarction. The levels peak within 12–16 hours after the onset of infarction and return to baseline within 5–9 days. Although measurement of serum LDH fractions was once considered the ideal marker for onset and severity of a heart attack, the high specificity of troponin I to heart muscle necrosis makes this protein the preferred marker to measure in patients suspected of suffering a myocardial infarct.

Lactate Dehydrogenases: The measurement of lactate dehydrogenase (LDH) is especially diagnostic for myocardial infarction because this enzyme exists in five closely related, but slightly different forms (isozymes). These five isoforms are generated by combinations of two different subunits encoded by two different genes. The subunits are identified as the M form for muscle-specific (encoded by the LDHA gene) and the H form for heart-specific (encoded by the LDHB gene). Humans also express two additional LDH genes: LDHC (expression restricted to testis) and LDHD (mitochondrial enzyme specific for D-lactate). Following a myocardial infarction, the serum levels of LDH rise within 24–48 hours reaching a peak by 2–3 days and return to normal in 5–10 days. Especially diagnostic is a comparison of the LDH-1/LDH-2 ratio. Normally, this ratio is less than 1. A reversal of this ratio is referred to as a "flipped LDH." Following an acute myocardial infarction, the flipped LDH ratio will appear in 12–24 hours and is definitely present by 48 hours in more than 80% of patients. Also important is the fact that persons suffering chest pain due to angina only will not likely have altered LDH levels.

Creatine Kinases: Creatine kinase is found primarily in heart and skeletal muscle as well as the brain. Therefore, measurement of serum CK (CPK) levels is a good diagnostic for injury to these tissues. The levels of CPK will rise within 6 hours of injury and peak by around 18 hours. If the injury is not persistent the level of CPK returns to normal within 2–3 days. Like LDH, there are tissue-specific isoforms of CPK derived from the expression of two distinct creatine kinase genes. The muscle CPK isoform is expressed from the creatine kinase, muscle (CKM) gene while the brain isoform is expressed from the CKB gene. Dependent on the tissue of expression, three major CPK isoforms are found in human tissues. CPK1 (CPK-BB) is a homodimer of two CKB encoded proteins and is the characteristic isoform in brain and is in significant amounts in smooth muscle and several other tissues and is 0% of the normal serum total. CPK2 (CPK-MB) is a heterodimer of the CKM and CKB encoded proteins and this

CLINICAL BOX 4–1 (CONTINUED)

form accounts for about 35% of the CPK activity in cardiac muscle, but less than 5% in skeletal muscle and is 0% of the normal serum total. CPK3 (CPK-MM) is a homodimer of two CKM encoded proteins and is the predominant isoform in muscle and is 100% of the normal serum total.

Carbonic Anhydrases: Carbonic anhydrases (CA) are enzymes that catalyze the formation of carbonic acid (H_2CO_3) from CO_2 and H_2O. Humans express 15 isoforms of CA with 12 of these isoforms exhibiting functional enzymatic activity. Carbonic anhydrases play an important role in renal control of acid-base balance and as pharmacologic targets in the control of certain hypertensive states, glaucoma, and epilepsy. The principal drugs used as diuretics are acetazolamide and methazolamide. The carbonic anhydrase, CA IX is one of only two tumor-associated carbonic anhydrases with CA XII being the other. Expression of CA IX is associated with renal cell carcinomas (RCC) but it is not expressed at all in normal renal tissues which makes it a useful diagnostic marker for this disease.

Gamma-glutamyltranferase: Gamma-glutamyltranferase (GGT, γ-glutamyltransferase; also called gamma-glutamyl transpeptidase) is involved in glutathione (GSH) metabolism and also in amino acid transport across membranes. Normal plasma levels of GGT are 15–85 IU/L for males and 5–55 IU/L for women. Elevated serum GGT levels are found in diseases of the liver, biliary system, and pancreas. Slight elevations in serum GGT levels are also seen in cardiovascular disease, in particular, GGT accumulates in atherosclerotic plaques. GGT-containing protein aggregates circulate in the blood in certain pathologies such as metabolic syndrome, alcohol addiction, and chronic liver disease.

specified time period. Reaction rate is always dependent on the concentration of the chemicals involved in the process and on rate constants that are characteristic of the reaction. For example, the reaction in which A is converted to B is written as follows:

$$A \rightarrow B$$

The rate of this reaction is expressed algebraically as either a decrease (denoted by a negative sign) in the concentration of reactant A, where k is the rate constant for the reaction:

$$-[A] = k[B]$$

or an increase in the concentration of product B:

$$[B] = k[A]$$

Rate constants are simply proportionality constants that provide a quantitative connection between chemical concentrations and reaction rates. The rate constant for the forward reaction is defined as k_{+1} and the reverse as k_{-1}. At equilibrium, the rate (v) of the forward reaction (A → B) is, by definition, equal to that of the reverse or back reaction (B → A). At equilibrium, the rate of the forward reaction is equal to the rate of the reverse reaction leading to the equilibrium constant of the reaction and is expressed by:

$$K_{eq} = \frac{K_{+1}}{K_{-1}} = \frac{[B]}{[A]}$$

MICHAELIS-MENTEN KINETICS

The kinetics of simple enzyme catalyzed reactions were first characterized by the German biochemists Leonor Michaelis and Maud Menten. The Michaelis-Menten equation is a quantitative description of the relationship among the rate of an enzyme catalyzed reaction [v_1], the concentration of substrate [S], and two constants, V_{max} and K_m (which are set by the particular equation).

$$v_1 = \frac{V_{max}[S]}{\{K_m + [S]\}}$$

Rearranging the Michaelis-Menten equation leads to:

$$K_m = [S]\left\{\left[\frac{V_{max}}{V_1}\right] - 1\right\}$$

HIGH-YIELD CONCEPT

The Michaelis-Menten equation can be used to demonstrate that at the substrate concentration that produces exactly half of the maximum reaction rate (½V_{max}), the substrate concentration is numerically equal to K_m.

Graphical analysis of enzymes functioning with Michaelis-Menten kinetics, where reaction rate (v) is plotted versus substrate concentration [S], will produce a hyperbolic rate plot (Figure 4–1). The key features of the plot are marked by points A,

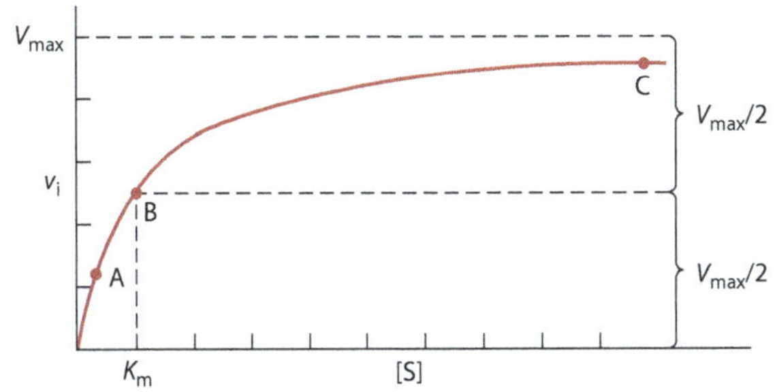

FIGURE 4–1 Effect of substrate concentration on the initial velocity of an enzyme-catalyzed reaction. (Reproduced with permission from Rodwell VW, Bender DA, Botham KM, et al: *Harper's Illustrated Biochemistry*, 31st ed. New York, NY: McGraw Hill; 2018.)

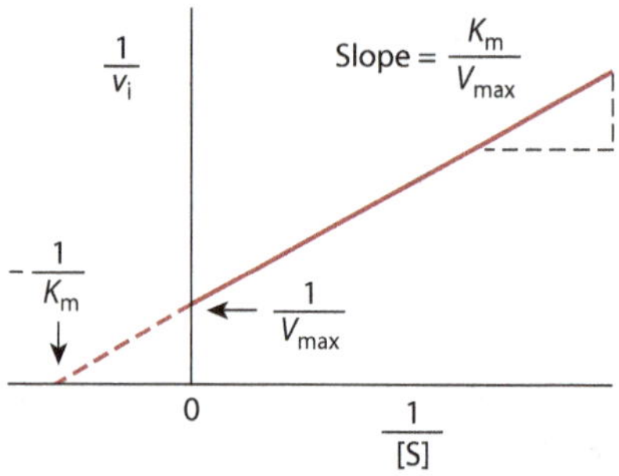

FIGURE 4–2 Double-reciprocal or Lineweaver–Burk plot of $1/v_i$ versus $1/[S]$ used to evaluate K_m and V_{max}. (Reproduced with permission from Rodwell VW, Bender DA, Botham KM, et al: *Harper's Illustrated Biochemistry*, 31st ed. New York, NY: McGraw Hill; 2018.)

B, and C. At substrate concentrations near point A, the reaction rate is directly proportional to substrate concentration, and the reaction rate is said to be first order. At the substrate concentration denoted by point B, the reaction is exactly half of V_{max} which defines K_m. At high substrate concentrations the rate represented by point C is essentially equal to V_{max}. When the reaction rate becomes independent of substrate concentration, or nearly so, the rate is said to be zero order.

Biochemists Hans Lineweaver and Dean Burk introduced an analysis of enzyme kinetics utilizing a double reciprocal rearrangement of the Michaelis-Menten equation such that straight line plots of $1/v$ versus $1/[S]$ are obtained (Figure 4–2), where the slope reflects K_m/V_{max} and the y-intercept is $1/V_{max}$.

INHIBITION OF ENZYME-CATALYZED REACTIONS

Enzyme inhibitors fall into two broad classes: those causing irreversible inactivation of enzymes and those whose inhibitory effects can be reversed. Irreversible inhibitors usually cause an inactivating, covalent modification of enzyme structure. Reversible inhibitors (Table 4–2) can be divided into two main categories; competitive inhibitors and noncompetitive inhibitors, with a third category, uncompetitive inhibitors, rarely encountered in the clinical setting.

Plotting enzyme activity in the presence and absence of reversible inhibitors using Lineweaver-Burk plots (Figure 4–3) demonstrates the characteristic features of these inhibitors as outlined in Table 4–2.

HIGH-YIELD CONCEPT PROBLEM-SOLVING ENZYME INHIBITION QUESTIONS

In most cases, the solving of examination problems related to enzyme inhibition is just a matter of understanding what effects various inhibitors exert and how to quickly recognize the type of inhibitor used in the context of the question. The vast majority of clinically relevant drugs exert their effects through either competitive or noncompetitive inhibition of enzyme activity. As such, these reflect the two most commonly encountered types of examination questions.

With respect to problems that contain a table of V_{max} and K_m values, in the absence and presence of an inhibitor, the question being asked is likely the identification of which kind of inhibitor is used. Remember that for competitive inhibitors, ONLY K_m changes. Yes, the value of K_m increases, but for these types of problems that is not the important concept to remember; it is that K_m changes while V_{max} does NOT change. Conversely, for noncompetitive inhibitors K_m does not change, ONLY V_{max} changes. Yes, for noncompetitive inhibitors V_{max} decreases, but for these types of problems it is only important to remember that V_{max} changes while K_m does NOT change for noncompetitive inhibitors.

The second common type of problem may also include a table of kinetic values but will also contain a Lineweaver-Burk plot. In these types of problems the key is to look immediately at the plot and determine if the lines cross or not. In these types of problems if the lines **C**ross the inhibitor is a **C**ompetitive inhibitor, whereas, if the lines do **N**ot cross then the inhibitor is a **N**oncompetitive inhibitor.

TABLE 4–2 Characteristics of enzyme inhibition.

Inhibitor Type	Binding Site on Enzyme	Kinetic Effect
Competitive inhibitor	Specifically at the catalytic site, where it competes with substrate for binding in a dynamic equilibrium-like process. Inhibition is reversible by substrate.	V_{max} is unchanged; K_m, as defined by [S] required for ½ maximal activity, is increased.
Noncompetitive inhibitor	Binds E or ES complex other than at the catalytic site. Substrate binding unaltered, but ESI complex cannot form products. Inhibition cannot be reversed by substrate.	K_m appears unaltered; V_{max} is decreased proportionately to inhibitor concentration.
Uncompetitive inhibitor	Binds only to ES complexes at locations other than the catalytic site. Substrate binding modifies enzyme structure, making inhibitor-binding site available. Inhibition cannot be reversed by substrate.	Apparent V_{max} decreased; K_m, as defined by [S] required for ½ maximal activity, is decreased.

Reproduced with permission from King MW: *Integrative Medical Biochemistry Examination and Board Review*. New York, NY: McGraw Hill; 2014.

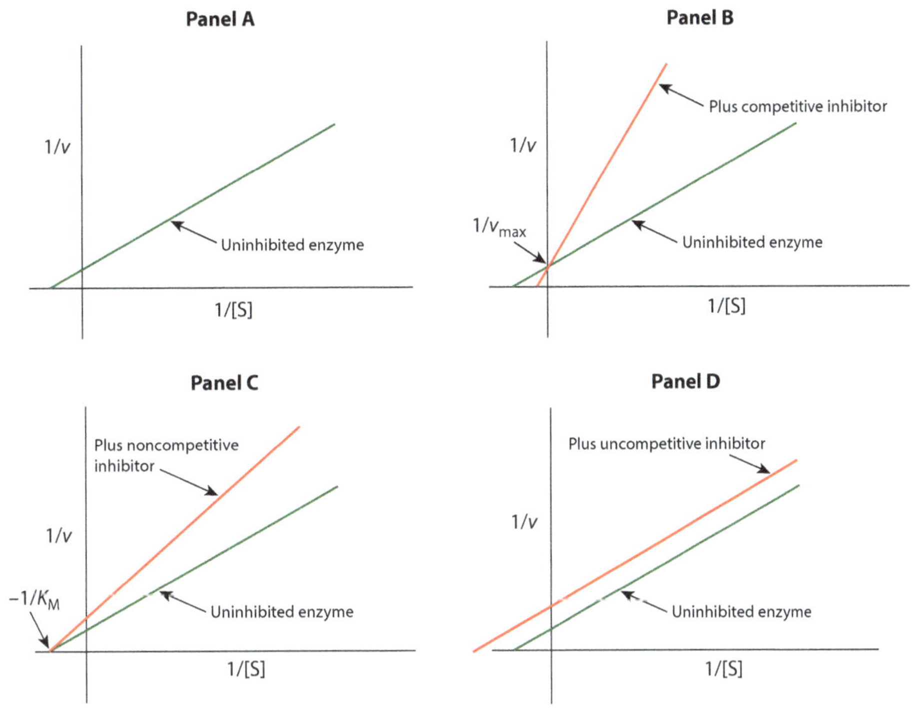

FIGURE 4–3 Lineweaver-Burk (L-B) plots of inhibited enzymes. Panel A shows the L-B plot for a hypothetical enzyme in the absence of any inhibitor. Panel B shows the L-B results when a competitive inhibitor is added to the hypothetical enzyme reaction. Panel C shows the L-B results when a noncompetitive inhibitor is added to the hypothetical enzyme reaction. Panel D shows the L-B results when an uncompetitive inhibitor is added to the hypothetical enzyme reaction. Note that for competitive inhibitors the two lines cross at the y-axis indicative of NO change in V_{max}. For noncompetitive inhibitors, the two lines essentially meet on the x-axis indicating that there is NO change in K_m. In the case of an uncompetitive inhibitor the lines end up parallel to one another indicating that both V_{max} and K_m change. (Reproduced with permission from themedicalbiochemistrypage, LLC.)

REGULATION OF ENZYME ACTIVITY

Enzyme concentration is continually modulated in response to physiologic needs. Three principal mechanisms are known to regulate the concentration of active enzyme in tissues:

1. Regulation of gene expression controls the quantity and rate of enzyme synthesis.
2. Proteolytic enzyme activity determines the rate of enzyme degradation.
3. Covalent modification of preexisting pools of inactive proenzymes produces active enzymes.

ALLOSTERIC ENZYMES

Many enzymes, in particular the critical rate-limiting enzymes of metabolic pathways, interact with molecules that are distinct from substrates. The interactions result in modulation of enzyme activity. These types of enzymes are known as allosteric enzymes and the regulatory molecules that bind to these enzymes are known as allosteric effectors.

HIGH-YIELD CONCEPT

Allosteric effectors bring about catalytic modification by binding to the enzyme at allosteric sites distinct from the catalytic site. The binding causes conformational changes that are transmitted through the bulk of the protein to the catalytically active site(s). Effectors that increase catalytic activity are known as positive effectors and effectors that reduce or inhibit catalytic activity are negative effectors. Their single defining feature is that they are not identical to the substrate.

CHECKLIST

- ☑ Enzymes are biological catalysts that, like inorganic catalysts, decrease the energy required to drive a reaction forward without themselves being consumed or permanently altered in the process.
- ☑ Enzymes are specific for both the type of reaction catalyzed and the substrate, or a small subset of closely related substrates, acted upon.
- ☑ Enzymes are divided into six classifications based on substrates involved and type of reaction catalyzed.
- ☑ Many enzymes are complexes consisting of both protein and organic or inorganic prosthetic groups, the latter being termed coenzymes. Many coenzymes are vitamins or vitamin derivatives.
- ☑ The study of enzyme kinetics allows for an understanding of the steps by which an enzyme can convert a substrate into product.
- ☑ The ratio of reaction rate constants is represented by the equilibrium constant, K_{eq}, which can be calculated from the concentration of substrates and products when a reaction has reached equilibrium.
- ☑ The rate of enzyme-catalyzed reactions is influenced by enzyme and substrate concentration, temperature, and pH, as well as the presence of inhibitors.
- ☑ The Michaelis-Menten equation illustrates the mathematical relationship between the initial reaction velocity and the substrate concentration.
- ☑ Linear forms of the Michaelis-Menten equation simplify the determination of K_m and V_{max} for a given enzyme catalyzed reaction.
- ☑ The Michaelis-Menten constant, K_m, is defined as the concentration of substrate required for an enzyme catalyzed reaction to attain half the maximal reaction velocity, V_{max}. Therefore, it becomes obvious that an enzyme with a lower K_m will carry out a reaction more efficiently than another enzyme with a higher K_m for the same substrate.
- ☑ Physiologically significant forms of enzyme inhibitor include competitive and noncompetitive inhibitors.
- ☑ Competitive inhibitors bind the same site as substrate resulting in an increase in K_m while having no effect on V_{max}.
- ☑ Noncompetitive inhibitors bind to sites on the enzyme other than substrate resulting in a decrease in V_{max} with no change in K_m.
- ☑ Analysis of the inhibition of enzyme catalysis reveals potentially important clinically relevant information for use in the design of pharmaceutical compounds.
- ☑ Ribozymes are RNA-based enzymes that represent a unique class of nonprotein enzyme.
- ☑ Analysis of the changes of the levels of enzymes in the blood aids in the diagnosis of various diseases and disorders such as in the case of liver disease and myocardial infarction.

REVIEW QUESTIONS

1. A 27-year-old migrant farm worker is admitted to the hospital in a comatose state. Physical examination shows excessive salivation and muscle twitching. History reveals that this worker was in the field at the time of aerial crop spraying. Suspecting pesticide exposure, the attending physician orders an assay of acetylcholinesterase activity in the patient's blood. The results of this assay, comparing the patient's activity to a normal control, are shown. Which of the following types of inhibition is most consistent with these findings?

	Velocity (μmol/min/mg)	
Substrate Concentration (μM)	**Normal Control**	**Patient**
1.0	1.6	1.4
3.0	4.9	4.0
5.0	6.2	5.8
10.0	10.0	6.0
20.0	11.7	6.7
30.0	12.0	6.9

(A) Allosteric
(B) Competitive
(C) Mixed
(D) Noncompetitive
(E) Uncompetitive

2. A 57-year-old man comes to the emergency department because of experiencing severe substernal chest pain approximately 18 hours ago. He has just returned from an overseas trip. Which of the following is the most appropriate laboratory test to order for this patient?
(A) Aspartate aminotransferase
(B) Creatine kinase, MB fraction
(C) Gamma-glutamyltransferase
(D) Lactate dehydrogenase, LD1 fraction
(E) Troponin I

3. Equimolar amounts of two carbohydrates of glycolysis (glucose-6-phosphate and fructose-6-phosphate) are incubated with the enzyme phosphohexose isomerase which catalyzes their interconversion. The reaction is allowed to proceed until equilibrium is attained at which time assay for the concentration of the two carbohydrates is undertaken. Results of this assay reveal that the concentration of glucose-6-phosphate is four times that of fructose-6-phosphate. Based on these findings, which one of the following values would most accurately represent the Gibbs free energy of the reaction as written?

Glucose-6-phosphate → Fructose-6-phosphate
(A) $\Delta G^{0'} = -7.3$ kJ/mol
(B) $\Delta G^{0'} = -1.72$ kJ/mol
(C) $\Delta G^{0'} = 0$
(D) $\Delta G^{0'} = +1.72$ kJ/mol
(E) $\Delta G^{0'} = +7.3$ kJ/mol

4. Experiments are being conducted on a novel compound designed to inhibit a cell cycle check point kinase. The compound was designed to act as a noncompetitive inhibitor of the kinase. In assaying the compound, which of the following kinetic parameters would most likely be found, in comparison to the absence of the compound, if the compound indeed functions as predicted?
(A) K_m decreased, V_{max} increased
(B) K_m decreased, V_{max} unchanged
(C) K_m increased, V_{max} decreased
(D) K_m unchanged, V_{max} decreased
(E) K_m unchanged, V_{max} unchanged

5. The standard free energy change ($\Delta G^{0'}$) for the hydrolysis of phosphoenolpyruvate (PEP) is −14.8 kcal/mol. The $\Delta G^{0'}$ for the hydrolysis of ATP is −7.3 kcal/mol. Which of the following most closely defines the $\Delta G^{0'}$ for the following coupled reaction?

Phosphoenolpyruvate + ADP → pyruvate + ATP
(A) −22.1 kcal/mol
(B) −14.8 kcal/mol
(C) −7.5 kcal/mol
(D) +7.5 kcal/mol
(E) +14.8 kcal/mol
(F) +22.1 kcal/mol

6. Experiments are being conducted on a novel compound designed to inhibit a cell cycle check point kinase. The compound was designed to act as a noncompetitive inhibitor of the kinase since these types of inhibitors are more effective as chemotherapeutics than are competitive inhibitors. Which of the following best explains why this latter statement is valid?
(A) Their inhibitory activity is unaffected by substrate concentration
(B) They affect only K_m and not V_{max}
(C) They bind to the same site as the substrate
(D) They increase the rate of degradation of the target enzyme
(E) They irreversibly inhibit the enzyme

7. Experiments are being conducted on a novel compound designed to inhibit a cell cycle check point kinase. The compound was designed to act as a competitive inhibitor of the kinase. In assaying the compound, which of the following kinetic parameters would most likely be found, in comparison to the absence of the compound, if the compound indeed functions as predicted?
(A) Decrease both V_{max} and K_m
(B) Decrease K_m but no effect on V_{max}
(C) Decrease V_{max} but no change on K_m
(D) Increase both V_{max} and K_m
(E) Increase K_m but no change in V_{max}
(F) Increase V_{max} but no increase in K_m

8. The activity of glycogen phosphorylase was assessed under standard conditions and the kinetic data were plotted as a linear Lineweaver-Burk graph as shown. The activity of the enzyme in the presence of glycogen is represented by the line identified as control. The dashed line indicated by 2 is most likely obtained by addition of which of the following to this enzyme assay?

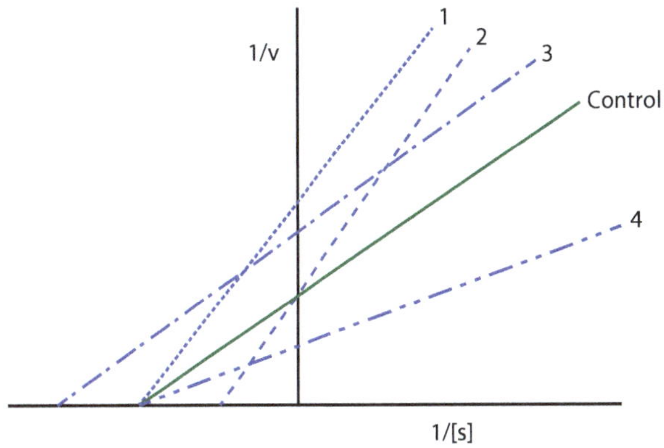

(A) Allosteric activator
(B) Competitive inhibitor
(C) Double the amount of enzyme
(D) Half the amount of enzyme
(E) Noncompetitive inhibitor

9. Experiments are being conducted on breast cancer cells in culture to test the efficacy of a novel potential chemotherapeutic compound that inhibits the activity of the kinase activity of the HER2 receptor. Addition of the compound to the cultures results in an increase in the K_m of the reaction but does not affect the V_{max}. Which of the following most closely defines the inhibitory action of the compound?
(A) Competitive
(B) Mixed function
(C) Noncompetitive
(D) Suicide
(E) Uncompetitive

10. For the reaction A → B, $\Delta G^{0'} = -5$ kcal/mol. The reaction is started with 10 mmol of A and there is no B present. After 24 hours, analysis reveals the presence of 2 mmol of B and 8 mmol of A. Which of the following is the most likely explanation?
(A) A and B have reached equilibrium concentrations
(B) An enzyme has shifted the equilibrium toward A
(C) B formation is kinetically slow; equilibrium has not been reached by 24 hours
(D) Formation of B is thermodynamically unfavorable
(E) The result described is impossible, given the fact that $\Delta G'^{o}$ is −5 kcal/mol

11. The standard free-energy changes for the reactions below are given.

Phosphocreatine → creatine + P_i	$\Delta G^{0'} = -43.0$ kJ/mol
ATP → ADP + P_i	$\Delta G^{0'} = -30.5$ kJ/mol

What is the most likely $\Delta G^{0'}$ for the following coupled reaction?

Phosphocreatine + ADP → creatine + ATP
(A) −73.5 kJ/mol
(B) −12.5 kJ/mol

(C) −2.7 kJ/mol
(D) +2.7 kJ/mol
(E) +12.5 kJ/mol
(F) +73.5 kJ/mol

12. A screening test for galactosemia is positive in a newborn female. Genetic studies determine that the infant harbors a missense mutation in the GALT gene. This mutation impairs the activity of the encoded galactose-1-phosphate uridylyltransferase enzyme. As a result of the impaired enzyme activity galactose-1-phosphate accumulates and affects the activity of UTP-dependent glucose-1-phosphate pyrophosphorylase 2 (encoded by the UGP2 gene). Which of the following actions, by galactose-1-phosphate, most closely demonstrates that it functions as a competitive inhibitor of the UGP2 encoded enzyme?
(A) Decreases both the V_{max} and the apparent K_m for glucose-1-phosphate
(B) Decreases the apparent K_m for glucose-1-phosphate
(C) Decreases the V_{max} for glucose-1-phosphate
(D) Increases both the V_{max} and the apparent K_m for glucose-1-phosphate
(E) Increases the apparent K_m for glucose-1-phosphate
(F) Increases the V_{max} for glucose-1-phosphate

13. Experiments are being conducted on the activity of a novel drug designed to inhibit the activity of the LDL receptor metabolizing enzyme, PCSK9. Kinetic assays are performed in the presence and absence of the compound and the resultant data are presented in the table. These data demonstrate that the drug is most likely acting as which of the following types of inhibitors?

	Velocity (μmol/min/mg)	
Substrate Concentration (μM)	**Normal Control**	**Patient**
1.0	1.6	0.4
3.0	4.9	2.2
5.0	6.2	2.8
10.0	10.0	3.9
20.0	11.7	7.4
30.0	12.0	11.8

(A) Allosteric
(B) Competitive
(C) Mixed
(D) Noncompetitive
(E) Uncompetitive

14. Experiments are being conducted on the activity of ceruloplasmin in a sample of blood drawn from a patient. The activity of the enzyme is tested in the undiluted blood sample and plotted on a Lineweaver-Burke plot giving the line identified as control. The blood sample is diluted, and the assay is performed again. Which of the following lines on the graph most likely represents the data for the diluted sample?
(A) 1
(B) 2
(C) 3
(D) 4
(E) Same as Control

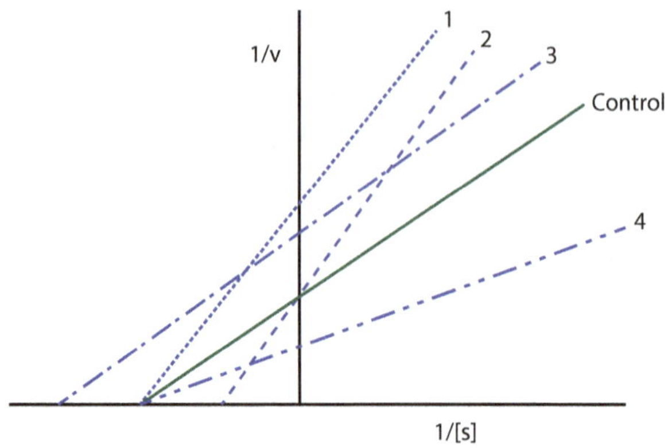

15. Experiments are being conducted on the activity of a novel drug designed to inhibit the activity of the LDL receptor metabolizing enzyme, PCSK9. Kinetic assays are performed in the presence and absence of the compound and the resultant data are presented in the table. These data are plotted using the Lineweaver-Burke transformation with the data for the enzyme with no compound present indicated as control. Which of the other lines on the graph is most likely representative of the kinetic data obtained in the presence of the drug?

	Velocity (μmol/min/mg)	
Substrate Concentration (μM)	**Normal Control**	**Patient**
1.0	1.6	0.4
3.0	4.9	2.2
5.0	6.2	2.8
10.0	10.0	3.9
20.0	11.7	7.4
30.0	12.0	11.8

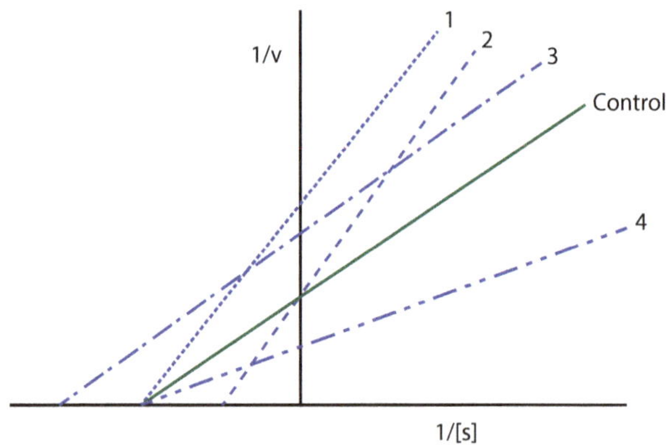

(A) 1
(B) 2
(C) 3
(D) 4
(E) Same as Control

ANSWERS

1. Correct answer is **D**. The most significant inhibitors, from a clinical perspective, are competitive and noncompetitive because the majority of drugs exhibit one or the other of these characteristics. One of the things that causes problems for many students is trying to solve examination problems related to enzyme inhibition. Now certainly in many cases, students will be required to carry out calculations that are aimed at determining the changed values of K_m and/or V_{max} in these types of problems. However, many times it is just a matter of understanding what effect various inhibitors exert and how to quickly recognize the type of inhibitor used in the context of the question. This is quite easily accomplished for two types of problems. In one case the problem may contain a table of V_{max} and/or K_m values in the absence and presence of an inhibitor and the question asks for identification of which kind of inhibitor is used. This can be easily discerned by determining which one of the two kinetic parameters is changing. For competitive inhibitors, ONLY K_m changes. True, the value of K_m increases but for these types of problems that is not the important concept to remember, it is that K_m and NOT V_{max} changes. Conversely, for noncompetitive inhibitors K_m does not change, ONLY V_{max} changes. For noncompetitive inhibitors V_{max} decreases, but for these types of problems it is only important to remember that V_{max} changes while K_m does not for noncompetitive inhibitors. From the table in this question, it can be seen that the V_{max} values are different between control and patient and thus, K_m must be unchanged. The data could be graphed to prove this point, but it is not necessary. None of the other types of inhibition (choices A, B, C, and E) fit the data that are presented.
2. Correct answer is **E**. Troponin I is now the method of choice for the laboratory diagnosis of myocardial infarction. There is a detectable increase within 4–8 hours of the infarction and the peak level is reached within 12–16 hours. Levels do not return to baseline for 3–10 days making it an appropriate test for this patient who was 3 days postinfarction. Aspartate aminotransferase (choice A) was the first serum enzyme marker used for the diagnosis of myocardial infarction, but it has poor specificity and sensitivity compared to newer markers and is no longer used for this purpose. Creatine kinase (choice B) total is not used for the diagnosis of myocardial infarction since the cardiac fraction (MB) can be overwhelmed by the presence of the skeletal muscle fraction. Creatine kinase-MB is still being used in some institutions, but it returns to baseline in 2–3 days and would not be useful for this patient. Elevated levels of gamma-glutamyltransferase, GGT (choice C) are found in diseases of the liver, biliary system, and pancreas. Slight elevations in serum GGT levels are also seen in cardiovascular disease, in particular, GGT accumulates in atherosclerotic plaques. GGT-containing protein aggregates circulate in the blood in certain pathologies such as metabolic syndrome, alcohol addiction, and chronic liver disease. The LD1 fraction of lactate dehydrogenase (choice D) is found in heart and red-blood cells and is 17–27% of the normal serum total. Following a myocardial infarct, the serum levels of LDH rise within 24–48 hours reaching a peak by 2–3 days and return to normal in 5–10 days. Especially diagnostic is a comparison of the LDH-1/LDH-2 ratio. Normally, this ratio is less than 1. A reversal of this ratio is referred to as a "flipped LDH." Following an acute myocardial infarct, the flipped LDH ratio will appear in 12–24 hours and is definitely present by 48 hours in over 80% of patients. However, the LDH1 levels return to baseline later than creatine kinase but has been replaced by troponin I and is seldom used for diagnostic purposes in suspected myocardial infarction.
3. Correct answer is **E**. Since there is more substrate than product when the reaction has reached equilibrium, the reaction can be assumed to be less than favorable when proceeding in the direction as written. Therefore, the free energy change value for the reaction is most likely to be positive. Since the amount of glucose-6-phosphate at equilibrium is found to be significantly higher than that of fructose-6-phosphate the most likely Gibbs free energy of the reaction, as written, would be the larger of the two positive free energy values and not the lower (choice D). The two negative free energy values (choices A and B) are indicative of reactions that are favorable in the direction as written and thus, there would be more product than substrate at equilibrium. A free energy of zero (choice C) is indicative of a reaction where there would be equal amounts of substrate and product at equilibrium.
4. Correct answer is **D**. Noncompetitive inhibitors bind to enzyme at a site that is not the catalytic site and thus, have no effect on substrate binding. However, the resultant ESI complex cannot form products. This type of inhibition cannot be reversed by the addition of more substrate. Because noncompetitive inhibitors effectively reduce the amount of active enzyme molecules, V_{max} is decreased proportionately to inhibitor concentration but K_m remains unchanged. None of the other options (choices A, B, C, and E) correspond changes in K_m and V_{max} that occur with noncompetitive inhibitors.
5. Correct answer is **C**. The reaction, as written, represents the coupling of two distinct reactions. One is the hydrolysis of PEP to pyruvate and the other is the synthesis of ATP from ADP. Each of the two reactions has their own $\Delta G^{o'}$. To simplify, a coupled biochemical reaction is one where the free energy of a thermodynamically favorable reaction (PEP to pyruvate) is used to drive a thermodynamically unfavorable one (the formation of ATP from ADP), by coupling the two reactions. The coupling in this case is carried out by the enzyme pyruvate kinase. When two reactions are coupled, the resultant free energy change is simply the mathematical sum of the two $\Delta G^{o'}$ values for each reaction. In the case of the formation of ATP from ADP, the $\Delta G^{o'}$ for the reaction in that direction is equal to, but mathematically opposite of, the reciprocal reaction and therefore, for this coupled reaction would be +7.3 kcal/mol. None of the other options (choices A, B, D, E, and F) represent the sum of the free energies for the two coupled reactions.
6. Correct answer is **A**. Pharmaceuticals that are designed to inhibit an enzyme in a noncompetitive manner are much more effective than inhibitors that function competitively since any increase in substrate will have no effect on the level of inhibition exerted by the pharmaceutical. Some pharmaceuticals do act as competitive inhibitors (choice B) but for the reasons stated are not as effective in many situations as are noncompetitive inhibitors. Noncompetitive inhibitors do not bind to the same site as substrate (choice C). Although some pharmaceuticals may increase the rate of degradation of their targets (choice D), this is not the primary goal of drug discovery and development. Some pharmaceuticals, such as aspirin, do irreversibly inhibit their targeted enzyme (choice E) by covalent attachment to sites that are not the substrate binding

site and as such are forms of noncompetitive inhibitors. However, it is much easier to generate noncompetitive chemicals that block function through noncovalent means.

7. Correct answer is **E**. Competitive inhibitors bind enzyme at the catalytic site, thereby competing with substrate for binding in a dynamic equilibrium-like process. This type of inhibition is reversible by the addition of higher concentrations of substrate. With competitive inhibitors the maximum velocity (V_{max}) of the reaction is unchanged, while the apparent affinity of the substrate to the binding site is decreased. In other words, K_m, as defined by the substrate concentration required for half maximal activity, is increased. None of the other options (choices A, B, C, D, and F) correspond changes in K_m and V_{max} that occur with competitive inhibitors.

8. Correct answer is **B**. Competitive inhibitors bind enzyme at the catalytic site thereby, competing with substrate for binding in a dynamic equilibrium-like process. This type of inhibition is reversible by the addition of higher concentrations of substrate. With competitive inhibitors the maximum velocity (V_{max}) of the reaction is unchanged, while the apparent affinity of the substrate to the binding site is decreased. In other words, K_m, as defined by the substrate concentration required for half maximal activity, is increased. These changes are visible in Lineweaver-Burk plots where the Y-axis intercept is unchanged while the X-axis intercept is closer to the Y-axis indicative of a larger value for K_m. One key feature of the interpretation of inhibitor type with questions that include Lineweaver-Burk plots is to determine if the lines cross or not. In these types of problems if the lines **C**ross the inhibitor is a **C**ompetitive inhibitor, whereas, if the lines **N**o cross then the inhibitor is a **N**oncompetitive inhibitor. Addition of an allosteric activator (choice A) would lead to a decrease in K_m which is not observed for line 2. Doubling the amount of enzyme (choice C) would double the value of V_{max} while having no effect on K_m, as is indicated by line 4 in the plot. Using half the amount of enzyme (choice D) and noncompetitive inhibitors (choice E) both would decrease the V_{max} of the reaction but would not affect K_m, both of which are indicated by line 1 in the plot.

9. Correct answer is **A**. Competitive inhibitors bind enzyme at the catalytic site, thereby competing with substrate for binding in a dynamic equilibrium-like process. This type of inhibition is reversible by the addition of higher concentrations of substrate. With competitive inhibitors the maximum velocity (V_{max}) of the reaction is unchanged, while the apparent affinity of the substrate to the binding site is decreased. In other words, K_m, as defined by the substrate concentration required for half maximal activity, is increased. Mixed function inhibitors (choice B) will result in changes to both V_{max} and K_m. Noncompetitive inhibitors (choice C) decrease the V_{max} of the reaction but do not affect K_m. Suicide inhibitors (choice D) are a form of noncompetitive inhibitor that exert their effects by covalent attachment to their target enzyme and thus, permanently inhibit the enzyme. Uncompetitive inhibitors (choice E) only bind to ES complexes at locations other than the catalytic site. Substrate binding modifies enzyme structure, making the inhibitor binding site available. Uncompetitive inhibitors decrease both K_m and V_{max} so that when plotted using the Lineweaver-Burk method yield a line that is parallel to the untreated enzyme.

10. Correct answer is **C**. When this reaction is at equilibrium the amount of product (B) would be greater than that of substrate (A) since the reaction proceeds favorably from A to B. Since the amount of B is still less than that of A the reaction has not yet reached equilibrium even after 24 hours. The reaction is still thermodynamically favorable since the free energy change for the reaction as written has a negative value. In addition, since equilibrium has not yet been reached in the time frame of the analysis it is implied that the reaction proceeds with slow kinetics. Although it could be argued that the results of the analysis indicate that the enzyme used did not favor A as its substrate (choice A), there is no indication in the question that this is a valid or most likely explanation for the results. The reaction, as written, would result in more B than A at equilibrium (choice B) since the free energy value is negative and thus thermodynamically favorable. Since the free energy value is negative the reaction, as written, is thermodynamically favorable (choice D). An enzyme catalyzed reaction with a Gibbs free energy of –5 kcal/mol represents a biochemically feasible reaction (choice E).

11. Correct answer is **B**. When two reactions are coupled the resultant free energy change is the arithmetic sum of the $\Delta G^{0'}$ values for the coupled reactions. In the case of the coupled reaction, instead of energy input from the hydrolysis of ATP the opposite reaction is being coupled. The $\Delta G^{0'}$ value for a given reaction is its reciprocal value when the reaction is running in the opposite direction to that for which the $\Delta G^{0'}$ value is denoted. Thus, for ATP synthesis from ADP the $\Delta G^{0'}$ value would be +30.5 kJ/mol. When the two reactions are coupled, there is sufficient energy released from the hydrolysis of phosphocreatine to drive the synthesis of ATP from ADP. The $\Delta G^{0'}$ value for the coupled reactions is the simple arithmetic sum of the $\Delta G^{0'}$ values for the individual reactions. None of the other options (choices A, C, D, E, and F) represents correct free energy values for the coupled reactions.

12. Correct answer is **E**. Competitive inhibitors affect only the K_m of the inhibited enzyme. Specifically, the inhibitor binds to the substrate binding site. It, therefore, takes more substrate to displace the inhibitor and lead to enzyme catalysis. Because more substrate is required the effect is observable as an apparent reduction in the affinity of the enzyme for the substrate, and since the K_m is a measure of substrate affinity (the concentration of substrate required to attain half the maximal velocity of the catalyzed reaction), the consequences of competitive inhibitors is an apparent increase in the K_m. Uncompetitive inhibitors (choice A) bind only to enzyme-substrate complexes at locations other than the catalytic site. Substrate binding modifies enzyme structure, which results in the inhibitor binding site being made available. Inhibition cannot be reversed by substrate and the number of active enzyme molecules is reduced. Therefore, the presence of uncompetitive inhibitors leads to decreases in both V_{max} and K_m. A decrease in the apparent K_m of an enzyme (choice B) would most likely be associated with the addition of an allosteric activator of the enzyme. This would result in increased enzyme activity, not decreased activity. Noncompetitive inhibitors (choice C) affect enzyme activity by binding to a site on the enzyme that is distinct from the substrate binding site. This effectively removes the enzyme from the active enzyme pool. Since the maximum velocity (V_{max}) of enzyme catalyzed reactions is solely correlated to the number of active enzyme molecules in the

reaction, the V_{max} decreases in the presence of noncompetitive inhibitors. A substance that increased apparent V_{max} (choice D) would be a compound that could both induce the expression of the gene while simultaneously binding to the substrate binding site, thereby resulting in an increase in the K_m of the enzyme. This phenomenon is not associated with typical competitive inhibitors. Substances that increase the V_{max} of enzyme catalyzed reactions (choice F) most likely increase the expression of the gene encoding the enzyme resulting in a higher number of active enzyme molecules in the reaction.

13. Correct answer is **B**. The most significant inhibitors, from a clinical perspective, are competitive and noncompetitive because the majority of drugs exhibit one or the other of these characteristics. One of the things that causes problems for many students is trying to solve examination problems related to enzyme inhibition. Now certainly in many cases, students will be required to carry out calculations that are aimed at determining the changed values of K_m and/or V_{max} in these types of problems. However, many times it is just a matter of understanding what effect various inhibitors exert and how to quickly recognize the type of inhibitor used in the context of the question. This is quite easily accomplished for two types of problems. In one case the problem may contain a Table of V_{max} and/or K_m values in the absence and presence of an inhibitor and the question asks for identification of which kind of inhibitor is used. This can be easily discerned by determining which one of the two kinetic parameters is changing. For competitive inhibitors ONLY K_m changes. True, the value of K_m increases but for these types of problems that is not the important concept to remember; it is that K_m and NOT V_{max} changes. Conversely, for noncompetitive inhibitors K_m does not change, ONLY V_{max} changes. For noncompetitive inhibitors V_{max} decreases, but for these types of problems it is only important to remember that V_{max} changes while K_m does not for noncompetitive inhibitors. From the table in this question, it can be seen that the V_{max} values are different between control and patient and thus, K_m must be unchanged. The data could be graphed to prove this point, but it is not necessary. None of the other types of inhibition (choices A, C, D, and E) fit the data that are presented.

14. Correct answer is **A**. Diluting the sample means less enzyme molecules so V_{max} goes down, but the enzymes are still the same, so their K_m is unchanged. The plot has the same K_m but lower V_{max} and thus, is not the same as control (choice E). It is tempting to think about V_{max} as an absolute enzyme constant, but V_{max} is a rate and therefore dependent on enzyme concentration. Lowering the concentration of enzyme by dilution decreases the V_{max}. Competitive inhibitors decrease K_m but do not affect V_{max} and are represented by line 2 (choice B) in the graph. Uncompetitive inhibitors decrease both K_m and V_{max} and when plotted against control show a parallel line (choice C). Doubling the amount of enzyme would double the value of V_{max} while having no effect on K_m, as is indicated by line 4 in the plot (choice D).

15. Correct answer is **B**. The data show that the drug functions as a competitive inhibitor. Competitive inhibitors bind enzyme at the catalytic site thereby, competing with substrate for binding in a dynamic equilibrium-like process. This type of inhibition is reversible by the addition of higher concentrations of substrate. With competitive inhibitors the maximum velocity (V_{max}) of the reaction is unchanged, while the apparent affinity of the substrate to the binding site is decreased. In other words, K_m, as defined by the substrate concentration required for half maximal activity, is increased. These changes are visible in Lineweaver-Burk plots where the Y-axis intercept is unchanged while the X-axis intercept is closer to the Y-axis indicative of a larger value for K_m. One key feature of the interpretation of inhibitor type with questions that include Lineweaver-Burk plots is to determine if the lines cross or not. In these types of problems if the lines **C**ross the inhibitor is a **C**ompetitive inhibitor, whereas, if the lines **N**o cross then the inhibitor is a **N**oncompetitive inhibitor (choice A). Using a noncompetitive inhibitor both would decrease the V_{max} of the reaction but would not affect K_m, which is indicated by line 1 in the plot (choice A). Uncompetitive inhibitors decrease both V_{max} and K_m and are evidenced by line parallel to the control uninhibited enzyme as depicted by line 3 (choice C). Doubling the amount of enzyme would double the value of V_{max} while having no effect on K_m, as is indicated by line 4 in the plot (choice D). Inhibitors affect either K_m or V_{max}, or both, and thus would not be seen as identical to control in a Lineweaver-Burk plot (choice E).

PART II METABOLIC BIOCHEMISTRY

CHAPTER 5

Glucose, Fructose, and Galactose Metabolism

High-Yield Terms

Hexokinase/Glucokinase	Glucose phosphorylating enzymes, differential tissue expression and regulatory properties; humans express four distinct hexokinase/glucokinase genes
PFK1	6-phosphofructo-1-kinase, major rate-limiting enzyme of glycolysis
PFK2	Bifunctional enzyme that is responsible for the synthesis of the major allosteric regulator of glycolysis via PFK1 and gluconeogenesis via fructose-1,6-bisphosphatase (F1,6-BPase)
Pyruvate kinase	Multiple forms with tissue-specific distribution and regulation
PKM2	Isoform of pyruvate kinase expressed in proliferating and cancer cells, participates in the Warburg effect
Substrate-level phosphorylation	Refers to the formation of ATP via the release of energy from a catabolic substrate as opposed to through oxidative phosphorylation
Intestinal glucose homeostasis	In addition to regulating glucose uptake from the diet and delivery to the blood, in times of fasting or compromised liver function the small intestine provides up to 20% of blood glucose via gluconeogenesis using glutamine and glycerol as substrates
Renal glucose homeostasis	Kidneys regulate circulating glucose levels through efficient resorption of plasma glucose as well as by being able to carry out gluconeogenesis using glutamine as a carbon source
Fructokinase	Encoded by the ketohexokinase (*KHK*) gene; produces two isoforms KHK-A and KHK-C catalyze phosphorylation of fructose to fructose-1-phosphate
Aldolase B	Enzyme catalyzing hydrolysis of fructose-1-phosphate to glyceraldehyde and dihydroxyacetone phosphate (DHAP)
Hereditary fructose intolerance	Potentially fatal infant disorder resulting from defect in the level of aldolase B activity
β-galactosidase	Intestinal enzyme complex involved in the hydrolysis of lactose to glucose and galactose. Commonly called lactase
Leloir pathway	Primary pathway for the conversion of galactose to glucose
Galactosemia	Results from defects in any of the three primary genes involved in conversion of galactose to glucose

DIGESTION AND UPTAKE OF DIETARY CARBOHYDRATE

Key features of the digestive processes are outlined in Chapter 28. Dietary carbohydrates enter the body in complex forms, such as disaccharides and polysaccharides. Sucrose and lactose represent the major dietary disaccharides. Through the actions of various salivary, intestinal, and pancreatic enzymes, these complex sugars are broken down into monosaccharides consisting primarily of glucose, fructose, and galactose.

Intestinal absorption of carbohydrates occurs via passive diffusion, facilitated diffusion, and active transport. The primary transporter involved in the intestinal uptake of glucose is the sodium-glucose cotransporter 1 (SGLT1). Galactose is also absorbed from the gut via the action of SGLT1. Fructose is absorbed from the intestine via GLUT5-mediated transport. The GLUT proteins belong to a large subfamily of carbohydrate transporters that belong to the solute carrier (SLC) family of transporters.

GLUCOSE TRANSPORTERS

The GLUT family of glucose transporters comprises a family of at least 14 members. Important members of this family include GLUT1 (SLC2A1), GLUT2 (SLC2A2), GLUT3 (SLC2A3), GLUT4 (SLC2A4, and GLUT5 (SLC2A5). Two additional glucose transporters that do not belong to the GLUT family are sodium-glucose co-transporter 1 (SGLT1) and SGLT2. SGLT2 is the major glucose transporter in the proximal tubule of the kidney and is responsible for more than 90% of glucose reabsorption from the glomerular filtrate.

GLUT1 is ubiquitously distributed in various tissues with highest levels of expression seen in erythrocytes. In fact in erythrocytes GLUT1 accounts for almost 5% of total protein. Although widely expressed GLUT1 is not expressed in hepatocytes.

GLUT2 is found primarily in intestine, pancreatic β-cells, kidney, and liver. The K_m of GLUT2 for glucose (17 mM) is the highest of all the sugar transporters. The high K_m ensures a fast equilibrium of glucose between the cytosol and the extracellular space ensuring that liver and pancreas do not metabolize glucose until its levels rise sufficiently in the blood. GLUT2 molecules can transport both glucose and fructose. When the concentration of blood glucose increases in response to food intake, pancreatic GLUT2 molecules mediate an increase in glucose uptake which leads to increased insulin secretion. For this reason, GLUT2 is thought to be a "glucose sensor."

GLUT3 is found primarily in neurons but also found in the intestine. GLUT3 binds glucose with high affinity (has the lowest K_m of the GLUTs) which allows neurons to have enhanced access to glucose especially under conditions of low blood glucose.

GLUT4 predominates in insulin-sensitive tissues, such as skeletal muscle and adipose tissue. Mobilization of GLUT4 to the plasma membrane is a major function of insulin in these tissues.

GLUT5 and the closely related transporter GLUT7 are involved in fructose transport. GLUT5 is expressed in intestine, kidney, testes, skeletal muscle, adipose tissue, and brain.

Although GLUT2, -5, -7, 8, -9, -11, and -12 can all transport fructose, GLUT5 is the only transporter that exclusively transports fructose.

GLYCOLYSIS

Glycolysis represents the pathway of glucose oxidation to pyruvate (Figure 5–1). Depending on the availability of oxygen and the mitochondrial pathway of pyruvate oxidation, pyruvate can be reduced to lactate. Since red blood cells (erythrocytes) lack mitochondria, they are a major source of the lactate present in the blood.

HIGH-YIELD CONCEPT

Glycolysis is a major pathway for the utilization of carbohydrate carbons for redistribution into biomass as well as being oxidized for the production of ATP. The unique, and highly significant, feature of glycolysis is that it can occur in the presence (aerobic) or absence (anaerobic) of oxygen.

Critical Reactions of Glycolysis

A. Hexokinases

The ATP-dependent phosphorylation of glucose to form glucose-6-phosphate (G6P) is the first reaction of glycolysis. This phosphorylation step is catalyzed by tissue-specific isoenzymes known as hexokinases. Four mammalian isozymes of hexokinase are known (Types I–IV), with the Type IV isozyme more commonly referred to as glucokinase. Glucokinase is the form of the enzyme found predominantly in hepatocytes and pancreatic β-cells.

There are two major differences between hexokinases I, II, and III and glucokinase. Hexokinases have low K_m for glucose (0.3–0.003 mM), are allosterically inhibited by physiologic concentrations of glucose-6-phosphate, and can utilize other hexoses (eg, fructose, mannose, glucosamine) as substrate. In contrast, glucokinase has a high K_m for glucose (5–8 mM), is not feedback inhibited by glucose-6-phosphate, and physiologically only recognizes glucose as a substrate. Although not product inhibited, hepatic glucokinase is allosterically inhibited by long-chain fatty acids (LCFA). In contrast, LCFAs do not inhibit the other forms of hexokinase. The kinetic properties of hepatic glucokinase allow the liver to effectively buffer blood glucose since most dietary glucose will pass through the liver and remain in the circulation for use by other tissues.

B. 6-Phosphofructo-1-Kinase (Phosphofructokinase-1, PFK1)

The highly regulated and principal rate-limiting reaction of glycolysis is the reaction catalyzed by 6-phosphofructo-1-kinase, better known as phosphofructokinase-1 or PFK1. PFK1 catalyzes the phosphorylation of the 1-carbon of fructose-6-phosphate generating fructose-1,6-bisphophate.

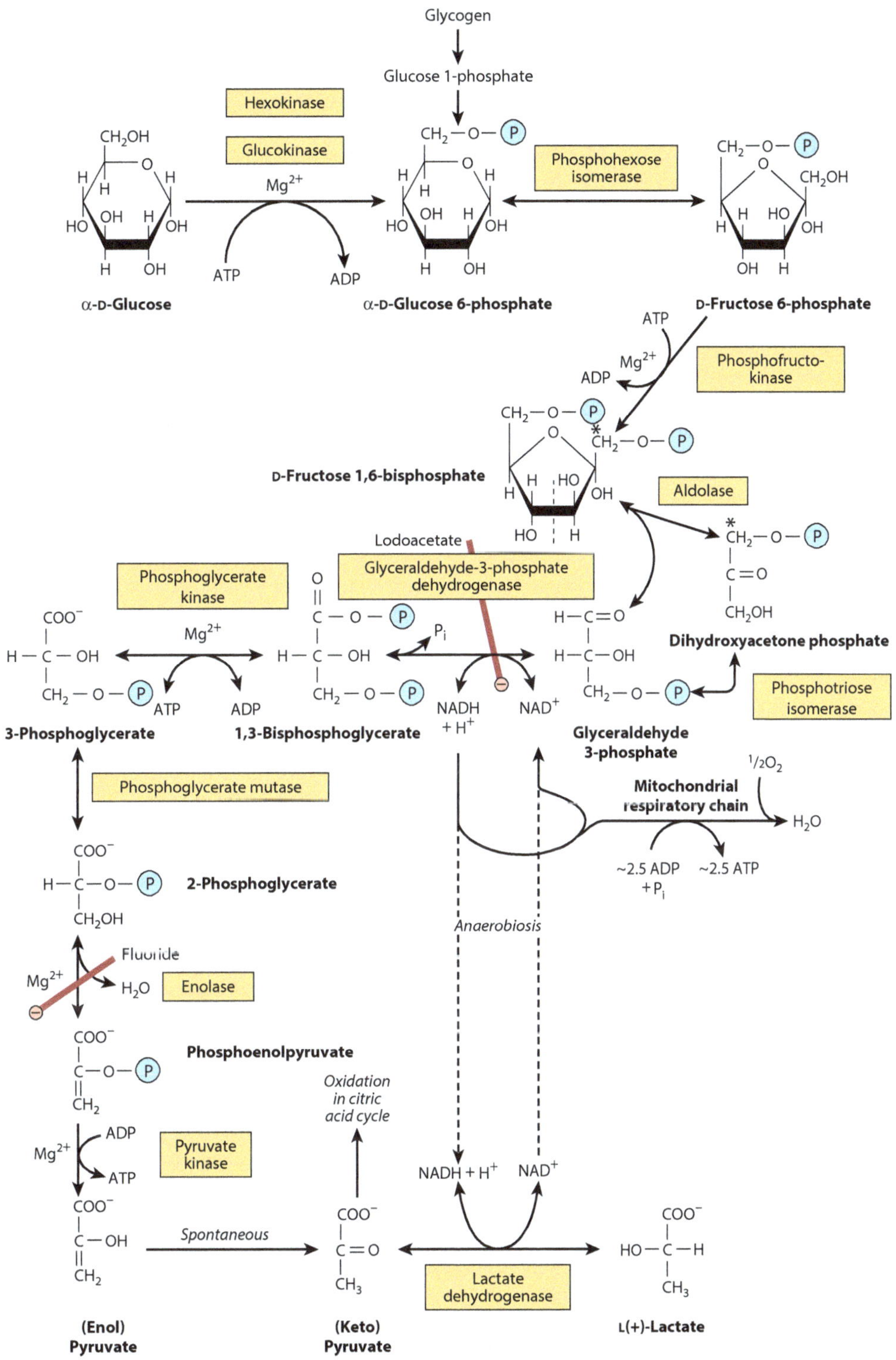

FIGURE 5–1 The pathway of glycolysis. (P, —PO_3^{2-}; Pi, $HOPO_3^{2-}$;⊖, inhibition.) *Carbons 1–3 of fructose bisphosphate form dihydroxyacetone phosphate, and carbons 4–6 form glyceraldehyde-3-phosphate. The term "bis-," as in bisphosphate, indicates that the phosphate groups are separated, whereas the term "di-," as in adenosine diphosphate, indicates that they are joined. (Reproduced with permission from Murray RK, Bender DA, Botham KM, et al: *Harper's Illustrated Biochemistry*, 29th ed. New York, NY: McGraw Hill; 2012.)

C. Pyruvate Kinase

The final reaction of aerobic glycolysis is catalyzed by the highly regulated enzyme, pyruvate kinase (PK). There are two distinct genes encoding PK activity. One encodes the liver and erythrocyte PK proteins (identified as the *PKLR* gene) and the other encodes the PKM proteins. Mutations in the *PKLR* gene result in the disorder referred to as erythrocyte PK deficiency (see Clinical Box 5–1).

CLINICAL BOX 5-1 ERYTHROCYTE PK DEFICIENCY

Erythrocyte pyruvate kinase (PK) deficiency is the most common enzyme deficiency resulting in inherited nonspherocytic hemolytic anemia. Pyruvate kinase deficiency is inherited as an autosomal recessive disorder and mutations in the *PKLR* (pyruvate kinase, liver, and red blood cell) gene occur with a frequency of 1 in 10,000. The disorder is characterized by lifelong chronic hemolysis of variable severity. Red blood cells from heterozygous individuals possess only 40–60% of the pyruvate kinase activity of normal individuals yet these individuals are almost always clinically normal. Numerous mutations (130 to date) have been identified in the *PKLR* gene resulting in erythrocyte PK deficiency. In persons of European descent, more than 50% of individuals with PK deficiency harbor a nucleotide change at position 1529 (encoding amino acid 510) that results in an Arg to Gln change in the protein and is identified as the R510Q mutation. The clinical severity of the anemia resulting from PKLR deficiencies varies from mild and fully compensated hemolysis to severe cases that require transfusions for survival. In the most severe cases an affected fetus will die *in utero*. Most PKLR deficient patients are diagnosed in infancy or early childhood. Severely affected patients may require multiple transfusions or splenectomy. The requirement for transfusion in many infants will diminish during childhood or following splenectomy. There are many patients with mild PKLR deficiency who do not manifest symptoms until adulthood. In these individuals, the symptoms, that include mild to moderate splenomegaly, mild chronic hemolysis, and jaundice, often manifest incidental to an acute viral infection or during an evaluation in pregnancy. Clinical evaluation of blood from patients with PKLR deficiency will show normocytic anemia (sometimes macrocytic) which is reflective of the reticulocytosis that is invariably present. In normal individuals, reticulocytes comprise 0.5–1.7% of the total erythrocytes. An increase in the percentage of reticulocytes (reticulocytosis) is an important sign in any patient suffering from anemia. In PKLR deficiency, the level of reticulocytosis results in a reticulocyte level of 4–15%. In association with the reticulocytosis there is a reduction in hematocrit (packed cell volume) to around 17–37% where it ranges from 41% to 50% in normal individuals. Hemoglobin measurement also shows a decrease to 6–12 g/dL, whereas the normal range is 12–16.5 g/dL. Examination of bone marrow from PKLR deficient patients will show normoblastic erythroid hyperplasia.

The *PKM* gene directs the synthesis of two isoforms of PK termed PKM1 and PKM2. The *PKM* gene was originally identified as the muscle pyruvate kinase gene, hence the nomenclature *PKM*. However, it is now known that the PKM1 protein is expressed in many tissues, whereas the PKM2 protein is most highly expressed in proliferating cells and all types of cancer (see Clinical Box 5–2).

CLINICAL BOX 5-2 GLYCOLYSIS IN CANCER: THE WARBURG EFFECT

In 1924, Otto Warburg made an observation that cancer cells metabolise glucose in a manner that was distinct from the glycolytic process of cells in normal tissues. Warburg discovered that, unlike most normal tissues, cancer cells tended to "ferment" glucose into lactate even in the presence of sufficient oxygen to support mitochondrial oxidative phosphorylation. This observation is known as the **Warburg Effect**. In the presence of oxygen, most differentiated cells primarily metabolize glucose to CO_2 and H_2O by oxidation of glycolytic pyruvate in the mitochondrial tricarboxylic acid (TCA) cycle. Proliferating cells, including cancer cells, require altered metabolism to efficiently incorporate nutrients such as glucose into biomass. The ultimate fate of glucose depends not only on the proliferative state of the cell but also on the activities of the specific glycolytic enzymes that are expressed. This is particularly true for pyruvate kinase, the terminal enzyme in glycolysis. In mammals, two genes encode a total of four pyruvate kinase (PK) isoforms: the *PKLR* gene and the *PKM* gene. The *PKM* gene encodes the PKM1 and PKM2 isoforms. Most tissues express either PKM1 or PKM2. PKM2 is expressed in most proliferating cells, including all cancer cell lines and tumors. PKM2 is much less active than PKM1 but is allosterically activated by the upstream glycolytic metabolite fructose 1,6-bisphosphate (FBP). PKM2 is also unique in that it can interact with phosphotyrosine in tyrosine phosphorylated proteins such as those resulting from growth factor stimulation of cells. The interaction of PKM2 with tyrosine phosphorylated proteins results in the release of FBP leading to reduced activity of the enzyme. Low PKM2 activity, in conjunction with increased glucose uptake, facilitates the diversion of glucose carbons into the anabolic pathways that are derived from glycolysis. Also, in cells expressing PKM2 there is increased phosphorylation of an active site histidine (His11) in the upstream glycolytic enzyme phosphoglycerate mutase (PGAM1) which increases its mutase activity. The phosphate donor for His11 phosphorylation of PGAM1 is phospho*enol*pyruvate (PEP) which is the substrate for pyruvate kinases. Phosphate transfer from PEP to PGAM1 yields pyruvate without concomitant generation of ATP. This alternate pathway allows for a high rate of glycolysis that is needed to support the anabolic metabolism observed in many proliferating cells. Targeting PKM2 for the treatment of cancers is a distinct possibility. Recent work has demonstrated that small molecule PKM2-specific activators are functional in tumor growth models in mice. These new drugs have been shown to constitutively activate PKM2 and the activated enzyme is resistant to inhibition by tyrosine phosphorylated proteins. PKM2-specific activators reduce the incorporation of glucose into lactate and lipids. In addition, PKM2 activation results in decreased pools of nucleotide, amino acid, and lipid precursors, and these effects may account for the suppression of tumorigenesis observed with these drugs.

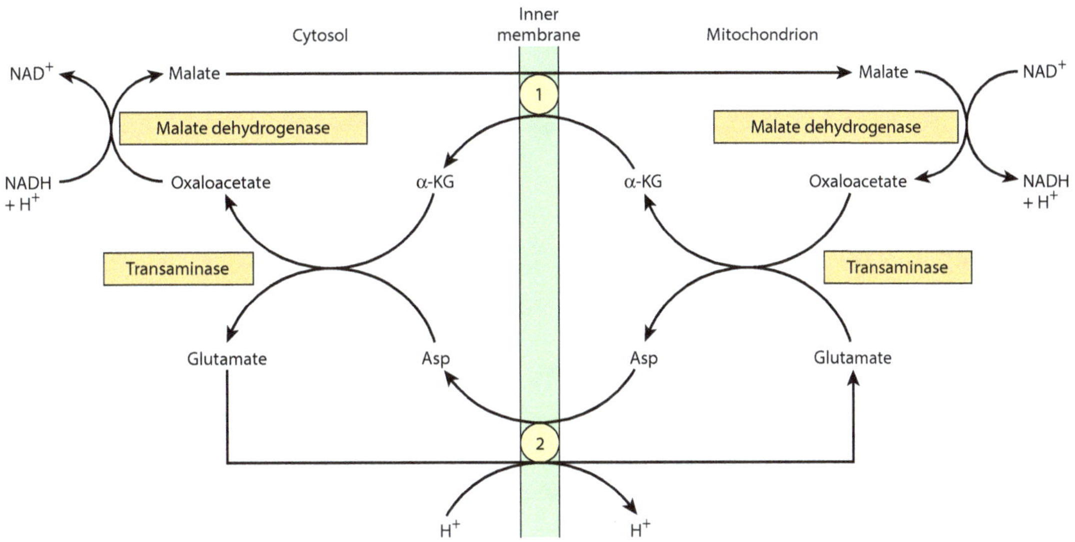

FIGURE 5–2 Malate shuttle for transfer of reducing equivalents from the cytosol into the mitochondrion. ① α-Ketoglutarate transporter and ② glutamate/aspartate transporter (note the proton symport with glutamate). (Reproduced with permission from Rodwell VW, Bender DA, Botham KM, et al: *Harper's Illustrated Biochemistry*, 31st ed. New York, NY: McGraw Hill; 2018.)

ATP Generation During Glycolysis

Glycolysis can produce ATP via glucose oxidation in the absence of oxygen and the need for mitochondrial oxidative phosphorylation. The two reactions of glycolysis that generate ATP are catalyzed by phosphoglycerate kinase (encoded by the *PGK1* gene) and pyruvate kinase. These ATP-generating reactions of glycolysis are referred to as substrate-level phosphorylations and generate a net yield of 2 moles of ATP per mole of free glucose.

Cytoplasmic NADH

The NADH (a reduced electron carrier) generated during glycolysis is used to fuel mitochondrial ATP synthesis via oxidative phosphorylation. The electrons carried by cytosolic NADH are transported into the mitochondria either by the malate-aspartate shuttle or the glycerol phosphate shuttle (Figures 5–2 and 5–3). The glycerol phosphate shuttle is the principal shuttle mechanism used in adipose tissue, skeletal muscle, and brain, whereas the liver, heart, and kidneys primarily utilize the malate-aspartate shuttle.

Lactate Metabolism

During anaerobic glycolysis, the reoxidation of NADH occurs via the coupled reduction of pyruvate to lactate. Pyruvate reduction is catalyzed by the enzymes of the lactate dehydrogenase (LDH) family. The lactate produced during anaerobic glycolysis diffuses from the tissues and is transported to the liver as well as cardiac muscle. The lactate is then oxidized to pyruvate by LDH and the pyruvate is further oxidized in the TCA cycle. In the liver, the pyruvate may be diverted into glucose biosynthesis via gluconeogenesis (see Chapter 6).

Mammalian cells contain two distinct types of LDH subunits, termed M (encoded by the *LDHA* gene) and H (encoded by the *LDHB* gene). Combinations of these different subunits generate LDH isozymes with different characteristics. The H-type subunit

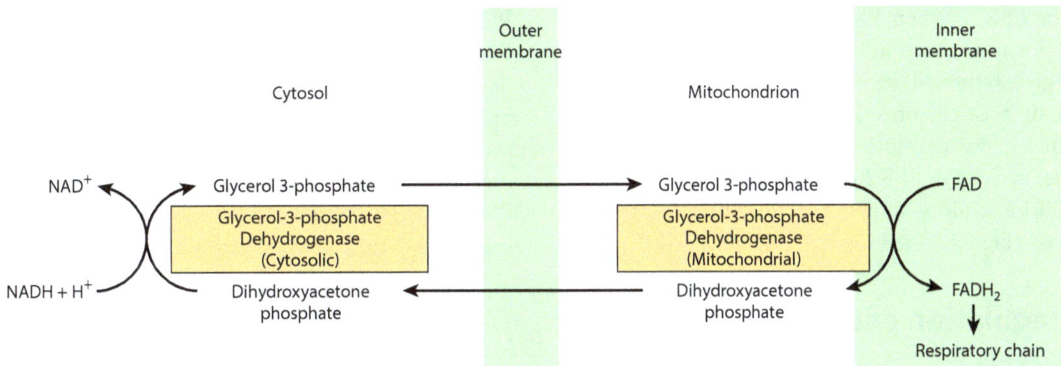

FIGURE 5–3 Glycerophosphate shuttle for transfer of reducing equivalents from the cytosol into the mitochondrion. (Reproduced with permission from Rodwell VW, Bender DA, Botham KM, et al: *Harper's Illustrated Biochemistry*, 31st ed. New York, NY: McGraw Hill; 2018.)

predominates in aerobic tissues such as heart muscle (as the H4 tetramer) while the M subunit predominates in anaerobic tissues such as skeletal muscle (as the M4 tetramer). H4 LDH has a low K_m for pyruvate and also is inhibited by high levels of pyruvate. The M4 LDH enzyme has a high K_m for pyruvate and is not inhibited by pyruvate.

Regulation of Glycolysis

The reactions catalyzed by hexokinase, PFK1, and PK represent the major regulated reactions of glycolysis. All three enzymes are allosterically regulated. However, neither regulation of hexokinase nor pyruvate kinase represent the major control point in glycolysis. Regulation of PK is important for reversing glycolysis when ATP levels are high in order to activate gluconeogenesis. The major rate-limiting step in glycolysis is the reaction catalyzed by PFK1.

The activity of PFK1 is regulated by numerous allosteric effectors including AMP, ATP, citrate, and fructose-2,6-bisphosphate (F2,6BP). ATP and citrate inhibit PFK1, whereas AMP and F2,6BP activate the enzyme. Indeed, F2,6BP is so potent at activating PFK1 that it can do so, particularly in hepatocytes, in the presence of ATP. Synthesis of F2,6BP is catalyzed from fructose-6-phosphate and ATP via the action of 6-phosphofructo-2-kinase/fructose-2,6-bisphosphatase (simply abbreviated PFK2). Because of the role of PFK2 in the control of F2,6BP levels it represents another critical regulatory step in glycolysis. F2,6BP also serves as a potent inhibitor of the gluconeogenic (see Chapter 6) enzyme, fructose-1,6-bisphosphatase. Therefore, PFK2 represents a critical control enzyme in overall hepatic glucose homeostasis.

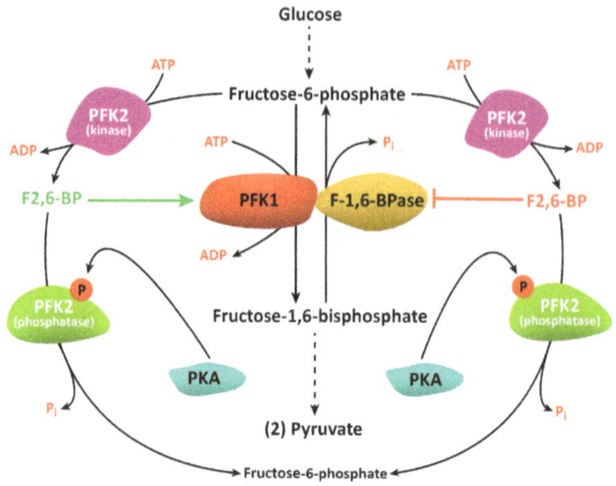

FIGURE 5–4 Regulation of glycolysis and gluconeogenesis by fructose-2,6-bisphosphate (F2,6BP). The major sites for regulation of glycolysis and gluconeogenesis are the phosphofructokinase-1 (PFK1) and fructose-1,6-bisphosphatase (F1,6BPase)-catalyzed reactions. PFK2 is the kinase activity and F2,6BPase is the phosphatase activity of the bifunctional regulatory enzyme, phosphofructokinase-2/fructose-2,6-bisphosphatase (PFK2). PKA is cAMP-dependent protein kinase, which phosphorylates PFK2 turning on the phosphatase activity. (+ve) and (−ve) refer to positive and negative activities, respectively. (Reproduced with permission from themedicalbiochemistrypage, LLC.)

Regulation of Glycolysis by PFK2

PFK2 is a bifunctional enzyme that can act as a kinase and phosphorylate fructose-6-phosphate with the use of ATP, generating F2,6BP, or it can act as a phosphatase and hydrolyze F2,6BP to fructose-6-phosphate and inorganic phosphate (P_i). Rapid, short-term regulation of the kinase and phosphatase activities of PFK2 is exerted by phosphorylation/dephosphorylation events. The phosphorylation of PFK2 is catalyzed by cAMP-dependent protein kinase, PKA. This PKA-mediated phosphorylation results in inhibition of the kinase activity while at the same time leading to activation of the phosphatase activity of PFK2. When PKA is active, for example, via glucagon or epinephrine action in the liver, there will be little F2,6BP and glycolysis will be reduced while simultaneously there will be enhanced gluconeogenesis. Conversely, when PKA activity is reduced, for example, due to insulin action on the liver, the kinase activity of PFK2 will be enhanced and the level of F2,6BP will rise resulting in increased glycolysis and reduced gluconeogenesis (Figure 5–4).

Hepatic Regulation of Blood Glucose Levels

The predominant tissue responding to signals that indicate reduced or elevated blood glucose levels is the liver. Both elevated and reduced levels of blood glucose trigger hormonal responses to initiate pathways designed to restore glucose homeostasis. Low blood glucose triggers release of glucagon from pancreatic α-cells and release of epinephrine from adrenal medullary chromaffin cells. High blood glucose triggers release of insulin from pancreatic β-cells. Glucocorticoids also act to increase blood glucose levels by inhibiting glucose uptake. Cortisol, the major glucocorticoid released from the adrenal cortex, is secreted in response to increased circulating ACTH.

The glucagon receptor is a G_s-type G-protein–coupled receptor (GPCR; see Chapter 26), the activation of which triggers an increase in adenylate cyclase activity leading to increased cAMP production. The cAMP in turn activates PKA which phosphorylates numerous substrates including PFK2. Phosphorylated PFK2 functions as a phosphatase that removes phosphate from F2,6BP. Reduced F2,6BP results in increased hepatic gluconeogenesis and reduced glycolysis. PKA also phosphorylates phosphorylase kinase (PHK) leading to increased phosphorylation of glycogen phosphorylase increasing its activity and thus, increased removal of glucose from glycogen (see Chapter 7). PKA and PHK also phosphorylate glycogen synthase making it less active such that less glucose incorporated into glycogen.

Epinephrine binds to both α_1- and β_2-adrenergic receptors on hepatocytes. The β_2-adrenergic receptor is coupled to a G_s-type G-protein and thus, elicits the same effects in the liver as glucagon. The α_1-type adrenergic receptor is coupled to a G_q-type G-protein whose activation leads to release of intracellularly stored Ca^{2+}. The release of Ca^{2+} to the cytosol directly activates

PHK and the resultant effects on glycolysis, gluconeogenesis, and glycogen metabolism.

In opposition to the cellular responses to glucagon and epinephrine on hepatocytes, insulin stimulates extrahepatic uptake of glucose from the blood and inhibits glycogenolysis in extrahepatic cells and conversely stimulates glycogen synthesis. These effects of insulin on the liver are exerted primarily via the activation of a phosphodiesterase (specifically PDE3B) that degrades cAMP and to the activation of protein phosphatase 1 (PP1).

Role of the Kidney and Small Intestines in Blood Glucose Control

Although the liver is the major site of glucose homeostasis, the kidneys and the small intestines do participate in the overall process of regulating blood glucose levels. These two tissues carry out gluconeogenesis utilizing the carbon skeleton of glutamine. The nitrogens are removed from glutamine by glutaminase and then glutamate dehydrogenase, and the resulting α-ketoglutarate (2-oxoglutarate) enters the TCA cycle (see Chapter 9) where the carbons can be diverted from malate into the pathway of gluconeogenesis. In addition to carrying out gluconeogenesis, the kidney regulates blood glucose levels via its ability to excrete glucose via glomerular filtration as well as to reabsorb the filtered glucose in the proximal convoluted tubules.

Fructose Entry Into Glycolysis

The pathway to utilization of fructose (Figure 5–5) differs in liver and most nonhepatic tissues due to the differential distribution

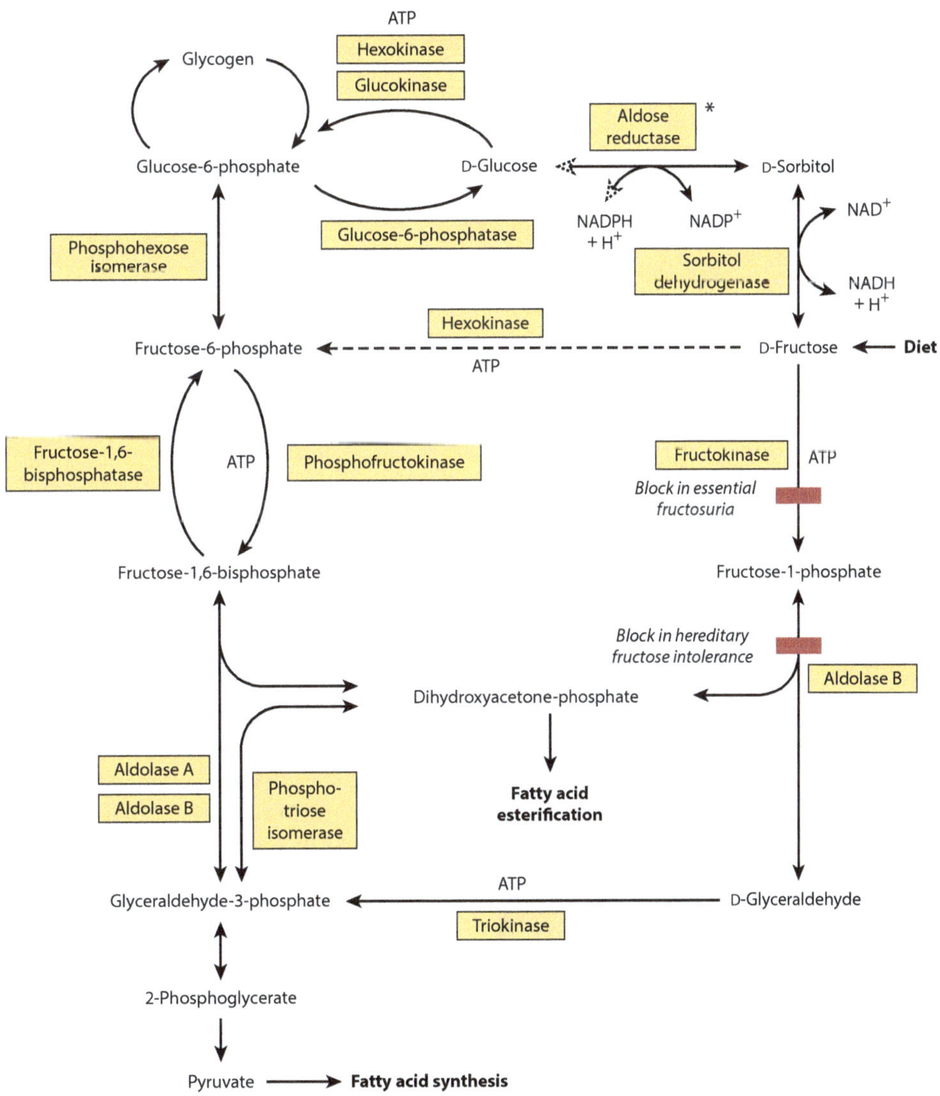

FIGURE 5–5 Metabolism of fructose. Aldolase A is found in all tissues, whereas aldolase B is the predominant form in liver. (*Not found in liver.) (Reproduced with permission from Rodwell VW, Bender DA, Botham KM, et al: *Harper's Illustrated Biochemistry*, 31st ed. New York, NY: McGraw Hill; 2018.)

of fructose phosphorylating enzymes. Hexokinases are a family of enzymes that phosphorylate hexose sugars such as glucose and fructose. In addition to hexokinases, fructose can be phosphorylated by fructokinases. Fructokinases are formally referred to as ketohexokinases (KHK). Mutations in several of the fructose metabolizing enzymes are associated with potentially fatal disorders (see Clinical Box 5–3).

The liver contains mostly glucokinase (hexokinase type IV), which exhibits substrate specificity for glucose, and thus, there is the requirement for fructokinase to utilize fructose in hepatic glycolysis. Hepatic fructokinase phosphorylates fructose on C-1 yielding fructose-1-phosphate (F1P). In liver (as well as in kidney and intestine), the form of aldolase that predominates (aldolase B, also called fructose-1,6-bisphosphate aldolase B) can utilize both F1,6BP and F1P as substrates. Therefore, when presented with F1P the enzyme generates dihydroxyacetone phosphate (DHAP) and glyceraldehyde. The DHAP is converted, by triose phosphate isomerase, to glyceraldehyde-3-phosphate (G3P) and enters glycolysis. The glyceraldehyde can be phosphorylated to G3P by triokinase (also called glyceraldehyde kinase) or converted to glycerate or glycerol.

HIGH-YIELD CONCEPT

Because hepatic fructose metabolism directly produces triose phosphates, its metabolism bypasses the hormonal regulation that is exerted on glucose metabolism at PFK1 and in addition, there is no allosteric regulation of the process such as occurs at the PFK1 and hexokinase reactions.

Galactose Entry Into Glycolysis

Galactose, which is predominantly derived from the metabolism of the milk sugar, lactose (a disaccharide of glucose and galactose), enters glycolysis by its conversion to glucose-1-phosphate (G1P). This occurs through a series of steps that is referred to as the Leloir pathway (Figure 5–6). Although galactose can be fully oxidized via glycolysis, up to 30% of ingested galactose is incorporated into glycogen following its conversion to G1P. Mutations in several of the galactose metabolizing enzymes are associated with potentially fatal disorders (see Clinical Box 5–4).

HIGH-YIELD CONCEPT

Galactose is an essential carbohydrate needed in the formation of glycolipids and glycoproteins that when present on the surfaces of cells enables cell-cell communication, immune recognition, growth factor-receptor interactions involved in signal transduction events, and many other critical cellular processes.

CLINICAL BOX 5-3 FRUCTOSE METABOLISM DISORDERS

There are three primary inherited disorders in fructose metabolism: essential fructosuria, hereditary fructose 1,6-bisphosphatase deficiency, and hereditary fructose intolerance. Essential fructosuria is a relatively benign autosomal-recessive disorder resulting from defects in hepatic fructokinase (KHK-C). Hyperfructosemia and fructosuria are the principal signs associated with this metabolic defect. Hereditary fructose-1,6-bisphosphatase deficiency is an extremely rare autosomal-recessive disorder characterized by episodes of hypoglycemia, ketosis, lactic acidosis, and hyperventilation. Hereditary fructose intolerance (HFI) is the more common and more severe form of inherited disorders in fructose metabolism. HFI is an autosomal-recessive disorder characterized by severe hypoglycemia and vomiting shortly after the intake of fructose resulting from mutations in the gene (*ALDOB*) encoding aldolase B whose expression predominates in liver, kidney cortex, and small intestine. Most of the aldolase B gene mutations are point mutations resulting in single amino acid changes that decrease stability or catalytic activity. The result is an inability to metabolize fructose, sucrose, and sorbitol correctly, manifesting as sugar toxicity that can lead to severe organ damage if untreated. The incidence of HFI is reportedly around 1/20,000–30,000 newborns and no cure is available. If appropriately diagnosed and treated, it constitutes a relatively benign disease, but without early intervention, it can be lethal. Prolonged fructose ingestion in infants leads to poor feeding, vomiting, hepatomegaly, jaundice, hemorrhage, proximal renal tubular syndrome, and finally, hepatic failure and death. Patients develop a strong distaste for noxious food. Hypoglycemia after fructose ingestion is caused by accumulation of F1P which simultaneously depletes phosphate pools thereby inhibiting glycogenolysis at the level of glycogen phosphorylase which requires inorganic phosphate for activity. Aldolase B deficiency also impairs hepatic gluconeogenesis at the level of the DHAP and G3P condensation to F1,6BP. Patients remain healthy on a fructose-, sucrose-, and sorbitol-free diet. The need for sorbitol restriction is important since fructose can be derived endogenously from sorbitol. Additionally, significant in the setting of HFI is that sorbitol can be synthesized in the body from glucose. Glucose is converted to sorbitol via the action of aldose reductase (also called aldehyde reductase 1). Sorbitol is then converted to fructose via sorbitol dehydrogenase. In the management of HFI this conversion has important clinical implications since sorbitol is found in numerous processed foods as a sweetener or conditioning agent and in the pharmaceutical industry as a bodying and emulsion agent.

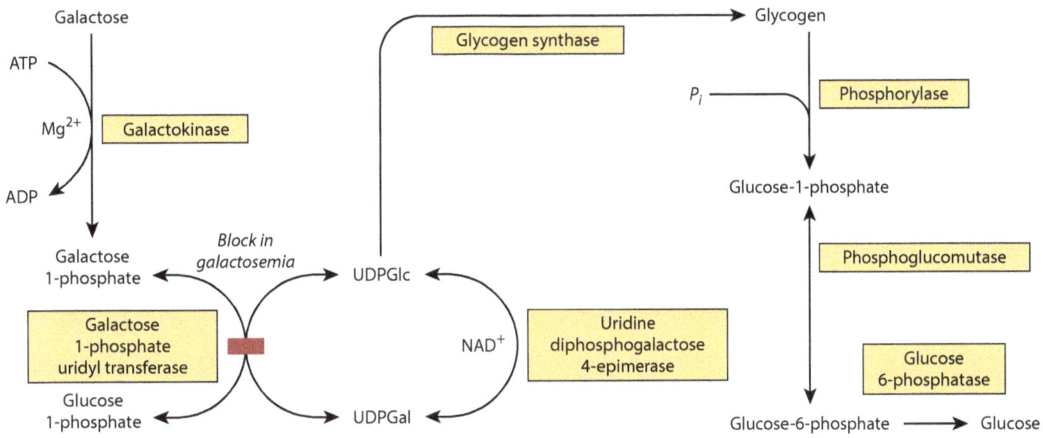

FIGURE 5–6 Pathway of conversion of (A) galactose to glucose in the liver. (Reproduced with permission from Rodwell VW, Bender DA, Botham KM, et al: *Harper's Illustrated Biochemistry*, 31st ed. New York, NY: McGraw Hill; 2018.)

CLINICAL BOX 5–4 GALACTOSE METABOLISM DISORDERS

Three inherited disorders of galactose metabolism have been identified that result in galactosemia of varying degrees. The most common disorder of galactose metabolism is referred to as classic galactosemia or type 1 galactosemia. Type 1 galactosemia is caused by mutations in the gene (*GALT*) encoding galactose-1-phosphate uridylyltransferase that result in severe reductions in enzyme activity. The disease occurs with a frequency of between 1:30,000 to 1:60,000 live births. Over 230 different mutations have been described in the gene encoding human GALT resulting in type 1 galactosemia. The most commonly detected mutation in Caucasians results in the Q188R allele defined by the substitution of arginine (R) for glutamine (Q) at amino acid 188 which lies close to the active site of the enzyme. Homozygotes for the Q188R allele show very little to no GALT activity in their erythrocytes. The majority of heterozygotes are found to have no GALT activity, while others exhibit a low level of enzyme activity generally no more than 20% of the wild type. Whereas the Q188R allele is most common in Caucasians, the most commonly detected mutations in European populations are K285N, S135L, and N314D. The K285N mutation is associated with 0% and 50% GALT activity in homozygous and heterozygous individuals, respectively. Classic galactosemia most often presents within the first weeks after birth and manifests by a failure of neonates to thrive. Vomiting and diarrhea occur following ingestion of milk, hence individuals are erroneously termed lactose intolerant. Clinical findings of these disorders include impaired liver function (which if left untreated leads to severe cirrhosis), hypergalactosemia, hyperchloremic metabolic acidosis, urinary galactitol excretion, and hyperaminoaciduria. On physical examination, infants will be jaundiced and have hepatomegaly. Due to the involvement of the liver, patients will exhibit prolonged bleeding after venous or arterial sampling or will show excessive bruising. Unless controlled by exclusion of galactose from the diet, these galactosemias can go on to produce blindness and fatal liver damage. Blindness is due to the conversion of circulating galactose to the sugar alcohol galactitol, by an NADPH-dependent aldose reductase that is present in neural tissue and in the lens of the eye. At normal circulating levels of galactose this enzyme activity causes no pathologic effects. However, a high concentration of galactitol in the lens causes osmotic swelling, with the resultant formation of cataracts and other symptoms. The principal treatment of these disorders is to eliminate lactose from the diet. Even on a galactose-restricted diet, GALT-deficient individuals exhibit urinary galactitol excretion and persistently elevated erythrocyte galactose-1-phosphate levels. In addition, even with life-long restriction of dietary galactose, many patients with classic galactosemia go on to develop serious long-term complications. These long-term complications include ovarian failure in female patients, cognitive impairment, and ataxic neurologic disease. The second form of galactosemia, termed type 2, results from deficiency of galactokinase (GALK1). This form of galactosemia is quite rare with a frequency of less than 1:100,000 live births. Infants with GALK1 deficiency, who continue to consume a milk-based diet, accumulate abnormally high levels of galactose in their blood and tissues, similar to infants with classic galactosemia. Like classic galactosemia patients, GALK1 deficiency often present with cataracts that will resolve on dietary restriction of galactose. However, unlike patients with classic galactosemia, patients with GALK1 deficiency who keep to a galactose-restricted diet experience no known long-term complications. This difference is biochemically and clinically quite significant because it provides compelling evidence that it is not the accumulation of galactose, but rather galactose-1-phosphate (Gal-1P), or possibly some metabolic derivative Gal-1P, that is the primary cause of the complications, in addition to cataracts, that are observed in classic galactosemia patients and the rarer severe form of GALE deficiency. The third disorder of galactose metabolism, termed type 3 galactosemia, results from a deficiency of UDP-galactose-4-epimerase (GALE). Two different forms of this deficiency have been identified. The more commonly occurring deficiency affects only red and white blood cells and is relatively benign. The other form of GALE deficiency is extremely rare and is characterized by profound enzyme impairment affecting multiple tissues and manifesting with symptoms similar to those seen with GALT deficiency (classic galactosemia).

CHECKLIST

- ☑ Glucose activated for oxidation by hexokinase/glucokinase and PFK1 phosphorylation.
- ☑ Hexokinase, but not glucokinase, can phosphorylate several 6-carbon sugars.
- ☑ K_m for glucose of glucokinase is high to prevent hepatic trapping of glucose, thus allowing for hepatic regulation of blood glucose.
- ☑ PFK1 is rate-limiting enzyme of glycolysis, regulated by multiple allosteric effectors.
- ☑ PFK2 critical bifunctional enzyme is responsible for regulating levels of F2,6BP, a significant allosteric regulator of PFK1.
- ☑ PK isozymes control whether or not glucose oxidation proceeds from pyruvate into the TCA cycle or is reduced to lactate.
- ☑ Glucose oxidation can proceed aerobically whereby pyruvate is completely oxidized by entry into the TCA cycle or oxidation can occur anaerobically with the reduction of pyruvate to lactate.
- ☑ Insulin and glucagon are major counter-regulatory hormones influencing overall glucose storage and oxidation.
- ☑ Fatty acid oxidation interferes with glucose oxidation and can thus exacerbate the hyperglycemia typical of type 2 diabetes.
- ☑ The interrelationship between glucose and fatty acid oxidation is referred to as the glucose-fatty acid cycle.
- ☑ Cancer cells are said to "ferment" glucose to lactate even under conditions of plentiful oxygen, referred to as the Warburg effect.
- ☑ Loss of PK-R activity is the leading cause of inherited nonspherocytic anemia.
- ☑ Dietary fructose is absorbed by the intestine via GLUT5-mediated uptake.
- ☑ Metabolism of fructose in the intestine, liver, and kidneys involves fructokinase (ketohexokinase, KHK).
- ☑ Fructose can be metabolized by most tissues but its utilization within the liver is most significant physiologically.
- ☑ Fructose metabolism in the glycolytic pathway, following fructokinase phosphorylation to fructose-1-phosphate, effectively bypasses all of the hormonal and allosteric regulations imposed on glucose metabolism.
- ☑ Fructose metabolism in the hypothalamus results in enhanced desire to consume food due to depletion of ATP with resultant activation of AMPK and subsequent altered metabolic processes.
- ☑ Defects in fructose metabolic genes can lead to a spectrum of disorders from relatively benign hyperfructosemia and fructosuria to neonatal fatal hypoglycemia and lacticacidemia.
- ☑ The primary source of galactose is milk sugar, lactose.
- ☑ Galactose is absorbed from the gut via the SGLT1 sugar transporter and enters the blood via the intestinal GLUT2 transporter.
- ☑ *N*-acetylgalactosamine (GalNAc) cannot be supplied in the diet and thus, humans require galactose in the diet to serve as a precursor for this amino sugar which is a critical component of cellular function.
- ☑ Galactose carbons can be completely oxidized for ATP production following conversion to glucose or stored as glucose in glycogen polymers.
- ☑ Defects in galactose conversion to glucose result in galactosemias with classic galactosemia, caused by defects in the *GALT* gene, being the most severe form.

REVIEW QUESTIONS

1. An 11-year-old type 1 diabetic female patient self-administered her afternoon insulin dose but forgot to eat afterwards. Upon becoming very weak and lightheaded her mother used a glucose monitor to find that the patient's serum glucose level was 28 mg/dL (N nonfasting = 70–120 mg/dL). Which of the following statements most correctly defines the metabolic situation in this patient?

(A) A reversal of the muscle hexokinase reaction converts glucose-6-phosphate to glucose for oxidation in glycolysis
(B) Hepatic glycogen releases glucose in response to insulin-mediated dephosphorylation of glycogen phosphorylase
(C) Hepatic glycogen releases glucose through a reversal of the glycogen synthase reaction
(D) Phosphorylation of hepatic glycogen synthase prevents glucose incorporation into glycogen
(E) The activity of muscle glycolysis is inhibited by the phosphorylation of PFK1

2. A 37-year-old woman visits her physician with complaints of shortness of breath and rapid fatigue during her exercise routine. Laboratory studies show normocytic and slightly macrocytic erythrocytes indicative of reticulocytosis. Brilliant cresyl blue staining of peripheral blood shows reticulocytes containing a fine basophilic network. Hematocrit is 22% (N = 36–44%) and hemoglobin is 10 g/dL (N = 12–15 g/dL).

Which of the following would most likely be elevated in the blood of this patient?

(A) 2,3-Bisphosphoglycerate (2,3BPG)
(B) Heinz bodies
(C) Lactate
(D) Oxidized glutathione (GSSG)
(E) Pyruvate

3. An experimental compound has been studied using a hepatocyte cell culture system. The effects of this compound on overall glucose homeostasis closely mimics the expected effects from increased cytosolic citrate. This novel compound is most likely altering the rate of glycolysis by which of the following mechanisms?

(A) Inhibiting phosphodiesterase (PDE)
(B) Inhibiting phosphofructokinase-1 (PFK1)
(C) Inhibiting pyruvate kinase
(D) Stimulating phosphoenolpyruvate carboxykinase (PEPCK)
(E) Stimulating phosphofructokinase-1 (PFK1)
(F) Stimulating pyruvate kinase

4. A patient, exhibiting frequent episodes of moderate hypoglycemia, is being examined by his physician. Measurement of circulating insulin and glucagon levels indicate that they are normal and responsive to cycles of feeding and fasting. *In vitro* studies with liver biopsy tissue from the patient demonstrates that there are normal levels of both the insulin and glucagon receptors and that these cells bind the hormones with normal kinetics. Given the findings in this patient, which of the following would most likely explain the recurrent hypoglycemia?

(A) A constitutively inactive hepatic glycogen synthase
(B) Glycogen synthase that lacks the phosphorylase kinase target site
(C) Hepatic glucokinase with a K_m equal to that of muscle hexokinase
(D) Pancreatic β-cell glucokinase with a K_m equal to that of hepatic glucokinase
(E) Phosphofructokinase-1 (PFK1) that is nonresponsive to the allosteric effects of frustose-2,6-bisphosphate

5. Laboratory studies are being conducted to examine the effects of an experimental compound on the metabolic activities of primary hepatocytes in culture. These studies demonstrate that addition of the compound to cultures of these cells leads to metabolic changes that are highly similar to those induced by addition of the hormone glucagon. Determination of phosphate incorporation shows that several proteins become hyperphosphorylated following addition of the compound. Which of the following laboratory findings is most likely?

(A) Glycogen phosphorylase activity will be increased
(B) Phosphofructokinase-1 (PFK1) kinase activity will be unaffected
(C) Phosphofructokinase-2 (PFK2) kinase activity will be increased
(D) Phosphoprotein phosphatase-1 (PP-1) activity will be increased
(E) Phosphorylase kinase activity will be decreased

6. Experiments are being performed to assess the effects of an unknown chemical compound on glucose metabolism in laboratory animals. The test compound is administered orally by addition to the food. When this modified food is consumed, it is observed that there is a significant decrease in glucose output by the liver of the test animals. Analysis of fractionated liver biopsy cells isolated 2-days following compound addition indicates decreased cytoplasmic citrate in the test animal cells compared to control animal liver cells. Which of the following changes in enzyme activity is most likely in the liver cells of the test animals?

(A) Decreased glycogen synthase
(B) Decreased glyceraldehyde-3-phosphate dehydrogenase
(C) Decreased phosphofructokinase-2 (PFK2)
(D) Increased phosphofructokinase-1 (PFK1)
(E) Increased glycogen phosphorylase
(F) Increased pyruvate kinase

7. Laboratory studies on carbohydrate metabolism are conducted using primary myocyte cultures derived from the rectus femoris. Glucose is added to the cells in culture under anaerobic and aerobic conditions. Which of the following would show the greatest concentration difference between the two metabolic conditions?

(A) Acetate
(B) Acetyl-CoA
(C) Alanine
(D) Lactate
(E) Oxaloacetate

8. The enzymatic activities of hepatic PFK2 (phosphofructokinase-2/fructose bisphosphatase-2) are reciprocally regulated under various physiological conditions. In an examination of these activities, which of the following is most likely to be true in a comparison of the well-fed versus the fasting states?

	Physical State	Predominant Hormone	Predominant Product
A.	Fasting	Cortisol	Fructose-6-phosphate
B.	Fasting	Glucagon	Fructose-2,6-bisphosphate
C.	Fasting	Insulin	Fructose-2,6-bisphosphate
D.	Fed	Cortisol	Fructose-6-phosphate
E.	Fed	Glucagon	Fructose-6-phosphate
F.	Fed	Insulin	Fructose-2,6-bisphosphate

(A)
(B)
(C)
(D)
(E)
(F)

9. A 1-year-old boy is brought to the physician because of a 3-month history of intermittent vomiting, shakiness, and a failure to thrive. The symptoms began when breastfeeding stopped and fruit and vegetables were added to his diet. He is currently below the 5th percentile for length and weight. Physical examination shows jaundice and hepatomegaly. Laboratory studies show hypoglycemia and hypophosphatemia. Given these signs and symptoms this patient is most likely suffering from which of the following?

(A) Classic galactosemia
(B) Hereditary fructose intolerance
(C) Hunter syndrome

(D) Medium-chain acyl-CoA dehydrogenase deficiency (MCADD)
(E) Pompe disease
(F) Tay-Sachs disease

10. A 28-year-old woman comes to the physician because of intermittent right upper quadrant pain that extends to the inferior tip of her scapula. Laboratory studies show mild anemia with the presence of relatively normal shaped erythrocytes that appear normocytic and normochromic. Additional blood work shows elevated levels of 2,3-bisphosphoglycerate (2,3BPG). Ultrasonic examination of the abdomen shows cholelithiasis. Following removal of her gallbladder, the stones are examined and shown to contain high concentrations of bilirubin. A defect in which of the following metabolic pathways most likely exists in this patient?
(A) Glycogen synthesis
(B) Glycolysis
(C) Heme biosynthesis
(D) Pentose phosphate pathway
(E) Protein synthesis

11. A 1-year-old girl is brought to the hospital because of fatigue, nausea, and a yellowing of her skin and eyes. Her family, who lives in New York City, recently had a vacation at an apple orchard. The child began to experience her symptoms a few days after consuming the homemade apple sauce her parents had prepared. Laboratory studies show nonfasting glucose is 57 mg/dL (N = 100–180 mg/dL), direct bilirubin is 0.85 mg/dL (N = 0.1–0.3 mg/dL), and lactic acid is 3.4 mM (N = 0.5–2.2 mM). Analysis of urine indicates elevated levels of carbohydrate, but it is shown not to be glucose. A defect in which of the following enzymes is the most likely cause of these findings?
(A) Aldolase B
(B) Fructokinase
(C) Fructose-1,6-bisphosphatase
(D) Galactokinase
(E) Galactose-1-phosphate uridylyltransferase

12. A 1-year-old boy is brought to the physician because of a 3-month history of intermittent vomiting, shakiness, and a failure to thrive. The symptoms began when breastfeeding stopped and solid foods were added to his diet. He is currently below the 5th percentile for length and weight. Physical examination shows jaundice and hepatomegaly. Laboratory studies show hypoglycemia and hypophosphatemia. Ingestion of which of the following is the most likely cause of this patient's symptoms?
(A) Glycogen
(B) Lactose
(C) Maltose
(D) Starch
(E) Sucrose

13. A patient is being examined by his physician with complaints of cramping in the lower belly, bloating, gas, and diarrhea. These symptoms appear within 30 minutes to 2 hours after the ingestion of dairy products. On the advice of his physician, so as to avoid repeated episodes, the patient should most likely avoid the consumption of foods that contain which of the following?
(A) Fructose
(B) Galactose
(C) Glucose
(D) Lactose
(E) Sucrose

14. Metabolism of fructose, within cells of the hypothalamus, is associated with an increased desire for food intake. The changes in behavior caused by fructose metabolism are most likely to be the result of changing levels of which of the following metabolic intermediates?
(A) Acetyl-CoA
(B) Citrate
(C) Fructose-2,6-bisphosphate
(D) Malonyl-CoA
(E) Pyruvate

15. A 2-week-old girl is brought to the physician because of diarrhea, frequent vomiting, and yellowing of the skin and eyes. She appeared healthy for a few days after birth at which time she began to experience these symptoms. Physical examination shows hepatomegaly, jaundice, and early cataract formation. The infant is at the 10th percentile for appropriate developmental milestones. Which of the following is the most likely diagnosis?
(A) Galactosemia
(B) Hurler syndrome
(C) Pyloric stenosis
(D) Tay-Sachs disease
(E) von Gierke disease

16. A 23-year-old male is being examined by his physician with complaints of intermittent right upper quadrant pain that extends to the inferior tip of his scapula. Analysis of blood reveals mild anemia with the presence of normocytic and normochromic nonspherical erythrocytes. Additional blood work shows elevated levels of glucose-6-phosphate (G6P) and 2,3-bisphosphoglycerate (2,3BPG). Ultrasonic examination of the abdomen shows cholelithiasis. Following removal of his gallbladder the stones are examined and shown to contain bilirubin. A deficiency in which of the following metabolic processes would most explain the signs and symptoms in this patient?
(A) Erythrocyte redox maintenance
(B) Erythrocyte glycolysis
(C) Hepatic bile acid synthesis
(D) Hepatic LDL uptake
(E) Renal bicarbonate reabsorption
(F) Renal ammoniagenesis

17. Laboratory studies are being conducted to examine the effects of an experimental compound on the metabolic activities of primary hepatocytes in culture. These studies demonstrate that addition of the compound to cultures of these cells leads to metabolic changes that are highly similar to those induced by addition of the hormone insulin. Phosphoprotein analysis shows that several proteins become hypophosphorylated following addition of the compound. Which of the following laboratory findings is most likely?
(A) Glycogen phosphorylase activity will be increased
(B) Phosphofructokinase-1 (PFK1) activity will be unaffected
(C) Phosphofructokinase-2 (PFK2) kinase activity will be increased
(D) Phosphoprotein phosphatase-1 (PP-1) activity will be decreased
(E) Phosphorylase kinase activity will be increased

18. Biopsy-derived cells from a skeletal muscle tumor are being studied and compared to normal muscle cells. The primary experiments are aimed at comparing the effects of high levels of fatty acids on glucose oxidation within the two types of cells. Results from these studies find that exposing the normal cells to high levels of palmitic acid results in impaired levels of glucose oxidation. However, the tumor-derived cells do not exhibit reduced glycolysis under these same conditions. These tumor cells are most likely to exhibit which of the altered activities?

(A) Acetyl-CoA carboxylase that is insensitive to citrate resulting in reduced conversion of acetyl-CoA to malonyl-CoA and the acetyl-CoA then activates phosphoenolpyruvate carboxykinase
(B) ATP-citrate lyase that is more active causing significant reductions in mitochondrial citrate resulting in loss of citrate-mediated inhibition of PFK1
(C) Carnitine palmitoyltransferase 1 that restricts mitochondrial uptake of fatty acids which then build up in the cytosol leading to allosteric inhibition of PFK1
(D) Phosphofructokinase-1 (PFK1) that is insensitive to allosteric activation by fructose-2,6-bisphophate
(E) Phosphofructokinase-1 (PFK1) that is insensitive to allosteric inhibition by citrate

19. Under conditions of anaerobic glycolysis, the NAD^+ required by glyceraldehyde-3-phosphate dehydrogenase is most likely to be supplied by a reaction catalyzed by which of the following enzymes?

(A) Glycerol-3-phosphate dehydrogenase
(B) α-Ketoglutarate (2-oxoglutarate) dehydrogenase
(C) Lactate dehydrogenase
(D) Malate dehydrogenase
(E) Pyruvate dehydrogenase

20. A novel compound has been designed to study the effects on the regulation of glycolysis. The compound is being tested in a hepatocyte cell line in culture. Addition of the compound results in an increased rate of ATP production from glucose while simultaneously reducing glucose output into the culture medium. Your experimental compound is most likely mimicking which of the following?

(A) Fructose-1,6-bisphosphate
(B) Fructose-2,6-bisphosphate
(C) Fructose-1-bisphosphate
(D) Glucose-1-phosphate
(E) Glucose-6-bisphosphate

21. Which of the following are most likely to result in an enhanced rate of hepatic glycolysis?

(A) AMP, citrate, and fructose-2,6-bisphosphate
(B) AMP, inorganic phosphate, and fructose-2,6-bisphosphate
(C) ATP, citrate, and inorganic phosphate
(D) ATP, inorganic phosphate, and fructose-1,6-bisphosphate
(E) Inorganic phosphate, citrate, and fructose-2,6-bisphosphate

22. Reduction in the activity of lactate dehydrogenase in erythrocytes will result in a reduced capacity to carry out glycolysis. This effect is most likely to be associated with the depletion in which of the following intermediates in this metabolic pathway?

(A) ADP
(B) Citrate
(C) Glucose-6-phosphate
(D) NAD^+
(E) Pyruvate

23. Experiments are being conducted to determine the effects of a novel compound on the overall rate of glycolysis in laboratory animals. The compound is added to the water consumed by the animals resulting in an increase in the rate of glucose oxidation to pyruvate compared to that in control animals. Given these findings, it is most likely that the compound causes an increase in the ratio of which of the following hormones?

(A) Cortisol to insulin
(B) Epinephrine to glucagon
(C) Glucagon to epinephrine
(D) Glucagon to insulin
(E) Insulin to glucagon

24. Experiments are being conducted to determine the effects of a novel compound on the overall rate of glycolysis in laboratory animals. The compound is added to the water consumed by the animals resulting in an increase in the rate of glucose oxidation to pyruvate compared to that in control animals. Examination of hepatocytes isolated from the livers of the test animals demonstrates that the compound induces a rapid decrease in the ATP/ADP ratio. Which of the following most likely represents the consequences of the effects of this compound?

(A) Decreased isocitrate dehydrogenase activity
(B) Decreased phosphofructokinase-1 (PFK1) activity
(C) Decreased rate of electron transport
(D) Increased glycogen synthase activity
(E) Increased glycolytic pathway flux
(F) Increased pyruvate carboxylase activity

25. A 17-year-old female, suffering from intermittent pain in her right upper quadrant that also extends to the inferior tip of her scapula, is being attended to in the emergency department. Analysis of blood reveals mild anemia with the presence of normocytic and normochromic nonspherical erythrocytes Serum studies find an elevated level of glucose-6-phosphate (G6P). Ultrasonic examination of the abdomen shows cholelithiasis. Serum analysis for elevation in which of the following would be most useful in making a correct diagnosis in this patient?

(A) 2,3-Bisphosphoglycerate
(B) Glucose
(C) Glutamine
(D) Lactate
(E) Urea
(F) Uric acid

26. During the oxidation of glucose there are reactions whose standard free energies are sufficient to drive the synthesis of ATP from ADP and Pi. Which of the following enzymes is the most likely candidate for catalyzing such a reaction?

(A) Glucose-1-phopsphate
(B) Glucose-6-phosphate
(C) Glycerol-1-phosphate
(D) Phosphoenolpyruvate
(E) 3-Phosphoglycerate

27. A 27-year-old man complains of intermittent right upper quadrant pain that extends to the inferior tip of his scapula. Analysis of blood reveals mild anemia with the presence of normocytic and normochromic erythrocytes. Additional blood work shows elevated levels of glucose-6-phosphate (G6P) and

2,3-bisphosphoglycerate (2,3BPG). A deficiency in which of the following metabolic processes would most explain the signs and symptoms in this patient?
(A) Erythrocyte redox maintenance
(B) Erythrocyte glycolysis
(C) Hepatic bile acid synthesis
(D) Hepatic LDL uptake
(E) Renal ammoniagenesis
(F) Renal bicarbonate reabsorption

28. The Warburg effect refers to the process of glycolysis that leads to increased lactate formation even in the presence of functional mitochondria. Which of the following enzymes is most likely to be responsible for the observations accounting for the Warburg effect?
(A) Glucokinase
(B) Glyceraldehyde-3-phosphate dehydrogenase
(C) Phosphofructokinase 1 (PFK1)
(D) Phosphofructokinase 2 (PFK2)
(E) Pyruvate kinase

29. When an experimental compound is added to hepatocyte cell cultures there is a dramatic increase in the levels of cytosolic cAMP. Which of the following is most likely to be the initial response to the effect of this compound?
(A) Binding of the cAMP to the regulatory subunits of cAMP-dependent protein kinase (PKA)
(B) cAMP-mediated desensitization of the β_2-adrenergic receptor
(C) Dissociation of the α-subunit from a G_s-type G-proteins
(D) Increase in cytosolic Ca^{2+}
(E) Inhibition of glycogen synthase

30. A 9-month-old child is presented to the emergency department by his parents who report that he has been vomiting and has severe diarrhea. The episodes of vomiting began when the parents started feeding their child cow's milk. The infant exhibits signs of failure to thrive, weight loss, hepatomegaly, and jaundice. Laboratory tests show the infant has an anion gap of 14 mEq/L (N = 8 mEq/L–12 mEq/L) and a prothrombin time of 13.7 sec (N = 11.0–12.5 sec). These clinical and laboratory findings are most consistent with a deficiency in which of the following processes?
(A) Fructose metabolism
(B) Galactose metabolism
(C) Glycogen synthesis
(D) Long-chain fatty acid oxidation
(E) Peroxisomal phytanic acid oxidation

31. Chronic consumption of ethanol contributes to hepatic steatosis. Altered activity of which of the following enzymes is most likely to contribute to this pathology?
(A) Fatty acyl-CoA dehydrogenase
(B) Glucose-6-phosphate dehydrogenase
(C) Glycerol-3-phosphate dehydrogenase
(D) Lactate dehydrogenase
(E) Pyruvate dehydrogenase

32. As a result of sympathetic outflow from the brain, such as in response to fear, epinephrine is released from the adrenal medullary chromaffin cells. The tissue responses to this released epinephrine are inhibited glycolysis and stimulated gluconeogenesis in the liver by stimulated glycolysis in cardiac muscle. Which of the following is the most likely reason for these observed tissue-specific differences?
(A) Different adrenergic receptors to which epinephrine bind in the liver and heart
(B) Different isozymes of adenylate cyclase and cAMP phosphodiesterase in the heart versus liver
(C) Different isoforms of phosphofructokinase-2 (PFK2) in the heart versus liver
(D) Different isoforms of protein kinase A (PKA) in the heart versus liver
(E) Different receptor associated G-proteins with liver inhibiting and heart activating adenylate cyclase

33. Experiments are being designed with the aim of altering anaerobic energy production in cancer cells. Enhancement in the activity of which of the following enzymes would be most useful to this aim?
(A) Glyceraldehyde-3-phosphate dehydrogenase
(B) Hexokinase
(C) Phosphofructokinase-1 (PFK1)
(D) Phosphofructokinase-2 (PFK2) kinase activity
(E) Pyruvate kinase

34. A patient is being treated in the emergency department for severe abdominal pain, diarrhea, and vomiting. Physical examination finds the patient is severely dehydrated, a urine sample very dark, and the patient's breath has an odor of garlic. Given the signs and symptoms, the attending physician suspects the patient has ingested an environmental toxin. The production of which of the following is most likely reduced, accounting for the pathologic action of the toxic substance?
(A) Acetyl-CoA
(B) Glycogen
(C) Lactate
(D) Methionine
(E) Pyruvate
(F) Tyrosine

35. Increased activity of which of the following is most likely to be responsible for the enhanced glucose metabolism found in tumor cells in the brain?
(A) Glucokinase
(B) GLUT3
(C) GLUT4
(D) Glycogen phosphorylase
(E) Pyruvate kinase

36. A 6-month-old girl is brought to the emergency department because of increased crying, sweating, and shaking chills. The mother states that until recently the child had been exclusively breast-fed but she was now trying to see whether the child might enjoy other foods. The symptoms started soon after feeding the child applesauce and puréed pears, which at first, she ate eagerly. Onset of symptoms began approximately 1 hour later. Based on the signs and symptoms in the infant and the history, a tentative diagnosis is made. Which of the following metabolic pathways is most likely defective in this patient?
(A) Hepatic fructose metabolism
(B) Hepatic galactose metabolism
(C) Hepatic gluconeogenesis
(D) Renal ammoniagenesis
(E) Renal galactose metabolism
(F) Renal gluconeogenesis

37. A 1-year-old girl is brought to the hospital because of lethargy, nausea, and vomiting. Physical examination shows the patient to have yellowish coloration to her skin and icteric sclera.

The child began to experience her symptoms a few days after consuming a large amount of honey. Laboratory studies show nonfasting glucose is 57 mg/dL (N = 100–180 mg/dL), direct bilirubin is 0.85 mg/dL (N = 0.1–0.3 mg/dL), and lactic acid is 3.4 mM (N = 0.5–2.2 mM). Given the signs and symptoms in this patient, which of the following is most likely to be defective?

(A) Carbohydrate metabolism
(B) Glycosaminoglycan synthesis
(C) Lysosomal hydrolase activity
(D) Mitochondrial fatty acid oxidation
(E) Peroxisomal fat metabolism

38. Hereditary fructose intolerance is associated with rapid and severe hypoglycemia upon consumption of fructose. Which of the following best explains this metabolic defect associated with fructose ingestion?

(A) Activation of AMPK which phosphorylates and inhibits glycogen phosphorylase
(B) Allosteric activation of glycogen synthase by fructose-1-phosphate
(C) Allosteric inhibition of phosphorylase by fructose-1-phosphate
(D) Depletion of the inorganic phosphate pool required by glycogen phosphorylase
(E) Trapping of ATP in the form of fructose-1-phosphate

39. Patients with hereditary fructose intolerance are required to avoid certain foods as their consumption can lead to significant hypoglycemia. Which of the following carbohydrates most likely represents a substance to be avoided by these patients?

(A) Amylose
(B) Cellulose
(C) Lactose
(D) Maltose
(E) Sorbitol

40. Hypothalamic metabolism of fructose rapidly depletes the ATP pool resulting in increased levels of AMP. These energy changes alter metabolic processes leading to an increased desire for food intake. Which of the following metabolic changes is the most likely contributor to the changes in feeding behavior?

(A) Decreased fatty acid synthesis
(B) Decreased glycogen synthesis
(C) Decreased glycolysis
(D) Increased fatty acid synthesis
(E) Increased gluconeogenesis
(F) Increased glycogen synthesis

41. A 10-month-old infant is presented to the emergency department by his parents who report that he has been vomiting and has severe diarrhea. History reveals that the mother was unable to breastfeed the infant and that the episodes of vomiting began when she started preparing the infants formula with cow's milk. Laboratory tests show metabolic acidosis, albuminuria, and hyperaminoaciduria. These clinical findings are most consistent with which of the following disorders?

(A) Classic galactosemia
(B) Hereditary fructose intolerance
(C) Hers disease
(D) Pompe disease
(E) von Gierke disease

42. A 3-month-old infant is being examined by her pediatrician due to concerns from the parents that the infant's eyes began to look cloudy. The infant was born at home and the mother has been continuously breastfeeding the infant. Given the limited information available, which of the following is the most likely pathway contributing the observations in this infant?

(A) Erythrocyte glycolysis
(B) Fatty acid oxidation
(C) Fructose metabolism
(D) Galactose metabolism
(E) Gluconeogenesis
(F) Hepatic glycogen synthesis

43. Studies are being conducted to assess the effects of a novel compound on the rate of glycolysis in hepatocytes. Results from these studies demonstrate that addition of the compound decreases the kinase activity of phosphofructokinase-2 (PFK2) while simultaneously increasing the phosphatase activity of the enzyme. This response most closely reflects which of the following naturally occurring controls exerted on PFK2?

(A) Allosteric inhibition by insulin
(B) Dephosphorylation by the appropriate protein phosphatase
(C) Increased AMP concentrations
(D) Increased glucose-6-phosphate concentrations
(E) Phosphorylation by cAMP-dependent protein kinase (PKA)

44. Patients suffering from hereditary fructose intolerance experience severe hypoglycemia and can also have hyperuricemia following the consumption of foods containing fructose. Activation of which of the following enzymes is the most likely contributor to the hyperuricemia in these patients?

(A) Adenosine deaminase
(B) Adenylosuccinate lyase
(C) AMP deaminase
(D) Hypoxanthine-guanine phosphoribosyltransferase
(E) Purine nucleotide phosphorylase

45. A portion of the energy derived from glucose oxidation is generated from the electrons carried in NADH. The NADH generated by glycolysis is in the cytosol requiring the electrons to be transferred to the mitochondria. With respect to this process, a deficiency in which of the following is most likely to result in lost ATP production from glycolysis?

(A) Active transport of NADH into the mitochondrion
(B) Passive diffusion of NADH into the mitochondrion
(C) Transfer of electrons from NADH to NADH reductase at the mitochondrial surface
(D) Transfer of electrons to oxaloacetate with transport of malate into the mitochondrion
(E) Transfer of electrons to pyruvate with transport of lactate into the mitochondrion

46. A 3-month-old infant is being examined by her pediatrician due to concerns from the parents that the infant's eyes began to look cloudy. The infant was born at home and the mother has been continuously breastfeeding the infant. The pediatrician suspects a specific metabolic defect in the metabolism of carbohydrate. Given the limited information available, measurement for the activity of which of the

following would be most useful in confirming the pediatrician's diagnosis?
(A) Blood galactokinase
(B) Blood pyruvate kinase
(C) Hepatic glucose-6-phosphatase
(D) Hepatic glycogen branching enzyme
(E) Skeletal muscle galactose-1-phosphate uridylyltransferase
(F) Skeletal muscle glycogen phosphorylase

47. A healthy 28-year-old woman exhibits a peak serum glucose concentration of 220 mg/dL within 30 minutes of the consumption of 75 g of glucose. Two hours after ingestion, her serum glucose concentration decreased to 100 mg/dL. Which of the following enzymes is most likely contributing to the change in serum glucose concentration?
(A) cAMP-dependent protein kinase (PKA)
(B) Glucokinase
(C) Glycogen synthase
(D) Phosphofructokinase-1 (PFK1)
(E) Pyruvate kinase

48. Hypoxia, a condition associated with reduced levels of oxygen, leads to decreased mitochondrial ATP production and increased lactic acid production resulting in lactic acidosis. Which of the following metabolic conditions most accurately explains the lactic acidosis associated with hypoxia?
(A) Low ATP levels result in allosteric activation of lactate dehydrogenase by AMP
(B) Low ATP levels result in allosteric activation of PFK1 by AMP increasing the rate of glycolysis
(C) Low ATP levels inhibit lactate dehydrogenase from reducing lactate to pyruvate
(D) Low oxygen levels inhibit the ability of lactate dehydrogenase to oxidized lactate to pyruvate
(E) Low oxygen levels activate hexokinase, causing increased glycolysis and lactate production
(F) Low oxygen levels result in allosteric activation of pyruvate kinase enhancing lactate production from the pyruvate

49. A 12-year-old boy is being examined by his pediatrician as a routine for participation in middle school basketball. When blood and urine are examined, it is discovered that both contain elevated levels of fructose and normal levels of glucose. The patient presented with no complaints and no significant medical history. Physical examination shows a healthy, normal appearing male who is at the 90th percentile for both height and weight. Given the laboratory results in this patient, which of the following enzymes is most likely to be found to be impaired?
(A) Aldolase A
(B) Aldolase B
(C) Fructokinase
(D) Galactokinase
(E) Hexokinase

50. A 10-day-old female infant is brought to the Emergency Department by her parents because they are concerned about her persistent vomiting and lack of desire to breastfeed. The infant was born at home at 40 weeks gestation to a healthy primigravida female. She has not received recommended newborn screening. The parents report that their infant has only had two wet diaper changes in the past 24 hours. Physical examination finds scleral icterus and bilateral cataracts. There is palpable hepatomegaly. Laboratory studies show a normocytic anemia, elevated liver enzymes, hypoglycemia, and normal levels of ammonia. Given the signs and symptoms in this patient, the activity of which of the following enzymes is most likely to be deficient?
(A) Aldolase B
(B) Galactose-1-phosphate uridylyltransferase
(C) Glucocerebrosidase
(D) Glucose-6-phosphate dehydrogenase
(E) Phenylalanine hydroxylase

51. A 7-day-old male infant is being examined by his pediatrician for a routine newborn examination. The infant was delivered at term following a normal pregnancy. The infant's mother tells the pediatrician that she feels her son is not eating enough breast milk and that he has had frequent vomiting episodes. Physical examination shows that the infant is now below his original birth weight, has a palpable liver edge of 3.7 cm, is lethargic, does not respond appropriately to stimulation, has scleral icterus, and clouding in both lenses. Given these signs and symptoms, which of the following is the most likely disorder affecting this infant?
(A) Classic galactosemia
(B) Erythrocyte pyruvate kinase deficiency
(C) Hereditary fructose intolerance
(D) Maple syrup urine disease
(E) Phenylketonuria

52. A 3-year-old girl is brought to her pediatrician by her mother. The mother indicates that her daughter began complaining of severe stomach pains and nausea this morning. Physical examination finds the presence of mild hepatomegaly, and the child is lethargic, diaphoretic, and tachypneic. The mother reports that the child had ricotta cheese with a large serving of honey for dessert following the previous evening's dinner, the first time her daughter had eaten either. Laboratory studies ordered by the pediatrician show elevated anion gap metabolic acidosis and moderate hypoglycemia. Urine is of normal color, and there are no evident abnormalities. Given the most likely diagnosis in this patient, elevated levels of which of the following are the most likely cause of the observed hypoglycemia?
(A) Fructose
(B) Fructose-1-phosphate
(C) Galactose
(D) Galactose-1-phosphate
(E) Glyceraldehyde

53. A 6-year-old girl is brought to the hospital by her parents because they are concerned about her complaint of upper abdominal pain that is radiating to her right shoulder. The child was born at home at 39 weeks following an uncomplicated pregnancy. The parents indicate that no newborn screening tests were performed on their daughter. They indicated that she has had no recent infections nor been treated with antibiotics. Physical examination shows a well-developed and well-nourished child that exhibits scleral icterus, conjunctival pallor, and a palpable spleen. Abdominal ultrasound finds the presence of calculi within the bile duct. The attending physician orders an analysis of hemoglobin composition and finds that the levels of Hb_{A1}, Hb_{A2}, and HbF are within expected norms. The results of blood studies are shown:

	Patient Values	Normal Values
Hemoglobin	9.8 g/dL	11.5–14 g/dL
Hematocrit	30.1%	35–45%
Reticulocytes	17%	0.5–1.5%

The signs and symptoms in this patient are most likely the result of which of the following disorders?

(A) Chronic granulomatous disease
(B) Glucose-6-phosphate dehydrogenase deficiency
(C) Hereditary fructose intolerance
(D) Pyruvate dehydrogenase deficiency
(E) Pyruvate kinase deficiency

54. A 3-year-old boy is brought to his pediatrician by his mother because she is concerned about the yellowish coloration of his skin. The pediatrician's records indicate that the child was jaundiced at birth and required phototherapy. The boy's mother states that she experienced an episode of jaundice while she was pregnant with her son. The pediatrician orders blood work to be performed. Analysis of a peripheral blood smear shows the presence of polychromatic echinocytes. The results of the laboratory studies show:

	Patient Values	Normal Values
Hemoglobin	8.4 g/dL	11.5–13.5 g/dL
Hematocrit	17%	35–40%
Reticulocyte count	10%	0.6–1.85%
Total bilirubin	6 mg/dL	< 1.0 mg/dL
Direct bilirubin	0.3 mg/dL	< 0.3 mg/dL

Given the most likely diagnosis in this patient, which of the following substances is most likely to be found at elevated levels in the blood?

(A) Alloisoleucine
(B) 2,3-Bisphosphoglycerate
(C) Delta-aminolevulinic acid
(D) Glucose-6-phosphate
(E) Methylmalonyl-CoA

55. A 3-year-old girl is brought by her mother to her pediatrician. The mother indicates that her daughter began complaining of severe stomach pains and nausea this morning. Physical examination finds the presence of mild hepatomegaly and the child is lethargic, diaphoretic, and tachypneic. The mother reports that the child had ricotta cheese with a large serving of honey for dessert following the previous evening's dinner, the first time her daughter had eaten either. Laboratory studies ordered by the pediatrician show elevated anion gap metabolic acidosis and moderate hypoglycemia. Urine is of normal color and there are no evident abnormalities. Given the most likely diagnosis in this patient, consumption of which of the following should most likely be avoided by this patient?

(A) Glucose
(B) Isoleucine
(C) Lactose
(D) Phenylalanine
(E) Sucrose

ANSWERS

1. Correct answer is **D.** As the level of blood glucose falls, the pancreas will secrete glucagon and the adrenal glands will secrete epinephrine in order to stimulate hepatic gluconeogenesis. Within hepatocytes, glucagon activation of its G_s-type G-protein–coupled receptor, and epinephrine binding to G_s-type G-protein coupled β_2-adrenergic receptors on hepatocytes will result in the activation of the kinase, PKA. Activation of PKA will then lead to the phosphorylation of numerous substrates. One of the substrates for PKA is phosphorylase kinase which results in activation of this PKA substrate. Activation of phosphorylase kinase results in the phosphorylation of both glycogen synthase and glycogen phosphorylase. When glycogen synthase is phosphorylated its level of activity is decreased resulting in reduced incorporation of glucose into glycogen. Hexokinase (choice A) cannot remove phosphate from glucose-6-phosphate. Under conditions of fasting the level of insulin (choice B) is low preventing dephosphorylation of glycogen phosphorylase. Glycogen synthase (choices C) does not remove glucose from glycogen; this is the function of glycogen phosphorylase. Muscle PFK1 (choice E) is not phosphorylated as a regulatory mechanism of glycolysis.

2. Correct answer is **A.** The signs and symptoms in this patient are highly suggestive of erythrocyte pyruvate kinase (PK) deficiency. The reduced PK activity leads to increased levels of its substrate, phosphoenolpyruvate, as well as the other intermediates in the glycolytic pathway above the PK reaction. This ultimately results in increased concentrations of 1,3-bisphosphoglycerate which then serves as a substrate for the 2,3-bisphosphoglycerate mutase (BPGM) reaction resulting in increased levels of erythrocyte 2,3-bisphosphoglycerate, 2,3-BPG. The formation of Heinz bodies (choice B) occurs in erythrocytes when there is a disturbance in the glutathione reductase and glutathione peroxidase system of reactive oxygen species removal. Heinz bodies result from the oxidation of cysteine sulfhydryl groups, primarily in hemoglobin, resulting in the cross-linking of large amounts of hemoglobin, as well as sulfated glycolipids. The ability to observe Heinz bodies in erythrocytes is demonstrative of the histopathology associated with deficiencies in glucose-6-phosphate dehydrogenase, G6PD. The major source of blood lactate (choice C) is erythrocyte glycolysis. Since erythrocytes lack mitochondria, they cannot fully oxidize pyruvate to acetyl-CoA. Instead, the pyruvate from glycolysis is reduced to lactate and the lactate is then delivered to the liver for use as a substrate for gluconeogenesis. Since the erythrocytes have a deficiency in PK, there would be reduced production of lactate, not increased. In addition, since the processes of hepatic gluconeogenesis are not disturbed in patients with erythrocyte

PK deficiencies, the conversion of lactate to glucose is unaffected and, therefore, there would be no significant increase in blood lactate. In patients with erythrocyte PK deficiency, there is no defect in the glutathione reductase and glutathione peroxidase system of reactive oxygen species removal. Therefore, there would not be any significant increases in serum oxidized glutathione (choice D) in this patient. Since the processes of hepatic gluconeogenesis are not disturbed in patients with erythrocyte PK deficiencies, the conversion of the pyruvate to glucose in the liver would not be disturbed and, therefore, there would be no significant increase in blood pyruvate (choice E).

3. Correct answer is **B.** The predominant subcellular location for citrate is in the mitochondria, being generated by the citrate synthase reaction of the TCA cycle. Citrate, present in the cytosol, serves as a signal for a high energy charge and inhibition of the TCA cycle. During periods of high energy in hepatocytes TCA cycle activity declines and the accumulating mitochondrial citrate is transported to the cytosol as a means of acetyl-CoA transport out of the mitochondria. Within the cytosol, the citrate will serve to allosterically inhibit the rate-limiting enzyme of glycolysis, PFK1. The experimental compound, if functioning similar to citrate, would, therefore, be inhibiting the activity of PFK1 as opposed to stimulating the activity of PFK1 (choice E). The effects of citrate on the rate of glycolysis do not involve any of the other actions (choices A, C, D, and F).

4. Correct answer is **C.** The K_m, for glucose, of each of the hexokinases is significantly lower than that of glucokinase. The average K_m for hexokinases is around 0.1 mM. The K_m for glucose of glucokinase is variously reported to be around 8 mM. This difference in glucose affinity ensures that non-hepatic tissues (which contain hexokinase) rapidly and efficiently trap blood glucose within their cells by converting it to glucose-6-phosphate. One major function of the liver is to deliver glucose to the blood, and this is ensured by having a glucose phosphorylating enzyme (glucokinase) whose K_m for glucose is sufficiently higher that of the normal circulating concentration of glucose. Normal fasting plasma glucose is around 5 mM (90 mg/dL). Therefore, in an individual with a variant glucokinase that exhibits a K_m for glucose equivalent to that of hexokinase, there would be increased trapping of glucose within hepatocytes which would be apparent as episodic mild to moderate hypoglycemia, particularly during periods of fasting. In an individual with a constitutively inactive hepatic glycogen synthase (choice A), there would be a reduced capacity to divert glucose into the synthesis of glycogen and this would in turn result in increased levels of glucose remaining in the blood, thereby, reducing the potential for hypoglycemia. Glycogen synthase (choice B) is regulated by its state of phosphorylation. In the dephosphorylated state the enzyme is more active. The phosphorylation of glycogen synthase is catalyzed by phosphorylase kinase (PHK). The result of phosphorylation is reduced incorporation of glucose into glycogen. Therefore, a glycogen synthase that cannot be inhibited by phosphorylation would allow for unregulated glucose incorporation into glycogen. Although this could theoretically contribute to the hypoglycemia in the patient, there is a limiting capacity for glucose storage as glycogen and thus, any excess glucose would be diverted into the glycolytic pathway, the pentose phosphate pathway, or remain in the blood. Therefore, the potential and the level of hypoglycemia in the case of an unregulated glycogen synthase would be much less than that associated with a hepatic glucokinase with a reduced K_m for glucose. The form of hexokinase expressed within pancreatic β-cells (choice D) is the same as that expressed in hepatocyte, that is, the glucokinase form. Therefore, there would be no pathology associated with this option. The allosteric effector, fructose-2,6-bisphosphate, is a powerful activator of the glycolytic enzyme PFK1. If this enzyme were unresponsive to the effects of fructose-2,6-bisphosphate, the liver would be unable to divert glucose into the glycolytic pathway at any significant rate and, therefore, a higher level of glucose would potentially be found in the blood, not a reduced level (choice E) as found in this patient.

5. Correct answer is **A.** When glucagon binds to its receptor on hepatocytes the result is an increase in the production of cAMP which in turn leads to increased levels of active PKA. PKA phosphorylates numerous substrates, many of which are enzymes involved in the regulation of carbohydrate and lipid metabolism. One of the substrates of PKA is phosphorylase kinase, PHK. Phosphorylation of PHK makes it much more active toward its two primary substrates, glycogen synthase and glycogen phosphorylase. The effect of PHK-mediated phosphorylation of glycogen phosphorylase is an increase in its activity, whereas the activity of glycogen synthase is decreased by PHK-mediated phosphorylation. One of the substrates for PKA is the enzyme PFK2. When PFK2 is phosphorylated by PKA it is active as a phosphatase and it removes a phosphate from the 2-position of the potent allosteric regulator, fructose-2,6-bisphosphate, F2,6BP. Reduction in the level of F2,6BP results in a significantly lower level of activity of PFK1 (choice B), which is the rate-limiting enzyme in the pathway of glycolysis. As indicated, PKA-mediated phosphorylation of PFK2 renders the enzyme more active as a phosphatase and much less active as a kinase (choice C). One of the substrates for PKA is the regulatory subunit of phosphoprotein phosphatase-1 (PP-1). When the regulatory subunit is phosphorylated it is released from PP-1 resulting in reduced, not increased (choice D) activity of PP-1. As indicated for the correct choice (choice A) one of the substrates of PKA is phosphorylase kinase, PHK. Phosphorylation of PHK, via the action of PKA, makes it much more active, not less active (choice E) toward its two primary substrates, glycogen synthase and glycogen phosphorylase.

6. Correct answer is **D.** Increases in cytosolic citrate primarily result from an increase in the ATP/ADP and NADH/NAD^+ ratios that signifies an increased energy charge in the cell. Normally citrate is high in the mitochondria, but under high energy charge it is transported into the cytosol. Cytosolic citrate exerts allosteric effects at the level of glycolysis and at the level of fatty acid synthesis. Within the context of glycolysis, citrate functions as an allosteric inhibitor of PFK1, therefore, reductions in cytosolic citrate would lead to concomitant increases in the activity of the enzyme. Changes in the levels of cytosolic citrate have no significant effect on the activities of the other enzymes (choices A, B, C, E, and F), each of which could contribute to changes in glucose output by the liver, either positively or negatively.

7. Correct answer is **D.** Under aerobic conditions, glucose can be completely oxidized to CO_2 and H_2O following the oxidative decarboxylation of pyruvate into acetyl-CoA which then enters the TCA cycle for further oxidation. The absence of oxygen (anaerobic metabolism) results in the increased

reduction of skeletal muscle pyruvate to lactate, via the action of lactate dehydrogenase. Within the context of the body, the increased lactate is released to the blood and delivered to the liver where it serves as a substrate for gluconeogenesis. Under normal conditions the levels of acetate (choice A) in human serum is less than 0.2 mM. Normal physiologic sources of acetate include bacterial fermentation in the colon which increases significantly when consuming a high-fiber diet. This intestinal acetate enters the portal circulation and is taken up by the liver where it is converted to acetyl-CoA. Intracellular generation of acetate is the consequence of the ubiquitously expressed cytosolic enzyme acetyl-CoA hydrolase. The acetate can then be salvaged by reactivation to acetyl-CoA through the action of acetyl-CoA synthetases. In the nervous system, the neurotransmitter acetylcholine (ACh) is degraded to acetate by acetylcholinesterase. In addition, following the consumption of ethanol, acetate levels can be elevated by as much as 20-fold. None of these sources of acetate correlate to glucose metabolism in skeletal muscle and, therefore, there would be no measurable changes in this metabolite under the conditions of this experiment. When using glucose as a substrate, the production of acetyl-CoA (choice B) requires an active pyruvate dehydrogenase complex, PDHc. The activity of the PDHc will be reduced under anaerobic conditions as a result of increased levels of NADH. The level of NADH increases under anaerobic conditions because of inhibited oxidative phosphorylation. The primary source of skeletal muscle alanine (choice C) is from the transamination of pyruvate via the action of alanine transaminase, ALT. This reaction is an important reaction for the disposal of waste nitrogen during skeletal muscle protein breakdown during periods of fasting and starvation. Since the conditions of this experiment involve the use of glucose there would be no demonstrable increase in protein breakdown and thus, no increased release of alanine from the cells. Oxaloacetate (choice E) is an intermediate in the TCA cycle and its formation requires continued input of acetyl-CoA. Since the PDHc would be inhibited (see choice A) under anaerobic conditions, the production of acetyl-CoA will be reduced and the TCA cycle activity will also be reduced limiting the production of oxaloacetate.

8. Correct answer is **F.** In the well-fed state there will be an increased level of insulin released from the pancreas, concomitant with a reduction in the level of glucagon release, not increased (choice E), from the pancreas and a reduction in cortisol production, not increased (choice D), by the adrenal glands. The effect of insulin on the liver is activation of a phosphodiesterase leading to decreased levels of cAMP and thus, reduced levels of active PKA. In addition, inulin activates protein phosphatase 1 (PP1) which removes phosphate from numerous substrates, with PFK2 being one of the PP1 substrates. Removal of phosphate from PFK2 results in the activation of its kinase activity. When PFK2 is active as a kinase, fructose-6-phosphate is phosphorylated to fructose-2,6-bisphosphate (F2,6BP). Thus, the fed state, not the fasting state (choice C) increases insulin and increases F2,6BP. In the fasted stated there will be an increased level of glucagon release from the pancrease and a decreased level of insulin release from the pancreas. Fasting also results in increased levels of cortisol release from the adrenal glands. Cortisol (choices A and D) is a steroid hormone and as such does not exert direct effects on the kinase and phosphatase activities of PFK2. In the fasted stated when glucagon is the predominant pancreatic hormone, it will bind to its receptors on hepatocytes triggering the activation of adenylate cyclase leading to increased production of cAMP and consequent activation of PKA. One of the targets of PKA is PFK2. When phosphorylated, PFK2 functions as a phosphatase which results in the removal of phosphate from fructose-2,6-bisphosphate, yielding fructose-6-phosphate and decreasing, not increasing (choice B) the levels of fructose-2,6-bisphosphate.

9. Correct answer is **B.** The patient is most likely suffering from the consequences of hereditary fructose intolerance, HFI. HFI is a potentially lethal disorder resulting from a lack of aldolase B which is normally present in the liver, small intestine, and kidney. The disorder is characterized by severe hypoglycemia and vomiting following fructose intake. Prolonged intake of fructose by infants with this defect leads to vomiting, poor feeding, jaundice, hepatomegaly, hemorrhage, and eventually hepatic failure and death. The primary cause of the manifesting symptoms in HFI is the trapping of inorganic phosphate (P_i) in fructose-1-phosphate and the consequent reduction in the pool of ATP via the fructokinase reaction. The trapping of the P_i pool and ATP depletion leads to global reduction in all cellular processes that rely on phosphorylation or ATP. The reduction in P_i impairs glycogen breakdown due to its role as a substrate for the phosphorolytic action of hepatic glycogen phosphorylase. This, therefore, contributes to the severe hypoglycemia upon ingestion of fructose or sucrose. Also contributing to the severe hypoglycemia in HFI patients is the increased levels of fructose-1-phosphate (F1P). Hepatic glucose is phosphorylated by glucokinase. The activity of glucokinase is regulated by the protein identified as glucokinase regulatory protein, GKRP. During the fasting state, glucokinase is "held" in the nucleus by interaction with GKRP. This localization prevents glucokinase access to cytosolic glucose until it is released from GKRP. Fructose-1-phosphate, derived from the action of hepatic fructokinase phosphorylating fructose, stimulates the release of glucokinase from GKRP. Indeed, the ability of F1P to stimulate release of glucokinase from GKRP ultimately contributes to the potentially lethal hypoglycemia associated with HFI. This latter effect results from inappropriate release of glucokinase to the cytosol leading to the phosphorylation of glucose, thereby, trapping the glucose within hepatocytes. HFI patients remain relatively symptom free on a diet devoid of fructose and sucrose. Classic galactosemia (choice A) results from mutations in the galactose metabolizing enzyme, galactose-1-phosphate uridylyltransferase (GALT). Classic galactosemia manifests by poor feeding behavior, a failure of neonates to thrive, bleeding problems, and *Escherichia coli*-associated sepsis in untreated infants. In classic galactosemia, infants will exhibit vomiting and diarrhea rapidly following ingestion of lactose from breast milk or from lactose-containing formula. Hunter syndrome (choice C) is a lysosomal storage disease resulting from mutations in the lysosomal hydrolase, iduronate sulfatase. Symptoms of Hunter syndrome include developmental delay, hepatosplenomegaly, and coarse facial features. Medium-chain acyl-CoA dehydrogenase (MCAD) deficiency (choice D) is a disorder of mitochondrial fatty acid oxidation resulting from mutations in MCAD. Characteristic features of MCAD deficiency are severe hypoglycemia and hypoketonemia upon fasting. Pompe disease (choice E) is a glycogen storage disease resulting from mutations in the lysosomal hydrolase, acid α-glucosidase (acid maltase). The clinical presentation of Pompe disease encompasses a wide range of phenotypes but all include various degrees of cardiomegaly. Tay-Sachs disease (choice F) is a lysosomal storage disease resulting from mutations in hexosaminidase A. Tay-Sachs is a debilitating lethal disorder, usually by 2 years of age, resulting from progressive neurodegeneration.

10. Correct answer is **B.** The patient most likely has a deficiency in erythrocyte pyruvate kinase. Deficiency of erythrocyte pyruvate kinase, PK (encoded by the *PKLR* gene) is the most common enzyme deficiency resulting in inherited nonspherocytic hemolytic anemia. The disorder is characterized by lifelong chronic hemolysis of variable severity. Red blood cells from heterozygous individuals possess only 40–60% of the pyruvate kinase activity of normal individuals yet these individuals are almost always clinically normal. The clinical severity of the anemia resulting from erythrocyte PK deficiencies varies from mild and fully compensated hemolysis to severe cases that require transfusions for survival. There are many patients with mild erythrocyte PK deficiency who do not manifest symptoms until adulthood. In these individuals, the symptoms, that include mild to moderate splenomegaly, mild chronic hemolysis, and jaundice, often manifest incidental to an acute viral infection or during an evaluation in pregnancy. Clinical evaluation of blood from patients with erythrocyte PK deficiency will show normocytic anemia (sometimes macrocytic) which is reflective of the reticulocytosis that is invariably present. The hemolysis results in increased heme metabolism in the liver generating bilirubin in excess which then accumulates in the gallbladder resulting in the stones present in this patient. The presence of elevated levels of serum 2,3BPG and glucose-6-phosphate is indicative of anemia due to erythrocyte PK deficiency as opposed to the more common cause due to glucose-6-phosphate dehydrogenase deficiency. The reduced activity of erythrocyte PK leads to increased levels of upstream glycolytic intermediates which are diverted into the 2,3BPG pathway. Defects in the processes of glycogen synthesis (choice A), heme biosynthesis (choice C), the pentose phosphate pathway (choice D), or protein synthesis (choice E) would not be associated with mild anemic states nor to increases in serum 2,3BPG levels.

11. Correct answer is **A.** The patient is most likely suffering from the consequences of hereditary fructose intolerance, HFI. HFI is a potentially lethal disorder resulting from a lack of aldolase B which is normally present in the liver, small intestine, and kidney. The disorder is characterized by severe hypoglycemia and vomiting following fructose intake. Prolonged intake of fructose by infants with this defect leads to vomiting, poor feeding, jaundice, hepatomegaly, hemorrhage, and eventually hepatic failure and death. The primary cause of the manifesting symptoms in HFI is the trapping of inorganic phosphate (P_i) in fructose-1-phosphate and the consequent reduction in the pool of ATP via the fructokinase reaction. The trapping of the P_i pool and ATP depletion leads to global reduction in all cellular processes that rely on phosphorylation or ATP. The reduction in P_i impairs glycogen breakdown due to its role as a substrate for the phosphorolytic action of hepatic glycogen phosphorylase. This, therefore, contributes to the severe hypoglycemia upon ingestion of fructose or sucrose. Also contributing to the severe hypoglycemia in HFI patients is the increased levels of fructose-1-phosphate (F1P). Hepatic glucose is phosphorylated by glucokinase. The activity of glucokinase is regulated by the protein identified as glucokinase regulatory protein, GKRP. During the fasting state, glucokinase is "held" in the nucleus by interaction with GKRP. This localization prevents glucokinase access to cytosolic glucose until it is released from GKRP. Fructose-1-phosphate, derived from the action of hepatic fructokinase phosphorylating fructose, stimulates the release of glucokinase from GKRP. Indeed, the ability of F1P to stimulate release of glucokinase from GKRP ultimately contributes to the potentially lethal hypoglycemia associated with HFI. This latter effect results from inappropriate release of glucokinase to the cytosol leading to the phosphorylation of glucose, thereby, trapping the glucose within hepatocytes. HFI patients remain relatively symptom free on a diet devoid of fructose and sucrose. Essential fructosuria is a benign metabolic disorder caused by the lack of fructokinase (choice B) which is normally present in the liver, pancreatic islets, and kidney cortex. Hereditary fructose-1,6-bisphosphatase (F1,6BPase) deficiency (choice C) results in severely impaired hepatic gluconeogenesis and leads to episodes of hypoglycemia, apnea, hyperventilation, ketosis, and lactic acidosis. One of the forms of galactosemia, termed type 2 galactosemia, results from deficiency of galactokinase (choice D). Patients with galactokinase deficiency often present with cataracts that will resolve upon dietary restriction of galactose. Classic galactosemia refers to a disorder arising from profound deficiency of the enzyme galactose-1-phosphate uridylyltransferase (choice E) and is termed type 1 galactosemia. Classic galactosemia manifests by poor feeding behavior, a failure of neonates to thrive, bleeding problems, and *E. coli*-associated sepsis in untreated infants.

12. Correct answer is **E.** The patient is manifesting symptoms associated with the ingestion of fructose in the context of hereditary fructose intolerance, HFI. HFI is a potentially lethal disorder resulting from a lack of aldolase B (also known as fructose-1-phosphate aldolase) which is normally present in the liver, small intestine, and kidney cortex. The disorder is characterized by severe hypoglycemia and vomiting following fructose intake. Ingestion of foods containing sucrose or fructose will lead to the manifesting symptoms of HFI. The primary cause of the manifesting symptoms in HFI is the trapping of inorganic phosphate (P_i) in fructose-1-phosphate and the consequent reduction in the pool of ATP via the fructokinase reaction. The trapping of the inorganic phosphate pool and ATP depletion leads to global reduction in all cellular processes that rely on phosphorylation or ATP. The loss of the inorganic phosphate (P_i) pool impairs glycogen breakdown due to the role of P_i as a substrate for phosphorolytic action of hepatic glycogen phosphorylase. This, therefore, contributes to the severe hypoglycemia upon ingestion of fructose or sucrose. Glycogen (choice A), maltose (choice C), and starch (choice D) each represent polymers of glucose. Glucose was present in the milk sugar, lactose (choice B), during the breastfeeding period in this patient and, therefore, cannot be a contributor to the manifesting symptoms.

13. Correct answer is **D.** The patient is most likely deficient in intestinal lactase and is thus, lactose intolerant. The signs and symptoms of lactose intolerance usually begin 30 minutes to 2 hours after eating or drinking foods that contain lactose and include nausea, vomiting, diarrhea, bloating, gas, and painful abdominal cramping. Consumption of none of the other carbohydrates (choices A, B, C, and E) would result in the observed gastrointestinal disturbances in this patient.

14. Correct answer is **D.** Unlike the regulation of the rate-limiting enzyme of glycolysis, PFK1, which is highly regulated by energy charge, the metabolism of fructose escapes these regulatory processes. As a consequence of the unregulated activity of fructokinase, hypothalamic fructose metabolism rapidly depletes ATP levels resulting in increased AMP levels. The rise in AMP results in activation of AMP-activated protein kinase, AMPK which, in turn leads to phosphorylation and inhibition of acetyl-CoA carboxylase (ACC). Inhibition of acetyl-CoA carboxylase results in decreased malonyl-CoA levels in the hypothalamus. Although the brain does not readily oxidize fatty acids for energy production, the major enzymes of the fatty acid biosynthetic pathway, such as acetyl-CoA carboxylase and fatty acid synthase (FAS), are expressed in neuronal regions of the hypothalamus that are involved in energy homeostasis. Various hormones and metabolic fuels affect hypothalamic malonyl-CoA levels and malonyl-CoA is considered a key satiety inducing signal in the brain. Changes in hypothalamic malonyl-CoA levels are followed quickly by changes in expression of orexigenic (hunger-inducing) and anorexigenic (satiety-inducing) neuropeptides. During periods of fasting, hypothalamic levels of malonyl-CoA rapidly decrease and act as a signal of hunger triggering the release of orexigenic neuropeptides. Conversely, during feeding, hypothalamic levels of malonyl-CoA rapidly rise and act as a signal to stop eating through the release of anorexigenic neuropeptides. The decrease in malonyl-CoA that result from the metabolism of fructose leads to increased desire to consume food even in the well-fed state. None of the other metabolic intermediates (choices A, B, C, and E) affect neuropeptide synthesis and release from the hypothalamus.

15. Correct answer is **A.** The patient is exhibiting the symptoms of classic galactosemia. Classic galactosemia results from profound deficiency of the enzyme galactose-1-phosphate uridylyltransferase (GALT) and is termed type 1 galactosemia. Classic galactosemia manifests by poor feeding behavior, a failure of neonates to thrive, bleeding problems, and *E. coli*-associated sepsis in untreated infants. In classic galactosemia, infants will exhibit vomiting and diarrhea rapidly following ingestion of lactose from breast milk or from lactose-containing formula. Clinical findings in infants with classic galactosemia who consume lactose or galactose containing meals include impaired liver function (which if left untreated leads to severe cirrhosis), hypoglycemia, hyperbilirubinemia, elevated blood galactose, hypergalactosemia, hyperchloremic metabolic acidosis, urinary galactitol excretion, and hyperaminoaciduria. Unless controlled by exclusion of galactose from the diet, these galactosemias can go on to result in fatal liver failure, brain damage, and blindness. Blindness is due to the conversion of circulating galactose to the sugar alcohol galactitol, by an NADPH-dependent aldose reductase that is present in neural tissue and in the lens of the eye. Hurler syndrome (choice B) is a progressive disorder manifesting with multiple organ and tissue involvement leading to death in early childhood. Most Hurler infants succumb to cardiomyopathy. Infants with pyloric stenosis (choice C) manifest with frequent episodes of vomiting, often with force. These episodes occur most often after feedings. Vomiting is the main symptom of pyloric stenosis. Infants with pyloric stenosis normally do not exhibit any other significant untoward signs. Infants with Tay-Sachs disease (choice D) appear normal at birth. Symptoms usually begin with mild motor weakness by 3–5 months of age and infants begin to show regression of prior acquired motor and mental skills, progressing to severe psychomotor deterioration. von Gierke disease (choice E) presents during the neonatal period with lactic acidosis and hypoglycemia. The hallmark features of this disease are hypoglycemia, lactic acidosis, hyperuricemia, and hyperlipidemia.

16. Correct answer is **B.** Deficiency of pyruvate kinase is one of the most common enzyme deficiencies resulting in inherited nonspherocytic hemolytic anemia. The disorder is characterized by lifelong chronic hemolysis of variable severity. Red blood cells from heterozygous individuals possess only 40–60% of the pyruvate kinase activity of normal individuals yet these individuals are almost always clinically normal. The clinical severity of the anemia resulting from pyruvate kinase deficiencies varies from mild and fully compensated hemolysis to severe cases that require transfusions for survival. The hemolysis results in increased heme metabolism in the reticuloendothelial system generating excessive bilirubin. The increased bilirubin delivery to the liver can result in accumulation in the gallbladder resulting in the calculi present in this patient. The presence of elevated levels of serum 2,3BPG and glucose-6-phosphate is indicative of anemia due to erythrocyte PK deficiency as opposed to glucose-6-phosphate dehydrogenase deficiency. Pyruvate kinase deficiency leads to increased levels of glycolytic intermediates which are diverted into the synthesis of 2,3BPG accounting for the elevated levels of this metabolite in this patient. Deficiency in none of the other processes (choices A, C, D, E, and F) would be associated with the signs and symptoms in this patient.

17. Correct answer is **C.** Within hepatocytes, insulin activation of its receptor results in numerous changes in metabolism that lead to the storage of carbon from the diet such as glucose and fat. Insulin mediates these effects through the concerted activation of phosphatases, in particular protein phosphatase-1 (PP-1) and a phosphodiesterase that hydrolyzes cAMP to AMP. The removal of phosphate from PFK2 activates the kinase activity of this enzyme resulting in increased production of the potent allosteric activator fructose-2,6-bisphosphate, F2,6BP. Removal of phosphate from glycogen phosphorylase (choice A) decreases its activity as opposed to increases. The production of F2,6BP, by the activated kinase of PFK2, strongly allosterically activates PFK1 (choice B) as opposed to this enzyme being unaffected. As indicated, PP-1 activity is increased, not decreased (choice D) via the actions of insulin. The removal of phosphate from phosphorylase kinase renders this enzyme less active not more active (choice E).

18. Correct answer is **E.** The reciprocal regulation of fuel metabolism between lipids and carbohydrates is defined by what is referred to as the glucose fatty acid cycle. According to the glucose-fatty acid cycle, glucose and fats reciprocally antagonize the utilization of each other. In other words, glucose oxidation can restrict fatty acid metabolism and fatty acid oxidation leads to reduced utilization of glucose. There are two major mechanisms by which fatty acid oxidation can restrict the flow of glucose through glycolysis. High levels of fat oxidation lead to generation of acetyl-CoA in excess of the cells ability to fully oxidize it in the TCA cycle. Some of this acetyl-CoA is converted to citrate via the citrate synthase reaction of the TCA cycle but the citrate cannot be further oxidized so it is transported to the cytosol where it allosterically inhibits the PFK1 reaction. In addition, the acetyl-CoA allosterically activates pyruvate dehydrogenase complex (PDHc) kinases that, when activated, phosphorylate the PDHc. Phosphorylated PDHc is less capable of oxidizing acetyl-CoA and leads to increased levels of pyruvate in the cytosol. The increased pyruvate restricts the ability of pyruvate kinase to oxidize phosphoenolpyruvate resulting in reduced flow through glycolysis. The metabolic regulation explained by the glucose fatty acid cycle implies that the cancer cells are expressing a version of PFK1 that is resistant to the inhibitory effects of citrate. None of the other mechanisms (choices A, B, C, and D) adequately explain why fat oxidation in the cancer cells does not lead to restriction of glucose metabolism.

19. Correct answer is **C.** During aerobic glycolysis, the NADH generated by the glyceraldehyde-3-phosphate dehydrogenase catalyzed reaction is ultimately reoxidized to NAD^+ in the mitochondria via the oxidative phosphorylation pathway. The transfer of the electrons from cytoplasmic NADH to mitochondrial NADH occurs via two shuttles mechanism resulting in the continued oxidation of NADH to NAD^+ keeping the glyceraldehyde-3-phosphate dehydrogenase reaction supplied with necessary NAD^+ for glycolysis. However, during anaerobic glycolysis pyruvate is not oxidized in the TCA cycle but is reduced to lactate via the action of lactate dehydrogenase, LDH. The reduction of pyruvate by LDH, within the cytosol, results in the oxidation of NADH to NAD^+ thus, supplying the NAD^+ required for the glyceraldehyde-3-phosphate dehydrogenase and allowing glycolysis to continue. Although cytoplasmic malate dehydrogenase (choice D) is used to reduce oxaloacetate to malate, while simultaneously oxidizing NADH to NAD^+, this reaction is limited by the amount of cytoplasmic oxaloacetate and, therefore, cannot contribute to the reoxidation of NADH to the degree required to maintain anaerobic glycolysis. None of the other enzymes (choices A, B, and E) can oxidize NADH to NAD^+.

20. Correct answer is **B.** The rate-limiting, and highly regulated, enzyme of glycolysis is phosphofructokinase-1, PFK1. Allosteric regulation of PFK1 is exerted by ATP, citrate, and fructose-2,6-bisphosphate. Fructose-2,6-bisphosphate (F2,6BP) is the most potent allosteric activator of PFK1 resulting in activation of glycolysis. Simultaneously, F2,6BP allosterically inhibits the gluconeogenic enzyme fructose-1,6-bisphosphatase. Given the findings in these hepatocyte cell cultures the experimental compound is most likely similar to and mimicking the effects of F2,6BP. None of the other carbohydrates (choices A, C, D, and E) would exert simultaneous effects on glycolysis and gluconeogenesis such as is the case for F2,6BP.

21. Correct answer is **B.** Activation of hepatic glycolysis occurs predominantly through allosteric regulation of the rate-limiting enzyme, phosphofructokinase-1 PFK1. Allosteric activation of PFK1 would be expected to occur under conditions of low energy charge. Thus, as the level of ATP drops there will be a concomitant rise in both AMP and inorganic phosphate levels. Both serve to allosterically activate PFK1. PFK1 is also allosterically activated by fructose-2,6-bisphosphate. Citrate (choices A, C, and E) and ATP (choices C and D) both function as allosteric inhibitors of PFK1 and would, therefore, result in reduced hepatic glycolysis.

22. Correct answer is **D.** Erythrocytes do not contain mitochondria and therefore, only oxidize glucose via anaerobic metabolism. Instead of oxidation of pyruvate via the pyruvate dehydrogenase complex the pyruvate generated by glycolysis in erythrocytes is reduced to lactate via lactate dehydrogenase. The benefit of this reaction is that the NADH produced by the glyceraldehyde-3-phosphate dehydrogenase reaction is oxidized to NAD^+ which can then be utilized for glycolysis. The coupling of NADH, produced by the glycolytic enzyme glyceraldehyde-3-phosphate dehydrogenase, and the reoxidation of the NADH to NAD^+ via lactate dehydrogenase is necessary for continued energy generation via glycolysis. Therefore, a loss of lactate dehydrogenase activity would lead to rapid depletion of NAD^+ within the cell and cessation of glycolysis. The lack of glycolysis would result in a rapid depletion of ATP as opposed to ADP (choice A). Citrate (choice B) is generated in the mitochondria by citrate synthase, and therefore, is not produced in erythrocytes. The lack of lactate dehydrogenase would result in an increase in pyruvate (choice E), not depletion.

23. Correct answer is **E.** Insulin, glucagon, epinephrine, and cortisol are the major regulators of glucose oxidation, and in hepatocytes, glucose synthesis. The primary goal of insulin is to stimulate carbon storage. Within the liver insulin stimulates glycogen synthesis as well as glycolysis. The latter allows for excess glucose to be oxidized to acetyl-CoA for fatty acid biosynthesis. Conversely glucagon, epinephrine, and cortisol will stimulate the synthesis of glucose via gluconeogenesis. Epinephrine and glucose will also stimulate the removal of glucose from glycogen. As the level of insulin rises there will be a concomitant increase in the activity of phosphodiesterase within responsive cells, such as the liver. The phosphodiesterase will hydrolyze cAMP leading to reduced activity of PKA. As the activity of PKA falls the level of phosphorylation of phosphofructokinase-2 (PFK2) will fall which reduces its phosphatase activity. When functioning as a phosphatase, PFK2 hydrolyzes fructose-2,6-bisphosphate (F2,6BP) to fructose-6-phosphate. When PFK2 is not phosphorylated, such as via insulin stimulation, it acts as a kinase and will, therefore lead to increased levels of F2,6BP. Conversely, as the level of glucagon and epinephrine increases during fasting, or via sympathetic outflow, the activity of PKA increases leading to increased phosphorylation of PFK2. This in turn results in decreased F2,6BP levels due to the phosphatase activity of PFK2. As the ratio of insulin to glucagon increases the level of F2,6BP also increases driving glycolysis. An increase in cortisol (choice A) would result in inhibited glycolysis. An increased level of epinephrine (choice B) or glucagon (choices C and D) would both inhibit glycolysis and stimulate gluconeogenesis.

24. Correct answer is **E.** As the level of ATP falls the level of ADP and AMP will increase. AMP functions as an allosteric activator of the rate-limiting enzyme of glycolysis, phosphofructokinase-1 (PFK1). Thus, as the level of ATP falls the rate of flux through PFK1 will increase, not decrease (choice B) and glycolysis will increase. As the level of ATP falls TCA cycle activity will increase, not decrease (choice A). Decreasing ATP results in more ADP and glycolysis and the TCA cycle will provide more NADH; therefore, the rate of electron transport will increase not decrease (choice C). An increased need for ATP synthesis via glycolysis will prevent glycogen synthesis and therefore glycogen synthase activity will be decreased not increased (choice D). Pyruvate carboxylase is activated by acetyl-CoA and under conditions of reduced ATP gluconeogenesis decreased, therefore pyruvate carboxylase activity would be decreased not increased (choice F).

25. Correct answer is **A.** The patient is most likely manifesting the symptoms of erythrocyte pyruvate kinase deficiency. Deficiency of pyruvate kinase is one of the most common enzyme deficiencies resulting in inherited nonspherocytic hemolytic anemia. The disorder is characterized by lifelong chronic hemolysis of variable severity. Red blood cells from heterozygous individuals possess only 40–60% of the pyruvate kinase activity of normal individuals yet these individuals are almost always clinically normal. The clinical severity of the anemia resulting from pyruvate kinase deficiency varies from mild and fully compensated hemolysis to severe cases that require transfusions for survival. Clinical evaluation of blood from patients with pyruvate kinase deficiency will show normocytic anemia (sometimes macrocytic) which is reflective of the reticulocytosis that is invariably present. The hemolysis results in increased heme metabolism in the reticuloendothelial system with consequent increase in the level of bilirubin delivered to the liver. When bilirubin is in excess of hepatic capacity to conjugate and excrete it there can be accumulation in the gallbladder resulting in the stones present in this patient. The presence of elevated levels of serum glucose-6-phosphate is indicative of anemia due to erythrocyte pyruvate kinase deficiency as opposed to glucose-6-phosphate dehydrogenase deficiency. The reduced pyruvate kinase leads to increased levels of glycolytic intermediates and in erythrocytes results in increased production of 2,3-bisphosphoglycerate. Since the erythrocytes block pyruvate kinase activity there is less pyruvate generated and therefore there would be less lactate generated (choice D). Although the liver is receiving more bilirubin than normal, due to the hemolysis, its function is not likely to be impaired or altered to the extent that there would be a significant increase in glucose (choice B), glutamine (choice C), urea (choice E), or uric acid (choice F) in this patient.

26. Correct answer is **D.** Only two compounds of glycolysis contain sufficient energy to drive the synthesis of ATP from ADP and thus, have $\Delta G^{0'}$ values more negative than the hydrolysis of ATP. These are 1,3-bisphosphoglycerate and phosphoenolpyruvate. None of the other intermediates of glycolysis (choices A, B, C, and E) possess sufficient energy to contribute to ATP synthesis during glycolysis.

27. Correct answer is **B.** The patient is most likely manifesting the symptoms of erythrocyte pyruvate kinase deficiency. Deficiency of pyruvate kinase is one of the most common enzyme deficiencies resulting in inherited nonspherocytic hemolytic anemia. The disorder is characterized by lifelong chronic hemolysis of variable severity. Red blood cells from heterozygous individuals possess only 40–60% of the pyruvate kinase activity of normal individuals yet these individuals are almost always clinically normal. The clinical severity of the anemia resulting from pyruvate kinase deficiency varies from mild and fully compensated hemolysis to severe cases that require transfusions for survival. Clinical evaluation of blood from patients with pyruvate kinase deficiency will show normocytic anemia (sometimes macrocytic) which is reflective of the reticulocytosis that is invariably present. The presence of elevated levels of serum glucose-6-phosphate and 2,3-bisphosphoglycerate is indicative of anemia due to erythrocyte pyruvate kinase deficiency as opposed to glucose-6-phosphate dehydrogenase deficiency. The reduced pyruvate kinase leads to increased levels of glycolytic intermediates and in erythrocytes results in increased production of 2,3-bisphosphoglycerate. Deficiencies in none of the other processes (choices A, C, D, E, and F) would be associated with the signs and symptoms in this patient.

28. Correct answer is **E.** In mammals, two genes encode a total of four pyruvate kinase (PK) isoforms. The *PKM* gene, so called originally due to initial characterization in muscle tissues, encodes the PKM1 and PKM2 isoforms. PKM1 and PKM2 are derived via alternative splicing of the *PKM* gene encoded mRNA. PKM2 can exist as a homodimeric or as a homotetrameric enzyme. The tetrameric form of PKM2 exhibits high catalytic activity in the conversion of phosphoenolpyruvate (PEP) to pyruvate and this is associated with ATP synthesis and catabolic metabolism of glucose. In contrast, the dimeric form of PKM2 has low catalytic activity and this low activity, in part, facilitates the diversion of glycolytic intermediates into glucose metabolic branch pathways that including glycerol synthesis and the pentose phosphate pathway. Of significance to proliferating cells, as well as cancer, is that the NADPH produced by the pentose phosphate pathway is used to reduce the level of reactive oxygen species (ROS) and is used in numerous reductive biosynthetic pathways. In addition, the ribose-5-phosphate is used for nucleotide synthesis. None of the other enzymes (choices A, B, C, and D) substantially contributed to the Warburg effect.

29. Correct answer is **A.** The production of cAMP is stimulated by certain hormones binding to their receptors that are coupled to G_s-type G-proteins. G_s-type G-proteins stimulate adenylate cyclase which generates cAMP from ATP. The primary function of cAMP is to bind to the regulatory subunits of PKA which leads to the activation of the catalytic subunits. The result of activation of PKA is the phosphorylation of numerous substrates. None of the other responses (choices B, C, D, and E) are associated with the effects of cAMP.

30. Correct answer is **B.** The patient is exhibiting the symptoms of classic galactosemia. Classic galactosemia results from profound deficiency of the enzyme galactose-1-phosphate uridylyltransferase (GALT) and is termed type 1 galactosemia. Classic galactosemia manifests by poor feeding behavior, a failure of neonates to thrive, bleeding problems, and *E. coli*-associated sepsis in untreated infants. In classic glactosemia, infants will exhibit vomiting and diarrhea rapidly following ingestion of lactose from breast milk or from lactose-containing formula. Clinical findings in infants with classic galactosemia who consume lactose or galactose containing meals include impaired liver function (which if left untreated leads to severe cirrhosis), hypoglycemia, hyperbilirubinemia, elevated blood galactose, hypergalactosemia, hyperchloremic metabolic acidosis, urinary galactitol excretion, and hyperaminoaciduria. Deficiency in fructose metabolism (choice A) is found associated with hereditary fructose intolerance. Deficiency in glycogen synthesis (choice C) is most likely to be found associated with defects in glycogen-branching enzyme as in Anderson disease. Deficiency in long-chain fatty acid oxidation (choice D) is associated with potentially severe hypoglycemia. Deficiency in peroxisomal phytanic acid oxidation (choice E) is the cause of Refsum disease.

31. Correct answer is **C.** The metabolism of ethanol, which occurs almost exclusively by the liver, leads to a large increase in both cytosolic and mitochondrial NADH. This increase in NADH disrupts the normal processes of metabolic regulation such as hepatic gluconeogenesis, TCA cycle function, and fatty acid oxidation. Concomitant with reduced fatty acid oxidation is enhanced fatty acid synthesis and increased triglyceride production by the liver. The end product of ethanol metabolism is acetate which is converted to acetyl-CoA in both the mitochondria and the cytosol via the action of acetyl-CoA synthetases. Since the increased generation of mitochondrial NADH also reduces the activity of the TCA cycle, the acetyl-CoA is diverted to fatty acid synthesis and ketones. The increased cytosolic NADH drives the activity of glycerol-3-phosphate dehydrogenase in the direction of the reduction of dihydroxyacetone phosphate to glycerol-3-phosphate. The resulting increased levels of glycerol-3-phosphate promote the synthesis of triglycerides. Both of these two events lead to fatty acid deposition in the liver leading to fatty liver syndrome and excessive levels of lipids in the blood, referred to as hyperlipidemia. The activity of none of the other enzymes (choices A, B, D, and E) contributes to hepatic steatosis during the process of alcohol metabolism.

32. Correct answer is **C.** There are four PFK2 isozymes in mammals, each coded for by a different gene. Each PFK2 gene also encodes several different isoforms via alternative splicing. The four different PFK2 isoforms are expressed in the liver, heart, brain (or placenta), and testis and each differs by the sequences of their bifunctional catalytic cores and their N-terminal amino acid sequences. Rapid, short-term regulation of the kinase and phosphatase activities of PFK2 are exerted by phosphorylation and dephosphorylation events. The liver isoform is phosphorylated at the N-terminus by PKA. This PKA-mediated phosphorylation results in inhibition of the kinase activity of PFK2 activity while at the same time leading to activation of the phosphatase activity. In contrast, the heart isoform is phosphorylated at the C-terminus by several protein kinases in different signaling pathways, resulting in enhancement of the kinase activity of PFK2 activity. None of the other mechanisms (choices A, B, D, and E) correctly explains the heart and liver differences in response to epinephrine at the level of glycolysis.

33. Correct answer is **E.** The only pathway for the production of ATP, under anaerobic conditions, is glycolysis. Therefore, targeting enzymes of the glycolytic pathway would potentially be useful in the interference with the growth of cancer cells. However, there would be limited specificity to these approaches. One glycolytic enzyme, pyruvate kinase, is expressed in a specific isoform, PKM2, in cancer cells, therefore, targeting this glycolytic enzyme would most likely be of benefit in the treatment of cancer. Recent work has demonstrated that small molecule PKM2-specific activators are functional in reducing tumor growth. Drugs that constitutively activate PKM2 are functional in reducing tumor growth. This is, in part, because the activated enzyme is resistant to inhibition by tyrosine phosphorylated proteins. PKM2-specific activators reduce the incorporation of glucose into lactate and lipids. In addition, PKM2 activation results in decreased pools of nucleotide, amino acid, and lipid precursors and these effects account for the suppression of tumorigenesis observed with PKM2 activating drugs. Activation of none of the other glycolytic enzymes (choices A, B, C, and D) would result in repression of cancer cell growth, on the contrary it would result in enhanced cancer cell growth.

34. Correct answer is **A.** The patient has most likely been exposed to arsenate as evidenced from the garlic odor of the patient's breath and the attendant pathology. Arsenates inhibit glycolysis and the TCA cycle, in particular the pyruvate dehydrogenase catalyzed reaction. The inhibition of pyruvate dehydrogenase would be the major contributor to a reduced ability to generate acetyl-CoA. Reductions in none of the other compounds (choices B, C, D, E, and F) would be parent in an individual poisoned with arsenate.

35. Correct answer is **B.** Enhanced glycolysis can result from increased activity of glycolytic enzymes, altered allosteric regulation of glycolysis, and by increased levels of glucose within the cell. Enhanced access to glucose would be a predominant contributor to increase glucose metabolism in tumor cells. Transport of glucose into the cells of the brain is carried out by both GLUT3 and GLUT1. Therefore, an increased activity of GLUT3 would be the most significant mechanism to provide brain tumor cells with the increased amount of glucose that promotes their rapid growth. Increased activity of glucokinase (choice A) and pyruvate kinase (choice E) would contribute to enhanced glucose metabolism. However, the more likely contributor to enhanced glycolysis in brain tumor cells would be enhanced transport of glucose into the cells. GLUT4 (choice C) is only expressed in adipocytes and skeletal muscle, and therefore, would not contribute to increased glucose transport in the brain. Although the brain does store glucose as glycogen the amount is not significant to account for the high rate of glycolysis in brain tumor cells. Therefore, increased glycogen phosphorylase (choice D) would not support increased tumor cell metabolism of glucose.

36. Correct answer is **A.** The patient is most likely suffering from the consequences of hereditary fructose intolerance, HFI. HFI is a potentially lethal disorder resulting from a lack of aldolase B which is normally present in the liver, small intestine, and kidney. The disorder is characterized by severe hypoglycemia and vomiting following fructose intake. Prolonged intake of fructose by infants with this defect leads to vomiting, poor feeding, jaundice, hepatomegaly, hemorrhage, and eventually hepatic failure and death. Defects in none of the other pathways (choices B, C, D, E, and F) would account for the observations in this patient.

37. Correct answer is **A.** The patient is most likely suffering from the consequences of hereditary fructose intolerance, HFI. HFI is a potentially lethal disorder resulting from a lack of aldolase B which is normally present in the liver, small intestine, and kidney. The disorder is characterized by severe hypoglycemia and vomiting following fructose intake. The carbohydrate in honey is almost exclusively fructose. Prolonged intake of fructose by infants with this defect leads to vomiting, poor feeding, jaundice, hepatomegaly, hemorrhage, and eventually hepatic failure and death. Defects in none of the other processes (choices B, C, D, and E) would account for the observations in this patient.

38. Correct answer is **D.** The primary cause of the manifesting symptoms in hereditary fructose intolerance is the trapping of inorganic phosphate (P_i) in fructose-1-phosphate and the consequent reduction in the pool of ATP via the fructokinase reaction. The trapping of the P_i pool and ATP depletion leads to global reduction in all cellular processes that rely on phosphorylation or ATP. The reduction in P_i impairs glycogen breakdown due to its role as a substrate for the phosphorolytic action of hepatic glycogen phosphorylase. This, therefore, contributes to the severe hypoglycemia upon ingestion of fructose or sucrose. Also contributing to the severe hypoglycemia in HFI patients is the increased levels of fructose-1-phosphate (F1P). Hepatic glucose is phosphorylated by glucokinase. The activity of glucokinase is regulated by the protein identified as glucokinase regulatory protein, GKRP. During the fasting state, glucokinase is "held" in the nucleus by interaction with GKRP. This localization prevents glucokinase access to cytosolic glucose until it is released from

GKRP. Fructose-1-phosphate, derived from the action of hepatic fructokinase phosphorylating fructose, stimulates the release of glucokinase from GKRP. Indeed, the ability of F1P to stimulate release of glucokinase from GKRP ultimately contributes to the potentially lethal hypoglycemia associated with HFI. This latter effect results from inappropriate release of glucokinase to the cytosol leading to the phosphorylation of glucose, thereby, trapping the glucose within hepatocytes. None of the other options (choices A, B, C, and E) correctly explain the severe hypoglycemia associated with hereditary fructose intolerance.

39. Correct answer is **E.** Patients with hereditary fructose intolerance must avoid any carbohydrate that contains fructose or any foods that contain fructose. Typical carbohydrates to avoid would be sucrose which is a disaccharide of glucose and fructose. Foods that contain fructose include most fruits and honey. Sorbitol is a carbohydrate often used in the pharmaceutical and food industries as a thickener or for the production of transparent gels such in certain toothpastes. Sorbitol can be metabolized to fructose via the action of sorbitol dehydrogenase. Therefore, it is important that patients with hereditary fructose intolerance monitor food and pharmaceuticals for the presence of sorbitol as ingestion can lead to significant health complications. None of the other carbohydrates (choices A, B, C, and D) contain fructose and therefore need not be avoided by patients with hereditary fructose intolerance.

40. Correct answer is **A.** Unlike the regulation of the rate-limiting enzyme of glycolysis, PFK1, which is highly regulated by energy charge, the metabolism of fructose escapes these regulatory processes. As a consequence of the unregulated activity of fructokinase, hypothalamic fructose metabolism rapidly depletes ATP levels resulting in increased AMP levels. The rise in AMP results in activation of AMP-activated protein kinase, AMPK which, in turn leads to phosphorylation and inhibition of acetyl-CoA carboxylase (ACC). Inhibition of acetyl-CoA carboxylase results in decreased malonyl-CoA levels and, consequently, decreased fatty acid synthesis in the hypothalamus, as opposed to increased synthesis (choice D). Although the brain does not readily oxidize fatty acids for energy production, the major enzymes of the fatty acid biosynthetic pathway, such as acetyl-CoA carboxylase and fatty acid synthase (FAS), are expressed in neuronal regions of the hypothalamus that are involved in energy homeostasis. Various hormones and metabolic fuels affect hypothalamic malonyl-CoA levels and malonyl-CoA is considered a key satiety inducing signal in the brain. Changes in hypothalamic malonyl-CoA levels are followed quickly by changes in expression of orexigenic (hunger-inducing) and anorexigenic (satiety-inducing) neuropeptides. During periods of fasting, hypothalamic levels of malonyl-CoA rapidly decrease and act as a signal of hunger triggering the release of orexigenic neuropeptides. Conversely, during feeding, hypothalamic levels of malonyl-CoA rapidly rise and act as a signal to stop eating through the release of anorexigenic neuropeptides. The decrease in malonyl-CoA that result from the metabolism of fructose leads to increased desire to consume food even in the well-fed state. None of the other metabolic changes (choices B, C, E, and F) occur in the hypothalamus as a result of fructose metabolism.

41. Correct answer is **A.** This patient is most likely suffering from the symptoms of classic (type 1) galactosemia. Classic galactosemia refers to a disorder arising from profound deficiency of the enzyme, galactose-1-phosphate uridylyltransferase, GALT. Classic galactosemia manifests with poor feeding behavior, a failure of neonates to thrive, bleeding problems, and *E. coli*-associated sepsis in untreated infants. In classic galactosemia, infants will exhibit vomiting and diarrhea rapidly following ingestion of lactose from breast milk or from lactose-containing formula. Clinical findings include impaired liver function (which if left untreated leads to severe cirrhosis), elevated blood galactose, hypergalactosemia, hyperchloremic metabolic acidosis, urinary galactitol excretion, and hyperaminoaciduria. Unless controlled by exclusion of galactose from the diet, these patients can go on to develop blindness and fatal liver damage. Blindness is due to the conversion of circulating galactose to the sugar alcohol galactitol, by an NADPH-dependent aldose reductase that is present in neural tissue and in the lens of the eye. Hereditary fructose intolerance (choice B) is due to mutations in the aldolase B gene. The disorder is characterized by severe hypoglycemia and vomiting following fructose intake. Hers disease (choice C) is a glycogen storage disease resulting from mutations in the gene (PGYL) encoding the liver isoform of phosphorylase. Hers disease is associated with hepatomegaly, mild fasting hypoglycemia, hyperlipidemia, and ketosis. Pompe disease (choice D) is a glycogen storage disease that results from mutations in the lysosomal hydrolase, acid α-glucosidase gene (acid maltase). The clinical presentation of Pompe disease encompasses a wide range of phenotypes but all include various degrees of cardiomegaly. von Gierke disease (choice E) is a glycogen storage disease resulting from mutations in the glucose-6-phosphatase gene. The hallmark features of von Gierke disease are hypoglycemia, lactic acidosis, hyperuricemia, and hyperlipidemia.

42. Correct answer is **D.** The patient is most likely exhibiting the symptoms of classic galactosemia. Classic galactosemia results from profound deficiency of the enzyme galactose-1 phosphate uridylyltransferase (GALT) and is termed type 1 galactosemia. Classic galactosemia manifests by poor feeding behavior, a failure of neonates to thrive, bleeding problems, and *E. coli*-associated sepsis in untreated infants. In classic galactosemia, infants will exhibit vomiting and diarrhea rapidly following ingestion of lactose from breast milk or from lactose-containing formula. The primary disorder associated with erythrocyte glycolysis (choice A) is erythrocyte pyruvate kinase deficiency. Numerous disorders of fatty acid oxidation (choice B) are known but the most common manifesting in the neonatal period is medium chain acyl-CoA dehydrogenase deficiency, MCADD. MCADD is associated with severe hypoglycemia and hypoketonemia during periods of fasting. Disorders of fructose metabolism (choice C) are primarily related to deficiency in aldolase B, the cause of hereditary fructose intolerance. Disorders related to gluconeogenesis (choice E) are most likely the result of mutations in pyruvate carboxylase, PC. PC deficiency is an infantile onset disease characterized by mild metabolic acidosis, delayed motor development, intellectual disability, failure to thrive, hypotonia, ataxia, ocular disorder (nystagmus), and convulsions. Hepatic glycogen synthesis (choice F) related disorders that would most likely be evident in the neonatal period would be the glycogen storage disease, Andersen disease, that results from mutations in the glycogen branching enzyme. Classic Andersen disease is a rapidly progressive disorder that will result in early lethality as a result of liver failure.

43. Correct answer is **E.** Phosphofructokinase-2 is a bifunctional enzyme that possesses both phosphatase and kinase activities. These two activities of PFK2 are regulated by the state of phosphorylation of the enzyme. When PFK2 is phosphorylated, via the action of PKA, its activity shifts from a kinase to a phosphatase. Within hepatocytes changes in the catalytic activity of PFK2 occur in response to the effects of insulin, glucose, and epinephrine. Insulin activates a phosphatase that removes phosphate from PFK2-activating Disse kinase activity. Conversely glucagon and epinephrine lead to activation of PKA which phosphorylates PFK2 inducing the phosphatase activity. Since the compound decreases the kinase activity of PFK2 in these hepatocyte cell cultures it is most likely mimicking the effects of PKA-mediated phosphorylation. None of the other activities (choices A, B, C, and D) are correlated to the changing catalytic activity of PFK2.

44. Correct answer is **A.** The depletion of the inorganic phosphate pool in patients with hereditary fructose intolerance (HFI) results in the activation of AMP deaminase. Enhanced levels of AMP deaminase activity result in increased nucleotide catabolism. This latter effect is the cause of the hyperuricemia associated with HFI. None of the other enzymes (choices B, C, D, and E) is activated as a result of depletion of the inorganic phosphate pool in patients with HFI.

45. Correct answer is **D.** The electrons from reduced cytosolic NADH enter the mitochondria via either the malate-aspartate shuttle or the glycerol phosphate shuttle. In the context of the malate-aspartate shuttle, the electrons from cytosolic NADH are transferred to oxaloacetate forming malate via the action of cytosolic malate dehydrogenase. The malate is then actively transported into the mitochondria where it enters the TCA cycle. In the TCA cycle malate is oxidized to oxaloacetate by the mitochondrial malate dehydrogenase, while simultaneously transferring electrons to NAD^+ reducing it to NADH. The now mitochondrial NADH can transfer the energy of these electrons to oxidative phosphorylation at complex I. None of the other processes (choices A, B, C, and E) correctly relate to the mechanism of transfer of cytoplasmic NADH electrons to the mitochondria.

46. Correct answer is **A.** The infant is most likely suffering from the consequences of galactokinase (GALK) deficiency. Patients with GALK deficiency often present with cataracts that will resolve upon dietary restriction of galactose. Testing for GALK deficiency involves the assay for enzyme activity in whole blood. Although patients with classic galactosemia (GALT deficiency) also develop cataracts, the prevalence is markedly less than among GALK-deficient patients. In addition, the symptoms of classic galactosemia are much more severe than those associated with galactokinase deficiency. Measurement of blood pyruvate kinase (choice B) would be appropriate for assessing erythrocyte pyruvate kinase deficiency. Measurement of hepatic glucose-6-phosphatase (choice C) would be beneficial when von Gierke disease was suspected. Measurement of hepatic glycogen branching enzyme (choice D) would be beneficial in assessing for the glycogen storage disease, Anderson disease. Assessment of skeletal muscle galactose-1-phosphate uridylyltransferase, GALT (choice E) would be beneficial in assessment of classic galactosemia; however, the standard assay is to measure blood samples for GALT activity or the level of galactose-1-phosphate. Measurement of skeletal muscle glycogen phosphorylase (choice F) would be beneficial when the glycogen storage disease, McArdle disease was suspected.

47. Correct answer is **B.** Hepatic glucokinase has a high K_m for glucose in order to ensure that the liver does not trap glucose before sufficient levels are obtained in the blood for use by peripheral tissues, in part particular the brain and red blood cells. As the level of blood glucose increases, glucokinase will become more active resulting in phosphorylation of more glucose thus, trapping it in hepatocytes leading to a gradual reduction in blood glucose levels. Although not one of the options, when blood glucose levels rise significantly the pancreas secretes insulin. One of the effects of insulin is mobilization of vesicles containing plasma membrane of adipocytes and skeletal muscle further contributing to reductions in circulating blood glucose. Activation of PKA (choice A) would stimulate the liver to release glucose to the blood as a result of activated gluconeogenesis, therefore, blood glucose levels would increase as opposed to decrease. Activation of glycogen synthase (choice C) in the liver does contribute to removal of glucose from the blood, but it must first be phosphorylated by glucokinase prior to incorporation into glycogen. PFK1 (choice D) and pyruvate kinase (choice E) would drive glycolysis reducing intracellular levels of glucose allowing for glucose to be removed from the blood. However, the glucose from the blood must first be phosphorylated by glucokinase.

48. Correct answer is **B.** The total amount of adenosine nucleotides does not vary much in a cell, but the ratio of ATP to ADP+AMP varies significantly depending on the energy state of the cell. By far, most of the ATP generated in cells is produced during oxidative phosphorylation which utilizes the energy of the electrons carried by the reduced electron carriers, NADH and $FADH_2$, to drive ATP synthesis. These reduced electron carriers are formed by aerobic pathways, such as glycolysis, the TCA cycle, and mitochondrial β-oxidation of fatty acids. Glycolysis is the only ATP-generating metabolic pathway that can function anaerobically. The key issue is the regeneration of NADH in any pathway. Most of the pathways regenerate NADH back to NAD^+ by the mitochondrial electron transport chain that depends on the presence of oxygen as the ultimate electron acceptor. Without sufficient oxygen, all the pathways are inoperable except for glycolysis. The NADH generated by the glyceraldehyde-3-phosphate dehydrogenase reaction can be recycled back to NAD^+ aerobically or anaerobically via the lactate dehydrogenase enzyme that reduces pyruvate to lactate. In tissue hypoxia, there will be high AMP (low ATP), which is an allosteric activator of PFK1 leading to increased glycolysis. However, during hypoxia the pyruvate cannot be oxidized by pyruvate dehydrogenase resulting in reduction of pyruvate to lactate as the means to oxidize NADH to NAD^+ which is required to ensure continued anaerobic glycolysis. The result is the lactic acidosis resulting from hypoxia. None of the other mechanisms (choices A, C, D, E, and F) correctly explains the lactic acidosis associated with hypoxia.

49. Correct answer is **C.** The patient is most likely manifesting the benign symptom of a deficiency in fructokinase, a disorder referred to as essential fructosuria. The only significant issue with this disorder is increased fructose in the urine. Deficiency in none of the other enzymes (choices A, B, D, and E) would be associated with normal serum and urine glucose levels and increased serum and urine fructose. Deficiency in aldolase B (choice B) is the cause of hereditary fructose intolerance. Deficiency in galactokinase (choice D) results in a form of galactosemia which is typified by early onset cataracts.

50. Correct answer is **B.** The patient is most likely exhibiting the symptoms of classic galactosemia. Classic galactosemia results from profound deficiency of the enzyme galactose-1-phosphate uridylyltransferase (GALT) and is termed classic (type 1) galactosemia. Classic galactosemia manifests with poor feeding behavior, a failure of neonates to thrive, bleeding problems, and *E. coli*-associated sepsis in untreated infants. In classic galactosemia, infants will exhibit vomiting and diarrhea rapidly following ingestion of lactose from breast milk or from lactose-containing formula. Clinical findings include impaired liver function (which, if left untreated, leads to severe cirrhosis), elevated blood galactose, hypergalactosemia, hyperchloremic metabolic acidosis, urinary galactitol excretion, and hyperaminoaciduria. Unless controlled by exclusion of galactose from the diet, these patients can go on to develop blindness and fatal liver damage. Blindness is due to the conversion of circulating galactose to the sugar alcohol galactitol by an NADPH-dependent aldose reductase that is present in neural tissue and in the lens of the eye. Deficiency in aldolase B (choice A) is the cause of hereditary fructose intolerance. Deficiency in glucocerebrosidase (choice C) is the cause of Gaucher disease. Although there are younger patients that exhibit the symptoms of Gaucher disease, over 95% of patients do not exhibit symptoms until the second or third decade of life. Deficiency in glucose-6-phosphate dehydrogenase (choice D) is the leading cause of inherited nonspherocytic anemia. Deficiency in phenylalanine hydroxylase (choice E) is the cause of phenylketonuria, PKU.

51. Correct answer is **A.** The patient is most likely exhibiting the symptoms of classic galactosemia. Classic galactosemia results from profound deficiency of the enzyme galactose-1-phosphate uridylyltransferase (GALT) and is termed classic (type 1) galactosemia. Classic galactosemia manifests with poor feeding behavior, a failure of neonates to thrive, bleeding problems, and *E. coli*-associated sepsis in untreated infants. In classic galactosemia, infants will exhibit vomiting and diarrhea rapidly following ingestion of lactose from breast milk or from lactose-containing formula. Clinical findings include impaired liver function (which, if left untreated, leads to severe cirrhosis), elevated blood galactose, hypergalactosemia, hyperchloremic metabolic acidosis, urinary galactitol excretion, and hyperaminoaciduria. Unless controlled by exclusion of galactose from the diet, these patients can go on to develop blindness and fatal liver damage. Blindness is due to the conversion of circulating galactose to the sugar alcohol galactitol, by an NADPH-dependent aldose reductase that is present in neural tissue and in the lens of the eye. Erythrocyte pyruvate kinase deficiency (choice B) is one of the two leading causes of inherited nonspherocytic anemia. Hereditary fructose intolerance, HFI (choice C) results from a deficiency in aldolase A. HFI is characterized by severe hypoglycemia and vomiting following fructose intake. Prolonged intake of fructose by infants with this defect leads to vomiting, poor feeding, jaundice, hepatomegaly, hemorrhage, and eventually hepatic failure and death. Maple syrup urine disease, MSUD (choice D) is caused by mutations in genes encoding subunits of branched-chain keto acid dehydrogenase (BCKD) responsible for the catabolism of leucine, isoleucine, and valine. Classic MSUD is defined by neonatal onset of encephalopathy and is the most severe form of the disorder. Phenylketonuria, PKU (choice E) results from mutations in phenylalanine hydroxylase. The major clinical manifestation associated with PKU is impaired cognitive development and function.

52. Correct answer is **B.** The patient is most likely suffering from the effects of hereditary fructose intolerance, HFI. HFI results from a lack of aldolase B which is normally expressed in the liver, small intestine, and kidney cortex. The disorder is characterized by severe hypoglycemia and vomiting following fructose intake. Prolonged intake of fructose by infants with this defect leads to vomiting, poor feeding, jaundice, hepatomegaly, hemorrhage, and eventually hepatic failure and death. Contributing to the severe hypoglycemia in HFI patients is the increased levels of fructose-1-phosphate (F1P). Hepatic glucose is phosphorylated by glucokinase, a member of the hexokinase family of enzymes, which is specific for glucose as its substrate. The activity of glucokinase is regulated by the protein identified as glucokinase regulatory protein (GKRP). During the fasting state, glucokinase is "held" in the nucleus by interaction with GKRP. This localization prevents glucokinase access to cytosolic glucose until it is released from GKRP. Fructose-1-phosphate, derived from the action of hepatic fructokinase phosphorylating fructose, stimulates the release of glucokinase from GKRP. Indeed, the ability of F1P to stimulate release of glucokinase from GKRP ultimately contributes to the potentially lethal hypoglycemia associated with HFI. Elevation in the level of none of the other carbohydrates (choices A, C, D, and E) will lead to the severe hypoglycemia associated with HFI.

53. Correct answer is **E.** The patient is most likely exhibiting the signs and symptoms of the hemolytic anemia caused by deficiency in erythrocyte pyruvate kinase. The clinical severity of the anemia resulting from pyruvate kinase deficiency varies from mild and fully compensated hemolysis to severe cases that require transfusions for survival. Biochemically, the loss of fully functional pyruvate kinase in erythrocytes results in impaired production of ATP which leads to cessation of all active processes in the cell. As a result of the loss of ATP, plasma membrane Na^+,K^+-ATPases are some of the first activities to cease functioning, resulting in loss of intracellular K^+. The erythrocyte becomes hypotonic leading to loss of water and shrinkage of the cell contributing to hemolysis. In addition to loss of ATP production impaired pyruvate kinase activity leads to the accumulation of upstream glycolytic intermediates, in particular 2,3-biphosphoglycerate (2,3-BPG). Accumulation of 2,3-BPG further impairs glycolytic flux as a result of the inhibition of the hexokinase reaction. Chronic granulomatous disease, CGD (choice A) is caused by loss of function of leukocyte NADPH oxidase activity. Glucose-6-phosphate dehydrogenase (G6PDH) deficiency (choice B), like erythrocyte PK deficiency, is associated with the potential for severe hemolytic anemia. However, the anemia caused by G6PDH deficiency is very often associated with infections and the use of certain antibiotics, circumstances that are not found in the patient. Hereditary fructose intolerance (HFI) (choice D) is characterized by severe hypoglycemia and vomiting following fructose intake. Prolonged intake of fructose by infants with this defect leads to vomiting, poor feeding, jaundice, hepatomegaly, hemorrhage, and eventually hepatic failure and death. Pyruvate dehydrogenase deficiency (choice D) can result from mutations in any of the genes encoding subunits of the pyruvate dehydrogenase complex, PDHc. In patients with PDHc deficiency, the major presentations encompass metabolic and neurologic pathologies with both occurring with equal frequency. The metabolic form presents with severe lactic acidosis in the newborn period which very often leads to lethality. PDHc deficiency accounts for about 15% of known causes of congenital lactic acidosis.

54. Correct answer is **B.** The patient is most likely exhibiting the signs and symptoms of the hemolytic anemia caused by deficiency in erythrocyte pyruvate kinase. The clinical severity of the anemia resulting from pyruvate kinase deficiency varies from mild and fully compensated hemolysis to severe cases that require transfusions for survival. Biochemically, the loss of fully functional pyruvate kinase in erythrocytes results in impaired production of ATP which leads to cessation of all active processes in the cell. As a result of the loss of ATP, plasma membrane Na^+,K^+-ATPases are some of the first activities to cease functioning resulting in loss of intracellular K^+. The erythrocyte becomes hypotonic leading to loss of water and shrinkage of the cell contributing to hemolysis. In addition to loss of ATP production, impaired pyruvate kinase activity leads to the accumulation of upstream glycolytic intermediates, in particular 2,3-biphosphoglycerate (2,3-BPG). Accumulation of 2,3-BPG further impairs glycolytic flux as a result of the inhibition of the hexokinase reaction. Elevation of serum alloisoleucine (choice A) is found in patients with maple syrup urine disease, MSUD. Elevation in serum levels of delta-aminolevulinic acid (choice C) occurs in patients with defects in enzymes of heme biosynthesis. Since glucose-6-phosphate (choice D) is trapped inside cells, it is unlikely that levels in the blood would increase but hepatocyte levels do increase in von Gierke disease. Elevation in serum levels of methylmalonyl-CoA (choice E) is primarily associated with deficiency of vitamin B_{12}.

55. Correct answer is **E.** The patient is most likely experiencing the signs and symptoms of hereditary fructose intolerance (HFI). HFI results from a lack of aldolase B which is normally expressed in the liver, small intestine, and kidney cortex. The disorder is characterized by severe hypoglycemia and vomiting following fructose intake. Prolonged intake of fructose by infants with this defect leads to vomiting, poor feeding, jaundice, hepatomegaly, hemorrhage, and eventually hepatic failure and death. Since sucrose is a disaccharide of glucose and fructose, consumption of food containing sucrose, as well as common table sugar, should be avoided. Avoidance of none of the other substances (choices A, B, C, and D) would have a positive benefit to patients with HFI.

CHAPTER

6

Gluconeogenesis

High-Yield Terms

Cori cycle	Describes the interrelationship between lactate production during anaerobic glycolysis and the use of lactate carbons to produce glucose via hepatic gluconeogenesis
Endogenous glucose production	Designated as EGP, refers to the process of glucose production via gluconeogenesis
Glucose-alanine cycle	Describes the interrelationship between pyruvate transamination to alanine during skeletal muscle glycolysis and delivery to the liver where the alanine is deaminated back to pyruvate which is then diverted into hepatic gluconeogenesis

PATHWAY OF GLUCONEOGENESIS

Gluconeogenesis is the biosynthesis of new glucose (ie, not glucose from glycogen). The production of glucose from other carbon skeletons is necessary for certain cell types as well as during periods of fasting and starvation. This is acutely true for erythrocytes since these cells exclusively depend on glucose oxidation for ATP production. The primary carbon skeletons used for hepatic gluconeogenesis are derived from pyruvate, lactate, alanine but can also include glycerol and glutamine (Figure 6–1). The liver is the major site of gluconeogenesis; however, as discussed later, the kidney and the small intestine utilize glutamine as the carbon source for gluconeogenesis.

HIGH-YIELD CONCEPT

The three reactions of glycolysis that proceed with a large negative free energy change are bypassed during gluconeogenesis by using different enzymes. The bypass reactions represent the reversal of glycolysis at the pyruvate kinase, phosphofructokinase-1 (PFK1), and hexokinase-/glucokinase-catalyzed reactions.

Pyruvate to Phosphoenolpyruvate, Bypass 1

Conversion of pyruvate to phosphoenolpyruvate (PEP) requires the action of two enzymes. The first is an ATP-requiring reaction catalyzed by pyruvate carboxylase, (PC) which catalyzes the carboxylation of pyruvate to the TCA cycle intermediate, oxaloacetic acid (OAA). The second enzyme of bypass 1 is the GTP-dependent PEP carboxykinase (PEPCK) which converts OAA to PEP. Human cells contain almost equal amounts of mitochondrial and cytosolic PEPCK (designated PEPCK-m and PEPCK-c, respectively), so this second reaction can occur in either cellular compartment.

The net result of the PC and PEPCK reactions is:

$$\text{Pyruvate} + \text{ATP} + \text{GTP} + H_2O \rightarrow \text{PEP} + \text{ADP} + \text{GDP} + \text{Pi} + 2H^+$$

Fructose-1,6-bisphosphate to Fructose-6-phosphate, Bypass 2

Fructose-1,6-bisphosphate (F1,6BP) conversion to fructose-6-phosphate (F6P) is the reverse of the rate-limiting step of glycolysis. The reaction, a simple hydrolysis, is catalyzed by fructose-1,6-bisphosphatase (F1,6BPase). Like the regulation of glycolysis occurring at the PFK1 reaction, the F1,6BPase reaction is a major point of control of gluconeogenesis (see later).

Glucose-6-phosphate (G6P) to Glucose (or Glycogen), Bypass 3

G6P is converted to glucose through the action of glucose-6-phosphatase (G6Pase). This reaction is also a simple hydrolysis reaction like that of F1,6BPase. In the kidney, muscle, and especially the liver, G6P can be shunted toward glycogen if blood glucose levels are adequate.

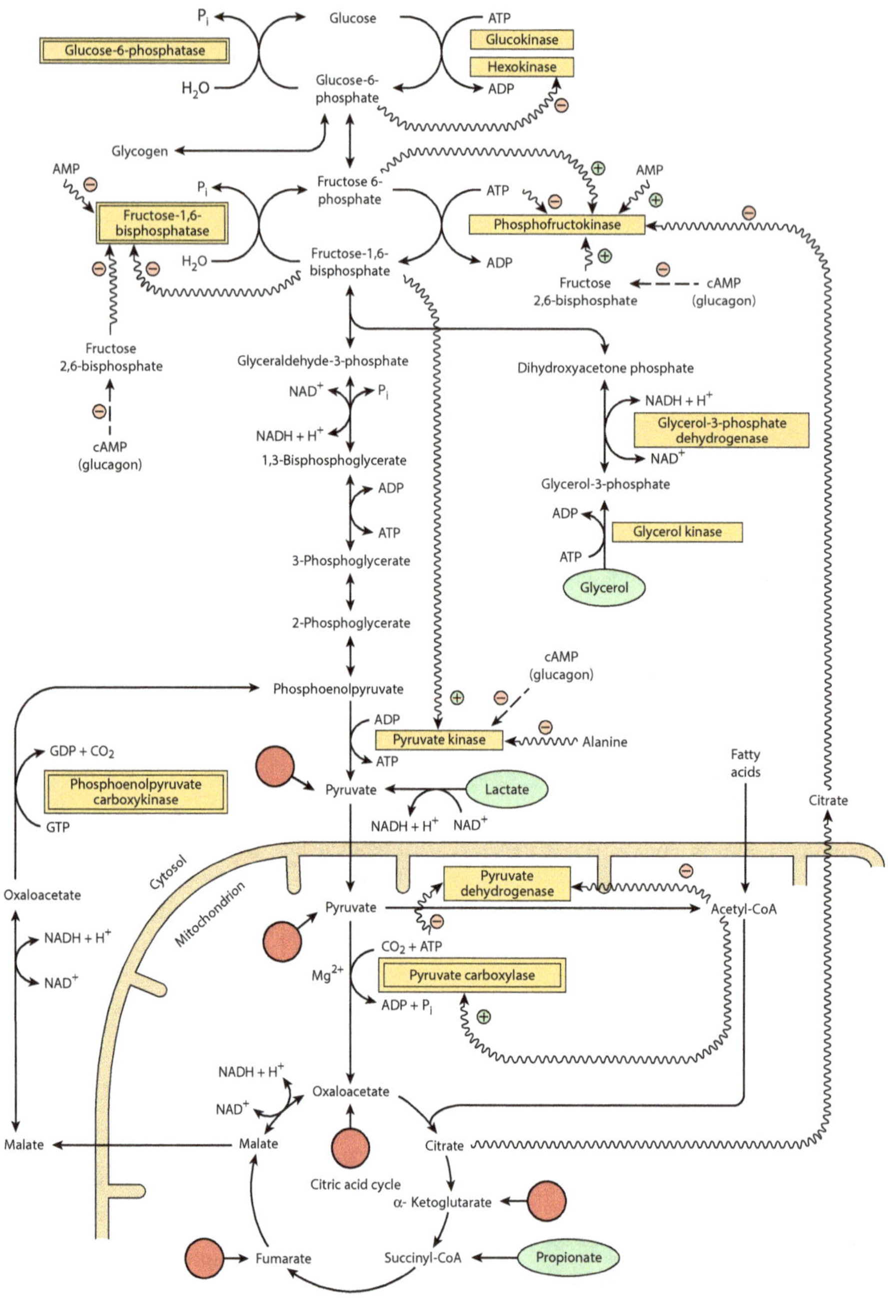

FIGURE 6–1 Major pathways and regulation of gluconeogenesis and glycolysis in the liver. Entry points of glucogenic amino acids after transamination are indicated by arrows extended from circles. The key gluconeogenic enzymes are enclosed in double-bordered boxes. The ATP required for gluconeogenesis is supplied by the oxidation of fatty acids. Propionate is of quantitative importance only in ruminants. Arrows with wavy shafts signify allosteric effects; dash-shafted arrows signify covalent modification by reversible phosphorylation. High concentrations of alanine act as a "gluconeogenic signal" by inhibiting glycolysis at the pyruvate kinase step. (Reproduced with permission from Rodwell VW, Bender DA, Botham KM, et al: *Harper's Illustrated Biochemistry*, 31st ed. New York, NY: McGraw Hill; 2018.)

SUBSTRATES FOR GLUCONEOGENESIS

Lactate

Lactate is a major source of carbon atoms for hepatic gluconeogenesis. The primary source of this lactate is erythrocyte anaerobic glycolysis with anaerobic skeletal muscle glycolysis the next major source. During anaerobic glycolysis, pyruvate is reduced to lactate by lactate dehydrogenase (LDH) encoded by the *LDHA* gene. This reaction serves the critical function of yielding not only lactate, which can be utilized in hepatic gluconeogenesis, but also NAD^+ which is then available for use by the GAPDH reaction of glycolysis allowing anaerobic glycolysis to continue. The process of lactate release from erythrocytes and muscle and conversion to glucose in the liver is termed the Cori cycle (Figure 6–2).

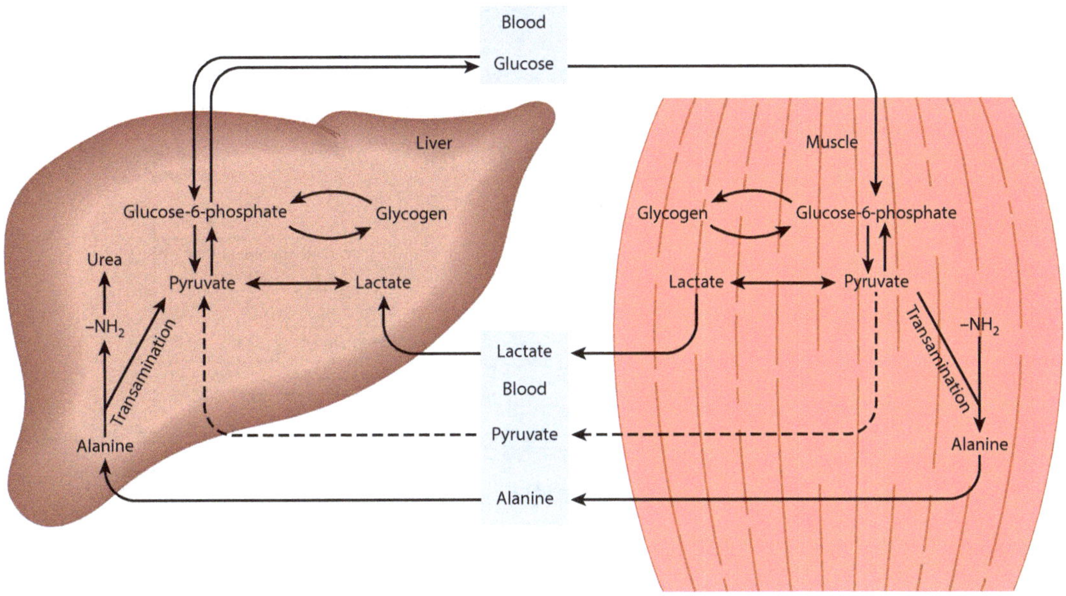

FIGURE 6–2 The lactic acid (Cori cycle) and glucose-alanine cycles. (Reproduced with permission from Rodwell VW, Bender DA, Botham KM, et al: *Harper's Illustrated Biochemistry*, 31st ed. New York, NY: McGraw Hill; 2018.)

Pyruvate

Pyruvate generated in nonhepatic tissues (particularly skeletal muscle) can be transaminated to alanine, via the action of alanine transaminase (ALT), and then delivered to the liver for gluconeogenesis. This pathway is termed the glucose-alanine cycle (see Figure 6–2). The glucose-alanine cycle serves a critical mechanism for muscle to eliminate waste nitrogen from amino acid catabolism while replenishing its energy supply as glucose. Within the liver the alanine is deaminated via ALT and the resultant pyruvate used as a gluconeogenic substrate or oxidized in the TCA cycle. The amino nitrogen is converted to urea in the urea cycle (see Chapter 17) and excreted by the kidneys.

Amino Acids

All of the amino acids present in proteins, except leucine and lysine, can be degraded to TCA cycle intermediates (see Chapter 18) which allows the carbon skeletons ultimately to be converted to pyruvate. The pyruvate thus formed can be utilized by the gluconeogenic pathway. Of all the amino acids utilized for gluconeogenesis, glutamine is the most important as this amino acid is critical for glucose production by the kidneys and small intestine.

Glycerol

The glycerol backbone of triglycerides can be used for gluconeogenesis. Indeed, the glycerol released from adipose tissue during periods of fasting (see Chapter 13) provides a major source of carbon atom for hepatic gluconeogenesis. The glycerol is first phosphorylated to glycerol-3-phosphate by glycerol kinase followed by oxidation to dihydroxyacetone phosphate (DHAP) by glycerol-3-phosphate dehydrogenase (GPD).

Propionate

Oxidation of fatty acids with an odd number of carbon atoms and the amino acids methionine, isoleucine, valine, and threonine generates propionyl-CoA. Propionyl-CoA is converted to the TCA intermediate, succinyl-CoA (Figure 6–3).

INTESTINAL AND RENAL GLUCONEOGENESIS

The gut, in particular the small intestine, and the kidneys play critical roles in the overall regulation of endogenous glucose synthesis via gluconeogenesis. Glutamine serves as the major precursor of glucose formed within the small intestine and the kidney. Indeed, during periods of fasting, the small intestine accounts for approximately 20% of whole body endogenous glucose by 48 hours and up to 35% by 72 hours.

HIGH-YIELD CONCEPT

Protein-rich diets are known to reduce hunger and subsequent food intake in both humans and experimental animals. In addition, protein-rich, carbohydrate-free diets have been shown to strongly induce the expression of G6Pase, PEPCK-c, and glutaminase in the intestine.

Within the proximal tubules of the nephron in the kidney the process of glutamine utilization in gluconeogenesis serves two important functions. The ammonia (NH_3) that is liberated via the concerted actions of glutaminase and glutamate dehydrogenase, spontaneously ionizes to ammonium ion (NH_4^+) and is excreted

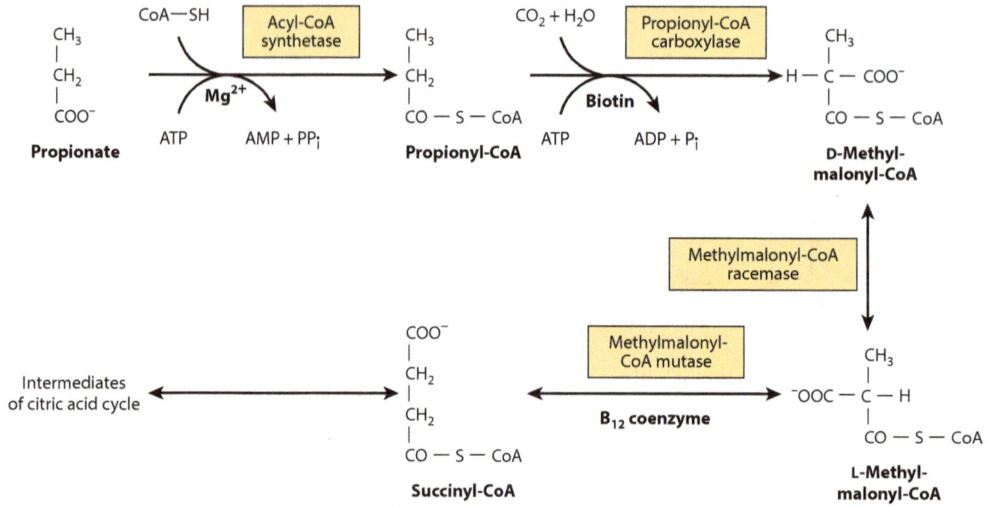

FIGURE 6–3 Metabolism of propionate. (Reproduced with permission from Rodwell VW, Bender DA, Botham KM, et al: *Harper's Illustrated Biochemistry*, 31st ed. New York, NY: McGraw Hill; 2018.)

in the urine effectively buffering the hydrogen ions in the urine. In addition, the glucose that is produced via gluconeogenesis can provide the brain and erythrocytes with critically needed energy. Another physiologically relevant consequence of renal glutamine metabolism is that the α-ketoglutarate (2-oxoglutarate) generated by the glutaminase and glutamate dehydrogenase reactions can be oxidized in the TCA cycle releasing CO_2 that contributes to renal bicarbonate homeostasis and thus, the role of the kidneys in acid-base homeostasis.

REGULATION OF GLUCONEOGENESIS

Insulin increases glycolysis and decreases gluconeogenesis, whereas glucagon and epinephrine exert the opposite effects. These effects are exerted through the regulation of cAMP levels, the activity of PKA, and the production and hydrolysis of F2,6BP (see Figure 5–4). With respect to allosteric regulation, in general the negative effectors of glycolysis are positive effectors of gluconeogenesis.

CHECKLIST

- ☑ Gluconeogenesis is carried out primarily within the liver as a means to ensure normal glucose homeostasis during periods of fasting.
- ☑ The primary sources of carbon for hepatic gluconeogenesis are lactate, pyruvate, and alanine.
- ☑ The primary source of carbon for intestinal and renal gluconeogenesis is glutamine.
- ☑ Gluconeogenesis is regulated at the level of pyruvate carboxylase (which is absolutely dependent on acetyl-CoA as an allosteric activator), PEPCK, and F1,6-BPase.
- ☑ Regulation of gluconeogenesis at the level of F1,6-BPase represents a reciprocal regulation to that of the glycolytic enzyme PFK1.
- ☑ Delivery of lactate from the blood to the liver with the liver subsequently delivering glucose to the blood is referred to as the Cori cycle.
- ☑ Delivery of alanine, primarily from skeletal muscle, to the liver with subsequent delivery of glucose back to muscle via the blood is referred to as the glucose-alanine cycle.
- ☑ Intestinal gluconeogenesis contributes to overall endogenous glucose production.
- ☑ Intestinal glucose delivery to the portal circulation influences feeding behaviors via afferent circuits to the hypothalamus.
- ☑ Renal reabsorption of glucose and renal gluconeogenesis contribute to the maintenance of endogenous glucose production.

REVIEW QUESTIONS

1. A 30-year-old man has been on a hunger strike for 1 week. During this period, he has consumed only vitamin supplements and water. In spite of the lack of food intake, a routine blood test, carried out by a physician monitoring his health, finds his serum glucose concentration to be 55 mg/dL (normal fasting plasma glucose = 60–110 mg/dL). Which of the following processes is most likely contributing to the level of glucose in his blood?
   (A) Adipocyte triglyceride metabolism
   (B) Hepatic glycogen metabolism
   (C) Intestinal fructose metabolism
   (D) Skeletal muscle amino acid metabolism
   (E) Skeletal muscle glycogen metabolism

2. Which of the following processes is most likely contributing to the activation of gluconeogenesis at the level of pyruvate carboxylase?
   (A) Hepatic fatty acid oxidation
   (B) Hepatic glycogen breakdown
   (C) Hepatic triglyceride metabolism
   (D) Skeletal amino acid metabolism
   (E) Skeletal muscle fatty acid oxidation
   (F) Skeletal muscle glycogen breakdown

3. A 7-month-old infant, who suffered a seizure following an acute episode of vomiting, was diagnosed with a defect in pyruvate carboxylase. Treatment of the infant included a diet supplemented with triheptanoin, a triglyceride containing three 7-carbon saturated fatty acids. Which of the following best explains the benefits of this therapeutic intervention?
   (A) Odd-chain fatty acid oxidation represses glycolysis
   (B) Odd-chain fatty acid oxidation yields a substrate for gluconeogenesis
   (C) Odd-chain fatty acid oxidation yields a substrate for ketogenesis
   (D) Odd-chain fatty acids activate glycogen phosphorylase
   (E) Odd-chain fatty acids stimulate glucagon secretion by the pancreas

4. A 37-year-old man is being treated in the emergency department following his rescue from a mine cave-in. The patient was trapped for 6 days. Which of the following represents the most likely mechanism taking place in the liver of this patient as a means to ensure sufficient levels of blood glucose?
   (A) Activation of glucose-6-phosphatase by insulin
   (B) Activation of pyruvate kinase by glucagon
   (C) Activation of phosphoenolpyruvate carboxykinase synthesis by cortisol
   (D) Inhibition of fructose-1,6-bisphosphatase by fructose-1,6-bisphosphate
   (E) Inhibition of glucokinase by glucagon
   (F) Inhibition of phosphofructokinase-1 (PFK1) by insulin

5. Experiments are being conducted utilizing a cultured hepatic cell line isolated from a patient with hepatocellular carcinoma. It is discovered that the rate of endogenous glucose production by these cells is not affected by changes to the level of acetyl-CoA when compared to normal hepatocytes. Given these findings, which of the following enzymes in this cell line is most likely to harbor a mutation?
   (A) Fructose-1,6-bisphosphatase
   (B) Glyceraldehyde-3-phosphate dehydrogenase
   (C) Phosphoenolpyruvate carboxykinase (PEPCK)
   (D) Phosphofructokinase-2 (PFK2)
   (E) Pyruvate carboxylase

6. Experiments are being conducted on cells in culture that harbor a mutant form of lactate dehydrogenase (LDH). The level of activity of this enzyme is only 20% that of normal LDH. Results from these cells find that utilization of pyruvate as a gluconeogenic substrate does not rescue 100% of the glucose synthesizing capacity of normal cells. In addition, it is found that the NAD^+/NADH ratio is elevated when compared to normal cells. A defect in which of the following enzymes is most likely to explain the observed results in these cells?
   (A) Glucose-6-phosphate dehydrogenase
   (B) Malate dehydrogenase
   (C) Phosphoenolpyruvate carboxykinase
   (D) Pyruvate carboxylase
   (E) Pyruvate dehydrogenase

7. Which of the following processes best explains why the carbon atoms from fatty acids with an even number of carbon atoms cannot be used for net synthesis of glucose in the liver?
   (A) Oxidation occurs in the mitochondria and gluconeogenesis occurs in the cytosol
   (B) States of catabolism and anabolism are never concurrently active
   (C) Storage of fats occurs in adipose tissue and gluconeogenesis occurs primarily in the liver
   (D) The carbons from fat oxidation are lost as CO_2 in the TCA cycle
   (E) The carbons from fat oxidation inhibit conversion of pyruvate to oxaloacetate

8. A 4-day-old infant presents with severe lactic acidemia, hyperammonemia, citrullinemia, hyperlysinemia, and 2-oxoglutaric (α-ketoglutarate) aciduria. Genetic and metabolic studies determine that the infant does not harbor a defect in the process of urea synthesis. Given these finding, which of the following is most likely to be defective in this infant?
   (A) Acetyl-CoA carboxylase
   (B) Fructose-1,6-bisphophatase
   (C) Glucose-6-phosphate dehydrogenase
   (D) Medium-chain acyl-CoA dehydrogenase
   (E) Pyruvate carboxylase

9. A 9-month-old infant is being examined in the emergency department after repeated episodes of vomiting followed by a seizure. Physical examination showed hypotonia, ataxia, and nystagmus. Laboratory results demonstrated a high anion gap metabolic acidosis and elevated serum levels of lactate, pyruvate, and alanine. Before a definitive diagnosis could be made, the infant lapsed into a coma and died. Which of the following was the most likely defective process in the infant contributing to the pathology and outcomes?
   (A) Fatty acid oxidation
   (B) Gluconeogenesis
   (C) Glycogen processing
   (D) Glycogen synthesis
   (E) Peroxisomal fatty acid metabolism

10. Which of the following processes is most likely to contribute to the maintenance of serum glucose following depletion of hepatic glycogen stores?
(A) Adipose tissue fatty acid oxidation
(B) Liver fatty acid oxidation
(C) Proximal tubule glucose reabsorption
(D) Skeletal muscle glycogen breakdown
(E) Skeletal muscle protein breakdown

11. A 30-year-old man has been on a hunger strike for 2 weeks. During this period, he has consumed only vitamin supplements and water. In spite of the lack of food intake, a routine blood test, carried out by a physician monitoring his health, finds his serum glucose concentration to be 55 mg/dL (normal fasting plasma glucose = 60–110 mg/dL). Which of the following compounds is the most likely source of the carbon atoms contributing to this patient's blood glucose?
(A) Alanine
(B) Glutamine
(C) Glycerol
(D) β-Hydroxybutyrate
(E) Palmitate

12. A 3-month-old infant is being examined in the emergency department following a seizure. Physical examination finds the infant has hepatomegaly. Blood work finds hypoglycemia, lactic acidosis, hyperuricemia, and hyperlipidemia. Given these signs and symptoms, which of the following enzymes is most likely defective in this infant?
(A) Fructose-1,6-bisphosphatase
(B) Glucose-6-phosphatase
(C) Phosphofructokinase-1 (PFK1)
(D) Pyruvate carboxylase
(E) Pyruvate kinase

13. A 37-year-old man is being treated in the emergency department following his rescue from a mine cave-in. The patient was trapped for 5 days. Blood work finds the patients serum glucose to be 85 mg/dL. Which of the following processes is the most likely explanation for the maintenance of a normal serum glucose concentration in this patient?
(A) Hepatic gluconeogenesis
(B) Hepatic glycogen breakdown
(C) Renal gluconeogenesis
(D) Skeletal muscle glycogen breakdown
(E) Skeletal muscle protein breakdown

14. Renal nitrogen handling increases significantly during a long-term fast when compared to the level following consumption of a normal diet. A portion of this nitrogen is excreted as urea which is most likely elevated as a consequence of which of the following processes?
(A) Amino acid oxidation coupled to hepatic gluconeogenesis
(B) Amino acid transport into skeletal muscle
(C) Enhanced activity of carbamoyl phosphate synthetase 1 (CPS 1)
(D) Fatty acids oxidation in skeletal muscle
(E) Hepatic synthesis of ketone bodies

15. In a healthy individual, who does not consume food overnight, measurement of serum glucose in the morning will find the concentration to be in the normal reference range. Which of the following processes best explains this observation?
(A) Hepatic gluconeogenesis in response to glucagon
(B) Hepatic gluconeogenesis in response to insulin
(C) Hepatic ketogenesis in response to glucagon
(D) Hepatic ketogenesis in response to insulin
(E) Hepatic glycogenolysis in response to insulin
(F) Hepatic protein breakdown in response to glucagon

16. An 18-month-old infant is brought to the emergency department by his parents due to severe vomiting and a convulsion. History reveals that the infant was recently treated for an infection. Physical examination finds hypotonia, tachypnea, nystagmus, and physical signs of failure to thrive. Laboratory studies are consistent with severe hypoglycemia and metabolic acidosis. Given the signs and symptoms in this infant, the attending physician suspects an inherited metabolic disorder. Which of the following compounds would be most useful in this infant to provide the necessary carbon atoms for gluconeogenesis?
(A) Alanine
(B) Glutamine
(C) Glycerol
(D) Lactate
(E) Pyruvate

17. A 27-year-old man, who is 70 inches tall with a BMI of 28 has started a high-fat low carbohydrate diet as a means to lose weight. On a diet such as this, which of the following is most likely to serve as a substrate for the maintenance of the man's serum glucose levels?
(A) Acetoacetate
(B) Alanine
(C) Glycerol
(D) β-Hydroxybutyrate
(E) Palmitate

18. A newborn experienced several episodes of hypoglycemia, apnea, hyperventilation, ketosis, and lactic acidosis. A diet high in glucose was able to reduce the episodes and the infant developed at a near normal rate. At the age of 6 years, the child had an infection resulting in a high fever and a loss of appetite. During this episode, the child experienced severe lactic acidosis. Which of the following is the most likely enzyme deficiency in this child?
(A) Aldolase B
(B) Fructose-1,6-bisphosphatase
(C) Glucose-6-phosphate dehydrogenase
(D) Phosphofructokinase-1 (PFK1)
(E) Pyruvate kinase

19. A 2-year-old girl is being examined in the emergency department, being brought in by her parents due to their inability to rouse her that morning. History reveals that the infant recently had the flu and was not eating well. Physical examination finds the infant is small for her age. Blood and urine analyses find marked hypoglycemia, ketonemia, and ketonuria, as well as low levels of alanine. Serum insulin levels were found to be low as expected during a period of fasting. Intravenous administration of alanine results in a rapid rise in the infant's serum glucose level. Based upon the signs and symptoms in this patient which of the following processes is most likely to be impaired?
(A) Gluconeogenesis
(B) Glycogenolysis
(C) Mitochondrial fatty acid oxidation
(D) Protein catabolism in muscle
(E) Triglyceride hydrolysis in adipose tissue

ANSWERS

1. Correct answer is **D.** During periods of fasting the liver is the major organ tasked with ensuring the rest of the body has adequate energy first in the form of glucose and then ketone bodies and glucose, the latter primarily for use by red blood cells. Early during a fast the liver is stimulated to break down its glycogen stores (choice B) for delivery of the glucose to the blood. This source of hepatic glucose is depleted within several hours. During the next period, that ranges up to one week to 10 days, the liver utilizes the carbon skeleton of various amino acids derived from skeletal muscle protein breakdown to produce glucose via gluconeogenesis. As a fast progresses beyond this secondary period the source of carbon atom for hepatic ketone body synthesis comes from the fatty acids released from adipose tissue triglycerides (choice A). Metabolism of fructose by the small intestine (choice C) is predominantly for its own energy requirements and does not contribute to blood glucose. Skeletal muscle glycogen metabolism (choice E) cannot contribute to blood glucose due to the very high affinity of hexokinase for glucose resulting in immediate phosphorylation of any free glucose removed from glycogen by the debranching enzyme.
2. Correct answer is **A.** Pyruvate carboxylase activity is absolutely dependent on acetyl-CoA and hepatic fatty acid oxidation is the primary source of this acetyl-CoA. The major source of the fatty acids being oxidized, under conditions where the liver is hormonally stimulated to carry out gluconeogenesis, is the free fatty acids released from adipose tissue triglycerides. Hepatic glycogen breakdown (choice B) is an early source of free glucose for delivery to the blood during periods of fasting and stress, but it is not contributory to gluconeogenesis. Hepatic triglyceride metabolism (choice C) could contribute to fatty acid oxidation but in general the liver makes triglycerides for export of excess carbon atoms from glucose as fat for storage in adipose tissue; it does not metabolize triglycerides for energy generation. Oxidation of some skeletal muscle amino acids (choice D) does yield acetyl-CoA but this does not contribute to the activation of hepatic pyruvate carboxylase. Skeletal muscle fatty acid oxidation (choice E) does not result in release of acetyl-CoA as it is all consumed by the TCA cycle as a means to produce the energy necessary for ATP synthesis in this tissue. Skeletal muscle glycogen metabolism (choice F) cannot contribute to hepatic gluconeogenesis, nor blood glucose, due to the very high affinity of hexokinase for glucose resulting in immediate phosphorylation of any free glucose removed from glycogen by the debranching enzyme.
3. Correct answer is **B.** Fatty acids with odd numbers of carbon atoms are oxidized to propionyl-CoA and acetyl-CoA. The propionyl-CoA is converted to succinyl-CoA which then serves to generate malate in the TCA cycle. The malate can be transported to the cytosol and oxidized to oxaloacetate (OAA). The OAA is then converted to phosphoenolpyruvate, by PEPCK, and ultimately to glucose. This process bypasses the need for the pyruvate carboxylase reaction in the process of hepatic gluconeogenesis. Odd-chain length fatty acids do not repress glycolysis (choice A). Oxidation of odd-chain length fatty acids will yield acetyl-CoA that can contribute to ketogenesis (choice C); however, the major benefit of these fats is their contribution to endogenous glucose production via the resultant succinyl-CoA. Odd-chain fatty acids do not activate glycogen phosphorylase (choice D) nor do they stimulate glucagon release by the pancreas (choice E).
4. Correct answer is **B.** When blood glucose levels fall the pancreas releases glucagon to stimulate the liver to carry out gluconeogenesis. The effects of glucagon on hepatic metabolism are exerted both short term and long term. Prolonged fasting and starvation lead to long-term glucagon effects which are exerted at the level of gene expression. A major hepatic target of these long-term effects is the activation of increased transcription of the genes that encode mitochondrial (PCK2) and cytoplasmic (PCK1) PEPCK. Both of these genes are induced by glucagon receptor-mediated signaling via PKA. Activated PKA phosphorylates the transcription factor, cAMP response element-binding protein (CREB), which then enhances transcription of these PEPCK encoding genes. During a prolonged fast, blood glucose levels will be low and thus insulin release from the pancreas will be negligible (choices A and F). Although low blood glucose and stress result in increased release of cortisol which exerts some of its effects through activation of expression of the PCK1 and PCK2 genes (choice C), the primary mechanisms stimulating hepatic gluconeogenesis in this case are glucagon and epinephrine-mediated activation of PKA activity. Glucagon-mediated signaling does not result in the inhibition of glucokinase (choice E). Fructose-1,6-bisphosphate does not inhibit fructose-1,6-bisphosphatase (choice D). Insulin stimulates the activity of PFK1 (choice F); it does not inhibit the enzyme. In addition, insulin levels would be low during a prolonged fast.
5. Correct answer is **E.** Pyruvate carboxylase activity is normally absolutely dependent on allosteric activation by acetyl-CoA. Since gluconeogenesis is not affected by changes in acetyl-CoA levels it is most likely that the cells harbor a mutation in the pyruvate carboxylase gene rendering the activity of the encoded enzyme independent of acetyl-CoA effects. None of the other enzymes (choices A, B, C, and D) are affected by the cellular levels of acetyl-CoA.
6. Correct answer is **B.** In order for gluconeogenesis to occur, the NADH needed by the reversal of the glycolytic glyceraldehyde-3-phosphate dehydrogenase reaction, must be supplied by either lactate dehydrogenase or the action of cytosolic malate dehydrogenase. Since there is a deficit in the reduction of NAD^+ to NADH, the additional defective enzyme must be cytosolic malate dehydrogenase. None of the other enzymes contributes to the cytoplasmic pool of NADH (choices A, C, D, and E).
7. Correct answer is **D.** When the carbons of fatty acids are oxidized for energy production, the by-product of that process is the two-carbon compound, acetyl-CoA. Acetyl-CoA can then enter the TCA cycle for complete oxidation. Although the malate generated by the TCA cycle can be directed into the gluconeogenic pathway of glucose synthesis, the carbons of acetyl-CoA cannot provide a net source of carbon in that latter pathway. This is due to the fact that following entry of the two carbons of acetyl-CoA into the TCA cycle, two carbons are lost as CO_2 during the subsequent reactions of the cycle at the isocitrate dehydrogenase and α-ketoglutarate (2-oxoglutarate) dehydrogenase catalyzed reactions. As stated, mitochondrial TCA cycle-derived malate carbons can be used for gluconeogenesis which occurs following transport of malate to the cytosol. Thus, there is a direct connection between mitochondrial and cytosolic processes (choice A). Anabolic reactions and catabolic reactions (choice B) are always occurring concurrently; it is only the absolute rate of either process that changes depending on energy states. Although the primary site of fatty acid storage

is in adipose tissue (choice C), during fasting and stress they are released to the blood and picked up by the liver to be oxidized to provide the energy necessary to carry out gluconeogenesis. The carbons of fat oxidation, at the level of acetyl-CoA stimulate, as opposed to inhibit (choice E), the conversion of pyruvate to oxaloacetate.

8. Correct answer is **E.** Mutations in the pyruvate carboxylase gene result in three types of pyruvate carboxylase deficiency syndromes. The type A form is the infantile form and most afflicted individuals will die in infancy or early childhood. The type B form is the severe neonatal form and afflicted patients will die before 3 months of age. The type C form is referred to as the intermittent or benign form. Individuals with the type C form of pyruvate carboxylase deficiency experience either normal or delayed neurologic development and episodic metabolic acidosis. Pyruvate carboxylase is the first enzyme in the gluconeogenic conversion of pyruvate, lactate, and alanine carbons into glucose. A defect in pyruvate carboxylase would restrict the conversion of lactate into pyruvate and then subsequently to glucose. This would lead to severe lactic academia. The consequent liver damage in pyruvate carboxylase deficiency is the primary contributor to the other symptoms seen in this patient. Deficiency of acetyl-CoA carboxylase (choice A) is associated with severe brain damage, persistent myopathy, and poor growth. Deficiency in fructose-1,6-bisphosphatase (choice B) results in severely impaired hepatic gluconeogenesis and leads to episodes of hypoglycemia, apnea, hyperventilation, ketosis, and lactic acidosis. Deficiency in glucose-6-phosphate dehydrogenase (choice C) results in hemolytic anemia. Deficiency in medium-chain acyl-CoA dehydrogenase (choice D) is associated with episodic hypoketotic hypoglycemia brought on by fasting. Symptoms appear within the first 2 years of life. Clinical crisis is characterized by an infant presenting with episodes of vomiting and lethargy that may progress to seizures and ultimately coma.

9. Correct answer is **B.** The infant is most likely suffering from the effects of a defect in pyruvate carboxylase, a critical enzyme required for the initiation of hepatic gluconeogenesis from alanine, lactate, and pyruvate. Mutations in the pyruvate carboxylase gene results in three types of pyruvate carboxylase deficiency syndromes. The type A form is the infantile form and most afflicted individuals will die in infancy or early childhood. Type A PCD is characterized by mild metabolic acidosis, delayed motor development, intellectual disability, failure to thrive, hypotonia, ataxia, ocular disorder (nystagmus), and convulsions. These infants will experience episodes of metabolic acidosis, acute vomiting, and tachypnea as a result of metabolic stress or as a result of infections. Defective fatty acid oxidation (choice A) can represent a wide spectrum of different disorders but one of the most common infantile defects is medium-chain acyl-CoA dehydrogenase deficiency, MCADD. The most common symptom of MCADD is episodic hypoketotic hypoglycemia brought on by fasting. Symptoms appear within the first 2 years of life. Clinical crisis is characterized by an infant presenting with episodes of vomiting and lethargy that may progress to seizures and ultimately coma. Numerous disorders of glycogen processing (choice C) and synthesis (choice D) are known and are collectively referred to as glycogen storage diseases. Infantile presenting glycogen storage diseases include von Gierke disease, Pompe disease, and Anderson disease. Many different disorders of peroxisomal fatty acid metabolism (choice E) have been identified with the most common being Refsum disease. Refsum disease results from defects in peroxisomal fatty acid α-oxidation of phytanic acid.

10. Correct answer is **E.** During periods of fasting and starvation, when liver glycogen levels are depleted, the major source of carbon atom for hepatic gluconeogenesis is from the amino acids released during protein degradation within skeletal muscle. Adipose tissue fatty acid oxidation (choice A) cannot contribute carbon atoms for hepatic gluconeogenesis. However, when adipose tissue is stimulated by glucagon and epinephrine during fasting and/or stress the stimulated breakdown of triglycerides does lead to the release of glycerol that can be used by the liver to make glucose. Fatty acid oxidation in the liver (choice B) yields predominantly acetyl-CoA whose carbons cannot contribute to net synthesis of glucose carbons. In the much less common oxidation of fatty acids with odd numbers of carbon atoms the resultant propionyl-CoA is converted to succinyl-CoA and via the TCA cycle will yield malate that, when transported out of the mitochondria, can contribute to net glucose synthesis. Renal reabsorption of glucose (choice C) is efficient, resulting in the reabsorption of 80–90% of the glucose in the glomerular filtrate but this represents the levels of glucose already in the blood and therefore, does not contribute to the maintenance of glucose levels when liver glycogen stores are depleted. The glucose from skeletal muscle glycogen breakdown (choice D) will be utilized in the glycolytic pathway of these cells and cannot contribute to the maintenance of blood glucose.

11. Correct answer is **C.** In the absence of adequate carbohydrate the body will begin to divert stored fats in adipose tissue into the metabolic pool in order to allow for adequate energy production. In addition, the liver will oxidize fatty acids to acetyl-CoA and then divert the acetyl-CoA into ketone synthesis to ensure the brain receives adequate amounts of an oxidizable energy source. When adipose tissue is stimulated to release fatty acids stored in triglycerides the glycerol backbone diffuses into the blood and is delivered to the liver. Within the liver glycerol is phosphorylated and is converted to dihydroxyacetone phosphate (DHAP) which is then diverted into the glucose production via gluconeogenesis. Alanine and glutamine (choices A and B) could represent amino acids derived from skeletal muscle protein degradation, but this process is self-limiting for supplying carbon atoms for hepatic gluconeogenesis such that after 6–10 days of fasting no longer serves the major role in this process. Beta-hydroxybutyrate (choice D) is a ketone body derived from hepatic oxidation of fatty acids. The ketones cannot be diverted into the gluconeogenesis pathway since they are oxidized to acetyl-CoA. Palmitic acid (choice E) is the major fatty acid in the circulation but when it is oxidized in tissues, such as the liver, it will yield acetyl-CoA which cannot contribute to net glucose synthesis.

12. Correct answer is **B.** Deficiencies in glucose-6-phosphatase represent the causes of type 1 glycogen storage disease, more commonly called von Gierke disease. The hallmark features of this disease are hypoglycemia, lactic acidosis, hyperuricemia, and hyperlipidemia. When the liver is unable to release free glucose, it is diverted into other metabolic pathways including the pentose phosphate pathway. The result of this shunting of glucose-6-phosphate is increased ribose-5-phosphate production. Ribose-5-phosphate ultimately stimulates purine nucleotide biosynthesis, and the excess nucleotides are catabolized to uric acid accounting for the hyperuricemia in this patient. Deficiency in fructose-1,6-bisphosphatase (choice A) results in severely impaired hepatic gluconeogenesis and leads to episodes of hypoglycemia, apnea, hyperventilation, ketosis, and lactic acidosis. Deficiency in PFK1 is found in the muscle-specific subunit of PFK1 and is associated with the glycogen storage disease originally called Tarui disease. In the classic form of PFK1 deficiency patients exhibit symptoms in early childhood, not in early infancy. Mutations in the pyruvate carboxylase gene (choice D) result in three types of deficiency syndromes. The type A form is the infantile form and most afflicted individuals will die in infancy or early childhood. Type A PCD is characterized by mild metabolic acidosis, delayed motor development, intellectual disability, failure to thrive, hypotonia, ataxia, ocular disorder (nystagmus), and convulsions. Deficiency in pyruvate kinase (choice E) is most commonly manifest with hemolytic anemia.

13. Correct answer is **A.** During periods of prolonged fasting the body will begin to divert stored fats into the hepatic metabolic pool in order to allow for adequate energy production for the purposes of carrying out gluconeogenesis. When adipose tissue is stimulated to release fatty acids stored in triglycerides the glycerol backbone diffuses into the blood and is delivered to the liver. Within the liver glycerol is phosphorylated and converted to dihydroxyacetone phosphate (DHAP) which is then diverted into glucose production via gluconeogenesis. Hepatic glycogen breakdown (choice B) will only sustain blood glucose levels for several hours. Renal gluconeogenesis (choice C) can contribute up to 5% of the daily endogenous glucose pool but alone cannot maintain normal fasting plasma glucose levels during starvation. Skeletal muscle glycogen breakdown (choice D) cannot contribute to blood glucose since all of the released glucose is phosphorylated or the small amounts of free glucose released by the debranching enzyme are rapidly phosphorylated by hexokinase. This ensures that the glucose stored in skeletal muscle is used solely for the energy needs of this tissue. The breakdown of skeletal muscle protein (choice E) will provide the liver with carbon atoms for glucose synthesis, but this is hepatic gluconeogenesis.

14. Correct answer is **A.** Protein breakdown into constituent amino acids provides an important source of carbon for oxidative energy production. When amino acids are oxidized, the nitrogen is first transferred to a suitable α-keto acid acceptor such as α-ketoglutarate (2-oxoglutarate). Eventually the waste nitrogen from hepatic amino acid metabolism is diverted into the urea cycle for excretion in a nontoxic form. This accounts for the increased plasma urea concentrations following fasting. During fasting amino acids would be transported out of skeletal muscle not into the cells of this tissue (choice B). Although the urea cycle requires the activity of CPS-1 (choice C) to incorporate waste ammonium ion (NH_4^+), this nitrogen is derived from amino acid oxidation. The products of skeletal muscle fatty acid oxidation (choice D) would fuel the TCA cycle in the cells of this tissue and would not contribute to hepatic urea synthesis. Ketone body synthesis (choice E) does not involve nitrogenous compounds and therefore, cannot contribute to urea synthesis.

15. Correct answer is **A.** When blood glucose levels fall during the overnight period the pancreas secretes glucagon. Glucagon binds to receptors on hepatocytes and triggers a series of metabolic changes that shift hepatic metabolism to glucose synthesis via gluconeogenesis. Insulin (choice B) inhibits gluconeogenesis primarily through activation of the production of fructose-2,6-bisphosphate, a potent allosteric inhibitor of the gluconeogenic enzyme, fructose-1,6-bisphosphatase. Although glucagon stimulates adipose tissue triglyceride breakdown and the resultant oxidation of the released fatty acids will contribute to hepatic ketone body synthesis (choice C), this does not contribute to the maintenance of blood glucose. Fatty acid oxidation is repressed by insulin (choice D) so ketone body synthesis would be reduced. Insulin stimulates hepatic glycogen synthesis as opposed to glycogenolysis (choice E). The breakdown of protein (choice F) does contribute amino acid carbon atoms for hepatic gluconeogenesis, but this process is not stimulated by the actions of glucagon.

16. Correct answer is **C.** The infant most likely has a defect in pyruvate carboxylase which would restrict the use of carbons from pyruvate, alanine, and lactate for glucose synthesis via gluconeogenesis. Therefore, the burden is shifted to the use of the glycerol backbone of stored triglycerides. Glycerol is phosphorylated within hepatocytes to glycerol-3-phosphate and then converted to dihydroxyacetone phosphate (DHAP) via the action of glycerol-3-phosphate dehydrogenase. The DHAP then can be used for glucose production via gluconeogenesis. In order for alanine (choice A), lactate (choice D), and pyruvate (choice E) to be utilized for gluconeogenesis there needs to be functional pyruvate carboxylase. Glutamine (choice B) serves as a major form of waste nitrogen delivery from the liver to the kidney and as such does not contribute to hepatic gluconeogenesis. Glutamine does serve as a carbon source for renal and intestinal gluconeogenesis, but this would not suffice to treat a patient with a pyruvate carboxylase deficiency.

17. Correct answer is **C.** In the absence of adequate carbohydrate the body will begin to divert stored fats in adipose tissue into the metabolic pool in order to allow for adequate energy production. In addition, the liver will oxidize fatty acids to acetyl-CoA and then divert the acetyl-CoA into ketone synthesis to ensure the brain receives adequate amounts of an oxidizable energy source. When adipose tissue is stimulated to release fatty acids stored in triglycerides the glycerol backbone diffuses into the blood and is delivered to the liver. Within the liver glycerol is phosphorylated and is converted to dihydroxyacetone phosphate (DHAP) which is then diverted into the glucose production via gluconeogenesis. Alanine (choices B) could represent an amino acid derived from skeletal muscle protein degradation and can contribute to hepatic gluconeogenesis, but it is not as important as the glycerol backbone of adipose tissue triglycerides. Acetoacetate (choice A) and β-hydroxybutyrate (choice D) are the ketone bodies derived from hepatic oxidation of fatty acids. The ketones cannot be diverted into the gluconeogenesis pathway since they are oxidized to acetyl-CoA. Palmitic acid (choice E) is the major fatty acid in the circulation but when it is oxidized in tissues, such as the liver, it will yield acetyl-CoA which cannot contribute to net glucose synthesis.

18. Correct answer is **B.** During normal hepatic gluconeogenesis the major substrates for glucose synthesis are alanine, pyruvate, and lactate. Defective fructose-1,6-bisphosphatase would restrict the flow of alanine and lactate conversion to pyruvate and the subsequent input of pyruvate into gluconeogenesis. The net effect would be a significant increase in circulating levels of lactate. Deficiency in aldolase B (choice A) is the cause of hereditary fructose intolerance, HFI. HFI is characterized by severe hypoglycemia and vomiting following fructose intake.

Prolonged intake of fructose by infants with this defect leads to vomiting, poor feeding, jaundice, hepatomegaly, hemorrhage, and eventually hepatic failure and death. Glucose-6-phosphate dehydrogenase deficiency (choice C) represents the most common cause of inherited hemolytic anemia. Deficiency in PFK1 (choice D) is found the muscle-specific subunit of PFK1 and is associated with the glycogen storage disease originally called Tarui disease. In the classic form of PFK1 deficiency patients exhibit symptoms in early childhood, not in early infancy. Deficiency in pyruvate kinase (choice E) is most commonly manifest with hemolytic anemia.

19. Correct answer is **D.** The hypoglycemia and ketonemia occurring following an overnight fast suggests that there may be a defect in gluconeogenesis or in a pathway providing substrates for gluconeogenesis. Under fasting conditions, the primary substrates for hepatic gluconeogenesis are alanine derived from muscle protein, lactate from red blood cell metabolism, which is oxidized to pyruvate in hepatocytes, as well as glycerol from adipose tissue triglyceride breakdown. During fasting skeletal muscle proteins can be degraded releasing the amino acids which are oxidized for ATP generation in this tissue. Skeletal muscle pyruvate can be transaminated to alanine, thereby allowing for the waste nitrogen to be delivered to the liver while also delivering the carbons of pyruvate which can enter the gluconeogenesis pathway. This process is referred to as the glucose-alanine cycle (also known as the Cahill cycle). Alanine levels in the patient were found to be abnormally low, and infusion of alanine rapidly increased blood glucose indicating that hepatic gluconeogenesis (choice A) was indeed functional. The results of the alanine administration are most consistent with a defect in protein catabolism in muscle. A defect in glycogenolysis (choice B) would not produce a severe hypoglycemia as a result of the normal process of hepatic gluconeogenesis. The presence of ketonemia and ketonuria indicates that the processes of mitochondrial fatty acid oxidation are indeed functional (choice C). Adipose tissue triglyceride hydrolysis (choice E) is also functional as the released fatty acids are oxidized in hepatocytes to provide energy for gluconeogenesis and also contribute to ketone body production.

CHAPTER

7

Glycogen Metabolism

High-Yield Terms

Glycosidic linkage	Covalent bond that joins a carbohydrate (sugar) molecule to another group such as another sugar typical of the bonds between glucose molecules in glycogen
Glycogenin	Protein with self-glucosylating activity that serves as the primer molecule for initiation of glycogen synthesis
Phosphorylase kinase	This enzyme is critical for the regulation of the flux of glucose into and out of glycogen as it reciprocally regulates the two key enzymes of glycogenolysis and glycogen synthesis and is itself the target of regulation by insulin, glucagon, and epinephrine
Glycogen storage disease	Disorders that result from defects in genes encoding enzymes involved in the process of glycogen synthesis or breakdown, primarily affecting muscles and liver

GLYCOGEN COMPOSITION

Glycogen is a polymer of glucose residues linked by α-(1,4)- and α-(1,6)-glycosidic bonds (Figure 7–1). Glycogen serves as a readily available source of glucose for oxidation when ATP synthesis is required. The major sites of glycogen synthesis and storage are hepatocytes of the liver and skeletal muscle cells.

The major site of daily glucose consumption (75%) is within the brain. Most of the remainder of it is utilized by erythrocytes, skeletal muscle, and cardiac muscle, but all cells can carry out glycolysis (see Chapter 5). The body obtains glucose from three principal sources: directly from the diet (see Chapter 28), from the breakdown of glycogen, or via gluconeogenesis (see Chapter 6). Stores of glycogen in the liver are considered the main buffer of blood glucose levels.

Normal glycogen polymers contain small amounts of phosphate at positions C2, C3, and C6 of the glucose residues in the molecule. Removal of the phosphates from glycogen occurs within the lysosomes and is catalyzed by the dual specificity phosphatase encoded by the *EPM2A* gene (EPM2A glucan phosphatase). The protein encoded by the *EPM2A* gene is called laforin (also known as laforin glycogen phosphatase) since loss of the enzyme is associated with the lethal neurodegenerative disease called Lafora disease (see Clinical Box 7–1).

GLYCOGEN SYNTHESIS (GLYCOGENESIS)

De novo glycogen synthesis is initiated by the attachment of the first glucose residue to a tyrosine residue in the protein known as glycogenin. The attached glucose then serves as the primer required by glycogen synthase to attach additional glucose molecules (Figure 7–2).

Glycogen synthase polymerizes glucose (using UDP-glucose as the substrate) via α-1,4 glycosidic bonds. The α-1,6 branches in glycogen are introduced by amylo-(1,4–1,6)-transglycosylase, more commonly just called branching enzyme. This enzyme transfers a terminal fragment of 6–7 glucose residues (from a polymer at least 11 glucose residues long) to an internal glucose residue at the C-6 hydroxyl position (Figure 7–3). Mutations in the gene (*GBE1*) that encodes glycogen branching enzyme result in the potentially lethal glycogen storage disease identified as Andersen disease (see Clinical Box 7–2).

REGULATION OF GLYCOGEN SYNTHESIS

Glycogen synthase is a tetrameric enzyme consisting of four identical subunits. The liver and muscle glycogen synthase proteins are derived from different genes and share only 46% amino acid identity. The activity of glycogen synthase is influenced by phosphorylation of serine residues in the subunit proteins as well as via allosteric regulation.

Phosphorylation of glycogen synthase reduces its activity toward UDP-glucose. When phosphorylated, glycogen synthase activity can be increased by binding the allosteric activator, glucose-6-phosphate (G6P). Activation by G6P does not occur when glycogen synthase is not phosphorylated.

The two forms of glycogen synthase are identified by the use of "a" and "b" such that the nonphosphorylated, and most active form, is called glycogen synthase-*a* and the phosphorylated less active glucose-6-phosphate-dependent form is called glycogen synthase-*b*.

Numerous kinases have been shown to phosphorylate and regulate both hepatic and muscle forms of glycogen synthase (Figure 7–4). The most significant glycogen synthase kinases

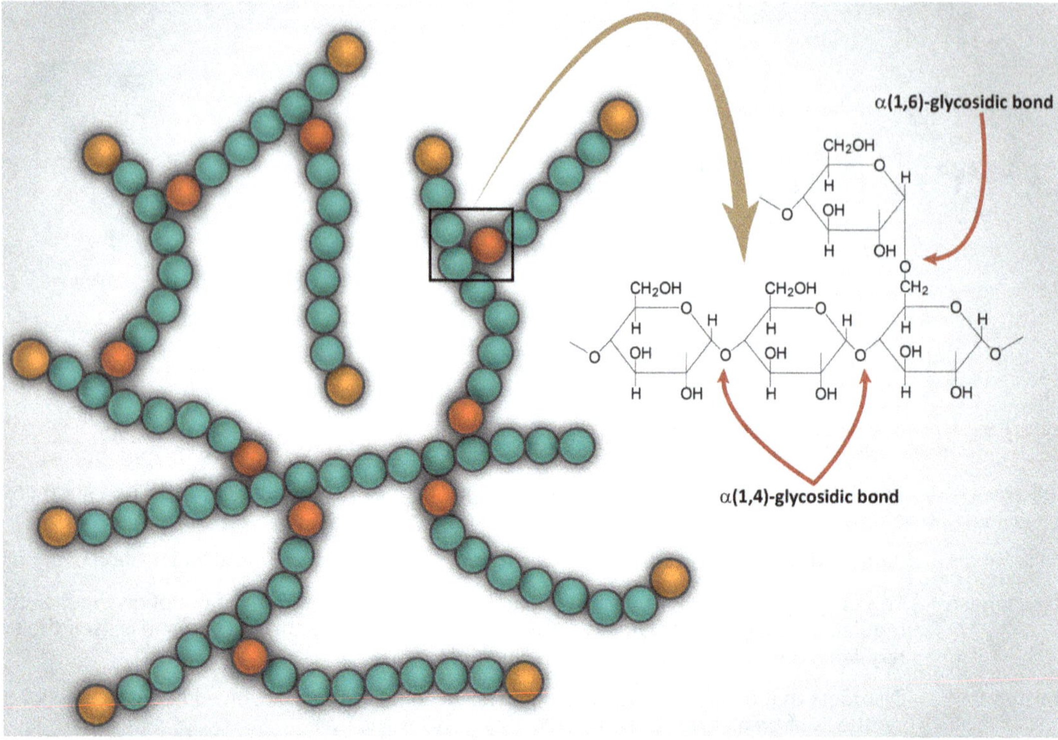

FIGURE 7–1 Glycogen structure: Highly simplified section of a glycogen granule depicting glucose monomers as colored balls. The blue balls represent glucose linked by α1,4 glycosidic bonds. The red balls represent glucose at branch points where there are both α1,4 and α1,6 glycosidic bonds. The orange balls represent the reducing ends of the polymeric chains of α1,4-linked glucose residues. The area in the box is expanded to show the actual structure of the glucose monomers in both α-1,4- and α-1,6 glycosidic linkages. Within the cells glycogen exists in what is referred to as the glycosome, a complex of proteins and glycogen. (Reproduced with permission from themedicalbiochemistrypage, LLC.)

CLINICAL BOX 7–1 LAFORA DISEASE

Lafora disease is a fatal autosomal recessive disease that is the result of a defect in glycogen metabolism. The disease gets its name from the Spanish neuropathologist, Gonzalo Rodriguez Lafora, who initially characterized the disorder. Lafora disease is characterized by the presence of inclusion bodies (the composition of which is glycogen), called Lafora bodies, in the cytoplasm of the cells of numerous tissues including neurons, heart, skeletal muscle, and liver. Essentially Lafora bodies are found in all tissues that form glycogen, while the pathology of Lafora disease results from the massive accumulation of precipitated glycogen in neuronal cell bodies. Lafora disease is a late-onset neurodegenerative disease associated with myoclonus epilepsy (irregular and uncontrollable jerks of a muscle or group of muscles associated with epileptic seizures) and death within a few years of diagnosis. Loss-of-function mutations in either of two genes are the cause of Lafora disease. One gene (*EPM2A*) encodes the EPM2A glucan (glycogen) phosphatase, which is commonly called laforin (also known as laforin glycogen phosphatase). The other gene (*NHLRC1*) encodes the NHL repeat containing E3 ubiquitin protein ligase 1, which is commonly called malin. The *NHLRC1* gene was also known as EPM2B. Mutations in EPM2A account for 50% of Lafora disease cases, and mutations in NHLRC1 account for the other 50% of cases. Laforin is a dual specificity phosphatase that removes phosphate from carbohydrates, primarily glycogen. The lack of laforin activity in Lafora disease leads to hyperphosphorylation of glycogen. Hyperphosphorylated glycogen disrupts the processes of branching and debranching leading to longer glucose chains than in a normal glycogen molecule. These abnormal glycogens (called polyglucans) are insoluble and ultimately lead to the formation of Lafora bodies. The incorporation of phosphate into glycogen is a function of glycogen synthase which is capable of transferring the β-phosphate of UDP-glucose to glycogen. Normal laforin functions to maintain the low level of phosphomonoesters in glycogen which prevents the molecule from precipitating. Malin is a ubiquitin ligase whose precise function in the process of glycogen dephosphorylation is incompletely understood However, evidence indicates that malin ubiquitylates the regulatory subunit of protein phosphatase 1 (PP1) which was originally identified as PTG for protein targeting glycogen. Malin has been shown to ubiquitylate PPP1R3A (the version of PTG found in skeletal muscle) and PPP1R3D. The malin-mediated ubiquitylation occurs in a laforin-dependent manner. Together laforin and malin interact to regulate glycogen phosphorylation and chain length pattern, the latter of which is crucial to the solubility of glycogen in the cell. The typical Lafora disease patient will begin to manifest symptoms in the second decade of life. The onset of symptoms is accompanied with vague symptoms of headaches and difficulties concentrating. Shortly after the onset of symptoms myoclonus appears along with generalized tonic-clonic seizures. Patients commonly develop visual

CLINICAL BOX 7-1 (CONTINUED)

hallucinations. Medications such as valproic acid, perampanel, levetiracetam, and zonisamide are used to treat Lafora disease with valproic acid being the mainstay in therapeutic intervention. However, the seizures and especially the myoclonus become intractable. Atypical and myoclonic absences set in, and they become so constant that a patient's every thought and spoken words are constantly interrupted and incomplete. Within a short period of a few years the patients are unable to attend school or work and become unable to walk because of frequent myoclonic and atonic attacks. Most Lafora patients will die in status epilepticus (defined as a continuous seizure lasting more than 30 minutes, or two or more seizures without full recovery of consciousness between any of them) or from aspiration pneumonia secondary to the loss of neurological control of secretions.

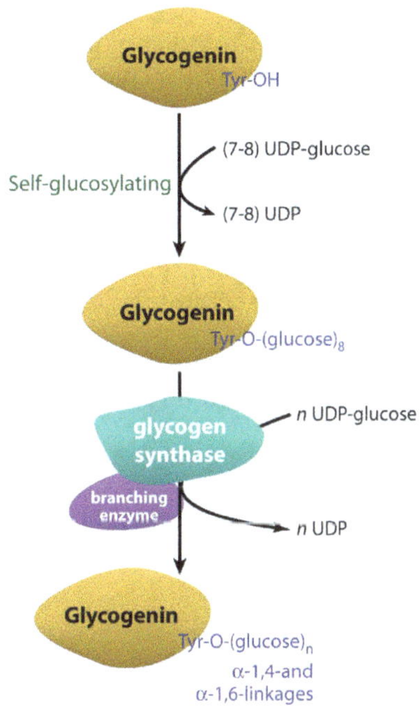

FIGURE 7–2 Role of glycogenin in the synthesis of glycogen: Beginning with free glucose, several reactions are required to initiate and then produce glycogen polymers. Glucose is first phosphorylated by hexokinases (e.g. muscle) or glucokinase (liver) generating glucose-6-phosphate (G6P). G6P is then converted to glucose-1-phosphate (G1P) via the action of phosphoglucomutase (PGM). G1P is then activated for glycogen synthesis via the addition of uridine nucleotide catalyzed by UDP-glucose pyrophosphorylase 2 (UGP2). The resultant UDP-glucose can then be used as a substrate for the self-glucosylating reaction of glycogenin. (Reproduced with permission from themedicalbiochemistrypage, LLC.)

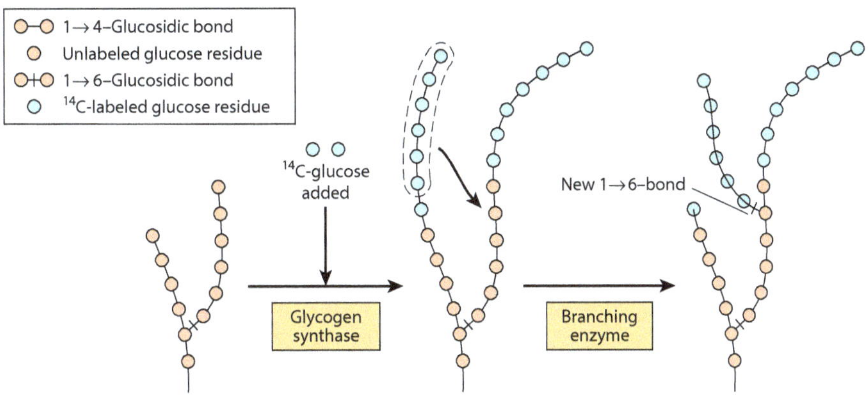

FIGURE 7–3 The biosynthesis of glycogen. The mechanism of branching as revealed by feeding 14C-labeled glucose and examining liver glycogen at intervals. (Reproduced with permission from Rodwell VW, Bender DA, Botham KM, et al: *Harper's Illustrated Biochemistry*, 31st ed. New York, NY: McGraw Hill; 2018.)

CLINICAL BOX 7-2 ANDERSEN DISEASE

Glycogen storage disease type IV (GSD IV) is more commonly known as Andersen disease or also as amylopectinosis. Andersen disease is inherited as an autosomal recessive disorder. This disease was originally described by the American pediatrician and pathologist, Dorothy Hansine Andersen in 1956, hence the association of her name with the disease. The disease is associated with the storage of an abnormal glycogen with few branch points and with long outer chains containing more α-1,4-linked glucose than normal glycogen. This structure is similar to that of amylopectin (the structure of starch in plants), thus the associated name of amylopectintosis. Andersen disease results from mutations in the gene (*GBE1*) encoding glycogen-branching enzyme, also called amylo-(1,4–1,6) transglycosylase. The *GBE1* gene is located on chromosome 3p12.2 and is composed of 16 exons that encode a protein of 702 amino acids. Classic Andersen disease is a rapidly progressive disorder that will result in early lethality as a result of liver failure. Liver transplantation is the only means of survival with this form of the disease. Other mutations in the *GBE1* gene have been identified in patients with the milder nonprogressive hepatic form of the disease. In addition to the classic lethal form of Andersen disease and the milder hepatic form, several other variant forms of the disease have been reported. There is a variant form that consists of multisystem involvement including skeletal and cardiac muscle, nerve, and liver. There is a juvenile polysaccharidosis form that manifests with multisystem involvement but patients with this form have normal GBE1 enzyme activity. There is a fetal neuromuscular form that results in death within the first few months of life that results from a splice site mutation in the *GBE1* gene. The clinical presentation of the classic form of Andersen disease usually occurs in the first few months of life and is characterized by hepatosplenomegaly and failure to thrive. The disease progresses to liver cirrhosis, portal vein hypertension, esophageal varices (dilated submucosal veins in the lower third of the esophagus), and ascites. Death will usually ensue by 5 years of age due to liver failure. Because of the similarities in symptoms between Andersen disease and other causes of cirrhosis in infancy it is necessary to carry out a biopsy of the liver and examine for the presence of the associated abnormal glycogen. In addition, assay for branching enzyme deficiency in muscle, leukocytes, erythrocytes, or fibroblasts can be carried out to determine the exact defect resulting in the hepatomegaly. The treatment of Andersen disease normally involves maintenance of normal blood glucose along with adequate nutrient intake both of which will improve liver function and muscle strength. In cases of progressive liver failure, liver transplant is the only effective option.

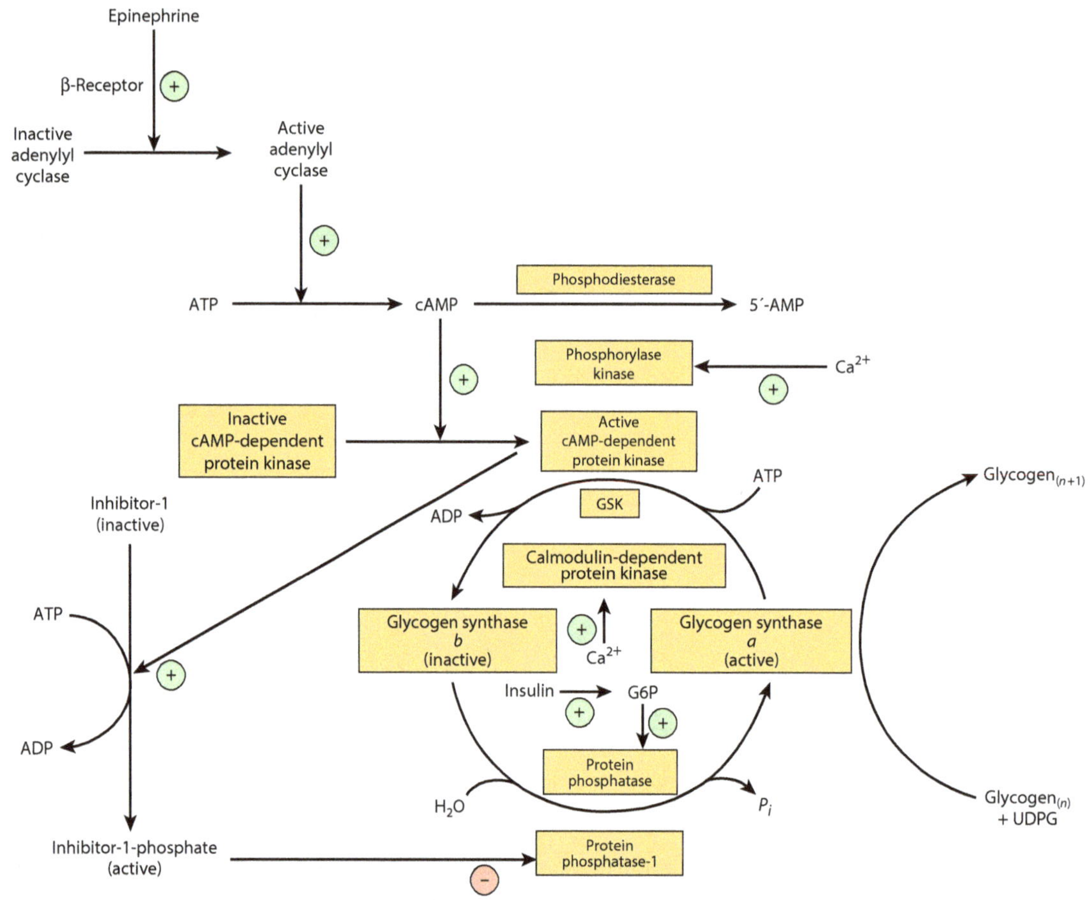

FIGURE 7–4 Control of glycogen synthase in muscle. (GSK, glycogen synthase kinase; G6P, glucose-6-phosphate; *n*, number of glucose residues.) (Reproduced with permission from Rodwell VW, Bender DA, Botham KM, et al: *Harper's Illustrated Biochemistry*, 31st ed. New York, NY: McGraw Hill; 2018.)

are cAMP-dependent protein kinase (PKA) and phosphorylase kinase, PHK (also known as glycogen synthase-phosphorylase kinase). Phosphorylase kinase is a multi-subunit enzyme with one of the subunits being the Ca^{2+}-binding protein, calmodulin.

Glucagon binds its receptor (a G_s-type G-protein coupled receptor, GPCR) on hepatocytes leading to the activation of adenylate cyclase. Activation of adenylate cyclase leads to a large increase in the formation of cAMP which then binds to and activates PKA. In addition, PKA phosphorylates PHK increasing its activity which in turn phosphorylates glycogen synthase at one of the same sites as PKA. During sympathetic nervous outflow from the brain (the "fight-or-flight" response), adrenal medullary chromaffin cells release epinephrine which bind to both α_1- and β_2-adrenergic receptors on hepatocytes. The α_1-receptor activates a G_q-type G-protein leading to increased release of intracellular Ca^{2+} and the activation of PHK. The β_2-receptor activates a G_s-type G-protein leading to the same PKA-mediated responses as glucagon.

The role of insulin is to stimulate the liver to store glucose as glycogen. In order to exert these effects insulin exerts effects that are counter to those of glucagon and epinephrine. The action of insulin, at the level of PKA, is to increase the activity of a phosphodiesterase which hydrolyzes cAMP to AMP thereby reducing the level of active PKA. Insulin also activates protein phosphatase-1 (PP-1) which removes the activating phosphate from PHK and the inhibitory phosphates from glycogen synthase.

GLYCOGENOLYSIS

Degradation of stored glycogen, termed glycogenolysis, occurs through the action of glycogen phosphorylase (commonly referred to simply as phosphorylase). The action of phosphorylase is to remove single glucose residues from α-(1,4) linkages within the glycogen molecule via phosphorolysis. The product of this reaction is glucose-1-phosphate (Figure 7–5).

Humans express three genes encoding proteins with glycogen phosphorylase activity. One gene (*PYGL*) expresses the hepatic form of the enzyme, a second (*PYGM*) expresses the muscle form (referred to as myophosphorylase), and the third (*PYGB*) expresses the brain form. Mutations in the *PYGM* gene are the cause of the glycogen storage disease identified as McArdle disease (see Clinical Box 7–3).

Glycogen phosphorylase cannot remove glucose residues from the branch points (α-1,6 linkages) in glycogen. The activity of phosphorylase ceases four glucose residues from the branch point.

CLINICAL BOX 7-3 MCARDLE DISEASE

Glycogen storage disease type V (GSD V) is also known as McArdle disease. This disease was originally described by B. McArdle in 1951, hence the association of his name with the disease. The disease was seen in a 30-year-old patient who was suffering from muscle weakness, pain, and stiffness following slight exercise. It was observed that blood lactate fell in this patient during exercise instead of the normal rise that would be seen. This indicated the patient had a defect in the ability to convert muscle glycogen to glucose and ultimately lactate. The identification that the deficiency causing these symptoms was the result of a muscle phosphorylase defect was not made until 1959. Glycogen phosphorylase (most commonly just called phosphorylase) exists in multiple tissue-specific isoforms. The muscle, brain, and liver forms are encoded by separate genes. The muscle form is the only isozyme found expressed in mature muscle. The clinical presentation of GSD V is usually seen in young adulthood and is charac terized by exercise intolerance and muscle cramps following slight exercise. Attacks of myoglobinuria frequently accompany the muscle symptoms of GSD V. About half of GSD V patients will exhibit burgundy colored urine after exercise. Diagnosis of muscle glycogenoses such as GSD V can be made by the observation of a lack of increased blood lactate upon ischemic exercise testing. In addition, there will be an associated large increase in blood ammonia levels. In order to distinguish GSD V from other muscle defects along the pathway from glycogen to glucose to lactate, an enzymatic evaluation of muscle phosphorylase must be done. Also, molecular analysis for known mutations in the muscle phosphorylase gene can be accomplished using DNA extracted from leukocytes.

HIGH-YIELD CONCEPT

The conversion of glucose-6-phosphate to free glucose occurs via the action of glucose-6-phosphatase. This enzyme is expressed in the liver, intestine, and kidney (key gluconeogenic tissues) but not in skeletal muscle. Therefore, any glucose released from glycogen stores of muscle will be oxidized in the glycolytic pathway. Mutations in the gene (*G6PC*) encoding glucose-6-phosphatase are the cause of the potentially lethal glycogen storage disease identified as von Gieke disease (see Clinical Box 7–4).

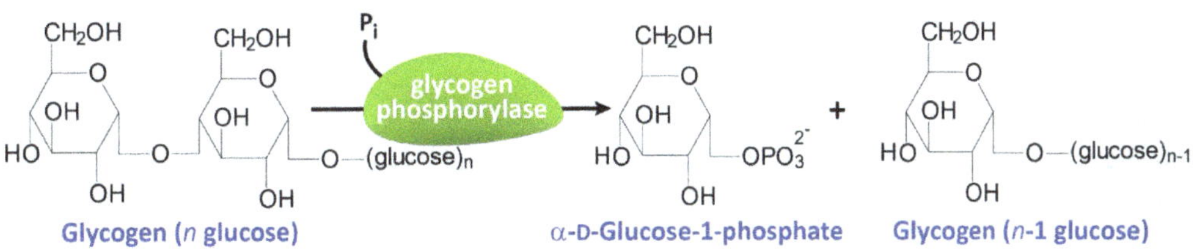

FIGURE 7–5 Phosphorylase catalyzed reaction showing the release of glucose-1-phosphate from glycogen. (Reproduced with permission from themedicalbiochemistrypage, LLC.)

The removal of these branch point glucose residues requires the action of glycogen debranching enzyme (also called glucan transferase) which possesses two activities: glucotransferase and glucosidase. The transferase activity removes the terminal three glucose residues of one branch and attaches them to a free C-4 end of a second branch. The glucose in α-(1,6) linkage at the branch is then removed by the action of glucosidase as free glucose (Figure 7–6). Mutations in the gene (*AGL*) that encodes glycogen debranching enzyme result in the glycogen storage disease identified as Cori disease (see Clinical Box 7–5).

Increased phosphorylation of glycogen polymers makes them less soluble inducing their degradation via the lysosomal pathway. Lysosomal glycogen degradation is catalyzed by the enzyme lysosomal acid α-glucosidase (also called acid maltase) which is encoded by the *GAA* gene. The significance of this pathway for glycogen degradation is evidenced from the lethal disorder, Pompe disease (see Clinical Box 7–6), that is the result of mutations in the *GAA* gene.

The disorder is associated with the accumulation of an abnormally structured glycogen having very short outer chains. This structure is similar to what would be seen in a phosphorylase-limit

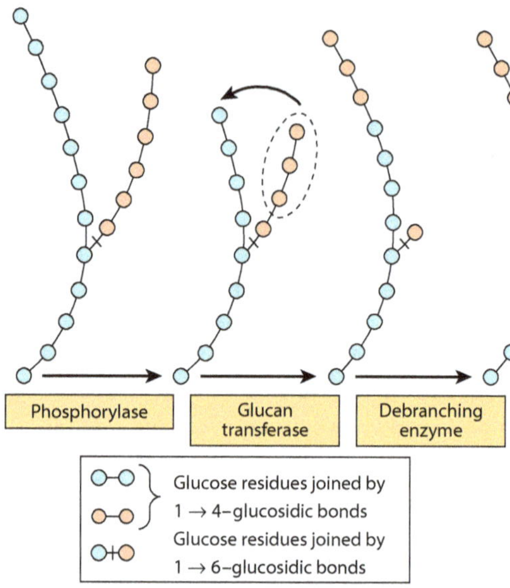

FIGURE 7–6 Steps in glycogenolysis. (Reproduced with permission from Rodwell VW, Bender DA, Botham KM, et al: *Harper's Illustrated Biochemistry*, 31st ed. New York, NY: McGraw Hill; 2018.)

CLINICAL BOX 7–4 von GIERKE DISEASE

Type I glycogen storage disease (GSD I) was first described in 1929 by E. von Gierke as a "hepato-nephromegalia glycogenica." For this reason the disease is still more commonly referred to von Gierke disease. In 1952, G. Cori and C. Cori identified that the absence of glucose-6-phosphatase activity was the cause of von Gierke disease. This discovery was the first ever identification of an enzyme defect in a metabolic disorder. Subsequent to the identification of the pathway of glucose release from glucose-6-phosphate, additional patients with similar clinical manifestations to von Gierke disease were identified. However, these patients were not deficient in glucose-6-phosphatase. These latter patients were identified as having type Ib GSD. Type Ia GSD is caused by a defect in the ER-localized glucose-6-phosphatase. Type Ib disease results from defects in the glucose-6-phosphate transporter 1. Type Ic GSD was identified in 1983 and found to be the result of defects in the microsomal pyrophosphate transporter. This form of type I GSD has only been found in few cases. As shown in the Figure 7–8, there are four enzyme activities that function in the release of free glucose in the cell and as such there is the theoretical possibility that type Id GSD would be caused by defects in the microsomal glucose transporter. However, no individuals have been reported to exist with a defect in this latter enzyme activity. In order to gain access to glucose-6-phosphatase, glucose-6-phosphate must pass through a specific translocase in the ER membrane (Figure 7–8). Mutation of either the phosphatase or the translocase makes transfer of glucose from liver glycogen to the blood a very limited process. Thus, mutation of either gene leads to symptoms associated with von Gierke disease, which occurs at a rate of about 1 in 200,000 people.

The metabolic consequences of the hepatic glucose-6-phosphate deficiency of von Gierke disease extend well beyond just the obvious hypoglycemia that result from the deficiency in liver being able to deliver free glucose to the blood. The inability to release the phosphate from glucose-6-phopsphate results in diversion into glycolysis and production of pyruvate as well as increased diversion onto the pentose phosphate pathway. The production of excess pyruvate, at levels above the capacity of the TCA cycle to completely oxidize it, results in its reduction to lactate resulting in lactic acidemia. In addition, some of the pyruvate is transaminated to alanine leading to hyperalaninemia. Some of the pyruvate will be oxidized to acetyl-CoA which can't be fully oxidized in the TCA cycle and so the acetyl-CoA will end up in the cytosol where it will serve as a substrate for triglyceride and cholesterol synthesis resulting in hyperlipidemia. The oxidation of glucose-6-phophate via the pentose phosphate pathway leads to increased production of ribose-5-phosphate which then activates the *de novo* synthesis of the purine nucleotides. In excess of the need, these purine nucleotides will ultimately be catabolized to uric acid resulting in hyperuricemia and consequent symptoms of gout. The interrelationships of these metabolic pathways are shown in Figure 7–9.

Patients with type I glycogen storage disease can present during the neonatal period with lactic acidosis and hypoglycemia. More commonly though, infants of 3–4 months of age will manifest with hepatomegaly and hypoglycemic seizures. The hallmark features of this disease are hypoglycemia, lactic acidosis, hyperuricemia, and hyperlipidemia. The severity of the hypoglycemia and lactic acidosis can be such that in the past affected individuals died in infancy. Infants often have a doll-like facial appearance due to excess adipose tissue in the cheeks. In addition, patients have thin extremities, a short stature, and protuberant abdomens (due to the severe hepatomegaly).

CLINICAL BOX 7–4 (CONTINUED)

Long-term complications are usually only seen now in adults whose disease was poorly treated early on. The main problem is associated with liver function, but multiple organ systems are also involved, in particular the intestines and kidneys. Growth will continue to be impaired, and puberty is often delayed. Affected female patients will have polycystic ovaries, but none of the other symptoms of polycystic ovarian syndrome (PCOS) such as hirsutism.

The common treatment for type I glycogen storage disease is to maintain normal blood glucose concentration. With normoglycemia will come reduced metabolic disruption and a reduced morbidity associated with the disease. To attain normoglycemia, patients are usually treated in infancy with nocturnal nasogastric infusion of glucose. Total parenteral nutrition or the oral feeding of uncooked cornstarch can also achieve the desired results.

In the past, the prognosis for type I glycogen storage disease patients was poor. However, with proper nutritional intervention growth will improve and the lactic acidosis, cholesterol, and lipidosis will decrease.

CLINICAL BOX 7–5 CORI DISEASE

Glycogen storage disease type III (GSD III) is more commonly known as Cori disease. Cori disease is also known as Forbes disease and limit dextrinosis. Cori disease is inherited as an autosomal recessive disorder. The symptoms associated with Cori disease were first described in 1952 by B. Illingworth and G.T. Cori and the disease was studied clinically by G.B. Forbes, hence the associated names for this disorder.

dextrin. The disorder was predicted, and later shown, to be the result of a deficiency of amylo-α-1,6-glucosidase, 4-α-glucanotransferase (encoded by the *AGL* gene), also known more simply as the glycogen debranching enzyme (GDE). The glycogen debranching enzyme has two distinct catalytic activities, amylo-α-1,6-glucosidase and 4-α-glucanotransferase. The two activities encompass distinct catalytic sites on the enzyme and can function independent of each other. However, both activities, as well as the binding of glycogen, are required for complete function. Deficiency in glycogen debranching activity causes hepatomegaly, ketotic hypoglycemia, hyperlipidemia, variable skeletal myopathy, cardiomyopathy, and

CLINICAL BOX 7–6 POMPE DISEASE

Glycogen storage disease type II (GSD II) is also known as Pompe disease or acid maltase deficiency (AMD). This disease was originally referred to as Pompe disease since Joannes Cassianus Pompe (published in 1932) made the important observation of a massive accumulation of glycogen within the vacuoles of all tissues in a 7-month-old girl who died suddenly from idiopathic hypertrophy of the heart. Through the investigations carried out by the Cori's (Gerty T. Cori and Carl F. Cori) this disease was classified as glycogen storage disease type II. GSD II is the most severe of all of the glycogen storage diseases. The excess storage of glycogen in the vacuoles is the consequence of defects in the lysosomal hydrolase, acid α-glucosidase which removes glucose residues from glycogen in the lysosomes. The acid α-glucosidase enzyme is encoded by the *GAA* gene. GSD II has been shown to be caused by missense, nonsense, and splice-site mutations, partial deletions and insertions. Some mutations are specific to certain ethnic groups. There are three common allelic forms of acid α-glucosidase that segregate in the general population. These forms are designated GAA1, GAA2, and GAA4. The normal function of acid α-glucosidase is to hydrolyze both α-1,4- and α-1,6-glucosidic linkages at acid pH. The activity of the enzyme leads to the complete hydrolysis of glycogen which is its natural substrate. As would be expected from this activity, deficiency in acid α-glucosidase leads to the accumulation of structurally normal glycogen in numerous tissues, most notably in cardiac and skeletal muscle. The clinical presentation of GSD II encompasses a wide range of phenotypes but all include various degrees of cardiomegaly. Additional clinical manifestations associated with idiopathic cardiomegaly accompanied by storage of glycogen are indicative of Pompe disease. These symptoms included hepatomegaly, marked hypotonia, muscular weakness, and death before 1 year of age. The different phenotypes can be classified dependent upon age of onset, extent of organ involvement and the rate of progression to death. The infantile-onset form is the most severe and was the phenotype described by JC Pompe. The other extreme of this disorder is a slowly progressing adult onset proximal myopathic disease. The late onset disease usually presents as late as the second to sixth decade of life and usually only involves the skeletal muscles. There is also a heterogeneous group of GSD II disorders that are classified generally by onset after early infancy and called the juvenile or childhood form. In addition to classical symptoms that can lead to a diagnosis of GSD II, analysis for the level and activity of acid α-glucosidase in muscle biopsies is used for confirmation. The infantile onset form of GSD II presents in the first few months of life. Symptoms include marked cardiomegaly, striking hypotonia (leading to the designation of "floppy baby syndrome") and rapid progressive muscle weakness. Patients will usually exhibit difficulty with feeding and have respiratory problems that are frequently complicated by pulmonary infection. The prominent cardiomegaly that can be seen on chest X-ray is normally the first indication leading to a preliminary diagnosis of GSD II. There is currently no cure for GSD II. In 2006 the US FDA approved the use of Myozyme® (alglucosidase alpha) as an enzyme replacement therapy (ERT) for treatment of infantile-onset Pompe disease. Supportive therapy with attention to treatment of respiratory function can impact the course of the disease in the late-onset form.

results in short stature. Patients with both liver and muscle involvement have GSD IIIa, and those with only liver involvement (~15% of GSD III patients) are classified as GSD IIIb. Because hepatomegaly, hypoglycemia, hyperlipidemia, and growth impairment are common symptoms in both von Gierke disease (GSD I; Clinical Box 7–4) and Cori disease, it is difficult to initially determine from which disease an infant is suffering. Definitive diagnosis is only made by examining the structure of the glycogen in patients as well as assaying for the level of activity of the debranching enzyme. This diagnosis is best accomplished from liver and/or muscle biopsy. The hepatic symptoms of Cori disease usually resolve after puberty. However, liver failure due to cirrhosis may occur. Cori disease is treated with frequent high carbohydrate meals with cornstarch supplements. A high protein diet is also an effective treatment as this drives gluconeogenesis. There is currently no effective treatment for the progressive cardiomyopathy.

HIGH-YIELD CONCEPT

The activity of hexokinase in muscle is so high that any free glucose is immediately phosphorylated and enters the glycolytic pathway. Indeed, the precise reason for the temporary appearance of the free glucose from glycogen is the need of the skeletal muscle cell to generate energy from glucose oxidation, thereby, precluding any chance of the glucose entering the blood.

HIGH-YIELD CONCEPT

Within skeletal muscle cells calcium ions play a crucial role in the regulation of glycogenolysis. Calcium ions bind to the calmodulin subunit of phosphorylase kinase. Binding induces a conformational change in calmodulin which in turn enhances the catalytic activity of the phosphorylase kinase toward its substrate, phosphorylase-*b*. This activity is crucial to the enhancement of glycogenolysis in muscle cells where muscle contraction is induced via acetylcholine stimulation at the neuromuscular junction.

REGULATION OF GLYCOGENOLYSIS

Glycogen phosphorylase is regulated both by phosphorylation and by allosteric effectors. The allosteric activator is AMP and the allosteric inhibitors are ATP and glucose-6-phosphate. Phosphorylase is less active in the unphosphorylated state. The kinase that phosphorylates and activates phosphorylase is PHK.

Glucagon binding to its receptors on hepatocytes results in activation of PKA which then phosphorylates and activates PHK. In the liver and in skeletal muscle, similar effects are exerted by epinephrine binding to β-adrenergic receptors (Figure 7–7). Activated PHK in turn phosphorylates phosphorylase greatly enhancing its activity toward glycogen breakdown.

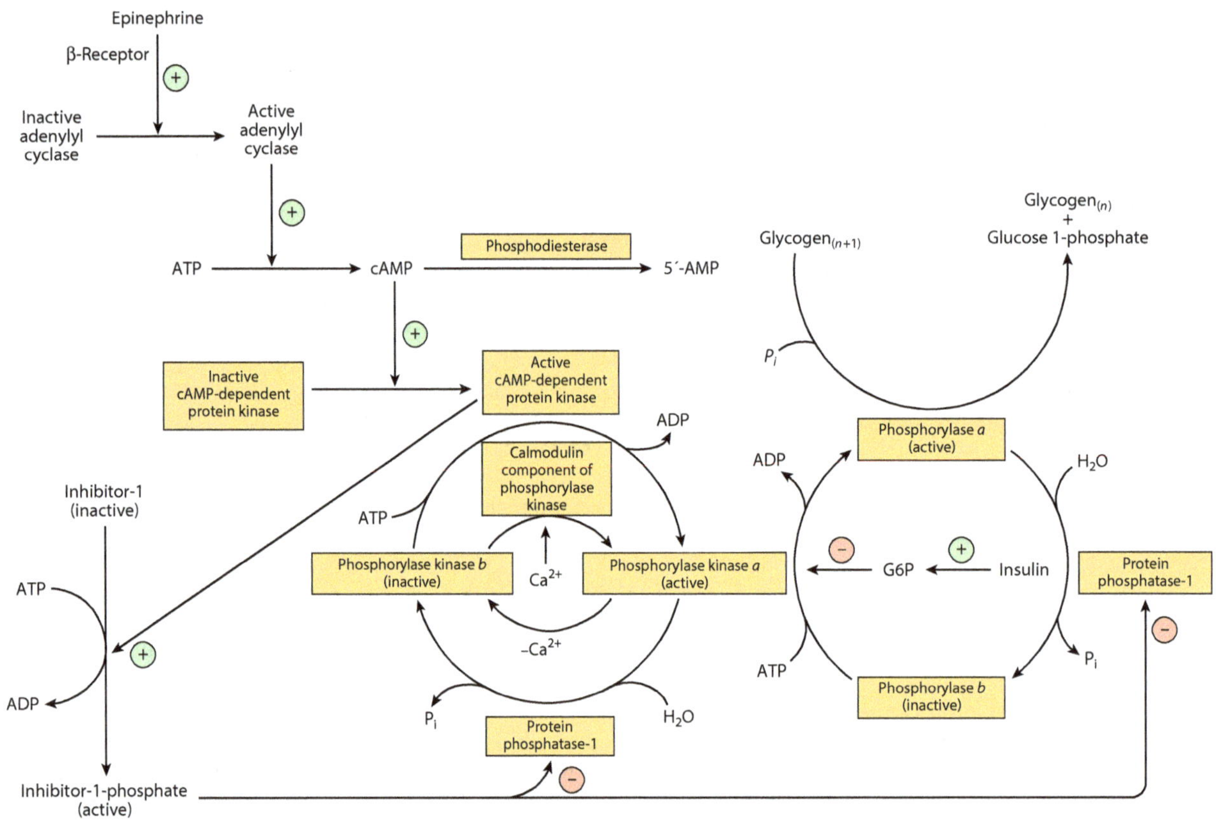

FIGURE 7–7 Control of phosphorylase in muscle. The sequence of reactions arranged as a cascade allows amplification of the hormonal signal at each step. (G6P, glucose 6-phosphate; *n*, number of glucose residues.) (Reproduced with permission from Rodwell VW, Bender DA, Botham KM, et al: *Harper's Illustrated Biochemistry*, 31st ed. New York, NY: McGraw Hill; 2018.)

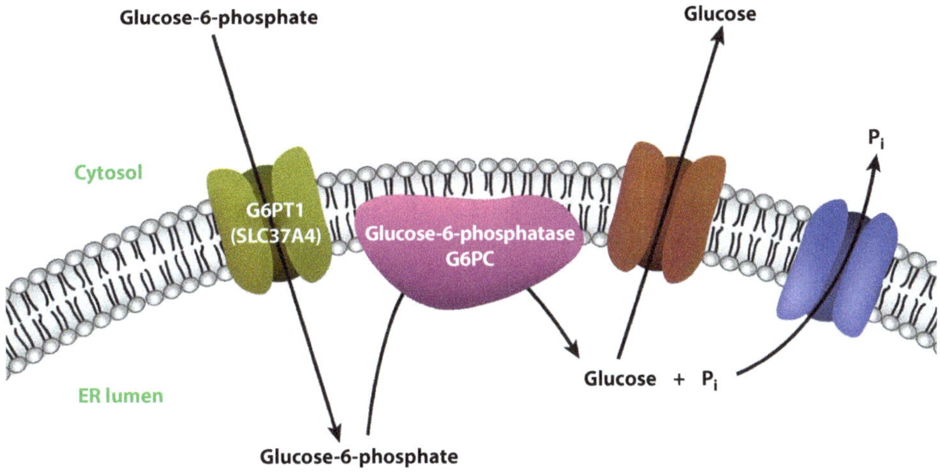

FIGURE 7–8 Mechanism of glucose-6-phosphate conversion to free glucose. Glucose-6-phosphate is transported from the cytosol into the lumen of the endoplasmic reticulum (ER) through the actions of the glucose-6-phosphate transporter 1 (G6PT1). The removal of phosphate from glucose-6-phosphate is catalyzed by the ER membrane-localized glucose-6-phosphatase encoded by the G6PC gene. Following removal of the phosphate, the free glucose is transported out of the ER lumen to the cytosol. Evidence indicates that this glucose transport occurs via GLUT2 (in the liver) as this glucose transporter is transiting the ER to the plasma membrane following its synthesis. (Reproduced with permission from themedicalbiochemistrypage, LLC.)

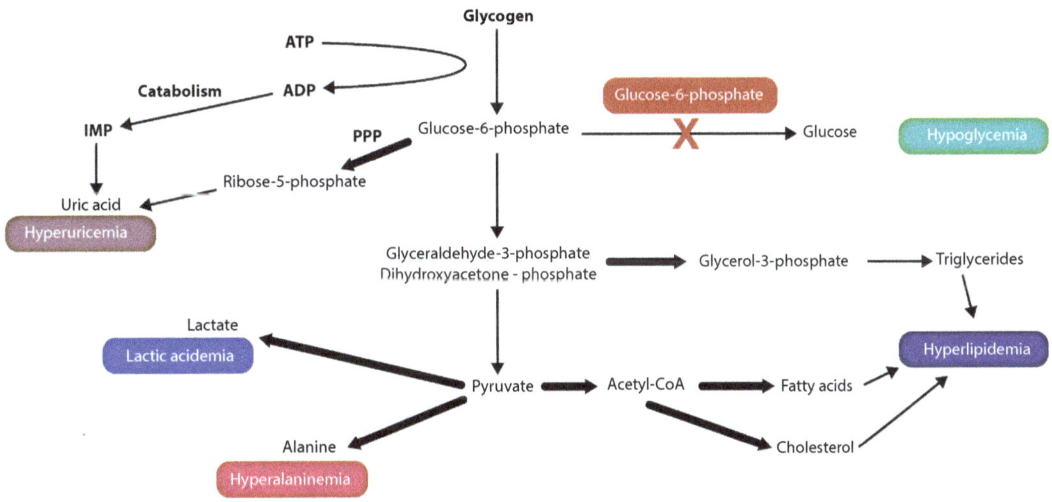

FIGURE 7–9 Interrelationships of metabolic pathway disruption in von Gierke disease. In the absence of glucose-6-phosphatase activity, free glucose cannot be released from the liver contributing to severe fasting hypoglycemia. In addition, the increased glucose-6-phosphate levels lead to increased pentose phosphate pathway (PPP) activity as well as increased glycolysis to pyruvate. Increase PPP activity results in excessive purine nucleotide synthesis, the products of which are catabolized to uric acid resulting in hyperuricemia. The increased levels of pyruvate lead to increased lactate production via lactate dehydrogenase (LDH) and alanine via alanine transaminase (ALT). In addition, the increased pyruvate is oxidized via the pyruvate dehydrogenase complex (PDHc) leading to increased production of acetyl-CoA which is, in turn, used for the synthesis of fatty acids and cholesterol. The excess glycolysis also results in increased production of glycerol-3-phosphate (G3P) from dihydroxyacetone phosphate (DHAP) via the action of glycerol-3-phosphate dehydrogenase (GPD1). Increased G3P and fatty acids leads to increased triglyceride synthesis which, in conjunction with the increased cholesterol, leads to hyperlipidemia as well as fatty infiltration in hepatocytes contributing to hepatomegaly and cirrhosis. (Reproduced with permission from themedicalbiochemistrypage, LLC.)

CHECKLIST

- ☑ Glycogen constitutes the primary storage form of carbohydrate from which glucose can be released during periods of fasting, starvation, and aerobic metabolism particularly within skeletal muscle.
- ☑ The two major sites for glycogen storage are the liver and skeletal muscle. Hepatic glycogen allows the liver to respond to low blood glucose levels and readily release its stored glucose to the blood for use by extrahepatic tissues. Within skeletal muscle, glycogen allows this tissue to respond to periods of aerobic metabolism by readily releasing the glucose into the glycolytic pool.
- ☑ Release of glucose from glycogen does not require the input of energy since the release is a phosphorylytic reaction catalyzed by phosphorylase.
- ☑ The primary hormone-mediated regulator of glycogen synthesis and breakdown is cAMP which activates PKA. Glucagon stimulates cAMP production leading to inhibition of glycogen synthesis and activation of glycogenolysis. Conversely, insulin stimulates the hydrolysis of cAMP reversing the effects of glucagon.
- ☑ Epinephrine also stimulates glycogenolysis via the activation of β-adrenergic receptors that results in increased cAMP production.
- ☑ Skeletal muscle twitch leads to release of stored calcium from the sarcoplasmic reticulum. The calcium then activates phosphorylase kinase resulting in phosphorylation and inhibition of glycogen synthase while simultaneously phosphorylating and activating phosphorylase.
- ☑ Deficiencies in many of the enzymes of glycogen synthesis and breakdown result in mild to severe disorders. These disorders primarily affect the liver and/or skeletal muscle and therefore, manifest with symptoms associated with defects in metabolic functions in these two tissues.

REVIEW QUESTIONS

1. Studies are being conducted to examine the biochemical characteristics of a liver dysfunction in a patient exhibiting signs of a glycogen storage disease. The microsomal fraction (contains the endoplasmic reticulum) of a liver biopsy homogenate from the patient, as well as from a control individual are being utilized in these studies. Incubation of the microsomal fractions with ^{32}P-glucose-6-phosphate results in an increase in isotope associated with the microsomes from control samples but no increase in association with the microsomes from the patient samples. These results are best explained by a defect in which of the following microsomal activities?
   (A) Aldolase A
   (B) Frucose-1,6-bisphosphatase
   (C) Glucose-6-phosphatase
   (D) Glucose-6-phosphate transporter
   (E) Glucose transporter
   (F) Inorganic phosphate transporter

2. An 8-month-old female infant is being examined by her pediatrician due to concerns by her parents of a failure sit alone, hold her head, and to engage with them. Physical examination indicates the infant is hypotonic with muscle weakness and atrophy. Palpation of the abdomen shows significant hepatomegaly. A liver biopsy is ordered and shows the presence of amylopectin-like carbohydrates and the onset of cirrhosis. Given the signs and symptoms in this infant, which of the following is most suited to the treatment of her disorder?
   (A) Glucose restricted diet
   (B) High fat, low carbohydrate diet
   (C) High glucose diet
   (D) High protein diet
   (E) Lactose restricted diet
   (F) Sucrose restricted diet

3. A 9-month-old infant is brought to the physician by his parents with concerns about their difficulty getting him to feed. Physical examination shows hypotonia, a bulging abdomen, and a demonstrably palpable liver. Chest X-ray shows prominent cardiomegaly. Prior to diagnosis, the patient lapses into a coma and dies. An H&E-stained heart section obtained at autopsy shows enlarged vacuoles in almost all cardiac myocytes. Given the observations and outcomes in this case, which of the following metabolic processes was most likely defective in the patient prior to his death?
   (A) Cardiac myocyte glycosaminoglycan synthesis
   (B) Hepatic bile acid synthesis
   (C) Lysosomal glycogen metabolism
   (D) Mitochondrial branched-chain amino acid metabolism
   (E) Mitochondrial fatty acid oxidation

4. A 6-month-old boy is brought to the physician because of failure to thrive. Physical examination shows hepatosplenomegaly, muscle weakness and atrophy, hypotonia, and decreased deep tendon reflexes. Laboratory studies show a serum glucose concentration of 95 mg/dL. A liver biopsy shows the initial stages of cirrhosis and accumulation of abnormally structured glycogen. Which of the following metabolic processes is most likely to be defective in this patient?
   (A) Glucose catabolism
   (B) Glucose synthesis
   (C) Glycogen catabolism
   (D) Glycogen synthesis
   (E) Fatty acid oxidation
   (F) Fatty acid synthesis

5. Biochemical studies are being conducted on a 9-month-old female infant manifesting signs and symptoms suggestive of a liver disorder. Liver biopsy derived hepatocytes have been homogenized and the microsomal fraction purified and compared to the similar fraction from normal hepatocytes. Incubation of the microsomes with radioactive phosphate labeled glucose-6-phosphate results in an increase in isotope associated with the microsomal membranes from the patient's hepatocytes but no increase in association with the microsomal membranes from normal hepatocytes. These results are best explained by a defect in activity of which of the following?
(A) Glucose 6-phosphatase
(B) Glucose-6-phosphate transport
(C) Glucose transport
(D) Glycogen-branching enzyme
(E) Glycogen-debranching enzyme

6. A 7-month-old infant is being examined in the emergency department because his parents are concerned about his problems with eating. Physical examination finds a palpable liver, generalized muscle weakness, and hypotonia. A chest X-ray finds significant cardiomegaly. The infant is admitted to the hospital but before a definitive diagnosis can be made, he lapses into a coma and dies. Postmortem tissue analysis finds a skeletal muscle pathology that includes fiber destruction, lysosomal vacuolation, and autophagic abnormalities. Given the findings from this case, which of the following is the most likely diagnosis?
(A) Andersen disease
(B) Cori (Forbes) disease
(C) McArdle disease
(D) Pompe disease
(E) von Gierke disease

7. Experiments are being conducted on a hepatic cell line derived from biopsy tissue of a patient with hepatocellular carcinoma. The activity of the phosphorylated form of glycogen phosphorylase, purified from these cells, is found to be unresponsive to a known allosteric inhibitor when compared to the enzyme from normal hepatocytes. Given this result, it is most likely that the enzyme has sustained a mutation in the binding site for which of the following?
(A) AMP
(B) Calcium ion
(C) cAMP
(D) cAMP-dependent protein kinase (PKA)
(E) Glucose-6-phosphate

8. A 4-month-old boy is brought to the physician because of listlessness, vomiting, watery stools, and a 2-day history of fever. His temperature is 38.4°C (101.1°F). Physical examination shows the infant has a protuberant abdomen and thin extremities. Laboratory studies show serum glucose is 40 mg/dL (N = 70-150 mg/dL), lactate is 3.2 mEq/L (N = 1.0-3.3 mEq/L), uric acid is 7.3 mg/dL (N = 2.0–6.2 mg/dL), and triglycerides are 143 mg/dL (N under 10 years of age = <75 mg/dL). Intravenous administration of 5% dextrose improves the infant's attentiveness. Given the signs and symptoms in this infant, which of the following is most likely to be elevated in his liver?
(A) Dicarboxylic acids
(B) Fructose-1-phosphate
(C) Glucocerebrosides
(D) Glucose-6-phosphate
(E) G_{M2} gangliosides

9. A 7-year-old boy is examined by his pediatrician because of complaints of severe cramping pain in his legs whenever he rides his bike. In addition, he experiences nausea and vomiting during these attacks. Clinical studies undertaken following a treadmill test demonstrate myoglobinuria, hyperuricemia, elevated serum creatine kinase (CK), and unconjugated hyperbilirubinemia. Analysis of muscle biopsy tissue shows PAS positive staining and normal levels of glycogen phosphorylase activity. A deficiency in which of the following would most likely account for the symptoms observed in this patient?
(A) Glucose-6-phosphatase
(B) Glycogen synthase
(C) Liver glycogen-debranching enzyme
(D) Lysosomal acid maltase
(E) Muscle phosphofructokinase-1 (PFK1)

10. A 6-month-old boy is brought to the physician because of failure to thrive. Physical examination shows hepatosplenomegaly, muscle weakness and atrophy, hypotonia, and decreased deep tendon reflexes. Laboratory studies show a serum glucose concentration of 95 mg/dL. A liver biopsy shows the initial stages of cirrhosis and accumulation of glycogen molecules that resemble amylose. Based upon the signs and symptoms in this infant, which of the following represents the most likely diagnosis?
(A) Andersen disease
(B) Cori disease
(C) McArdle disease
(D) Tarui disease
(E) von Gierke disease

11. An 8-month-old girl has died due to cardiorespiratory failure. Physical findings that were apparent prior to her death included feeding difficulties, cardiomegaly, macroglossia, mild hepatomegaly, hypotonia, and a rapidly progressing muscle weakness. Autopsy findings show marked intralysosomal accumulation of a substance that stains with PAS. These signs and symptoms are most likely associated with which of the following disorders?
(A) Erythrocyte pyruvate kinase deficiency
(B) Medium-chain acyl-CoA dehydrogenase deficiency
(C) Pompe disease
(D) Porphyria cutanea tarda
(E) Zellweger syndrome

12. A 4-month-old Caucasian boy is brought to the physician because of listlessness, vomiting, watery stools, and a 4-day history of fever. His temperature is 38.4°C (101.1°F). Physical examination shows the infant has a protuberant abdomen, thin extremities, and a doll-like face. Laboratory studies show serum glucose is 35 mg/dL (N = 70-150 mg/dL), pH is 7.30 (N = 7.35–7.45), bicarbonate is 16 mEq/L (N = 22–26 mEq/L), lactate is 3.2 mEq/L (N = 1.0-3.3 mEq/L), and triglycerides are 143 mg/dL (N under 10 years of age = <75 mg/dL). Intravenous administration of 5% dextrose improves the infant's attentiveness. Which of the following enzyme activities is most likely defective in this infant?
(A) Glucose-6-phosphatase
(B) Glycogen synthase
(C) Muscle phosphofructokinase 1
(D) Muscle phosphorylase
(E) Pyruvate kinase

13. A 5-month-old girl is brought by her parents to see her pediatrician where they report that they are concerned about her problems with eating. Upon physical examination the pediatrician notes significant hypotonia and a bulging abdomen with a demonstrably palpable liver. The infant shows difficulty breathing, so the pediatrician orders a chest X-ray which shows prominent cardiomegaly. Prior to diagnosis, the infant lapses into a coma and dies. An H&E-stained heart section obtained at autopsy shows the presence of numerous large vacuoles. A defect in which of the following enzymes was the most likely cause of the infant's mortality?
(A) Glucose-6-phosphatase
(B) Glycogen-branching enzyme
(C) Glycogen-debranching enzyme
(D) Lysosomal acid maltase
(E) Liver phosphorylase
(F) Muscle phosphorylase

14. A 24-year-old man comes to his doctor because of a 3-month history of pain in the arms and legs after strenuous exercise. He also had severe cramps and passed red urine after digging out several bushes from his front yard. Physical examination shows no abnormalities. This patient most likely has an inherited deficiency in which of the following enzymes?
(A) Glucocerebrosidase
(B) Glucose-6-phosphatase
(C) Hexosaminidase A
(D) Muscle phosphorylase
(E) Sphingomyelinase

15. A 6-month-old boy is brought to the physician because of failure to thrive. Physical examination shows hepatosplenomegaly, muscle weakness and atrophy, hypotonia, and decreased deep tendon reflexes. Laboratory studies show a serum glucose concentration of 95 mg/dL. A liver biopsy shows the initial stages of cirrhosis and accumulation of abnormally structured glycogen. Which of the following metabolic processes is most likely to be defective in this patient?
(A) Glucose catabolism
(B) Glucose synthesis
(C) Glycogen catabolism
(D) Glycogen synthesis
(E) Fatty acid oxidation
(F) Fatty acid synthesis

16. A 19-year-old man who has a severe allergy to bee stings has injected himself with his EpiPen following being stung while mowing the lawn. Measurement of serum glucose in this individual would be expected to be elevated, most likely due to which of the following processes?
(A) Absorption of carbohydrate from the digestive tract
(B) Hepatic glycogenesis
(C) Hepatic glycogenolysis
(D) Proteolysis in muscle and release of amino acids
(E) Synthesis of glucose from odd-chain fatty acids

17. A 4-month-old white male infant with a temperature of 38.4°C is examined by his pediatrician. His mother indicates that he has had the fever for the past 4 days, been listless, vomiting, and has watery stools. Blood work indicates the infant is hypoglycemic, but this condition does not respond to either epinephrine or glucose administration. In addition, his blood pH is slightly acidic and shows reduced bicarbonate. Other untoward blood chemistry includes elevated triglycerides, cholesterol, and liver enzymes. The child has a protuberant abdomen, thin extremities, and a doll-like face. The pediatrician suspects a specific condition, and in order to confirm his diagnosis he would most likely need to assay for which of the following enzyme activities?
(A) Erythrocyte pyruvate kinase
(B) Hepatic glucose-6-phosphatase
(C) Hepatic glycogen synthase
(D) Hepatic pyruvate kinase
(E) Muscle glycogen phosphorylase
(F) Muscle glycogen synthase

18. A 17-year-old boy has a history of intermittent muscle pain, weakness, and stiffness following training for the high school track team. Following these episodes, he experiences a pink coloration to his urine. During a treadmill test, serum analysis found no increase in the levels of lactate compared to those measured prior to the test. Which of the following is the most likely deficiency in the skeletal muscles of this individual accounting for these findings?
(A) Creatine kinase
(B) Creatine phosphate
(C) Glucose-6-phosphatase
(D) Glycogen phosphorylase
(E) Glycogen synthase

19. A 21-year-old woman comes to the physician because of a 3-month history of pain in the arms and legs after strenuous exercise. She reports that she also has severe cramps and passes reddish-purple urine following exertion. Physical examination is unremarkable. This patient most likely has an inherited deficiency of which of the following enzymes?
(A) Glucocerebrosidase
(B) Glucose-6-phosphatase
(C) Hexosaminidase A
(D) Muscle phosphorylase
(E) Sphingomyelinase

20. A 9-month-old infant is brought to the physician by his parents with concerns about their difficulty getting him to feed. Physical examination shows hypotonia, a bulging abdomen, and a demonstrably palpable liver. Chest X-ray shows prominent cardiomegaly. Prior to diagnosis, the patient lapses into a coma and dies. Histopathology sections of the heart obtained at autopsy show enlarged vacuoles in almost all cardiac myocytes. Given the observations and outcomes in this case, which of the following metabolic processes was most likely defective in the patient prior to his death?
(A) Fructose metabolism
(B) Galactose metabolism
(C) Gluconeogenesis
(D) Glycogen metabolism
(E) Glycolysis

21. A 20-year-old man comes to the physician because of a 3-month history of progressive, painful muscle cramps, and intolerance to exercise. He says that on one occasion, he passed burgundy-colored urine. Laboratory studies show that there is no evidence of increased serum lactate in blood samples taken during a forearm ischemic exercise test (FIET). A biopsy specimen of muscle shows an increased concentration of PAS-positive staining material. Which of the following enzymes is most likely deficient in this patient?
(A) Acid α-glucosidase
(B) Glucose-6-phosphatase
(C) Glycogen-debranching enzyme
(D) Glycogen phosphorylase
(E) UDP-glucose pyrophosphorylase

22. A common practice among long-distance runners is high carbohydrate loading. Following the consumption of such a diet, which of the following enzymes is most likely to be stimulated in hepatocytes?
(A) Glucokinase
(B) Glucose-6-phosphatase
(C) Glycogen phosphorylase
(D) Hexokinase
(E) Lactate dehydrogenase

23. A 9-month-old girl has a 6-month history of progressive muscle weakness and congestive heart failure accompanied by significant cardiomegaly. The infant can no longer roll over, is hypotonic, and her head flops back when she is lifted. She remains alert and engaged in her environment. A muscle biopsy shows lysosomal accumulation of PAS staining material. The most likely cause of these symptoms is a deficiency of which of the following enzymes?
(A) Acid maltase
(B) Glucose-6-phopshatase
(C) α-Glucosidase
(D) Muscle phosphofructokinase-1 (PFK1)
(E) Muscle phosphorylase

24. A 2-year-old girl is brought to the physician because of irritability and failure to thrive. Physical examination shows hepatomegaly. Laboratory studies show her fasting plasma glucose is 48 mg/dL (N = 65–99 mg/dL). A high-protein diet or intravenous administration of fructose results in an increased serum glucose concentration. Biopsy of hepatic tissue demonstrates increased amounts of amylopectin-like material. The most likely cause of this condition is a defect in which of the following enzymes?
(A) Glucokinase
(B) Glucose-6-phosphatase
(C) Glycogen-debranching enzyme
(D) Glycogen phosphorylase
(E) Glycogen synthase

25. Hepatic metabolism of glycogen can be stimulated by both cAMP-dependent and cAMP-independent pathways. Activation of which of the following is most likely to be associated with the latter mechanism of glycogen metabolism?
(A) α_1-Adrenergic receptors
(B) β_2-Adrenergic receptors
(C) Cortisol receptors
(D) Glucagon receptors
(E) Insulin receptors

26. An experimental compound is being developed to mimic the actions of glucose-6-phosphate in the regulation of hepatic glycogen metabolism. Which of the following responses to this compound would most likely be found if the effects are as expected?
(A) Activation of glycogen synthase
(B) Activation of phosphorylase kinase
(C) Activation of protein phosphatase 1 (PP1)
(D) Inhibition of dephosphorylated glycogen phosphorylase
(E) Inhibition of phosphorylase kinase
(F) Inhibition protein phosphatase 1 (PP1)

27. Sympathetic outflow from the hindbrain, as is typical during periods of exercise, will most likely exert which of the following effects on skeletal muscle glycogen metabolism?
(A) Activation of glycogen-debranching enzyme
(B) Activation of glycogen synthase
(C) Activation of phosphorylase kinase
(D) Inhibition of glycogen-debranching enzyme
(E) Inhibition of glycogen phosphorylase
(F) Inhibition of phosphorylase kinase

28. Muscle membrane will depolarize in response to acetylcholine binding its receptors at the neuromuscular junction. Which of the following represents the most likely changes in enzyme activity that will be the result of this depolarization?
(A) Decreased phosphorylase kinase activity due to an increase in calcium binding to its calmodulin subunit
(B) Decreased phosphorylation of, and inhibited activity of phosphorylase kinase
(C) Decreased phosphorylase kinase activity due to an activation of phosphoprotein phosphatase
(D) Increased phosphorylase kinase activity due to an activation of phosphoprotein phosphatase
(E) Increased phosphorylase kinase activity due to an increase in calcium binding to its calmodulin subunit
(F) Increased phosphorylation of, and inhibited activity of phosphorylase kinase

29. An increase in the state of phosphorylation, in hepatocytes in response to glucagon action, will be most accurately reflected by which of the following statements?
(A) Glycogen phosphorylase activity will be increased
(B) PFK1 activity will be unaffected
(C) PFK2 will exhibit an increased level of kinase activity
(D) Phosphorylase kinase activity will be decreased
(E) Phosphoprotein phosphatase-1 activity will be increased

30. Hepatic glycogen synthesis is inhibited by the actions resulting from glucagon binding its receptor. Which of the following most correctly defines these actions?
(A) Decreased activity of phosphoprotein phosphatase 1 (PP1)
(B) Decreased level of phosphorylated phosphoprotein phosphatase inhibitor-1 (PPI-1)
(C) Decreased level of phosphorylated phosphorylase kinase
(D) Increased activity of the kinase activity of phosphofructokinase-2 (PFK2)
(E) Increased level of the dephosphorylated form of glycogen synthase
(F) Increased level of the phosphorylated form of glycogen synthase

31. Hepatic glycogen homeostasis is regulated by changes in the serum levels of several different hormones. Which of the following is most correct with respect to increased hepatic glycogen content?

	Epinephrine	Cortisol	Glucagon
A.	↓	↓	↓
B.	↓	↓	↑
C.	↓	↑	↓
D.	↑	↓	↑
E.	↑	↑	↓

(A)
(B)
(C)
(D)
(E)

32. The response of the liver to insulin includes the activation of protein phosphatase 1 (PP1). In response to these effects, which of the following enzymes is most likely to be enhanced?
(A) cAMP-dependent protein kinase (PKA)
(B) Glucose-6-phosphatase
(C) Glycogen phosphorylase
(D) Glycogen synthase
(E) UDP-glucose pyrophosphorylase

33. A 17-year-old boy has a history of intermittent muscle pain, weakness, and stiffness following training for the high school track team. Following these episodes, he experiences a pink coloration to his urine. During a treadmill test, serum analysis found no increase in the levels of lactate compared to those measured prior to the test. This patient is most likely to be deficient in acquiring energy from the metabolism of which of the following?
(A) Glucose
(B) Glycerol
(C) Glycogen
(D) Lactate
(E) Pyruvate

34. With respect to carbohydrate metabolism, the activity of which of the following is most likely to be increased in hepatocytes as a result of sympathetic outflow from the hindbrain?
(A) Glycogen phosphorylase
(B) Glycogen synthase
(C) Phosphofructokinase 1 (PFK1)
(D) Pyruvate carboxylase
(E) Pyruvate kinase

35. A 19-year-old man comes to the physician because of frequent light-headedness and upper abdominal pain and discomfort. Laboratory studies show a fasting plasma glucose concentration of 58 mg/dL (N = 60–100 mg/dL), total serum cholesterol of 230 mg/dL (N = <200 mg/dL), plasma triglyceride concentration of 220 mg/dL (N = <150 mg/dL), elevated levels of AST and ALT, and ketonemia. Liver biopsy results show normal activities of glycogen phosphorylase, glycogen-debranching enzyme, and glucose-6-phosphatase. A deficiency in which of the following enzymes is most likely in this patient?
(A) Glycogen-branching enzyme
(B) Glycogen synthase
(C) Hexokinase
(D) Phosphoprotein phosphatase 1
(E) Phosphorylase kinase

36. Which of the following is most correct with respect to the regulation of hepatic glycogen synthase in response to glucagon activation of its receptor?
(A) Allosteric inhibition by bound AMP
(B) Binding of intracellular glucose-1-phosphate with a lower K_m
(C) Dephosphorylation by a glucagon-dependent phosphatase
(D) Increased amounts of the enzyme due to the CREB protein
(E) Phosphorylation on serine residues

37. A 4-month-old boy is brought to the physician because of listlessness, vomiting, watery stools, and a 4-day history of fever. His temperature is 38.4°C (101.1°F). Physical examination shows the infant has a protuberant abdomen, thin extremities, and a doll-like face. Blood chemistry shows serum glucose is 45 mg/dL (N = 70-150 mg/dL), pH is 7.30 (N = 7.35 – 7.45), bicarbonate is 16 mEq/L (N = 22 – 26 mEq/L), lactate is 3.2 mEq/L (N = 1.0-3.3 mEq/L), uric acid is 7.3 mg/dL (N = 2.0–6.2 mg/dL), and triglycerides are 143 mg/dL (N under 10 years of age = <75 mg/dL). Additional studies would most likely show which of the following sets of laboratory results?

	Serum Glucose	Serum Lactate	Serum Pyruvate
A.	↑	↑	↑
B.	↑	↑	↓
C.	↑	↓	↓
D.	↓	↑	↑
E.	↓	↓	↓

(A)
(B)
(C)
(D)
(E)

38. An 11-year-old boy is being examined by his pediatrician because his parents are concerned that he has been complaining of muscle pain and cramping in his legs after riding his bike around with his friends. He says that this has been happening a lot lately but that it usually goes away, especially after he eats his lunch or dinner. His mother states that another concern she has is that the prior morning, she noticed that her son had a reddish tinge to his urine. Physical examination shows that the boy is well within developmental parameters and appears otherwise healthy. Which of the following is the most likely deficiency contributing to this patient's primary complaint?
(A) Acid α-glucosidase
(B) 1,4-α-Glucan branching enzyme 1
(C) Glucose-6-phosphate dehydrogenase
(D) Glycogen phosphorylase
(E) Pyruvate kinase

39. A 4-month-old girl is being examined by pediatrician because her mother is concerned that she is not feeding well and that she seems to be having trouble breathing, especially during feeding. The infant was born at 38 weeks gestation following an uneventful and uncomplicated pregnancy. Physical examination finds that the infant is hypotonic, has macroglossia, and a palpable liver. The infant has a temperature of 37.2°C (98.8°F) and respirations of 60 breaths per minute (N =24–40 breaths per minute). Cardiac auscultation finds S4 sounds prior to S1 sounds indicative of ventricular hypertrophy. Given the signs and symptoms in this patient, which of the following is most likely?
(A) Cori disease
(B) Hurler syndrome
(C) Hunter syndrome
(D) McArdle disease
(E) Pompe disease
(F) Tay-Sachs disease
(G) von Gierke disease

40. A 2-month-old male infant is brought to the Emergency Department by his parents because they are concerned about their difficulty in arousing him. Upon questioning, the parents state that their baby sleeps through the night and that over the past week it has been progressively more difficult for them to arouse him in the mornings. Physical examination finds the infant to be afebrile, has a palpable liver, and is manifesting generalized hypotonia. All other vital signs appear normal. The infant is at the 15th percentile for length and weight and at the 50th percentile for head circumference. History reveals that the infant was at the 35th percentile for both length and weight when born. The attending orders laboratory studies which find a normal CBC, and normal serum lactate, Na^+, Cl^-, and K^+ levels. Serum glucose is 57 mg/dL and there is moderate elevation in the levels of AST, ALT, and creatinine kinase. Despite the patient's most likely metabolic defect, a metabolic pathway is contributing to a reduction in the severity resulting from the primary dysfunction. The initial reaction of this pathway most likely requires which of the following vitamin-derived cofactors?

(A) Biotin
(B) Folate
(C) Niacin
(D) Thiamine
(E) Pyridoxine

41. A 3-month-old female infant is rushed to the Emergency Department by her mother following the onset of a seizure. The infant is stabilized, and a physical examination shows a demonstrably palpable liver, thin extremities, and that she is at the 10th percentile for both weight and length. The mother reports that her daughter has slept through the night for the past week and that it is difficult to rouse her in the mornings. She indicates that her daughter feeds frequently but does not stay awake for long after feeding. History reveals that the infant was born at 38 weeks gestation following an uncomplicated pregnancy. Blood is drawn for laboratory studies with the following serum findings:

Na^+	140 mEq/L (N = 135–145 mEq/L)
Cl^-	103 mEq/L (N = 95–110 mEq/L)
HCO_3^-	12 mEq/L (N = 16–24 mE/L)
Glucose	35 mg/dL (N = 70–150 mg/dL)
Lactate	7.6 mmol/L (N = 0.22–2.98 mmol/L)
Total cholesterol	205 mg/dL (N = < 170 mg/dL)
Triglycerides	457 mg/dL (N = < 150 mg/dL)

Given the most likely diagnosis in this patient, which of the following organelles is most likely to be involved in the pathogenesis of the disease?

(A) Endoplasmic reticulum
(B) Lysosomes
(C) Mitochondria
(D) Nucleus
(E) Peroxisomes

42. A 5-month-old boy is brought to the Emergency Department by his mother due to concerns about his rapid noisy breathing. Physical examination finds that the infant is afebrile, has a respiration rate of 75 breaths per minute associated with retractions, and has a bluish tinge to his lips. Cardiac auscultation reveals a mid-systolic murmur. EKG finds a shortened PR interval which, combined with the results of the cardiac auscultation indicated to the attending physician that the infant is exhibiting the signs of cardiomyopathy. The signs and symptoms exhibited by this infant are most likely the result of a deficiency in which of the following?

(A) 1,4-α-Glucan branching enzyme 1
(B) Glucose-6-phosphatase
(C) Homogentisic acid oxidase
(D) Lysosomal acid α-glucosidase
(E) Myophosphorylase
(F) Phenylalanine hydroxylase

43. A 3-month-old female infant is rushed to the Emergency Department by her mother following the onset of a seizure. The infant is stabilized, and a physical examination shows a demonstrably palpable liver, thin extremities, and that she is at the 10th percentile for both weight and length. The mother reports that her daughter has slept through the night for the past week and that it is difficult to rouse her in the mornings. She indicates that her daughter feeds frequently but does not stay awake for lnog after feeding. Blood is drawn for laboratory studies and reveals two striking findings, a glucose level of 48 mg/dL, despite the infant feeding shortly after arrival to the Emergency Department, and a lactate level of 3.8 mmol/L (N = 0.22–2.98 mmol/L). Given the signs and symptoms presenting in this infant, which of the metabolic processes is most likely to be found to be abnormal?

(A) Branched-chain amino acid catabolism
(B) Glycogen synthesis
(C) Medium-chain length fatty acid oxidation
(D) Microsomal branched-chain fatty acid oxidation
(E) Purine nucleotide synthesis

44. A 13-year-old girl is being examined by her pediatrician because her parents are concerned that she has been complaining of muscle pain and cramping in his legs and severe fatigue following involvement in school sports activities. She says that this has been happening a lot lately but that it usually goes away, especially after she eats her dinner. The patient reports that she has also noticed that on some occasions she notices what she thinks is blood in her urine. History is unremarkable with no evidence of any significant illnesses beyond common colds. Physical examination shows that the girl is well within developmental parameters and appears otherwise healthy. Suspecting a metabolic problem, the pediatrician orders a forearm ischemic exercise test (FIET), the results of which find that the level of lactate produced is well below the expected value with a normal level of detectable ammonia. Given the most likely diagnosis in this patient, which of the following complications is most likely to affect this patient?

(A) Cataracts
(B) Cirrhosis
(C) Nephrolithiasis
(D) Retinal pigment epithelial (RPE) dystrophy
(E) Ventricular cardiomyopathy

45. A 2-month-old male infant is brought to the Emergency Department by his parents because they are concerned about their difficulty in arousing him. Upon questioning, the parents state that their baby sleeps through the night and that over the past week it has been progressively more difficult for them to arouse him in the mornings. Physical examination finds the infant to be afebrile, has a palpable liver, and is manifesting generalized hypotonia. All other vital signs appear normal. The infant is at the 15th percentile for length and weight and at the 50th percentile for head circumference. History reveals that the infant was at the 35th percentile for both length and weight when born. The attending orders laboratory studies which find a normal CBC, and normal serum lactate, Na^+, Cl^-, and K^+ levels. Serum glucose is 37 mg/dL and there is moderate elevation in the levels of AST, ALT, and creatinine kinase. The physician suspects the infant is showing the signs and symptoms of a metabolic defect in carbohydrate homeostasis which is most likely due to a deficiency in which of the following?

(A) Branching of glycogen polymers
(B) Carboxylation of pyruvate
(C) Debranching of glycogen polymers
(D) Erythrocyte production of pyruvate
(E) Lysosomal catabolism of glycogen
(F) Release of free glucose

ANSWERS

1. Correct answer is **D.** The patient is suffering from a form of type I glycogen storage disease (GSD I). The most common form of the disorder is referred to as von Gierke disease (also called type Ia) and results from a defect in the gene encoding glucose-6-phosphatase (choice C). However, some type I patients, although exhibiting identical symptoms, turn out not to be deficient in glucose-6-phosphatase. These latter patients are identified as having type Ib GSD. The mechanism by which free glucose is released from glucose-6-phosphate involves several different steps. Glucose-6-phosphate must first be transported from the cytosol into the lumen of the endoplasmic reticulum, ER. Inside the ER the phosphate is removed through the action of ER localized glucose-6-phosphatase. Type Ib disease results from defects in the glucose-6-phosphate transporter 1. Thus, liver cells from type Ib patients will not accumulate glucose inside the membranes of the ER. Deficiency in aldolase A (choice A) results in the fructose metabolic disorder, hereditary fructose intolerance. Deficiency in fructose-1,6-bisphosphatase results in severely impaired hepatic gluconeogenesis and leads to episodes of hypoglycemia, apnea, hyperventilation, ketosis, and lactic acidosis. The glucose transporter GLUT2 (choice E) is responsible for transport of free glucose out of the ER to the cytosol where it can then be transported out of the hepatocyte into the blood, also via the action of GLUT2. The inorganic phosphate transporter (choice F), NPT4 encoded by the *SLC17A3* gene, is responsible for transport of the phosphate released from glucose-6-phosphate from the lumen of the ER to the cytosol. Although it has been postulated that deficiency in NPT4 function could result in a form of type I GSD, suggested to be type Ic, there is no evidence for this.

2. Correct answer is **D.** The patient is most likely suffering the consequences of Andersen disease (type IV glycogen storage disease). Andersen disease, also referred to as amylopectinosis, results from mutations in the glycogen branching enzyme. Since infants with Andersen disease cannot properly branch glycogen, it is poorly soluble, especially within hepatocytes, resulting in rapid development of hepatic fibrosis (cirrhosis). There is no cure for Andersen disease, but dietary modification can help ameliorate the pathology. The most useful diet for Andersen disease infants is high in protein to ensure both growth and energy demands via amino acid oxidation. Since infants do not carry out gluconeogenesis as efficiently as older children and adults, they need a certain amount of glucose in their diet and thus it cannot be restricted (choice A). A high-fat, low carbohydrate diet (choice B) could provide much of the energy demands of a neonate; however, infants and children require adequate protein intake for growth. Feeding these infants high amounts of glucose containing carbohydrates (choice C) would only lead to exacerbation of the production of the insoluble glycogen. Lactose restriction (choice E) would be beneficial in infants with classic galactosemia but not in Andersen disease. Restriction of sucrose (choice F) may be somewhat beneficial in infants with fructose metabolic disorders but not in Andersen disease infants.

3. Correct answer is **C.** The infant most likely suffered from the effects of the glycogen storage disease known Pompe disease. Pompe disease results from defects in the gene (*GAA*) encoding acid α-glucosidase, also known as lysosomal acid maltase. Due to defects in acid maltase function, there is massive accumulation of glycogen within the vacuoles of all tissues. Pompe disease was the first lysosomal storage disease to be characterized. The clinical presentation of Pompe disease encompasses a wide range of phenotypes but all include various degrees of cardiomegaly. Additional clinical manifestations associated with idiopathic cardiomegaly accompanied by storage of glycogen are indicative of Pompe disease. These symptoms include hepatomegaly, marked hypotonia, muscular weakness and death before 1 year of age. The different phenotypes can be classified dependent upon age of onset, extent of organ involvement and the rate of progression to death. The infantile-onset form is the most severe and was the phenotype described by Joannes Pompe. Defects in cardiac muscle glycosaminoglycan synthesis (choice A) represent one of pathologies of mucopolysaccharidotic disease known as Hurler syndrome. Defects in hepatic bile acid synthesis (choice B) are associated with numerous disorders with the most common being associated with progressive jaundice, hepatomegaly, pruritis, and fat malabsorption. Defects in mitochondrial branched-chain amino acid metabolism (choice D) is the basis of the disease known as maple syrup urine disease, MSUD. Defects in mitochondrial fatty acid oxidation (choice E) are associated with numerous disorders with medium-chain acyl-CoA dehydrogenase (MCAD) deficiency exhibiting serious pathology in the neonate.

4. Correct answer is **D.** The patient is most likely suffering the consequences of Andersen disease (type IV glycogen storage disease). Andersen disease, also referred to as amylopectinosis, results from mutations in the glycogen branching enzyme. Since infants with Andersen disease cannot properly branch glycogen, it is poorly soluble, especially within hepatocytes, resulting in rapid development of hepatic fibrosis (cirrhosis). Defects in the other metabolic processes (choices A, B, C, E, and F) do not manifest with the symptoms appearing in this infant.

5. Correct answer is **A.** The patient is most likely suffering from von Gierke disease. von Gierke disease (also called type Ia glycogen storage disese) results from a defect in the gene encoding glucose-6-phosphatase. The mechanism by which free glucose is released from glucose-6-phosphate involves several different steps. Glucose-6-phosphate must first be transported from the cytosol into the lumen of the endoplasmic reticulum, ER. Inside the ER the phosphate is removed through the action of ER localized glucose-6-phosphatase. The lack of glucose-6-phosphatase activity would result in the radioctive glucose remaining associated with the microsomal fraction whereas in normal hepatocytes the radioactive phosphate would be released, transported out of the microsomal fraction and thus no longer be associated with the membrane fraction. A deficiency in the glucose-6-phosphate transporter (choice B) would prevent transport of radioactive glucose-6-phosphate into the microsomes and there would be no radioactivity associated with this membrane fraction of hepatocytes. Free glucose is transported out of the ER (choice C) after removal of the phosphate from glucose-6-phosphate. A defect in this glucose transport process would not prevent the free radioactive inorganic phosphate from being transported out of the microsomes. Defects in glycogen branching enzyme (choice D) and glycogen debranching enzyme (choice E) would not affect microsomal distribution of glucose-6-phosphate.

6. Correct answer is **D.** The infant most likely succumbed to the glycogen storage disease known as Pompe disease. Pompe disease (glycogen storage disease type II, GSD II) results from defects in the gene (*GAA*) encoding acid α-glucosidase, also known as lysosomal acid maltase. Thus, the disease is also referred to as acid maltase deficiency (AMD). The clinical presentation of GSD II encompasses a wide range of phenotypes but all include various degrees of cardiomegaly. Additional clinical manifestations associated with idiopathic cardiomegaly accompanied by storage of glycogen are indicative of Pompe disease. These symptoms included hepatomegaly, marked hypotonia, muscular weakness, and death before 1 year of age. The different phenotypes can be classified dependent upon age of onset, extent of organ involvement, and the rate of progression to death. Andersen disease (choice A), also known as glycogen storage disease type IV, is characterized by hepatosplenomegaly and failure to thrive. The disease progresses to liver cirrhosis and portal vein hypertension, and death usually by 5 years of age due to liver failure. Cori disease (choice B), also known as glycogen storage disease type III, is associated with hepatomegaly, ketotic hypoglycemia, hyperlipidemia, variable skeletal myopathy, cardiomyopathy, and short stature. McArdle disease (choice C), also known as glycogen storage disease type V, is usually seen in young adulthood and is characterized by exercise intolerance and muscle cramps following bursts of muscle activity such as during sprint training. The hallmark features of von Gierke disease (choice E), manifest in infants of 3–4 months of age and includes hypoglycemia, lactic acidosis, hyperuricemia, and hyperlipidemia.

7. Correct answer is **E.** Glycogen homeostasis is controlled by regulating the rate of glycogen synthesis and breakdown. Release of glucose from stored glycogen is the role of glycogen phosphorylase (commonly just called phosphorylase). The rate of glucose liberation from glycogen by phosphorylase is controlled primarily by short-term phosphorylation and dephosphorylation events. When phosphorylase is phosphorylated phosphorylase kinase is more active in releasing glucose. This phosphorylation occurs in hepatocytes when stimulation by glucagon or epinephrine leads to increased activity of PKA which in turn phosphorylates, and activates, phosphorylase kinase. Active phosphorylase liberates glucose-1-phosphate from glycogen which is converted to glucose-6-phosphate. The glucose-6-phosphate is either oxidized in the glycolytic pathway or the phosphate is removed by glucose-6-phosphatase and the free glucose flows into the blood. When glucose-6-phosphate levels rise in hepatocytes, due to reduced utilization, it acts as an allosteric inhibitor of the phosphorylated and active form of phosphorylase. AMP (choice A) acts to allosterically activate the dephosphorylated, less active form of phosphorylase. Calcium ions (choice B) will bind to the calmodulin subunit of phosphorylase kinase making the enzyme more active at phosphorylating and activating phosphorylase. cAMP (choice C) will activate PKA which, in turn, phosphorylates and activates phosphorylates. PKA (choice D) phosphorylates phosphorylase kinase enhancing its activity and thus, increased phosphorylation of phosphorylase.

8. Correct answer is **D.** This child is manifesting the classic signs and symptoms of von Gierke disease which results from mutations in the gene encoding glucose-6-phosphatase. Patients with von Gierke disease can present during the neonatal period with lactic acidosis and hypoglycemia. The hallmark features of this disease are hypoglycemia, lactic acidosis, hyperuricemia, and hyperlipidemia. The severity of the hypoglycemia and lactic acidosis can be such that in the past affected individuals died in infancy. The metabolic consequences of the hepatic glucose-6-phosphatase deficiency of von Gierke disease extend well beyond just the obvious hypoglycemia that results from the deficiency in liver being able to deliver free glucose to the blood. The inability to release the phosphate from glucose-6-phopsphate results in diversion into the pentose phosphate pathway. The oxidation of glucose-6-phosphate via the pentose phosphate pathway leads to increased production of ribose-5-phosphate which then activates the *de novo* synthesis of the purine nucleotides. In excess of hepatic needs, these purine nucleotides will ultimately be catabolized to uric acid resulting in hyperuricemia and consequent symptoms of gout. Elevated levels of dicarboxylic acids (choice A) are a hallmark sign of medium-chain acyl-CoA dehydrogenase (MCAD) deficiency. Elevated fructose-1-phosphate (choice B) occurs in hereditary fructose intolerance due to mutations in the gene encoding aldolase A. Glucocerebrosides (choice C) accumulate in cells of the macrophage lineage in Gaucher disease as a result of mutations in the gene encoding glucocerebrosidase. G_{M2} gangliosides (choice E) accumulate, predominantly in neural tissues, in Tay-Sachs disease as a result of mutations in the *HEXA* gene encoding the α-subunit of hexosaminidase A.

9. Correct answer is **E.** This patient is exhibiting symptoms of Tarui disease (glycogen storage disease type VII). Tarui disease is caused by mutations in the gene (*PKFM*) encoding muscle and erythrocyte PFK1. The symptoms of this disease are very similar to those observed in patients suffering from McArdle disease which results from mutations in the gene (*PYGM*) encoding the muscle isoform of phosphorylase. Similarities in the symptoms of Tarui disease and McArdle disease are exercise-induced pain and myoglobinuria. However, since Tarui disease also involves a defect in erythrocyte PFK1 there are associated mild forms of jaundice, resulting from accelerated destruction of erythrocytes and evidenced by the elevated serum levels of unconjugated bilirubin. Defects in glucose-6-phosphatase (choice A) result in von Gierke disease

whose hallmark features, manifesting in infants of 3–4 months of age, include hypoglycemia, lactic acidosis, hyperuricemia, and hyperlipidemia. Defects in glycogen synthase (choice B) are associated with mutations in the liver isoform encoded by the *GYS2* gene. This particular glycogen storage disease is known as type 0A (GSD0A) and is associated with hyperketonemia, hypoglycemia, and early death. Defects in liver glycogen branching enzyme (choice C) result in Andersen disease which is characterized by hepatosplenomegaly and failure to thrive. The disease progresses to liver cirrhosis and portal vein hypertension, and death usually by 5 years of age due to liver failure. Defects in lysosomal acid maltase (choice D) result in Pompe disease, the hallmarks of which are varying degrees of cardiomegaly. In the most common form of Pompe, children usually do not live beyond the age of two due to heart failure.

10. Correct answer is **A.** The infant is most likely experiencing the symptoms of Andersen disease. Andersen disease (glycogen storage disease type IV) is also known as amylopectinosis. The disease results from defects in the gene (*GBE1*) encoding glycogen-branching enzyme. The disease manifests with progressive hepatosplenomegaly along with the storage of an abnormal glycogen that exhibits poor solubility in the liver. The abnormal glycogen is characterized by few branch points with long outer chains containing more α-1,4-linked glucose than normal glycogen. This resultant structure is similar to that of amylopectin (the structure of starch in plants), thus the associated name of amylopectinosis. Cori disease (choice B), also known as glycogen storage disease type III, is associated with hepatomegaly, ketotic hypoglycemia, hyperlipidemia, variable skeletal myopathy, cardiomyopathy, and short stature. McArdle disease (choice C), also known as glycogen storage disease type V, is usually seen in young adulthood and is characterized by exercise intolerance and muscle cramps following bursts of muscle activity such as during sprint training. Tarui disease (choice D) manifests with symptoms that are similar to those of McArdle disease but results from mutations in the muscle and erythrocyte isoform of PFK1. The involvement of erythrocyte pathology in Tarui results in the added pathology of jaundice and hyperbilirubinemia as a result of hemolysis. The hallmark features of von Gierke disease (choice E), manifest in infants of 3–4 months of age and includes hypoglycemia, lactic acidosis, hyperuricemia, and hyperlipidemia.

11. Correct answer is **C.** The infant most likely succumbed to the glycogen storage disease known as Pompe disease. Pompe disease (glycogen storage disease type II, GSD II) results from defects in the gene (*GAA*) encoding acid α-glucosidase, also known as lysosomal acid maltase. Thus, the disease is also referred to as acid maltase deficiency (AMD). The clinical presentation of GSD II encompasses a wide range of phenotypes, but all include various degrees of cardiomegaly. Additional clinical manifestations associated with idiopathic cardiomegaly accompanied by storage of glycogen are indicative of Pompe disease. These symptoms included hepatomegaly, marked hypotonia, muscular weakness and death before 1 year of age. Erythrocyte pyruvate kinase deficiency (choice A) is one of the most common inherited causes of hemolytic anemia with varying degrees of severity ranging from mild and fully compensated hemolysis to severe cases that require transfusions for survival. In the most severe cases an affected fetus will die in utero. Medium-chain acyl-CoA dehydrogenase deficiency (choice B) manifests with episodic hypoketotic hypoglycemia brought on by fasting. Symptoms appear within the first 2 years of life. Clinical crisis is characterized by an infant presenting with episodes of vomiting and lethargy that may progress to seizures and ultimately coma. Porphyria cutanea tarda (choice D) is an adult-onset disorder resulting from mutations in the heme biosynthetic enzyme, uroporphyrinogen decarboxylase (UROD) and is characterized by blistering skin lesions on sun-exposed areas of the skin. Zellweger syndrome (choice E) represents a spectrum of disorders resulting from mutations in at least 12 genes responsible for peroxisomal biogenesis and/or function. The disorder is a severe neonatal presenting disease where infants display severe hypotonia, weakness, and seizures.

12. Correct answer is **A.** This child is manifesting the classic signs and symptoms of von Gierke disease which results from mutations in the gene encoding glucose-6-phosphatase. Patients with von Gierke disease can present during the neonatal period with lactic acidosis and hypoglycemia. The hallmark features of this disease are hypoglycemia, lactic acidosis, hyperuricemia, and hyperlipidemia. The severity of the hypoglycemia and lactic acidosis can be such that in the past affected individuals died in infancy. Infants often have a doll-like facial appearance due to excess adipose tissue in the cheeks. The metabolic consequences of the hepatic glucose-6-phosphate deficiency of von Gierke disease extend well beyond just the obvious hypoglycemia that results from the deficiency in liver being able to deliver free glucose to the blood. The inability to release the phosphate from glucose-6-phopsphate results in diversion into glycolysis and production of pyruvate as well as increased diversion into the pentose phosphate pathway. The production of excess pyruvate, at levels above of the capacity of pyruvate dehydrogenase to oxidize it, results in its reduction to lactate resulting in lactic acidemia. In addition, some of the pyruvate is transaminated to alanine leading to hyperalaninemia. Some of the pyruvate will be oxidized to acetyl-CoA which can't be fully oxidized in the TCA cycle and so the acetyl-CoA will end up in the cytosol where it will serve as a substrate for triglyceride and cholesterol synthesis resulting in hyperlipidemia. The oxidation of glucose-6-phosphate via the pentose phosphate pathway leads to increased production of ribose-5-phosphate which then activates the *de novo* synthesis of the purine nucleotides. In excess of hepatic needs, these purine nucleotides will ultimately be catabolized to uric acid resulting in hyperuricemia and consequent symptoms of gout. Defects in glycogen synthase (choice B) are associated with mutations in the liver isoform encoded by the *GYS2* gene. This particular glycogen storage disease is known as type 0A and is associated with hyperketonemia, hypoglycemia, and early death. Deficiency in muscle PFK1 (choice C) results in Tarui disease, also known as glycogen storage disease type VII. This defect also impacts erythrocyte PFK1 activity resulting in increased hemolysis and the associated hyperbilirubinemia. Deficiency in muscle phosphorylase (choice D) results in McArdle disease, also known as glycogen storage disease type V. The pathology of McArdle disease is usually seen in young adulthood and is characterized by exercise intolerance and muscle cramps following bursts of muscle activity such as during sprint training. Deficiency in pyruvate kinase (choice E) manifests with pathology of red blood cells and is one of the most common forms of inherited hemolytic anemia.

13. Correct answer is **D.** The infant suffered from the glycogen storage disease known as Pompe disease. Pompe disease (glycogen storage disease type II, GSD II) results from defects in the gene (*GAA*) encoding acid α-glucosidase, also known as lysosomal acid maltase. Thus, the disease is also referred to as acid maltase deficiency (AMD). The clinical presentation of GSD II encompasses a wide range of phenotypes but all include various degrees of cardiomegaly. Deficiency in glucose-6-phosphatase (choice A) results in von Gierke disease, also known as glycogen storage disease type Ia. The hallmark features of von Gierke disease are hypoglycemia, lactic acidosis, hyperuricemia, and hyperlipidemia in the first few months of life. Defects in glycogen branching enzyme (choice B) result in the glycogen storage disease called Andersen disease. Andersen disease is characterized by hepatosplenomegaly and failure to thrive. The disease progresses to liver cirrhosis and portal vein hypertension, and death usually by 5 years of age due to liver failure. Deficiency in glycogen debranching enzyme (choice C) result in the glycogen storage disease known as Cori disease. Cori disease is associated with hepatomegaly, ketotic hypoglycemia, hyperlipidemia, variable skeletal myopathy, cardiomyopathy, and results in short stature. Deficiency in the liver isoform of phosphorylase (choice E) results in the glycogen storage disease known as Hers disease. Hers disease is associated with hepatomegaly, mild fasting hypoglycemia, hyperlipidemia, and ketosis. Deficiency in the muscle isoform of phosphorylase (choice F) results in McArdle disease, also known as glycogen storage disease type V. The pathology of McArdle disease is usually seen in young adulthood and is characterized by exercise intolerance and muscle cramps following bursts of muscle activity such as during sprint training.

14. Correct answer is **D.** The patient is experiencing the symptoms of the glycogen storage disease known as McArdle disease which results from mutations in the gene (*PYGM*) encoding the muscle isoform of phosphorylase. The clinical presentation of McArdle disease is usually seen in young adulthood and is characterized by exercise intolerance and muscle cramps following shorts burst of muscle activity. Attacks of myoglobinuria frequently accompany the muscle symptoms and about half of McArdle disease patients will exhibit burgundy colored urine after exercise. Deficiency in glucocerebrosidase (choice A) is the cause of the lysosomal storage disease known as Gaucher disease. Deficiency in glucose-6-phosphatase (choice B) results in von Gierke disease, also known as glycogen storage disease type Ia. The hallmark features of von Gierke disease are hypoglycemia, lactic acidosis, hyperuricemia, and hyperlipidemia in the first few months of life. Deficiency in hexosaminidase A (choice C) results in the lysosomal storage disease known as Tay-Sach disease, a disease for which there is no cure and results in death, usually by the age of 2. Deficiency in sphingomyelinase (choice E) results in the lysosomal storage disease known as Niemann-Pick disease, a disease in which the most common form (type A) results in death by 2 to 3 years of age.

15. Correct answer is **D.** The infant is most likely suffering from the effects of Andersen disease (glycogen storage disease type IV) which is also known as amylopectinosis. Andersen disease results from mutations in the gene (*GBE1*) encoding glycogen branching enzyme, also called amylo-(1,4 to 1,6) transglycosylase. The disease manifests with progressive hepatosplenomegaly along with the storage of an abnormal glycogen that exhibits poor solubility in the liver. The abnormal glycogen is characterized by few branch points with long outer chains containing more α-1,4-linked glucose than normal glycogen. This resultant structure is similar to that of amylopectin (the structure of starch in plants), thus the associated name of amylopectinosis. Defects in none of the other metabolic processes (choices A, B, C, E, and F) are related to the symptoms experienced by the infant.

16. Correct answer is **C.** Epinephrine can bind and activate both α-adrenergic and β-adrenergic receptors. Hepatocytes express both the α_1- and β_2-adrenergic receptors. When epinephrine binds α_1-adrenergic receptors there is an activation of the associated G_q-type G protein which then activates the membrane-associated enzyme phospholipase Cβ (PLCβ). PLCβ hydrolyzes membrane PIP_2 into diacylglycerol (DAG) and inositol trisphosphate (IP_3). The IP_3 then binds to receptors present in membranes of the endoplasmic reticulum (ER) resulting in release of stored calcium ion. The released calcium binds to the calmodulin subunit of phosphorylase kinase (PHK) resulting in its activation. Phosphorylase kinase then phosphorylates both phosphorylase and glycogen synthase which activates the former and inhibits the later (choice B). When epinephrine binds the hepatic β_2-adrenergic receptors there is activation of adenylate cyclase resulting in increased cAMP with consequent activation of PKA. PKA phosphorylates and activates phosphorylase kinase with the results being the same as for the activation of the α_1-adrenergic receptor. Epinephrine does not stimulate carbohydrate absorption from the gut (choice A) nor enhance muscle proteolysis (choice D). Epinephrine actions will result in stimulation of gluconeogenesis in the liver and the propionyl-CoA derived from the oxidation of fatty acids (choice E) with an odd number of carbon atoms can be used for glucose synthesis. However, the level of fatty acids with odd numbers of carbon atoms in humans represents less than 1% of the total and the resultant propionyl-CoA from their oxidation represents a fraction of the total carbon that could be used for glucose synthesis.

17. Correct answer is **B.** This child is manifesting the classic signs and symptoms of von Gierke disease (glycogen storage disease type Ia) which results from deficiency in glucose 6-phosphatase activity. Patients with von Gierke disease can present during the neonatal period with lactic acidosis and hypoglycemia. The hallmark features of this disease are hypoglycemia, lactic acidosis, hyperuricemia, and hyperlipidemia. The severity of the hypoglycemia and lactic acidosis can be such that in the past affected individuals died in infancy. Infants often have a doll-like facial appearance due to excess adipose tissue in the cheeks. The metabolic consequences of the hepatic glucose-6-phosphate deficiency of von Gierke disease extend well beyond just the obvious hypoglycemia that results from the deficiency in liver being able to deliver free glucose to the blood. The inability to release the phosphate from glucose-6-phopsphate results in diversion into glycolysis and production of pyruvate as well as increased diversion onto the pentose phosphate pathway. The production of excess pyruvate, at levels above of the capacity of the TCA cycle to completely oxidize it, results in its reduction to lactate resulting in lactic acidemia. In addition, some of the pyruvate is transaminated to alanine leading to hyperalaninemia. Some of the pyruvate will be oxidized to acetyl-CoA which can't be fully oxidized in the TCA cycle and so the acetyl-CoA will end up in the cytosol where it will serve as a substrate for triglyceride and cholesterol synthesis resulting in hyperlipidemia. The oxidation of glucose-6-phophate via the pentose phosphate pathway leads to increased production of ribose-5-phosphate which then activates the *de novo* synthesis of the purine nucleotides. In excess of the need, these purine nucleotides will ultimately be catabolized to uric acid resulting in hyperuricemia and consequent symptoms of gout. Erythrocyte pyruvate kinase deficiency (choice A) is one of the most common inherited causes of hemolytic anemia with varying degrees of severity ranging from mild and fully compensated hemolysis to severe cases that require transfusions for survival. In the most severe cases an affected fetus will die in utero. Deficiency in the liver isoform of glycogen synthase (choice C) is the cause of glycogen storage disease type 0A. This glycogen storage disease is associated with hypoglycemia, hyperketonemia, and early death. Deficiency in hepatic pyruvate kinase (choice D) has not been detected. Deficiency in the muscle isoform of phosphorylase (choice E) results in McArdle disease. Deficiency in muscle glycogen synthase (choice F) is the cause of glycogen storage disease type 0B which is associated with sudden cardiac arrest particularly after physical activity.

18. Correct answer is **D.** This patient is most likely experiencing the symptoms of McArdle disease. Deficiency in muscle phosphorylase activity is associated with the development of McArdle disease (glycogen storage disease type V). The clinical presentation of McArdle disease is usually seen in young adulthood and is characterized by exercise intolerance and muscle cramps following burst of aerobic exercise, such as during sprint training. Attacks of myoglobinuria frequently accompany the muscle symptoms of McArdle disease and about half of all patients will exhibit burgundy colored urine after exercise. Deficiency in muscle creatine kinase (choice A), which would lead to deficiency in creatine phosphate (choice B), however, the incidence of creatine kinase deficiency is extremely rare but will be associated with death from myocardial infarction in middle age. Muscle cells do not express glucose-6-phosphatase (choice C). Deficiency in muscle glycogen synthase (choice E) is the cause of glycogen storage disease type 0B which is associated with sudden cardiac arrest particularly after physical activity.

19. Correct answer is **D.** This patient is most likely experiencing the symptoms of McArdle disease. Deficiency in muscle phosphorylase activity is associated with the development of McArdle disease (glycogen storage disease type V). The clinical presentation of McArdle disease is usually seen in young adulthood and is characterized by exercise intolerance and muscle cramps following burst of aerobic exercise, such as during sprint training. Attacks of myoglobinuria frequently accompany the muscle symptoms of McArdle disease and about half of all patients will exhibit burgundy colored urine after exercise. Deficiency in glucocerebrosidase (choice A) results in the lysosomal storage disease called Gaucher disease. Deficiency in glucose-6-phosphatase (choice B) results in von Gierke disease, also known as glycogen storage disease type Ia. The hallmark features of von Gierke disease are hypoglycemia, lactic acidosis, hyperuricemia, and hyperlipidemia in the first few months of life. Deficiency in hexosaminidase A (choice C) results in the lysosomal storage disease known as Tay-Sach disease, a disease for which there is no cure and results in death, usually by the age of 2. Deficiency in sphingomyelinase (choice E) results in the lysosomal storage disease known as Niemann-Pick disease, a disease in which the most common form (type A) results in death by 2 to 3 years of age.

20. Correct answer is **D.** The infant suffered from the glycogen storage disease known as Pompe disease. Pompe disease (glycogen storage disease type II, GSD II) results from defects in the gene (*GAA*) encoding acid α-glucosidase, also known as lysosomal acid maltase. Thus, the disease is also referred to as acid maltase deficiency (AMD). The clinical presentation of GSD II encompasses a wide range of phenotypes but all include various degrees of cardiomegaly. Defects in fructose metabolism are most severe when the defect is in the aldolase B gene which is the cause of hereditary fructose intolerance. Defects in galactose metabolism can occur due to mutations in several of the genes encoding enzymes in this process, but the most significant is classic galactosemia which results from mutations in the gene (*GALT*) encoding galactose-1-phosphate uridyltransferase. Defects in gluconeogenesis (choice C) predominantly occur with mutations in pyruvate carboxylase or fructose-1,6-bisphosphatase. Defects in glycolysis (choice E) would be associated with severe pathology most likely resulting in early lethality.

21. Correct answer is **D.** The signs and symptoms in this patient are typical of those associated with McArdle disease. McArdle disease results from deficiency in muscle glycogen phosphorylase activity. The clinical presentation of GSD V is usually seen in young adulthood and is characterized by exercise intolerance and muscle cramps following slight exercise. Attacks of myoglobinuria frequently accompany the muscle symptoms of McArdle disease and about half of these individuals will exhibit burgundy colored urine after exercise. Deficiency in acid α-glucosidase, also known as lysosomal acid maltase (choice A), results in the glycogen storage disease known as Pompe disease. Pompe disease is associated with hepatomegaly, marked hypotonia, muscular weakness and death before 1 year of age. Deficiency in glucose-6-phosphatase (choice B) results in von Gierke disease, also known as glycogen storage disease type Ia. The hallmark features of von Gierke disease are hypoglycemia, lactic acidosis, hyperuricemia, and hyperlipidemia in the first few months of life. Deficiency in glycogen-debranching enzyme (choice C) results in the glycogen storage disease known as Cori disease. Cori disease is associated with hepatomegaly, ketotic hypoglycemia, hyperlipidemia, variable skeletal myopathy, cardiomyopathy, and results in short stature. Deficiency in UDP-glucose pyrophosphorylase (choice E) is not found in humans.

22. Correct answer is **A.** High carbohydrate loading, as is typical for distance runners, results in an increased level of insulin release from the pancreas. Insulin effects on the liver include changes in the activities of several enzymes, such as that of glucokinase. Glucokinase is the hepatic form of the glucose phosphorylating family of enzymes known as hexokinases (choice D). Within the liver insulin activates glycolysis and inhibits gluconeogenesis so the activity of glucose-6-phosphatase (choice B) and lactate dehydrogenase (choice E) would be reduced, not stimulated. Insulin stimulates the formation of glycogen, in liver and skeletal muscle, by activating glycogen synthase and inhibiting phosphorylase (choice C).

23. Correct answer is **A.** The infant suffered from the glycogen storage disease known as Pompe disease. Pompe disease (glycogen storage disease type II, GSD II) results from defects in the gene (*GAA*) encoding acid α-glucosidase, also known as lysosomal acid maltase. Thus, the disease is also referred to as acid maltase deficiency (AMD). The clinical presentation of Pompe disease encompasses a wide range of phenotypes but all include various degrees of cardiomegaly. Deficiency in glucose-6-phosphatase (choice B) results in von Gierke disease, also known as glycogen storage disease type Ia. The hallmark features of von Gierke disease are hypoglycemia, lactic acidosis, hyperuricemia, and hyperlipidemia in the first few months of life. Deficiency in the liver isoform of phosphorylase (choice C) results in the glycogen storage disease known as Hers disease. Hers disease is associated with hepatomegaly, mild fasting hypoglycemia, hyperlipidemia, and ketosis. Deficiency in muscle PFK1 (choice D) results in Tarui disease, also known as glycogen storage disease type VII. This defect also impacts erythrocyte PFK1 activity resulting in increased hemolysis and the associate hyperbilirubinemia. Deficiency in the muscle isoform of phosphorylase (choice E) results in McArdle disease, also known as glycogen storage disease type V. The pathology of McArdle disease is usually seen in young adulthood and is characterized by exercise intolerance and muscle cramps following bursts of muscle activity such as during sprint training.

24. Correct answer is **C.** The child is suffering from Cori disease, glycogen storage disease type III (GSD III) which is also known as Forbes disease and limit dextrinosis. Cori disease results from defects in the gene (*AGL*) encoding glycogen-debranching enzyme, also known as amylo-1,6-glucosidase. Deficiency in glycogen debranching activity causes hepatomegaly, ketotic hypoglycemia, hyperlipidemia, variable skeletal myopathy, cardiomyopathy, and results in short stature. Patients with both liver and muscle involvement have GSD IIIa and those with only liver involvement (~15% of GSD III patients) are classified as GSD IIIb. Because hepatomegaly, hypoglycemia, hyperlipidemia, and growth retardation are common symptoms in both von Gierke disease (GSD Ia) and Cori disease, it is difficult to initially determine from which disease an infant is suffering. Definitive diagnosis is only made by examining the structure of the glycogen in patients as well as assaying for the level of activity of the debranching enzyme. Deficiency in glucokinase results in the inherited form of maturity onset type diabetes of the young (MODY) known as MODY2. Deficiency in glucose-6-phosphatase (choice B) results in von Gierke disease, also known as glycogen storage disease type Ia. The hallmark features of von Gierke disease are hypoglycemia, lactic acidosis, hyperuricemia, and hyperlipidemia in the first few months of life. Deficiency in the liver isoform of phosphorylase (choice D) results in the glycogen storage disease known as Hers disease. Hers disease is associated with hepatomegaly, mild fasting hypoglycemia, hyperlipidemia, and ketosis. Defects in glycogen synthase (choice E) are associated with mutations in the liver isoform encoded by the GYS2 gene. This particular glycogen storage disease is known as type 0A and is associated with hyperketonemia, hypoglycemia, and early death.

25. Correct answer is **A.** Epinephrine can bind and activate both α-adrenergic and β-adrenergic receptors. Hepatocytes express both the α_1- and β_2-adrenergic receptors. When epinephrine binds α_1-adrenergic receptors there is an activation of the associated G_q-type G protein which then activates the membrane-associated enzyme phospholipase Cβ (PLCβ) as a result of the activation of the receptor-associated G_q-type G protein. PLCβ hydrolyzes membrane PIP_2 into diacylglycerol (DAG) and inositol trisphosphate (IP_3). The IP_3 then binds to receptors present in membranes of the endoplasmic reticulum (ER) resulting in release of stored calcium ion. The released calcium binds to the calmodulin subunit of phosphorylase kinase (PHK) resulting in activation of this regulatory enzyme. PHK will then phosphorylate both phosphorylase and glycogen synthase. The net effect is enhanced activity of phosphorylase and inhibited activity of glycogen synthase. The β-adrenergic receptors (choice B) and the glucagon receptor (choice D) are coupled to G_s-type G proteins that activate adenylate cyclase resulting in increased cAMP production. The cortisol receptor (choice C) is the glucocorticoid receptor that is a member of the nuclear receptor family of ligand-activated transcription factors. The effect of activation of nuclear receptors is direct alteration of gene expression and is technically independent of cAMP action but does not represent the more correct choice. The insulin receptor (choice E) exerts its effects in response to receptor tyrosine phosphorylation. The effect of activation of the insulin receptor is technically independent of cAMP action but does not represent the more correct choice.

26. Correct answer is **A.** Regulation of the activity of glycogen synthase is altered by both covalent modification and allosteric effectors. When glycogen synthase is phosphorylated by phosphorylase kinase it is rendered less active (referred to as the glycogen synthase-*b* state). When in this less active state the enzyme activity can be enhanced by the positive allosteric effector glucose-6-phosphate. The more active state of glycogen synthase, referred to as the glycogen synthase-a state, is the dephosphorylated state of the enzymes and this state of the enzyme does not respond to changing levels of glucose-6-phosphate. Glycogen phosphorylase is inhibited by glucose-6-phosphate (choice D) but only when the enzyme is in the phosphorylated state. None of the other options (choices B, C, E, and F) are associated with glucose-6-phosphate-mediated effects.

27. Correct answer is **C.** Epinephrine, released from adrenal medullary cells in response to sympathetic outflow, can bind and activate both α-adrenergic and β-adrenergic receptors. When epinephrine binds α_1-adrenergic receptors there is an activation of the associated G_q-type G protein which then activates the membrane-associated enzyme, phospholipase Cβ (PLCβ). PLCβ hydrolyzes membrane PIP_2 into diacylglycerol (DAG) and inositol trisphosphate (IP_3). The IP_3 then binds to receptors present in membranes of the endoplasmic reticulum (ER) resulting in release of stored calcium ion. The released calcium binds to the calmodulin subunit of phosphorylase kinase (PHK) resulting in activation of this regulatory enzyme as opposed to inhibition (choice F). Activated phosphorylase kinase will then phosphorylate and inhibit, not activate (choice B) glycogen synthase and phosphorylate and activate, not inhibit phosphorylase (choice E). When epinephrine binds β-adrenergic receptors there is activation of adenylate cyclase resulting in increased cAMP with consequent activation of PKA. PKA phosphorylates and activates phosphorylase kinase with the results being the same as for α_1-adrenergic receptor activation. The activity of the glycogen debranching enzyme (choices A and D) is independent of any epinephrine-mediated effects.

28. Correct answer is **E.** Acetylcholine binding to nictotinic acetylcholine receptors in the neuromuscular junction results in depolarization of the muscle cell membrane and an influx of calcium ion. This calcium influx triggers muscle contraction. Muscle contraction results in release of stored calcium ion from sarcoplasmic reticulum. The calcium that is taken up by skeletal muscle in response to acetylcholine-mediated depolarization and the released calcium bind to the calmodulin subunit of glycogen phophorylase kinase resulting in activation of this regulatory enzyme. Activated phosphorylase kinase will then phosphorylate and inhibit glycogen synthase and phosphorylate and activate phosphorylase. None of the other options (choices A, B, C, D, and F) correspond to the changes in skeletal muscle in response to acetylcholine binding its receptors.

29. Correct answer is **A.** When glucagon binds to its receptors on hepatocytes there is activation of the associated G_s-type G protein which, in turn, activates adenylate cyclase resulting in increased production of cAMP with consequent activation of PKA. PKA phosphorylates and activates phosphorylase kinase (PHK) as opposed to inhibiting the enzyme (choice D). Activated phosphorylase kinase will phosphorylate and activate phosphorylase while also phosphorylating and inhibiting glycogen synthase. PKA-mediated phosphorylation of PFK2, in response to glucagon binding its receptor on hepatocytes, activates the phosphatase activity of the enzyme while simultaneously inhibiting its kinase activity (choice C). The effect of this change will result in hydrolysis of fructose-2,6-bisphosphate which is a potent allosteric activator of PFK1, thus the activity of PFK1 will be decreased, as opposed to unaffected (choice B). The activity of phosphoprotein phosphatase 1 (PP1) is controlled by the association of a regulator protein identified as protein targeting glycogen (PTG). In the liver this regulatory subunit is encoded by the *PPP1R3B* gene. Phosphorylation of PTG by PKA releases it from PP1 rendering PP1 less active, as opposed to more active (choice E).

30. Correct answer is **F.** Conditions of low blood glucose result in glucagon release from the pancreas. When glucagon binds to its receptors on hepatocytes there is activation of the associated G_s-type G protein which, in turn, activates adenylate cyclase resulting in increased production of cAMP with consequent activation of PKA. PKA phosphorylates and activates phosphorylase kinase (PHK), thus the level of the phosphorylated enzyme is increased not decreased (choice C). Activated phosphorylase kinase will phosphorylate and activate phosphorylase while also phosphorylating and inhibiting glycogen synthase. Thus, the level of the dephosphorylated from of glycogen synthase is reduced not increased (choice E). The activity of glucokinase (choice A) is not affected by glucagon-mediated signaling in hepatocytes. The activity of phosphoprotein phosphatase 1 (PP1) is controlled by the association of a regulator protein identified as protein targeting glycogen (PTG). In the liver this regulatory subunit is encoded by the *PPP1R3B* gene. Phosphorylation of PTG by PKA releases it from PP1 rendering PP1 less active not more active (choice D). PP1 is not subjected to PKA-mediated phosphorylation (choice B).

31. Correct answer is **C.** Glucagon and catecholamines such as epinephrine stimulate the mobilization of glycogen by triggering the cAMP cascade. Hormones that increase liver cell cAMP promote glycogen breakdown, and hormones that decrease liver cell cAMP promote glycogen synthesis. Cortisol, the main glucocorticoid, regulates the metabolism of proteins, fats, and carbohydrates. It acts on most organs catabolically. However, on the liver it has anabolic effects, increasing glycogen synthesis and accumulation in the liver. None of the other hormone levels (choices A, B, D, and E) correctly associate with their roles in glycogen homeostasis.

32. Correct answer is **D.** The activity of glycogen synthase is inhibited when the enzyme undergoes phosphorylation. There are a number of kinases that target this enzyme for inhibition including phosphorylase kinase (PHK), PKA, PKC, and GSK3. Thus, removal of the phosphate added by any of these enzymes would result in increased glycogen synthase activity. The primary phosphatase responsible for dephosphorylating glycogen synthase is PP1. Dephosphorylation of glycogen phosphorylase by PP1 renders the enzyme less active nor enhanced (choice C). None of the other enzymes (choices A, B, and E) is regulated by phosphorylation/dephosphorylation.

33. Correct answer is **C.** The patient is experiencing the signs and symptoms of McArdle disease. McArdle disease is a glycogen storage disease of the muscle glycogenosis family. A deficiency in muscle phosphorylase results in defective release of glucose from glycogen stores preventing energy production from glucose oxidation in skeletal muscle during brief periods of intense exertion. Metabolism of glucose (choice A), acquired from the blood, and the metabolism of the byproduct of glycolysis, pyruvate (choice E) is not impaired in McArdle disease. Glycerol (choice B) and lactate (choice D) do not provide energy for muscle activity.

34. Correct answer is **A.** Epinephrine, released from adrenal medullary cells in response to sympathetic outflow, can bind and activate both α-adrenergic and β-adrenergic receptors. When epinephrine binds β_2-adrenergic receptors on hepatocytes there is an activation of the associated G_s-type G protein which then activates adenylate cyclase resulting in increased cAMP with consequent activation of PKA. PKA phosphorylates and activates phosphorylase kinase. Phosphorylase kinase will phosphorylate and activate glycogen phosphorylase. Phosphorylase kinase will also phosphorylate and inhibit glycogen synthase (choice B). PKA also phosphorylates PFK2 which activates its phosphatase activity and inhibits its kinase activity. The phosphatase activity of PFK2 will result in reduced levels of the potent allosteric activator of PFK1, fructose-2,6-bisphosphate. The net effect of this will be decreased activity of PFK1 (choice C). The activity of pyruvate carboxylase (choice D) is not directly responsive to the actions of epinephrine binding to its hepatocyte receptors. PKA also phosphorylates and inhibits the hepatic isoform of pyruvate kinase (choice E).

35. Correct answer is **E.** Given that liver glycogen phosphorylase, debranching enzyme, and glucose-6-phosphatase activities were normal, coupled with the patients age, one can rule out Hers disease, Cori disease, and von Gierke disease, respectively. A deficiency in the activity of the hepatic form of phosphorylase kinase results in a glycogen storage disease (GSD9A1/A2) whose symptoms include hepatomegaly, hypercholesterolemia, hypertriglyceridemia, fasting hyperketosis, and elevated plasma AST and ALT. These symptoms are similar to, but less severe than those exhibited in patients with Hers disease. Deficiency in glycogen branching enzyme (choice A) results in Andersen disease which is characterized by hepatosplenomegaly and failure to thrive. Andersen disease progresses to liver cirrhosis and portal vein hypertension, and death usually by 5 years of age due to liver failure. Deficiency in hepatic glycogen synthase (choice B) is associated with hypoglycemia, hyperketonemia, and early death. Deficiencies in hexokinase (choice C) and phosphoprotein phosphatase 1 (choice D) have not been described in humans.

36. Correct answer is **E.** During periods of fasting the pancreas releases glucagon to stimulate the liver to deliver glucose to the blood via activation of gluconeogenesis. When glucagon binds to its receptors on hepatocytes there is activation of the associated G_s-type G protein which then activates adenylate cyclase. Adenylate cyclase produces cAMP which then activates PKA. PKA phosphorylates and activates phosphorylase kinase (PHK) which will phosphorylate and activate phosphorylase while also phosphorylating and inhibiting glycogen synthase. Glycogen synthase activity is not affected by AMP (choice A). Glycogen synthase utilizes UDP-glucose as its substrate, not glucose-1-phosphate (choice B). Glycogen phosphorylase is phosphorylated in response to glucagon, not dephosphorylated (choice C). The activity of the transcription factor CREB (choice D) is enhanced by glucagon action in hepatocytes, but the glycogen synthase gene is not a target for the factor.

37. Correct answer is **D.** The infant is most likely suffering from the effects of von Gierke disease. von Gierke disease, the most common of the glycogen storage diseases, results from mutations in the gene encoding glucose-6-phosphatase. The defective enzyme prevents release of phosphate from glucose-6-phosphate which then accumulates resulting in inhibition of phosphorylase. The reduced activity of phosphorylase leads to reduced release of glucose from glycogen. Combined, these effects result in severe hypoglycemia. An additional consequence of von Gierke disease is impaired gluconeogenesis such that serum pyruvate and lactate levels rise. The lactic acidemia can result in severe complications associated with metabolic acidosis. None of the other options (choices A, B, C, and E) correctly correspond to the laboratory findings in von Gierke disease.

38. Correct answer is **D.** The patient is most likely experiencing the symptoms of McArdle disease (glycogen storage disease V, GSD V). McArdle disease is the result of mutations in the *PYGM* gene that expresses the muscle form (referred to as myophosphorylase) of glycogen phosphorylase. The clinical presentation of McArdle disease is usually seen in young adulthood and is characterized by exercise intolerance and muscle cramps following bursts of muscle activity such as during sprint training and bicycle riding, or other forms of brief strenuous exercise. Attacks of rhabdomyolysis with myoglobinuria frequently accompany the muscle symptoms of McArdle disease. About half of McArdle disease patients will exhibit burgundy colored urine after exercise due to the myoglobinuria. In addition, these patients will present with significant increases in serum creatine kinase. Diagnosis of muscle glycogenoses such as McArdle disease was originally made by the observation of a lack of increased blood lactate upon ischemic exercise testing. Mutations in the gene encoding acid α-glucosidase (choice A) are the cause of Pompe disease. Mutations in the gene encoding 1,4-α-glucan branching enzyme 1, commonly known as glycogen branching enzyme (GBE) are the cause of Andersen disease. Mutations in the gene encoding glucose-6-phosphate dehydrogenase (choice C) result in a form of hemolytic anemia that is one of the most common forms of inherited nonspherocytic anemia. Mutations in the gene encoding pyruvatre kinase (choice E) are the cause of the second most common form of inherited nonspherocytic anemia, referred to as erythrocyte pyruvate kinase deficiency.

39. Correct answer is **E.** The infant is most likely experiencing the symptoms of Pompe disease (glycogen storage disease II, GSD II). Pompe disease is the result of mutations in the *GAA* gene that encodes the lysosomal hydrolase, acid α-glucosidase. About 25% of Pompe disease patients have the infantile lethal form of the disease. The infantile onset form of Pompe disease presents in the first few months of life. Symptoms include marked cardiomegaly, striking hypotonia (leading to the designation of "floppy baby syndrome") and rapid progressive muscle weakness. Patients will usually exhibit difficulty with feeding and have respiratory problems that are frequently complicated by pulmonary infection. The prominent cardiomegaly that can be seen on chest X-ray and/or detected by shortened PR intervals and heightened QRS complexes on an ECG are normally the first indications leading to a preliminary diagnosis of Pompe disease. Although Cori disease (choice A) and Hurler syndrome (choice B) are associated with cardiomyopathy, which can lead to cardiomegaly, cardiomegaly is uncommon in either of these diseases. Neither Hunter syndrome (choice C), McArdle disease (choice D), Tay-Sachs disease (choice F), nor von Gierke disease (choice G) are characterized by prominent cardiomegaly in infancy.

40. Correct answer is **A.** The infant is most likely experiencing the symptoms of Cori disease (glycogen storage disease type III, GSD III). Cori disease results from mutations in the gene encoding amylo-α-1,6-glucosidase, 4-α-glucanotransferase, also known more simply as the glycogen debranching enzyme (GDE). The disease is associated with the accumulation of an abnormally structured glycogen having very short outer chains. Deficiency in glycogen debranching activity causes hepatomegaly, ketotic hypoglycemia, hyperlipidemia, variable skeletal myopathy, cardiomyopathy, and results in short stature. Although glucose release from glycogen is impaired, glucose delivery to the blood can still be provided by gluconeogenesis. Hepatic gluconeogenesis is initiated by the pyruvate carboxylase-catalyzed reaction and this enzyme is dependent on biotin for activity. Gluconeogenesis requires niacin (choice C), as NADH, at the glyceraldehyde-3-phosphate dehydrogenase catalyzed reaction, this is not the initial reaction of gluconeogenesis. None of the other vitamins (choices B, D, and E) are required for gluconeogenesis.

41. Correct answer is **A.** The patient is most likely manifesting the signs and symptoms of von Gieke disease (glycogen storage disease I, GDSI). The hallmark features of this disease are hypoglycemia, lactic acidosis, hyperuricemia, and hyperlipidemia. The severity of the hypoglycemia and lactic acidosis can be such that, in the past, affected individuals died in infancy. Infants often have a doll-like facial appearance due to excess adipose tissue in the cheeks. In addition, patients have thin extremities, a short stature, and protuberant abdomens (due to the severe hepatomegaly). von Gierke disease is the result of mutations in the gene encoding the enzyme glucose-6-phosphatase (G6Pase). G6Pase is localized to the inner leaflet of the endoplasmic reticulum. None of the other intracellular organelles (choices B, C, D, and E) are involved in the pathogenesis of von Gierke disease.

42. Correct answer is **D.** The infant is most likely experiencing the symptoms of Pompe disease (glycogen storage disease II, GSD II). Pompe disease is the result of mutations in the *GAA* gene that encodes the lysosomal hydrolase, acid α-glucosidase. About 25% of Pompe disease patients have the infantile lethal form of the disease. The infantile onset form of Pompe disease presents in the first few months of life. Symptoms include marked cardiomegaly, striking hypotonia (leading to the designation of "floppy baby syndrome") and rapid progressive muscle weakness. Patients will usually exhibit difficulty with feeding and have respiratory problems that are frequently complicated by pulmonary infection. The prominent cardiomegaly that can be seen on chest X-ray and/or detected by shortened PR intervals and heightened QRS complexes on an ECG, are normally the first indications leading to a preliminary diagnosis of Pompe disease. Deficiency in 1,4-α-glucan branching enzyme 1 (choice A) is the cause of Andersen disease. Deficiency in glucose-6-phosphatase (choice B) is the cause of von Gierke disease. Deficiency in homogentisate oxidase (choice C) is the cause of the relatively benign amino acid metabolic disorder, alkaptonuria. Deficiency in myophosphorylase (choice E), the muscle-specific form of glycogen phosphorylase, is the cause of McArdle disease. Deficiency in phenylalanine hydroxylase (choice F) is the cause of the amino acid metabolic disorder, phenylketonuria, PKU.

43. Correct answer is **E.** The patient is most likely manifesting the signs and symptoms of von Gieke disease (glycogen storage disease I, GDSI). The hallmark features of this disease are hypoglycemia, lactic acidosis, hyperuricemia, and hyperlipidemia. The severity of the hypoglycemia and lactic acidosis can be such that, in the past, affected individuals died in infancy. Infants often have a doll-like facial appearance due to excess adipose tissue in the cheeks. In addition, patients have thin extremities, a short stature, and protuberant abdomens (due to the severe hepatomegaly). von Gierke disease is the result of mutations in the gene encoding the enzyme, glucose-6-phosphatase (G6Pase). Deficiency in G6Pase results in glucose-6-phosphate being diverted into glycolysis and the pentose phosphate pathway, PPP. As a result of increased PPP activity, there is increased ribose-5-phosphate production which activates the enzyme PRPP synthetase leading to increased production of PRPP, that activated form of ribose-5-phosphate. The increased PRPP in turn, activates the rate-limiting enzyme of purine nucleotide biosynthesis resulting in excessive purine nucleotide synthesis. The unnecessary purine nucleotides are catabolized generating increased levels of uric acid. None of the other metabolic processes (choices A, B, C, and D) is significantly, or at all, affected by a deficiency in G6Pase.

44. Correct answer is **D.** The patient is most likely experiencing the complications associated with McArdle disease (glycogen storage disease V, GSD V). McArdle disease is the result of mutations in the *PYGM* gene that expresses the muscle form (referred to as myophosphorylase) of glycogen phosphorylase. The clinical presentation of McArdle disease is usually seen in young adulthood and is characterized by exercise intolerance and muscle cramps following bursts of muscle activity, such as during sprint training and bicycle riding, or other forms of brief strenuous exercise. Attacks of rhabdomyolysis with myoglobinuria frequently accompany the muscle symptoms of McArdle disease. About half of McArdle disease patients will exhibit burgundy colored urine after exercise due to the myoglobinuria. In addition, these patients will present with significant increases in serum creatine kinase. Diagnosis of muscle glycogenoses, such as McArdle disease, was originally made by the observation of a lack of increased blood lactate upon ischemic exercise testing. As McArdle disease progresses, degeneration in the retinal pigment epithelium (RPE) occurs leading to RPE atrophy. This ocular pathology in McArdle disease is seen as a granular appearance to the fundus of the eye on ophthalmoscopic examination. Although visual issues are associated with McArdle disease, cataracts (choice A) are not characteristic of the disease. Many, but not all, McArdle disease patients can develop renal failure, but this is not related to the formation of kidney stones, nephrolithiasis (choice C). Cirrhosis (choice B) and ventricular cardiomyopathy (choice E) are not symptoms associated with McArdle disease.

45. Correct answer is **C.** The infant is most likely exhibiting the signs and symptoms of Cori disease (glycogen storage disease type III, GSD III). Cori disease results from mutations in the gene encoding amylo-α-1,6-glucosidase, 4-α-glucanotransferase, also known more simply as the glycogen debranching enzyme (GDE). The disease is associated with the accumulation of an abnormally structured glycogen having very short outer chains. Deficiency in glycogen debranching activity causes hepatomegaly, ketotic hypoglycemia, hyperlipidemia, variable skeletal myopathy, cardiomyopathy, and results in short stature. Deficiency in glycogen branching (choice A) is characteristic of Andersen disease (GSD IV). Deficiency in pyruvate carboxylation (choice B) is the result of mutations in the gene encoding pyruvate carboxylase, the initial enzyme of hepatic gluconeogenesis. Deficiency in erythrocyte pyruvate production (choice D), due to mutations in the *PKLR* gene is the cause of the hemolytic anemia identified as erythrocyte pyruvate kinase deficiency. Deficiency in lysosomal glycogen catabolism (choice E) is the cause of Pompe disease (GSD II). Although glucose release from glycogen is impaired in Cori disease, free glucose delivery to the blood (choice F) can still be provided by gluconeogenesis.

CHAPTER

8

Pentose Phosphate Pathway

High-Yield Terms

Glucose-6-phosphate dehydrogenase	Primary rate-limiting, oxidative enzyme of the PPP; numerous mutations in this gene are associated with hemolytic anemia, yet protect individuals from malaria
Transketolase	Enzyme of the nonoxidative stage of the PPP that transfers two-carbon units
Transaldolase	Enzyme of the nonoxidative stage of the PPP that transfers three-carbon units
Oxygen burst	Phagocytic cells of the immune system utilize NADPH generated via the PPP to generate superoxide radicals to kill phagocytized microorganisms, this requires a dramatic increase in O_2 consumption referred to as the oxygen burst

THE PENTOSE PHOSPHATE PATHWAY

The pentose phosphate pathway (PPP) consists of a series of interconnected reactions that serve as an alternate route for the metabolism of glucose (Figure 8–1). The major functions of the PPP are to generate the NADPH required as a cofactor for reductive biosynthetic reactions, as well as in antioxidant functions, and to generate the ribose-5-phosphate required for nucleotide biosynthesis (see Chapter 20).

Cells of the liver, adipose tissue, adrenal cortex, testis, and lactating mammary gland have high levels of the PPP enzymes. In fact, 30% of the oxidation of glucose in the liver occurs via the PPP. Additionally, erythrocytes utilize the reactions of the PPP to generate large amounts of NADPH used in the reduction of glutathione (see later).

Although the PPP operates in all cells, with high levels of expression in the earlier indicated tissues, the highest levels of PPP enzymes (in particular glucose-6-phosphate dehydrogenase) are found in neutrophils and macrophages. These leukocytes are the phagocytic cells of the immune system and they utilize NADPH to generate reactive oxygen species (ROS) from molecular oxygen in a reaction catalyzed by one of the NADPH oxidase complexes, specifically the NOX2 system. These ROS are then used to kill phagocytized microorganisms (see Clinical Box 8–1).

HIGH-YIELD CONCEPT

Following exposure to bacteria and other foreign substances there is a dramatic increase in O_2 consumption by phagocytes in a phenomenon referred to as the oxygen burst.

THE PPP IN THE CONTROL OF OXIDATIVE STRESS

Oxidative stress within cells is controlled primarily by the action of the peptide, glutathione (GSH; see Chapter 19). GSH is a tripeptide composed of γ-glutamate, cysteine, and glycine. The sulfhydryl side chains of the cysteine residues of two glutathione molecules form a disulfide bond (GSSG) during the course of being oxidized in reactions with various ROS and lipid hydroperoxides (LOOH) in cells. Reduction of oxidized glutathione involves the NADPH-dependent enzyme, glutathione reductase (Figure 8–2).

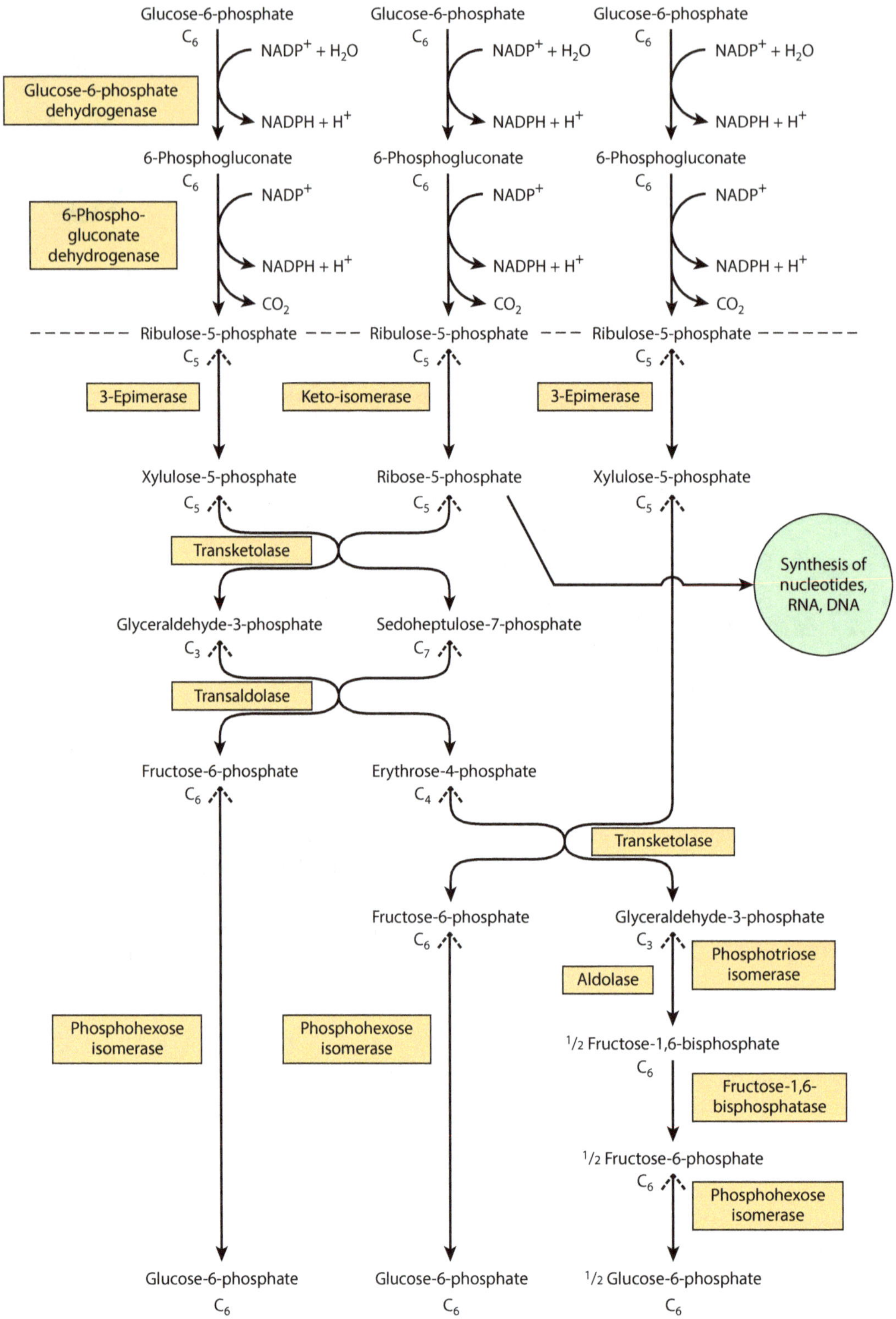

FIGURE 8–1 Flow chart of pentose phosphate pathway and its connections with the pathway of glycolysis. The full pathway, as indicated, consists of three interconnected cycles in which glucose-6-phosphate is both substrate and end product. The reactions above the broken line are nonreversible, whereas all reactions under that line are freely reversible apart from that catalyzed by fructose-1,6-bisphosphatase. (Reproduced with permission from Rodwell VW, Bender DA, Botham KM, et al: *Harper's Illustrated Biochemistry*, 31st ed. New York, NY: McGraw Hill; 2018.)

CLINICAL BOX 8–1 CHRONIC GRANULOMATOUS DISEASE

Because of the need for NADPH in phagocytic cells, by the NADPH oxidase system, any defect in enzymes in this process can result in impaired killing of infectious organisms. Chronic granulomatous disease (CGD) is a syndrome that results in individuals harboring defects in the NADPH oxidase system. There are several forms of CGD involving defects in various components of the NADPH oxidase system. Individuals with CGD are at increased risk for specific recurrent infections. The most common are pneumonia, abscesses of the skin, tissues, and organs, suppurative arthritis (invasion of the joints by infectious agent leading to generation of pus), and osteomyelitis (infection of the bone). The majority of patients with CGD harbor mutations in an X-chromosome gene that encodes a component of the NADPH oxidase system. The encoded protein is the β-subunit of cytochrome b^{245} (gene symbol *CYBB*), also called p91-PHOX or NOX2. This form of the disorder is referred to as cytochrome *b*-negative X-linked CGD. There is an autosomal recessive cytochrome *b*-negative form of CGD due to defects in the α-subunit of cytochrome b^{245} (gene symbol *CYBA*), also called p22-PHOX or NOX1. There are also two autosomal recessive cytochrome *b*-positive forms of CGD identified as cytochrome *b*-positive CGD type I and type II. The type I form is caused by mutation in the neutrophil cytosolic factor 1 (*NCF1*) gene, which encodes the p47-PHOX (phagocyte oxidase) protein. The type II form is caused by mutation in the *NFC2* gene which encodes the p67-PHOX (phagocyte oxidase) protein. Given the role of NADPH in the process of phagocytic killing it should be clear that individuals with reduced ability to produce NADPH (such as those with G6PDH deficiencies) may also manifest with symptoms of CGD.

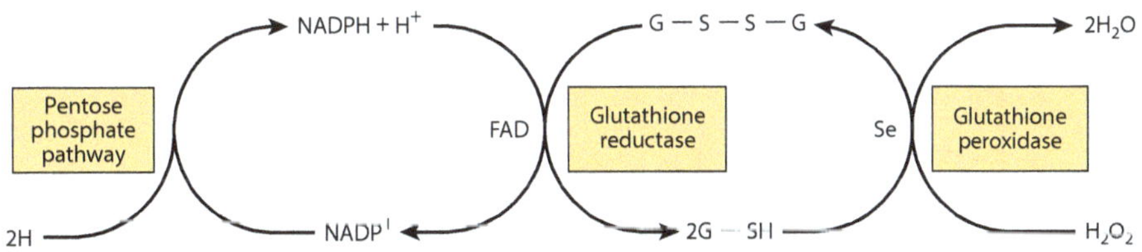

FIGURE 8–2 Role of the pentose phosphate pathway in the glutathione peroxidase reaction of erythrocytes. (G-SH, reduced glutathione; G-S-S-G, oxidized glutathione; Se, selenium-containing enzyme.) (Reproduced with permission from Rodwell VW, Bender DA, Botham KM, et al: *Harper's Illustrated Biochemistry*, 31st ed. New York, NY: McGraw Hill; 2018.)

ERYTHROCYTE OXIDATION AND THE PENTOSE PHOSPHATE PATHWAY

The PPP supplies the erythrocyte with NADPH needed to maintain the reduced state of glutathione. The inability to maintain reduced glutathione in erythrocytes leads to increased accumulation of peroxides, predominantly H_2O_2, (see Figure 8–3) that in turn results in oxidation of hemoglobin causing it to precipitate which is visible by histology as Heinz bodies. The increase in ROS also oxidizes lipids in the plasma membrane, weakening the membrane resulting in a concomitant hemolysis (see Clinical Box 8–2).

Deficiency in the level of activity of G6PDH is the basis of favism, primaquine (an antimalarial drug) sensitivity, and several other drug-sensitive hemolytic anemias, anemia and jaundice in the newborn, and chronic nonspherocytic hemolytic anemia. In addition, G6PDH deficiencies are associated with resistance to the malarial parasite, *Plasmodium falciparum*, among individuals of Mediterranean and African descent. The basis for this resistance is the weakening of the erythrocyte membrane such that it cannot sustain the parasitic lifecycle long enough for productive growth.

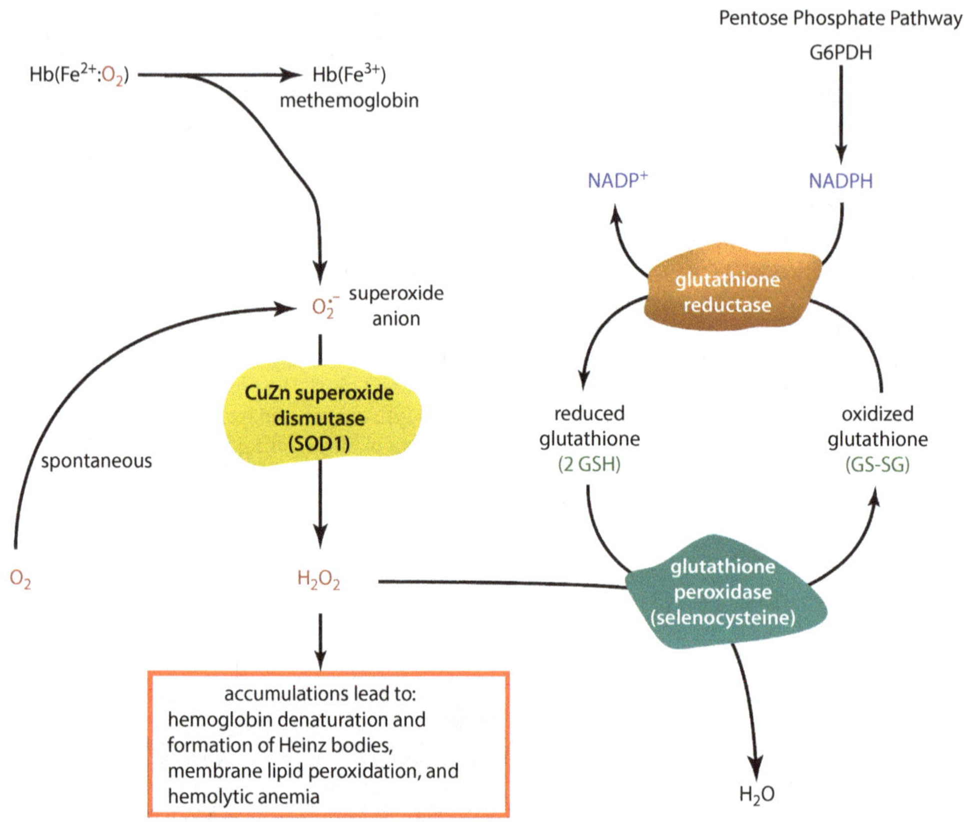

FIGURE 8–3 Pathway for reactive oxygen species (ROS) removal in erythrocytes. Formation of the reactive oxygen species (ROS), H_2O_2, occurs by two primary mechanisms in red blood cells. One mechanism is a spontaneous process by which superoxide anion is formed and then reduced to H_2O_2 via superoxide dismutase (SOD). The other is a result of O_2 oxidation of the ferrous iron (Fe^{2+}) to ferric iron (Fe^{3+}) in hemoglobin resulting in superoxide anion formation followed by reduction to H_2O_2 via SOD. The Fe^{3+} form of iron does not bind O_2; however, the presence of at least one Fe^{3+} in the hemoglobin tetramer results in enhanced binding of the O_2 to the remaining Fe^{2+} irons causing reduced delivery of the O_2 to the tissues with potential for cyanosis. The NADPH produced in the PPP, and the antioxidant glutathione (GSH), are both necessary for the continual removal of ROS from within the erythrocyte. The enzyme glutathione peroxidase (GPx) utilizes reduced glutathione (GSH) as the electron donor in the process of reducing H_2O_2 to H_2O while simultaneously generating oxidized glutathione (GS-SG). Oxidized glutathione is then reduced via the action of the NADPH-requiring enzyme, glutathione reductase. (Reproduced with permission from themedicalbiochemistrypage, LLC.)

CLINICAL BOX 8–2 GLUCOSE-6-PHOSPHATE DEHYDROGENASE DEFICIENCY

Deficiencies in glucose-6-phosphate dehydrogenase (G6PDH) are inherited as X-linked recessive disorders. Humans express two genes that generate glucose-6-phosphate dehydrogenase activity, the X-linked gene and an autosomal gene identified as H6PD (hexose-6-phosphate dehydrogenase/glucose 1-dehydrogenase). Glucose-6-phosphate dehydrogenase of the PPP is encoded by the *G6PD* gene that is located on the X chromosome (Xq28) and is composed of 14 exons that generate three alternatively spliced mRNAs. These three mRNAs encode two distinct G6PDH proteins identified as isoform a (545 amino acids) and isoform b (515 amino acids). The first exon of the gene is a noncoding exon with the translational initiation codon present in exon 2. The 545 amino acid isoform a protein is inactive but posttranslational processing results in a 515 amino acid functional protein containing an acetylated alanine residue at the N-terminus. Biologically active G6PDH is functional as either a homodimer or a homotetramer and both forms coexist in equal proportions at neutral pH. Deficiencies in G6PDH are the most commonly inherited enzyme deficiencies (enzymopathies) worldwide with estimates of greater than 400 million affected individuals. The incidence of deficiency approaches 25% of the population of persons of Mediterranean, tropical African, and tropical and sub-tropical Asian descent. In fact, the incidence of G6PDH deficiency is so high in some populations that the occurrence of homozygous females is not at all rare as would normally be expected for an X-linked disorder. The inheritance of G6PDH deficiency is clinically classified as an X-linked recessive disorder; however, because heterozygous females can develop hemolytic episodes the disorder is not truly recessive in the Mendelian sense. The phenomenon of symptom manifesting heterozygous females is

CLINICAL BOX 8–2 (CONTINUED)

explained by the coexistence of populations of G6PDH positive and negative cells in the same female as a result of X-chromosome inactivation. Deficiency in G6PDH represents one of the most genetically heterogeneous disorders. There are over 400 different variants of G6PDH defined by their diverse biochemical characteristics. To date, a total of 130 different point mutations have been identified in the G6PD gene. Complete loss of G6PDH activity is associated with embryonic lethality. G6PDH deficiency cannot be classified by a single mutation but is manifest as a consequence of numerous structural allelic mutants. In addition, G6PDH deficiencies are also classifiable by a variety of physicochemical parameters including chromatographic properties, thermostability, pH dependence, K_M for glucose-6-phosphate, and K_M for $NADP^+$. *G6PD* gene variants are currently divided into five classifications dependent on enzyme activity and clinical manifestations. In addition, the deficiencies are classified as to whether or not they are sporadic or polymorphic. Mutations in the *G6PD* gene that result in nonspherocytic hemolytic anemia have all been found to cluster near the C-terminal end of the protein, whereas the mutations that result in clinically mild symptoms are clustered near the N-terminal end of the protein. Nearly all G6PD mutations are single nucleotide missense mutations resulting in the substitution of a single amino acid. The acute hemolysis that is the only common clinical manifestation in G6PD mutations can rapidly be compensated for and thus may remain undetectable. The most common symptoms of G6PDH deficiency are neonatal jaundice and acute hemolytic anemia. The acute hemolytic attacks are the result of reduced antioxidant capacity of red blood cells with the result being membrane lipid peroxidation and consequent cell lysis. The accumulation of reactive oxygen species in G6PDH deficiency also leads to aberrant oxidation of the cysteine sulfhydryl groups in the globin proteins in hemoglobin. This results in significant cross-linking of hemoglobin tetramers which can be visualized microscopically. The cross-linked hemoglobin forms what is referred to histologically as Heinz bodies. The presence of Heinz bodies is diagnostic for G6PDH deficiency versus erythrocyte pyruvate kinase deficiency (Clinical Box 5–1), which is not associated with the formation of these inclusion bodies. Red blood cells containing Heinz bodies interact with splenic macrophages which remove the membrane-localized Heinz bodies generating cells that, histopathologically, look like there has been a "bite" taken out of them. For this reason, bite cells (also known as degmacytes) are another characteristic feature of G6PDH deficiency. In addition, red cell deficiency in G6PDH is the basis of favism, primaquine sensitivity (a drug used in the treatment of malaria similar to quinine), and some other drug-sensitive hemolytic anemias (eg, due to sulfonamides used to treat bacterial infections). Favism is a term relating to a hemolytic anemia that results from the ingestion of the fava bean (*Vicia faba*) also known as broad beans. Aside from favism and drug-induction of hemolytic anemia, infection is the most common cause of hemolysis in G6PDH-deficient individuals.

CHECKLIST

- ☑ The PPP reactions occur in the cytosol and oxidize glucose while producing NADPH and CO_2, but they do not generate ATP energy.
- ☑ The oxidative reactions of the PPP are irreversible, whereas, the nonoxidative reactions are reversible.
- ☑ Major tissues utilizing the reactions of the PPP have a high need for NADPH for reductive biosynthesis pathways or a high need for ribose-5-phosphate for nucleic acid synthesis.
- ☑ Erythrocytes have a critical need for the oxidative reactions of the PPP to generate NADPH for use in the regeneration of oxidized glutathione (GSH), via the glutathione peroxidase reaction, in order that it can be used to continuously repair oxidized membrane lipids.
- ☑ Generation of NADPH via the PPP is critical for the function of phagocytic cells. Mutations in G6PDH can lead to chronic granulomatous disease whose symptoms are reflective of the lack of phagocytic killing of pathogens.
- ☑ Inherited mutations in G6PDH can cause hemolytic anemia in afflicted individuals who are exposed to high oxidizing conditions in the blood or following the ingestion of certain pharmaceuticals. However, G6PDH deficiencies also protect afflicted individuals from the harmful effects of the malarial parasite.

REVIEW QUESTIONS

1. A 28-year-old man comes to the physician because of intermittent right upper quadrant pain that extends to the inferior tip of his scapula. Laboratory studies show mild anemia with the presence of relatively normal shaped erythrocytes that appear normocytic and normochromic. Laparoscopic cholecystectomy shows an accumulation of bilirubin diglucuronide. A defect in which of the following metabolic pathways most likely exists in this patient?
   (A) Glycogen synthesis
   (B) Heme degradation
   (C) Homocysteine metabolism
   (D) Pentose phosphate pathway
   (E) Urea synthesis

2. A clinic physician sees many transient workers. The physician finds that almost 30% of the patients show significantly reduced erythrocyte transketolase activity. Examination of liver function in these individuals would most likely show deficiency in which of the following metabolic processes?
   (A) Biosynthesis of fatty acids from acetyl-CoA
   (B) Biosynthesis of ketone bodies
   (C) Conversion of glycerol to glucose during fasting
   (D) Conversion of pyruvate to acetyl-CoA
   (E) Incorporation of dietary glucose into hepatic glycogen

3. A 22-year-old man of Mediterranean descent is being examined by his physician with complaints of fatigue and shortness of breath for the past 3 days. He recently had a urinary tract infection treated with trimethoprim-sulfamethoxazole. Physical examination shows pallor and scleral icterus. Laboratory studies show a decreased erythrocyte count and an increased serum bilirubin concentration that is mainly indirect. A deficiency in which of the following is most likely contributing to the pathology in this patient?
   (A) Bone marrow production of reticulocytes
   (B) Erythrocyte glucose-6-phosphate dehydrogenase activity
   (C) Erythrocyte production of NADH
   (D) Erythrocyte pyruvate kinase activity
   (E) Reticulocyte synthesis of heme

4. A 37-year-old man from Genoa, Italy is admitted to the hospital with complaints of fatigue, shortness of breath, and concern about his yellowing skin. Physical examination shows pallor, tachycardia, and splenomegaly. Laboratory studies find the patient has a decreased red cell count and an increased reticulocyte count along with elevated urinary concentrations of hemoglobin and bilirubin. The patient reports that he has been taking sulfamethoxazole for a urinary tract infection for the past 2 weeks. Based on the findings in this patient, it is most likely that he is deficient in which of the following enzymes?
   (A) Acid sphingomyelinase
   (B) Glucocerebrosidase
   (C) Glucose-6-phosphate dehydrogenase
   (D) Lysyl oxidase
   (E) Pyruvate kinase

5. A clinic physician sees many transient workers. The physician finds that almost 30% of the patients show significantly reduced erythrocyte transketolase activity. A deficiency in which of the following would most likely account for these observations?
   (A) Ascorbate
   (B) Biotin
   (C) Folate
   (D) Linoleic acid
   (E) Thiamine

6. A 29-year-old man is admitted to the hospital with complaints of fatigue, shortness of breath, and concern about his yellowing skin. Physical examination shows pallor, tachycardia, and splenomegaly. Laboratory studies find the patient has a decreased red cell count and an increased reticulocyte count along with elevated urinary concentrations of hemoglobin and bilirubin. The patient reports that he has been taking sulfamethoxazole for a urinary tract infection for the past 2 weeks. Which of the following tissues would most likey be the least affected by the likely deficiency in this patient?
   (A) Adipose tissue
   (B) Adrenal cortical tissue
   (C) Erythrocytes
   (D) Hepatocytes
   (E) Skeletal muscle

7. A patient is being examined with complaints of redness and swelling in his mouth, diarrhea, vomiting, and pains in his chest upon inhalation. Physical examination finds swollen lymph nodes in the neck and fever. History reveals the patient has had frequent bouts. The physician suspects a particular disorder and orders a dihydrorhodamine 123 (DHR 123) test for confirmation. Assuming the physician is correct in his diagnosis, a defect in which of the following would most likely contribute to the pathology in this patient?
   (A) Acid sphingomyelinase
   (B) Glucocerebrosidase
   (C) Glucose-6-phosphatase
   (D) Glucose-6-phosphate dehydrogenase
   (E) Pyruvate kinase

8. A 32-year-old man has been taking primaquine while on an expedition on the Amazon River. Several days into the expedition he begins to feel dizzy, has a fever, and notes that his urine is darker than usual. A deficiency in which of the following is most likely contributing to his symptoms?
   (A) Ascorbate
   (B) Glucose-6-phosphate dehydrogenase
   (C) β-Hexosaminadase A
   (D) Pyruvate kinase
   (E) Thiamine
   (F) Vitamin K

9. A 2-year-old child experiences a mild hemolytic anemia following the consumption of fava beans. Given the most likely underlying defect in this child, which of the following symptoms might also be most likely to present in this child?
   (A) Coarse facial features and bulging forehead
   (B) Dermatitis, diarrhea, and dementia
   (C) Hypoglycemia and galactosemia
   (D) Ocular stomatitis
   (E) Xerophthalmia

10. A 50-year-old alcoholic male presents with pain, numbness, tingling, and weakness in his hands and feet. The activity of which of the following enzymes is most likely decreased as a result of the nutritional deficiency contributing to this patient's pathology?
    (A) Fructose-1,6-bisphosphatase
    (B) Glucose-6-phosphatase
    (C) Glucose-6-phosphate dehydrogenase
    (D) Pyruvate kinase
    (E) Transketolase

11. Which of the following represents the best explanation for the reduced activity of the pentose phosphate pathway in skeletal muscle?
    (A) Skeletal muscle does not require NADPH
    (B) Skeletal muscle expresses low levels of the dehydrogenases of the pathway
    (C) Skeletal muscle expresses low levels of the enzymes of the nonoxidative phase of the pathway
    (D) The glutathione reductase enzyme is not present in skeletal muscle
    (E) The pentose sugars generated by the pathway are not required by muscle tissue

12. A 29-year-old woman is consuming a high carbohydrate diet in preparation for an upcoming marathon race. When she begins the race, a major biochemical change will be cessation of fatty acid synthesis from the excess glucose carbons present in her diet. A decrease in which of the following processes provides the best explanation for this biochemical change?
    (A) Adipocyte triglyceride synthesis
    (B) Gluconeogenesis
    (C) Glycogenolysis
    (D) Oxidative phosphorylation
    (E) Pentose phosphate pathway

13. A 23-year-old man of Italian origin, comes to the physician because of a 5-day history of fatigue and shortness of breath. He recently had a urinary tract infection treated with trimethoprim-sulfamethoxazole. Physical examination shows pallor and scleral icterus. Laboratory studies show a hematocrit of 38% (N = 41–50%), MCV of 83 fL (N = 82–98 fL), and an indirect bilirubin concentration of 4.8 mg/dL (N = 0.2–0.7 mg/dL). This patient's laboratory findings are most likely due to failure of which of the following?
    (A) Bone marrow production of leukocytes
    (B) Bone marrow production of reticulocytes
    (C) Erythrocyte production of lactic acid
    (D) Erythrocyte protection against membrane oxidation
    (E) Reticulocyte maturation
    (F) Reticulocyte synthesis of heme

14. A 2-year-old child experiences a mild hemolytic anemia following the consumption of fava beans. A peripheral blood smear obtained from the patient is shown:

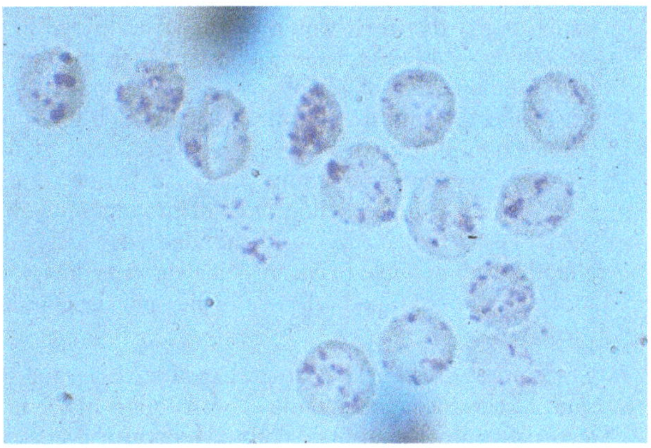

Given the most likely underlying defect in this child, which of the following would be the most likely additional finding?
    (A) Decreased pyruvate concentration
    (B) Decreased reduced glutathione concentration
    (C) Decreased transketolase activity
    (D) Increased glutathione reductase activity
    (E) Increased lactate concentration
    (F) Increased transketolase activity

15. A 23-year-old man of Italian origin comes to the physician because of a 2-day history of fatigue and shortness of breath. He recently had a urinary tract infection treated with trimethoprim-sulfamethoxazole. His pulse is 100/min. Physical examination shows pallor and scleral icterus. Laboratory studies show a hematocrit of 32% (N = 41–50%), MCV of 75 fL (N = 82–98 fL), and an indirect bilirubin concentration of 4.8 mg/dL (N = 0.2–0.7 mg/dL). Which of the following changes is most likely contributing to the laboratory values in this patient?
    (A) Decreased H_2O_2 concentration
    (B) Decreased NADPH concentration
    (C) Decreased pyruvate dehydrogenase activity
    (D) Increased glucose-6-phosphate dehydrogenase activity
    (E) Increased lactate concentration
    (F) Increased pyruvate kinase activity

ANSWERS

1. Correct answer is **D.** The patient is most likely suffering from the symptoms of deficiency in the pentose phosphate pathway enzyme, glucose-6-phosphate dehydrogenase (G6PD). The acute hemolysis that is the only common clinical manifestation in G6PD mutations can rapidly be compensated for and thus, may remain undetectable. The most common symptoms of G6PD deficiency are jaundice and acute hemolytic anemia. The acute hemolytic attacks are the result of reduced antioxidant capacity of red blood cells with the result being membrane lipid peroxidation and consequent cell lysis. The heme released from hemoglobin as a result of hemolysis results in increased conjugation of glucuronate to the heme degradation byproduct, bilirubin, in the liver. In excess, this process can lead to swelling of the gallbladder with bilirubin-diglucuronide which explains the right upper quadrant pain. Numerous diseases of glycogen synthesis (choice A) constitute some of the glycogen storage diseases such as Pompe disease and von Gierke disease. A defect in heme degradation (choice B) would prevent formation of bilirubin and thus, would not be associated with increased levels of bilirubin-diglucuronide. Defects in homocysteine metabolism (choice C) are associated with homocysteinemia and homocystinuria. The homocysteinemia impairs proper collagen processing at the level of lysyl oxidase which contributes to lens dislocations and also results in the potential for increased atherosclerosis and the potential for deep vein thrombotic episodes and stroke. Numerous disorders of urea synthesis (choice E) are known with the most common being associated with serious neonatal complications such as the neural toxicity of hyperammonemia.

2. Correct answer is **D.** The observation that the level of transketolase activity is reduced is a strong indication that the workers examined by the physician were suffering from a deficiency in thiamine. Transketolase requires the active cofactor form of thiamine, thiamine pyrophosphate (TPP) as do the pyruvate dehydrogenase complex (PDHc), the 2-oxoglutarate dehydrogenase complex (OGDH; commonly referred to as α-ketoglutarate dehydrogenase), and the branched-chain keto acid dehydrogenase complex (BCKD). A deficiency in

thiamine would have a negative impact on the function of each of these dehydrogenases and with PDHc would mean reduced oxidation of pyruvate to acetyl-CoA. Biosynthesis of fatty acids (choice A) is rate-limiting at the level of acetyl-CoA carboxylase, a biotin-dependent enzyme. Biosynthesis of ketones (choice B) requires the nicotinic acid-derived cofactor NADH as does the glycerol-3-phosphate dehydrogenase reaction that is involved in getting glycerol carbons into glucose (choice C) via gluconeogenesis. Incorporation of dietary glucose into glycogen (choice E) is dependent on uridine nucleotide activation of glucose to UDP-glucose, the substrate for glycogen synthase.

3. Correct answer is **B.** The patient is most likely suffering from the symptoms of deficiency in the pentose phosphate pathway enzyme, glucose-6-phosphate dehydrogenase (G6PD). The acute hemolysis that is the only common clinical manifestation in G6PD mutations can rapidly be compensated for and thus, may remain undetectable. The most common symptoms of G6PD deficiency are jaundice and acute hemolytic anemia. The acute hemolytic attacks are the result of reduced antioxidant capacity of red blood cells with the result being membrane lipid peroxidation and consequent cell lysis. The heme released from hemoglobin as a result of hemolysis results in increased levels of indirect (unconjugated) bilirubin in the blood as well as increased conjugation of glucuronate to bilirubin, in the liver. The oxidative crisis in red blood cells can result from the ingestion of certain drugs such as sulfonamides like sulfamethoxazole. Hemolytic anemia will lead to reticulocytosis (choice A) but this is a consequence of the hemolysis not a cause. Erythrocyte production of NADH (choice C) is associated with the glyceraldehyde-3-phosphate dehydrogenase reaction of glycolysis and if this reaction is reduced there would be decreased ATP production and increased levels of methemoglobin, the latter the result of reduced methemoglobin reductase activity due to its requirement for NADH. Deficiency of erythrocyte pyruvate kinase (choice D) is the second most common cause of inherited hemolytic anemia, with G6PD deficiency being the main cause. Although pyruvate kinase deficiency is associated with hemolytic anemia, it is not triggered by drugs such as sulfamethoxazole. A deficiency in reticulocyte heme synthesis (choice E) would result in the cessation of protein synthesis due to heme-regulated inhibitor-mediated phosphorylation of eIF-2. The reduced level of protein synthesis results in small erythrocytes not reduced numbers.

4. Correct answer is **C.** The patient is most likely suffering from the symptoms of deficiency in the pentose phosphate pathway enzyme, glucose-6-phosphate dehydrogenase (G6PD). The acute hemolysis that is the only common clinical manifestation in G6PD mutations can rapidly be compensated for and thus, may remain undetectable. The most common symptoms of G6PD deficiency are jaundice and acute hemolytic anemia. The acute hemolytic attacks are the result of reduced antioxidant capacity of red blood cells with the result being membrane lipid peroxidation and consequent cell lysis. The heme released from hemoglobin as a result of hemolysis results in increased levels of indirect (unconjugated) bilirubin in the blood as well as increased conjugation of glucuronate to bilirubin, in the liver. The increased hemolysis results in increased reticuloendothelial cell metabolism causing the splenomegaly. The increased bilirubin is the cause of the yellowing (jaundice) of his skin. Deficiency of acid sphingomyelinase (choice A) is the cause of the lysosomal storage disease, Nieman-Pick disease types A and B. Deficiency in glucocerebrosidase (choice B) is the cause of Gaucher disease. Deficiency in lysyl oxidase (choice D) would result in defective extracellular processing of collagen. Deficiency of erythrocyte pyruvate kinase (choice E) is the second most common cause of inherited hemolytic anemia, with G6PD deficiency being the main cause. Although pyruvate kinase deficiency is associated with hemolytic anemia, it is not triggered by drugs such as sulfamethoxazole.

5. Correct answer is **E.** Transketolase requires the active cofactor form of thiamine, thiamine pyrophosphate (TPP) as do the pyruvate dehydrogenase complex (PDHc), the 2-oxoglutarate dehydrogenase complex (OGDH; commonly referred to as α-ketoglutarate dehydrogenase), and the branched-chain keto acid dehydrogenase complex (BCKD). A deficiency in ascorbate (choice A) would result in defective collagen processing, reduced iron uptake into cells, and reduced antioxidant capacity of tissues. Biotin (choice B) is required for carboxylase enzymes such as pyruvate carboxylase of gluconeogenesis, acetyl-CoA carboxylase of fatty acid synthesis, and propionyl-CoA carboxylase which is required for the conversion of propionyl-CoA to succinyl-CoA. Folate (choice C) is the precursor for the various tetrahydrofolate derivatives that are required for numerous pathways such as thymidine nucleotide synthesis, purine nucleotide synthesis, and metabolism of methionine. Linolenic acid (Choice D) serves as a cofactor for dehydrogenase complexes such as pyruvate dehydrogenase and 2-oxoglutarate dehydrogenase (α-ketoglutarate dehydrogenase).

6. Correct answer is **E.** The patient is most likely suffering from the symptoms of deficiency in the pentose phosphate pathway enzyme, glucose-6-phosphate dehydrogenase, G6PD. The acute hemolysis that is the only common clinical manifestation in G6PD mutations can rapidly be compensated for and thus, may remain undetectable. The most common symptoms of G6PD deficiency are jaundice and acute hemolytic anemia. The reactions of fatty acid biosynthesis and steroid biosynthesis utilize large amounts of NADPH with the pentose phosphate pathway and G6PD making significant contributions to the pool of NADPH. Skeletal muscle, although active at *de novo* fatty acid synthesis, has the lowest levels of expression of enzymes of the pentose phosphate pathway and therefore, would be the least affected by deficiencies in G6PD. As a consequence of their high levels of lipid synthesis, cells of adipose tissue (choice A), adrenal cortex (choice B), and liver (choice D) have high levels of the pentose phosphate pathway enzymes. Erythrocytes (choice C) also have high levels of pentose phosphate pathway enzymes to ensure adequate reduction of oxidized glutathione by the NADPH-dependent enzyme, glutathione reductase. Reduced glutathione is required to ensure oxidative stress does not lead to damage of red blood cell membranes and the consequent hemolysis.

7. Correct answer is **D.** The patient has all the signs and symptoms of chronic granulomatous disease. Some of the highest levels of pentose phosphate pathway enzymes (in particular glucose-6-phosphate dehydrogenase) are found in neutrophils and macrophages. These leukocytes are the phagocytic cells of the immune system, and they utilize NADPH to generate superoxide radicals from molecular oxygen in a reaction catalyzed by NADPH oxidase. Therefore, deficiency in the

activity of glucose-6-phosphate dehydrogenase can result in defective function in the NADPH oxidase system in these cells. A defect in none of the other enzymes (choices A, B, C, and E) would contribute to the symptoms in the patient.

8. Correct answer is **B.** The patient is most likely suffering from the symptoms of deficiency in the pentose phosphate pathway enzyme, glucose-6-phosphate dehydrogenase (G6PD). The acute hemolysis that is the only common clinical manifestation in G6PD mutations can rapidly be compensated for and, thus, may remain undetectable. The most common symptoms of G6PD deficiency are jaundice and acute hemolytic anemia. The oxidative crisis in red blood cells can result from the ingestion of certain drugs such as primaquine. Primaquine is used to treat malaria since it causes lysis of erythrocytes that have been weakened by the presence of the parasite. When administered to humans, primaquine is metabolized into an arylhydroxylamine metabolite that exerts the hemotoxic effects. Primaquine causes methemoglobinemia in all patients. However, dangerous levels of methemoglobinemia only occur in patients with glucose-6-phosphate dehydrogenase deficiency and thus, this drug should not be administered to anyone with a deficiency in this enzyme. A deficiency in ascorbate (choice A) would result in defective collagen processing, reduced iron uptake into cells, and reduced antioxidant capacity of tissues. Deficiency in β-hexosaminidase A (choice C) results in Tay-Sachs disease, a lethal disorder of early childhood and thus would not be found in a 32-year-old patient. Deficiency of erythrocyte pyruvate kinase (choice D) is the second most common cause of inherited hemolytic anemia, with G6PD deficiency being the main cause. Although pyruvate kinase deficiency is associated with hemolytic anemia, it is not triggered by drugs such as primaquine. Deficiency in thiamine would exert its effects through reduced activity of critical dehydrogenase complexes such as pyruvate dehydrogenase. Typical signs and symptoms of thiamine deficiency include ataxic gate, nystagmus, and cognitive decline. Vitamin K deficiency (choice E) would result in loss of activity of the blood coagulation factors, prothrombin, factors VII, IX, X, protein C, and protein C.

9. Correct answer is **A.** The infant is most likely suffering the symptoms of deficiency in the pentose phosphate pathway enzyme, glucose-6-phosphate dehydrogenase (G6PD). The acute hemolysis that is the only common clinical manifestation in G6PD mutations can rapidly be compensated for and thus, may remain undetectable. The most common symptoms of G6PD deficiency are jaundice and acute hemolytic anemia. The oxidative crisis in red blood cells can result from the ingestion of certain foods such as fava beans. Favism is the term associated with the hemolytic anemia that results from the consumption of fava beans in individuals with deficiencies in glucose-6-phosphate dehydrogenase (G6PDH). The deficiency prevents erythrocytes from coping with the oxidative stress induced by metabolism of substances in fava beans. The continued hemolysis leads to hyperbilirubinemia, splenomegaly, and skeletal abnormalities in infants. The facial anomalies associated with favism are due to repeated episodes of intracranial hemorrhage. The symptoms of niacin deficiency (choice B) are referred to as pellagra and include dermatitis, diarrhea, and neurological defects that in the adult would be termed dementia. Hypoglycemia and galactosemia (choice C) are associated with defects in the galactose metabolizing enzyme, galactose-1-phosphate uridylyltransferase (GALT). Ocular (angular) stomatitis (choice D) and xerophthalmia (choice E) are pathologies of the eye that are associated with deficiency in vitamin A.

10. Correct answer is **E.** Alcoholics often do not adhere to a diet sufficient in nutrients, particularly vitamins. The signs and symptoms in this patient are typical of Wernicke-Korsakoff syndrome which are predominantly the result of reduced nervous system activity of the pyruvate dehydrogenase complex (PDHc). The PDHc is dependent on several vitamin-derived cofactors including thiamine pyrophosphate (TPP). The transketolase enzyme of the pentose phosphate pathway is also a TPP-dependent enzyme and its activity would, therefore, be reduced in this patient due to the deficiency of thiamine in his diet. None of the other enzymes (choices A, B, C, and D) would be functionally affected by thiamine deficiency.

11. Correct answer is **B.** The enzymes of the pentose phosphate pathway are expressed at highest levels in tissues that carry out high rates of lipid biosynthesis, such as the liver, adrenal glands, gonads, and adipose tissue. Skeletal muscle, although active at *de novo* fatty acid synthesis, does not require high rates of fatty acid synthesis because it can acquire them readily from the blood. Therefore, expression of the oxidative enzymes of the pathway are at low levels in this tissue. Skeletal muscle requires NADPH (choice A) for reductive biosynthesis and oxidative stress control. The level of glutathione production (choice C) in any given cell type would not correlate to the activity of the pentose phosphate pathway given that there are numerous pathways, in addition to oxidative stress reduction, that require the NADPH. Glutathione reductase (choice D) is expressed in all tissues. Skeletal muscle cells require nucleotides for RNA synthesis and, therefore, require some level of pentose phosphate pathway activity for the generation or ribose-5-phoshate (choice E).

12. Correct answer is **E.** Fatty acid synthesis requires NADPH derived from the pentose phosphate pathway via glucose-6-phosphate dehydrogenase and the 6-phosphogluconate dehydrogenase catalyzed reactions. During strenuous exercise, all skeletal muscle glucose is shunted into glycolysis for complete oxidation. Therefore, little glucose-6-phosphate is available for oxidation via the pentose phosphate pathway. During exercise fatty acids will be released from triglycerides stored in adipose tissue (choice A); however, these fatty acids were predominantly synthesized in the liver prior to transport to adipose tissue for storage. As blood glucose levels fall during her running, and the associated increased epinephrine release from adrenal glands, the liver will be stimulated to carry out gluconeogenesis (choice B), but this does not directly contribute to cessation of fatty acid synthesis. The epinephrine released due to exercise will stimulate live glycogen breakdown (choice C) but this does not directly affect fatty acid synthesis. Oxidative phosphorylation (choice D) in several tissues will increase during running but the potential effects on fatty acid synthesis will be indirect.

13. Correct answer is **D.** The patient is most likely suffering from the symptoms of deficiency in the pentose phosphate pathway enzyme, glucose-6-phosphate dehydrogenase (G6PD). The acute hemolysis that is the only common clinical manifestation in G6PD mutations can rapidly be compensated for and thus, may remain undetectable. The most common symptoms of G6PD deficiency are jaundice and acute hemolytic anemia. The oxidative crisis in red blood cells can result from the ingestion of certain drugs such as sulfamethoxazole.

Erythrocytes require a continuous source for NADPH to ensure that oxidized glutathione can be reduced by the glutathione peroxidase/glutathione reductase system. Glutathione is oxidized when it scavenges reactive oxygen species and by reducing oxidized membrane lipids. Administration of oxidizing drugs such as those of the sulfonamide class, can lead to weakening of erythrocyte plasma membranes due to rapid depletion of reduced glutathione levels and inadequate NADPH-dependent reduction of the oxidized form. Failure of bone marrow production of white (choice A) and red (choice B) blood cells would be associated with immunocompromised pathologies and severe life-threatening anemia, respectively. Erythrocytes have no option but to reduce pyruvate to lactate (choice C) in order to reoxidize NADH to NAD^+ to allow continued glycolysis, the only metabolic pathway for ATP generation in these cells. Maturation of reticulocytes (choice D) is not significantly affected in G6PD deficiency, so the MCV value is usually normal as in this patient. A deficiency in reticulocyte heme synthesis (choice F) would result in the cessation of protein synthesis due to heme regulated inhibitor-mediated phosphorylation of eIF-2. The reduced level of protein synthesis results in small erythrocytes, not reduced numbers.

14. Correct answer is **B.** The infant is most likely suffering from the symptoms of deficiency in the pentose phosphate pathway enzyme, glucose-6-phosphate dehydrogenase (G6PD). A deficiency in this enzyme results in oxidative crisis in red blood cells precipitating hemolytic anemia. In the absence of G6PD the activity of the enzyme, glutathione reductase, is significantly impaired. The result is that the levels of oxidized glutathione increase, and reduced glutathione levels decrease (see Figure 8–3). The lack of sufficient levels of glutathione lead to increased levels of H_2O_2 which in turn leads to increased rates of cysteine sulfhydryl oxidation in hemoglobin. The oxidation of the cysteines in hemoglobin results in the formation of cross-linked complexes of denatured hemoglobin. These large complexes of denatured hemoglobin can be visualized by light microscopy and are referred to as Heinz bodies which are visible in peripheral blood smears treated with a hypotonic solution of crystal violet. Due to a reduced level of functional red blood cells during a hemolytic crisis there may be decreased levels of pyruvate (choice A), but this would not be a significant finding in patients with G6PD deficiency. Since the pentose phosphate pathway enzyme, transketolase, is dependent on thiamine and not NADPH for its activity, there would not likely be a change, either down (choice C) or up (choice F), in the activity of this enzyme in red blood cells deficient in G6PD. Glutathione reductase (choice D) requires NADPH for its activity and so in the presence of a deficiency in G6PD its activity would be reduced not increased. Due to a reduced level of functional red blood cells during a hemolytic crisis there may be decreased levels of lactate but not an increase (choice E).

15. Correct answer is **B.** The patient is most likely suffering from the symptoms of deficiency in the pentose phosphate pathway enzyme, glucose-6-phosphate dehydrogenase (G6PD), as opposed to increased G6PD activity (choice D). The acute hemolysis that is the only common clinical manifestation in G6PD mutations can rapidly be compensated for and thus, may remain undetectable. The most common symptoms of G6PD deficiency are jaundice and acute hemolytic anemia. The oxidative crisis in red blood cells can result from the ingestion of certain drugs such as sulfamethoxazole. Deficiency in G6PD activity will lead to reduced red blood cell NADPH synthesis. Due to the progressive oxidation of glutathione resulting from lack of NADPH required by glutathione reductase, there will be an increase in the level of H_2O_2, not a decrease (choice A). Red blood cells do not possess mitochondria and as such do not contain any pyruvate dehydrogenase (choice C). A deficiency in G6PD is associated with hemolytic crises and would most likely be associated with a decrease in lactate production as opposed to an increase (choice E) due to poor red blood cell survival. Increased pyruvate kinase activity (choice F) would actually be biochemically beneficial to red blood cells as this is the only reaction of red blood cell metabolism that results in a net yield of ATP.

CHAPTER

9

Pyruvate Dehydrogenase Complex and the TCA Cycle

High-Yield Terms

Substrate-level phosphorylation	The succinyl-CoA synthetase catalyzed reaction involves the use of the high-energy thioester of succinyl-CoA to drive synthesis of a high-energy nucleotide phosphate (GTP); this process is referred to as substrate-level phosphorylation

THE PYRUVATE DEHYDROGENASE COMPLEX

The fate of pyruvate depends not only on the cell energy charge but also on the tissue. For example, in erythrocytes the fate of pyruvate is exclusively reduction to lactate. In liver and most tissues, when the energy charge is low, pyruvate is preferentially oxidized to acetyl-CoA via the pyruvate dehydrogenase complex, PDHc. The acetyl-CoA is then completely oxidized to CO_2 and H_2O in the TCA cycle. Conversely, in the liver under conditions of adequate energy the activity of the TCA cycle is inhibited and as a result acetyl-CoA accumulates and allosterically activates pyruvate carboxylase (PC), directing pyruvate toward gluconeogenesis (see Chapter 6).

The PDHc is comprised of multiple copies of three separate enzymes (Figure 9–1): pyruvate dehydrogenase (PDH, referred to as E1), dihydrolipoamide *S*-acetyltransferase, (DLAT, referred to as E2), and dihydrolipoamide dehydrogenase, (DLD, referred to as E3). The PDHc also requires five different coenzymes: CoA, NAD^+, FAD^+, lipoic acid, and thiamine pyrophosphate (TPP). The coenzymes of the PDHc can be remembered using the mnemonic Tender (TPP) Loving (lipoic acid) Care (CoA) For (FAD) Nancy (NAD^+).

The net result of the reactions of the PDHc is:

$$\text{Pyruvate} + \text{CoA} + \text{NAD}^+ \rightarrow \text{CO}_2 + \text{acetyl-CoA} + \text{NADH} + \text{H}^+$$

Mutations in several of the genes encoding the subunits of the PDHc have been identified resulting in several disorders (see Clinical Box 9–1). The most common mutations are in the X-linked gene (*PDHA1*) encoding the α-subunit of the E1 activity of the complex.

REGULATION OF THE PDH COMPLEX

The activity of the PDHc is highly regulated by a variety of allosteric effectors and by covalent modification. The activity of the E1 subunits of the PDHc is rapidly regulated by phosphorylation and dephosphorylation events that are catalyzed by PDH kinases (PDK) and PDH phosphatases (PDP), respectively. Phosphorylation of the E1 subunits results in inhibition of activity, whereas, dephosphorylation increases it.

Four PDK isozymes have been identified in humans: PDK1, PDK2, PDK3, and PDK4. These PDK are inhibited by pyruvate. In contrast to inhibition of the PDK by pyruvate, products of the PDHc, namely acetyl-CoA and NADH, allosterically activate the PDK. The ratio of NADH to NAD^+ also exerts allosteric regulation of PDK (Figure 9–2).

Energy charge, reflected in ATP/ADP and NADH/NAD ratios, influences the activity of the PDK. High ATP levels result in allosteric activation of the PDK to ensure the excess carbon atoms can be diverted into anabolic synthesis pathways instead of into the TCA cycle. Conversely, as the ATP/ADP ratio falls, the increasing ADP will exert an allosteric inhibition on the activity of the PDK.

NADH and acetyl-CoA are also negative allosteric effectors of the nonphosphorylated and active form of the PDHc. Both effectors reduce the affinity of the enzyme for pyruvate, thus limiting the flow of carbon through the PDHc.

Phosphate removal from the PDHc is catalyzed by two genetically and biochemically distinct PDP isoforms, PDP1 and PDP2. PDP1 is considered a major regulator of PDHc activity. The role of Ca^{2+} in stimulating the phosphatase activity of PDP1 toward the PDHc is by increasing its interaction with the PDHc.

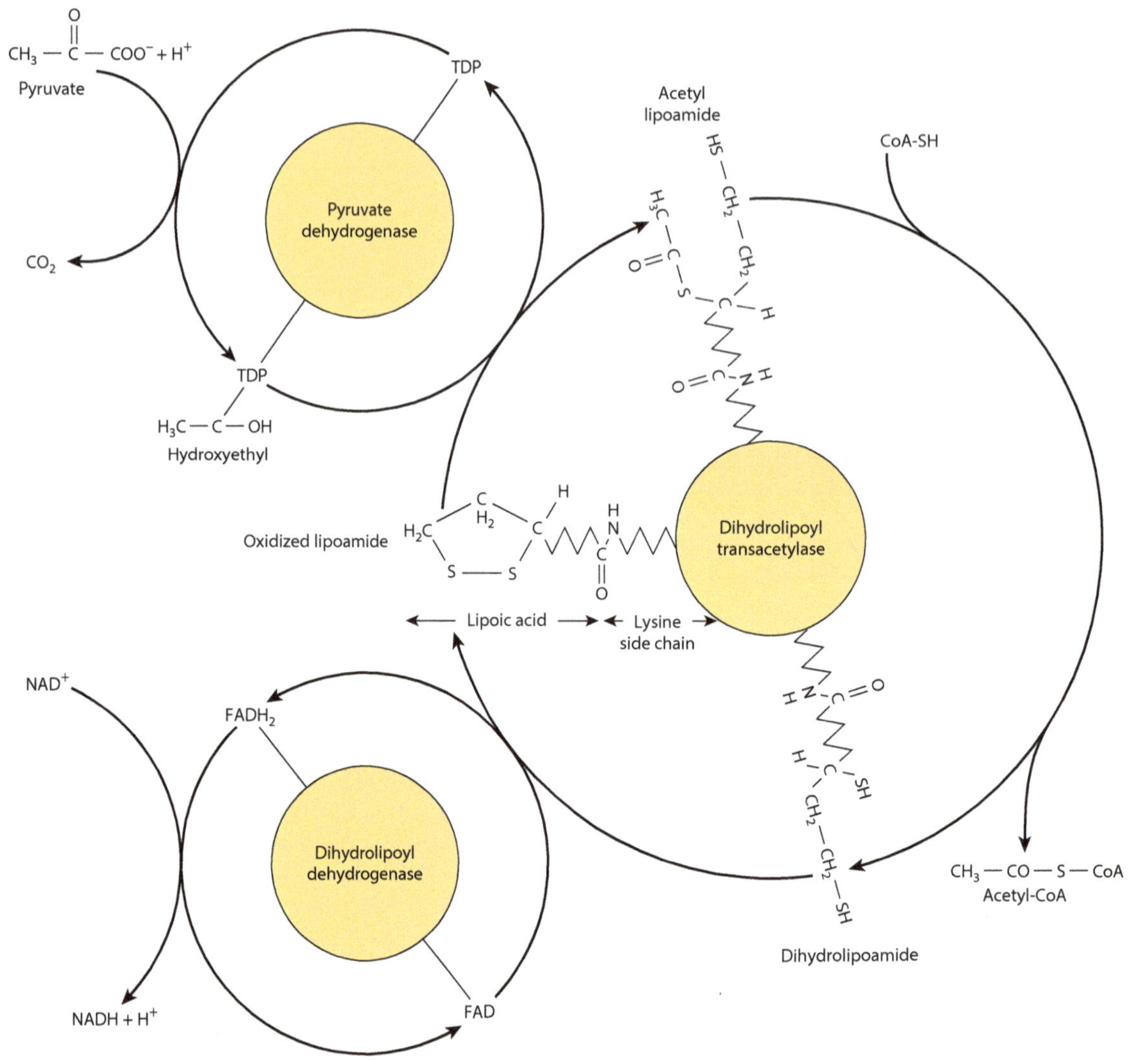

FIGURE 9–1 Oxidative decarboxylation of pyruvate by the pyruvate dehydrogenase complex. Lipoic acid is joined by an amide link to a lysine residue of the transacetylase component of the enzyme complex. It forms a long flexible arm, allowing the lipoic acid prosthetic group to rotate sequentially between the active sites of each of the enzymes of the complex. (FAD, flavin adenine dinucleotide; NAD^+, nicotinamide adenine dinucleotide; TDP, thiamin diphosphate.) (Reproduced with permission from Murray RK, Bender DA, Botham KM, et al: *Harper's Illustrated Biochemistry*, 29th ed. New York, NY: McGraw Hill; 2012.)

CLINICAL BOX 9–1 PDH COMPLEX DEFICIENCIES

All of the components of the PDHc are encoded by nuclear genes and, thus, deficiencies of PDHc activity are referred to as nuclear-encoded mitochondrial disorders. PDHc deficiencies represent a major cause of neonatal encephalopathies associated with primary lactic acidosis. Elevated lactate accompanied by elevated pyruvate with a normal lactate-to-pyruvate ratio is a hallmark of PDHc deficiency. PDHc deficiency can be caused by mutations in any of the genes encoding the principal subunits of the complex: the E1α encoding *PDHA1* gene, the E1 β encoding *PDHB* gene, the E2 encoding *DLAT* gene, or the E3 encoding *DLD* gene. In addition, PDHc deficiency is associated with mutations in the *PDHX* gene, the pyruvate dehydrogenase phosphatase catalytic subunit 1 (PPM2C) encoding gene *PDP1*, and the lipoic acid synthase encoding gene *LIAS*. The most common (84%) causes of PDHc deficiency are mutations in the *PDHA1* gene that encodes the E1α subunit. The *PDHA1* gene is localized to the X chromosome (Xp22.12) and is composed of 12 exons that generate four alternatively spliced mRNAs. The predominant PDHA1 derived mRNA (isoform 1) encodes a precursor protein of 390 amino acids. PDHA1 deficiency is considered an X-linked dominant condition given that both males and females manifest the symptoms of PDHc deficiency. More than 20 different mutations, including deletions, insertions, and point mutations have been identified in the *PDHA1* gene. Most missense mutations are found in exons 1 to 9 and most frameshift mutations are found in exons 10 and 11. Males and females with PDHA1 mutations

CLINICAL BOX 9–1 (CONTINUED)

have been found to be equally represented. However, almost all of the missense mutations have been identified in males and almost all of the deletions or insertions have been identified in females. It is speculated that insertions and deletions in hemizygous males may cause intrauterine death. With respect to the *PDHA1* gene, the most frequently reported mutations were found at amino acid positions 263, 302, and 378 with most of the mutations being missense mutations. Again, males account for the majority (83%) of patients harboring missense mutations in PDHA1. One of the most significant amino acid positions in PDHA1, with respect to disease, is amino acid position 378. Mutations in this amino acid may be particularly lethal resulting in death within the first two years of life. In contrast, patients harboring missense mutations at either position 263 or 302 appeared to have the lowest rate of lethality. In cells from PDHc-deficient patients it was found that there is overexpression of hypoxia inducible factor 1α (HIF1α). HIF1α is a transcription factor that regulates the expression of numerous genes involved in critical pathways of growth control and cell metabolism such as those encoding glucose transporters and most enzymes in the pathway of glycolysis. The increased levels of HIF1α create a positive feedback loop in PDHc deficiency due to the HIF1α-mediated increase in glycolytic flux. In patients with PDHc deficiency the major presentations encompass metabolic and neurologic pathologies with both occurring with equal frequency. The metabolic form presents as severe lactic acidosis in the newborn period which very often leads to lethality. PDHc deficiency accounts for about 15% of known causes of congenital lactic acidosis. The common neurologic pathologies in PDH-deficient patients are hypotonia, lethargy, spasticity, intellectual impairment, and the development of seizures. Between these two extremes of metabolic lethality and severe neurologic deficit there is a continuous spectrum of intermediate forms characterized by intermittent episodes of lactic acidosis associated with cerebellar ataxia. The symptoms of many patients with PDHc deficiency fit into the category of Leigh syndrome. Leigh syndrome represents a large family of related disorders characterized by subacute necrotizing encephalopathy. Leigh syndrome patients present in the first year of life with and characteristically develop rapidly progressing psychomotor retardation and death within the first 2–3 years of life. With respect to PDHc deficiency, the more severe the molecular defect, the more severe is the accompanying clinical illness. In addition, the earlier the onset of symptoms of PDHc deficiency, the more rapid will be the progression of the disease resulting in more widespread damage in the central nervous system. Patients with less than 15–20% of normal PDHc activity generally present with lactic acidosis of infancy and severe neurologic deficits. Patients with 40–50% residual PDHc activity have a milder illness in which intermittent ataxia is the most prominent neurologic symptom. There is currently no effective treatment for patients with PDHc deficiency. One strategy that has had variable success is the use of a ketogenic diet, supplementation with thiamine, and administration of dichloroacetate. In typical ketogenic diets the majority of fat is in the form of long-chain saturated fatty acids in triglycerides. The reduced glucose intake in the ketogenic diet result in a shift away from glycolysis, particularly in the brain, and toward the utilization of the ketones. The high fat content of the ketogenic diet drives ketone synthesis in the liver. The benefit of thiamine supplementation is in maximizing any residual PDHc activity, a complex that requires thiamine pyrophosphate in addition to several other vitamin-derived cofactors. Dichloroacetate inhibits the pyruvate dehydrogenase kinases (PDK) which normally phosphorylate and inhibit the PDHc. Thus, inhibition of the PDKs will prevent any inhibition of residual PDH activity.

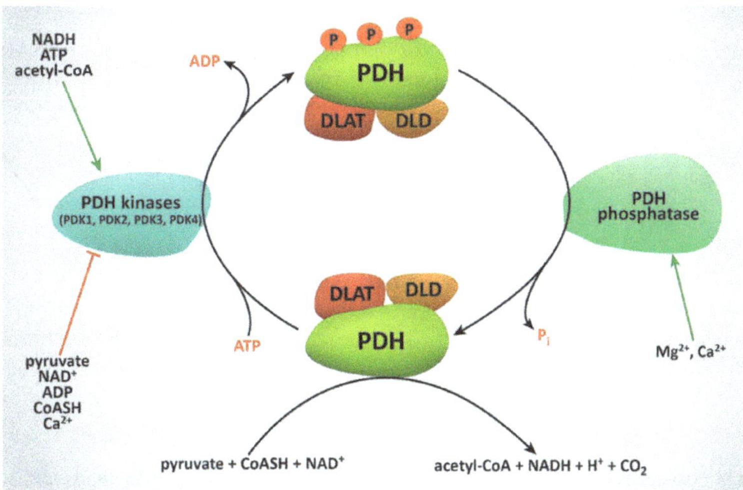

FIGURE 9–2 Factors regulating the activity of the PDHc. PDH activity is regulated by its state of phosphorylation; being most active in the dephosphorylated state. Phosphorylation of PDH is catalyzed by four specific PDH kinases, designated PDK1, PDK2, PDK3, and PDK4. The activity of these kinases is enhanced when cellular energy charge is high, which is reflected by an increase in the level of ATP, NADH, and acetyl-CoA. Conversely, an increase in pyruvate strongly inhibits PDH kinases. Additional negative effectors of PDH kinases are ADP, NAD^+, and CoASH, the levels of which increase when energy levels fall. The regulation of PDH phosphatases (PDPs) is less well understood but it is known that Mg^{2+} and Ca^{2+} activate the enzymes and that they are targets of insulin action. In adipose tissue, insulin increases PDH activity and in cardiac muscle PDH activity is increased by catecholamines. (Reproduced with permission from themedicalbiochemistrypage, LLC.)

THE TCA CYCLE

A key feature of the TCA cycle that distinguishes this metabolic pathway from the majority of other metabolic pathways is that there is no direct hormonal regulation of this pathway. This means that the major metabolic regulating hormones, insulin, glucagon, and epinephrine, do not directly lead to changes in the activity of any of the enzymes of the cycle via changes in cAMP levels or states of phosphorylation as is the case for other major metabolic pathways (Figure 9–3).

The net effect of the TCA cycle is the complete oxidation of acetyl-CoA to CO_2 and H_2O with the simultaneous generation of four moles of reduced electron carrier (three NADH and one $FADH_2$) and one mole of GTP. The acetyl-CoA can be derived from the oxidation of pyruvate via the PDHc, via the oxidation of numerous amino acids, and via the oxidation of fatty acids.

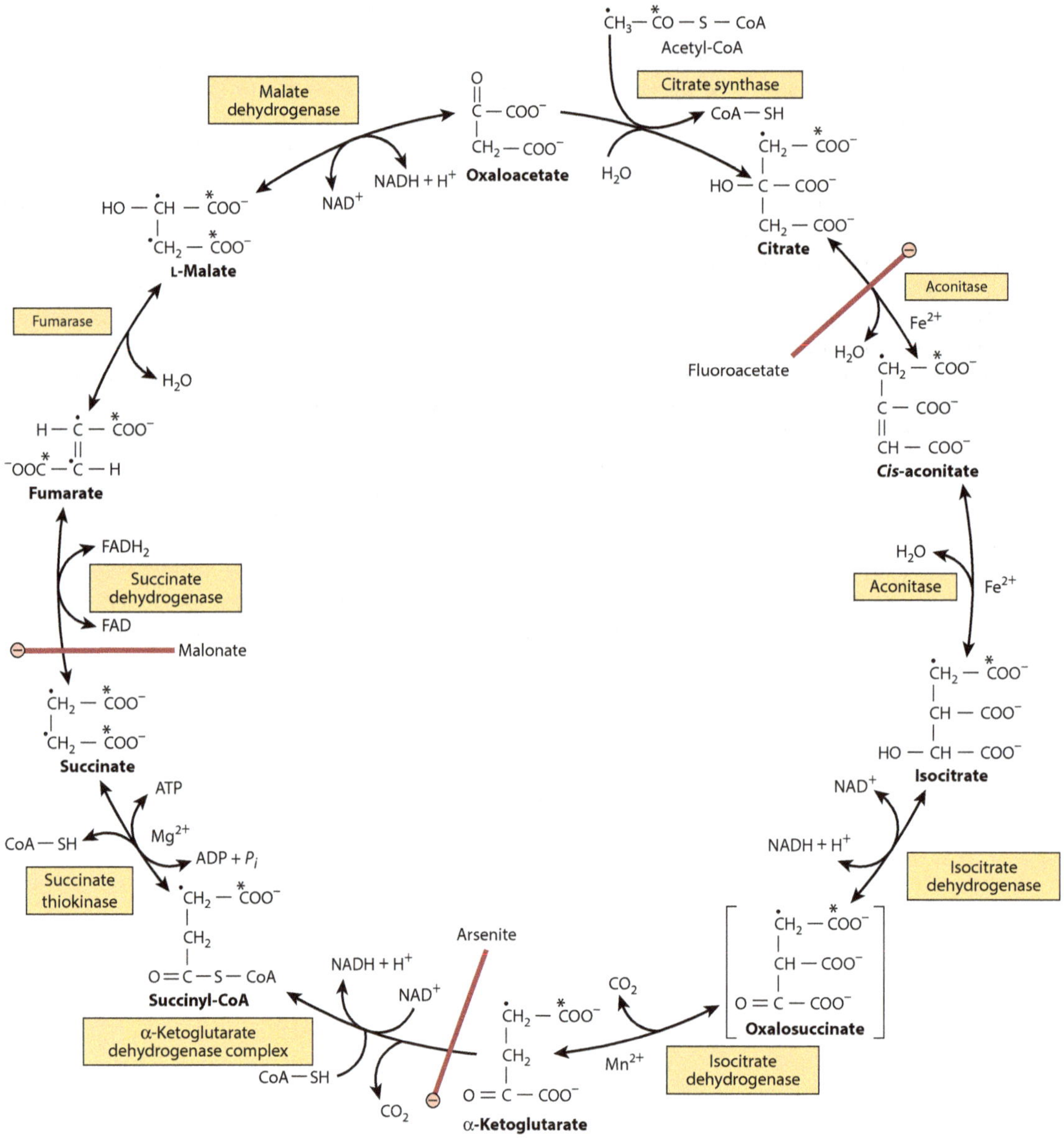

FIGURE 9–3 The citric acid (Krebs) cycle. Oxidation of NADH and FADH2 in the respiratory chain leads to the formation of ATP via oxidative phosphorylation. In order to follow the passage of acetyl-CoA through the cycle, the two carbon atoms of the acetyl radical are shown labeled on the carboxyl carbon (*) and on the methyl carbon (·). Although two carbon atoms are lost as CO_2 in one turn of the cycle, these atoms are not derived from the acetyl-CoA that has immediately entered the cycle, but from that portion of the citrate molecule that was derived from oxaloacetate. However, on completion of a single turn of the cycle, the oxaloacetate that is regenerated is now labeled, which leads to labeled CO_2 being evolved during the second turn of the cycle. Because succinate is a symmetric compound, "randomization" of label occurs at this step so that all four carbon atoms of oxaloacetate appear to be labeled after one turn of the cycle. During gluconeogenesis, some of the label in oxaloacetate is incorporated into glucose and glycogen. The sites of inhibition (⊖) by fluoroacetate, malonate, and arsenite are indicated. (Reproduced with permission from Rodwell VW, Bender DA, Botham KM, et al: *Harper's Illustrated Biochemistry*, 31st ed. New York, NY: McGraw Hill; 2018.)

The metabolic utility of the TCA cycle is not only the generation of large amounts of reduced electron carriers that can drive the synthesis of ATP but also to serve as a source of intermediates for gluconeogenesis (see Chapter 6), fatty acid biosynthesis (see Chapter 11), cholesterol and bile acid synthesis (see Chapter 15), and heme biosynthesis (see Chapter 21).

Mutations in several genes encoding enzymes, or subunits of enzymes, of the TCA cycle have been shown to be associated with the development of certain types of cancer (see Clinical Box 9–2).

REACTIONS GENERATING REDUCED ELECTRON CARRIERS

Four reactions of the TCA cycle yield reduced electron carriers. In order these reactions are catalyzed by isocitrate dehydrogenase (NADH), α-ketoglutarate (2-oxoglutarate) dehydrogenase (NADH), succinate dehydrogenase ($FADH_2$), and malate dehydrogenase (NADH). The α-ketoglutarate dehydrogenase complex is structurally and functionally very similar to the PDHc. Succinate dehydrogenase is also referred to as Complex II of oxidative phosphorylation (see Chapter 10).

DIRECT SYNTHESIS OF ATP: SUBSTRATE-LEVEL PHOSPHORYLATION

Nucleoside triphosphate, in the form of GTP, is synthesized during the course of the succinyl-CoA synthetase reaction. Succinyl-CoA synthetase is also called succinate thiokinase or succinyl-CoA ligase. As a result of the ubiquitous activity of nucleoside diphosphate kinases, the GTP serves as a donor of phosphate for the conversion of ADP to ATP.

CLINICAL BOX 9–2 DISORDERS ASSOCIATED WITH TCA CYCLE ENZYMES

Mutations in genes that encode TCA cycle enzymes (or homologues of TCA cycle enzymes) have been identified in certain types of familial cancer syndromes. Mutations in two of the three isocitrate dehydrogenase genes (*IDH1* and *IDH2*), but not the TCA cycle gene (*IDH3*), have been identified in gliomas in the brain. The succinate dehydrogenase (SDH) complex is composed of four subunits encoded by four distinct genes, *SDHA, SDHB, SDHC*, and *SDHD*. Mutations in all four of these genes are associated with several familial cancer syndromes. In addition to the four functional components of the SDH complex, mutations in the SDH assembly factor gene, *SDHAF2*, are also found in certain forms of cancers. Mutations in SDH complex encoding genes are found in paragangliomas, pheochromocytomas, gastrointestinal stromal tumors (GIST), and an aggressive form of renal cancer identified as SDH-RCC (SDH-deficient renal cell carcinoma). Cancer syndromes have also been associated with mutations in the fumarate hydratase (FH; also called fumarase) gene. The *FH* gene mutation-associated cancers are cutaneous and uterine leiomyomas and an aggressive form of type 2 papillary renal cancer. The type 2 renal papillary carcinoma is characterized by a metabolic shift to aerobic glycolysis and glutamine-dependent reductive carboxylation. Because loss of function of any of these genes results in the progression to cancer, all have been classified as tumor suppressors.

Mutations in the genes encoding the SDH complex result in a pathophysiologic state defined as pseudohypoxia. This pathophysiologic state leads to a subsequent increase in angiogenesis, via activation of the hypoxia-induced factor 1 (HIF-1) transcription factor complex, resulting in the ability of tumors to acquire nutrients encouraging their aberrant growth. Activation of HIF-1 in SDH-deficient tumors is the result of accumulating levels of succinate which is then transported into the cytosol via the action of the mitochondrial dicarboxylate transporter. Accumulation of cytosolic succinate inhibits the 2-oxoglutarate and Fe^{2+}-dependent dioxygenases [prolyl hydroxylase domain (PDH) enzymes] responsible for the hydroxylation of the α-subunit (HIF-1α) of HIF-1. The hydroxylation of HIF-1α normally occurs continuously under normoxic conditions which stimulates ubiquitylation and proteasomal degradation of HIF-1α, thereby restricting the transcription factor function of HIF-1. The loss of HIF-1α hydroxylation results in stabilization of the protein and consequent activation of the transcription factor activity of HIF-1 in the absence of hypoxia. Activation of HIF-1 in the absence of hypoxia leads to increased angiogenesis within the SDH-deficient tumor environment promoting the growth of the tumor cells. Since their initial characterization, the SDH-deficient GIST have been shown to account for up to 7.5% of these forms of cancer in adult patients and represent the vast majority of these types of tumors that are found in childhood.

Mutations in the fumarate hydratase (FH) gene have been shown to be associated with hereditary leiomyomatosis and renal cell carcinoma (HLRCC). HLRCC is an autosomal dominant hereditary cancer syndrome that is characterized by a predisposition to the development of cutaneous and uterine leiomyomas and a very aggressive form of papillary kidney cancer. HLRCC-associated renal tumors readily metastasize to both regional and distant lymph nodes making this form of renal cancer significantly more aggressive than other forms of genetically defined renal cancer. The FH mutations found in HLRCC are missense, frameshift, partial deletions, or complete deletions. Similar to the alterations that occur in the metabolic programs in SDH-deficient cancers, FH-deficient cells exhibit a substantial metabolic reorganization. FH-deficient tumor cells satisfy their need for high rates of ATP production by developing high rates of glucose uptake and higher rates of glucose oxidation via glycolysis. The reduced entry of glycolytic intermediates into the TCA cycle, due to FH deficiency, results in diversion of glucose to lactate as well as into other metabolic pathways of biomass production. All of these shifts in metabolism are not unique to FH-deficient tumors but are a common occurrence in most tumors. Similar to SDH-deficient tumors, FH-deficient tumors are associated with activation of the HIF-1 transcriptional program. When fumarate accumulates in the mitochondria of FH-deficient cells the metabolite is transported to the cytosol by the dicarboxylate transporter. Within the cytosol the accumulating fumarate, similar to the effect of accumulating succinate, results in the inhibition of 2-oxoglutarate and Fe^{2+}-dependent dioxygenases that are responsible for the hydroxylation of HIF1α. Additional metabolic changes in FH-deficient tumors have been shown to be the result of reduced activation and reduced expression of the master metabolic regulatory kinase, AMPK. The loss of AMPK activity results in increased rates of lipid and protein synthesis in the tumor cells.

HIGH-YIELD CONCEPT

The conversion of succinyl-CoA to succinate, by succinyl-CoA synthetase, drives synthesis of a high-energy nucleotide phosphate (GTP) in a process known as substrate-level phosphorylation.

TCA CYCLE STOICHIOMETRY

The overall stoichiometry of the TCA cycle, beginning and ending with acetyl-CoA, can be written:

$$\text{acetyl-CoA} + 3NAD^+ + FAD + GDP + P_i + 2H_2O \rightarrow 2CO_2 + 3NADH + FADH_2 + GTP + 2H^+ + HSCoA$$

REGULATION OF THE TCA CYCLE

Regulation of the TCA cycle occurs at both the level of substrate availability as well as through allosteric regulation of several enzymes of the cycle. Since three reactions of the TCA cycle utilize NAD^+ as cofactor, it is not difficult to understand why the cellular ratio of $NADH/NAD^+$ has a major impact on the flux of carbon through the TCA cycle. The primary site of allosteric control of TCA cycle activity is at the isocitrate dehydrogenase (IDH) reaction and as such this reaction is considered the rate-limiting reaction of the TCA cycle. Allosteric stimulation of IDH occurs through ADP, whereas NADH inhibits the enzyme.

CHECKLIST

- ☑ The entry of carbohydrate carbons into the TCA cycles occurs via the oxidative decarboxylation of pyruvate, catalyzed by the pyruvate dehydrogenase complex, PDHc.
- ☑ The PDHc is a large multi-subunit enzyme complex that requires five distinct cofactors, four of which are derived from vitamins.
- ☑ Regulation of the PDHc is complex involving both covalent modification (phosphorylation/dephosphorylation) and numerous allosteric effectors.
- ☑ The TCA cycle is the terminal pathway for the complete oxidation of the byproducts of carbohydrate, fatty acid, and amino acid metabolism. The common end-product of catabolism of these three types of compound is acetyl-CoA.
- ☑ The acetyl-CoA, derived from carbohydrate, fatty acid, and amino acid oxidation, reacts with oxaloacetate forming citrate. Citrate then undergoes a series of oxidation and decarboxylation steps in the context of the TCA cycle to regenerate oxaloacetate while simultaneously generating reducing equivalents as NADH and $FADH_2$, as well as releasing CO_2.

REVIEW QUESTIONS

1. A low-birth-weight newborn infant is being examined for the cause of her hypotonia, tachypnea, and abnormal eye movements. Laboratory studies find severe lactic acidosis, hyperammonemia, and elevated levels of alanine in the urine. The infant developed a seizure and died. Postmortem analysis of the brain found atrophy and underdevelopment of the corpus callosum. Which of the following is the most likely process that was defective in this infant resulting in the lethality?
(A) Hepatic glycogen metabolism
(B) Lysosomal ganglioside metabolism
(C) Metabolism of branched-chain amino acids
(D) Peroxisomal phytanic acid oxidation
(E) Pyruvate oxidation

2. A 38-year-old woman has been diagnosed with a type 2 papillary renal cell carcinoma and uterine leiomyomas. Given the most likely cause of this patient's cancer, which of the following is most likely to be found elevated in cells isolated from the cancerous tissues?
(A) Fumarate
(B) Isocitrate
(C) Malate
(D) Pyruvate
(E) Succinate

3. A 12-year-old woman is being treated for glioblastoma. Molecular studies performed on cells isolated from biopsy tissue discovers the presence of an altered arginine codon in the gene encoding isocitrate dehydrogenase 1 (IDH1). Given these findings, which of the following intermediates would most likely be found at elevated levels in the cancer cells of this patient?
(A) Fumarate
(B) 2-Hydroxyglutarate
(C) α-Ketoglutarate
(D) Oxaloacetate
(E) Succinate

4. A teenage patient is being treated in the ER following a reported suicide attempt. The teen ingested rat poison and has diarrhea and severe vomiting which has resulted in hypovolemic shock. Outward signs include a strong odor of garlic on the patient's breath. Which of the following is the most likely action of the toxic substance in the rat poison resulting in the observed symptoms?
(A) It activates pyruvate dehydrogenase
(B) It enhances the rate of gluconeogenesis
(C) It increases reduced glutathione production
(D) It inhibits pyruvate dehydrogenase
(E) It reduces the concentration of pyruvate

5. A 2-day-old male infant, who has exhibited extreme lethargy and poor feeding, has required ventilation due to severely reduced breathing. Laboratory studies show hypotonia, severe lactic acidosis, and elevated blood alanine. These observations are most indicative of a deficiency in which of the following enzymes?
   (A) Isocitrate dehydrogenase
   (B) α-Ketoglutarate dehydrogenase (2-oxoglutarate dehydrogenase)
   (C) Lactate dehydrogenase
   (D) Pyruvate dehydrogenase
   (E) Succinate dehydrogenase

6. A 25-year-old woman is participating in a marathon. While she is running which of the following mechanisms is most likely contributing to enhanced pyruvate oxidation?
   (A) Allosteric activation of pyruvate dehydrogenase by NADH
   (B) Allosteric activation of α-ketoglutarate dehydrogenase by NAD^+
   (C) Increased feedback activation of pyruvate dehydrogenase by oxaloacetate
   (D) Phosphorylation of α-ketoglutarate dehydrogenase to an inactive form
   (E) Stimulation of pyruvate dehydrogenase activity by Ca^{2+}

7. Which of the following is most likely to exert a positive effect on the oxidation of pyruvate?
   (A) Acetyl-CoA
   (B) ATP
   (C) Enzyme dephosphorylation
   (D) Enzyme phosphorylation
   (E) NADH

8. A 2-year-old boy is being examined in the emergency department following a period of vomiting and a seizure. Physical examination finds the infant has significant hypotonia, drooping eyelids, and limited eye mobility. Molecular studies carried out on muscle biopsy cells find that the cofactor binding site of one of the subunits of succinate dehydrogenase has sustained a deletion. Given these results, which of the following is most likely no longer capable of participating in the function of the enzyme?
   (A) Ascorbate
   (B) Biotin
   (C) Lipoic acid
   (D) Niacin
   (E) Riboflavin

9. A low-birth-weight newborn infant is being examined for the cause of her hypotonia, tachypnea, and abnormal eye movements. Laboratory studies find severe lactic acidosis, hyperammonemia, and elevated levels of alanine in the urine. Which of the following is most likely to be elevated in the serum of this patient?
   (A) Acetoacetate
   (B) Fumarate
   (C) Glutamine
   (D) β-Hydroxy butyrate
   (E) Lactate

10. A 24-year-old woman comes to the physician because of diarrhea, dysphagia, jaundice, and white transverse lines on the fingernails. This patient is most likely suffering from chronic poisoning by a compound that inhibits which of the following enzymes?
   (A) Aconitase
   (B) Citrate synthase
   (C) α-Ketoglutarate dehydrogenase (2-oxoglutarate dehydrogenase)
   (D) Malate dehydrogenase
   (E) Succinate dehydrogenase

11. A 47-year-old man is being examined by his physician with the complaint that he frequently urinates red-purple colored urine. History and physical examination indicate numerous dry scaly patches of skin and recurrent blistering rash upon sun exposure. Given these signs and symptoms, which of the following TCA cycle intermediates is required for the metabolic pathway most likely disrupted in this patient?
   (A) Fumarate
   (B) Malate
   (C) Pyruvate
   (D) Succinate
   (E) Succinyl-CoA

12. A 2-year-old boy is brought to the emergency department after a series of convulsions. The child is diagnosed with ammonia intoxication due to a urea cycle disorder. Reduced formation of the inhibitory neurotransmitter, γ-aminobutyrate (GABA) is the most likely cause of the patient's convulsions. Which of the following TCA cycle intermediates is most likely deficient in this patient?
   (A) Isocitrate
   (B) α-Ketoglutarate (2-oxoglutarate)
   (C) Malate
   (D) Pyruvate
   (E) Succinate

13. A 3-year-old child was rushed to emergency department after accidently consuming portions of a wallflower bush, a plant containing the compound fluoroacetate. Which of the following activities would most likely be impaired in this child?
   (A) Aconitase
   (B) Glucose-6-phosphate dehydrogenase
   (C) Malate dehydrogenase
   (D) Pyruvate kinase
   (E) Succinate dehydrogenase

14. A 62-year-old chronic alcoholic has been brought to the emergency department in a semiconscious state. Blood biochemistry reveals a blood glucose level of 35 mg/dL (normal for fasting = 60–100 mg/dL). Which of the following, if administered to this patient, would most likely contribute directly to the mobilization of mitochondrial carbon atoms into the cytoplasmic pathway of gluconeogenesis?
   (A) Isocitrate
   (B) α-Ketoglutarate (2-oxoglutarate)
   (C) Malate
   (D) Pyruvate
   (E) Succinate

15. Which of the following best explains why the carbons of acetyl-CoA, generated from glucose, cannot contribute to the net synthesis of glucose via the pathway of gluconeogenesis?
   (A) Insufficient NADH for gluconeogenesis is produced in the mitochondrial matrix
   (B) Oxidative decarboxylation reactions result in the release of acetyl-CoA carbons as CO_2
   (C) The acetyl-CoA carbons are used to generate succinyl-CoA which is used for heme synthesis
   (D) The mitochondrial membrane is impermeable to oxaloacetate which is trapped in the matrix
   (E) The two carbons of acetyl-CoA are perpetually utilized in the TCA cycle

ANSWERS

1. Correct answer is **E.** The signs and symptoms in the infant are most likely the result of a deficiency in the function of the pyruvate dehydrogenase complex, PDHc. In patients with PDHc deficiency, the major presentations encompass metabolic and neurologic pathologies with both occurring with equal frequency. The metabolic form presents as severe lactic acidosis in the newborn period which very often leads to lethality. The most common cause of PDHc deficiency is mutation in the gene, *PDHA1*, encoding the α-subunit of the E1 portion of the complex. Although the *PDHA1* gene is located on the X chromosome, females are nearly equally likely to inherit the disease as are males. This is due to the phenomenon where the X chromosome harboring the wild-type *PDHA1* gene is almost always the chromosome that is subjected to inactivation. There are several disorders associated with hepatic glycogen metabolism (choice A) with von Gierke disease having some similar symptoms to those presented in this case, such as lactic acidosis and hyperammonemia; however, there is no brain development issues with the disorder. Defective lysosomal ganglioside metabolism (choice B) is the cause of Tay-Sachs disease. Infants with Tay-Sachs disease appear normal at birth. Symptoms usually begin with mild motor weakness by 3–5 months of age. Defective metabolism of branched-chain amino acids (choice C) results in the disorder known as maple syrup urine disease, MSUD. Classic MSUD is defined by neonatal onset of encephalopathy and is the most severe form of the disorder but there is no lactic acidosis of hyperammonemia associated with the disorder. Defective peroxisomal phytanic acid oxidation (choice D) results in Refsum disease. The cardinal clinical features of Refsum disease are retinitis pigmentosa, chronic polyneuropathy, cerebellar ataxia, and elevated protein levels in cerebrospinal fluid.

2. Correct answer is **A.** Mutations in the fumarate hydratase (FH: also called fumarase) gene have been shown to be associated with hereditary leiomyomatosis and renal cell carcinoma (HLRCC). Leiomyoma is a form of smooth muscle tumor that can develop in any organ but is most commonly found in the uterus, esophagus, and small intestine. When fumarate accumulates in the mitochondria of FH-mutant cells the metabolite is transported to the cytosol by the dicarboxylate transporter. Within the cytosol the accumulating fumarate results in the inhibition of the family of 2-oxoglutarate and Fe^{2+}-dependent dioxygenases (2OG-oxygenases) that play critical roles in numerous reaction pathways including epigenetic modification of DNA and histones. Accumulation of isocitrate (choice B), malate (choice C), or pyruvate (choice D) are not common to the development of cancers. Accumulation of succinate (choice E) occurs in cancers that include paragangliomas, pheochromocytomas, gastrointestinal stromal tumors (GIST) as a result of mutations in any of the four subunits of the succinate dehydrogenase (complex II) complex.

3. Correct answer is **B.** Isocitrate is oxidatively decarboxylated to α-ketoglutarate (2-oxoglutarate) by isocitrate dehydrogenase, IDH. There are three different IDH enzymes in humans identified as IDH1, IDH2, and IDH3 with only the IDH3 isoform being involved in the TCA cycle. IDH1 and IDH2 normally convert isocitrate to α-ketoglutarate (2-oxoglutarate) while also generating NADPH. Mutations in the *IDH1* gene result in a loss of isocitrate binding while at the same time alter the catalytic activity of the enzyme such that it reduces α-ketoglutarate (2-oxoglutarate), the normal product, to 2-hydroxyglutarate (2-HG) while simultaneously oxidizing NADPH to $NAPD^+$. Indeed, in gliomas with IDH1 mutations the levels of 2-HG are elevated relative to normal cells. Fumarate (choice A) accumulates from mutations in the fumarate hydratase (also known as fumarase) which are associated with hereditary leiomyomatosis and renal cell carcinoma (HLRCC). Accumulation of α-ketoglutarate (choice C) and oxaloacetate (choice D) are not normally associated with cancers. Accumulation of succinate (choice E) occurs in cancers that includes paragangliomas, pheochromocytomas, gastrointestinal stromal tumors (GIST) as a result of mutations in any of the four subunits of the succinate dehydrogenase (complex II) complex.

4. Correct answer is **D.** The signs and symptoms in this patient are typical of arsenic poisoning. Although no longer used in rodent poisons it was, at one time, a common ingredient. The molecular mechanism of arsenic toxicity is believed to be due to the ability of arsenite [As(III)] to bind protein thiols. One of the major effects of arsenic poisoning is inhibition of the pyruvate dehydrogenase complex, PDHc. Arsenic inhibits, not activates (choice A), the PDHc and as such will result in increased, not reduced (choice E), pyruvate levels. Arsenate [As(V)] has been shown to be reduced to As(III) by glyceraldehyde-3-phosphate dehydrogenase. In so doing there would be less enzyme for carrying out gluconeogenesis and thus, the rate would be decreased not increased (choice B). Arsenic also increases oxidative stress in cells and will therefore result in an increase in oxidized glutathione as opposed to the reduced form (choice C).

5. Correct answer is **D.** The signs and symptoms in the infant are most likely the result of a deficiency in the function of the pyruvate dehydrogenase complex, PDHc. In patients with PDHc deficiency, the major presentations encompass metabolic and neurologic pathologies with both occurring with equal frequency. The metabolic form presents as severe lactic acidosis in the newborn period which very often leads to lethality. The most common cause of PDHc deficiency is mutation in the gene, *PDHA1*, encoding the α-subunit of the E1 portion of the complex. Mutations in two of the three isocitrate dehydrogenase (choice A) genes result in the development of gliomas. Deficiency in α-ketoglutarate dehydrogenase (2-oxoglutarate dehydrogenase) function (choice B) is associated with oxoglutaric aciduria, ataxia, hypertonia, and global developmental delay. Lactate dehydrogenase deficiency (choice C) manifests with two forms of disorder, one of which is benign and usually goes undetected. In one form, patients experience fatigue, muscle pain, and cramps during exercise (exercise intolerance). Deficiencies in succinate dehydrogenase (choice E) occur in cancers that includes paragangliomas, pheochromocytomas, and gastrointestinal stromal tumors (GIST) as a result of mutations in any of the four subunits of the succinate dehydrogenase (complex II) complex.

6. Correct answer is **E.** Muscle contraction results in release of stored calcium ion from sarcoplasmic reticulum. The released calcium ions activate pyruvate dehydrogenase phosphatase (PDHP) resulting in dephosphorylation of the pyruvate dehydrogenase complex (PDHc), thereby increasing the overall activity of the PDHc. The PDHc is allosterically inhibited, not activated (choice A) by NADH. Although NAD^+ is utilized by α-ketoglutarate (2-oxoglutarate) dehydrogenase in the oxidation of α-ketoglutarate (2-oxoglutarate), the enzyme is not allosterically activated by the cofactor (choice B). Oxaloacetate plays no role in the regulation of the PDHc

(choice C). The α-ketoglutarate (2-oxoglutarate) dehydrogenase complex is regulated by levels of Ca^{2+}, ATP, ADP, NADH, and inorganic phosphate, but it is not regulated by phosphorylation/dephosphorylation (choice D) such as is the case for the PDHc.

7. Correct answer is **C.** The activity level of the pyruvate dehydrogenase complex (PDHc) is controlled by its state of phosphorylation. The PDHc is phosphorylated by a family of enzymes called the PDH kinases. In order to return the PDHc to full activity following PDH kinase-mediated phosphorylation the phosphates are removed by one of two PDH phosphatases. Phosphorylation of the PDHc (choice D) results in inhibition of the complex and thus, reduces the rate of pyruvate oxidation. Acetyl-CoA (choice A), ATP (choice B), and NADH (choice E) all activate the PDH kinases which will phosphorylate the PDHc rendering it less active and thus, reduce the rate of pyruvate oxidation.

8. Correct answer is **E.** The conversion of succinate to fumarate is catalyzed by the enzyme succinate dehydrogenase (SDH). This enzyme requires FAD, derived from riboflavin, as a cofactor for the reaction. None of the other enzyme cofactors (choices A, B, C, and D) are required for the activity of the SDH.

9. Correct answer is **E.** The signs and symptoms in the infant are most likely the result of a deficiency in the function of the pyruvate dehydrogenase complex, PDHc. In patients with PDHc deficiency the major presentations encompass metabolic and neurologic pathologies with both occurring with equal frequency. The metabolic form presents as severe lactic acidosis in the newborn period which very often leads to lethality. None of the other substances (choices A, B, C, and D) would be appreciably elevated as a result of deficiency in the PDHc.

10. Correct answer is **C.** The signs and symptoms in this patient are typical of arsenic poisoning. Mee's lines (semilunar white bands on nails) are associated with a number of pathologies including arsenic poisoning, Hodgkin lymphoma, and from certain chemotherapies. The molecular mechanism of arsenic toxicity is believed to be due to the ability of arsenite [As(III)] to bind protein thiols. One of the major effects of arsenic poisoning is inhibition of the α-ketoglutarate (2-oxoglutarate) dehydrogenase complex and the pyruvate dehydrogenase complex of the TCA cycle. None of the other enzymes (choices A, B, D, and E) are appreciably or directly affected by arsenic poisoning.

11. Correct answer is **E.** The patient is displaying signs and symptoms of porphyria cutanea tarda (PCT) which is a disorder in the synthesis of heme resulting from defects in the activity of uroporphyrinogen decarboxylase (UROD). The initiation of heme biosynthesis requires glycine and the TCA cycle intermediate, succinyl-CoA. None of the other compounds (choices A, B, C, and D) is involved in the pathway of heme biosynthesis.

12. Correct answer is **B.** The enzyme glutamate dehydrogenase is an important metabolic regulatory enzyme. It catalyzes the interconversion of α-ketoglutarate (2-oxoglutarate) to glutamate under conditions of high energy charge. Depletion of α-ketoglutarate will not only result in reduced carbon flow through the TCA cycle but will also reduce the synthesis of glutamate. Glutamate is the precursor for the synthesis of GABA, via the actions of glutamate decarboxylase, and therefore, reduced levels of α-ketoglutarate (2-oxoglutarate) can lead to reduced levels of glutamate which in turn will result in reduced levels of GABA. None of the other compounds (choices A, C, D, and E) directly participates in the pool of glutamate required for the synthesis of GABA.

13. Correct answer is **A.** Fluoroacetate is a structural analog of citrate and acts as a strong competitive inhibitor of aconitase. None of the other enzymes (choices B, C, D, and E) is inhibited by the actions of fluoroacetate.

14. Correct answer is **C.** The TCA cycle intermediate, malate, can be directly transported to the cytosol for conversion to oxaloacetate which is then converted to phosphoenolpyruvate and subsequently to glucose via gluconeogenesis. Although the carbons of isocitrate (choice A), α-ketoglutarate (2-oxoglutarate) (choice B), and succinate (choice E) will eventually make their way to the formation of malate in the TCA cycle, none can be transported out of the mitochondria for direct incorporation into the gluconeogenesis pathway. Pyruvate (choice D) is oxidized to acetyl-CoA and the equivalent of the two carbons of this compound are lost at the isocitrate dehydrogenase and α-ketoglutarate (2-oxoglutarate) dehydrogenase reactions and, therefore, cannot directly contribute to glucose synthesis.

15. Correct answer is **B.** The two carbon atoms that enter the TCA cycle as acetyl-CoA are stoichiometrically released as CO_2 at the isocitrate dehydrogenase and α-ketoglutarate (2-oxoglutarate) dehydrogenase catalyzed reactions. Thus, there is no net carbon input into malate which is the major gluconeogenic precursor of the TCA cycle. The NADH produced by the reactions of the TCA cycle (choice A) cannot be transported out of the mitochondria for use by glyceraldehyde-3-phosphate dehydrogenase during gluconeogenesis. Although succinyl-CoA can be diverted to heme synthesis (choice C), as indicated for the correct choice, acetyl-CoA carbons are stoichiometrically released as CO_2. Oxaloacetate is trapped in the mitochondrial matrix (choice D) and must first be converted to malate for transport to the cytosol. However, as indicated acetyl-CoA carbons are stoichiometrically released as CO_2 and thus cannot participate in the net synthesis of glucose. The carbons of acetyl-CoA are released as CO_2 at the isocitrate dehydrogenase and 2-oxoglutarate dehydrogenase and are not perpetually utilized (choice E) in the TCA cycle.

CHAPTER

10

Mitochondrial Functions and Oxidative Phosphorylation

High-Yield Terms

Mitochondrial DNA, mtDNA	The circular genome found within mitochondria encompasses genes involved in respiratory functions of this organelle
Electrochemical half-cell	Consists of an electrode and an electrolyte, two half-cells compose an electrochemical cell that is capable of deriving energy from chemical reactions
Ubiquinone, CoQ	A mobile component of the electron transport chain that can undergo either 1- or 2-electron reactions, transfers electrons from complexes I and II to complex III
Chemiosmotic potential	More correctly referred to as proton motive force (PMF), refers to the electrochemical gradient formed across the inner mitochondrial membrane due to the transport of protons, H^+, whose energy is used to drive ATP synthesis
Reactive oxygen species	Any of a group of chemically reactive molecules containing oxygen, such as hydrogen peroxide and superoxide anion
Encephalomyopathy	A disorder most often resulting from a defect in mitochondrial function affecting both skeletal muscle and central nervous system function
Adaptive thermogenesis	The regulated production of heat in response to environmental changes in temperature and diet, for example, shivering in humans is adaptive thermogenesis

MITOCHONDRIA

Oxidative phosphorylation is a critical energy (ATP) generating metabolic pathway that occurs within the mitochondria. Mitochondria contain a 16-kb circular genome (mitochondrial DNA, mtDNA) that contains 37 genes critical for the processes of oxidative phosphorylation. However, the mtDNA does not encode all of the proteins in the mitochondria. Over 900 mitochondrial proteins are actually encoded by the nuclear genome. Thirteen of the mtDNA genes encode protein subunits of respiratory complexes I, III, IV, and ATP synthase (sometimes referred to as complex V). Only complex II is solely composed of proteins encoded by nuclear genes. The mtDNA genome also encodes 22 mitochondrial tRNAs and 2 rRNAs that are essential for translation of mtDNA transcripts.

HIGH-YIELD CONCEPT

Mitochondria are maternally inherited due to the transmission of mitochondria from the egg to the zygote. Paternal mitochondria from the sperm are selectively marked with ubiquitin and degraded.

Mitochondria are the major energy producing organelles of cells. As a result of mutations in many of the mtDNA genes, the ability to produce ATP can be severely compromised. Given that mitochondria harbor between 1,100 and 1,400 different proteins, mutations in numerous nuclear genome genes are also associated with dysfunction of oxidative phosphorylation and ATP production. The brain and skeletal muscle require large amounts of mitochondrial ATP and are, therefore, the most severely affected tissues as a result of mtDNA mutations. Because of the brain and skeletal muscle involvement, these mtDNA disorders are most often referred to as the mitochondrial encephalomyopathies (see Clinical Box 35–1).

HIGH-YIELD CONCEPT

Redox reactions involve the transfer of electrons from one chemical species to another. The oxidized plus the reduced forms of each chemical species are referred to as an electrochemical half-cell.

PRINCIPLES OF REDUCTION/ OXIDATION (REDOX) REACTIONS

Coupled electrochemical half-cells have the thermodynamic properties of other coupled chemical reactions. An example of a coupled redox reaction is the oxidation of NADH by the electron transport chain:

$$NADH + ½O_2 + H^+ \rightarrow NAD^+ + H_2O$$

The thermodynamic potential of a chemical reaction is defined as the standard electrode potential, E^o. If the pH of a standard cell is in the biological range, pH 7, its potential is defined as the standard biological electrode potential and designated as $E^{o\prime}$. By convention, standard electrode potentials are written as potentials for reduction reactions of half-cells. The free energy of a typical reaction is calculated directly from its $E^{o\prime}$ by the Nernst equation, where n is the number of electrons involved in the reaction and F is the Faraday constant (23.06 kcal/volt/mol or 94.4 kJ/volt/mol):

$$\Delta G^{o\prime} = -nF\Delta E^{o\prime}$$

ENERGY FROM CYTOSOLIC NADH

The oxidation of glucose is a major pathway for the generation of cellular energy both aerobically and anaerobically. When carried out aerobically the NADH derived from cytosolic glycolysis is transferred into the mitochondria where it can be reoxidized and coupled to ATP synthesis. Two shuttle mechanisms exist termed the malate-aspartate shuttle (see Figure 5–2) and the glycerol-phosphate shuttle (see Figure 5–3). The glycerol-phosphate shuttle is the principal shuttle mechanism used in adipose tissue, skeletal muscle, and brain, whereas the liver, heart, and kidneys primarily utilize the malate-aspartate shuttle.

COMPLEXES OF THE ELECTRON TRANSPORT CHAIN

The large quantity of NADH resulting from glycolysis (Chapter 5) and the NADH and $FADH_2$ generated from fatty acid oxidation (see Chapter 13) and the TCA cycle (see Chapter 9) are used to supply the energy for ATP synthesis via oxidative phosphorylation (Figure 10–1).

HIGH-YIELD CONCEPT

Classically, the description of ATP synthesis through oxidation of reduced electron carriers indicated three moles of ATP could be generated for every mole of NADH and two moles for every mole of $FADH_2$. However, direct chemical analysis has shown that for every two electrons transferred from NADH to oxygen, 2.5 equivalents of ATP are synthesized and 1.5 ATP equivalents for $FADH_2$.

The reduced electron carriers, NADH and $FADH_2$, are oxidized by a series of catalytic redox carriers that are integral proteins of the inner mitochondrial membrane. These electron

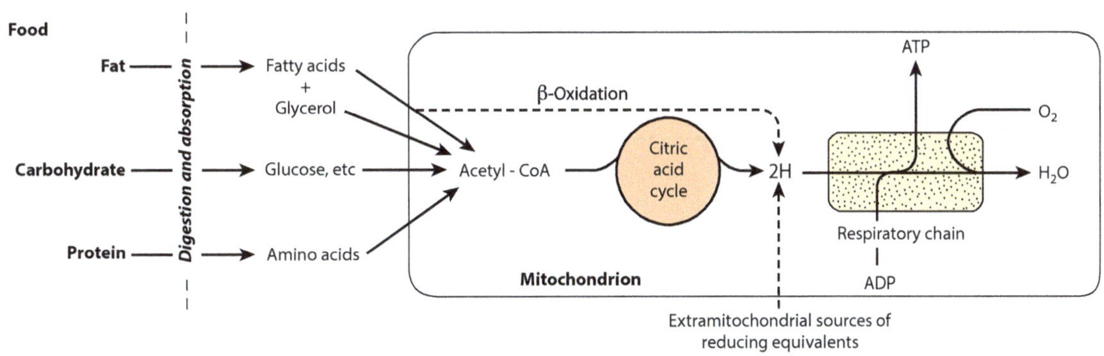

FIGURE 10–1 Role of the respiratory chain of mitochondria in the conversion of food energy to ATP. Oxidation of the major foodstuffs leads to the generation of reducing equivalents (2H) that are collected by the respiratory chain for oxidation and coupled generation of ATP. (Reproduced with permission from Rodwell VW, Bender DA, Botham KM, et al: *Harper's Illustrated Biochemistry*, 31st ed. New York, NY: McGraw Hill; 2018.)

carriers are termed complexes I, II, III, and IV. Coupled to these oxidation reduction steps is a transport process in which protons (H^+) from the mitochondrial matrix are transported to the space between the inner and outer mitochondrial membranes (Figure 10–2). The redistribution of protons leads to the formation of a proton gradient across the mitochondrial membrane. In the presence of ADP, protons flow down their thermodynamic gradient from outside the mitochondrial matrix back into the matrix. This process is facilitated by a proton carrier in the inner mitochondrial membrane known as ATP synthase. The energy of the proton gradient is utilized to drive the synthesis of ATP, hence the name of the proton carrier, ATP synthase.

Complex I is most commonly called NADH dehydrogenase but is also known as NADH:CoQ oxidoreductase or NADH-ubiquinone oxidoreductase. Complex II is most commonly called succinate dehydrogenase and is the same complex functioning in the TCA cycle (see Chapter 9). Complex II is also known as succinate:CoQ oxidoreductase or succinate:ubiquinone oxidoreductase.

Both complex I and complex II transfer electrons to coenzyme Q (CoQ: also known as ubiquinone). Because human CoQ possesses 10 isoprene units it is most often designated as CoQ_{10}. When reduced by electrons from complex I or II, CoQ (designated $CoQH_2$) donates its electrons to complex III.

Complex III is commonly called CoQ-cytochrome reductase but is also called ubiquinol-cytochrome *c* oxidoreductase. The electron carrier from complex III to complex IV is cytochrome *c*.

Complex IV is commonly called cytochrome *c* oxidase. This complex contains the hemeproteins known as cytochrome *a* and cytochrome *a3*, as well as copper-containing proteins in which the copper undergoes a transition from Cu^+ (cuprous) to Cu^{2+} (cupric) during the transfer of electrons through the complex. Oxygen (O_2) is the terminal electron acceptor, with water being the final product of oxygen reduction.

The free energy available as a consequence of transferring two electrons from NADH or $FADH_2$ to molecular oxygen is -57 and -36 kcal/mol, respectively. Oxidative phosphorylation utilizes some of this energy as in the formation of the high-energy phosphate of ATP via the activity of ATP synthase. However, not all of the energy is utilized in the work of ATP synthesis, the remainder of the energy is released as heat, the basis of the normal body temperature of 37°C.

ATP synthase is a multiple subunit complex that binds ADP and inorganic phosphate at its catalytic site inside the matrix of the mitochondria and requires a proton gradient for activity in the forward direction. ATP synthase is composed of three fragments: F_0, which is localized in the membrane; F_1, which protrudes from the inside of the inner membrane into the matrix; and oligomycin sensitivity-conferring protein (OSCP), which connects F_0 to F_1.

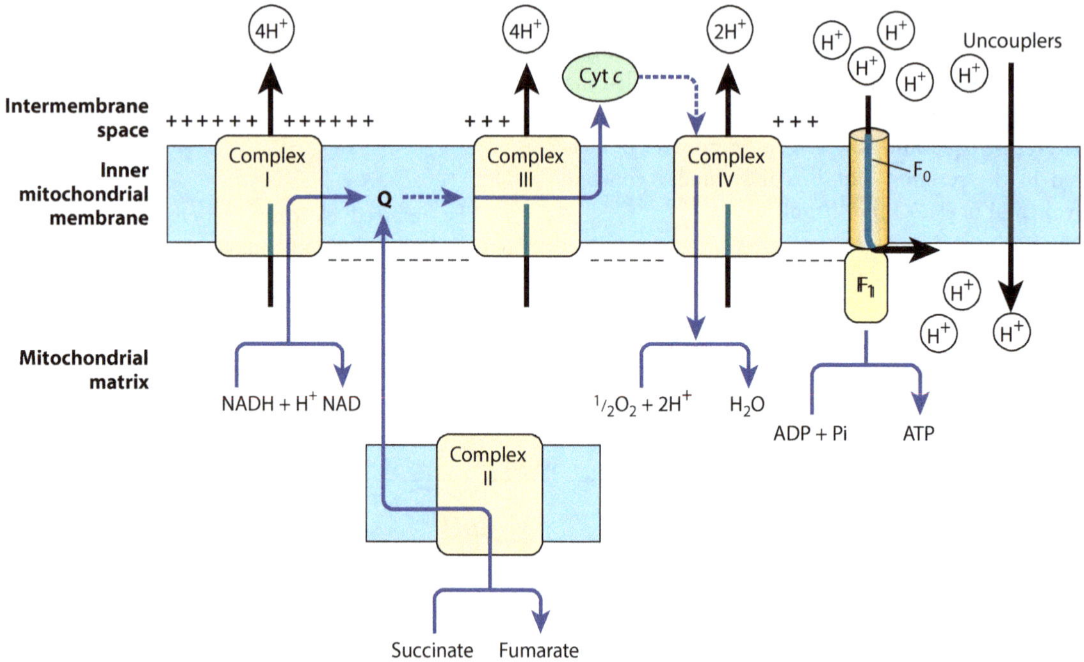

FIGURE 10–2 The chemiosmotic theory of oxidative phosphorylation. Complexes I, III, and IV act as proton pumps creating a proton gradient across the membrane, which is negative on the matrix side. The proton motive force generated drives the synthesis of ATP as the protons flow back into the matrix through the ATP synthase enzyme. Uncouplers increase the permeability of the membrane to ions, collapsing the proton gradient by allowing the H^+ to pass across without going through the ATP synthase, and thus uncouple electron flow through the respiratory complexes from ATP synthesis. (cyt, cytochrome; Q, coenzyme Q or ubiquinone.) (Reproduced with permission from Rodwell VW, Bender DA, Botham KM, et al: *Harper's Illustrated Biochemistry*, 31st ed. New York, NY: McGraw Hill; 2018.)

REGULATION OF OXIDATIVE PHOSPHORYLATION

Under resting conditions, with a high cell energy charge, the demand for new synthesis of ATP is limited. When energy demands are increased, such as during vigorous muscle activity, cytosolic ADP rises and is exchanged with intramitochondrial ATP via transmembrane ADP/ATP carriers (AAC) which are typical antiporters. Humans express three members of the AAC family of transporters. The concentration of ADP is the primary determinant of the rate of electron transport.

HIGH-YIELD CONCEPT

The rate of electron transport is usually measured by assaying the rate of oxygen consumption and is referred to as the cellular respiratory rate. The respiratory rate is known as the state 4 rate when the energy charge is high, the concentration of ADP is low, and electron transport is limited by ADP. When ADP levels rise and inorganic phosphate is available, the flow of protons through ATP synthase is elevated and higher rates of electron transport are observed; the resultant respiratory rate is known as the state 3 rate. Thus, under physiologic conditions mitochondrial respiratory activity cycles between state 3 and state 4 rates.

INHIBITION OF OXIDATIVE PHOSPHORYLATION

The experimental use of inhibitors of electron transport and oxidative phosphorylation were instrumental in the determination of the overall order of overall ATP synthesis. Some of these agents inhibit electron transport at specific sites in the electron transport assembly, while others stimulate electron transport by discharging the proton gradient (Figure 10–3). For example, antimycin A is a specific inhibitor of cytochrome *b*. In the presence of antimycin A, cytochrome *b* can be reduced but not oxidized. As expected, cytochrome *c* remains oxidized in the presence of antimycin A, as do the downstream cytochromes *a* and *a3*.

GENERATION OF REACTIVE OXYGEN SPECIES

The mitochondrial electron transport chain (ETC) of oxidative phosphorylation is the major site for the cellular generation of reactive oxygen species (ROS) (Figure 10–4).

HIGH-YIELD CONCEPT

As ATP demand decreases singlet electrons passing through the complexes of the ETC, particularly at complex I, can interact with molecular oxygen (O_2) resulting in the formation of superoxide anion. Superoxide anion is normally rapidly acted upon by superoxide dismutases (SOD). Humans express three SOD genes, *SOD1*, *SOD2*, and *SOD3*. The *SOD1* gene encodes a copper-zinc-superoxide dismutase (CuZn-SOD; also designated SOD1). The *SOD2* gene encodes a mitochondrial superoxide dismutase (Mn-SOD; also identified as SOD2). The SOD3 gene encodes an extracellular superoxide dismutase (EC-SOD; also identified as SOD3). All three SOD enzymes dismutate superoxide anion to yield hydrogen peroxide (H_2O_2).

Mitochondrial production of ROS contributes to the processes of aging as well as progression of numerous disorders such as type 2 diabetes and Parkinson disease. Dietary constituents can lead to increased ROS production which is evident in obesity and plays a major contributing role in the progression to insulin-resistance

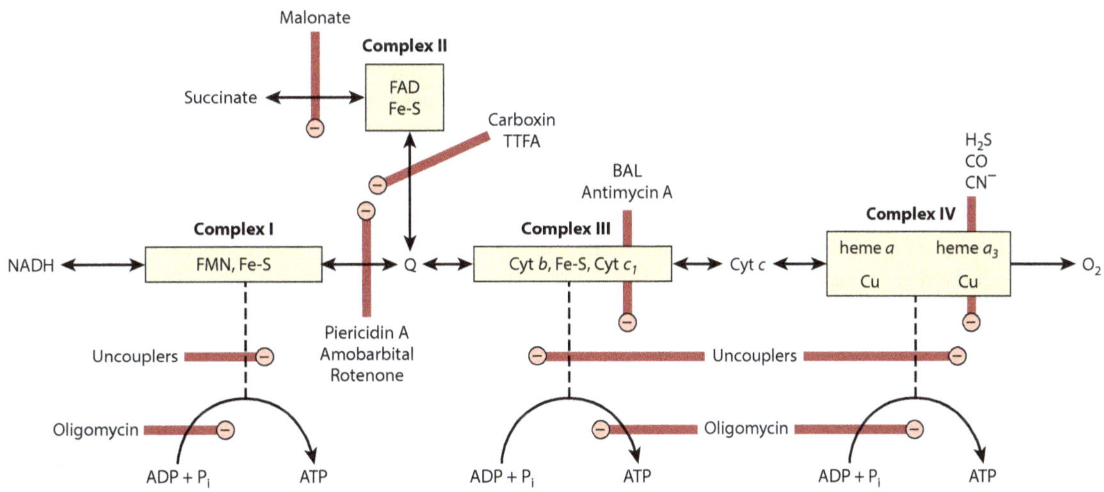

FIGURE 10–3 Sites of inhibition (⊖) of the respiratory chain by specific drugs, chemicals, and antibiotics. (BAL, dimercaprol; TTFA, an Fe-chelating agent. (Reproduced with permission from Rodwell VW, Bender DA, Botham KM, et al: *Harper's Illustrated Biochemistry*, 31st ed. New York, NY: McGraw Hill; 2018.)

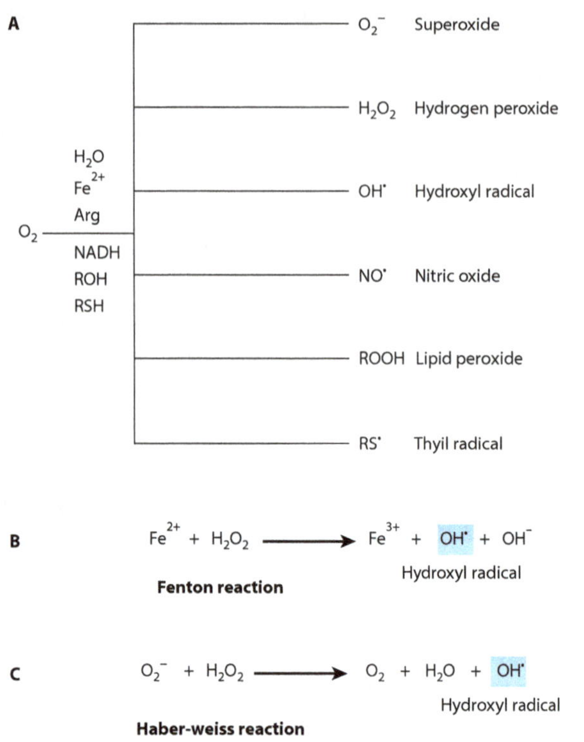

FIGURE 10–4 Reactive oxygen species (ROS) are toxic byproducts of life in an aerobic environment. (A) Many types of ROS are encountered in living cells. (B) Generation of hydroxyl radical via the Fenton reaction. (C) Generation of hydroxyl radical by the Haber-Weiss reaction. (Reproduced with permission from Rodwell VW, Bender DA, Botham KM, et al: *Harper's Illustrated Biochemistry*, 31st ed. New York, NY: McGraw Hill; 2018.)

and diabetes. Consumption of a high-fat diet results in a surplus of NADH and $FADH_2$ that then increases electron delivery to the ETC with a resultant increase in ROS generation. Indeed, a high-fat diet is known to increase the rate of H_2O_2 production in skeletal muscle mitochondria. Ultimately the increased rate of ROS production by the mitochondria results in mitochondrial dysfunction.

Most tissues are replete with enzymes to protect against the random chemical reactions that are triggered by ROS. Free-radical scavenging enzymes include the SOD, catalase, glutathione peroxidases (GPx), and peroxiredoxins (PRX). SODs convert superoxide anion to H_2O_2, thereby minimizing production of hydroxy radical which is the most potent of the oxygen-free radicals. Peroxides produced by SOD are also toxic. They are detoxified by conversion to water via the peroxidases such as the glutathione peroxidases. Catalase (located in peroxisomes) provides a reductant route for the degradation of H_2O_2.

BROWN ADIPOSE TISSUE AND ADAPTIVE THERMOGENESIS

The uncoupling of proton flow releases the energy of the electrochemical proton gradient as heat (Figure 10–5). This process is a normal physiologic function of brown adipose tissue (BAT) and is referred to as **adaptive thermogenesis**.

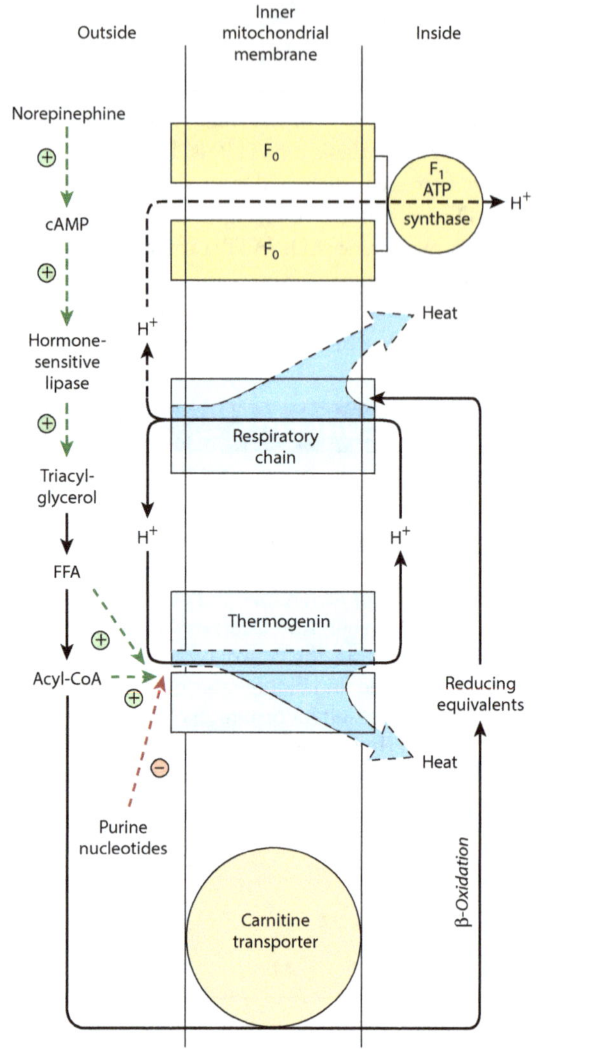

FIGURE 10–5 Thermogenesis in brown adipose tissue. Activity of the respiratory chain produces heat in addition to translocating protons. These protons dissipate more heat when returned to the inner mitochondrial compartment via thermogenin instead of via the F1 ATP synthase, the route that generates ATP. The passage of H^+ via thermogenin is inhibited by purine nucleotides when brown adipose tissue is unstimulated. Under the influence of norepinephrine, the inhibition is removed by the production of free fatty acids (FFA) and acyl-CoA. Note the dual role of acyl-CoA in both facilitating the action of thermogenin and supplying reducing equivalents for the respiratory chain. ⊕ and ⊖ signify positive or negative regulatory effects. (Reproduced with permission from Rodwell VW, Bender DA, Botham KM, et al: *Harper's Illustrated Biochemistry*, 31st ed. New York, NY: McGraw Hill; 2018.)

Newborn babies contain BAT in their neck and upper back that serves the function of nonshivering thermogenesis. The muscle contractions that take place in the process of shivering not only generate ATP but also produce heat. Nonshivering thermogenesis is a hormonally stimulated process for heat generation without the associated muscle contractions of shivering. The process of thermogenesis in BAT is initiated by norepinephrine-mediate release of fatty acids from the triglycerides stored in BAT.

The mitochondria in BAT contains a protein called uncoupling protein 1, UCP1 (also called thermogenin). There are three uncoupling protein genes in humans identified as *UCP1, UCP2,* and *UCP3.* Only UCP1 is involved in the process of adaptive thermogenesis.

UCP1 acts as a channel in the inner mitochondrial membrane to control the permeability of the membrane to protons. When norepinephrine is released in response to cold sensation, it binds to β_3-adrenergic receptors on the surface of brown adipocytes triggering the activation of adenylate cyclase. Activated adenylate cyclase leads to increased production of cAMP and the concomitant activation of PKA. PKA then phosphorylates, and activates, hormone-sensitive lipase (HSL). The released free fatty acids bind to UCP1 triggering an uncoupling of the proton gradient and the release of the energy of the gradient as heat.

CHECKLIST

- ☑ In biological systems the processes of oxidation and reduction refer to the loss and gain of electrons, respectively.
- ☑ Mitochondria is evolved from a symbiotic relationship between aerobic bacteria and primordial eukaryotic cells. The function of the mitochondria is to convert the energy from catabolic reaction into ATP via a process of electron transport.
- ☑ The energy released from the oxidation of carbohydrates, fats, and amino acids is made available to the mitochondria in the form of the educed electron carriers, NADH and $FADH_2$. The electrons from these compounds are then transferred through the electron transport chain to molecular oxygen.
- ☑ The electron transport chain is composed of four complexes. Three of these complexes utilize the energy of electron transport to pump protons across the inner mitochondrial membrane creating an electrochemical gradient between the inside of the mitochondria and the inner membrane space. This gradient is referred to as the proton motive force or the chemiosmotic potential and is the energy driving ATP synthesis.
- ☑ ATP synthase (sometimes referred to as complex V) is a rotary-type ATPase that spans the inner mitochondrial membrane and utilizes the energy of the proton gradient (proton motive force) to drive ATP synthesis from ADP and inorganic phosphate (P_i).
- ☑ Numerous poisons and chemicals interfere with the processes of oxidative phosphorylation, such as carbon monoxide and cyanide, both of which inhibit the activities of complex IV.
- ☑ Uncoupling agents create pores in the inner mitochondrial membrane thereby allowing protons to flow across the membrane preventing ATP synthesis and releasing the energy as heat. This process occurs naturally in brown adipose tissue (BAT) and is catalyzed by UCP1 in a process called adaptive thermogenesis.
- ☑ The electron transport chain is the major site for the generation of cellular reactive oxygen species (ROS) occurring mainly via complex I. Excess delivery of NADH to complex I can result in some electrons passing to molecular oxygen directly generating super oxide anion. Super oxide is neutralized via the action of mitochondrial and cytosolic superoxide dismutases (SOD).
- ☑ The excess oxidation of fatty acids, as is typical in obesity, drives an increase in ROS production leading to progressive mitochondrial dysfunction. Pancreatic β-cells are especially susceptible to ROS damage and mitochondrial-triggered apoptosis contributing to the development of diabetes in overweight and obese individuals.

REVIEW QUESTIONS

1. A laboratory analysis of isolated mitochondria demonstrates that oxygen consumption is normal when succinate is added but extremely low when pyruvate and malate are used. The mitchondria are subsequently shown to have normal cytochromes but a reduced iron content. The reduced pyruvate/malate oxidation is most likely to be due to a defect in which of the following respiratory components?
(A) Cytochrome c
(B) Cytochrome oxidase
(C) NADH dehydrogenase
(D) Succinate dehydrogenase
(E) Ubiquinone

2. A 27-year-old woman has undergone genetic testing to ascertain the cause of her persistent nausea, vomiting, shakiness, fever, and irregular heartbeat. These studies have ascertained that the symptoms are due to mitochondrial dysfunction and that the inheritance is strictly due to nuclear gene defects. Given these findings, oxidation of which of the following substrates would be most impaired in this patient?
(A) Alanine
(B) Lactate
(C) Malate
(D) Pyruvate
(E) Succinate

3. A family is being studied due to the presentation of severe symptoms and early lethality in several members. It is determined that the disease is transmitted as an autosomal recessive disorder. The characteristic features in affected family members include intellectual deterioration, weakness, ataxia, seizures, and death at a young age. Muscle biopsy studies

determine that there is a deficiency of cytochrome *c* oxidase activity. Postmortem pathology shows symmetric necrosis that affects the brain from the thalamus to the spinal cord. Which of the following cellular organelles is most likely to be defective in affected members of this family?
(A) Golgi apparatus
(B) Lysosomes
(C) Mitochondria
(D) Ribosomes
(E) Smooth endoplasmic reticulum

4. A 47-year-old man is rushed to the emergency department after being found unconscious outside his burning home. Laboratory studies show a serum pH of 7.27 (N = 7.35–7.45), bicarbonate of 14 mEq/L (N = 19–25 mEq/L), an anion gap of 15 mEq/L (N = 8–12 mEq/L), and lactic acidemia. The attending physician noted an odor of bitter almonds on his breath and immediately prescribed inhalation amyl nitrite followed by IV sodium nitrite. Given the symptoms and treatment protocol, which of the following was most likely to be inhibited in this patient?
(A) ATP synthase
(B) Complex I
(C) Complex II
(D) Complex III
(E) Complex IV

5. Studies are being undertaken to examine the effects of a compound on the respiratory activity of isolated mitochondria. Results from these experiments demonstrate that oxygen consumption is normal when pyruvate and malate are used as well as when succinate is added. However, the production of ATP is severely impaired with addition of the compound. These results most closely resemble the effects that would be seen by the addition of which of the following?
(A) Antimycin A
(B) Azide
(C) Dinitrophenol (DNP)
(D) Oligomycin
(E) Rotenone

6. A 9-year-old boy is being examined by his pediatrician following an episode of hemiparesis resulting in loss of motor skills. History reveals that the child has been suffering from persistent headaches, vision problems, loss of appetite, and vomiting. The parents note that their 5-year-old daughter has also recently shown signs of incoordination in her walking. Ophthalmoscopic examination reveals pigmentary retinopathy. Blood analysis shows elevated levels of lactic acid, and the ratio of lactate to pyruvate is high relative to normal values. Based upon family history and the signs and symptoms in this patient, which of the following is the most likely mode of inheritance?
(A) Autosomal dominant
(B) Autosomal recessive
(C) Mitochondrial
(D) X-linked dominant
(E) X-linked recessive

7. Studies are being undertaken to examine the effects of a compound on the respiratory activity of isolated mitochondria. Addition of the compound significantly reduces the oxidation of iron from the ferrous to the ferric state. Given these findings, this compound is most likely to be interfering with the activity of which of the following?
(A) Catalase
(B) Cytochrome *c* oxidase
(C) Cytochrome P450-associated ferredoxin 1
(D) Peroxidase
(E) Superoxide dismutase

8. Studies are being carried out to examine the effects of a compound on the respiratory activity of isolated mitochondria. Addition of the compound results in a significant increase in the rate of oxygen consumption regardless of whether pyruvate, malate, or succinate is used as a substrate. These results most closely resemble the effects that would be seen by the addition of which of the following?
(A) Antimycin A
(B) Carbon monoxide
(C) Cyanide
(D) Dinitrophenol
(E) Phenobarbitol

9. An 18-year-old woman is being examined by her physician because of increasing vision problems and a postural tremor. History reveals that she has an older brother and an older sister and both of them experienced similar deteriorating symptoms in their twenties. Her aunt and uncle on her mother's side were also similarly afflicted with variable manifestation of symptoms. Examination shows diminished eye movements and a pigmentary retinopathy. Her physician suspects the family suffers from a form of mitochondrial dysfunction. If this diagnosis is correct, mitochondrial electron transfer is most likely to be defective at which location?
(A) ATP synthase
(B) Complex I
(C) Complex III
(D) Complex IV
(E) Pyruvate dehydrogenase

10. A 37-year-old woman has been brought to the emergency department in an unconscious state. Upon taking blood for analysis the attending physician notices its intense cherry-red color. Results of the blood analysis show a high anion gap metabolic acidosis. Given these findings, the physician suspect poisoning as the cause of the pathology in this patient. Which of the following is the most likely target of the suspected poison?
(A) ATP synthase
(B) Complex I
(C) Complex II
(D) Complex IV
(E) Pyruvate dehydrogenase

11. A physician is examining a 6-year-old boy who has been experiencing progressive muscle weakness. Assays on muscle biopsy tissue from this patient find that mitochondrial oxidation of succinate is normal, but that pyruvate oxidation is severely impaired. Mitochondrial extracts demonstrate that the activity of the pyruvate dehydrogenase complex is normal as is the activity of malate dehydrogenase. These results are consistent with the patient harboring a defect in which of the following mitochondrial components?
(A) ATP-synthase
(B) Complex I
(C) Complex II

(D) Complex III
(E) Complex IV
(F) Mitochondrial pyruvate transporter
(G) Mitochondrial succinate transporter

12. Experiments are being carried out on isolated skeletal muscle mitochondria with malate as the oxidizable substrate. Following the addition of malate, potassium cyanide is added. Under these conditions which of the following components of the electron transport chain is most likely to be in an oxidized state?
(A) Coenzyme Q
(B) Complex I
(C) Complex II
(D) Complex III
(E) Cytochrome *c*

13. A 6-year-old boy is being examined by his pediatrician following an episode of hemiparesis resulting in loss of motor skills. History reveals that the child has been suffering from persistent headaches, vision problems, loss of appetite, and vomiting. Physical examination notes that the patient is short for his age and an ophthalmoscopic examination reveals pigmentary retinopathy. Blood analysis shows elevated levels of lactic acid and the ratio of lactate to pyruvate is high relative to normal values. These signs and symptoms are most indicative of which of the following disorders?
(A) Erythrocyte pyruvate kinase deficiency
(B) Kearns-Sayre syndrome (KSS)
(C) Leigh syndrome
(D) Mitochondrial myopathy, encephalopathy, lactic acidosis, and stroke-like episodes (MELAS)
(E) Type 1 diabetes

14. Experiments are being conducted to ascertain the mode of action of a potential novel pharmacologic agent. The experiments are being conducted with the use of isolated mitochondria extracted from muscle biopsy tissue. Addition of the agent significantly reduces ATP synthesis suggesting that it's most likely mode of action is which of the following?
(A) Activation of cytochrome *c*
(B) Disruption of the pH gradient across the inner mitochondrial membrane
(C) Increasing the rate of pyruvate transport across the mitochondrial membrane
(D) Inhibition of glyceraldehyde-3-phosphate dehydrogenase
(E) Inhibition of NADH generation by NADH dehydrogenase

15. A newborn is exposed to cold but does not shiver. Under these conditions, the infant maintains a normal core temperature of 37.2°C. This is most likely the result of which of the following actions of a specialized tissue present in the neonate?
(A) Blocking the actions of hepatic lipase
(B) Blocking the activation of adrenal medullary hormone production
(C) Increased cortisol production
(D) Increased thyroxine synthesis
(E) Uncoupling of chemiosmotic potential from ATP formation
(F) Uncoupling of gluconeogenesis from triglyceride hydrolysis

16. A 1-year-old infant is being examined in the emergency department following suffering a series of seizures. Physical examination finds icteric sclera and a yellowish hue to the infant's skin. Blood work finds elevated levels of both AST and ALT. Studies utilizing liver biopsy tissue finds that mitochondrial DNA replication is significantly impaired. This infant is most likely suffering from which of the following disorders?
(A) Alpers-Huttenlocher syndrome
(B) Kearns-Sayre syndrome (KSS)
(C) Leigh syndrome
(D) Mitochondrial myopathy, encephalopathy, lactic acidosis, and stroke-like episodes (MELAS)
(E) Myoclonic epilepsy and ragged red fiber disease (MERRF)

17. A 21-year-old man is brought to the emergency department after being found unconscious. There is evidence that he has vomited recently. Physical examination shows he is tachypneic and has an odor of bitter almonds on his exhaled breaths. Blood lactate concentration is 3.3 mmol/L (normal = 0.5–1 mmol/L). Which of the following processes is most likely inhibited in this patient contributing to his pathology?
(A) Conversion of pyruvate to alanine
(B) Glycolysis
(C) Mitochondrial electron transport
(D) Mobilization of fatty acids from adipose tissue
(E) Release of insulin from pancreas

18. Experiments are being conducted on the effects of a novel compound on respiratory function in mitochondria. Addition of the compound is shown to dissipate the normal proton gradient across the inner mitochondrial membrane. Based upon these finding which of the following is the most likely metabolic effect of this compound?
(A) Cessation of fatty acid oxidation
(B) Cessation of NADH oxidation
(C) Cessation of TCA cycle activity
(D) Loss of ATP production with normal O_2 consumption
(E) Loss of O_2 consumption with normal ATP production

19. Experiments are being conducted on the activity of succinate dehydrogenase in isolated mitochondria. The standard reduction potentials ($E^{0'}$) are provided for several reactions in this system. Succinate, fumarate, FAD, and $FADH_2$, all at 1M, are added to the mitochondria. Which of the following initial event is most likely to take place?

$$\text{Fumarate} + 2H^+ + 2^{e-} \rightarrow \text{succinate} \qquad E^{0'} = +0.031\text{ V}$$
$$\text{FAD} + 2H^+ + 2^{e-} \rightarrow FADH_2 \qquad E^{0'} = -0.219\text{ V}$$

(A) Fumarate and succinate would become oxidized; FAD and $FADH_2$ would become reduced
(B) Fumarate would become reduced, $FADH_2$ would become oxidized
(C) No reaction would occur because all reactants and products are already at their standard concentrations
(D) Succinate would become oxidized, and FAD would become reduced
(E) Succinate would become oxidized, and $FADH_2$ would be unchanged because it is a cofactor

20. A 1-year-old infant is being examined in the emergency department following suffering a series of seizures. Physical examination finds icteric sclera and a yellowish hue to the infant's skin. Blood work finds elevated levels of both AST and ALT. Studies utilizing liver biopsy tissue finds that mitochondrial

DNA replication is significantly impaired. Based upon the findings, in this case which of the following represents the most likely mode of inheritance of the disorder?

(A) Autosomal dominant
(B) Autosomal recessive
(C) Mitochondrial
(D) X-linked dominant
(E) X-linked recessive

ANSWERS

1. Correct answer is **C.** During the process of oxidative phosphorylation, electrons from reduced electron carriers enter the pathway at either complex I (NADH) or complex II ($FADH_2$). The reduced electron carrier, derived from the oxidation of pyruvate and malate (NADH), enters the oxidative phosphorylation machinery at complex I, NADH-coenzyme Q reductase (also identified as NADH dehydrogenase and NADH-ubiquinone oxidoreductase). The reduced electron carrier generated during the succinate dehydrogenase-mediated (choice D) oxidation of succinate ($FADH_2$) enters the oxidative phosphorylation machinery at complex II. Thus, a defect in the activity of complex I would inhibit oxygen consumption in the presence of pyruvate or malate but not succinate. Cytochrome c (choice A) is a component of complex III and thus is downstream of both complex I and complex II, so a defect in cytochrome c function would reduce oxygen consumption by all of the indicated substrates. Cytochrome oxidase (choice B) is also known as cytochrome c oxidase or complex IV which is downstream of both complex I and complex II so a defect in cytochrome oxidase function would reduce oxygen consumption by all of the indicated substrates. Electrons from complex I and complex II are transferred to ubiquinone, also called CoQ10, (choice E) so if this component was defective there would be no oxygen consumption with any of the indicated substrates.

2. Correct answer is **E.** The symptoms in this patient are highly indicative of paraganglioma which has been shown to be associated with mutations in any of the four genes encoding the subunits of succinate dehydrogenase (complex II). All four of these gene are strictly within the nuclear genome. Complex II accepts electrons from $FADH_2$. The principal sources of $FADH_2$ are oxidation of fatty acids by the various fatty acyl-CoA dehydrogenases, oxidation of succinate via succinate dehydrogenase (also known as complex II), and oxidation of glycerol-3-phosphate to dihydroxyacetone phosphate (DHAP) via mitochondrial glycerol-3-phosphate dehydrogenase (GPD2) as occurs in the glycerol phosphate shuttle. Metabolism of alanine (choice A) includes deamination to pyruvate and then oxidation of pyruvate via pyruvate dehydrogenase yielding NADH. The NADH generated by oxidation of lactate (choice B), malate (choice C), and pyruvate (choice D) would pass electrons to complex I and therefore bypass any defect in complex II.

3. Correct answer is **C.** The family members afflicted with the disorder are manifesting symptoms of a mitochondrial encephalomyopathy. Cytochrome *c* oxidase is also known as complex IV of the oxidative phosphorylation pathway which occurs within the inner mitochondrial membrane. None of the other organelles (choices A, B, D, and E) possess cytochrome *c* oxidase activity.

4. Correct answer is **E.** The patient has symptoms of cyanide poisoning. In house fires, cyanide anion (CN^-) is released during the combustion of furniture, rugs, plastics, and other construction materials. Cyanide anion has a very high affinity for iron in the ferric state (Fe^{3+}) as it exists in complex IV of the oxidative phosphorylation pathway. When CN^- is absorbed, it reacts with the Fe^{3+} of cytochrome oxidase in complex IV. As a consequence of decreased oxidative phosphorylation, glycolysis is increased and pyruvate oxidation is impaired, both of which result in lactic acidosis. The odor of bitter almonds is a distinctive feature of cyanide poisoning. Cyanide anion does not interfere with the activity of other components of oxidative phosphorylation (choices A, B, C, and D).

5. Correct answer is **C.** The normal flow of electrons, through the protein complexes of the oxidative phosphorylation machinery, is coupled with the establishment of a proton gradient across the inner mitochondrial membrane. The establishment of this pH gradient is the chemiosmotic potential that is coupled with the production of ATP. If the process of proton movement is uncoupled from the normal pathway through the ATP synthase complex, oxygen can be consumed but no ATP will be synthesized. This is the effect of uncoupling agents such as dinitrophenol, which act to discharge the proton gradient releasing the energy as heat instead of allowing it to be used for the work of ATP sythesis. Antimycin A (choice A) inhibits the flow of electrons from cytochrome *b* to cytochrome *c* within complex III and as such would interfere with the oxidation of all the substrate utilized in this study. Azide (choice B) inhibits the function of complex IV and as such would interfere with the oxidation of all the substrate utilized in this study. Oligomycin (choice D) directly inteferes with ATP synthase stopping the synthesis of ATP. Since the proton gradient cannot be utilized for ATP synthesis all of the other steps of oxidative phosphorylation will begin to cease in the presence of oligomycin. Rotenone (choice E) inhibits complex I which would be associated with a block to the oxidation of pyruvate and malate.

6. Correct answer is **C.** The patient is most likely suffering from the consequences of the mitochondrial encephalomyopathy known as MELAS (mitochondrial encephalopathy with lactic acidosis and stroke-like symptoms). MELAS, as the name implies, is characterized by severe lactic acidosis and stroke-like episodes. MELAS results from mutations in several mitochondrial genome (mtDNA) genes. Mitochondrial inheritance is near exclusively maternal and all of the children, regardless of their sex, of the mother will manifest varying degrees of the symptoms of MELAS. None of the other modes of inheritance (choices A, B, D, and E) conform to the mode of inheritance of MELAS.

7. Correct answer is **B.** The iron in the heme moiety of cytochrome *c* is oxidized from the ferrous (Fe^{2+}) to the ferric (Fe^{3+}) states by ubiquinone (CoQ10) which itself was oxidized by both complex I and complex II. Cytochrome c is associated with complex IV, also known as cytochrome *c* oxidase. Complex IV contains the hemeproteins known as cytochrome *a* and cytochrome *a*3, as well as copper-containing proteins in which the copper undergoes a transition from cuprous (Cu^+) to cupric (Cu^{2+}) during the reduction of the Fe^{3+} iron in cytochrome c back to the Fe^{2+} state allowing for more electrons to be transferred, ultimately to molecular oxygen. Catalase (choice A) catalyzes the reduction of hydrogen peroxide

(H_2O_2) to water (H_2O). The ferredoxin 1 component of many cytochrome P540 (CYP) enzymes (choice C) contributes to the overall process of substrate oxidation carried out by these enzymes. Peroxidase (choice D) is an enzyme that reduces peroxides such as hydrogen peroxide and hydroperoxides. The members of the glutathione peroxidase family are peroxides. Superoxide dismutase (choice E) catalyzes the dismutation of superoxide anion into molecular oxygen (O_2) and hydrogen peroxide.

8. Correct answer is **D.** Dinitrophenol, DNP, is a chemical uncoupler of electron transport. Uncouplers cause increased oxygen consumption. DNP exerts its effects by acting as a proton ionophore allowing protons to flow back into the matrix of the mitochondria through the inner mitochondrial membrane which dissipates the electrochemical gradient and preventing ATP synthesis. Since the proton motive force across the membrane is lost there is no longer a gradient to restrict the rate of electron flow, electron transport accelerates resulting in increased oxygen consumption. Antimycin A (choice A) inhibits the flow of electrons from cytochrome *b* to cytochrome *c* within complex III and as such would interfere with the oxidation of all the substrate utilized in this study. Carbon monoxide (choice B) and cyanide (choice C) inhibit the function of complex IV. Phenobarbitol (choice E) inhibits complex I and, thus, would prevent electrons from pyruvate and malate from being passed through the electron transport chain.

9. Correct answer is **B.** The signs and symptoms in this patient, coupled with the family history, strongly indicates that patient is suffering from the effects of Leber hereditary optic neuropathy (LHON). LHON is most commonly caused by mutations in one of the protein coding genes of the mitochondrial genome identified as MT-ND1. MT-ND1 encodes a subunit of NADH dehydrogenase (complex I) indicating that none of the other options (choices A, C, D, and E) are correct.

10. Correct answer is **D.** Exposure to carbon monoxide (CO) can be lethal, primarily as a result of the high affinity of hemoglobin for CO which binds to the same domain as oxygen (O_2) but with an affinity on the order of 100 times higher than O_2. Binding of CO forms carboxyhemoglobin, which imparts the cherry-red color to blood. In addition to blocking O_2 binding to hemoglobin, CO binds to other heme proteins, in particular within complex IV, thereby blocking its ability to transfer electrons to molecular oxygen. None of the other complexes (choices A, B, C, and E) are appreciably affected by carbon monoxide poisoning.

11. Correct answer is **B.** Since the activity of the pyruvate dehydrogenase complex (PDHc) of the patient's mitochondria was shown to be normal but the NADH produced by this reaction could not be oxidized via electron transport it suggests that the defect causing the muscle weakness is in mitochondrial complex I. Succinate oxidation was normal indicating that electron flow to complex II (choice C) is not impaired, further strengthening the argument that the defect lies in complex I. If ATP synthase (choice A), complex III (choice D), or complex IV (choice E) were defective neither pyruvate nor succinate oxidation would occur normally. If either mitochondrial pyruvate transporter (choice F) was defective there would be little measurable PDHc activity. If the mitochondrial succinate transporter (choice G) was defective, the oxidation of succinate would be impaired.

12. Correct answer is **C.** Cyanide inhibits the transfer of electrons through complex IV (cytochrome oxidase). In order for any of the components of electron transport to be in an oxidized state they must have either transferred electrons to the next component downstream or never have received electrons in the first place. Oxidation of malate generates NADH which is then reoxidized by donating its electrons to complex I. Complex I is reoxidized by donating its electrons to coenzyme Q. Coenzyme Q is then reoxidized by donating its electrons to complex III, then to cytochrome *c*, and finally they are passed to complex IV. Since cyanide blocks the transfer of electrons from complex IV to oxygen, all of the upstream electron acceptors (choices A, B, D, and E) will be "blocked" in the reduced state. Only complex II will have never accepted electrons and thus will be in the oxidized state under the conditions of this experiment.

13. Correct answer is **D.** Disorders of mitochondrial biogenesis and function are similar to lysosomal storage diseases in that there are symptom similarities between several different diseases of the class. Many of the mitochondrial encephalomyopathies are associated with hearing loss, vision problems such as pigmentary retinopathy, and neurologic dysfunction. MELAS is characterized by the fact that it is also associated with the potential for severe lactic acidosis and stroke-like episodes. Erythrocyte pyruvate kinase deficiency (choice A) is one of the most common enzyme deficiencies resulting in inherited nonspherocytic hemolytic anemia. It is most often diagnosed in infancy or early childhood. Symptoms of Kearns-Sayre syndrome (choice B) usually appear before age 20 and most commonly affect the eyes with characteristic symptoms including chronic progressive external ophthalmoplegia (PEO) which represents weakness or paralysis of the eye muscles impairing eye movement and causing drooping eyelids (ptosis). Leigh syndrome (choice C) is normally fatal before age 5 and so could be eliminated solely on the basis of the patient's age. Type 1 diabetes (choice E) is characterized by autoimmune destruction of the insulin secreting cells of the pancreas resulting in the potential for severe metabolic derangement characteristically manifesting as chronic hyperglycemia and frequent episodes of potentially fatal ketoacidosis.

14. Correct answer is **B.** The normal flow of electrons, through the proteins of the oxidative phosphorylation machinery, is coupled with the establishment of a proton gradient across the inner mitochondrial membrane. The establishment of this pH gradient is the chemiosmotic potential that is coupled with the production of ATP. Any disruption in this proton motive force, such as with the addition of an uncoupling agent, results in a dissipation of the energy of the pH gradient as heat instead of the energy being used for the work of ATP synthesis but does not prevent oxygen consumption. Activation of cytochrome *c* (choice A) would increase electron flow and contribute to an increase, not a decrease, in ATP synthesis. Increasing pyruvate transport (choice C) would increase its oxidation, ultimately increasing, not decreasing, ATP synthesis. Inhibition of glyceraldehyde-3-phosphate dehydrogenase (choice D) would impair the oxidation of glucose and reduce cytosolic NADH production, but it would not inhibit the oxidation of other substrates and thus, would not lead to loss of ATP synthesis. NADH dehydrogenase (complex I) oxidizes NADH to NAD^+ as opposed to generating NADH (choice E).

15. Correct answer is **E.** The uncoupling of proton flow releases the energy of the electrochemical proton gradient as heat.

This process is a normal physiologic function of brown adipose tissue (BAT). Newborn babies contain BAT in their neck and upper back that serves the function of nonshivering thermogenesis. The mitochondria in BAT contains a protein called uncoupling protein 1, UCP1 (also called thermogenein). UCP1 acts as a channel in the inner mitochondrial membrane to control the permeability of the membrane to protons. When norepinephrine is released in response to cold sensation it binds to β_3-adrenergic receptors on the surface of brown adipocytes triggering the activation of adenylate cyclase. Activated adenylate cyclase leads to increased production of cAMP and the concomitant activation of PKA with the result being phosphorylation and activation of hormone-sensitive lipase, HSL. The released free fatty acids, as a result of HSL activation, bind to UCP1 triggering an uncoupling of the proton gradient and the release of the energy of the gradient as heat. Blocking the actions of hepatic lipase (choice A) would exert no effect on adipose tissue thermogenesis. Blocking adrenal medullary hormone production (choice B) would result in less circulating norepinephrine and a reduction in BAT-mediated adaptive thermogenesis. Increased cortisol production (choice C) would result in enhanced triglyceride metabolism and fatty acid release but would not contribute to adaptive thermogenesis ion BAT. Increased thyroxine (T4) synthesis (choice D) would result in an increase in the rate of adaptive thermogenesis in BAT but this is not the mechanism that occurs in response to the sensation of cold in the neonate. Uncoupling of gluconeogenesis from triglyceride hydrolysis (choice F) would result in reduced serum glucose levels but not directly affect the process of adaptive thermogenesis.

16. Correct answer is **A.** The infant is most likely manifesting the signs and symptoms of Alpers-Huttenlocher syndrome. This disease, which usually manifests in infancy, is associated with intractable seizures and a failure to meet meaningful developmental milestones. Primary symptoms of the disease are developmental delay, progressive mental retardation, hypotonia (low muscle tone), spasticity (stiffness of the limbs), and progressive dementia. The typical seizures are of a type that consists of repeated myoclonic (muscle) jerks. Experimental evidence indicates that Alpers-Huttenlocher syndrome results from mutations in the nuclear gene (*POLG*) encoding mtDNA polymerase gamma. Kearns-Sayre syndrome (choice B) usually appears before age 20 and most commonly affects the eyes with characteristic symptoms including chronic progressive external ophthalmoplegia (PEO) which represents weakness or paralysis of the eye muscles impairing eye movement and causing drooping eyelids (ptosis). Leigh syndrome (choice C) can result from mutations in more than 80 different genes and is characterized by subacute necrotizing encephalomyelopathy. Early onset symptoms of Leigh syndrome include vomiting, diarrhea, dysphagia (difficulty swallowing) all of which result in growth retardation and failure to thrive. Symptoms of MELAS (choice D) usually appear in early childhood following a period of normal growth and include severe lactic acidosis, muscle weakness and pain, recurrent headaches, loss of appetite, vomiting, and seizures. Symptoms of MERFF (choice E) are characterized by myoclonus (muscle twitching), muscle weakness (myopathy), progressive stiffness (spasticity), seizures, ataxia, peripheral neuropathy, optic neuropathy, hearing loss, and dementia.

17. Correct answer is **C.** The patient is most likely suffering from the effects of cyanide poisoning. Cyanide is a poison that acts by inhibiting electron flow through complex IV of the oxidative phosphorylation pathway. The block in the function of complex IV prevents further mitochondrial electron transport leading to rapid decline in ATP synthesis capacity and ultimately cellular death. Inhibition of the conversion of pyruvate to alanine (choice A), as occurs predominantly in skeletal muscle could lead to increased lactate in the blood but would not be associated with the other signs and symptoms in the patient. Inhibition of glycolysis (choice B) would reduce the potential for lactate production, not lead to lactic acidosis. Inhibition of fatty acid mobilization from adipose tissue (choice D) would lead to reduced hepatic gluconeogenesis due to lack of sufficient energy from fatty acid oxidation. This would have an effect on the metabolism of lactate into glucose but would not be associated with the other signs and symptoms in this patient. Inhibited release of insulin (choice E) would result in hyperglycemia, not lactic acidemia, and would not be associated with the other symptoms seen in the patient.

18. Correct answer is **D.** The normal flow of electrons, through the proteins of the oxidative phosphorylation machinery, is coupled with the establishment of a proton gradient across the inner mitochondrial membrane. The establishment of this pH gradient is the chemiosmotic potential that is coupled with the production of ATP. If the process of proton movement is uncoupled from the normal pathway through the ATP synthase complex, oxygen can be consumed but no ATP will be synthesized. Since the proton motive force across the membrane is lost in the presence of the novel compound there is no longer a gradient to restrict the rate of electron flow, electron transport accelerates resulting in normal or possibly increased oxygen consumption. Since the novel compound does not inhibit the complexes of oxidative phosphorylation there would not be cessation of oxidation (choices A, B, and C). Dissipation of the proton gradient releases the energy of the proton gradient as heat instead of it being used for the work of ATP synthesis and does not impede oxygen consumption (choice E).

19. Correct answer is **B.** The reactions, as written, demonstrate that the free energy available from the oxidation of $FADH_2$ is sufficient to drive the succinate dehydrogenase reaction in the direction of fumarate reduction to succinate. None of the other options (choices A, C, D, and E) correctly correspond to the outcomes of the two reactions as they are written.

20. Correct answer is **B.** The infant is most likely manifesting the signs and symptoms of Alpers-Huttenlocher syndrome. This disease, which usually manifests in infancy, is associated with intractable seizures and a failure to meet meaningful developmental milestones. Primary symptoms of the disease are developmental delay, progressive mental retardation, hypotonia (low muscle tone), spasticity (stiffness of the limbs), and progressive dementia. Alpers-Huttenlocher syndrome results from mutation in the nuclear gene (*POLG*) encoding mtDNA polymerase gamma. This disorder is an example of a mitochondrial encephalomyopathy resulting from nuclear DNA mutations and, therefore, exhibits typical Mendelian inheritance, specifically autosomal recessive inheritance. None of the other options (choices A, C, D, and E) represent the correct mode of inheritance of Alpers-Huttenlocher syndrome.

CHAPTER

11

Fatty Acid, Triglyceride, and Phospholipid Synthesis

High-Yield Terms

ATP-citrate lyase, ACL	Cytosolic enzyme involved in the transport of acetyl-CoA from the mitochondria to the cytosol; a nuclear ACL is involved in delivery of acetyl-CoA to histone acetyltransferases (HAT) involved in modulating gene expression at the level of epigenetic marking
Acetyl-CoA carboxylase, ACC	Rate-limiting and highly regulated enzyme of *de novo* fatty acid synthesis
Fatty acid synthase, FAS	Homodimeric enzyme that carries out all of the reactions of *de novo* fatty acid synthesis generating palmitic acid as the final product
Carbohydrate-response element-binding protein	Major glucose-responsive transcription factor that is required for glucose-induced expression of L-PK and the lipogenic genes *ACC* and *FAS*
Stearoyl-CoA desaturase, SCD	Rate-limiting enzyme for the synthesis of monounsaturated fatty acids (MUFA), primarily oleate (18:1) and palmitoleate (16:1), both of which represent the majority of MUFA present in membrane phospholipids, triglycerides, and cholesterol esters.
Triglyceride	Also called triacylglyceride or triacylglycerol, major storage form of lipid in the body, composed of a glycerol backbone and three esterified fatty acids
Phospholipid	Major lipid component of all cell membranes, composed of a glycerol backbone esterified to two fatty acids with phosphate esterified to the sn3 position; the phosphate group, with an esterified alcohol, is referred to as the polar head group of phospholipids
Plasmalogen	Alkyl ether (–O–CH_2–) and alkenyl ether (–O–CH=CH–) glycerophospholipids, the plasmalogen platelet-activating factor (PAF) is one of the most potent biological lipids

FATTY ACID SYNTHESIS

The pathway for fatty acid synthesis occurs in the cytoplasm, utilizes the oxidation of NADPH, and requires an activated intermediate. The activated intermediate is malonyl-CoA which is derived via carboxylation of acetyl-CoA. The synthesis of malonyl-CoA represents the first committed step as well as the rate-limiting and major regulated step of fatty acid synthesis (Figure 11–1). This reaction is catalyzed by the biotin-requiring enzyme, acetyl-CoA carboxylase (ACC). Humans express two distinct ACC genes identified as *ACC1* and *ACC2*.

The reactions of fatty acid synthesis are catalyzed by fatty acid synthase, FAS. All of the reactions of fatty acid synthesis take place in distinct reactive centers within the enzyme as outlined in Figure 11–2. The primary fatty acid synthesized by FAS is palmitate. Palmitate is then released from the enzyme and can then undergo separate elongation and/or unsaturation to yield other fatty acid molecules.

ORIGIN OF CYTOPLASMIC ACETYL-COA

Acetyl-CoA is generated in the mitochondria via the oxidation of pyruvate, fatty acids, and several amino acids. Acetyl-CoA enters the cytoplasm in the form of citrate via the tricarboxylate transport system (Figure 11–3). In the cytoplasm, citrate is converted to oxaloacetate and acetyl-CoA by the ATP-citrate lyase (ACL) reaction. The resultant oxaloacetate is reduced to malate by cytoplasmic malate dehydrogenase (MDH). Malate is then oxidatively decarboxylated by cytosolic malic enzyme (ME1). The malic enzyme reaction represents a major pathway for the generation of NADPH.

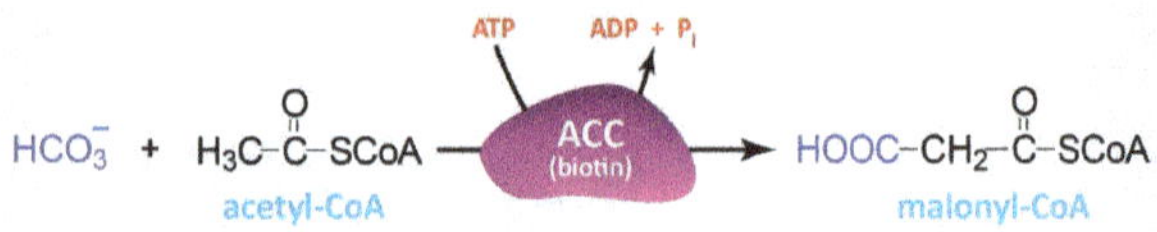

FIGURE 11–1 Synthesis of malonyl-CoA catalyzed by acetyl-CoA carboxylase. (Reproduced with permission from themedicalbiochemistrypage, LLC.)

REGULATION OF FATTY ACID SYNTHESIS

HIGH-YIELD CONCEPT

The ACC-catalyzed reaction is the rate-limiting and highly regulated step in fatty acid synthesis.

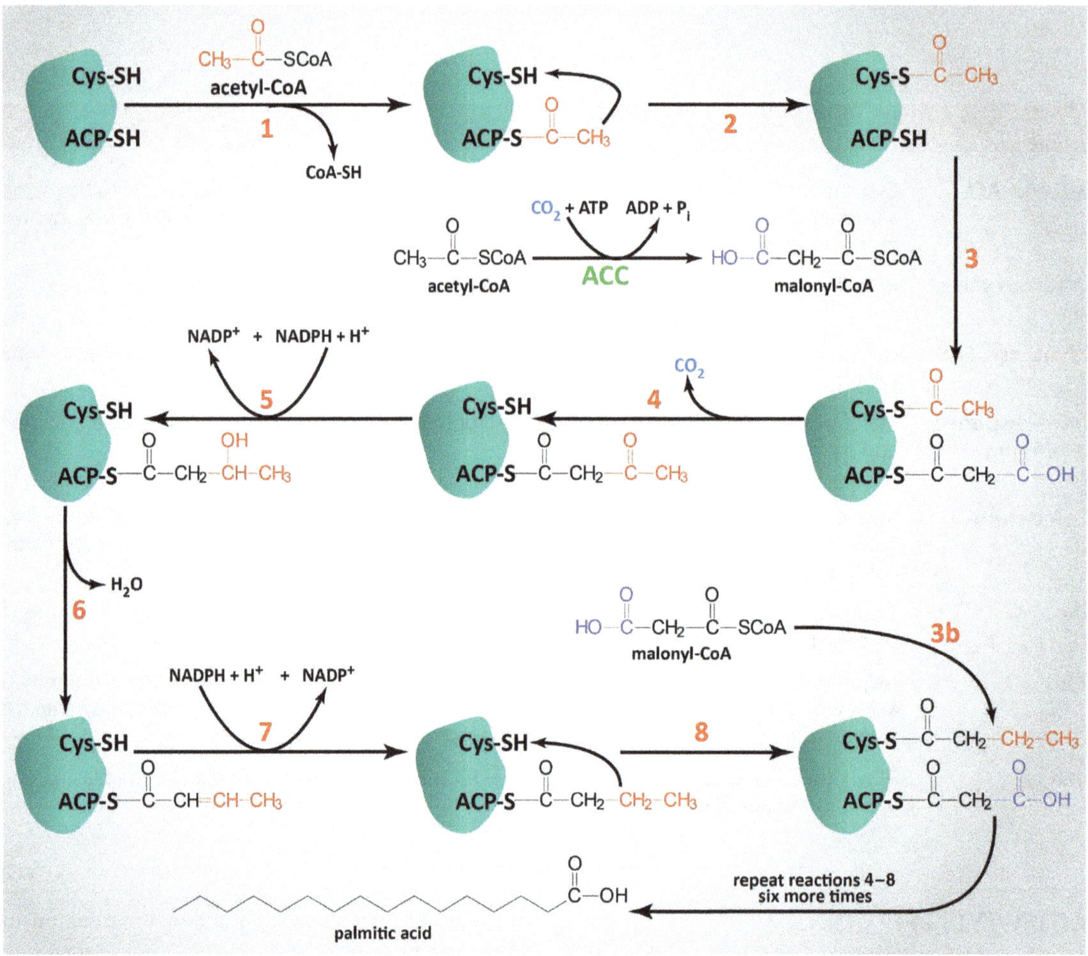

FIGURE 11–2 Reactions of fatty acid synthesis catalyzed by FAS. Only half of the normal head-to-tail (head-to-foot) dimer of functional FAS is shown. Synthesis of malonyl-CoA from CO_2 and acetyl-CoA is carried out by ACC as shown in Figure 11–1. The acetyl group is initially attached to the sulfhydryl of the 4′-phosphopantothenate of the acyl carrier protein portion of FAS (ACP-SH). This is catalyzed by malonyl/acetyl-CoA ACP transacetylase (reactions 1 and 2). This activating acetyl group represents the omega (ω) end of the newly synthesized fatty acid. Following transfer of the activating acetyl group to a cysteine sulfhydryl in the β-keto-ACP synthase portion of FAS (CYS-SH), the three carbons from a malonyl-CoA are attached to ACP-SH (reaction 3), also catalyzed by malonyl/acetyl-CoA ACP transacetylase. The acetyl group attacks the methylene group of the malonyl attached to ACP-SH catalyzed β-keto-ACP synthase (reaction 4) which also liberates the CO_2 that was added to acetyl-CoA by ACC. The resulting 3-ketoacyl group then undergoes a series of 3 reactions catalyzed by the β-keto-ACP reductase (reaction 5), 3-OH acyl-ACP dehydratase (reaction 6), and enoyl-CoA reductase (reaction 7) activities of FAS resulting in a saturated 4-carbon (butyryl) group attached to the ACP-SH. This butyryl group is then transferred to the CYS-SH (reaction 8) as for the case of the activating acetyl group. At this point another malonyl group is attached to the ACP-SH (3b) and the process begins again. Reactions 4 through 8 are repeated another 6 times, each beginning with a new malonyl group being added. At the completion of synthesis, the saturated 16-carbon fatty acid, palmitic acid, is released via the action of the thioesterase activity of FAS (palmitoyl ACP thioesterase) located in the C-terminal end of the enzyme. Not shown are the released CoASH groups. (Reproduced with permission from themedicalbiochemistrypage, LLC.)

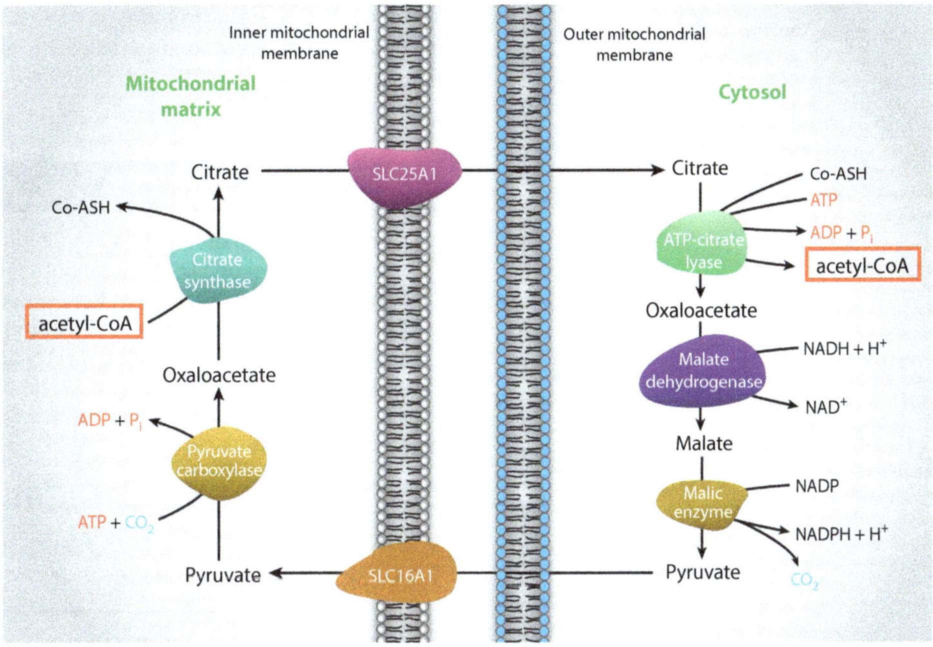

FIGURE 11–3 Pathway for the movement of acetyl-CoA units from within the mitochondrion to the cytoplasm for use in lipid and cholesterol biosynthesis. Note that the cytoplasmic malic enzyme-catalyzed reaction generates NADPH which can be used for reductive biosynthetic reactions such as those of fatty acid and cholesterol synthesis. (Reproduced with permission from themedicalbiochemistrypage, LLC.)

There are two major isoforms of ACC in mammalian tissues. These are identified as ACC1 and ACC2. ACC1 is strictly cytosolic and is enriched in liver, adipose tissue, and lactating mammary tissue. ACC2 expression occurs in the heart, liver, and skeletal muscle. ACC2 possesses a mitochondrial targeting motif and is found associated with carnitine palmitoyltransferase 1 (CPT1) involved in fatty acid oxidation (see Chapter 13). The synthesis of malonyl-CoA by ACC2 allows for rapid regulation of CPT1 and inhibition of fatty acid oxidation.

Both isoforms of ACC are allosterically activated by citrate and inhibited by palmitoyl-CoA and other short- and long-chain fatty acyl-CoAs. Citrate triggers the polymerization of ACC1 which leads to significant increases in its activity. Although ACC2 does not undergo significant polymerization (presumably due to its mitochondrial association), it is allosterically activated by citrate. Glutamate and other dicarboxylic acids can also allosterically activate both ACC isoforms.

ACC activity is also regulated by phosphorylation. Both ACC1 and ACC2 contain at least eight sites that undergo phosphorylation. Phosphorylation of ACC1 by AMP-activated protein kinase (AMPK) leads to inhibition of the enzyme (Figure 11–4). Glucagon- and epinephrine-mediated increases in PKA activity lead to phosphorylation of both ACC isoforms. Conversely, insulin action results in increased ACC activity via reduction in cAMP levels and via dephosphorylation of ACC.

Long-term regulation of fatty acid synthesis occurs at the level of gene expression primarily controlled by the circulating levels of insulin and glucagon. Insulin stimulates both ACC and FAS synthesis, whereas, starvation leads to decreased synthesis of these enzymes.

HIGH-YIELD CONCEPT

Carbohydrate response element-binding protein (ChREBP) is a major glucose-responsive transcription factor that is required for glucose-induced expression of the liver isoform of pyruvate kinase (L-PK) and the lipogenic genes *ACC* and *FAS*. ChREBP is encoded by the *MLXIPL* (MLX interacting protein-like) gene. Expression of the *MLXIPL* gene is induced in the liver in response to increased glucose uptake. In addition, the activity of ChREBP is regulated by posttranslational modifications as well as subcellular localization.

ELONGATION AND DESATURATION

Elongation and unsaturation of fatty acids occur in both the mitochondria and endoplasmic reticulum (ER). Elongation in the ER involves condensation of fatty acyl-CoA molecules with malonyl-CoA. The resultant product is two carbons longer which then undergoes reduction, dehydration, and reduction yielding a saturated fatty acid. The reduction reactions of elongation require NADPH as cofactor just as for the similar reactions catalyzed by FAS. Mitochondrial elongation involves acetyl-CoA units and is essentially a reversal of fatty acid oxidation.

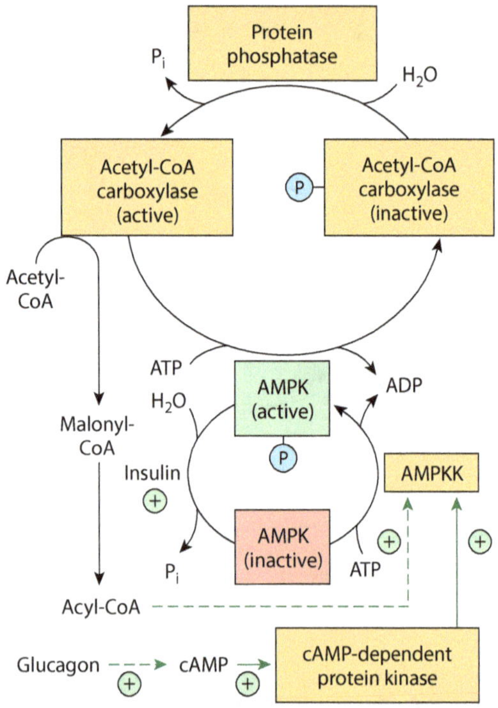

FIGURE 11–4 Regulation of acetyl-CoA carboxylase by phosphorylation/dephosphorylation. The enzyme is inactivated by phosphorylation by AMP-activated protein kinase (AMPK), which in turn is phosphorylated and activated by AMP-activated protein kinase kinase (AMPKK). Glucagon (and epinephrine) increase cAMP, and thus activate this latter enzyme via cAMP-dependent protein kinase. The kinase kinase enzyme is also believed to be activated by acyl-CoA. Insulin activates acetyl-CoA carboxylase via dephosphorylation of AMPK. (Reproduced with permission from Rodwell VW, Bender DA, Botham KM, et al: *Harper's Illustrated Biochemistry*, 31st ed. New York, NY: McGraw Hill; 2018.)

The desaturation of fatty acids occurs in the ER membranes as well. In mammalian cells, fatty acid desaturation involves three broad specificity fatty acyl-CoA desaturases that utilize NADH as a cofactor. These enzymes introduce unsaturation at C5, C6, or C9. The names of these enzymes are Δ^5-eicosatrienoyl-CoA desaturase (D5D), Δ^6-oleoyl(linolenoyl)-CoA desaturase (D6D), and Δ^9-stearoyl-CoA desaturase (SCD1).

HIGH-YIELD CONCEPT

SCD1 is the rate-limiting enzyme catalyzing the synthesis of monounsaturated fatty acids, primarily oleate (18:1) and palmitoleate (16:1). These two monounsaturated fatty acids represent the majority of monounsaturated fatty acids present in membrane phospholipids, triglycerides, and cholesterol esters.

The electrons transferred from the oxidized fatty acids during desaturation are transferred from the desaturases to cytochrome b_5 and then NADH-cytochrome b_5 reductase. These electrons are uncoupled from mitochondrial oxidative phosphorylation and, therefore, do not yield ATP.

HIGH-YIELD CONCEPT

Since mammalian desaturases cannot introduce sites of unsaturation beyond C9, they cannot synthesize either linoleic acid ($18{:}2^{\Delta 9,12}$) or α-linolenic acid (ALA; $18{:}3^{\Delta 9,12,15}$). These fatty acids must be acquired from the diet and are, therefore, referred to as **essential fatty acids.**

SYNTHESIS OF BIOLOGICALLY ACTIVE OMEGA-3 AND -6 POLYUNSATURATED FATTY ACIDS

The three major omega-3 polyunsaturated fatty acids (PUFA) utilized by human tissues are ALA, eicosapentaenoic acid (EPA), and docosahexaenoic acid (DHA) (see Chapter 12). Although ALA can serve as the precursor for EPA and DHA synthesis in humans (Figure 11–5) by pathway is limited in its capacity and also varies dramatically between males and females, as well as in conditions of disease. Therefore, direct dietary intake of foods rich in EPA and DHA are of the most benefit clinically.

BIOLOGICAL ACTIVITIES OF OMEGA-3 AND OMEGA-6 PUFAS

The most important omega-6 PUFA is arachidonic acid which serves as the precursor for the synthesis of the biologically active eicosanoids (see Chapter 12), the prostaglandins (PG), the thromboxanes (TX), the leukotrienes (LT), and the lipoxins (LX). The arachidonic acid-derived eicosanoids function in diverse biological phenomena such as platelet and leukocyte activation, signaling of pain, induction of bronchoconstriction, and regulation of gastric secretions. These activities are targets of numerous pharmacological agents such as the nonsteroidal anti-inflammatory drugs (NSAID), COX-2 inhibitors, and leukotriene antagonists.

The metabolic and clinical significances of the omega-3 PUFAs are due to the ability of these lipids to exert effects on numerous biologically important pathways as well as to serve as precursors for clinically important bioactive lipids (see Chapter 12). EPA and DHA compete with the inflammatory, pyretic (fever), and pain-promoting properties imparted by arachidonic acid, because they displace arachidonic acid from phospholipids present in cell membranes. In addition, EPA and DHA compete with the enzymes that convert arachidonic acid into the biologically active eicosanoids. An important effect of EPA and DHA is, therefore, a decrease in the potential for monocytes,

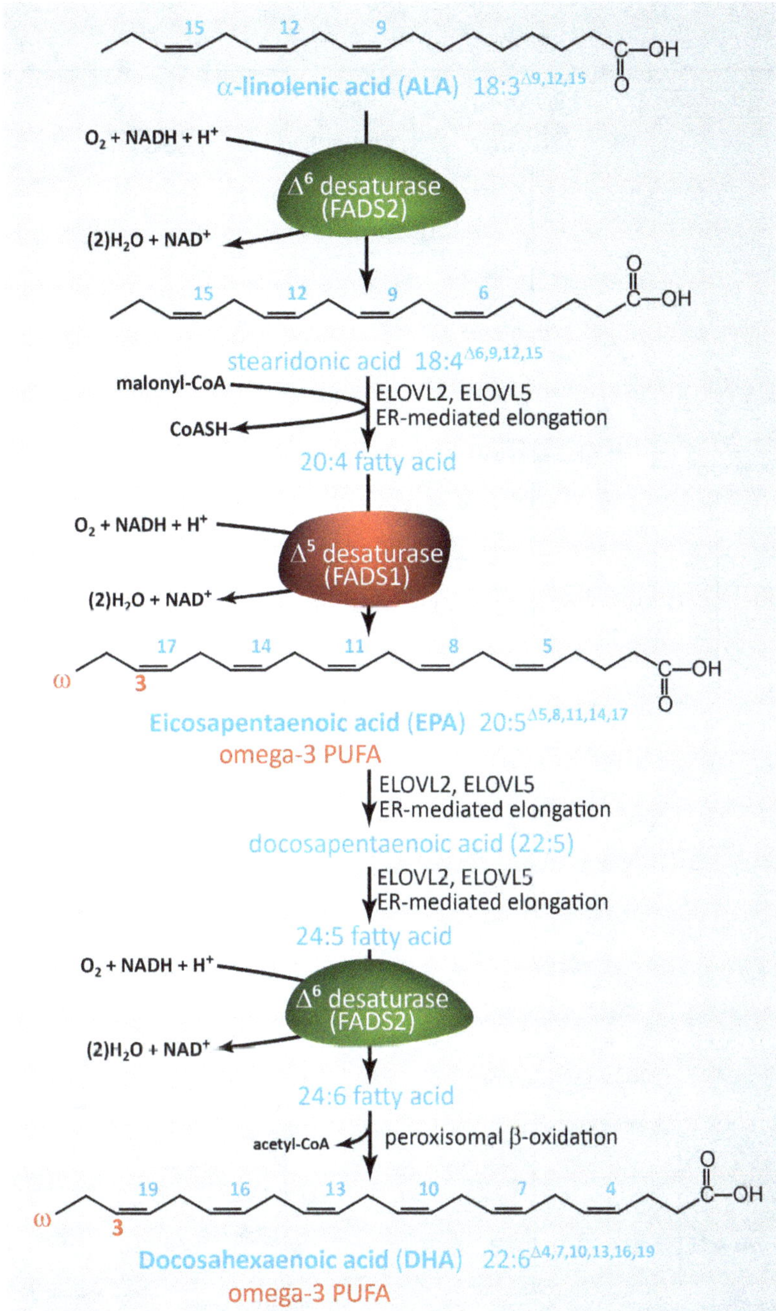

FIGURE 11–5 Pathway for ALA conversion to EPA and DHA: Alpha(α)-linolenic acid (ALA) is converted to the omega-3 polyunsaturated fatty acids (PUFA), eicosapentaenoic acid (EPA), docosapentaenoic acid (DPA), and docosahexaenoic acid (DHA), via the actions of a series of microsomal (endoplasmic reticulum, ER) enzymes. The final step in DHA synthesis involves peroxisomal β-oxidation to remove the 2-carbon acetyl-CoA from the 24:6 fatty acid called tetracosahexaenoic acid (also called nisinic acid). This pathway involves both the D5D and D6D desaturases encoded by the FADS1 and FADS2 genes, respectively. The microsomal elongation steps are carried out by four enzymes with the initiating 3-keto acyl-CoA synthases (ELOVL2 and ELOVL5) being indicated. The 20:4 fatty acid is called eicosatetraenoic acid. The 24:5 fatty acid is called tetracosapentaenoic acid. (Modified with permission from themedicalbiochemistrypage, LLC.)

neutrophils, and eosinophils to synthesize potent mediators of inflammation and to reduce the ability of platelets to release TXA_2, a potent stimulator of the coagulation process. One of the most important functions of EPA and DHA is that they serve as the precursors for potent inflammation resolving lipids called resolvins (Rv) and protectins (PD).

SYNTHESIS OF TRIGLYCERIDES

Triglycerides (TG) constitute molecules of glycerol to which three fatty acids have been esterified (Figure 11–6). The fatty acids present in TG are predominantly saturated. The major building block for the synthesis of TG, in tissues other than adipose tissue and

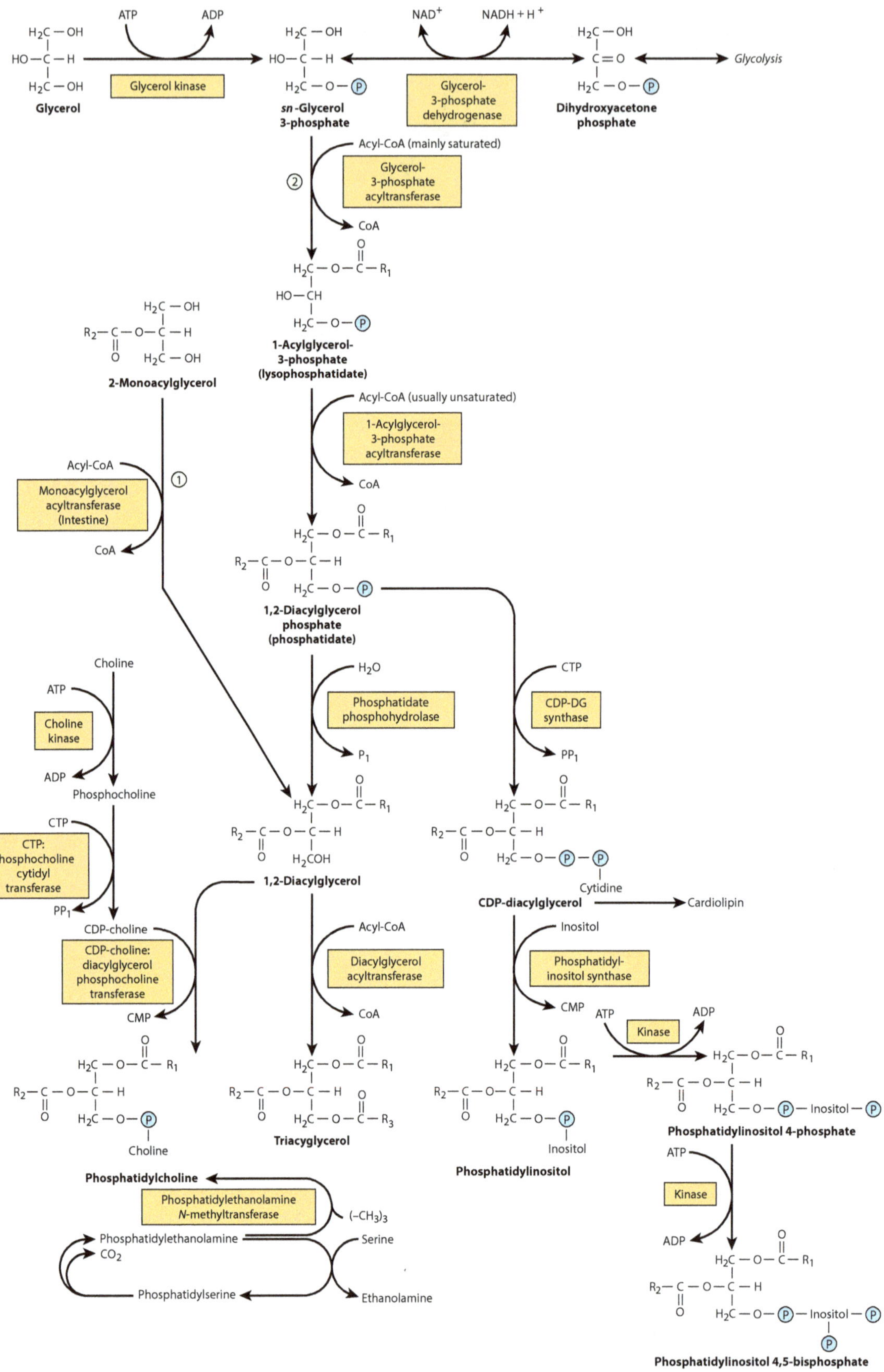

FIGURE 11–6 Biosynthesis of triacylglycerol and phospholipids. (1, Monoacylglycerol pathway; 2, glycerol phosphate pathway.) Phosphatidylethanolamine may be formed from ethanolamine by a pathway similar to that shown for the formation of phosphatidylcholine from choline. (Reproduced with permission from Rodwell VW, Bender DA, Botham KM, et al: *Harper's Illustrated Biochemistry*, 31st ed. New York, NY: McGraw Hill; 2018.)

intestinal enterocytes, is glycerol. Adipocytes lack glycerol kinase, therefore, dihydroxyacetone phosphate (DHAP), produced during glycolysis, is the precursor for TG synthesis in adipose tissue. This means that adipocytes must have glucose in order to store fatty acids in the form of TG. Within intestinal enterocytes, the precursors for TG synthesis are the monoacylglycerols that are derived through the action of pancreatic lipases on dietary TG.

The glycerol backbone of TG is activated by phosphorylation at the *sn*3 position by glycerol kinase. When DHAP is the starting molecule for TG synthesis, it is first converted to glycerol-3-phosphate through the action of glycerol-3-phosphate dehydrogenase.

The fatty acids incorporated into TG are activated to acyl-CoAs through the action of various acyl-CoA synthetases. Two molecules of acyl-CoA are esterified to glycerol-3-phosphate to yield 1,2-diacylglycerol phosphate (commonly identified as phosphatidic acid). The phosphate is then removed, by phosphatidic acid phosphatases, to yield 1,2-diacylglycerol, the substrate for addition of the third fatty acid.

PHOSPHOLIPID SYNTHESIS

Phospholipids are synthesized by esterification of an alcohol to the phosphate of phosphatidic acid (1,2-diacylglycerol 3-phosphate). Most phospholipids have a saturated fatty acid on C-1 and an unsaturated fatty acid on C-2 of the glycerol backbone.

The major classifications of phospholipids are the phosphatidylserines (PS), the phosphatidylethanolamines (PE), the phosphatidylcholines (PC; often referred to as lecithins), the phosphatidylinositols (PI), phosphatidylglycerols (PG; major components of pulmonary surfactant), and the diphosphatidylglycerols (DPG; more commonly called the cardiolipins).

Phospholipids are synthesized by two distinct mechanisms. The synthesis of PC, PE, and PS involves one pathway, while the synthesis of PI, PG, and the cardiolipins occurs via the second pathway (see Figure 11–6). PC, PE, and PS are freely interconvertible through polar head group exchange or via *S*-adenosylmethionine-dependent methylation.

Classifications of Major Phospholipids

Phosphatidylcholine, PC: This class of phospholipids is also called the lecithins. They contain primarily palmitic or stearic acid at carbon-1 and primarily oleic, linoleic, or linolenic acid at carbon-2. The lecithin dipalmitoyl lecithin is a component of lung or pulmonary surfactant. It contains palmitate at both carbon-1 and 2 of glycerol and is the major (80%) phospholipid found in the extracellular lipid layer lining the pulmonary alveoli. PC can serve as the precursor for PS via an exchange of serine for choline.

Phosphatidylethanolamine, PE: Phosphatidylethanolamines contain primarily palmitic or stearic acid on carbon-1 and a long-chain unsaturated fatty acid (eg, 18:2, 20:4, and 22:6) on carbon-2. PE can be derived from PS via a decarboxylation reaction. PE can serve as the precursor for PC via *S*-adenosylmethionine-dependent methylation.

Phosphatidylserine, PS: Phosphatidylserines are composed of fatty acids similar to the PEs. PS can be synthesized from PE through an exchange of serine for ethanolamine.

Phosphatidylinositol, PI: Phosphatidylinositols contain almost exclusively stearic acid at carbon-1 and arachidonic acid at carbon-2. These molecules exist in membranes with various levels of phosphate esterified to the hydroxyls of the inositol. Molecules with phosphorylated inositol are termed polyphosphoinositides. The polyphosphoinositides are important intracellular transducers of signals emanating from the plasma membrane. One polyphosphoinositide (phosphatidylinositol 4,5-bisphosphate, PIP_2) is a critically important membrane phospholipid involved in the transmission of signals for cell growth and differentiation from outside the cell to inside.

Phosphatidylglycerol, PG: Phosphatidylglycerols are found in high concentration in mitochondrial membranes and as components of pulmonary surfactant. Phosphatidylglycerol also is a precursor for the synthesis of cardiolipin. A vital role of PG is to serve as the precursor for the synthesis of diphosphatidylglycerols (DPGs).

Cardiolipins (diphosphatidylglycerols, DPG): Cardiolipins are primarily found in the inner mitochondrial membrane and also as components of pulmonary surfactant.

The fatty acid distribution at the C-1 and C-2 positions of glycerol within phospholipids is in continual flux, owing to phospholipid degradation and the phospholipid remodeling that occurs while these molecules are in membranes. Phospholipid degradation results from the action of phospholipases (Figure 11–7). The products of these phospholipases are called lysophospholipids and they can be substrates for acyl transferases utilizing different acyl-CoA groups. Lysophospholipids can also accept acyl groups from other phospholipids in an exchange reaction. Many lysophospholipids exert specific biological functions (see Chapter 12).

PLASMALOGENS

Plasmalogens are glycerol ether phospholipids (Figure 11–8). Three major classes of plasmalogen have been identified: choline, ethanolamine, and serine plasmalogens. Ethanolamine plasmalogen is prevalent in myelin. Choline plasmalogen is abundant in cardiac tissue.

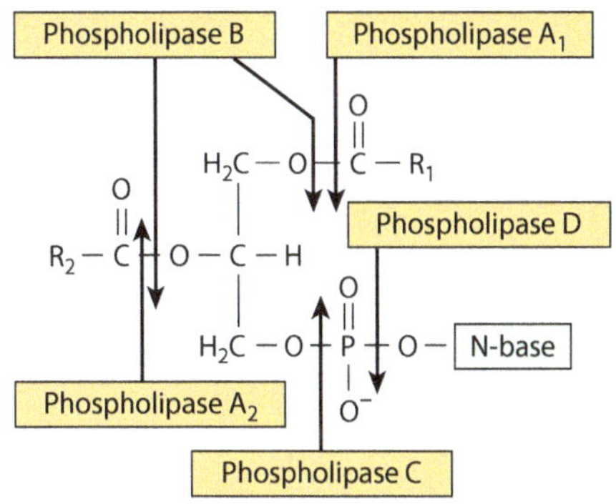

FIGURE 11–7 Sites of the hydrolytic activity of phospholipases on a phospholipid substrate. (Reproduced with permission from Rodwell VW, Bender DA, Botham KM, et al: *Harper's Illustrated Biochemistry*, 31st ed. New York, NY: McGraw Hill; 2018.)

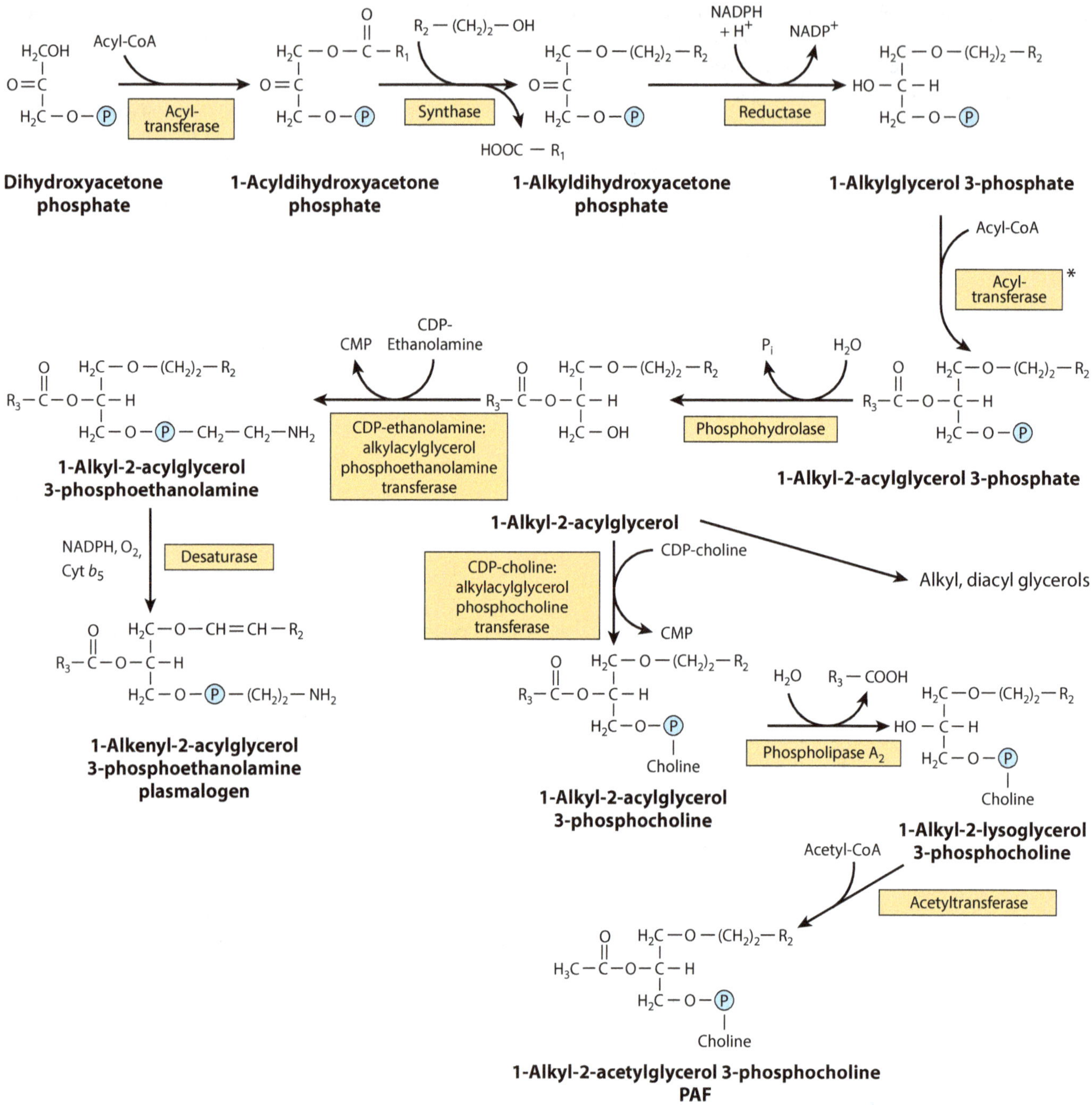

FIGURE 11–8 Biosynthesis of ether lipids, including plasmalogens and platelet-activating factor (PAF). In the *de novo* pathway for PAF synthesis, acetyl-CoA is incorporated at stage*, avoiding the last two steps in the pathway shown here. (Reproduced with permission from Rodwell VW, Bender DA, Botham KM, et al: *Harper's Illustrated Biochemistry*, 31st ed. New York, NY: McGraw Hill; 2018.)

One particular choline plasmalogen (1-*O*-1′-enyl-2-acetyl-*sn*-glycero-3-phosphocholine), identified as platelet-activating factor (PAF), is an extremely powerful biological mediator. PAF functions as a mediator of hypersensitivity, acute inflammatory reactions, and anaphylactic shock. PAF is synthesized by stimulated basophils, monocytes, polymorphonuclear neutrophils, platelets, and endothelial cells. The synthesis and release of PAF from cells leads to platelet aggregation and the release of serotonin from platelets. PAF also produces responses in liver, heart, smooth muscle, and uterine and lung tissues.

CHECKLIST

- ☑ Long-chain fatty acid synthesis occurs in the cytosol and requires the activities of acetyl-CoA carboxylase (ACC) and fatty acid synthase (FAS). The end-product of *de novo* fat synthesis is palmitic acid.
- ☑ ACC represents the rate-limiting step in fatty acid synthesis. The enzyme is subject to complex short-term and long-term regulation. Two forms of ACC exist, ACC1 and ACC2 with ACC1 being primarily responsible to initiate fat synthesis and ACC2 being primarily responsible for regulating fat entry into the mitochondria.
- ☑ ATP-citrate lyase (ACL) is critical for the delivery of acetyl-CoA to the cytosol from the mitochondria so that it can be used for fat synthesis. Nuclear activity of ACL is necessary for providing acetyl-CoA as a substrate for histone acetyltransferases required for regulating gene activity.
- ☑ Carbohydrate-response element-binding protein is a transcription factor critical for coordinating the expression of genes involved in lipogenesis as well as carbohydrate metabolism. The activity of ChREBP is itself regulated by the level of glucose within the cell.
- ☑ Fatty acid elongation and desaturation occurs in the membranes of the ER as well as in the mitochondria. Mammalian tissues express a limited set of desaturase enzymes and thus cannot introduce double bonds into fatty acids beyond carbon 9.
- ☑ Synthesis of omega-3 and omega-6 fatty acids and their derivatives play critical roles in the regulation of a wide range of biological activities.
- ☑ Triglycerides represent the major storage form of lipid in the body. These molecules are synthesized from glycerol and three fatty acids.
- ☑ Adipose tissue requires glycolysis coupled to triglyceride synthesis since adipocytes do not express glycerol kinase and must acquire glycerol-3-phosphate via the reduction of the glycolytic intermediate, dihydroxyacetone phosphate catalyzed by glycerol-3-phosphate dehydrogenase.
- ☑ Phospholipids represent the major lipid molecules present in plasma membranes of cells. In this capacity phospholipids serve as sources of precursor lipids for the synthesis of numerous bioactive lipid derivatives. Release of fatty acids from membrane phospholipids occurs most often in response to ligand-mediated receptor activation of PLA_2, but can also result from activation of PLD.
- ☑ Plasmalogens are a form of phospholipid containing an ether linked fatty acid at the *sn*1 position of the glycerol backbone. One of the most potent plasmalogens is platelet-activating factor, PAF. PAF is a unique plasmalogen in that it contains acetate esterified to the *sn*2 position instead of a long-chain fatty acid.

REVIEW QUESTIONS

1. A 16-hour-old neonate, who was born prematurely at 29 weeks gestation, is being cared for in the neonatal Intensive Care Unit. The infant is tachypneic and is exhibiting signs of cyanosis and breathing difficulty including nasal flaring, apnea, and inspirational stridor. Which of the following, normally produced by lung endothelium, is most likely to be deficient in this infant?
(A) Cardiolipin
(B) Phosphatidylcholine
(C) Phosphatidylethanolamine
(D) Phosphatidylinositol
(E) Phosphatidylserine

2. A 32-year-old woman has been consuming a low-fat, high-carbohydrate diet for the past week. The transcription rate of which of the following genes is most likely to be enhanced in this individual?
(A) Fatty acid synthase
(B) Hormone-sensitive lipase
(C) Phosphoenolpyruvate carboxykinase (PEPCK)
(D) Pyruvate carboxylase
(E) Stearoyl-CoA desaturase

3. Studies are being carried out on the process of mitochondrial fatty acid oxidation by utilizing a cell culture system. Results of these studies showed that the rate of fatty acid oxidation increased when the cells were stimulated by insulin. Which of the following enzymes involved in fatty acid metabolism is most likely to be abnormal in these cells allowing for fat oxidation to be enhanced in response to the actions of insulin?
(A) Acetyl-CoA carboxylase
(B) ATP-citrate lyase
(C) Carnitine palmitoyltransferase 1
(D) Fatty acid synthase
(E) Fatty acyl-CoA synthetase
(F) Stearoyl-CoA desaturase

4. Fatty acid metabolism is being studied in cells isolated from a hepatocellular carcinoma. Results with these cells demonstrate that they do not accelerate the rate of palmitic acid synthesis when glucose is added at high concentration as is the case in normal hepatocytes. Given these results, which of the following proteins, in the cancer cells, is most likely to be defective in its regulation, compared to normal cells?
(A) Acetyl-CoA carboxylase
(B) ATP-citrate lyase
(C) Carnitine palmitoyltransferase 1

(D) Fatty acid synthase
(E) Stearoyl-CoA desaturase

5. Experiments are being conducted on *de novo* triglyceride synthesis using a cell line derived from biopsy tissue of a hepatocellular carcinoma. Results of these experiments find that synthesis of palmitic acid is higher than in normal hepatocytes. Increased activity of which of the following is most likely to account for these observations?
(A) Glycerol kinase
(B) Glycerol-3-phosphate dehydrogenase
(C) Glyceraldehyde-3-phosphate dehydrogenase
(D) Lipoprotein lipase
(E) Hormone sensitive lipase

6. Gas chromatographic analysis of fatty acids present in cells isolated from a particular strain of mice shows little to no palmitoleic and oleic acid but expected levels of palmitic acid. A defect in which of the following proteins is most likely causing the absence of the two fatty acids?
(A) Acetyl-CoA carboxylase
(B) ATP-citrate lyase
(C) Carbohydrate response element-binding protein
(D) Fatty acid synthase
(E) Stearoyl-CoA desaturase

7. A 29-year-old woman comes to the physician because of redness of the skin, itching, and skin lesions, several of which are oozing pus. The patient also says that a bad scrape that resulted from a fall from a bicycle several weeks ago, has not properly healed. Patient history indicates that she started on a new fat-free diet 10 months ago. This patient is most likely deficient in which of the following?
(A) Ascorbate
(B) Leucine
(C) Linoleic acid
(D) Oleic acid
(E) Palmitic acid
(F) Thiamine

8. Experiments are being conducted on the activity of acetyl-CoA carboxylase in a cell-free system containing the enzyme and its substrate. Addition of which of the following substances is most likely to result in the largest decrease in production of malonyl-CoA?
(A) Acetyl-CoA
(B) Citrate
(C) Glucose-6-phosphate
(D) NAD^+
(E) Palmitic acid

9. A 14-year-old type 1 diabetic has self-injected his morning dose of insulin. Under these conditions, which of the following is most likely to exhibit an increase in the level of activity?
(A) Acetyl-CoA carboxylase
(B) ATP-citrate lyase
(C) Fatty acid synthase
(D) Malonyl-CoA decarboxylase
(E) Stearoyl-CoA desaturase

10. Experiments are being conducted on *de novo* fatty acid synthesis using a cell line derived from biopsy tissue of a hepatocellular carcinoma. Results of one assay find that a major contributor to the dramatically increased rate of fatty acid synthesis is an elevated pool of reduced electron carrier, NADPH. Which of the following enzymes is most likely to be contributing to these observations?
(A) Acetyl-CoA carboxylase
(B) Glyceraldehyde-3-phosphate dehydrogenase
(C) Malate dehydrogenase
(D) Malic enzyme
(E) Pyruvate dehydrogenase

11. Experiments are being conducted on hepatocytes derived from a biopsy of a liver tumor. Analysis of triglyceride synthesis demonstrates that production in these cells is significantly reduced compared to normal hepatocytes. Given these results, which of the following enzymes is most likely to exhibit reduced activity in the cancer cells?
(A) Glycerol kinase
(B) Glycerol-3-phosphate acyltransferase
(C) Glycerol-3-phosphate dehydrogenase
(D) Hepatic lipase
(E) Phosphatidic acid phosphatase

12. Experiments are being conducted on *de novo* triglyceride synthesis using a cell line derived from biopsy tissue of a hepatocellular carcinoma. Molecular studies discover that the gene encoding the transcription factor, ChREBP, has sustained a small deletion in the DNA-binding domain. Which of the following genes would most likely be transcribed at significantly reduced levels as a result of the identified mutation?
(A) Glycerol kinase
(B) Glycerol-3-phosphate acyltransferase
(C) Hepatic lipase
(D) Phosphatidic acid phosphatase
(E) Phospholipase A_2

13. Experiments are being conducted to ascertain the activity of protein kinase C (PKC) in human endothelial cells that have been exposed to UV irradiation. In control cells the addition of angiotensin II results in increased PKC activity. However, when added to the irradiated cells, angiotensin II elicits a significantly reduced level of PKC activation. Given these results, which of the following is most likely synthesized at reduced levels in the irradiated cells compared to normal cells?
(A) Cardiolipin
(B) Phosphatidylcholine
(C) Phosphatidylethanolamine
(D) Phosphatidylinositol-4,5-bisphosphate
(E) Phosphatidylserine

14. Experiments are being conducted on cells isolated from the biopsy of an adenocarcinoma. Results of these experiments find that the activity of phospholipase D (PLD) is dramatically reduced relative to that in normal cells. Production of which of the following would most likely be expected to be reduced in these adenocarcinoma-derived cells?
(A) Cardiolipin
(B) Diacylglycerol
(C) Lysolecithin
(D) Platelet-activating factor
(E) Phosphatidic acid

15. Adipocytes from type 2 diabetic patients do not mobilize the GLUT4 transporter to the plasma membrane in response to insulin binding its receptor. Associated with this defect in insulin signaling is a reduced capacity for triglyceride

synthesis. Which of the following is most likely to be significantly reduced in type 2 diabetic adipocytes accounting for the observed effects on lipid homeostasis?

(A) Acetyl-CoA
(B) Citrate
(C) Glycerol-3-phosphate
(D) Palmitate
(E) 6-Phosphogluconate

ANSWERS

1. Correct answer is **B.** A significant cause of death in premature infants and, on occasion, in full-term infants is respiratory distress syndrome (RDS) or hyaline membrane disease. This condition is caused by an insufficient amount of pulmonary surfactant. Under normal conditions the surfactant is synthesized by type II endothelial cells and is secreted into the alveolar spaces to prevent atelectasis following expiration during breathing. Surfactant is comprised primarily of dipalmitoyl lecithin; additional lipid components include phosphatidylglycerol and phosphatidylinositol along with proteins of 18 and 36 kDa (termed surfactant proteins). Phosphatidylcholines are a class of phospholipid also called lecithins. Infants born prior to 30 weeks of gestation have a significantly decreased capacity to synthesize surfactant and are thus highly susceptible to respiratory distress within minutes of birth. Although phosphatidylinositols (choice D) are components of the overall complex of surfactant, it is phosphatidylcholine that is the primary lipid constituent. None of the other lipid classes (choices A, C, and E) is a substantial component of lung surfactant.
2. Correct answer is **A.** Dietary composition can exert long-term effects on biochemical pathways and these effects are predominantly exerted at the level of the regulation of gene expression. A diet low in fat will trigger a need for increased *de novo* synthesis of fatty acids and thus, be reflected in an increased level of expression of fatty acid synthase. Since blood glucose levels will be elevated on a high-carbohydrate diet there is less chance for glucagon and epinephrine to be released to trigger fatty acid release from adipose tissue as a means to provide the liver with energy for gluconeogenesis. Therefore, hormone-sensitive lipase activity (choice B) will more likely be reduced. A high-carbohydrate diet will dramatically reduce the need for hepatic gluconeogenesis and thus, the expression of the genes encoding phosphoenolpyruvate carboxykinase (choice C) and pyruvate carboxylase (choice D). Stearoyl-CoA desaturase (choice E) gene expression is enhanced by a high fat diet but is not significantly altered by a low fat, high-carbohydrate diet.
3. Correct answer is **C.** Fatty acid synthesis is normally stimulated by insulin, a process mediated by activation of acetyl-CoA carboxylase (ACC). ACC is the rate-limiting enzyme of *de novo* fatty acid synthesis. During fatty acid synthesis the malonyl-CoA produced from acetyl-CoA carboxylase directly interacts with carnitine palmitoyltransferase 1 (CPT1) at the outer mitochondrial membrane to prevent fatty acyl-CoA movement into the mitochondria. The primary source of this CPT1 inhibiting malonyl-CoA is derived from the ACC2 isoform of the enzyme. A defect in CPT1-mediated inhibition by malonyl-CoA would, therefore, lead to reduced inhibition of regulated mitochondrial transport of fatty acyl-CoA resulting in increased fat oxidation from newly synthesized fatty acids produced in response to the actions of insulin. Although a defect in ACC (choice A) would reduce the level of malonyl-CoA and thus, the inhibition of CPT1, the more likely abnormal enzyme in this assay would by CPT1 since insulin stimulated fatty acid synthesis, thereby providing more substrate for transfer into the mitochondria for oxidation. An abnormality in none of the other activities (choices B, D, E, and F) would adequately account for increased fatty acid oxidation in cells responding to insulin.
4. Correct answer is **D.** Regulation of *de novo* fatty acid synthesis takes place primarily at the level of acetyl-CoA carboxylase (ACC) but also at the level of fatty acid synthase, FAS. FAS is regulated by both short-term and long-term mechanisms. Short-term regulation is primarily the result of the allosteric activation of FAS by phosphorylated sugars, such as glucose-6-phosphate. Increased levels of glucose will result in increased glucose-6-phosphate, which if in excess of energy needs, will stimulate fatty acid synthesis through activation of FAS. Acetyl-CoA carboxylase (choice A) is the rate-limiting enzyme in fatty acid synthesis, but it is not regulated by excess glucose as is the case for FAS regulation. None of the other enzymes (choices B, C, and E) are directly regulated by glucose or its metabolites.
5. Correct answer is **A.** The major building block for the synthesis of triglycerides, in tissues other than adipose tissue, is glycerol. The glycerol backbone of triglycerides is activated by phosphorylation at the *sn*3 position by glycerol kinase. Increased activity of glycerol kinase would lead to increased levels of glycerol-3-phosphate, the backbone of triglycerides. Increased levels of activity of glycerol-3-phosphate dehydrogenase (choice B) and glyceraldehyde-3-phosphate dehydrogenase (choice C) could result in increased levels of glycerol-3-phosphate from dihydroxyacetone phosphate and NADH, respectively but this would need to be coupled to increased glucose metabolism which was not indicated in the experiments. Lipoprotein lipase (choice D) is present only on the endothelial cells of the vasculature of skeletal and cardiac muscle and adipose tissue and therefore, would not be involved in lipid homeostasis in isolated hepatocytes. Hormone sensitive lipase (choice E) is expressed predominantly in adipocytes and therefore, would not participate in lipid homeostasis in isolated hepatocytes.
6. Correct answer is **E.** The desaturation of fatty acids in mammalian cells involves three broad specificity fatty acyl-CoA desaturases. Stearoyl-CoA desaturase (SCD1) is the rate-limiting enzyme catalyzing the synthesis of monounsaturated fatty acids, primarily palmitoleic acid (16:1) and oleic acid (18:1). These two monounsaturated fatty acids represent the majority of monounsaturated fatty acids present in membrane phospholipids, triglycerides, and cholesterol esters. Acetyl-CoA carboxylase (choice A) is the rate-limiting enzyme of fatty acid synthesis and since the levels of palmitic acid, the end-product of the action of fatty acid synthase (choice D), are normal in these cells there is not likely to be a defect in either of these two enzymes. ATP-citrate lyase activity is required to hydrolyze acetyl-CoA from cytosolic citrate and since this acetyl-CoA is the substrate for fatty acid synthesis and palmitic acid synthesis is normal in these cells there is not likely to be a defect in this enzyme. Carbohydrate response

element-binding protein (choice C) is a glucose-responsive transcription factor that activates the expression of numerous genes involved in lipid synthesis including acetyl-CoA carboxylase and fatty acid synthase. Since palmitic acid synthesis is normal, it is most likely that the activity of this transcription factor is also normal in these cells.

7. Correct answer is **C.** Linoleic is an essential fatty acid in that it must be acquired in the diet. Linoleic acid is especially important in that it required for the synthesis of arachidonic acid. Arachidonic acid is a precursor for the synthesis of the eicosanoids (prostaglandins, thromboxanes, and leukotrienes). It is this role of linoleic acid in eicosanoid synthesis that leads to poor growth, poor wound healing, and dermatitis in individuals consuming a fat-free diet. A deficiency in ascorbate (choice A) would contribute to poor wound healing due to lack of proper collagen processing but there is no indication that the patient's diet is deficient in any component other than fats. None of the other compounds (choices B, D, and E), when deficient, would contribute to the symptoms in this patient.

8. Correct answer is **E.** Both isoforms of acetyl-CoA carboxylase (ACC1 and ACC2) are allosterically activated by citrate and inhibited by palmitoyl-CoA and other short- and long-chain fatty acyl-CoAs. Citrate (choice B) triggers the polymerization of ACC1 which leads to significant increases in its activity. Although ACC2 does not undergo significant polymerization (presumably due to its mitochondrial association), it is allosterically activated by citrate. Glutamate and other dicarboxylic acids can also allosterically activate both isoforms of ACC. Acetyl-CoA (choice A) is the substrate for ACC and would increase the production of malonyl-CoA by the enzyme. Glucose-6-phosphate (choice C) activates fatty acid synthase which would increase the utilization of the product of the ACC reaction, thereby resulting in potential increases in ACC activity. There is no direct role for NAD^+ (choice D) in the *de novo* synthesis of fatty acids.

9. Correct answer is **A.** Acetyl-CoA carboxylase (ACC), the rate-limiting enzyme of fatty acid synthesis, is inhibited by phosphorylation. Both isoforms of ACC, ACC1 and ACC2, are phosphorylated in response to the actions of glucagon and epinephrine. Glucagon activates its G_s-coupled receptor and epinephrine activates the G_s-coupled β-adrenergic receptors, resulting in increased cAMP and subsequently to increased PKA activity. PKA phosphorylates and inhibits ACC. The activating effects of insulin on ACC are complex but are, in part, related to reductions in cAMP levels via the insulin-mediated activation of a phosphodiesterase and the activation of protein phosphatase 1 (PP1). The activity of none of the other enzymes (choices B, C, D, and E) is directly increased by the actions of insulin.

10. Correct answer is **D.** Contributing to increases in fatty acid synthesis is the transport of mitochondrial citrate to the cytosol. In the cytosol, citrate is converted to oxaloacetate and acetyl-CoA by the ATP driven, ATP-citrate lyase (ACL) reaction. This reaction is essentially the reverse of that catalyzed by the TCA enzyme citrate synthase except it requires the energy of ATP hydrolysis to drive it forward. The resultant oxaloacetate is oxidized to malate via the action of malate dehydrogenase (MDH). The malate produced by this pathway can undergo oxidative decarboxylation by malic enzyme. The coenzyme for the malic enzyme reaction is $NADP^+$ generating NADPH. The advantage of this series of reactions for converting mitochondrial acetyl-CoA into cytoplasmic acetyl-CoA is that the NADPH produced by the malic enzyme reaction can be a major source of reducing cofactor for the activities of fatty acid synthase. None of the other enzymes (choices A, B, C, and E) generate NADPH.

11. Correct answer is **A.** Hepatocytes predominantly utilize glycerol as the building block for the synthesis of triglycerides. The glycerol backbone is activated by phosphorylation at the *sn*3 position by glycerol kinase. Therefore, a loss of glycerol kinase activity in these cells would most likely explain the reduced capability to synthesize triglycerides. Members of the glycerol-3-phosphate acyltransferase family (choice B) and the phosphatidic acid phosphatase family (choice E) are involved in hepatic triglyceride synthesis so reduced activity of either enzyme could contribute to the observations in these cells. However, both enzymes function downstream of the glycerol kinase reaction and, therefore, reduced activity of glycerol kinase is the most likely contributor to the observations in this cell culture system. The other two enzymes (choices C and D) do not contribute to the synthesis of triglycerides.

12. Correct answer is **B.** The enzymes of the glycerol-3-phosphate acyltransferase (GPAT) family carry out the esterification of a fatty acyl-CoA to glycerol-3-phosphate generating the monoacylglycerol phosphate structure called lysophosphatidic acid (LPA). The expression of the GPAT genes is under the influence of the transcription factor ChREBP. Therefore, defective ChREBP activity would result in reduced expression of GPAT resulting in reduced capacity to synthesize triglycerides. Other important targets for transcriptional activation by ChREBP include stearoyl-CoA desaturase (SCD1), fatty acid synthase (FAS), acetyl-CoA carboxylase (ACC1 and ACC2), and ATP-citrate lyase (ACLY). None of the other enzymes (choices A, C, D, and E) are directly regulated by ChREBP.

13. Correct answer is **D.** Phosphatidylinositols are important intracellular transducers of signals emanating from the plasma membrane. Phosphatidylinositol 4,5-bisphosphate (PIP_2) is a critically important membrane phospholipid involved in the transmission of signals for cell growth and differentiation from outside the cell to inside. Numerous G_q-type G protein-coupled receptors, such as the angiotensin II receptor type 1 (AT1R), activate phospholipase Cβ (PLCβ) which releases diacylglycerol (DAG) and inositol 1,4,5-trisphosphate (IP_3) from PIP_2. The IP_3 binds to receptors, that are ligand-activated calcium channels, on endoplasmic reticulum (ER) membranes resulting in the release of stored calcium into the cytosol. Within smooth muscle cells, particularly of the arterioles, the released calcium activates a myosin light-chain kinase (MLCK) through its interactions with the calmodulin subunit of the enzyme. The activation of MLCK results in phosphorylation of myosin light chains and the initiation of smooth muscle contraction resulting in increased systolic and diastolic blood pressure. None of the other lipid classes (choices A, B, C, and E) participate in the activities of angiotensin II.

14. Correct answer is **E.** Phospholipase D (PLD) enzymes hydrolyze the alcohol esterified to the phosphate of various phospholipids. Humans express six genes of the PLD family, but not all (eg, *PLD3* and *PLD6*) exhibit the same catalytic activity. The major PLD family members in humans are PLD1 and PLD2. The products of the action of these PLD enzymes are phosphatidic acid and the original alcohol such as phosphoinositol or ethanolamine from

phosphatidylinositol-4,5-bisphosphate (PIP_2) and phosphatidylethanolamine, respectively. None of the other lipid classes (choices A, B, C, and D) are substrates for PLD enzymes.

15. Correct answer is **C.** Adipocytes do not express the glycerol kinase gene and are, therefore, incapable of phosphorylating glycerol to glycerol-3-phosphate. Instead, adipocytes are dependent on glycolysis to generate dihydroxyacetone phosphate (DHAP) which can then be reduced to glycerol-3-phosphate through the action of cytosolic glycerol-3-phosphate dehydrogenase (GPD1). The glycerol-3-phosphate generated by this process in adipocytes then serves as the backbone for triglyceride synthesis. In the insulin resistance typical of type 2 diabetes the reduced uptake of glucose by adipocytes, due to reduced mobilization of GLUT4 to the plasma membrane, significantly impairs the storage of fatty acids as triglycerides in adipose tissue. None of the other compounds (choices A, B, D, and E) directly or significantly contribute to adipose tissue triglyceride synthesis.

CHAPTER 12

Bioactive Lipids and Lipid Mediators

High-Yield Terms

Eicosanoids	A family of bioactive lipids derived via the oxidation of 20-carbon omega-3 or omega-6 polyunsaturated fatty acids, such as prostaglandins, thromboxanes, and leukotrienes
Cyclic pathway	Describes the pathway, initiated by prostaglandin G/H synthase, PGS (also called prostaglandin endoperoxide synthetase), for the synthesis of arachidonic acid-derived eicosanoids containing a cyclic moiety
Linear pathway	Describes the pathway, initiated through the action of lipoxygenases (LOXs), for the synthesis of arachidonic acid-derived eicosanoids with linear structure
Cyclooxygenase, COX	Common name for prostaglandin G/H synthase which possesses both cyclooxygenase and peroxidase activities; two principal COX enzymes exist in humans, COX1 and COX2
Peptidoleukotrienes	Also called the cysteinyl leukotrienes; LTC_4, LTD_4, LTE_4, and LTF_4 constitute this group of eicosanoids because of the presence of amino acids
Slow-reacting substance of anaphylaxis, SRS-A	Consists of the leukotrienes LTC_4, LTD_4, and LTE_4, secreted by mast cells during anaphylactic reaction; induces slow contraction of smooth muscle resulting in bronchoconstriction
Sphingolipid	A class of lipid composed of a core of the long-chain amino alcohol, sphingosine, to which is attached a polar head group (such as a sugar) and a fatty acid via *N*-acylation
Ceramide	A class of lipid composed of a sphingosine core and a single fatty acid but no polar head group as for sphingolipids
Sphingomyelins	A class of sphingolipid that contain phosphocholine as the polar head group and are, therefore, also a class of phospholipid
Saposin	A family (A, B, C, and D) of small glycoprotein activators of lysosomal hydrolases that are all derived from a single precursor, prosaposin
Hexosaminidases	Dimeric enzymes composed of two subunits, either the α subunit (encoded by the *HEXA* gene) and/or the β subunit (encoded by the *HEXB* gene); various isoforms of β-hexosaminidase result from the combination of α and β subunits.
Lysosomal storage disease	Any of a large family of disorder resulting from defects in lysosomal hydrolases resulting in accumulation of incompletely degraded complex lipids, particularly of the sphingolipid family
Cherry-red spot	A finding describing the appearance of a small circular deep-red choroid shape in the fovea centralis (fundus) of the eye in a variety of lipid storage diseases
Oleoylethanolamide	Amide derivative of oleic acid synthesized by intestinal cells following intake in the diet; functions by binding to the fat-sensing receptor, GPR119
Lysophospholipid	Represents class of phospholipid generated via the removal of the fatty acid esterified to the *sn*1 or *sn*2 position of the glycerol backbone catalyzed by either PLA_1 or PLA_2, respectively
Lipoxin	Anti-inflammatory and pro-resolution eicosanoids synthesized through lipoxygenase interactions
Aspirin-triggered lipoxin	Epimeric lipoxins synthesized as a result of aspirin-mediated acetylation of COX-2
Docosahexaenoic acid, DHA	An omega-3 polyunsaturated fatty acid that can exert numerous activities by binding to a specific G-protein–coupled receptor, also is a precursor for the synthesis of anti-inflammatory lipids
Polymorphonuclear leukocytes, PMN	Commonly refers to neutrophils (can be any of the granulocyte family of leukocytes); they are characterized by the varying shapes of the nucleus which is usually lobed into three segments

INTRODUCTION TO THE EICOSANOIDS

The principal eicosanoids consist of the prostaglandins (PG), the thromboxanes (TX), the leukotrienes (LT), and the lipoxins (LX) (Figure 12–1). The PG and TX are collectively identified as prostanoids. The nomenclature (series) of the prostanoids includes a subscript number which refers to the number of carbon-carbon double bonds that exist in the molecule. The majority of the biologically active PG and TX are referred to as series-2 molecules due to the presence of two double bonds. There are, however, important series-1 and series-3 PG and TX. The predominant LT are series-4 molecules due to the presence of four double bonds. The LX are synthesized through *lipox*ygenase *in*teractions (hence the derivation of the name). The major eicosanoids, their primary sites of synthesis, and their major biological activities are outlined in Table 12–1.

Confusion can result in the classification of eicosanoids due to the use of the terms "series" which designates the number of carbon-carbon double bonds, and "group" which defines the fatty acid from which individual eicosanoids are derived. Group 1 eicosanoids are all derived from dihomo-γ-linolenic acid (DGLA; a 20:3 omega-6 PUFA). DGLA is a substrate for COX-1 and two lipoxygenases,

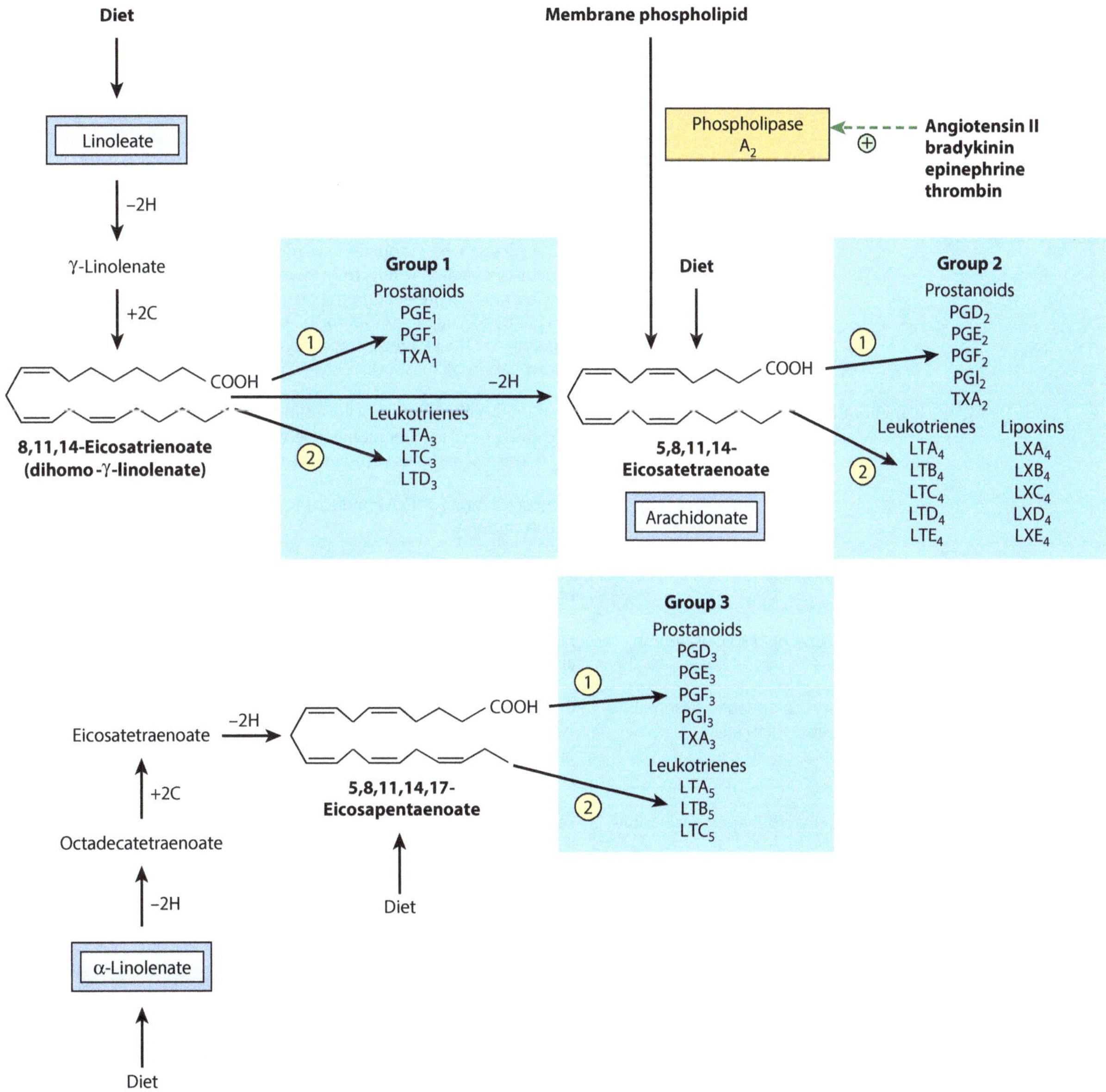

FIGURE 12–1 The three groups of eicosanoids and their biosynthetic origins. (1, cyclooxygenase pathway; 2, lipoxygenase pathway; LT, leukotriene; LX, lipoxin; PG, prostaglandin; PGI, prostacyclin; TX, thromboxane). Group 1 eicosanoids are all derived from dihomo-γ-linolenic acid (DGLA; a 20:3 omega-6 PUFA). Group 2 eicosanoids are all derived from arachidonic acid (a 20:4 omega-6 PUFA). Group 3 eicosanoids are all derived from eicosapentaenoic acid (EPA; a 20:5 omega-3 PUFA). The subscript denotes the total number of double bonds in the molecule. (Reproduced with permission from Rodwell VW, Bender DA, Botham KM, et al: *Harper's Illustrated Biochemistry*, 31st ed. New York, NY: McGraw Hill; 2018.)

TABLE 12–1 Biological activities of the major eicosanoids.

Eicosanoid	Major Site(s) of Synthesis	Major Biological Activities
LXA_4	Platelets, endothelial cells, mucosal epithelial cells, and other leukocytes via interactions with PMN	Prevents vascular permeability, reduces inflammation, blocks histamine and PGE2-mediated edema, accelerates resolution, protective in ischemia-reperfusion injury, reduces endothelial cell proliferation and migration thus, preventing atherosclerotic plaque rupture, attenuates proinflammatory gene expression in the gut reducing the severity of colitis, stimulates bone marrow and enhances growth of myeloid progenitors, reduces leukocyte adherence, decreases neutrophil recruitment, limits neovascularization and promotes host defense in the eye, protects against graft-versus-host diseases (GVHD)
LXB_4	Platelets, endothelial cells, mucosal epithelial cells, and other leukocytes via interactions with PMN	Same as LXA_4
PGD_2	Mast cells, eosinophils, brain	Inhibits platelet aggregation; induces inflammatory responses principally by recruiting eosinophils and basophils; induces bronchoconstriction; involved in androgenetic alopecia, inhibitors of PGD_2 being studied to treat male pattern baldness
PGE_1	Vascular endothelial cells, smooth muscle	Opposes actions of PGE2; induces vasodilation and inhibits platelet aggregation; binds to EP2 and EP4; alprostadil is drug version of PGE_1 used in the treatment of ductus arteriosus in neonates; alprostadil was formerly used in the treatment of erectile dysfunction
PGE_2	Kidney, spleen, heart, macrophages	Exerts a wide array of effects via binding to 1 of 4 different receptors: EP1, EP2, EP3, and EP4; modulates vascular tone and platelet reactivity; additional variability of action results from localized concentration differences; at low concentration platelet aggregation is potentiated while at high concentration it is inhibited; major contributor to arachidonic acid-mediated inflammation primarily via the EP3 receptor; enhances vascular permeability via EP3 receptor activation on mast cells
PGI_2	Heart, vascular endothelial cells	Commonly called prostacyclin; inhibits platelet and leukocyte aggregation, decreases T-cell proliferation and lymphocyte migration and secretion of IL-1α and IL-2; induces vasodilation and production of cAMP
TXA_1		Opposes actions of TXA2; induces vasodilation and inhibits platelet aggregation
TXA_2	Platelets	Induces platelet aggregation, vasoconstriction, lymphocyte proliferation, and bronchoconstriction
LTB_4	Monocytes, basophils, neutrophils, eosinophils, mast cells, epithelial cells	Powerful inducer of leukocyte chemotaxis and aggregation, vascular permeability, T-cell proliferation and secretion of INF-γ, IL-1, and IL-2
LTC_4	Monocytes and alveolar macrophages, basophils, eosinophils, mast cells, epithelial cells	Component of slow-reactive substance of anaphylaxis (SRS-A), microvascular vasoconstrictor, vascular permeability and bronchoconstriction and secretion of INF-γ, recruitment of leukocytes to sites of inflammation, enhance mucus secretions in gut and airway
LTD_4	Monocytes and alveolar macrophages, eosinophils, mast cells, epithelial cells	Same as LTC_4
LTE_4	Mast cells and basophils	Same as LTC_4

12-LOX and 15-LOX. DGLA serves as the substrate for the synthesis of PGD_1, PGE_1, $PGF_{1\alpha}$, and TXA_1. Group 2 eicosanoids are all derived from arachidonic acid (a 20:4 omega-6 PUFA). The major proinflammatory and/or prothrombotic eicosanoids derived from arachidonic acid include PGE_2, TXA_2, and LTB_4. Group 3 eicosanoids are all derived from eicosapentaenoic acid (EPA; a 20:5 omega-3 PUFA) which itself is synthesized from the essential fatty acid, α-linolenic (ALA). PGD_3 and PGI_3, both derived from EPA, decrease platelet aggregation and they counter the effects of PGD_2.

HIGH-YIELD CONCEPT

The eicosanoids produce a wide range of biological effects on inflammatory responses (predominantly those of the joints, skin, and eyes), on the intensity and duration of pain and fever, and on reproductive function (including the induction of labor). They also play important roles in inhibiting gastric acid secretion, regulating blood pressure through vasodilation or constriction, and inhibiting or activating platelet aggregation and thrombosis.

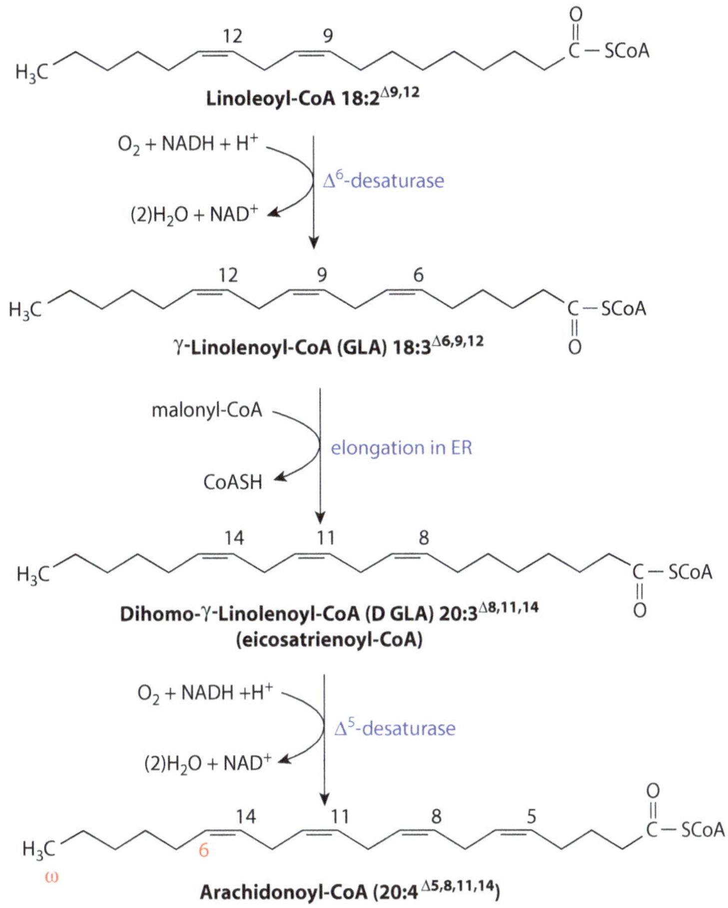

FIGURE 12–2 Synthesis of DGLA and arachidonic acid from linoleic acid. (Reproduced with permission from themedicalbiochemistrypage, LLC.)

ARACHIDONIC ACID SYNTHESIS

The principal eicosanoids of biological significance to humans are a group of molecules derived from the omega-6 polyunsaturated fatty acid (PUFA), arachidonic acid. Arachidonic acid itself is synthesized from the essential fatty acid, linoleic acid (Figure 12–2). Additional biologically significant eicosanoids are derived from dihomo-γ-linolenic acid (DGLA) which is produced in the reaction pathway leading to arachidonic acid from the essential fatty acid, linoleic acid. Within the cell, arachidonic acid resides predominantly at the C-2 position of membrane phospholipids and is released on the activation of phospholipase A_2, PLA_2 (see Figure 11–7).

SYNTHESIS OF PROSTAGLANDINS AND THROMBOXANES: THE CYCLIC PATHWAY

All mammalian cells, except erythrocytes, synthesize eicosanoids. All eicosanoids function locally at the site of synthesis, through G-protein–coupled receptor (GPCR) signaling pathways (see Chapter 26). Two main pathways are involved in the biosynthesis of eicosanoids. The PG and TX are synthesized by what is referred to as the cyclic pathway (Figure 12–3).

HIGH-YIELD CONCEPT

A widely used class of drugs, the nonsteroidal anti-inflammatory drugs (NSAIDs) such as aspirin, ibuprofen, indomethacin, naproxen, and phenylbutazone all act on the cyclooxygenase activity, inhibiting both COX-1 and COX-2.

The cyclic pathway is initiated through the action of prostaglandin G/H synthase, PGS (also called prostaglandin endoperoxide synthetase). This enzyme possesses two activities, cyclooxygenase (COX) and peroxidase. There are two forms of the COX activity in humans. COX-1 (PGS-1) is expressed constitutively in gastric mucosa, kidney, platelets, and vascular endothelial cells. COX-2 (PGS-2) is inducible and is expressed in macrophages and monocytes in response to inflammation.

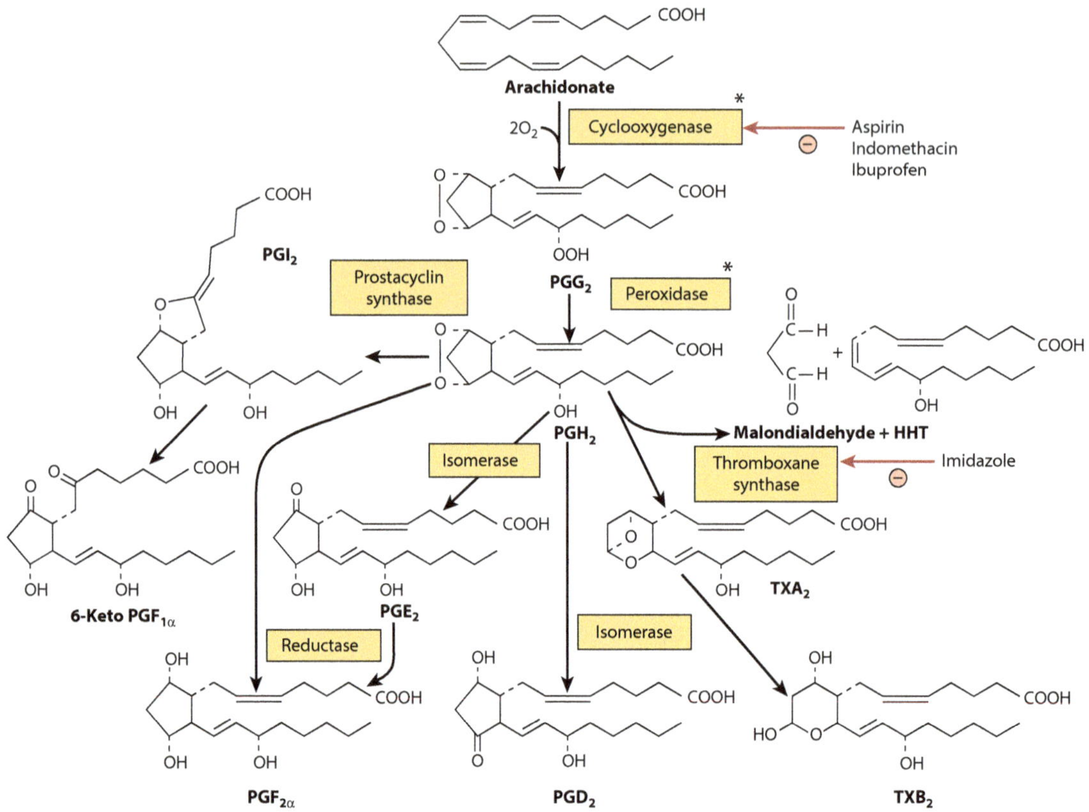

FIGURE 12–3 Conversion of arachidonic acid to prostaglandins and thromboxanes of series 2. (HHT, hydroxyheptadecatrienoate; PG, prostaglandin; PGI, prostacyclin; TX, thromboxane.) (*Both of these starred activities are attributed to the cyclooxygenase enzyme [prostaglandin H synthase]. Similar conversions occur in prostaglandins and thromboxanes of series 1 and 3.) (Reproduced with permission from Rodwell VW, Bender DA, Botham KM, et al: *Harper's Illustrated Biochemistry*, 31st ed. New York, NY: McGraw Hill; 2018.)

SYNTHESIS OF LEUKOTRIENES: THE LINEAR PATHWAY

The linear pathway of LT synthesis (Figure 12–4) is initiated through the action of the arachidonate lipoxygenase identified as 5-lipoxygenase (5-LOX). Humans express three different arachidonate lipoxygenase enzymes identified as 5-LOX, 12-LOX, and 15-LOX. The LT are synthesized by several different cell types including leukocytes, mast cells, lung, spleen, brain, and heart.

HIGH-YIELD CONCEPT

The primary endogenous lipid mediators that are released by cells that infiltrate the site of immune challenge are prostaglandin E_2 (PGE_2) and leukotriene B_4 (LTB_4). These molecules are important for host defense but can also inadvertently lead to tissue damage if inappropriately and/or excessively produced. Once initiated, an inflammatory response must be turned off following completion of the required processes triggered by the initiating challenge. This process is referred to as resolution of inflammation.

The addition of the amino acids from glutathione to leukotriene A4 (LTA_4) results in the generation of the peptidoleukotrienes (LTC_4, LTD_4, and LTE_4), also termed the cysteinyl leukotrienes. These latter leukotrienes are components of the slow-reacting substance of anaphylaxis (SRS-A) that produces a slow and sustained contraction of certain smooth muscle cells.

SYNTHESIS OF THE LIPOXINS: LIPID MEDIATORS OF INFLAMMATION

The lipoxins (LX), or the **lipox**ygenase **in**teraction products, represent a group of linear eicosanoids that are synthesized in response to inflammation and are responsible for the initiation of the resolution and termination sequences of the inflammatory process. The LX are generated from arachidonic acid via sequential actions of the different lipoxygenases (Figure 12–5). Epimeric forms of the lipoxins LXA_4 and LXB_4 are generated as a result of the actions of aspirin (acetylsalicylate) on the functions of COX-2 (Figure 12–6). These lipoxins are referred to as the aspirin-triggered lipoxins (ATL).

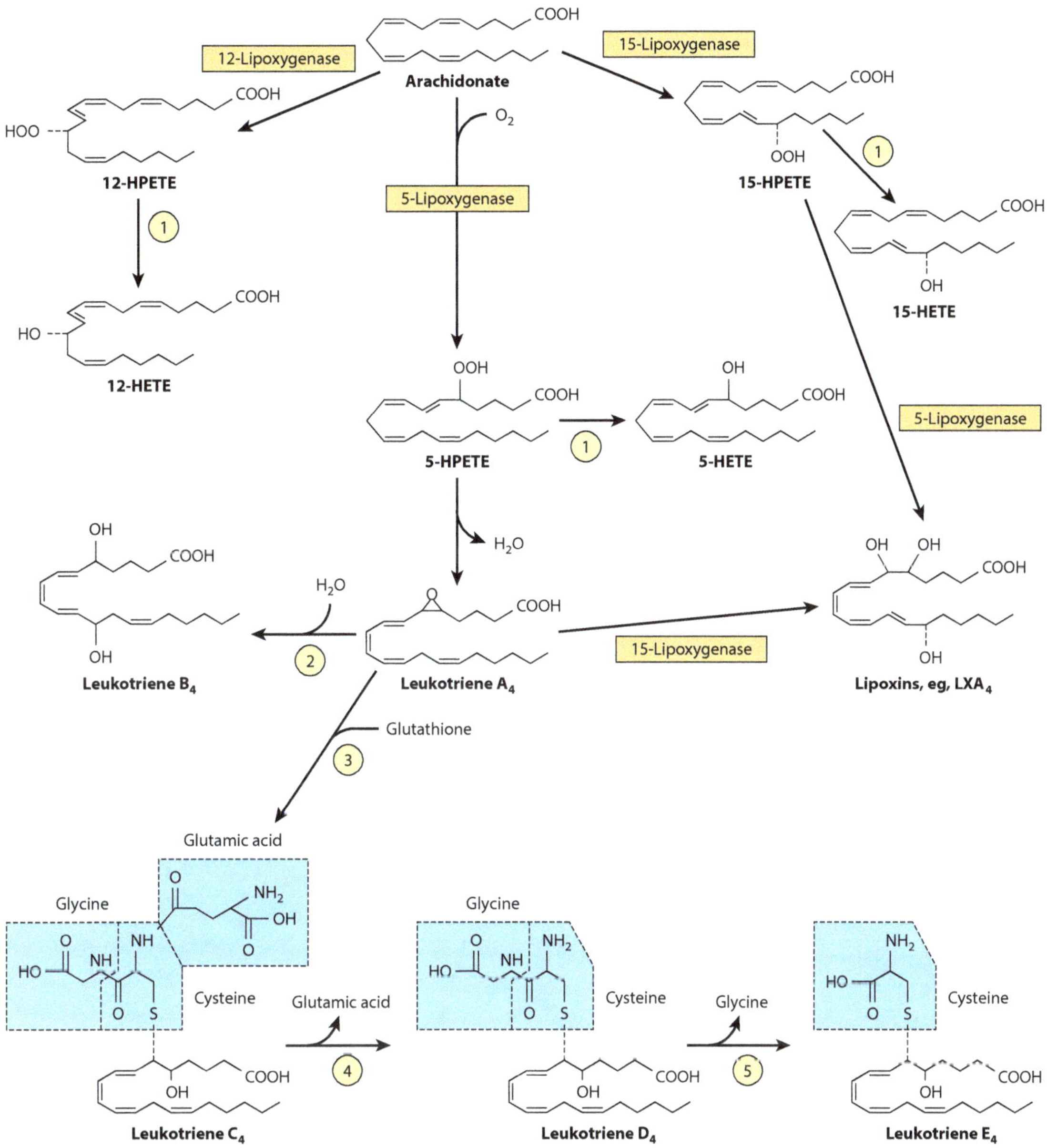

FIGURE 12–4 Conversion of arachidonic acid to leukotrienes and lipoxins of series 4 via the lipoxygenase pathway. Some similar conversions occur in series 3 and 5 leukotrienes. (1, peroxidase; 2, leukotriene A4 epoxide hydrolase; 3, glutathione S-transferase; 4, γ-glutamyltranspeptidase; 5, cysteinyl-glycine dipeptidase; HETE, hydroxyeicosatetraenoate; HPETE, hydroperoxyeicosatetraenoate.) (Reproduced with permission from Rodwell VW, Bender DA, Botham KM, et al: *Harper's Illustrated Biochemistry*, 31st ed. New York, NY: McGraw Hill; 2018.)

Lipoxin A_4 (LXA_4) and lipoxin B_4 (LXB_4) were the first recognized eicosanoid-related lipid mediators that display both potent anti-inflammatory and pro-resolving actions. The LX and their analogs exert important activities related to airway inflammation, asthma, arthritis, cardiovascular disorders, gastrointestinal disease, periodontal disease, kidney diseases and graft-vs-host disease (GVHD), and many other diseases/disorders where uncontrolled inflammation is a key mediator of disease pathogenesis.

SYNTHESIS OF SPHINGOSINE AND THE CERAMIDES

The sphingolipids represent a group of biologically active lipids that are composed of a polar head group and two nonpolar tails. The core of a sphingolipid is the long-chain amino alcohol, sphingosine (Figure 12–7). The sphingolipids include the

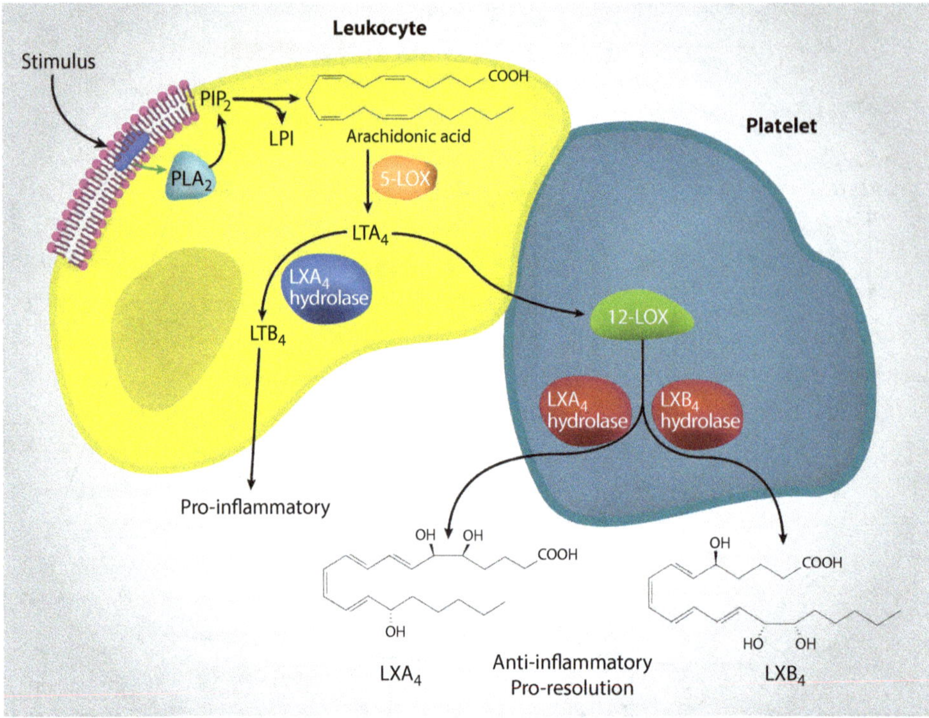

FIGURE 12–5 Synthesis of the lipoxins from arachidonic acid via transcellular interactions. Three pathways exist for the synthesis of the lipoxins. The "classic" pathway involves 5-LOX activity in leukocytes followed by 12-LOX action in platelets. The action of 15-LOX in epithelial cell (such as in the airway) followed by 5-LOX action in leukocytes is the second major lipoxin synthesis pathway. The action of aspirin on COX-2 in epithelial, or endothelial cells as well as in monocytes results in the eventual production of the 15 epi-lipoxins (also referred to as aspirin-triggered lipoxins, ATL). (Reproduced with permission from themedicalbiochemistrypage, LLC.)

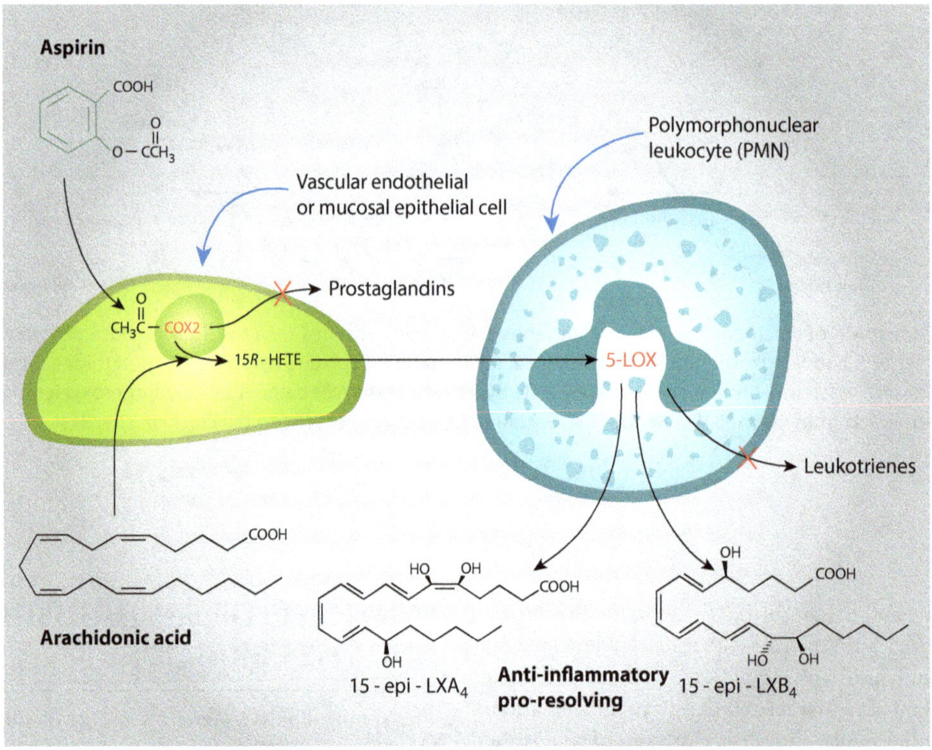

FIGURE 12–6 Synthesis of the aspirin-triggered lipoxins. Aspirin, at low doses, induces the acetylation of COX-2 resulting in an alteration in its activity such that arachidonic acid is converted to 15*R*-hydroxyeicosatetraenoic acid (15*R*-HETE). Following uptake by leukocytes the 15*R*-HETE is converted to the 15 epi-lipoxins (also referred to as aspirin-triggered lipoxins, ATL) via the action of 5-LOX. (Reproduced with permission from themedicalbiochemistrypage, LLC.)

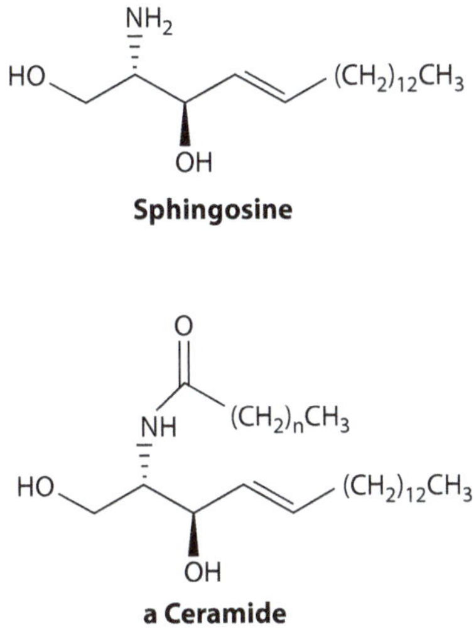

FIGURE 12–7 Structure of sphingosine and a ceramide. (Reproduced with permission from themedicalbiochemistrypage, LLC.)

sphingomyelins and glycosphingolipids (the cerebrosides, sulfatides, globosides, and gangliosides). Sphingomyelins are unique in that they are also phospholipids. Sphingolipids are components of all membranes but are particularly abundant in the myelin sheath.

The initiation of the synthesis of sphingosine, dihydrosphingosine, and ceramides takes place via the condensation of palmitoyl-CoA and serine (Figure 12–8). This reaction occurs on the cytoplasmic face of the endoplasmic reticulum (ER) and is catalyzed by serine palmitoyltransferase (SPT). The SPT reaction is the rate-limiting step in the sphingolipid biosynthesis pathway.

Following the conversion to ceramide, sphingosine is released via the action of ceramidase. Sphingosine can be reconverted to a ceramide by condensation with a fatty acyl-CoA catalyzed by the various ceramide synthases (CerS). There are at least two ceramidase genes in humans both of which are defined by their pH range of activity: acid and neutral. Acid ceramidase is encoded by the *ASAH1* gene. Defects in the human *ASAH1* gene result in Farber lipogranulomatosis (Clinical Box 12–1).

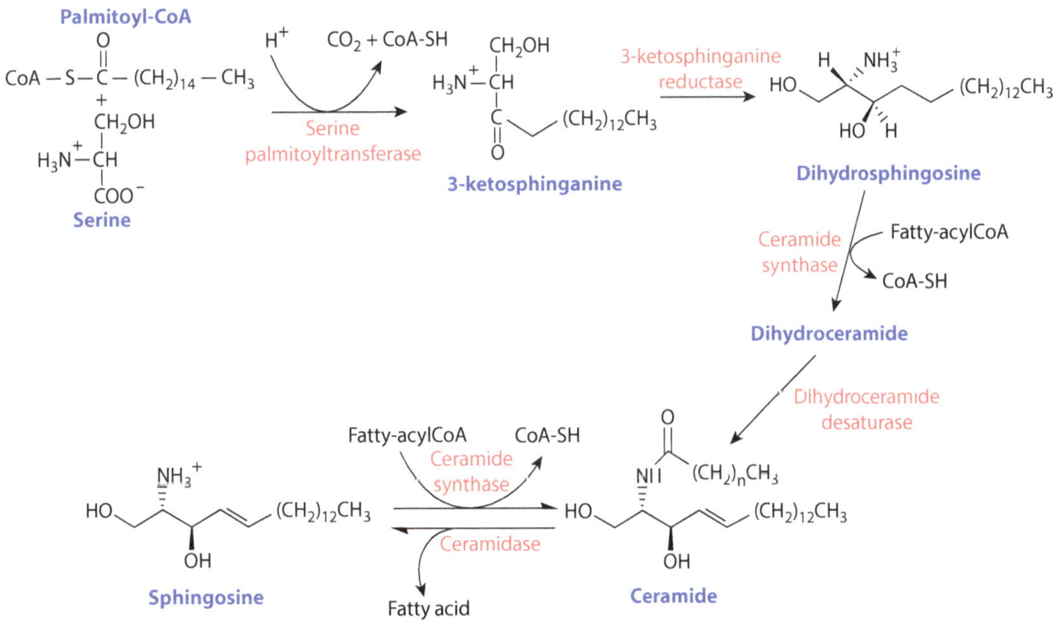

FIGURE 12–8 Pathway for sphingosine and ceramide synthesis. (Reproduced with permission from themedicalbiochemistrypage, LLC.)

CLINICAL BOX 12–1 FARBER LIPOGRANULOMATOSIS

Farber lipogranulomatosis belongs to a family of disorders identified as lysosomal storage diseases. This disorder is characterized by the lysosomal accumulation of ceramides. Farber lipogranulomatosis results from defects in the gene encoding the lysosomal hydrolase: acid ceramidase encoded by the *ASAH1* gene. Acid ceramidase catalyzes the hydrolysis of ceramides generating sphingosine and a free fatty acid. Symptoms of Farber lipogranulomatosis commonly appear during the first months after birth. The clinical manifestations are characterized by painful and progressively deformed joints, progressive hoarseness due to laryngeal involvement, and subcutaneous nodules particularly over the joints. The tissues in afflicted individuals contain granulomatous and lipid-laden macrophages. The liver, spleen, lungs, and heart are particularly affected with central nervous system involvement resulting in the progressive degeneration in psychomotor development. Farber lipogranulomatosis is a rapidly progressing disease often leading to death before 2 years of age. There are several clinical phenotypes associated with acid ceramidase deficiencies giving rise to seven subtypes of Farber lipogranulomatosis.

CLINICAL BOX 12–1 (CONTINUED)

Type 1 is the classic Farber disease. The characteristic clinical presentation of type 1 disease is painful swelling of the joints, especially the ankle, wrist, elbow, and knee and a hoarse cry. These symptoms are evident as early as 2 weeks of age. In many cases these patients will have an additional symptom characteristic of Tay-Sachs disease which is the "cherry-red spot" on the fundus of the eye.

Type 2 is the "intermediate" form and **type 3** is the "mild" form of the disease. These patients have longer survival times than do type 1 infants. In addition, the neurological involvement is much more mild than in type 1.

Type 4 is referred to as the "neonatal-visceral" form of the disease. Infants are extremely ill in the neonatal period. These patients will present with severe hepatosplenomegaly. In the severest cases, type 4 neonates will present as hydrops fetalis (severe fluid accumulation, usually in the brain) and die within days of birth. Unlike type 1 patients, infants with type 4 disease do not present with the characteristic features of deformed painful joints, thus, requiring biochemical assay for definitive diagnosis.

Type 5 is referred to as "neurologic progressive." As the name implies, the most striking clinical feature of type 5 disease is a progressive neurologic deterioration accompanied by seizures. Joint involvement is evident but to a lesser degree than in type 1 disease. Type 5 patients also exhibit the "cherry-red spot" seen in many type 1 patients.

Type 6 is characterized by patients exhibiting both Farber lipogranulomatosis as well as Sandhoff disease.

Type 7 disease results from a deficiency in prosaposin which is a precursor encoding the sphingolipid activator proteins called saposins (saposin A, B, C, and D).

SPHINGOMYELINS

Sphingomyelins are sphingolipids that are also phospholipids (Figure 12–9). Sphingomyelins are important structural components of nerve cell membranes. The predominant sphingomyelins contain palmitic or stearic acid *N*-acylated at carbon-2 of sphingosine. The sphingomyelins are synthesized by the transfer of phosphorylcholine from phosphatidylcholine to a ceramide in a reaction catalyzed by sphingomyelin synthases (SMS).

Sphingomyelins are degraded via the action of acid sphingomyelinase (ASMase) encoded for by the sphingomyelin phosphodiesterase-1 gene (*SMPD1*). Defects in the *SMPD1* gene result in the lysosomal storage disease known as Niemann-Pick disease (Clinical Box 12–2).

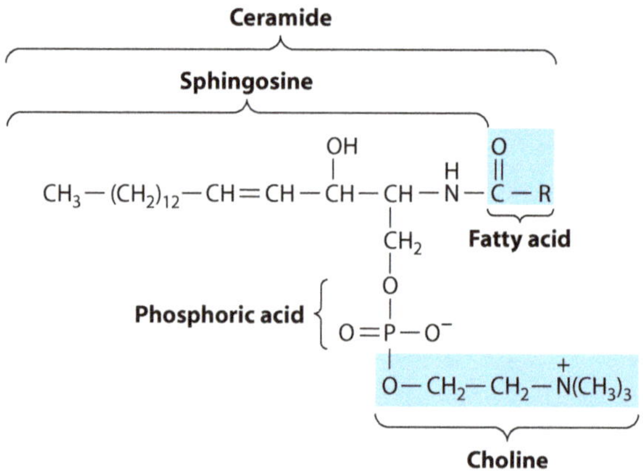

FIGURE 12–9 A sphingomyelin. (Reproduced with permission from Rodwell VW, Bender DA, Botham KM, et al: *Harper's Illustrated Biochemistry*, 31st ed. New York, NY: McGraw Hill; 2018.)

CLINICAL BOX 12–2 NIEMANN-PICK DISEASES

The Niemann-Pick (NP) diseases belong to a family of disorders identified as lysosomal storage diseases. There are two distinct subfamilies of NP diseases. NP type A (NPA) and type B (NPB) diseases are caused by defects in the acid sphingomyelinase gene (*SMPD1*). NP type C (NPC) diseases are caused by defects in a gene involved in LDL-cholesterol homeostasis identified as the *NPC1* gene. At least 95% of NPC patients contain mutations in the NPC1 locus with the remainder harboring mutations in a second gene identified as *NPC2*. Like the protein encoded by the NPC1 locus, the *NPC2* gene product also binds cholesterol esters.

Type A NP disease is associated with a rapidly progressing neurodegeneration leading to death by 2 to 3 years of age. In contrast, type B NP disease has a variable phenotype marked primarily by visceral involvement with little to no neurologic detriment. Diagnosis of type B NP disease is usually made in early childhood by the presence of hepatosplenomegaly. The most severely affected type B patients exhibit a progressive pulmonary involvement. Both type A and type B NP disease are

CLINICAL BOX 12–2 (CONTINUED)

characterized by the presence of the "Niemann-Pick" cell. This histologically distinct cell type is of the monocyte-macrophage lineage and is a characteristic lipid-laden foam cell. The course of type A NP disease is rapid. Infants are born following a typically normal pregnancy and delivery. Within 4–6 months the abdomen protrudes and hepatosplenomegaly will be diagnosed. The early neurologic manifestations include hypotonia, muscular weakness, and difficulty feeding. As a consequence of the feeding difficulties and the swollen spleen, infants will exhibit a decrease in growth and body weight. By the time afflicted infants reach 6 months of age the signs of psychomotor deterioration become evident. Ophthalmic examination reveals a cherry-red spot typical of patients with Tay-Sachs disease in about 50% of type A NP disease infants. As the disease progresses spasticity and rigidity increases and infants experience complete loss of contact with their environment.

Niemann-Pick disease type C (NPC) results from an error in the trafficking of exogenous cholesterol, thus it is more commonly referred to as a lipid trafficking disorder even though it belongs to the family of lysosomal storage diseases. The principle biochemical defect in patients with NPC is an accumulation of cholesterol, sphingolipids, and other lipids in the late endosomes/lysosomes (LE/L) of all cells. NPC is a disease characterized by fatal progressive neurodegeneration. The prevalence of NPC disease is more common than NPA and NPB disease combined. There can be significant clinical heterogeneity associated with NPC disease. Most afflicted individuals have progressive neurologic disease with early lethality. The characteristic phenotypes associated with "classic" NPC disease are variable hepatosplenomegaly, progressive ataxia, dystonia, dementia, and vertical supranuclear gaze palsy (VSGP). These individuals will present in childhood and death will ensue by the second or third decade. Because of the variable clinical phenotypes of NPC disease, it has been sub-divided into five presentation classifications: perinatal, early infantile, late infantile, juvenile, and adult. VSGP is a characteristic neurologic manifestation in NPC disease being found in virtually all juvenile and adult cases of the disease. Like NPA and NPB disease, NPC pathology is characterized by the presence of lipid-laden foam cells in the visceral organs and the nervous system.

A gene related to the *NPC1* gene, called Niemann-Pick type C1-like 1 (*NPC1L1*), is expressed in the brush border cells of the small intestine and is involved in intestinal absorption of cholesterol. The cholesterol-lowering action of the drug ezemitibe (Zetia®) stems from the fact that the drug binds to and interferes with the cholesterol absorption functions of *NPC1L1*.

SPHINGOSINE-1-PHOSPHATE, S1P

Sphingosine-1-phosphate (S1P) is a bioactive lipid that functions as a ligand for a family of five distinct GPCR. The activities initiated by S1P binding to its receptors include involvement in vascular system and central nervous system development, viability and reproduction, immune cell trafficking, cell adhesion, cell survival and mitogenesis, stress responses, tissue homeostasis, angiogenesis, and metabolic regulation.

Synthesis of S1P occurs exclusively from sphingosine via the action of sphingosine kinases. Humans express two related sphingosine kinases encoded by the *SPHK1* and *SPHK2* genes. Plasma levels of S1P are high with hematopoietic cells and vascular endothelial cells being the major sources. Lymphatic endothelial cells are also thought to secrete S1P into the lymphatic circulation. The majority of plasma S1P is bound to HDL (65%) with another 30% bound by albumin. Indeed, the ability of HDL to induce vasodilation and migration of endothelial cells, as well as to serve a cardioprotective role in the vasculature is dependent on S1P. Thus, the beneficial property of HDL to reduce the risk of cardiovascular disease may be due, in part, on its role as an S1P chaperone.

THE GLYCOSPHINGOLIPIDS

Glycosphingolipids, or glycolipids, are composed of a ceramide backbone with a wide variety of carbohydrate groups (mono- or oligosaccharides) attached to carbon-1 of sphingosine. The four principal classes of glycosphingolipids are the cerebrosides, sulfatides, globosides, and gangliosides.

One family of clinically important glycosphingolipids are the ABO blood group antigens. The ABO blood group antigens are the carbohydrates of glycosphingolipids on the surface of cells as well as the carbohydrates of secreted glycoproteins (Figure 12–10).

Cerebrosides have a single sugar group linked to ceramide with the most common being galactose forming the galactocerebrosides. Galactocerebrosides are synthesized from ceramide and UDP-galactose. Galactocerebrosides are found predominantly in neuronal cell membranes. Excess lysosomal accumulation of glucocerebrosides is observed in Gaucher disease (Clinical Box 12–3).

HIGH-YIELD CONCEPT

Glucocerebrosides are only intermediates in the synthesis of complex gangliosides or are found at elevated levels only in disease states such as Gaucher disease, where there is a defect in the catabolism of the complex gangliosides. Thus, the presence of high concentrations of glucocerebrosides in cells such as monocytes and macrophages is indicative of a metabolic defect.

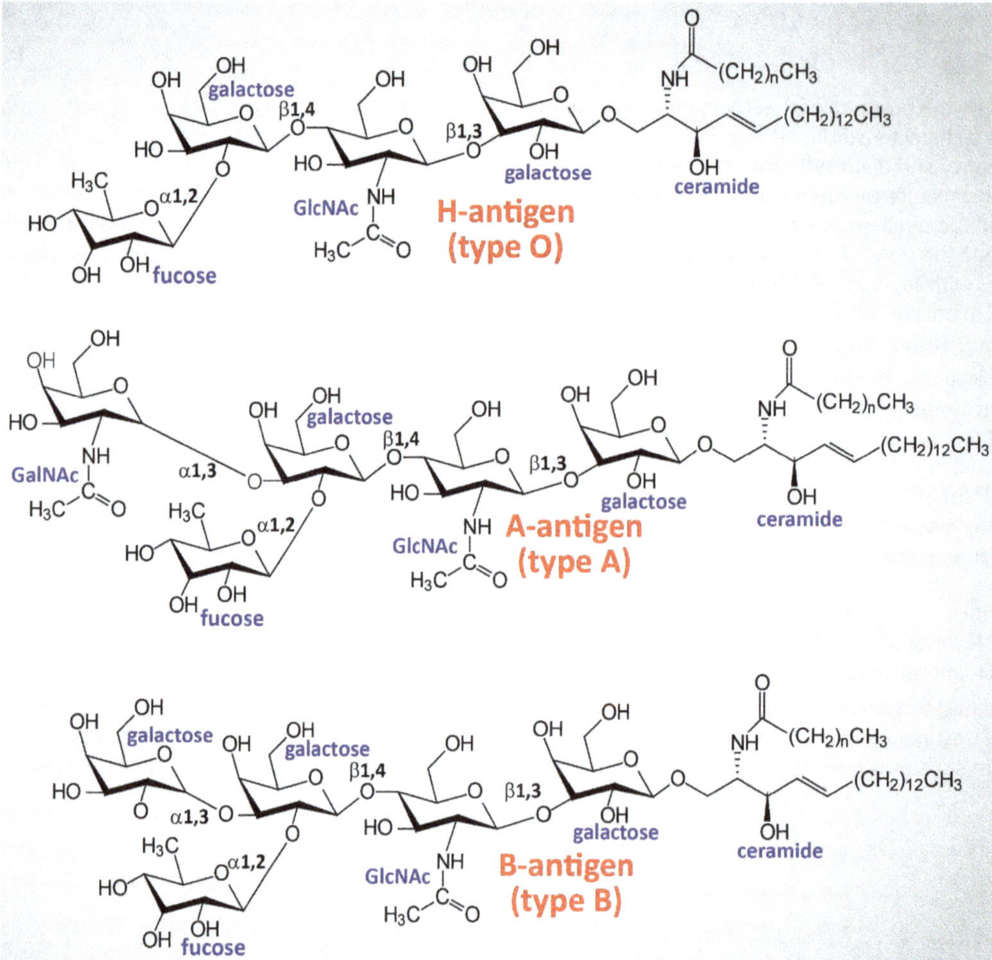

FIGURE 12–10 Structures of the ABO blood group antigens. The ABO blood group antigens are determined by the composition of the carbohydrates attached to ceramide in membrane glycolipids or to proteins in the secreted forms. The glycosidic bonds connecting the various carbohydrates to each other is indicated (eg, β1,4). GlcNAc: *N*-acetylglucosamine. GalNAc: *N*-acetylgalactosamine. (Reproduced with permission from themedicalbiochemistrypage, LLC.)

CLINICAL BOX 12–3 GAUCHER DISEASE

Gaucher disease (pronounced "go-shay") belongs to a family of disorders identified as lysosomal storage diseases. Gaucher disease is characterized by the lysosomal accumulation of glucosylceramide (glucocerebroside) which is a normal intermediate in the catabolism of globosides and gangliosides. Gaucher disease results from defects in the *GBA1* gene encoding the lysosomal hydrolase: acid β-glucosidase, also commonly called glucocerebrosidase. Acid β-glucosidase exists as a homodimer and the active hydrolytic complex requires an additional activator protein. The activator of acid β-glucosidase is saposin C, a member of the saposin family of small glycoproteins. The saposins (A, B, C, and D) are all derived from a single precursor, prosaposin. The mature saposins, as well as prosaposin, activate several lysosomal hydrolases involved in the metabolism of various sphingolipids. Prosaposin is proteolytically processed to saposins A, B, C and D, within lysosomes. The natural substrates for acid β-glucosidase are *N*-acyl-sphingosyl-1-*O*-β-D-glucosides, glucosylceramides, and various sphingosyl compounds. The physiologic significance of the role of saposin C in acid β-glucosidase activity is evident in patients with a saposin C deficiency exhibiting a Gaucher-like disease phenotype.

The hallmark of Gaucher disease is the presence of lipid-engorged cells of the monocyte/macrophage lineage with a characteristic appearance in a variety of tissues. These distinctive cells contain one or more nuclei and their cytoplasm contains a striated tubular pattern described as "wrinkled tissue paper." These cells are called Gaucher cells. Clinically, Gaucher disease is classified into three major types. These types are determined by the absence or presence and severity of neurologic involvement. Type 1 is the most commonly occurring form of Gaucher disease and is called the non-neuronopathic type (historically called the

CLINICAL BOX 12–3 (CONTINUED)

adult form). Type 1 Gaucher disease represents 95% of all cases of the disease. Both type 2 and type 3 Gaucher disease have neuronopathic involvement. Type 2 disease is the acute neuronopathic form, exhibits early onset of severe central nervous system dysfunction, and is usually fatal within the first 2 years of life. Type 3 Gaucher disease (subacute neuronopathic) patients have later onset neurologic symptoms with a more chronic course than type 2 patients. Enlargement of the liver is characteristic in all Gaucher disease patients. In severe cases the liver can fill the entire abdomen. Splenomegaly is present in all but the most mildly affected individuals and even in asymptomatic individuals spleen enlargement can be found. In addition to hepatosplenomegaly, bleeding is a common presenting symptom in Gaucher disease. The most common cause of the bleeding is thrombocytopenia (deficient production of platelets). There is no effective treatment for type 2 Gaucher disease. Current treatments for type 1 and type 3 Gaucher disease include enzyme replacement therapy (ERT), bone marrow transplantation (BMT), or oral medications. ERT replaces the deficient enzyme with artificial enzymes. The biotech company Genzyme, a unit of Sanofi SA, markets the drug imiglucerase (Cerezyme) for ERT treatment of Gaucher disease. Two additional ERT drugs prescribed for type 1 Gaucher patients are velaglucerase alfa (VPRIV) and taliglucerase alfa (Elelyso). These replacement enzymes are administered in an outpatient procedure through a vein (intravenously), typically in high doses at 2-week intervals. Although results can vary, treatment is frequently effective in people with type 1 Gaucher disease and, in some cases, type 3. In many people, enzyme replacement therapy can reduce the enlargement of the liver and spleen, help to resolve blood abnormalities, and improve bone density. It is unclear whether this therapy is effective for the neurologic problems of Gaucher disease. Occasionally people experience an allergic or hypersensitivity reaction to enzyme treatment. BMT has been used for severe cases of Gaucher disease. In this technique, blood-forming cells that have been damaged by Gaucher are removed and replaced, which can reverse many of Gaucher signs and symptoms. Because this is a high-risk approach, it is performed less often than is enzyme replacement therapy. The oral medication miglustat (Zavesca) has been approved for use in people with Gaucher disease. It appears to interfere with the production of glucocerebrosides in some people with type 1 disease. Diarrhea and weight loss are common side effects. This medication may also affect sperm production. Contraception is advised while using miglustat and for 3 months after stopping the drug.

DISORDERS OF SPHINGOLIPID METABOLISM

Some of the most devastating inborn errors in metabolism are those associated with defects in the enzymes responsible for the lysosomal degradation of membrane glycosphingolipids which are particularly abundant in the membranes of neural cells. Many of these disorders lead to severe psychomotor retardation and early lethality such as is the situation for Tay-Sachs disease (Clinical Box 12–4) or high potential for mortality as in Krabbe disease (Clinical Box 12–5). Some disorders of glycosphingolipid metabolism are less severe and can be treated through the use of enzyme replacement therapy, such as in the case of Fabry disease (see Clinical Box 12–6). Because the disorders are caused by defective lysosomal enzymes, with the result being lysosomal accumulation of pathway intermediates, these are often referred to as lysosomal storage diseases.

CLINICAL BOX 12–4 TAY-SACHS DISEASE

Tay-Sachs disease is a member of a family of disorders identified as the G_{M2} gangliosidoses. The G_{M2} gangliosidotic diseases are severe psychomotor developmental disorders caused by the inability to properly degrade membrane-associated gangliosides of the G_{M2} family (Figure 12–11). Because neural cell membranes are enriched in G_{M2} gangliosides, the inability to degrade this class of sphingolipid results in neural cell death. In addition to Tay-Sachs disease the family includes the Sandhoff diseases and the G_{M2} activator deficiencies. G_{M2} ganglioside degradation requires the enzyme β-hexosaminidase and the G_{M2} activator protein (encoded by the *GM2A* gene). β-Hexosaminidase is a dimer composed of two subunits, either the α subunit (encoded by the *HEXA* gene) and/or the β subunit (encoded by the *HEXB* gene). The various isoforms of β-hexosaminidase result from the combination of α and β subunits. The HexS protein is a homodimer of αα, HexA is a heterodimer of αβ, and HexB is a homodimer of ββ. It is the α-subunit that carries out the catalysis, and only the HexA form of β-hexosaminidase can catalyze the cleavage of G_{M2} gangliosides.

Tay-Sachs disease results from defects in the *HEXA* gene encoding the α-subunit of β-hexosaminidase. As such, Tay-Sachs disease and variants are defective in the HexA form of the enzyme but not the HexB form. Deficiencies in the *HEXB* gene result in Sandhoff disease and deficiencies in the *GM2A* gene result in G_{M2} activator deficiency disease, also referred to as the AB variant of Tay-Sachs disease. The eponym, Tay-Sachs disease, is reserved for the infantile forms of G_{M2} gangliosidotic diseases. The infantile forms are very severe and infants will not normally survive beyond 2 years of age. There are numerous variant mutants of the α-subunit that encompass a clinical spectrum from subacute to chronic forms of disease in which symptoms may be delayed for

CLINICAL BOX 12–4 (CONTINUED)

many years. The clinical phenotypes associated with the infantile forms of Tay-Sachs disease, Sandhoff disease, and G_{M2} activator deficiency disease are, for the most part, indistinguishable. In fact, the initial discrimination of Sandhoff disease from Tay-Sachs disease is only accomplished by enzyme assay not by clinical differential. Infants with Tay-Sachs disease appear normal at birth. Symptoms usually begin with mild motor weakness by 3–5 months of age. Parents will begin to notice that their afflicted child has a dull response to outside stimuli. Another early symptom is an exaggerated startle response (sudden extension of arms and legs) to sharp sounds. By 6–10 months of age infants will begin to show regression of prior acquired motor and mental skills. It is the loss of these activities that will normally prompt parents to seek a medical opinion. A progressive loss in visual attentiveness may lead to an ophthalmologic consultation which will reveal macular pallor and the presence of the characteristic "cherry-red spot" on the fundus of the eye (Figure 12–12). At around 8–10 months of age, the symptoms of Tay-Sachs disease begin to progress rapidly. Infants are progressively nonresponsive to parental stimulation. The exaggerated startle response becomes quite pronounced. Most frightening to parents is the onset of seizures which initially can be controlled by antiseizure medication. However, the seizures become progressively more severe and are very frequent by the end of the first year. Psychomotor deterioration increases by the second year and invariably leads to decerebrate posturing (typical of patients in persistent vegetative states), difficulty in swallowing, and increased seizure activity. Ultimately, the patient will progress to an unresponsive vegetative state with death resulting from bronchopneumonia resulting from aspiration in conjunction with a depressed cough.

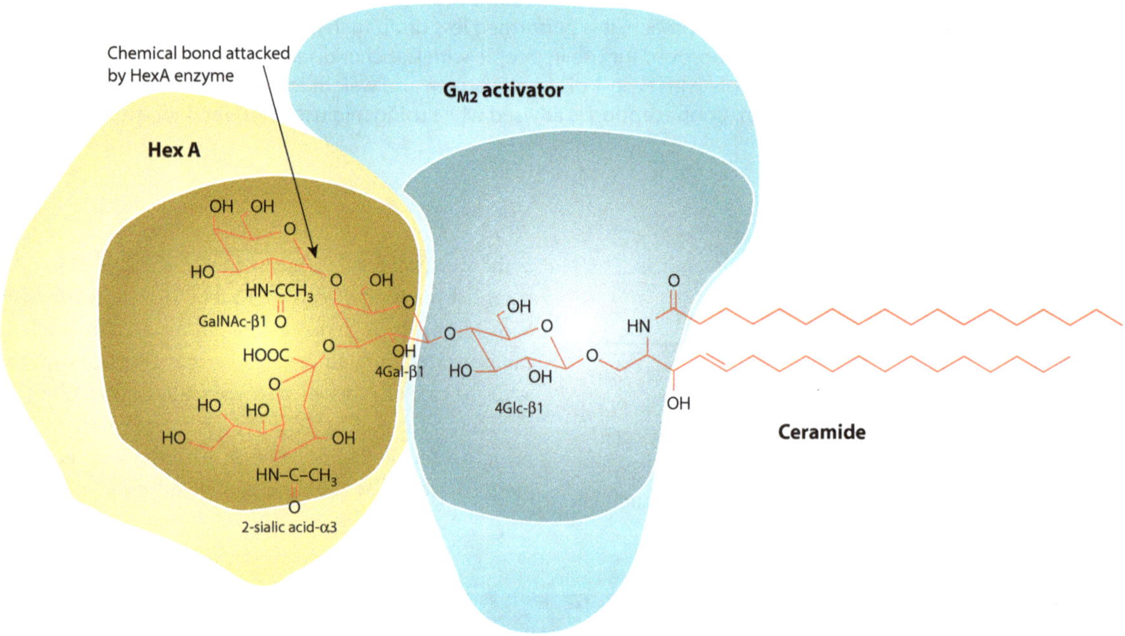

FIGURE 12–11 HexA and GM2 activator action on GM2 gangliosides. (Reproduced with permission from themedicalbiochemistrypage, LLC.)

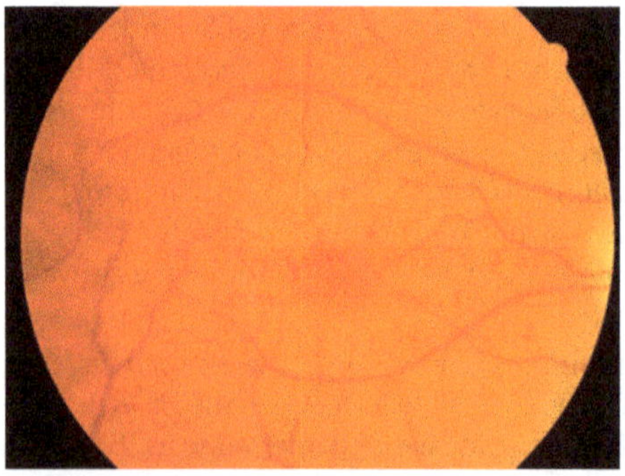

FIGURE 12–12 Typical "cherry-red spot" associated with Tay-Sachs disease. (Reproduced with permission from themedicalbiochemistrypage, LLC.)

BIOACTIVE LIPIDS AND LIPID-SENSING RECEPTORS

Originally fats were generally considered mere sources of energy and as components of biological membranes. Aside from the eicosanoids, few lipid-derived bioactive compounds had been characterized. However, research has now demonstrated a widely diverse array of biological activities associated with fatty acids and fatty acid derivatives as well as other lipid compounds. All bioactive lipids exert their effects through binding to specific receptors of the GPCR family. Bioactive lipids play important roles in energy homeostasis, cell proliferation, metabolic homeostasis, and regulation of inflammatory processes.

CLINICAL BOX 12–5 KRABBE DISEASE

Krabbe (pronounced "crab A") disease (also known as globoid cell leukodystrophy) is an autosomal recessive disorder of lysosomal glycosphingolipid metabolism. This disorder is characterized by the lysosomal accumulation of galactosylceramides as a consequence of defects in the lysosomal hydrolase, galactosylceramidase (Figure 12–13). Galactosylceramides are almost exclusively found in the myelin sheaths of nerve cells. Thus, defects in their metabolism lead to the severe neurologic involvement of Krabbe disease. The galactosylceramidase gene, formally identified as galactocerebroside β-galactosidase is encoded by the *GALC* gene. At least 60 different mutations have been identified in the *GALC* gene resulting in Krabbe disease. The frequency of Krabbe disease is 1 in 70,000 to 1 in 100,00 live births. Because a characteristic feature of Krabbe disease is the accumulation of multinucleated globoid cells in the white matter of the brain, the disease is also known as infantile globoid cell leukodystrophy (GLD). CT examination of the head in Krabbe disease patients typically shows hyperdense areas in the brain stem, cerebellum, and the caudate nucleus. This disease is a rapidly progressing disease that is invariably fatal before the end of the second year. There is a late-onset form of the disease that occurs in older children and adults of any age. The late-onset disease is characterized by blindness, dementia, and spastic paraparesis with a longer time frame of progression but yet is still a fatal disorder. Symptoms of the infantile form manifest around 3–6 months of age. Clinical manifestation of Krabbe disease is limited to the nervous system. In addition to the presence of the hematogenous globoid cells of macrophage lineage, there is near total loss of myelin and oligodendroglia as well as astrocytic gliosis. The earliest signs of Krabbe disease are hypersensitivity to external stimuli. The disease rapidly progresses to severe psychomotor deterioration. Infants become decerebrate, are blind and usually deaf, and have no contact with their surroundings. There is no treatment for the infantile form of Krabbe disease. Bone marrow transplantation (allogenic hematopoietic stem cells) has been effective in patients with minimal neurologic involvement and the late-onset form of the disease. Bone marrow transplantation has not proven to be effective in the treatment of the infantile-onset form of Krabbe disease. Although bone marrow transplantation does show promise for treating late-onset Krabbe disease, there is a high incidence of morbidity and mortality associated with this form of therapy. In addition, the high doses of chemotherapy, with or without radiation, required to ablate the patient's bone marrow prior to transplantation, the need for immunosuppressive therapy in conjunction with transplantation, and the immunological complications associated with graft-versus-host disease or graft rejection following bone marrow transplant markedly limit the effectiveness of this form of treatment.

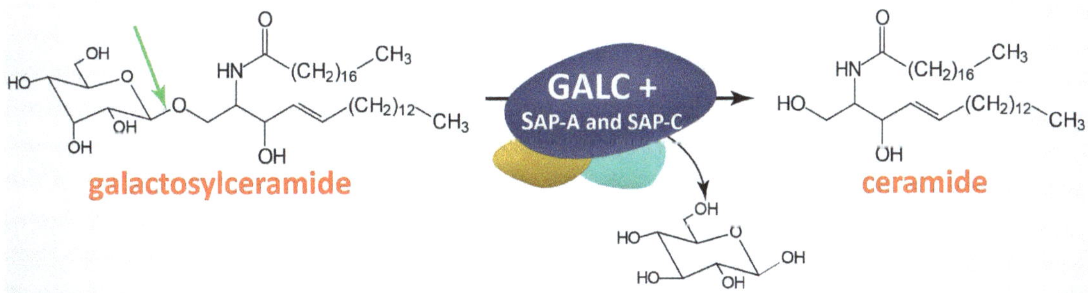

FIGURE 12–13 Reaction defective in Krabbe disease. The reaction catalyzed by galactosylceramidase and the cofactor proteins saposin A (SAP-A) and SAP-C hydrolyzes the galactose group from a galactosylceramide yielding free galactose and a ceramide. The green arrow indicates the bond that is the site of action of the GALC-encoded enzyme. Mutations in the *GALC* gene that encodes galactosylceramidase result in Krabbe disease. (Reproduced with permission from themedicalbiochemistrypage, LLC.)

CLINICAL BOX 12–6 FABRY DISEASE

Fabry disease is an X-linked recessive disorder that is characterized by the lysosomal accumulation of glycosphingolipids with terminal α-galactosyl residues. The predominant glycolipid is **globotriaosylceramide (Gb3)** and to a lesser extent blood group antigen B (of the **ABO blood group antigens**) derived compounds. Gb3 is commonly referred to as ceramide trihexoside. These glycolipids accumulate in the lysosomes as a consequence of defects in the lysosomal hydrolase, α-galactosidase A. The α-galactosidase A enzyme is encoded by the *GLA* (galactosidase alpha) gene. Like all enzymes destined for the lysosomes, the α-galactosidase A protein is co-translationally modified with mannose-6-phosphate residues. A portion of the phosphorylated enzyme is actually secreted from cells and then taken up by receptor-mediated endocytosis via mannose-6-phosphate receptors on the plasma membrane of cells. This secretion and reuptake of α-galactosidase A provides the basis for the rationale behind the enzyme replacement therapy (ERT) utilized in the treatment of Fabry disease. More than 300 different mutations have been identified in the *GLA* gene resulting in Fabry disease. Because the gene is X-linked most patients have a blood relative who

CLINICAL BOX 12–6 (CONTINUED)

is an affected male or a carrier female. The clinical manifestations of Fabry disease begin in childhood or adolescence. Classic symptoms include pain and paresthesia (burning or prickly sensation) in the extremities, gastrointestinal disturbances, cardiomyopathy, progressive renal impairment, corneal and lenticular opacities, and characteristic skin lesions called angiokeratoma (*angiokeratoma corporis diffusum*). These symptoms are all due to the deposition of Gb3 in the walls of small vessels, kidney tubules and glomerular cells, nerves, and dorsal root ganglia. The characteristic skin lesions of Fabry disease are the earliest signs that may lead to diagnosis in childhood. Death usually occurs in early adulthood from renal and cardiac complications of the vascular disease. Carrier females are usually asymptomatic but can, in rare cases, be as severely affected as hemizygous males. The most consistent clinical phenotype found in carrier females is corneal opacity. Current treatment for Fabry disease involves ERT with intravenous infusions of recombinant human α-galactosidase A. This therapeutic regimen consistently decreases Gb3 levels in plasma and clears lysosomal inclusions from vascular endothelial cells.

FREE FATTY ACID RECEPTORS

Humans express four GPCR that are activated by free fatty acids. These lipid-sensing receptors are encoded by the free fatty acid receptor 1 (FFAR1), FFAR2, FFAR3, and FFAR4. Each of these receptors was originally identified as an orphan GPCR with the original designations of GPR40 (FFAR1), GPR43 (FFAR2), GPR41 (FFAR3), and GPR120 (FFAR4). FFAR1 is activated by medium- and long-chain free fatty acids, whereas FFAR2 and FFAR3 are activated by short-chain free fatty acids. FFAR4 is the receptor for the omega-3 fatty acid, docosahexaenoic acid (DHA) but is also activated by long-chain nonesterified fatty acids (NEFA), in particular, in the intestines by α-linolenic acid (ALA).

In the small intestine the activation of FFAR4 results in increased GLP-1 secretion from enteroendocrine L cells (see Chapter 28). FFAR4 is highly expressed in adipose tissue, and proinflammatory macrophages and is inducible in liver-resident macrophage-like cells known as Kupffer cells.

The anti-inflammatory effects of DHA are the result of the activation of FFAR4 in macrophages (Figure 12–14). DHA stimulation

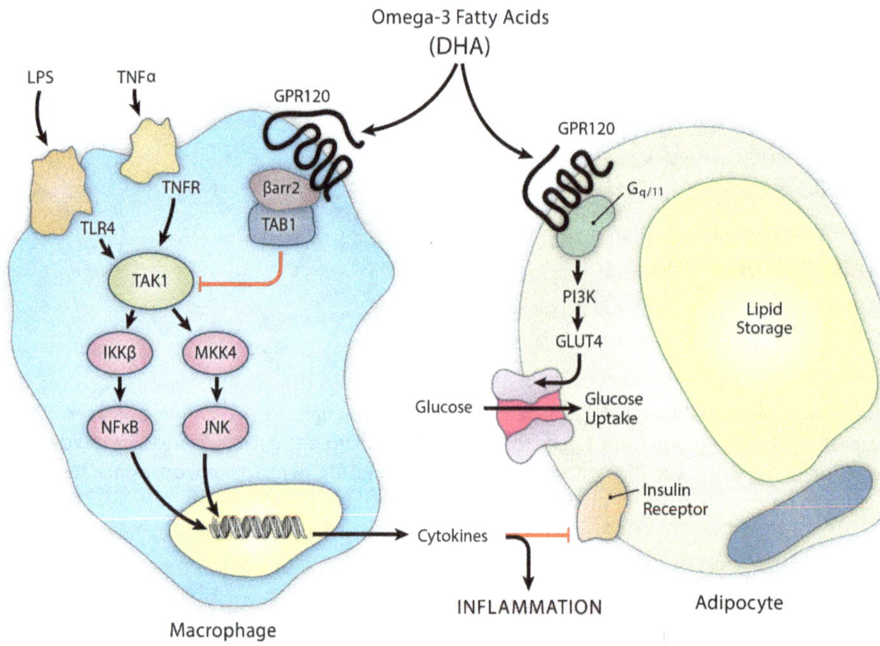

FIGURE 12–14 Diagrammatic representation of the signaling events initiated in response to DHA binding to GPR120 on macrophages and adipocytes. The mechanism of GPR120-mediated anti-inflammation involves inhibition of transforming growth factor-β–activated kinase 1 (TAK1) through a β-arrestin-2 (βarr2)–dependent effect. TAK1-binding protein (TAB1) is the activating protein for TAK1. Stimulation of GPR120 by DHA has been shown to inhibit both the Toll-like receptor 4 (TLR4) and TNF-α pro-inflammatory cascades via TAK1 inhibition. Activation of the kinases, inhibitor of nuclear factor kappa-B kinase subunit beta (IKKβ), and c-JUN N-terminal kinase (JNK), is common to TLR and TNF-α signaling. Nuclear factor kappa B (NFκB), one of the most important transcription factors regulating the expression of proinflammatory genes, is normally activated by IKKβ. JNK is normally activated by mitogen-activated protein kinase kinase 4 (MKK4). The effects of GRP120 activation in macrophages are reduced secretion of proinflammatory cytokines which would normally interfere with insulin effects on adipose tissue. Within adipose tissue, DHA-mediated activation of GRP120 results in enhanced mobilization of GLUT4 to the plasma membrane, thus, enhancing glucose uptake. (Reproduced with permission from King MW: *Integrative Medical Biochemistry Examination and Board Review,* New York, NY: McGraw Hill; 2014.)

of FFAR4 is also involved in glucose homeostasis in adipose tissue due to increased GLUT4 translocation to the cell surface with a subsequent increase in glucose transport into the cells. The effects of DHA on glucose uptake in adipocytes are additive to those of insulin.

HIGH-YIELD CONCEPT

Given the functions of omega-3 PUFA in inflammation, insulin sensitization, and lipid profiles mediated through activation of FFAR4 indicate that this GPCR is a critically important control point in the integration of anti-inflammatory and insulin sensitizing responses, which may prove useful in the future development of new therapeutic approaches for the treatment of diabetes.

OLEOYLETHANOLAMIDE AND GPR119

Oleoylethanolamide (OEA, Figure 12–15) is a member of the fatty-acid ethanolamide family that includes palmitoylethanolamide (PEA) and *N*-arachidonoylethanolamide (anandamide). Anandamide is an endogenous ligand (endocannabinoid) for the cannabinoid receptors. OEA is produced by mucosal cells in the proximal small intestine from dietary oleic acid. OEA activates the fatty acid-sensing GPCR identified as GPR119. The production of OEA is associated with a significant reduction in food intake and body weight gain.

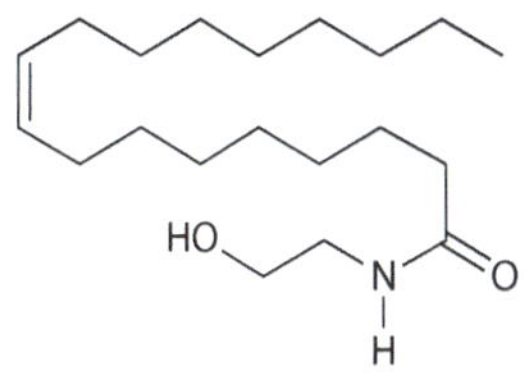

FIGURE 12–15 Structure of oleoylethanolamide (OEA). (Reproduced with permission from King MW: *Integrative Medical Biochemistry Examination and Board Review*, New York, NY: McGraw Hill; 2014.)

HIGH-YIELD CONCEPT

The observations that GPR119 activation is associated with reducing blood glucose suggest it may be a viable target in the treatment of type 2 diabetes. Indeed, currently there are several small molecule agonists of GPR119 in clinical trials being tested for their efficacy in treating the hyperglycemia of type 2 diabetes as well as for their efficacy in treating obesity.

CHECKLIST

- ☑ The eicosanoids consist of the prostaglandins (PG), thromboxanes (TX), leukotrienes (LT), and lipoxins (LX) and are synthesized from 20-carbon essential omega-3 or omega-6 polyunsaturated fatty acids (PUFA).
- ☑ All mammalian cells, except erythrocytes, synthesize eicosanoids.
- ☑ Eicosanoids are extremely potent bioactive lipids, able to induce physiologic effects at very dilute concentrations. All eicosanoids function locally at the site of synthesis, through binding to specific G-protein–coupled receptors (GPCR).
- ☑ The omega-6 fatty acid, arachidonic acid, serves as a primary precursor lipid for the synthesis of bioactive eicosanoids. It is found esterified to the *sn*2 position of membrane phospholipids and is released on receptor activation of PLA_2.
- ☑ Arachidonic acid synthesis is primarily initiated from the essential fatty acid, linoleic acid, but the pathway can also utilize dietary γ-linolenic acid (GLA).
- ☑ The primary prostaglandins and thromboxanes are synthesized from arachidonic acid via the cyclic pathway which involves the enzyme prostaglandin G/H synthase (more commonly called cyclooxygenase).
- ☑ The primary leukotrienes are synthesized from arachidonic acid via the linear pathway which involves the enzyme 5-lipoxygenase (5-LOX).
- ☑ Dihomo-γ-linolenic acid (DGLA) is an intermediate in arachidonic acid synthesis that can be diverted into membrane phospholipids where it competes with arachidonic acid. PLA_2-mediated release of DGLA results in synthesis of series 1 prostaglandins and thromboxanes which mediate effects opposite to those of arachidonic acid-derived molecules.
- ☑ The nonsteroidal anti-inflammatory (NSAID) class of pharmaceutical drugs all function by blocking the cyclooxygenase activity of prostaglandin G/H synthase.
- ☑ Sphingolipids are a class of lipid that includes the sphingomyelins and glycosphingolipids (the cerebrosides, sulfatides, globosides, and gangliosides). Sphingomyelins are the only sphingolipid class that are also phospholipids.
- ☑ Sphingosine is an amino alcohol that serves as the backbone of the ceramides and sphingolipids. Sphingosine is synthesized from palmitoyl-CoA and serine in a reaction initiated by serine palmitoyltransferase, SPT. SPT represents the rate-limiting step in sphingolipid synthesis.

- ☑ Ceramides and sphingosine can be interconverted through the actions of ceramidases and ceramide synthases (CerS). Humans express six distinct CerS genes. Sphingomyelins and ceramides can also be interconverted via the actions of sphingomyelin synthases and sphingomyelinase.
- ☑ Each CerS exhibits fatty acyl chain length specificity as well as differential tissue distribution.
- ☑ Cellular levels of ceramides depend on a balance between the need for sphingosine and sphingosine derivatives, such as sphingosine-1-phosphate (S1P), and the sphingomyelins.
- ☑ Increased levels of ceramides can induce insulin resistance by blocking the ability of the insulin receptor to activate the downstream kinase, PKB/Akt. Conversely, reduced synthesis of ceramides is associated with increased growth of certain types of cancers, whereas, enhanced expression of CerS1, in particular, is associated with increased efficacy of chemotherapeutic drugs.
- ☑ The glycosphingolipids are major constituents of all cellular membranes and they are the major glycans of the vertebrate brain, where more than 80% of glycoconjugates are in the form of glycosphingolipids.
- ☑ Sphigosine-1-phosphate (S1P) is a major biologically active lysophospholipid. S1P is derived by phosphorylation of sphingosine by two distinct sphingosine kinases. S1P binds to, and activates, five functionally distinct GPCR and eliciting activities that include involvement in vascular system and central nervous system development, viability and reproduction, immune cell trafficking, cell adhesion, cell survival and mitogenesis, stress responses, tissue homeostasis, angiogenesis, and metabolic regulation.
- ☑ Defects in lysosomal hydrolases, responsible for the degradation of membrane sphingolipids, results in potentially devastating clinical consequences. The disorders that arise due to these enzyme defects are referred to as lysosomal storage diseases.
- ☑ Bioactive lipids constitute a diverse array of fatty acid-derived molecules that exert their effects through binding to specific GPCR. The most potent bioactive lipids are those derived from the essential omega-3 and omega-6 polyunsaturated fatty acids.
- ☑ Oleoylethanolamide (OEA) is a member of the fatty-acid ethanolamide family that includes palmitoylethanolamide (PEA) and *N*-arachidonoylethanolamide (anandamide). OEA exerts its biological effects through activation of the GPCR, GPR119.
- ☑ The lipoxins are anti-inflammatory and proresolution eicosanoids synthesized from arachidonic acid through the concerted actions of cyclooxygenase and lipoxygenase via interactions between epithelial cells and leukocytes, or between leukocytes and platelets.
- ☑ Aspirin modifies the activities of COX-1 and COX-2 by acting as a suicide inhibitor at high doses; at low doses aspirin-mediated acetylation of COX-2 changes its activity toward the substrate, arachidonic acid such that instead of driving the synthesis of the prostaglandins and thromboxanes, it directs the lipid into the epimeric lipoxin synthesis pathway deriving the aspirin-triggered lipoxins.

REVIEW QUESTIONS

1. A 5-year-old boy is being examined by his pediatrician due to the rapid onset of severe psychomotor retardation. History shows that the child has suffered from numerous upper respiratory infections in the past 2 years. Physical examination shows several abnormalities in craniofacial development which includes pronounced gingival hyperplasia and the presence of hepatomegaly. The symptoms exhibited by this child are most likely due to a defect in which of the following processes?

(A) Production of the mannose-6-phosphate modifications in lysosomal enzymes
(B) Recycling of the lysosomal receptor for mannose-6-phosphate present on lysosomal enzymes
(C) Removal of mannose-6-phosphates from lysosomal enzymes prior to their transport to the lysosomes
(D) Synthesis of the mannose-6-phosphate receptor found in lysosomes
(E) Transport of mannose-6-phosphate receptors to lysosomes

2. An 8-month-old infant is being examined by his pediatrician due to concerns by his parents about deteriorating motor skills. The child was normal at birth, but the deteriorating signs began about 1 month ago. Ophthalmoscopic examination identifies a milky halo surrounding the fovea centralis. The enzyme, whose deficiency is resulting in the observed signs and symptoms in this child, normally performs which of the following functions?

(A) Degradation of glycolipids in skeletal muscle
(B) Degradation of glycolipids in the brain
(C) Degradation of glycolipids in the bone marrow
(D) Synthesis of glycolipids in smooth muscle
(E) Synthesis of glycolipids in the brain
(F) Synthesis of glycolipids in the liver

3. A 37-year-old man is being examined by his physician with complaints of chronic pain in his stomach area. Physical examination shows the patient to be mildly jaundiced. Palpation of his abdomen elicits a sharp pain response and indicates hepatosplenomegaly. Histological examination of a blood smear from the patient shows foamy fat-laden cells of the

granulocyte-macrophage lineage. The appearance of which of the following in the blood and/or urine would be most useful in making a correct diagnosis in this patient?
(A) Ceramides
(B) Glucocerebrosides
(C) GM_2 gangliosides
(D) Sphingomyelins
(E) Sulfatides

4. A 17-year-old boy is brought to the emergency department with complaints of dizziness, difficulty breathing, and swelling of his tongue. The patient reports that he believes he was stung by bees. Physical examination finds the patient has a rapid but weak pulse. Which of the following lipid-derived molecules is most likely contributing to the symptoms the patient is experiencing?
(A) Arachidonic acid
(B) Leukotriene B_4, LTB_4
(C) Platelet-activating factor, PAF
(D) Prostaglandin E_2, PGE_2
(E) Thromboxane A_2, TXA_2

5. A preterm infant whose birth weight was 1450 g (3 lb 2 oz) has difficulty feeding and has not gained weight or grown for 6 weeks. There are distinctive signs of pulmonary and systemic venous congestion and a continuous cardiac murmur. Diagnosis of the correct anatomical defect is determined, and therapy is begun which includes pharmacological intervention with a drug that is most likely designed to mimic the actions of which of the following class of molecule?
(A) Adrenal steroids
(B) Angiotensin
(C) Natriuretic factors
(D) Prostaglandins
(E) Vasopressin

6. Experiments are being performed on a novel compound that has been designed to act as an antagonist of the PGE_1 receptor. The compound is tested in an animal model system via intravenous injection. Which of the following activities is most likely reduced or absent in response to the novel compound?
(A) Activation of 5-LOX for leukotriene synthesis
(B) Enhancement of neutrophil adhesion
(C) Induction of slow cardiac contraction
(D) Platelet aggregation and activation
(E) Relaxation of vascular smooth muscle cells

7. Experiments are being conducted on the pathways of bioactive lipid synthesis from arachidonic acid. These experiments are being carried out with the use of peripheral blood mononuclear cells that have been treated with the chemotherapeutic, ethylnitrosourea. When arachidonic acid is metabolized by these cells there is detectable PGE_2 but no detectable LTA_4. Given these results, which of the following enzymes is most likely defective in these drug-treated cells?
(A) COX-1
(B) 5-Lipoxygenase
(C) LTC_4 synthase
(D) Prostacylin synthase
(E) Thromboxane synthase

8. Experiments are being conducted on a novel eicosanoid-like molecule. When this compound is administered to laboratory animals there is a demonstrable inhibition of platelet and leukocyte aggregation, induction of smooth muscle relaxation, decreased proliferation of T-cells, decreased lymphocyte migration, and decreased secretion of IL-1α and IL-2. The effects of this compound are most likely mimicking the activities of which of the following?
(A) LTB_4
(B) LTC_4
(C) PGE_2
(D) PGI_2
(E) TXA_2

9. Experiments are being carried out using a compound designed to mimic the activities of PGE_2 within the vasculature. If the compound is administered to laboratory animals at concentrations similar to the normal physiological concentration of PGE_2, which of the following effects would most likely confirm the expected activity?
(A) Inhibited endothelial permeability
(B) Decreased neutrophil adhesion
(C) Inhibited platelet aggregation
(D) Smooth muscle contraction
(E) Smooth muscle relaxation

10. A 64-year-old man is being examined by his physician with complaints of being tired and feeling weak. History reveals that he has been taking over-the-counter pain medications 6–8 times per day for the past 9 months due to severe pain in his left hip and shoulder. A fecal occult blood test is positive. Which of the following is the most likely activity of his medication that is contributing to the signs and symptoms in this patient?
(A) Activation of arachidonic acid synthesis
(B) Activation of bradykinin synthesis
(C) Activation of cyclooxygenase
(D) Inhibition of arachidonic acid synthesis
(E) Inhibition of bradykinin synthesis
(F) Inhibition of cyclooxygenase

11. Dietary studies are being undertaken to ascertain the optimal nutritional requirements needed for the production of the series 2 prostaglandins such as PGE_2. Results of these studies determined that daily ingestion of 10 g of a particular fatty acid was associated with maximal synthesis of PGE_2. Which of the following most likely represents that beneficial fatty acid?
(A) Linoleic
(B) Linolenic
(C) Myristic
(D) Palmitic
(E) Stearic

12. Aspirin is useful therapeutically in the treatment of fevers associated with viral infections. This activity of aspirin is most likely due to which of the following?
(A) Activation of adenylate cyclase
(B) Activation of nitric oxide synthase
(C) Activation of phospholipase Cβ (PLCβ)
(D) Inhibition of cyclooxygenase
(E) Inhibition of lipoxygenase
(F) Inhibition of PLA_2

13. A 4-month-old boy is brought to his pediatrician by his parents because they have noticed that he has developed a progressive lack of response to outside stimuli and that he does not seem to follow their voices with his eyes as he did the previous month. In addition, they say that their son exhibits an exaggerated startle response to sharp sounds and that

he seems to be losing previously acquired motor and mental skills. Accumulation of which of the following class of lipid is most likely contributing to the pathology in this patient?
(A) Glycosphingolipid
(B) Leukotriene
(C) Phospholipid
(D) Prostaglandin
(E) Thromboxane
(F) Sphingomyelin

14. A 5-month-old infant is brought to her pediatrician because she has had difficulty in feeding and frequently vomits following feedings. The parents indicate that their daughter had been able to sit by herself but now is incapable of doing so, seems to be unable to focus on them. Upon examination the doctor notes that the infant has obvious hypotonia, hepatosplenomegaly, and thin limbs. Given these signs and symptoms, analysis of the patient's monocytes for the presence of which of the following would be most useful in determining the cause of the pathology?
(A) Chondroitin sulfate
(B) Dermatan sulfate
(C) Globotriaosylceramide
(D) Glucocerebroside
(E) Heparan sulfate
(F) Sphingomyelin

15. A 23-year-old man died as a result of progressive heart failure. Results of his autopsy included the finding of significant cardiomyopathy (1100 g), cardiac storage of globotriaosylceramide (11 mg lipid/g wet weight), and restricted cardiocytes. A defect in which of the following processes is most likely to have contributing to this patients' death?
(A) Collagen synthesis
(B) Glycogen metabolism
(C) Glycosaminoglycan metabolism
(D) Glycosphingolipid metabolism
(E) Lipoprotein metabolism

16. A 4-month-old boy presents with painful progressive joint deformity (particularly the ankles, knees, elbows, and wrists), hoarse crying, and granulomatous lesions of the epiglottis and larynx leading to feeding and breathing difficulty. Analysis of liver biopsy tissue for the accumulation of which of the following would be most useful in the diagnosis of the disorder in this patient?
(A) Abnormal collagen
(B) Abnormal glycogen
(C) Ceramides
(D) Dermatan sulfates
(E) Triglycerides

17. A 2-month-old infant suffering from increased vomiting and diarrhea is seen in the hospital and observed to have significant abdominal distention due to hepatosplenomegaly. Unfortunately, the infant does not survive. Autopsy reveals calcification of the adrenals and massive accumulation of cholesteryl esters and triglycerides in most tissues. Accumulation of which of the following class of lipid is most likely contributing to the pathology in this patient?
(A) Glycosphingolipid
(B) Leukotriene
(C) Phospholipid
(D) Prostaglandin
(E) Thromboxane
(F) Triglycerides

18. A 42-year-old man presents with hepatomegaly, jaundice, refractory ascites, and renal insufficiency. A significant reduction in the activity of which of the following would most likely be correlated to the symptoms in this patient?
(A) Acid sphingomyelinase
(B) Glucocerebrosidase
(C) β-Hexosaminidase A
(D) Iduronate 2-sulfatase
(E) α-L-Iduronidase

19. A 4-month-old infant died following a brief period of severe psychomotor deterioration. The infant was born blind and deaf. Autopsy results found the presence of hematogenous globoid cells of macrophage lineage throughout the brain along with near total loss of myelin and oligodendroglia. Given the findings in this infant, which of the following metabolic processes was most likely defective?
(A) Glycogen metabolism
(B) Glycosaminoglycan metabolism
(C) Glycosphingolipid metabolism
(D) Lipoprotein metabolism
(E) Phospholipid metabolism

20. A 4-month-old infant exhibits an exaggerated startle response, hypotonia, and now only responds to loud voices and sounds indicative of a decrease in hearing acuity. Ophthalmoscopic examination shows a bright red center of the fovea centralis surrounded by a milky halo. Analysis of enzyme activity in peripheral blood cells shows lower than normal β-hexosaminidase A activity. Which of the following is most likely in this patient?
(A) Accumulation of undigested lipid intermediates in lysosomes
(B) Defective peroxisomal metabolism of lipid
(C) Failure to oxidize medium-chain fatty acids
(D) Impaired mitochondrial electron transport
(E) Reduced glucose oxidation via the pentose phosphate pathway

21. Experiments are being conducted on the effects of a novel compound on whole blood cell cultures. Results find that upon addition of the compound the activity of phospholipase A_2 (PLA_2) is identical to that in control cultures. However, the production of PGE_2 is significantly reduced relative to control cultures. Given these results, which of the following enzymes is most likely to be inhibited by the addition of the compound?
(A) Cyclooxygenase-1 (COX-1)
(B) 5-Lipoxygenase (5-LOX)
(C) Prostacyclin synthase
(D) Stearoyl-CoA desaturase 1 (SCD1)
(E) Thromboxane synthase

22. Experiments are being conducted with a novel compound to determine its effects on cultured vascular endothelial cells. Results from these experiments show that the compound induces the synthesis of 15-epi-LXA_4, an effect similar to the actions of acetylsalicylate. Given these results, which of the following enzymes is the most likely target of this novel compound?
(A) Cyclooxygenase-2
(B) Cyclooxygenase-1

(C) 5-Lipoxygenase
(D) 12-Lipoxygensase
(E) Prostacyclin synthase
(F) Thromboxane synthase

23. Experiments are being conducted on a novel compound using a cell line derived from a bone marrow aspirate. Addition of the compound to the culture prevents the release of arachidonic acid from membrane phospholipids. These results indicate that the compound is most likely interfering with the activity of which of the following?
(A) Cyclooxygenase
(B) Lipoprotein lipase
(C) 5-Lipoxygenase
(D) Phospholipase A_2
(E) Phospholipase D

24. A 5-month-old infant is brought to her pediatrician because she has had difficulty in feeding and frequently vomits following feedings. The parents indicate that their daughter had been able to sit by herself but now is incapable of doing so, seems to be unable to focus on them. Upon examination the doctor notes that the infant has obvious hypotonia, hepatosplenomegaly, and thin limbs. Ophthalmoscopic examination finds a pale halo surrounding the fovea centralis. These signs and symptoms are most likely indicative of a defect in which of the following processes?
(A) Collagen maturation
(B) Fatty acid oxidation
(C) Gluconeogenesis
(D) Glycogenolysis
(E) Phospholipid metabolism

25. Autopsy results performed on a 17-year-old boy who died as a result of progressive heart failure find significant cardiomyopathy, presence of restricted cardiocytes, and cardiac muscle accumulation of a complex lipid of the globoside family. A defect in which of the following processes is most likely to account for this patient's disorder?
(A) Adipose tissue triglyceride metabolism
(B) Lysosomal lipid degradation
(C) Mitochondrial fatty acid β-oxidation
(D) Peroxisomal fatty acid α-oxidation
(E) Sphingomyelin synthesis

26. A 4-month-old infant died following a brief period of severe psychomotor deterioration. The infant was born blind and deaf. Autopsy results found the presence of hematogenous globoid cells of macrophage lineage throughout the brain along with near total loss of myelin and oligodendroglia. The accumulation of which of the following class of molecule most likely contributed to the lethal course in this infant?
(A) Ceramide
(B) Ganglioside
(C) Plasmalogen
(D) Prostaglandin
(E) Sphingomyelin

27. Experiments are being conducted on human vascular endothelial cells in culture following their exposure to a known carcinogen. These cells were found to possess the histamine H1 receptor; however, addition of histamine to these cultures failed to elicit the expected changes in intracellular calcium. Based upon these results, which of the following enzymes is most likely defective?
(A) Phospholipase A_2
(B) Phospholipase Cβ
(C) Phospholipase D
(D) Protein kinase A
(E) Protein kinase C

28. A 6-month-old infant is being examined by her pediatrician due to concern by her parents about her lack of interaction with them or her surroundings. Physical examination shows the infant exhibits an exaggerated startle response and is hypotonic. Ophthalmoscopic examination shows a bright red center of the fovea centralis surrounded by a milky halo. Suspecting the infant has Tay-Sachs disease, the pediatrician orders a molecular analysis of the genes encoding α- and β-subunits of β-hexosaminidase A (HexA) in this infant. These results demonstrate that both genes are normal. Given these findings, which of the following is the most likely abnormal gene in this patient?
(A) Glucocerebrosidase
(B) G_{M2} activator
(C) Medium-chain acyl-CoA dehydrogenase
(D) Phytanoyl-CoA hydroxylase
(E) Sphingomyelinase

29. During fetal development, blood flow from the right ventricle bypasses the lungs via the ductus arteriosus. Closure of this structure following birth is most likely influenced by which of the following changes?
(A) Decreased serum calcium concentration
(B) Decreased serum lactate concentration
(C) Decreased serum prostaglandin concentration
(D) Increased serum calcium concentration
(E) Increased serum lactate concentration
(F) Increased serum prostaglandin concentration

30. An experimental compound is under investigation for its effects on the synthesis of series 2 prostaglandins in cultures of vascular endothelial cells. Addition of the compound results in a decrease in synthesis that is very nearly equivalent to that seen by addition of acetylsalicylate. These results indicate that the compound is most likely exerting its effects through the inhibition of which of the following reactions of prostaglandin synthesis?
(A) Acetyltransferase
(B) Desaturation
(C) Hydroxylation
(D) Oxygenation
(E) Peroxidation

31. A 1-year-old child is being examined for possible reasons for her failure to thrive. Physical examination finds jerking head movements, icteric sclera, hepatomegaly, and demonstrable vertical supranuclear gaze palsy. Given the most likely disorder in this child, which of the following processes would most likely be found to be impaired?
(A) Bilirubin conjugation
(B) Cholesterol trafficking
(C) Collagen maturation
(D) Glycogen synthesis
(E) Glycosphingolipid metabolism

32. Several bioactive lipids are involved in the pathology of asthma in the airway. These airway function modifying lipids are most likely to be associated with which of the following processes?
(A) Decreasing airway resistance
(B) Decreasing dead space volume
(C) Decreasing alveolar cell fluid density
(D) Increasing functional residual capacity
(E) Increasing lung compliance
(F) Increasing total lung capacity

33. Experiments are being performed to study the role of HDL-associated lipids on migration of endothelial cells in culture. HDL prepared from wild-type mice are found to result in a significant increase in cell migration, whereas HDL isolated from a mutant mouse line shows no increase in migration. Which of the following lipid classes is most likely to be reduced or missing from the HLD isolated from the mutant mice?
(A) Ceramide
(B) Galactocerebroside
(C) G_{M2} ganglioside
(D) Sphingomyelin
(E) Sphingosine-1-phosphate

34. Cells isolated from a squamous cell tumor of the neck are found to metabolize palmitic acid at a significantly reduced rate compared to cells isolated from normal tissue in the same region of the neck. Which of the following enzymes is most likely to be deficient in the cancer cells?
(A) Ceramide synthase
(B) Glucocerebrosidase
(C) β-Hexosaminidase A
(D) Serine palmitoyltransferase
(E) Sphingomyelinase

35. Studies are being carried out using a cell line derived from a cancerous tumor. Normal cells activate a pathway of apoptosis in response to tumor necrosis factor-α (TNF-α) but the cells derived from the tumor do not. Additional results show that the cancer cells take up serine and palmitic acid at a similar rate to normal cells but that the levels of sphingomyelins are elevated relative to normal cells. Given the responses of the cancer cells to TNF-α and the biochemical studies, the activity of which of the following enzymes is most likely to be reduced in the tumor cells?
(A) Acid sphingomyelinase
(B) Ceramidase
(C) β-Hexosaminidase A
(D) Serine palmitoyltransferase
(E) Sphingosine kinase

36. A 12-month-old infant exhibits severe developmental delay with associated macrocephaly, dysmorphic facies, hypotonia, and hepatosplenomegaly. Physical examination finds no significant ocular anomalies. Additional findings include a pebbly ivory-colored lesion over the infant's back. Analysis of the activity of which of the following enzymes would be most useful in the diagnosis in this patient?
(A) Acid sphingomyelinase
(B) Galactosylceramidase
(C) Glucocerebrosidase
(D) β-Hexosamindase A
(E) Iduronate 2-sulfatase

37. Experiments are being performed to ascertain the activity of a novel lipid molecule with respect to vascular function. Administration of the compound to experimental animals results in the induction of vasodilation and the aggregation of platelet aggregation to endothelial cells of the vasculature. The activities of this novel lipid compound are most likely the effects of which of the following lipids?
(A) Docosahexaenoic acid, DHA
(B) Eicosapentaenoic acid, EPA
(C) Lysophosphatidic acid, LPA
(D) Lysophosphatidylinositol, LPI
(E) Oleoylethaolamide, OEA

38. A 9-year-old boy is being examined by his pediatrician with a complaint of a dull burning pain in his hands and feet, which he has stated he most often experiences after playing soccer with his friends. Physical examination finds the patient has numerous small, raised purple spots on his thighs and around his umbilicus. Ophthalmoscopic examination finds the presence of cornea verticillata. Given the signs and symptoms in this patient, the most likely abnormal process is occurring in which of the following cellular locations?
(A) Cytosol
(B) Endoplasmic reticulum
(C) Lysosome
(D) Mitochondria
(E) Peroxisome

39. An 18-year-old woman is being examined by her physician with the primary complaint of severe pain during the period before and after her monthly menstrual cycle. Her physician prescribes a combination estrogen-progesterone oral contraceptive pill to help lessen the intensity of her periods as well as meloxicam for relief of her menstrual pain. Which of the following is the most likely consequence of the prescribed pain medication?
(A) Decreased ceramide synthesis
(B) Decreased leukotriene synthesis
(C) Decreased prostacyclin synthesis
(D) Increased ceramide synthesis
(E) Increased leukotriene synthesis
(F) Increased prostaglandin synthesis

40. A 5-month-old male infant is brought to the Emergency Department by his adoptive parents because he experienced a seizure following several days of having a fever. History reveals that the patient is frequently irritable and does not respond well or at all to voices or noise. Physical examination finds the patient is currently afebrile, is hypertonic with limb stiffness throughout all extremities, and has no palpable abdominal masses. Because of the seizure the attending physician orders a head CT scan, the results of which show increased density in the caudate nucleus, cerebellum, and brain stem. Additional testing would most likely be associated with which of the following histopathological findings?
(A) Increased abnormally branched glycogen in the liver
(B) Lipid-laden foam cells
(C) Liver infiltration with granulomatous macrophages
(D) Macrophages with coarse fibrillary cytoplasm
(E) Multinucleated globoid cells

41. A 4-month-old female infant is brought to the Emergency Department by her parents following a seizure. Physical examination shows the infant is in respiratory distress and has a demonstrably palpable liver. The parents indicate that they noticed their daughter's stomach bulging about a month ago. History reveals that the infant has had difficulty with feeding and does not appear to be attaining expected developmental milestones related to cognition and motor skills. Fundoscopic examination shows pallor around the fovea centralis. Blood studies find elevated levels of LDL cholesterol and triglycerides with decreased levels of HDL cholesterol. Biochemical analysis shows elevated blood levels of triglycerides and low-density lipoprotein, with low levels of high-density lipoprotein. Additional testing would most likely be associated with which of the following histopathological findings?

(A) Increased abnormally branched glycogen in the liver
(B) Lipid-laden foam cells
(C) Liver infiltration with granulomatous macrophages
(D) Macrophages with coarse fibrillary cytoplasm
(E) Multinucleated globoid cells

42. A 12-year-old boy is being examined by his pediatrician with a complaint of a dull burning pain in his hands and feet, which he has stated he most often experiences after he has played soccer with his friends. He also states that he does not think that he sweats as much as he used to while playing soccer. Physical examination finds the patient has numerous small, raised purple spots on his thighs and around his umbilicus. Ophthalmoscopic examination finds the presence of a swirling cloudiness in the lower portion of his corneas. Biochemical analysis of fibroblast activity is most likely to find a deficiency in which of the following?

(A) Acid ceramidase
(B) α-Galactosidase A
(C) Galactosylceramidase
(D) β-Hexosaminidase A
(E) Serine palmitoyltransferase

43. A 5-month-old female infant is brought to the Emergency Department by her parents because she experienced a seizure following several days of having a fever. History reveals that the patient is frequently irritable and does not respond well or at all to voices or noise. Physical examination finds the patient is currently afebrile, is hypertonic with limb stiffness throughout all extremities, and has no palpable abdominal masses. The patient was born at 39 weeks following an uncomplicated pregnancy. When the infant was born she was in the 40th percentile for both length and weight at birth, however, today the infant is at the 10th percentile for length and 5th percentile for weight. Fundoscopic examination shows optic atrophy in both eyes. A CT scan of the head shows increased density in the caudate nucleus, cerebellum, and brain stem. Given these signs and symptoms, this patient is most likely deficient in which of the following enzymes?

(A) Arylsulfatase A
(B) Galactosylceramidase
(C) β-Glucocerebrosidase
(D) β-Hexosaminidase A
(E) Sphingomyelinase

44. A 12-year-old boy is being examined by his pediatrician because his parents are concerned that he has been complaining about generalized pain that is particularly acute in his knees. Physical examination finds that the patient does not experience pain to palpation of the joints, however, the patient's spleen is palpable below the left costal margin. X-ray of the legs shows Erlenmeyer flask bone deformity in both distal femurs. A CBC reveals thrombocytopenia and leukopenia. The physician orders a bone marrow biopsy which reveals enlarged monocyte lineage cells that appear to be engorged with a coarse fibrillary substance. Given the signs and symptoms in this patient, which of the following is most likely to be found at elevated levels?

(A) Dermatan sulfate
(B) Galactocerebroside sulfate
(C) Globotriaosylceramide
(D) Glucocerebroside
(E) Sphingomyelin

45. A 10-year-old girl is being examined in the Emergency Department. History reveals that the patient was experiencing a fever, aches, cough, and sore throat for the past week. Her mother states that she gave her daughter over-the-counter pain and fever medication which seemed to help for a day or two but that this morning her daughter was sick again with vomiting, lethargy, and confusion. Physical examination shows her temperature is 38.4°C (101.1°F), her pulse is 112 beats per minute, her respirations are 16 per minute, and her blood pressure is 109/68 mm Hg. Physical examination finds a palpable liver and papilledema. Blood work finds elevated levels of both AST and ALT. The medication that was given to the patient, that is most likely contributing to the signs and symptoms observed, is most likely responsible for which of the following?

(A) Covalent modification of cyclooxygenase
(B) Covalent modification of lipoxygenase
(C) Enhanced turnover of cyclooxygenase
(D) Enhanced turnover of lipoxygenase
(E) Selective inhibition of cyclooxygenase in the neurons
(F) Selective inhibition of lipoxygenase in neurons

ANSWERS

1. Correct answer is **A.** The patient is most likely suffering from the disorder known as I-cell disease. I-cell disease (also called mucolipidosis IIA) results from defects in the process of phosphorylating mannose residues, in enzymes destined for the lysosomes, on the 6-position (mannose-6-phosphate. Man-6-P) while they are in the Golgi apparatus. This phosphorylation process requires the enzyme, UDP-*N*-acetylglucosamine. lysosomal-enzyme *N*-acetylglucosaminyl-1-phosphotransferase (GlcNAc-phosphotransferase; commonly called phosphotransferase). GlcNAc-phosphotransferase is an $\alpha_2\beta_2\gamma_2$ hexameric complex whose protein subunits are encoded by two genes. The α- and β-subunits of the phosphotransferase are encoded by the *GNPTAB* gene, and the γ-subunits are encoded by the *GNPTG* gene. The presence of the Man-6-P residues in lysosomal enzymes is recognized by a specific Man-6-P receptor (MPR) present in the membranes of the Golgi apparatus. I-cell disease results from mutations in the *GNPTAB* gene resulting in loss of correct localization of nearly all the enzymes of the lysosomes. None of the other options (choices B, C, D, and E) correctly correlates to the cause of the symptoms of I-cell disease.

2. Correct answer is **B.** The infant is most likely suffering from Tay-Sachs disease. Tay-Sachs disease is caused by mutations in the gene (*HEXA*) encoding the alpha subunit of β-hexosaminidase A. β-Hexosaminidase A is responsible for the lysosomal degradation of G_{M2} gangliosides, which are particularly enriched in the membranes of cells in the central nervous system. None of the other options (choices A, C, D, E, and F) correspond to the processes that would be defective in an infant with Tay-Sachs disease.

3. Correct answer is **B.** This patient is most likely exhibiting the signs and symptoms of Gaucher disease. Gaucher disease results from mutations in the enzyme, glucocerebrosidase, that is responsible for the lysosomal degradation of glucocerebrosides that are the products of the lysosomal degradation of more complex glycosphingolipids. As a result of the defective enzyme, elevated levels of glucocerebrosides are detectable in the blood and urine. The most common form of Gaucher disease, representing 95% of all cases, is the adult form identified as type 1 Gaucher disease. Enlargement of the liver is characteristic in all Gaucher disease patients. The hallmark of Gaucher disease is the accumulation of lipid-engorged cells of the monocyte/macrophage lineage with a characteristic appearance in a variety of tissues. The primarily affected tissues are bone, bone marrow, spleen, and liver. These distinctive cells contain one or more small nuclei, and their cytoplasm contains a coarse fibrillary material that forms a striated tubular pattern often described as "wrinkled tissue paper." These cells are called Gaucher cells. None of the other lipid molecules (choices A, C, D, and E) would be detectable elevated levels in the blood or urine of Gaucher disease patients.

4. Correct answer is **C.** The patient is most likely exhibiting the signs and symptoms of anaphylaxis. One of the potent bioactive lipids that contributes to the pathophysiology of anaphylaxis is platelet-activating factor, PAF. PAF is a unique complex lipid of the plasmalogen family. PAF functions in hypersensitivity, acute inflammatory reactions, and anaphylactic shock by inducing increased vasopermeability, vasodilation, and bronchoconstriction. Excessive production of PAF may be involved in the morbidity associated with toxic shock syndrome and strokes. None of the other bioactive lipids (choices A, B, D, and E) induce the symptoms of anaphylaxis seen in this patient.

5. Correct answer is **D.** The infant is most likely exhibiting the symptoms associated with a ductal-dependent congenital heart defect, most likely Tetralogy of Fallot. Pharmacologic intervention, prior to surgery, involves the use of the drug alprostadil (prostaglandin E1, PGE_1). PGE_1 induces vasodilation and inhibits platelet aggregation maintaining a patent ductus arteriosus. During fetal development, the aorta and the pulmonary artery are connected by a temporary blood vessel called the ductus arteriosus. While in the womb, the fetus receives oxygen from the mother's circulation, so blood does not need to flow through the lungs. The ductus arteriosus streamlines fetal circulation by flowing blood directly to the aorta, bypassing the lungs. After birth, the ductus arteriosus usually seals off so that blood from these two vessels does not mix. In infants with ductal-dependent congenital heart defects the maintenance of a patent ductus arteriosus prior to surgical intervention can relieve some of the symptoms. None of the other molecules (choices A, B, C, and E) are useful in the pharmacologic intervention of ductal-dependent congenital heart defects.

6. Correct answer is **E.** PGE_1 is a series 1 eicosanoid derived from linoleic acid or γ-linolenic acid (GLA). This lipid induces vasodilation through relaxation of smooth muscle cells, exhibits anti-inflammatory activity, and inhibits platelet aggregation. Antagonism of the receptor for PGE_1 would, therefore, interfere with the normal relaxation of vascular smooth muscle elicited by PGE_1 binding. None of the other activities (choices A, B, C, and D) would be associated with antagonism of the PGE_1 receptor.

7. Correct answer is **B.** As a consequence of appropriate signals that lead to activation of the phospholipid hydrolyzing enzyme PLA_2, arachidonic acid is released from these membrane lipids. Arachidonic acid serves as a substrate for both the lipoxygenase and the cyclooxygenase pathways of bioactive lipid synthesis. The lipoxygenase (linear) pathway is initiated through the action of one of three lipoxygenases (LOX), 5-LOX, 12-LOX, and 15-LOX. The lipoxygenase pathway generates the leukotrienes of which LTA_4 is a member. The cyclooxygenase pathway involves two enzymes, COX-1 and COX-2. The cyclooxygenase pathway leads to the generation of the prostaglandins, such as PGE_2, and the thromboxanes, such as TXA_2. The absence of LTA_4 synthesis would most likely be due to loss of 5-lipoxygenase (5-LOX) activity given that arachidonic acid was utilized effectively as a substrate for the synthesis of PGE_2 via the cyclooxygenase (choice A) pathway. Deficiency in none of the other enzymes (choices C, D, and E) would account for synthesis of PGE_2 and the lack of synthesis of LTA_4.

8. Correct answer is **D.** Prostacyclin (PGI_2) is primarily synthesized by cardiac and vascular endothelial cells. Activities associated with this bioactive lipid include inhibition of platelet and leukocyte aggregation, decreases in T-cell proliferation, decreases in lymphocyte migration, and decreased secretion of IL-1α and IL-2. Additional activities include smooth muscle relaxation leading to vasodilation. LTB_4 (choice A) is a potent proinflammatory bioactive lipid that functions as a chemokine promoting migration of macrophages and neutrophils into tissues. LTC_4 (choice B) is a member of the peptidoleukotriene (cysteinyl leukotriene) family of bioactive lipids. The peptidoleukotrienes are components of slow-reacting substance of anaphylaxis (SRS-A). PGE_2 (choice C) effects are complex and depend upon the cell type and receptor to which it binds. Generally, PGE_2 is considered a proinflammatory bioactive lipid. TXA_2 (choice E) is a major bioactive lipid released from activated platelets. The functions of TXA_2 include induction of platelet aggregation, vasoconstriction, lymphocyte proliferation, and bronchoconstriction.

9. Correct answer is **E.** PGE_2 is one of the most potent eicosanoids and it exhibits multiple activities. These multiple activities are in part, the result of the binding of PGE_2 to one of four receptors identified as EP1, EP2, EP3, and EPP4. The various activities of PGE_2 include the relaxation, not contraction (choice D) of smooth muscle cells resulting in increased vasodilation. Other effects exerted by PGE_2 include the enhancement of the effects of bradykinin and histamine, and induction of uterine contractions, and maintaining the open passageway of the fetal ductus arteriosus. The actions of PGE_2 in the vasculature include enhanced, not inhibited (choice A) endothelial permeability, increased, not decreased (choice B) neutrophil adhesion to the endothelium, and activation, not inhibition (choice C) of platelet aggregation.

10. Correct answer is **C.** The nonsteroidal anti-inflammatory drugs (NSAIDs) inhibit cyclooxygenase (COX), predominantly COX-1, and consequently inhibit the synthesis of the prostaglandins and the thromboxanes. In the stomach, prostaglandins have a cytoprotective effect through inhibition

of acid secretion, enhancement of mucosal blood flow, and stimulation of bicarbonate and mucus secretion. Inhibiting these processes can cause stomach ulcers and bleeding which has most likely occurred in this patient. The NSAIDs do not exert effects on arachidonate acid synthesis (choices A and D) nor on bradykinin synthesis (choices B and E). As indicated, NSAIDs inhibit cyclooxygenase as opposed to activating the enzyme (choice C).

11. Correct answer is **A.** The prostaglandins, such as PGE_2, are synthesized from the 20-carbon polyunsaturated fatty acid, arachidonic acid. Because arachidonic acid contains multiple sites of unsaturation, including at positions at which human desaturases are not functional, the synthesis of arachidonic acid requires the essential fatty acid, linoleic acid. Linoleic acid is termed as essential fatty acid because it contains sites of unsaturation that human tissues cannot introduce and the lipid must, therefore, be acquired in the diet. Linolenic acid (choice B) is the precursor for the polyunsaturated fatty acids of the omega-3 family such as eicosapentaenoic acid (EPA) and docosahexaenoic acid (DHA). None of the other fatty acids (choices C, D, and E) are essential fatty acids nor are they involved in the synthesis of prostaglandins.

12. Correct answer is **D.** The antipyretic (fever reducing) effects of aspirin (acetylsalicylate) are due to the ability of this drug to block the synthesis of proinflammatory and pyretic prostaglandins from arachidonic acid. The synthesis of the prostaglandins is initiated via the activity of cyclooxygenase (prostaglandin G/H synthase, PGS). This enzyme possesses two activities, cyclooxygenase (COX) and peroxidase. One of the actions of aspirin is the inhibition of the COX activity of this bifunctional enzyme. One of the additional effects of aspirin is the activation of nitric oxide synthase activity (choice B) in vascular endothelial cells. However, this activity is unrelated to the fever-reducing effects of aspirin. None of the other activities (choices A, B, C, E, and F) are directly affected by the action of aspirin.

13. Correct answer is **A.** The infant is most likely suffering the consequences of Tay-Sachs disease. Infants with Tay-Sachs disease appear normal at birth. Symptoms usually begin with mild motor weakness by 3–5 months of age. Parents will begin to notice that their afflicted child has a dull response to outside stimuli. Another early symptom is an exaggerated startle response. By 6–10 months of age infants will begin to show regression of prior acquired motor and mental skills. Tay-Sachs disease results from mutations in the gene encoding the α-subunit of the lysosomal hydrolase β-hexosaminidase A. The activity of β-hexosaminidase A is exerted on G_{M2} gangliosides which are enriched in cells of the central nervous system. Therefore, loss of β-hexosaminidase A activity results in the accumulation of G_{M2} gangliosides which are members of the glycosphingolipid class of bioactive lipids. None of the other lipid classes (choices B, C, D, E, and F) are found to be accumulating in Tay-Sachs disease.

14. Correct answer is **F.** The infant is most likely suffering the consequences of Niemann-Pick type IA disease. Niemann-Pick disease (NPD) comprises two distinct but related types of lipid storage disorder, type I and type II. In addition, both types comprise two subtypes. Type IA (NPA) and type IB (NPB) both result from defects in the lysosomal hydrolase, acid sphingomyelinase. Pathologic characteristics of the type I Niemann-Pick diseases are the accumulation of histiocytic cells that result from sphingomyelin deposition in cells of the monocyte-macrophage lineage. None of the other substances (choices A, B, C, D, and E) are found to accumulate in monocytes nor are they associated with the signs and symptoms of Niemann-Pick disease.

15. Correct answer is **D.** The signs and symptoms appearing in this patient prior to his death most likely indicate he was suffering from Fabry disease. Fabry disease is an X-linked disorder that results from a deficiency in the lysosomal hydrolase, α-galactosidase A. Deficiency in this enzyme leads to the deposition of neutral glycosphingolipids with terminal α-galactosyl moieties in most tissues and fluids. Most affected tissues are heart, kidneys, and eyes. The predominant glycosphingolipid accumulated is globotriaosylceramide [galactosyl-(α1→4)-galactosyl-(β1→4)-glucosyl-(β1→1')-ceramide], also referred to as ceramide trihexoside. With increasing age, the major symptoms of the disease are due to increasing deposition of glycosphingolipid in the cardiovascular system. Indeed, cardiac disease occurs in most hemizygous males. None of the other metabolic processes (choices A, B, C, and E), when defective, would account for the signs and symptoms in Fabry disease.

16. Correct answer is **C.** The patient is most likely exhibiting the signs and symptoms of Farber lipogranulomatosis. Farber lipogranulomatosis is a lysosomal storage disease that is characterized by painful and progressively deformed joints, and progressive hoarseness due to involvement of the larynx. Subcutaneous nodules form near the joints and over pressure points. Granulomatous lesions form in these tissues and there is an accumulation of lipid-laden macrophages. Significant accumulation of ceramide and gangliosides is observed, particularly in the liver. If these compounds accumulate in nervous tissue, there may be moderate nervous dysfunction. The illness often leads to death within the first few years of life, although milder forms of the disease have been identified. None of the other substances (choices A, B, D, and E) are found to be accumulating in Farber lipogranulomatosis.

17. Correct answer is **F.** The infant is most likely exhibiting the signs and symptoms of the disorder known as Wolman disease. Wolman disease results from a deficiency in the lysosomal hydrolase called cholesteryl ester hydrolase (also called lysosomal acid lipase) resulting in the massive infiltration of organs with macrophages filled with triglycerides and cholesteryl esters. Wolman disease is very nearly always a fatal disease of infancy. Clinical manifestations include hepatosplenomegaly leading to abdominal distention, gastrointestinal abnormalities, steatorrhea, and adrenal calcification. None of the other lipid classes (choices A, B, C, D, and E) would be found to be accumulating in a patient suffering from Wolman disease.

18. Correct answer is **A.** The patient is most likely exhibiting the signs and symptoms of Gaucher disease. Gaucher disease is characterized by the lysosomal accumulation of glucosylceramide (glucocerebroside) which is a normal intermediate in the catabolism of glycosphingolipids of the globoside and ganglioside subfamilies. Gaucher disease results from defects in the gene encoding the lysosomal hydrolase, acid β-glucosidase, also called glucocerebrosidase. The hallmark feature of Gaucher disease is the presence of lipid-engorged cells of the monocyte/macrophage lineage with a characteristic appearance in a variety of tissues. Metabolism of none of the other lipid classes (choices B, C, D, and E) is affected in patients with Gaucher disease.

19. Correct answer is **B.** The cause of the infant's early mortality was most likely a consequence of the lysosomal storage disease known as Krabbe disease. Krabbe disease (pronounced "crab A") is characterized by the lysosomal accumulation of galactosylceramides as a consequence of defects in the lysosomal hydrolase, galactosylceramidase. Galactosylceramides are almost exclusively found in the myelin sheaths of nerve cells. Thus, defects in their metabolism lead to the severe neurologic involvement of Krabbe disease. The characteristic feature of Krabbe disease is the accumulation of multinucleated globoid cells in the white matter of the brain; the disease is also known as infantile globoid cell leukodystrophy (GLD). This disease is a rapidly progressing disease that is invariably fatal before the end of the second year. Defects in none of the other processes (choices A, C, D, and E) are associated with the lethal course of Krabbe disease.

20. Correct answer is **A.** The infant is most likely suffering the consequences of Tay-Sachs disease. Infants with Tay-Sachs disease appear normal at birth. Symptoms usually begin with mild motor weakness by 3–5 months of age. Parents will begin to notice that their afflicted child has a dull response to outside stimuli. Another early symptom is an exaggerated startle response. By 6–10 months of age, infants will begin to show regression of prior acquired motor and mental skills. Tay-Sachs disease results from mutations in the gene encoding the α-subunit of the lysosomal hydrolase β-hexosaminidase A. The activity of β-hexosaminidase A is exerted on G_{M2} gangliosides which are enriched in cells of the central nervous system. Therefore, loss of β-hexosaminidase A activity results in the accumulation of undigested G_{M2} gangliosides in the lysosomes of all cells. None of the other options (choices B, C, D, and E) reflect the abnormal metabolism occurring in patients with Tay-Sachs disease.

21. Correct answer is **A.** As a consequence of appropriate signals that lead to activation of the phospholipid hydrolyzing enzyme PLA_2, arachidonic acid is released from these membrane lipids. Arachidonic acid serves as a substrate for both the lipoxygenase and the cyclooxygenase pathways of bioactive lipid synthesis. The lipoxygenase (linear) pathway is initiated through the action of one of three lipoxygenases (LOX), 5-LOX, 12-LOX, and 15-LOX. The lipoxygenase pathway generates the leukotrienes, such as of LTB_4. The cyclooxygenase pathway involves two enzymes, COX-1 and COX-2. The cyclooxygenase pathway leads to the generation of the prostaglandins, such as PGE_2, and the thromboxanes, such as TXA_2. The absence of PGE_2 synthesis would most likely be due to loss of cyclooxygenase-1 (COX-1) activity. Deficiency in none of the other enzymes (choices B, C, D, and E) would account for lack of synthesis of PGE_2.

22. Correct answer is **B.** At high doses aspirin functions to block the prostaglandin and thromboxane synthesizing activity of COX-1 which results in inhibition of the primary proinflammatory, pyretic, and pain-inducing action of these eicosanoids. At low doses aspirin will elicit its most important anti-inflammatory benefits. The low-dose anti-inflammatory effects of aspirin are due to its ability to trigger the synthesis of epimeric forms of the lipoxins (LXA_4 and LXB_4). Aspirin-induced acetylation of COX-2 alters the enzyme such that it converts arachidonic acid to 15*R*-hydroxyeicosatetraenoic acid (15*R*-HETE) instead of into prostaglandin H_2 (PGH_2). 15*R*-HETE is then rapidly metabolized to the epi-lipoxins (15-epi-LXA_4 and 15-epi-LXB_4) in monocytes and leukocytes through the action of 5-lipoxygenase (5-LOX). Cyclooxygenase-1 (choice A) does not contribute to the synthesis of the lipoxins. Although 5-LOX (choice C) is involved in the synthesis of the lipoxins it does not initiate the pathway as does aspirin at the level of COX-2. None of the other enzymes (choices D, E, and F) is involved in the synthesis of the epi-lipoxins.

23. Correct answer is **D.** Arachidonic acid is found esterified to the *sn*2 position of the glycerol backbone of membrane phospholipids. Signaling pathways that lead to activation of enzymes of the large phospholipase A_2 (PLA_2) family lead to the hydrolysis of the ester bond at the *sn*2 position in membrane phospholipids, thereby releasing whatever fatty acid is attached at this position, such as arachidonic acid and dihomo-γ-linoleic acid (DGLA). The inability to stimulate arachidonic acid release would, therefore, be most likely due to loss of PLA_2 activity. Phospholipase D (choice E) family enzymes hydrolyze the polar head group (eg, choline) from phospholipids generating a phosphatidic acid and the free polar head group. None of the other enzymes (choices A, B, and C) are involved in the release of arachidonic acid from membrane phospholipids.

24. Correct answer is **E.** The infant is most likely exhibiting the signs and symptoms of the lysosomal storage disease identified as Niemann-Pick disease (NPD). NPD comprises two distinct but related types of lipid storage disorder, type I and type II. In addition, both types comprise two subtypes. Type IA (NPA) and type IB (NPB) both result from a defect in the lysosomal hydrolase, acid sphingomyelinase. The sphingomyelins are a class of bioactive lipids that are also phospholipids that contain phosphocholine. Defects in none of the other metabolic processes (choices A, B, C, and D) are associated with Niemann-Pick disease.

25. Correct answer is **B.** The individual most likely died as a consequence of the pathology of Fabry disease. Fabry disease is an X-linked disorder that results from a deficiency in the lysosomal hydrolase, α-galactosidase A. This leads to the deposition of neutral glycosphingolipids with terminal α-galactosyl moieties in most tissues and fluids. Most affected tissues are heart, kidneys, and eyes. The predominant glycosphingolipid accumulated is a member of the globoside family, globotriaosylceramide (ceramide trihexoside). With increasing age, the major symptoms of the disease are due to increasing deposition of complex glycolipid in the cardiovascular system. Defects in none of the other processes (choices A, C, D, and E) are associated with the pathology of Fabry disease.

26. Correct answer is **A.** The cause of the infant's early mortality was most likely a consequence of the lysosomal storage disease known as Krabbe disease. Krabbe disease Krabbe (pronounced "crab A") disease is characterized by the lysosomal accumulation of galactosylceramides as a consequence of defects in the lysosomal hydrolase, galactosylceramidase. Galactosylceramides are almost exclusively found in the myelin sheaths of nerve cells. Thus, defects in their metabolism lead to the severe neurologic involvement of Krabbe disease. The characteristic feature of Krabbe disease is the accumulation of multinucleated globoid cells in the white matter of the brain, the disease is also known as infantile globoid cell leukodystrophy (GLD). This disease is a rapidly progressing disease that is invariably fatal before the end of the second year. None of the other classes of molecule (choices B, C, D, and E) are found to accumulate in patients with Krabbe disease.

27. Correct answer is **B.** The histamine H1 receptor is present on numerous cell types including endothelial cells and smooth muscle cells. This receptor is coupled to a G_q-type G-protein. The expected outcome from histamine binding to this receptor would be the activation of PLCβ and the generation of diacylglycerol (DAG) and inositol-1,4,5-trisphosphate (IP_3) from the membrane-localized phospholipid, phosphatidylinositol-4,5-bisphosphate (PIP_2). The IP_3 binds to receptors that are ligand-gated calcium channels in the endoplasmic reticulum, stimulating the release of stored calcium. The failure of histamine to stimulate changes in intracellular calcium, therefore, would be indicative of a failure of the receptor to activate PLCβ. None of the other enzymes (choices A, C, D, and E) are associated with the activation a G-protein–coupled receptor (GPCR) coupled to a G_q-type G-protein.

28. Correct answer is **B.** In addition to Tay-Sachs disease, two other disorders are associated with nearly identical signs and symptoms and disease course. These two other diseases are Sandhoff disease and G_{M2} activator deficiency syndrome. Sandhoff disease results from mutations in the gene encoding the β-subunit of β-hexosaminidase A, whereas G_{M2} activator deficiency, as the name implies, results from mutations in this required activator of β-hexosaminidase A. Given that the patient was found to have normal β-hexosaminidase A encoding genes, the most likely cause of the pathology is the loss of function of the G_{M2} activator protein. Deficiency in glucocerebrosidase (choice A) is the cause of the adult-onset disorder known as Gaucher disease. Deficiency in medium-chain acyl-CoA dehydrogenase (choice C) is the cause of the disorder identified as MCAD deficiency. Deficiency in phytanoyl-CoA hydroxylase (choice D) is the cause of Refsum disease. Deficiency in sphingomyelinase (choice E) is the cause of Niemann-Pick disease.

29. Correct answer is **C.** During fetal development, the aorta and the pulmonary artery are connected by a temporary blood vessel called the ductus arteriosus. While in the womb, the fetus receives oxygen from the mother's circulation, so blood does not need to flow through the lungs. The ductus arteriosus streamlines fetal circulation by flowing blood directly to the aorta, bypassing the lungs. After birth, the ductus arteriosus usually seals off so that blood from these two vessels does not mix. This occurs, in part, from the reduced levels of serum prostaglandins such as PGE_1. Due to the vasodilating action of PGE_1 it is used pharmaceutically (alprostadil) to treat newborn infants with ductal-dependent congenital heart disease. None of the other changes (choices A, B, D, E, and F) are associated with the normal closure of the fetal ductus arteriosus.

30. Correct answer is **D.** The synthesis of the prostaglandins is initiated via the activity of the enzymes commonly called cyclooxygenase-1 (COX-1) and COX-2. These enzymes are also known as prostaglandin G/H synthase, PGS (also called prostaglandin endoperoxide synthetase). These enzymes possess two activities, cyclooxygenase and peroxidase. One of the actions of aspirin (acetylsalicylate) is the inhibition of the oxygenation activity of the cyclooxygenase function of COX (PGS). Given that the experimental compound exhibits the same activity as aspirin, it is most likely that the oxygenation reaction is being inhibited. None of the other reactions (choices A, B, C, and E) are associated with the effects of aspirin on prostaglandin synthesis.

31. Correct answer is **B.** The infant is most likely exhibiting the signs and symptoms of the lysosomal storage disease identified as Niemann-Pick disease (NPD), specifically the type C form of the disease. Niemann-Pick comprises two distinct but related types of lipid storage disorder. The more common form of NPD is Niemann-Pick type C1 (NPC1) disease. NPC1 results from an error in the trafficking of exogenous cholesterol, thus it is more commonly referred to as a lipid trafficking disorder even though it belongs to the family of lysosomal storage diseases. The principal biochemical defect in patients with NPC1 is an accumulation of cholesterol, sphingolipids, and other lipids in the late endosomes/lysosomes (LE/L) of all cells. The characteristic phenotypes associated with NPC1 disease are variable hepatosplenomegaly, progressive ataxia, dystonia, dementia, and vertical supranuclear gaze palsy (VSGP). These individuals will present in childhood and death will ensue by the second or third decade. Disorders in none of the other processes (choices A, C, D, and E) are associated with the symptoms of NPC1.

32. Correct answer is **B.** Bronchiole volume contributes to dead space volume, so increasing bronchoconstriction would decrease bronchiolar volume and thus, would result in a decrease in dead space volume. Bronchoconstriction is a major determinant of airway resistance to air flow. The bioactive lipids of the leukotriene family, specifically the peptidoleukotrienes LTC_4, LTD_4, and LTE_4, are components of what is referred to as slow-reacting substance of anaphylaxis, SRS-A. Mast cell release of the peptidoleukotrienes is a significant contributor to bronchoconstriction and, therefore, leads to decreased dead space volume. None of the other processes (choices A, C, D, E, and F) are associated with the activities of the leukotrienes, specifically the peptidoleukotrienes.

33. Correct answer is **E.** Hematopoietic cells and vascular endothelial cells are the major sources of the high plasma concentrations of sphingosine-1-phosphate (S1P). Lymphatic endothelial cells are also thought to secrete S1P into the lymphatic circulation. The majority of plasma S1P is bound to HDL (65%) with another 30% bound by albumin. The ability of HDL to induce vasodilation and migration of endothelial cells, as well as to serve a cardioprotective role in the vasculature, is associated with the presence of S1P in these lipoprotein particles. Indeed, one of the beneficial properties of HDL in the reduction of the risk of cardiovascular disease is due to its role as an S1P chaperone. None of the other lipids (choices A, B, C, and D) are associated with the beneficial activities of HDL in the vasculature.

34. Correct answer is **D.** The initiation of the synthesis of the sphingoid bases (sphingosine, dihydrosphingosine, and ceramides) takes place via the condensation of palmitoyl-CoA and serine. This reaction is catalyzed by serine palmitoyltransferase (SPT). SPT is the rate-limiting enzyme of the sphingolipid biosynthesis pathway. Reduced activity of SPT would result in reduced synthesis of ceramides. Although decreased ceramide synthase 1 activity (choice A) is associated with more aggressive types of head and neck cancers, it is SPT that utilizes palmitic acid as a substrate and thus, reduced SPT activity would be associated with reduced palmitate metabolism in these cells. Deficiency in glucocerebrosidase (choice B) is associated with the lysosomal storage disease, Gaucher disease. Deficiency in β-hexosaminidase A (choice C) results in the lysosomal storage disease, Tay-Sachs disease. Deficiency in sphingomyelinase (choice E) is the cause of the lysosomal storage disease, Niemann-Pick disease.

35. Correct answer is **A.** Ceramides play a role in apoptotic processes via the activation of the aspartate protease, cathepsin D. Cathepsin D is associated with membranes, and when activated by ceramides, is released to the cytosol where it triggers the mitochondrial apoptosis pathway. Further evidence for the role of ceramides in negative growth responses is seen in cell cultures to which ceramide analogues are added. These types of assays demonstrate that ceramides induce oxidative stress, growth arrest, and apoptosis and/or necrosis. When derived from the sphingomyelins, ceramides are the products of the action of acid sphingomyelinase. The importance of sphingomyelin as a source of ceramide can be evidenced by the fact that the activation of the acid sphingomyelinase pathway is a shared response to the effects of cytokines, stress, radiation, chemotherapeutic drugs, and pathogenic and cytotoxic agents. The induction of acid sphingomyelinase in response to apoptotic triggers results in increased production of ceramides which then can initiate aspects of the apoptosis pathway. Deficiencies in none of the other enzymes (choices B, C, D, and E) would be associated with the observations in these tumor cells.

36. Correct answer is **E.** The infant is most likely suffering from the symptoms of Hunter syndrome. Hunter syndrome results from the lysosomal accumulation of dermatan and heparan sulfates as a consequence of deficiencies in the lysosomal hydrolase, iduronate 2-sulfatase. Hunter syndrome is characterized by progressive multiorgan failure and premature death. Hallmark features include enlargement of the spleen and liver, severe skeletal deformity, and coarse facial features which are associated with the constellation of defects referred to as dysostosis multiplex. Deficiency in acid sphingomyelinase (choice A) causes the disorder known as Niemann-Pick disease. Deficiency in galactosylceramidase (choice B) results in the disease identified as Krabbe disease. Deficiency in glucocerebrosidase (choice C) results in the disorder identified as Gaucher disease. Deficiency in β-hexosaminidase A (choice D) results in the disorder known as Tay-Sachs disease.

37. Correct answer is **C.** Removal of the fatty acid esterified to the *sn*2 position of phosphatidic acid results in the generation of lysophosphatidic acid, LPA. There can be several different types of LPA given that different fatty acids can be esterified to the *sn*1 position. LPA, although being simple in structure, exerts a wide variety of cellular responses in many different cell types. LPA is known to enhance platelet aggregation, smooth muscle contraction, cell proliferation, cell migration, neurite retraction, and the secretion of chemokines and cytokines. The effects of LPA are the result of binding to at least six specific receptors (LPA_1-LPA_6) that are members of the large family of G-protein–coupled receptors (GPCR). None of these other lipids (choices A, B, D, and E) are vasodilators and platelet aggregators.

38. Correct answer is **C.** The patient is most likely exhibiting the signs and symptoms of Fabry disease. Fabry disease is a lysosomal storage disease caused by deficiency in the lysosomal hydrolase, α-galactosidase A which is encoded by the *GLA* gene on the X chromosome. Classic symptoms of Fabry disease include pain and paresthesia (burning or prickly sensation) in the extremities, particularly the hands and feet, reduced capacity to sweat, gastrointestinal disturbances, cardiomyopathy, progressive renal impairment, corneal and lenticular opacities and characteristic skin lesions called angiokeratoma (angiokeratoma corporis diffusum). The typical corneal opacity seen via slit lamp examination is termed cornea verticillata, also known as vortex keratopathy, and is characterized by a distinctive swirling pattern of opacities in the lower cornea, primarily affecting the superficial corneal layer. Angiokeratoma, which are small dark red or purple raised papules that typically appear on the thighs and around the umbilicus. Angiokeratoma is caused by dilation of vessels near the surface of the skin. The activity of α-galactosidase A is not associated with any of the other cellular locations (choices A, B, D, and E).

39. Correct answer is **C.** Meloxicam is a member of the nonsteroidal anti-inflammatory (NSAID) class of pain medications. These drugs function by blocking the cyclooxygenase activity of the COX-1 and COX-2 enzyme complexes. The enzymes initiate the synthesis of the eicosanoids (prostaglandins and thromboxanes) from arachidonic acid. Certain eicosanoids are proinflammatory and as a result sensitize individuals to pain, thus, blocking, not increasing (choice F) their synthesis helps to relieve pain. The NSAIDs do not function by decreasing (choices A and B) or increasing (choices D and E) the synthesis of the leukotrienes or the ceramides.

40. Correct answer is **E.** The patient is most likely manifesting the classic signs and symptoms of Krabbe disease, also known as globoid cell leukodystrophy due to the accumulation of multinucleated globoid cells in the white matter of the brain. Krabbe disease is characterized by the lysosomal accumulation of galactosylceramides which are almost exclusively found in the myelin sheaths of nerve cells. Thus, defects in their metabolism lead to the severe neurologic involvement of Krabbe disease. Increased abnormally branched glycogen in the liver (choice A) is a characteristic finding in patients with Andersen disease which is a rapidly progressive disorder that will result in early lethality because of liver failure. Lipid-laden foam cells (choice B) are a characteristic finding in Niemann-Pick disease, type A. Nieman-Pick disease, type A is a rapidly progressing disease associated with hepatosplenomegaly and hypotonia. Liver infiltration with granulomatous macrophages (choice C) is a common finding in patients with Farber lipogranulomatosis which is characterized by painful and progressively deformed joints, progressive hoarseness due to laryngeal involvement, and subcutaneous nodules, particularly over the joints. Macrophages containing a coarse fibrillary substance in the cytoplasm (choice D) are characteristic of Gaucher disease. The striated tubular pattern of the accumulating substance is often described as "wrinkled tissue paper" inclusions. The most common form of Gaucher disease begins to manifest in the second or third decade of life.

41. Correct answer is **B.** The patient is most likely exhibiting the signs and symptoms of Niemann-Pick disease type A. Type A Niemann-Pick disease is associated with a rapidly progressing neurodegeneration leading to death by 2 to 3 years of age. Both type A and type B Niemann-Pick disease are characterized by the presence of the "Niemann-Pick" cell. This histologically distinct cell type is of the monocyte-macrophage lineage and is a characteristic lipid-laden foam cell. Patients with Niemann-Pick disease appear normal at birth but symptoms develop early, including significant hepatomegaly. Although pallor around the fovea centralis (characteristically described as a "cherry-red spot") is common in Tay-Sachs disease patients, it is also a frequent sign in Niemann-Pick type A patients. Increased abnormally branched glycogen in the liver (choice A) is a characteristic finding in patients with Andersen disease which is a rapidly progressive disorder that will result in early lethality because of liver failure. Liver infiltration with granulomatous macrophages (choice C) is a common finding in patients with Farber lipogranulomatosis which is characterized by painful and progressively deformed joints, progressive hoarseness due to laryngeal involvement, and subcutaneous nodules, particularly over the joints. Macrophages containing a coarse fibrillary substance in the cytoplasm (choice D) are characteristic of Gaucher disease. The striated tubular pattern of the accumulating substance is often described as "wrinkled tissue paper" inclusions. The most common form of Gaucher disease begins to manifest in the second or third decade of life. Multinucleated globoid cells (choice E) are a characteristic feature of Krabbe disease and as such the disease is also known as globoid cell leukodystrophy. Krabbe disease is characterized by the lysosomal accumulation of galactosylceramides which are almost exclusively found in the myelin sheaths of nerve cells. Thus, defects in their metabolism lead to the severe neurologic involvement of Krabbe disease.

42. Correct answer is **B.** The patient is most likely exhibiting the signs and symptoms of Fabry disease. Fabry disease is a lysosomal storage disease caused by deficiency in the lysosomal hydrolase, α-galactosidase A which is encoded by the *GLA* gene on the X chromosome. Classic symptoms of Fabry disease include pain and paresthesia (burning or prickly sensation) in the extremities, particularly the hands and feet, reduced capacity to sweat, gastrointestinal disturbances, cardiomyopathy, progressive renal impairment, corneal and lenticular opacities, and characteristic skin lesions called angiokeratoma (angiokeratoma corporis diffusum). The typical corneal opacity seen via slit lamp examination is termed cornea verticillata, also known as vortex keratopathy, and is characterized by a distinctive swirling pattern of opacities in the lower cornea, primarily affecting the superficial corneal layer. Angiokeratoma are small dark red or purple raised papules that typically appear on the thighs and around the umbilicus. Angiokeratoma is caused by dilation of vessels near the surface of the skin. Deficiency in acid ceramidase (choice A) causes Farber lipogranulomatosis, the symptoms of which most commonly appear during the first months after birth. The clinical manifestations are characterized by painful and progressively deformed joints, progressive hoarseness due to laryngeal involvement, and subcutaneous nodules particularly over the joints. Deficiency in galactosylceramidase (choice C) causes Krabbe disease which is characterized by the accumulation of multinucleated globoid cells in the white matter of the brain; hence, the disease is also known as infantile globoid cell leukodystrophy (GLD). Krabbe disease is a rapidly progressing disease that is invariably fatal before the end of the second year. Deficiency in β-hexosaminidase A (choice D) causes Tay-Sachs disease which is characterized by rapidly progressing psychomotor impairment ultimately leading to death before the age of three. Deficiency in serine palmitolyltransferase (choice E) is associated with a group of neurodegenerative and neurodevelopmental disorders as a consequence of the inability to synthesize ceramides.

43. Correct answer is **B.** The patient is most likely manifesting the signs and symptoms of Krabbe disease. Krabbe disease is caused by a deficiency in galactosylceramidase and is characterized by the accumulation of multinucleated globoid cells in the white matter of the brain; hence, the disease is also known as infantile globoid cell leukodystrophy (GLD). Krabbe disease is a rapidly progressing disease that is invariably fatal before the end of the second year. Deficiency in arylsulfatase A (choice A) is the cause of metachromatic leukodystrophy (MLD). In the infantile onset form of MLD, patients suffer from quadriparesis, peripheral neuropathy, loss of vision, and loss of speech as well as seizures. Deficiency in β-glucocerebrosidase (choice C) is the cause of Gaucher disease. The most common form of Gaucher disease is an adult-onset disease. The hallmark of Gaucher disease is the accumulation of lipid-engorged cells of the monocyte/macrophage lineage with a characteristic appearance in a variety of tissues. Deficiency in β-hexosaminidase A (choice D) is the cause of Tay-Sachs disease. Symptoms of Tay-Sachs disease usually begin with mild motor weakness by 3 to 5 months of age, along with a dull response to outside stimuli. Another early symptom is an exaggerated startle response (sudden extension of arms and legs) to sharp sounds. Deficiency in sphingomyelinase (choice E) is the cause of Niemann-Pick disease types A and B. Niemann-Pick disease is associated with a marked hepatosplenomegaly and a rapidly progressing neurodegeneration leading to death by 2 to 3 years of age. Both type A and type B Niemann-Pick disease are characterized by the presence of the "Niemann-Pick" cell. This histologically distinct cell type is of the monocyte-macrophage lineage and is a characteristic lipid-laden foam cell.

44. Correct answer is **D.** The patient is most likely suffering from the symptoms of Gaucher disease. Gaucher disease is an autosomal recessive disorder that is characterized by the lysosomal accumulation of glucocerebroside which is a normal intermediate in the catabolism of globosides and gangliosides. Due to the high levels of glucocerebrosides in the lysosomes of cells of the monocyte/macrophage lineage, these cells are the major contributors to the pathology of Gaucher disease. The hallmark of Gaucher disease is the accumulation of lipid-engorged cells of the monocyte/macrophage lineage with a characteristic appearance in a variety of tissues. The primarily affected tissues are bone, bone marrow, spleen, and liver. These distinctive cells contain one or more small nuclei, and their cytoplasm contains a coarse fibrillary material that forms a striated tubular pattern often described as "wrinkled tissue paper." These cells are called Gaucher cells. Gaucher cells also induce the production of proinflammatory cytokines resulting in enlargement of the liver and spleen (hepatosplenomegaly), destruction of bone, lung abnormalities, anemia, leukopenia, and thrombocytopenia. Accumulation of dermatan sulfate (choice A) occurs in cells of patients with Hunter syndrome and Hurler syndrome. The most common presentation of these two syndromes is evident by the age of 2 to 4 years and includes skeletal deformities, coarse facila features, and intellectual impairment. Accumulation of galactocerebroside sulfate (choice B) occurs in patients with metachromatic leukodystrophy (MLD). There is a wide degree of phenotypic variation in MLD, and as such, the disorder is divided into late infantile, early juvenile, late juvenile and adult forms. In the juvenile forms patients show gradual deterioration in scholastic performance, walking becomes difficult, and their speech slurs. There are also emotional and behavioral disturbances in these patients. Accumulation of globotriaosylceramide (choice C) occurs in patients with Fabry disease. Globotriaosylceramide (Gb3) is also identified as ceramide trihexoside. The clinical manifestations of Fabry disease begin in childhood or adolescence with the average age of presentation between 6 and 9 years of age. Classic symptoms include pain and paresthesia (burning or prickly sensation) in the extremities, particularly the hands and feet, reduced capacity to sweat, gastrointestinal disturbances, cardiomyopathy, progressive renal impairment, corneal and lenticular opacities, and characteristic skin lesions called angiokeratoma. Accumulation of sphingomyelin (choice E) occurs in patients with Niemann-Pick disease type A and type B. Type A Niemann-Pick disease is associated with a rapidly progressing neurodegeneration leading to death by 2 to 3 years of age. Both type A and type B Niemann-Pick disease are characterized by the presence of lipid-laden foam cells of the monocytic lineage.

45. Correct answer is **A.** The patient is most likely experiencing the signs and symptoms of Reye syndrome. Reye syndrome is associated with predominant pathology in the brain, liver, and blood. Typical symptoms of Reye syndrome in children include vomiting, lethargy, confusion, weakness, behavioral changes, and the potential for seizures and loss of consciousness. Reye syndrome can also be associated with hepatomegaly and papilledema; the latter being swelling of the optic disc due to increased intracranial pressure. The severity of the symptoms of Reye disease is such that the disorder needs to be diagnosed and treated with little delay. The mother of the patient most likely administered aspirin to her daughter as a means to bring down her fever and aches. Aspirin covalently acetylates the cyclooxygenase activity of the COX-1 and COX-2 enzymes that are the rate-limiting enzymes of synthesis of the eicosanoid class of bioactive lipids. Studies have shown a link between taking aspirin (acetylsalicylate) during a viral illness and the development of Reye syndrome. Because of the link between aspirin and Reye syndrome, healthcare professionals recommend acetaminophen or ibuprofen instead of aspirin for infants and children. Aspirin does not covalently modify lipoxygenases (choice B), nor does it enhance the turnover of cyclooxygenases (choice C), nor lipoxygenases (choice D). There is no tissue selectivity (choices E and F) to the actions of aspirin.

CHAPTER

13

Lipolysis, Fatty Acid Oxidation, and Ketogenesis

High-Yield Terms

Adipose tissue triglyceride lipase, ATGL	Primary rate-limiting enzyme involved in adipose tissue triglyceride metabolism
Hormone-sensitive lipase, HSL	An adipose tissue-specific hydrolase responsible for the release of fatty acids from stored triglycerides. Its activity is regulated by hormone-mediated phosphorylation
Alpha-oxidation	Peroxisomal oxidation pathway responsible for the oxidation of the methyl-substituted fatty acid, phytanic acid present at high concentration in the tissues of ruminants
Beta-oxidation	Major pathway for oxidation of fatty acids in both the mitochondria and the peroxisomes; peroxisomal β-oxidation is also important for metabolism of dicarboxylic acids generated via the ω-oxidation pathway
Omega-oxidation	A minor, but clinically significant, pathway for fatty oxidation initiated by microsomal ω-hydroxylation reactions; also involves the oxidation of dicarboxylic acids generated
Ketone body	Any of the compounds, β-hydroxybutyrate, acetoacetate, and acetone, generated during hepatic ketogenesis from the substrate, acetyl-CoA
Diabetic ketoacidosis, DKA	A condition of increased plasma ketone body concentration caused by excess adipose tissue fatty acid release and hepatic fatty acid oxidation resulting from unregulated glucagon release

DIETARY FATTY ACIDS

The predominant form of dietary lipid in the human diet is triglyceride (TG or TAG). Gastrointestinal lipid digestion and absorption is reviewed in Chapter 28. Following absorption of the products of lipid digestion, the resynthesis of TG, cholesterol esters, and phospholipids occurs within intestinal enterocytes. These lipid entities are then solubilized in lipoprotein complexes called chylomicrons. A review of the various lipoproteins present in human circulation is presented in Chapter 16.

As chylomicrons circulate in the vasculature, fatty acids are removed from the TG fraction through the action of endothelial cell-associated lipoprotein lipase (LPL) found exclusively in the vasculature of skeletal muscle, cardiac muscle, and adipose tissue. The free fatty acids are then absorbed by the cells and the glycerol is returned via the blood to the liver where it is utilized as a carbon skeleton for glucose synthesis via gluconeogenesis (see Chapter 6).

MOBILIZATION OF FAT STORES

The primary sources of fatty acids for oxidation are dietary and mobilization from cellular stores. Fatty acids are stored in the form of TGs within most cells but predominantly within adipocytes of adipose tissue. In response to energy demands, the fatty acids of stored TG can be mobilized for use by peripheral tissues. The release of these stored fatty acids is controlled by a complex series of interrelated cascades that result in the activation of TG hydrolysis. The primary intracellular lipases involved in the mobilization of stored fatty acids are adipose triglyceride lipase (ATGL, also called desnutrin), hormone-sensitive lipase (HSL), and monoacylglyceride lipase (MGL).

HIGH-YIELD CONCEPT

An additional lipase, lysosomal acid lipase (LAL), plays an important role in the intracellular degradation of cholesterol esters and TG taken into cells via endocytosis and transferred to the lysosomes. The importance of LAL in overall lipid homeostasis is evidenced by the fact that LAL deficiency results in the significant accumulation of cholesterol esters in tissues such as the spleen and liver. LAL deficiency is commonly called Wolman disease.

In adipose tissue, HSL activity is strongly induced by β-adrenergic receptor stimulation and to a lesser extent through

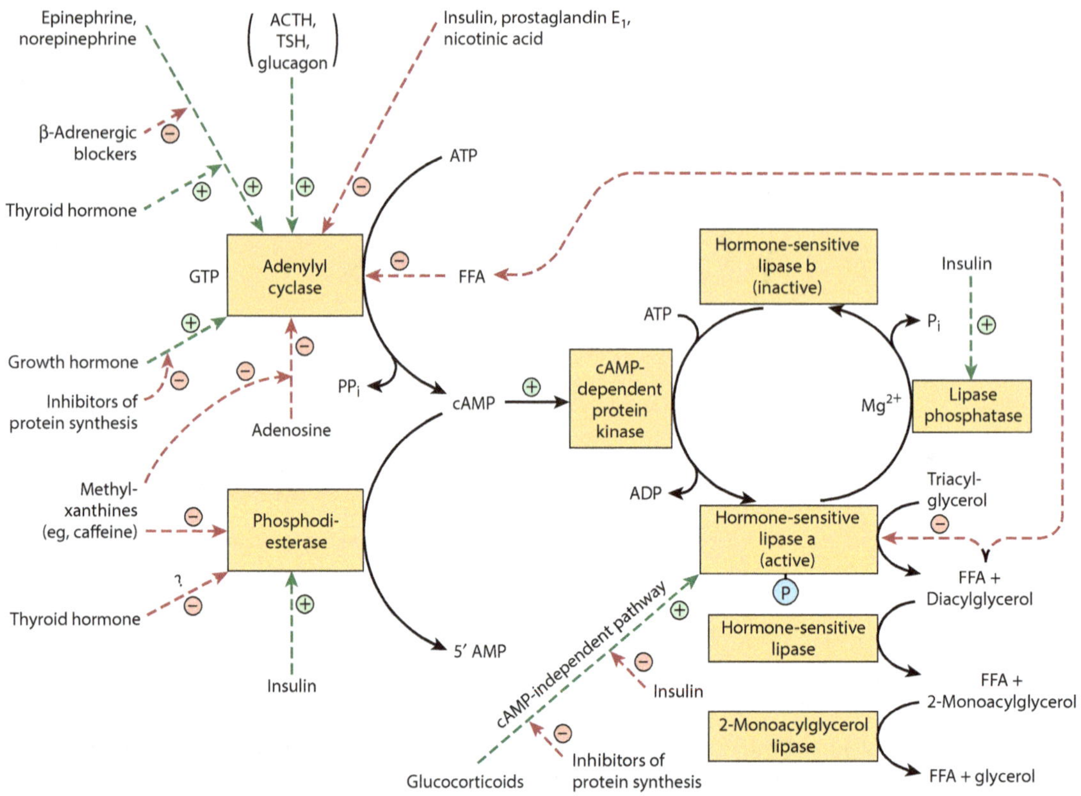

FIGURE 13–1 Control of adipose tissue lipolysis. (FFA, free fatty acids; TSH, thyroid-stimulating hormone.) Note the cascade sequence of reactions affording amplification at each step. The lipolytic stimulus is "switched off" by removal of the stimulating hormone; the action of lipase phosphatase; the inhibition of the lipase and adenylyl cyclase by high concentrations of FFA; the inhibition of adenylyl cyclase by adenosine; and the removal of Camp by the action of phosphodiesterase. ACTH, TSH, and glucagon may not activate adenylyl cyclase in vivo since the concentration of each hormone required in vitro is much higher than is found in the circulation. Positive ⊕ and negative ⊖ regulatory effects are represented by broken lines and substrate flow by solid lines. (Reproduced with permission from Rodwell VW, Bender DA, Botham KM, et al: *Harper's Illustrated Biochemistry*, 31st ed. New York, NY: McGraw Hill; 2018.)

the action of glucagon (Figure 13–1). Conversely insulin has a strong inhibitory effect. HSL is a major target for PKA-mediated phosphorylation. Insulin-mediated deactivation of lipolysis is associated with transcriptional downregulation of both ATGL and HSL expression. Insulin signaling also results in the activation of various phosphodiesterase (PDE) isoforms leading to PDE-catalyzed hydrolysis of cAMP which in turn results in reduced activation of PKA.

LIPID TRANSPORTERS AND CELLULAR UPTAKE OF FATS

When fatty acids are released from adipose tissue TG they enter the circulation as free fatty acids (FFA) and are bound to albumin for transport to peripheral tissues. When the fatty acid-albumin complexes interact with cell surfaces the dissociation of the fatty acid from albumin represents the first step of the cellular uptake process. Cellular uptake of fatty acids involves several members of the fatty acid receptor family that includes at least eight members.

Following uptake into cells, fatty acids must be activated to acyl-CoA intermediates. Several members of the fatty acid transporter family possess acyl-CoA synthetase activity. The overall process of cellular fatty acid uptake and subsequent intracellular utilization represents a continuum of dissociation from albumin by interaction with the membrane-associated transport proteins, activation to acyl-CoA followed by intracellular trafficking to sites of metabolic disposition.

MITOCHONDRIAL β-OXIDATION REACTIONS

The primary sites of fatty acid β-oxidation are the mitochondria and the peroxisomes. Fatty acids of between 4–8 and between 6–12 carbon atoms in length, referred to as short- and medium-chain fatty acids (SCFA and MCFA), respectively, are oxidized exclusively in the mitochondria. Long-chain fatty acids (LCFA: 10–16 carbons long) are oxidized in both the mitochondria and the peroxisomes with the peroxisomes exhibiting preference for 14-carbon and longer LCFA. Very-long-chain fatty acids

(VLCFA: C17–C26) are initially exclusively oxidized in the peroxisomes.

Prior to oxidation, fatty acids are activated by attachment to CoA. Activation is catalyzed by fatty acyl-CoA synthetases. The process of mitochondrial fatty acid oxidation is termed β-oxidation since it occurs through the sequential removal of two-carbon units by oxidation at the β-carbon position of the fatty acyl-CoA molecule.

The transport of fatty acyl-CoA into the matrix of the mitochondria for oxidation is accomplished by a multistep process involving carnitine attachment and removal. Fatty acyl-CoA molecules are converted to fatty acyl-carnitines via carnitine palmitoyltransferase 1 (CPT-1), an enzyme that resides in the outer mitochondrial membrane (Figure 13–2). There are three *CPT-1* genes in humans identified as CPT-1A, CPT-1B, and CPT-1C. Expression of CPT-1A predominates in the liver and is thus, referred to as the liver isoform. CPT-1B expression predominates in skeletal muscle and is thus, referred to as the muscle isoform. CPT-1C expression is exclusive to the brain and testes.

The fatty acyl-carnitine molecules are then transported into the matrix of the mitochondria through the action of the antiporter, carnitine acylcarnitine translocase (CACT). In exchange for the fatty acyl-carnitine CACT transports free carnitine out of the mitochondrial matrix. Within the matrix, fatty acyl-carnitines are converted back to fatty acyl-CoAs via the inner mitochondrial membrane-localized carnitine palmitoyltransferase 2 (CPT-2).

Defects in carnitine transport into cells represents the most common form of inherited carnitine deficiency (see Clinical Box 13–1). Defects in CPT-2 are the cause of several related disorders ranging from neonatal lethality to adult onset myopathy (see Clinical Box 13–2).

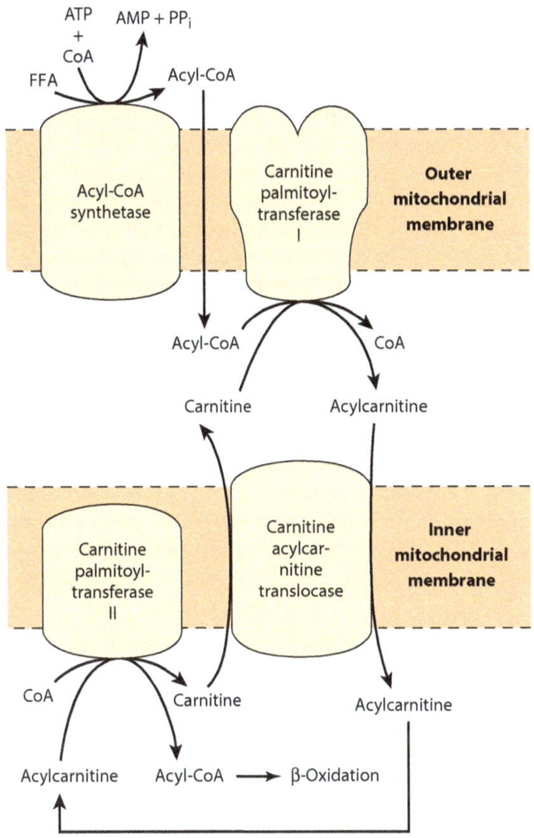

FIGURE 13–2 Role of carnitine in the transport of long-chain fatty acids through the inner mitochondrial membrane. Long-chain acyl-CoA cannot pass through the inner mitochondrial membrane, but its metabolic product, acylcarnitine, can. (Reproduced with permission from Rodwell VW, Bender DA, Botham KM, et al: *Harper's Illustrated Biochemistry*, 31st ed. New York, NY: McGraw Hill; 2018.)

CLINICAL BOX 13–1 PRIMARY CARNITINE DEFICIENCY

Carnitine deficiencies lead to an inability to transport long-chain fatty acids (as fatty acylcarnitine) into the mitochondria for oxidation. Carnitine deficiencies can occur in newborns and particularly in preterm infants. Carnitine deficiencies are also found in patients undergoing hemodialysis or those affected by any one of various organic acidemias/acidurias (eg, propionic acidemia or isovaleric acidemia). Deficiencies in carnitine are defined as either primary or secondary. Primary carnitine deficiencies are due to defects in carnitine transport into cells or due to defects in synthesis from lysine, although the latter are very rare with only a few cases identified worldwide. Mutations in the major carnitine transporter, encoded by the *SLC22A5* gene (also known as zwitterion/cation transporter 2 [OCTN2]), are the predominant causes of primary carnitine deficiency. This disorder is most correctly referred to as carnitine deficiency, systemic primary (CDSP). Primary carnitine deficiency (carnitine deficiency, systemic primary: CDSP) is an autosomal recessive disorder that result from the lack of functional OCTN2 carnitine transporters. Within the US, Europe, and Japan the estimated frequency of carnitine deficiency, primary systemic is 1:40,000 live births. The frequency in Australia has been estimated to be between 1:37,000 and 1:100,000. More than 100 mutations have been identified in the *SLC22A5* gene resulting in carnitine deficiency, systemic primary. The most commonly identified mutation is the change of the C residue at position 136 to a T. This mutation results in the change of proline at amino acid position 46 to a serine and this mutation is designated *P46S*. Due to loss of functional *OCTN2*, primary carnitine deficiency patients exhibit urinary carnitine wasting. The loss of carnitine in the urine leads to very low serum carnitine levels ranging from 0 mM to 5 mM where the normal value should be 25 mM–50 mM. In addition to low serum levels these patients have decreased intracellular carnitine accumulation. The major function of carnitine is to facilitate the transport of long-chain fatty acids (as fatty acylcarnitine) into the matrix of the mitochondria where the carnitine is subsequently exchanged for coenzyme A. Once inside the mitochondria, the fatty acyl-CoAs can be oxidized for energy production. Therefore, primary carnitine deficiency results in defective fatty acid oxidation. The lack of

CLINICAL BOX 13–1 (CONTINUED)

adequate energy production, particularly in the liver, leads to deficient glucose synthesis via gluconeogenesis. Coupled with an increase in glucose oxidation for energy production the result is potentially severe hypoglycemia. The hypoglycemia stimulates glucagon release from the pancreas and epinephrine release from the adrenal glands leading to increased fatty acid release from adipose tissue. Due to the lack of oxidation, the fatty acids accumulate in the liver, skeletal muscle, and heart resulting in hepatic steatosis, myopathy, and cardiomyopathy, respectively. The typical metabolic presentation in patients with primary carnitine deficiency occurs most frequently before 2 years of age. Infants with primary carnitine deficiency exhibit poor feeding and can become lethargic and minimally responsive. The presentation of primary carnitine deficiency is quite variable with respect to the age of onset, the severity of the symptoms, and the involved organs. The inability to utilize fat for energy during stress or fasting can trigger acute metabolic decompensation early in life. In most cases, due to the fatty infiltration of the liver, these infants will present with hepatomegaly. Blood laboratory studies will find hypoglycemia and hyperammonemia while urinalysis will show hypoketonuria. Liver function enzymes (AST and ALT) will be variably elevated and creatine kinase (CK) may also be found to be mildly elevated. Failure to treat primary carnitine deficiency infants promptly with intravenous glucose during periods of metabolic decompensation will result in progression to coma and death. In older patients with primary carnitine deficiency, there is a strong likelihood for skeletal myopathy, cardiomyopathy sometimes associated with hypotonia, and arrhythmias leading to sudden death. The key diagnostic for primary carnitine deficiency, systemic primary is the measurement of plasma carnitine levels. Free and acylated carnitine are extremely reduced where free carnitine is usually <5 mM (normal 25 mM–50 mM). Urine organic acids do not show any consistent anomaly, although in some patients a nonspecific dicarboxylic aciduria has been reported. Following assessment of serum carnitine levels, a diagnosis of carnitine deficiency, systemic primary is confirmed by demonstrating reduced carnitine transport in skin fibroblasts that have been isolated from the patient. The level of carnitine transport in cultured patient fibroblasts is correlated to the severity of the mutation in the *SLC22A5* gene. Nonsense mutations have been found to be associated with the absence of any carnitine transport activity. Treatment of primary carnitine deficiency patients with dietary carnitine supplementation (100–400 mg/kg/day) has been shown to be highly beneficial, particularly if started before irreversible organ damage occurs.

CLINICAL BOX 13–2 CARNITINE PALMITOYLTRANSFERASE 2 (CPT-2) DEFICIENCY

CPT-2 is one of a family of carnitine acyltransferases in humans that catalyzes the reversible transfer of acyl groups between coenzyme A (CoASH) and L-carnitine, converting fatty acyl-CoA esters into fatty acyl-carnitine esters. Inherited deficiencies of CPT-2 result in disorders that are divided into three clinical phenotypes according to the age of presentation. These three forms are a lethal neonatal form, severe infantile form involving the liver, heart, and skeletal muscle (referred to as the infantile hepatocardiomuscular form), and a myopathic form that exhibits a range of age of onset from infancy to adulthood. The lethal neonatal form of CPT-2 deficiency is characterized by hypoketotic hypoglycemia, cardiomyopathy, liver failure, and respiratory distress. Infants born with this form of the disorder present with hepatic calcifications and cystic dysplastic kidneys. Neuronal migration defects are also found resulting in cystic dysplasia of the basal ganglia. Additional symptoms seen in neonates with this form of CPT-2 deficiency include hydrocephalus, cerebral calcifications, agenesis of the corpus callosum, cerebellar vermian hypoplasia, polymicrogyria, pachygyria, as well as other neuronal migration defects. Characteristic blood work in this form of CPT-2 deficiency shows reduced serum concentrations of total and free carnitine, and increased serum concentrations of long-chain acylcarnitines and lipids. Infants with this form of CPT-2 deficiency usually die within days to months after birth. The most common mutations in the *CPT2* gene associated with the lethal neonatal form are null mutations that lead to truncated proteins or to mRNA degradation. Infants with the hepatocardiomuscular form of CPT-2 deficiency present with episodic hypoketotic hypoglycemia. The overall clinical presentation of the hepatocardiomuscular form of CPT-2 deficiency in infants is severe and includes cardiomyopathy and quite often is associated with sudden death. One particular mutation in the *CPT2* gene, the mutation of a phenylalanine at amino acid position 352 for cysteine (identified as the F352C mutation) has been associated with an increased likelihood for sudden death in infancy. Individuals with the infantile hepatocardiomuscular form of the disease are often compound heterozygotes. The adult form of CPT-2 deficiency, the myopathic form, is the most common form of CPT-2 deficiency. The myopathic form of CPT-2 deficiency is also the most common disorder of lipid metabolism that affects skeletal muscle as well as the most common cause of inherited myoglobinuria. This form of CPT-2 deficiency is characterized by recurrent episodes of muscle pain, rhabdomyolysis and myoglobinuria that is triggered by prolonged exercise. Metabolic studies done in patients with adult myopathic CPT-2 deficiency will show that oxidation of palmitic acid is normal at rest but severely impaired during prolonged low-intensity exercise. Palmitic acid is a 16 carbon saturated fatty acid representing the most abundant fatty acid in human blood. Often the symptoms of the myopathic form of CPT-2 deficiency are not apparent until an adolescent undertakes endurance training such as for track in middle school. The myopathic form of CPT-2 deficiency

CLINICAL BOX 13–2 (CONTINUED)

is a common cause of rhabdomyolysis and myoglobinuria in adults. Biopsy tissue taken from skeletal muscle will show lipid accumulation when analyzed with stains such as Sudan black or oil red O. Analysis of CPT-2 function in these biopsy samples will show reduced levels of activity. The capacity to oxidize medium-chain fatty acids via the mitochondrial β-oxidation pathway is partially preserved in patients with CPT-2 deficiency due to the lack of a strict requirement for medium-chain fatty acids to be attached to carnitine for entry into the mitochondrial matrix. In patients with the myopathic form of CPT-2 deficiency the utilization of medium-chain triglycerides results in dicarboxylic aciduria indicative of increased microsomal metabolism of fatty acids due to the limited capacity for mitochondrial fatty acid uptake in the absence of adequate CPT-2 function. The most common (60%) mutation in the *CPT2* gene observed in patients with the myopathic form of the disease is where the Ser at amino acid position 113 is mutated to a Leu (identified as the S113L mutation). Clinical intervention in patients with CPT-2 deficiency includes reducing the intake of long-chain fatty acids while still ensuring adequate intake of the essential fatty acids, linolenic and linoleic acid. Approximately one-third of the caloric intake by these patients should be from medium-chain triglycerides (MCT). Patients with CPT-2 deficiency should also follow a carbohydrate-rich diet while avoiding prolonged fasting. Carnitine supplementation will reduce the accumulation of toxic long-chain fatty acyl-CoAs. Some therapeutic benefit has been demonstrated in patients with mild forms CPT-2 deficiency with the use of the fibrate drug, bezafibrate. In these patients the use of bezafibrate is associated with increased *CPT2* gene expression and normalization of CPT-2 activity. The incidence of rhabdomyolysis was reduced in patients taking bezafibrate and their ability to undertake physical activity was greatly improved. Another avenue of therapy for myopathic CPT-2 deficiency patients is the inclusion of triglycerides with odd-chain fatty acids in their diets. The artificially produced triglyceride is called triheptanoin and it contains three 7-carbon saturated fatty acids. The released odd chain fatty acids provide anaplerotic substrates for the TCA cycle so this treatment is referred to as the anaplerotic diet. In addition to being used in the treatment of CPT-2 deficiency, triheptanoin has been used in patients with pyruvate carboxylase deficiency and with VLCAD deficiency. Metabolism of the 7-carbon fatty acids in triheptanoin also results in increased production of ketones (β-ketopentanoate and β-hydroxypentanoate) which easily cross the blood-brain barrier (BBB) and are utilized by neural tissues.

Each round of β-oxidation involves four steps that, in order, are oxidation, hydration, oxidation, and cleavage (Figure 13–3). The first oxidation step in mitochondrial β-oxidation involves a family of FAD-dependent acyl-CoA dehydrogenases. Each of these dehydrogenases has a range of substrate specificity determined by the length of the fatty acid. Short-chain acyl-CoA dehydrogenase (SCAD, also called butyryl-CoA dehydrogenase) prefers fats of 4–6 carbons in length. Medium-chain acyl-CoA dehydrogenase (MCAD) prefers fats of 4–16 carbons in length with maximal activity for C10 acyl-CoAs. Long-chain acyl-CoA dehydrogenase (LCAD) prefers fats of 6–16 carbons in length with maximal activity for C12 acyl-CoAs. Due to very low level of expression of LCAD in humans, this enzyme plays a limited, if any, role in mitochondrial fatty acid β-oxidation. Expression of LCAD is seen in alveolar type II pneumocytes which are the specialized cells of the alveolar epithelium that synthesize and secrete pulmonary surfactant. Within most tissues the oxidation of long-chain fatty acids is initiated through the action of very long-chain acyl-CoA dehydrogenase, VLCAD. VLCAD prefers fats of 16–24 carbons and is inactive on any fatty acid less than 12 carbons.

Deficiencies in several of the acyl-CoA dehydrogenases are known to result in impaired β-oxidation with MCAD deficiency being the most common form (Clinical Box 13–3).

Each round of β-oxidation produces one mole of $FADH_2$, one mole of NADH, and one mole of acetyl-CoA. The acetyl-CoA enters the TCA cycle (see Chapter 9), where it is further oxidized with the concomitant generation of three moles of NADH, one mole of $FADH_2$, and one mole of ATP. The NADH and $FADH_2$ enter the respiratory pathway for the production of ATP via oxidative phosphorylation (see Chapter 10).

OXIDATION OF FATTY ACIDS WITH ODD CARBON NUMBER

The majority of natural lipids contain an even number of carbon atoms. Most of the odd-chain fatty acids (OCFA) are found in milk and fat from ruminant animals with a small proportion of plant-derived fatty acids being OCFA. On complete β-oxidation of these OCFA there is the generation of a single mole of propionyl-CoA. The propionyl-CoA is converted, in an ATP-dependent pathway, to succinyl-CoA (Figure 13-4). The succinyl-CoA can then enter the TCA cycle for further oxidation (Chapter 9).

PEROXISOMAL α-OXIDATION PATHWAY

Phytanic acid is a fatty acid present in the tissues of ruminants and in dairy products and is, therefore, an important dietary component of fatty acid intake. Because phytanic acid is methylated, it cannot act as a substrate for the normal mitochondrial β-oxidation pathway. Phytanic acid is first converted to its CoA-ester and

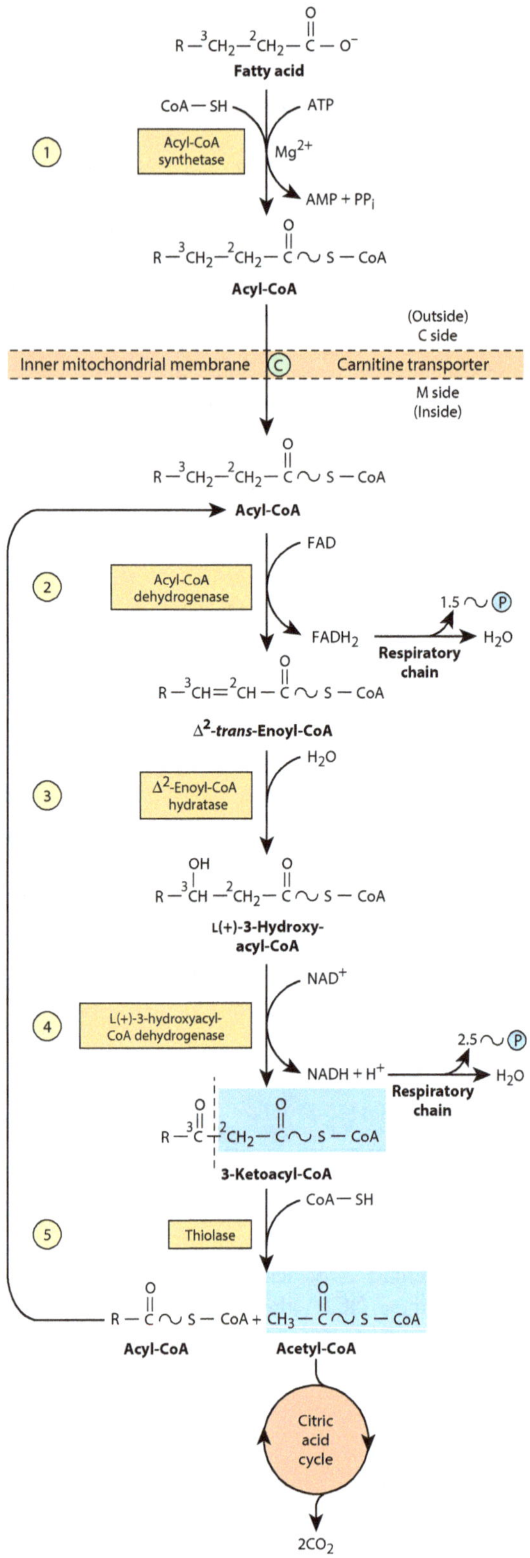

FIGURE 13–3 β-Oxidation of fatty acids. Long-chain acyl-CoA is cycled through reactions 2-5, acetyl-CoA being split off, each cycle, by thiolase (reaction 5). When the acyl radical is only 4-carbon atoms in length, 2 acetyl-CoA molecules are formed in reaction 5. (Reproduced with permission from Rodwell VW, Bender DA, Botham KM, et al: *Harper's Illustrated Biochemistry*, 31st ed. New York, NY: McGraw Hill; 2018.)

CLINICAL BOX 13–3 MEDIUM-CHAIN ACYL-COA DEHYDROGENASE DEFICIENCY (MCADD)

Deficiency in MCAD is the most common defect observed in the process of mitochondrial β-oxidation of fatty acids. In fact, MCAD deficiency is one of the most common inherited disorders of metabolism occurring with a frequency of approximately 1 in 10,000 live births. This disorder has been described in populations worldwide with the most frequently affected individuals being of northwestern European origin. MCAD deficiency (MCADD) is an autosomal recessive disorder that satisfies the criteria for newborn screening and is in fact one of the diseases that is screened for in the United States in all newborns. MCAD deficiency is a common inherited disorder with a frequency that approaches that of PKU. The disease can result in life-threatening complications and relatively simple dietary intervention can avert the clinical phenotype of MCAD deficiency. The MCAD enzyme is encoded by the acyl-CoA dehydrogenase, medium-chain (*ACADM*) gene. At least 340 mutations in the *ACADM* gene have been identified. By far, the most prevalent mutation (89%) found in MCAD deficiency patients is a single nucleotide substitution at position 985. This substitution is an A for G change that converts amino acid 329 from a lysine to a glutamic acid (K329E). This mutation alters the α-helical domain of the C-terminal portion of the enzyme. In addition to the A985G substitution mutation several additional nucleotide substitution mutations and insertion and deletion mutations have been identified in MCAD deficiency patients. The most common symptom of MCAD deficiency is episodic hypoketotic hypoglycemia brought on by fasting. Symptoms appear within the first 2 years of life. Clinical crisis is characterized by an infant presenting with episodes of vomiting and lethargy that may progress to seizures and ultimately coma. A prior upper respiratory or gastrointestinal viral infection will lead to reduced oral intake in these infants which can precipitate the acute crisis. The first episode in an infant may be fatal and the death ascribed to sudden infant death syndrome (SIDS). Autopsy results will often find marked fatty liver (hepatic steatosis) and cerebral edema. These findings are sometimes misdiagnosed as Reye syndrome especially in the circumstance where there is a prior infection reported. Because the capacity of the gluconeogenesis pathway is limited in newborn infants, they are highly susceptible to the lack of brain energy from the ketones that would normally be derived from fatty acid oxidation. The defect in fatty acid oxidation leads to the presence, in the plasma and urine, of toxic metabolic intermediates such as dicarboxylic acids as well as medium-chain acylcarnitines. The presence of the medium-chain dicarboxylic acids results from excess medium-chain fatty acids being oxidized via the microsomal ω-oxidation pathway. Normally dicarboxylic acids are oxidized in the peroxisomes but medium-chain dicarboxylic acids are not good substrates for the pathway and so these lipids end up accumulating in the blood and urine. Characteristic and diagnostic of MCAD deficiency is the presence of octanoylcarnitine (a medium-chain length

CLINICAL BOX 13-3 (CONTINUED)

acylcarnitine). Diagnosis can be made within 24–48 hours in specialized laboratories using tandem mass spectrometry (MS) of the blood for specific acylcarnitines. In MCAD deficiency the acylcarnitines that are found are highly diagnostic and specific for this disorder and include C6:0-, 4-cis-, and 5-cis-C8:1, C8:0, and 4-cis-C10:1 acylcarnitine species. The nomenclature C6:0, for example, refers to a fatty acid six carbons in length with no sites of unsaturation, whereas, C8:1 refers to a 8-carbon fatty acid with one site of unsaturation. When medium-chain length fatty acids are oxidized in the mitochondria there is no requirement for them first being attached to carnitine as is the case for long-chain length fatty acids. The lack of requirement for carnitine attachment is also true for short-chain length fatty acid oxidation. The mechanism that leads to the accumulation of medium-chain acylcarnitines in MCAD deficiency stems from the need for the mitochondria to replenish the CoASH pool for continued oxidation of long-chain fatty acids. When a long-chain fatty acyl-CoA is oxidized down to medium-chain length it can no longer be further oxidized due to the deficiency in MCAD. This results in the "trapping" of CoA as medium-chain acyl-CoAs. The inner mitochondrial membrane localized carnitine palmitoyltransferase 2 (CPT2) will exchange the CoA, from these accumulating medium-chain acyl-CoAs, for carnitine, thereby replenishing the CoASH pool for use by long-chain fatty acids. This mechanism results in the accumulation of the medium-chain acylcarnitines typically seen in MCAD deficient patient. The primary goal of treatment for MCAD deficiency patients is to provide adequate caloric intake, the avoidance of fasting, IV glucose to treat acute episodes, and aggressive therapy during periods of infection. Anorexia can develop during infections and fever leading to mobilization of stored fatty acids. The effect of increased lipid mobilization is the production of toxic intermediates from the accumulating medium-chain fatty acids, medium-chain acylcarnitines, and dicarboxylic acids which can lead to vomiting, lethargy, coma, and even death. Treatment with oral carnitine increases the removal of these toxic intermediates.

then phytanoyl-CoA serves as a substrate in pathway referred to as α-oxidation process; therefore, the process is referred to as α-oxidation (Figure 13–5). Loss of activity of phytanoyl-CoA hydroxylase (PhyH) results in the disorder known as Refsum disease (Clinical Box 13–4).

PEROXISOMAL β-OXIDATION REACTIONS

The peroxisomes play an important role in overall fatty acid metabolism. The oxidation of very-long-chain fatty acids (VLCFAs: C17–C26) begins exclusively in the peroxisomes. The peroxisomes also metabolize di- and trihydroxycholestanoic acids (bile acid intermediates); long-chain dicarboxylic acids that are produced by ω-oxidation of long-chain monocarboxylic acids; pristanic acid via the α-oxidation pathway (see earlier); certain polyunsaturated fatty acids (PUFA), and certain prostaglandins and leukotrienes.

The enzymatic processes of peroxisomal β-oxidation are very similar to those of mitochondrial β-oxidation with one major difference (Figure 13–6). In the peroxisome, the first oxidation step is catalyzed by acyl-CoA oxidases which are coupled to the reduction of O_2 to hydrogen peroxide (H_2O_2). Thus, the reaction is not coupled to energy production but instead yields a significant reactive oxygen species (ROS). Peroxisomes contain the enzyme catalase that degrades the hydrogen peroxide back to O_2.

HIGH-YIELD CONCEPT

The clinical significance of the activity of the acyl-CoA oxidases of peroxisomal β-oxidation is related to tissue specific oxidation processes. In the pancreatic β-cell there is little, if any, catalase expressed so that peroxisomal oxidation of VLCFA results in an increased release of ROS that can damage the β-cell contributing to the progressive insulin deficiency seen in obesity.

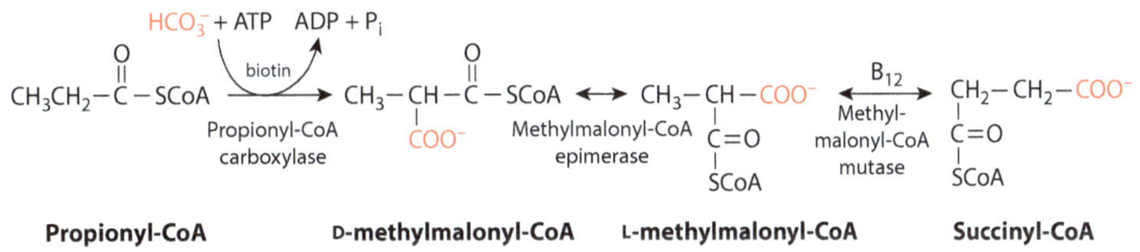

FIGURE 13–4 Conversion of propionyl-CoA to succinyl-CoA. (Reproduced with permission from themedicalbiochemistrypage, LLC.)

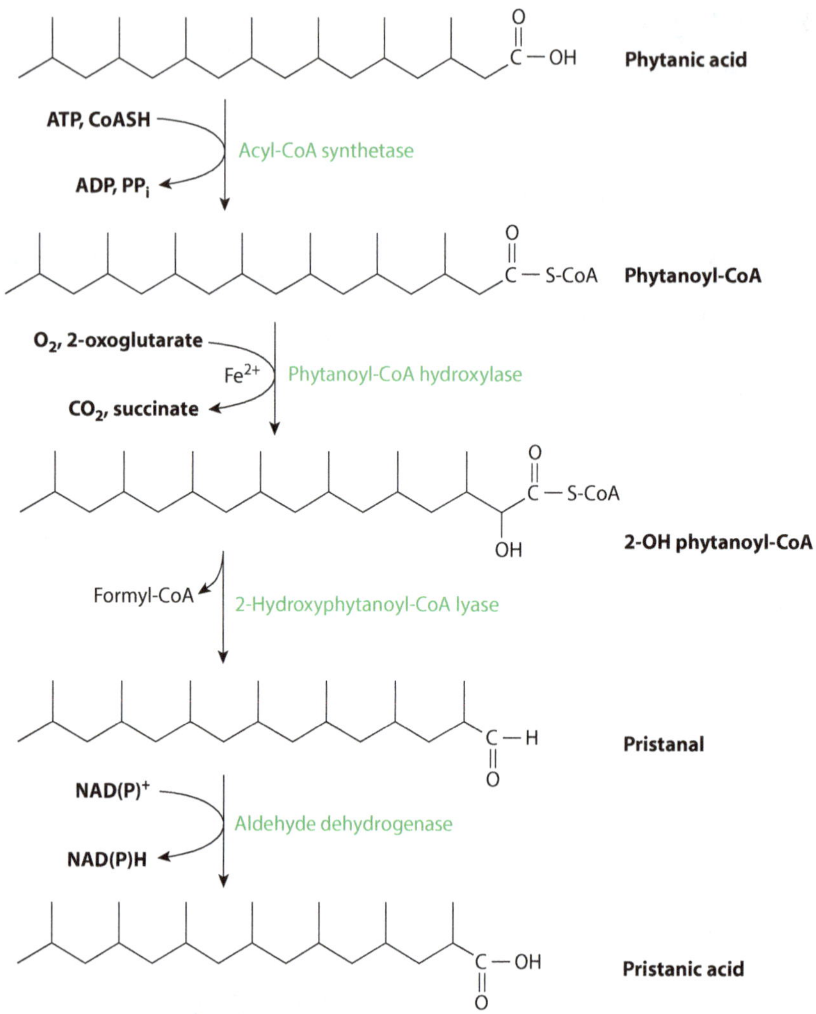

FIGURE 13–5 Phytanic acid oxidation pathway. Metabolism of phytanic acid occurs via a peroxisomal α-oxidation pathway. The 3-methyl substituted fatty acid is activated like all fatty acids via the action of acyl-CoA synthetases to yield phytanoyl-CoA. Phytanoyl-CoA is then decarboxylated via the action of the clinically significant enzyme, phytanoyl-CoA hydroxylase. Two additional reactions take place to yield pristanic acid which itself is activated for peroxisomal β-oxidation via the action of acyl-CoA synthetases. Through three cycles of peroxisomal β-oxidation, pristanoyl-CoA is metabolized to two moles of propionyl-CoA, one mole of acetyl-CoA, and one mole of 4,8-dimethylnonanoyl-CoA. All of these medium- and short-chain fats are then esterified to carnitine and transported to the mitochondria for further oxidation. (Reproduced with permission from themedicalbiochemistrypage, LLC.)

CLINICAL BOX 13–4 REFSUM DISEASE

Refsum disease (heredopathia atactica polyneuritiformis) is an autosomal recessive disorder named for Sigvald Refsum who initially characterized the cardinal clinical features of this disease that results from defects in fatty acid metabolism. Specifically, the disorder is due to deficiencies in the peroxisomal enzyme responsible for one of the initial steps in the oxidation of phytanic acid, a 3-methyl substituted fatty acid. This enzyme, phytanoyl-CoA hydroxylase, PhyH (also called phytanoyl-CoA dioxygenase), carries out an initial α-oxidation reaction generating the 19-carbon fatty acid, pristanic acid plus CO_2. Pristanic acid can then be oxidized by the remainder of the normal peroxisomal fatty acid β-oxidation pathway. Phytanic acid cannot be synthesized *de novo* in humans so dietary sources are the exclusive origin of this fatty acid. Dairy products, meat, ruminant fats, and fish are abundant sources of phytanic acid. The cardinal clinical features of Refsum disease are retinitis pigmentosa, chronic polyneuropathy, cerebellar ataxia, and elevated protein levels in cerebrospinal fluid. Most cases have electrocardiographic changes, and some have sensorineural hearing loss and/or ichthyosis. Multiple epiphyseal dysplasia (skeletal malformations) is a conspicuous feature in some cases. Refsum disease is a slowly developing, progressive peripheral neuropathy. Progression of the disease results in severe motor weakness and muscle wasting, particularly in the lower extremities.

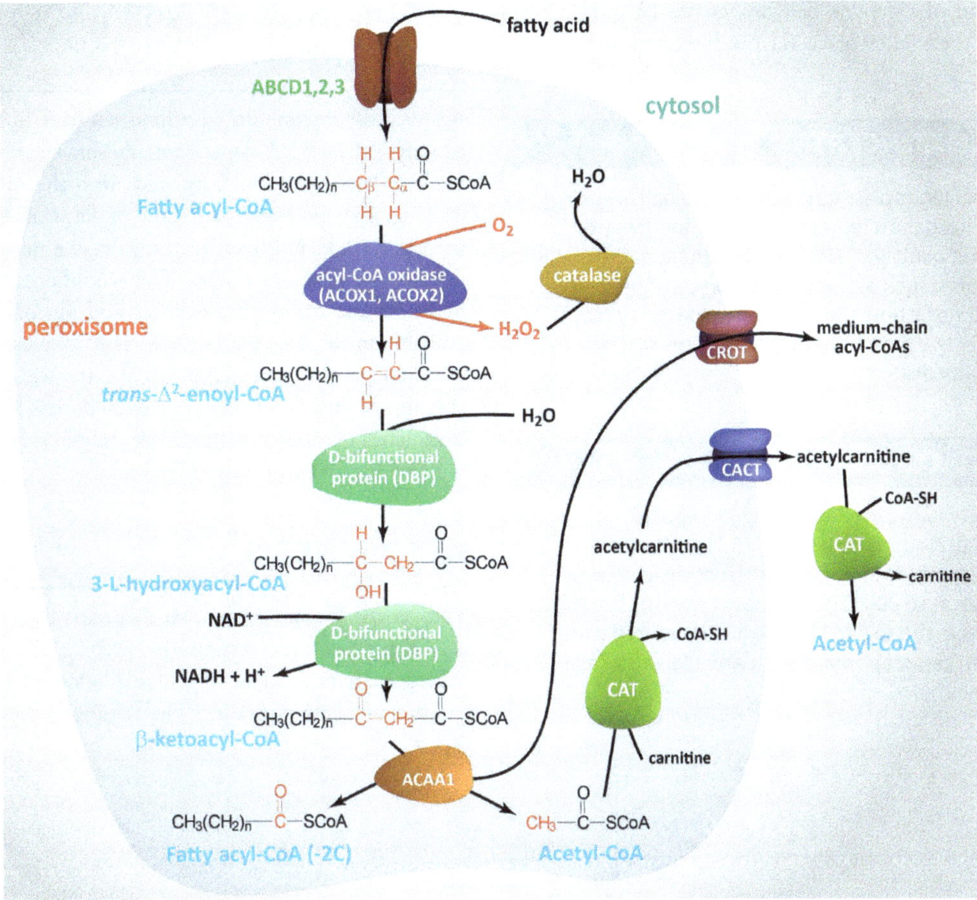

FIGURE 13–6 Pathway of peroxisomal fatty acid β-oxidation. Fatty acids are taken into the peroxisome and esterified to CoA by the solute carrier family member proteins ABCD1, ABCD2, or ABCD3. ABCD1 is also called VLCFA-CoA synthetase. DBP is D-bifunctional protein. The peroxisomal thiolase indicated in the figure is ACAA1 (acetyl-CoA C-acyltransferase 1, also known as peroxisomal 3-oxoacyl-CoA thiolase). The majority of the products of peroxisomal very long-chain fatty acid β-oxidation are long-chain and medium-chain fatty acyl-CoAs. These acyl-CoAs are transported to the cytosol through the action of the CROT (carnitine octanoyltransferase) encoded enzyme where they can then be taken up by the mitochondria for complete oxidation. Any acetyl-CoA generated by peroxisomal β-oxidation is transported out of the peroxisome after exchange of carnitine for the CoA. Peroxisomal and mitochondrial acetyl-carnitine is formed through the action of carnitine acetyltransferase (CAT). Acetyl-carnitine is transported out of the peroxisomes and mitochondria via the action of carnitine-acylcarnitine translocase (CACT which is encoded by the SLC25A20 gene). Once in the cytosol acetyl-carnitine is converted to acetyl-CoA via the action of cytosolic CAT. These acetyl-CoA units can be used for cytosolic fatty acid synthesis or imported into the mitochondria for oxidation in the TCA cycle. (Reproduced with permission from themedicalbiochemistrypage, LLC.)

MICROSOMAL ω-OXIDATION REACTIONS

The pathway refers to the fact that fatty acids first undergo a hydroxylation step at the terminal (omega, ω) carbon (Figure 13–7). Human ω-hydroxylases are all members of the cytochrome P450 family (CYP) of enzymes. CYP4A11 utilizes NADPH and O_2 to introduce an alcohol to the ω-CH_3– of several fatty acids including lauric (12:0), myristic (14:0), palmitic (16:0), oleic (18:1), and arachidonic acid (20:4). Following addition of the ω-hydroxyl, the fatty acid is a substrate for alcohol dehydrogenase (ADH) which generates an oxo-fatty acid, followed by generation of the corresponding dicarboxylic

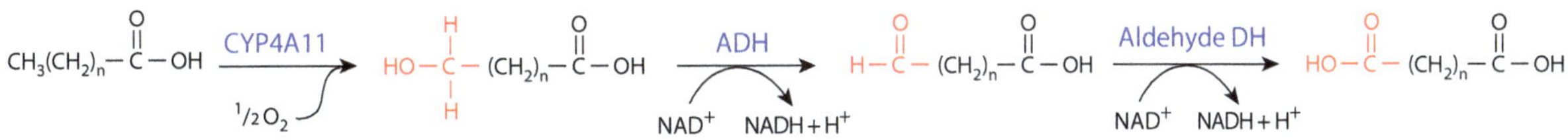

FIGURE 13–7 Pathway of microsomal ω-oxidation initiated by CYP4A11. The two subsequent reactions are catalyzed by an alcohol dehydrogenase (ADH) and an aldehyde dehydrogenase (ALDH), both of which require NAD^+ as a cofactor similar to these same reactions of hepatic alcohol metabolism (Chapter 14). (Reproduced with permission from themedicalbiochemistrypage, LLC.)

acid via the action of aldehyde dehydrogenases (ALDH). Further metabolism then takes place via the β-oxidation pathway in peroxisomes.

HIGH-YIELD CONCEPT

The microsomal (endoplasmic reticulum, ER) pathway of fatty acid ω-oxidation represents a minor pathway of overall fatty acid oxidation. However, in certain pathophysiologic states, such as diabetes, chronic alcohol consumption, and starvation, the ω-oxidation pathway may provide an effective means for the elimination of toxic levels of free fatty acids.

HIGH-YIELD CONCEPT

The formation of ω-hydroxylated arachidonic acid (20-hydroxyeicosatetraenoic acid, 20-HETE) by CYP4A11 plays an important role in the regulation of the cardiovascular system because 20-HETE is a known vasoconstrictor. Polymorphisms in the CYP4A11 gene are associated with hypertension in certain populations, particularly those of Asian heritage.

REGULATION OF FATTY ACID OXIDATION

Adipose tissue contains hormone-sensitive lipase (HSL), which is activated by PKA-dependent phosphorylation; this activation increases the release of fatty acids into the blood. This in turn leads to the increased oxidation of fatty acids in other tissues such as muscle and liver. In the liver, the net result is enhanced production of ketone bodies. This would occur under conditions in which the carbohydrate stores and gluconeogenic precursors available in the liver are not sufficient to allow increased glucose production. The increased levels of fatty acid that become available in response to glucagon or epinephrine are assured of being completely oxidized, because PKA also phosphorylates ACC leading to decreased synthesis of fatty acids.

KETOGENESIS

Ketogenesis (Figure 13–8), which occurs exclusively in the liver, is the process of diverting the acetyl-CoA, derived primarily during high rates of fatty acid oxidation in the liver, into the synthesis of ketone bodies. The ketone bodies are acetoacetate,

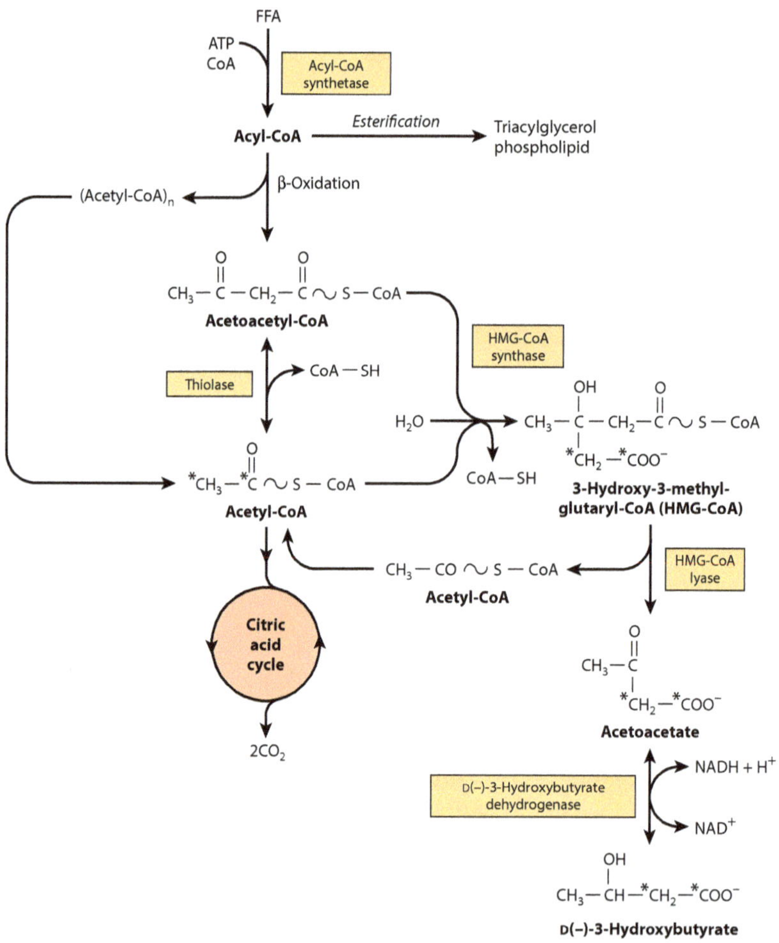

FIGURE 13–8 Pathways of ketogenesis in the liver. (FFA, free fatty acids.) (Reproduced with permission from Rodwell VW, Bender DA, Botham KM, et al: *Harper's Illustrated Biochemistry*, 31st ed. New York, NY: McGraw Hill; 2018.)

β-hydroxybutyrate, and acetone. The ketone bodies, principally β-hydroxybutyrate, can then be used for energy production during periods when glucose and gluconeogenesis are limiting. The synthesis of the ketone bodies occurs in the mitochondria allowing this process to be intimately coupled to rate of hepatic fatty acid oxidation. Conversely, the utilization of the ketones occurs in the cytosol.

HIGH-YIELD CONCEPT

The activity of HSL is inhibited via AMPK-mediated phosphorylation. Inhibition of HSL by AMPK may seem paradoxical since the release of fatty acids stored in triglycerides would seem necessary to promote the production of ATP via fatty acid oxidation and the major function of AMPK is to shift cells to ATP production from ATP consumption. This paradox can be explained if one considers that if the fatty acids that are released from triglycerides are not oxidized they will be recycled back into triglycerides at the expense of ATP consumption. Thus, inhibition of HSL by AMPK-mediated phosphorylation is a mechanism to ensure that the rate of fatty acid release does not exceed the rate at which they are utilized either by export or oxidation.

Acetoacetate can undergo spontaneous decarboxylation to acetone, or be enzymatically converted to β-hydroxybutyrate through the action of β-hydroxybutyrate dehydrogenase. The ketone bodies freely diffuse out of the mitochondria and hepatocytes and enter the circulation where they can be taken up by nonhepatic tissues such as the brain, heart, and skeletal muscle.

Ketone bodies are utilized by extrahepatic tissues via a series of cytosolic reactions that are essentially a reversal of ketone body synthesis (Figure 13–9). It is important to appreciate that under conditions where tissues are utilizing ketones for energy production their NAD^+/NADH ratios are going to be relatively high, thus driving the β-hydroxybutyrate dehydrogenase catalyzed reaction in the direction of acetoacetate synthesis. The second reaction of ketolysis involves the action of succinyl-CoA:3-oxoacid-CoA transferase (SCOT). The latter enzyme is present at high levels in most tissues except the liver. Importantly, very low level of SCOT expression in the liver allows the liver to produce ketone bodies but not to utilize them. This ensures that extrahepatic tissues have access to ketone bodies as a fuel source during prolonged fasting and starvation.

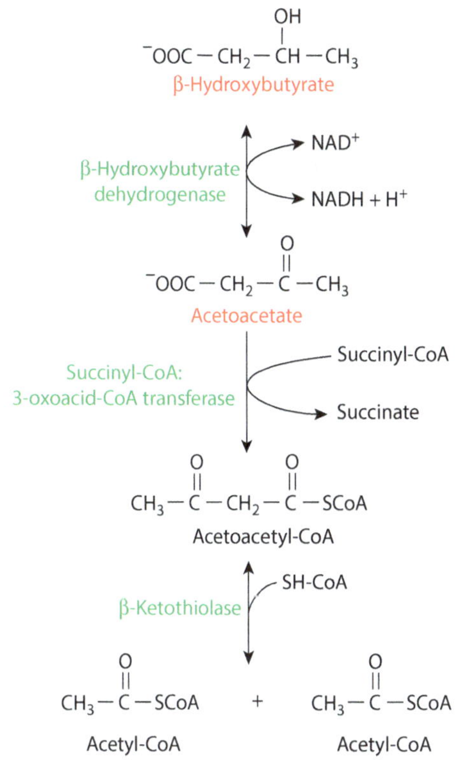

FIGURE 13–9 Reactions of ketone body utilization. Ketones are taken up by peripheral (non-hepatic) tissues and due to the relatively low energy charge in these tissues in the fasted state the NADH/NAD^+ ratio is quite low (in other words the NAD^+/NADH ratio is high) favoring the oxidation of β-hydroxybutyrate (BHB) back to acetoacetate. Acetaoacetate is then converted to acetoacetyl-CoA through the action of the OXCT1 encoded enzyme. The *OXCT1* gene is expressed at extremely low levels in hepatocytes, thus preventing those cells from utilizing the ketones they have synthesized. Acetoacetyl-CoA is then cleaved into two molecules of acetyl-CoA by the ACAA2 encoded enzyme. These acetyl-CoA units are then oxidized within the TCA cycle. (Reproduced with permission from themedicalbiochemistrypage, LLC.)

CHECKLIST

- ☑ Dietary fats are primarily in the form of triglycerides which are hydrolyzed by gastric and pancreatic lipases. The released fatty acids are then taken into intestinal enterocytes where triglycerides and phospholipids are formed and packaged into chylomicrons.
- ☑ Fatty acids are taken into cells via the actions of specific fatty acid transport proteins. Several transport proteins also possess acyl-CoA transferase activity, thus activating the fatty acids in conjunction with intracellular uptake.
- ☑ Fatty acids are stored for future use as triglycerides with the major storage location being adipose tissue. Adipose tissue releases stored fats on hormonal stimulation of the need for energy production. The fats are released through the concerted actions of ATGL, HSL, and MGL.

- ☑ Fatty acids are oxidized to produce large quantities of ATP. Oxidation takes place primarily within the mitochondria by a process referred to as β-oxidation that sequentially releases acetyl-CoA units that then enter the TCA cycle.
- ☑ Entry of fatty acyl-CoA into the mitochondria is controlled by malonyl-CoA-mediated inhibition of carnitine palmitoyltransferase I. This regulatory process connects fatty acid synthesis to fatty acid oxidation since malonyl-CoA is the product of the rate-limiting enzyme of fat synthesis.
- ☑ Long-chain fatty acids can undergo β-oxidation in the peroxisomes and very long-chain fatty acids are exclusively oxidized in the peroxisome. Peroxisomal β-oxidation generates hydrogen peroxide which is metabolized primarily by catalase. Excess peroxisomal oxidation in pancreatic β-cells leads to cellular dysfunction due to limiting amounts of catalase in these cells.
- ☑ Ruminant fats contain significant quantities of the methyl-substituted fatty acid, phytanic acid which is oxidized in the peroxisomes via an α-oxidation pathway. Defects in the α-oxidation pathway result in peroxisomal disorder called Refsum disease.
- ☑ Microsomal ω-oxidation is a minor fatty acid oxidation pathway that involves an initial hydroxylation step to the terminal ω-carbon. In certain pathophysiologic states, such as diabetes, chronic alcohol consumption, and starvation, the ω-oxidation pathway provides a route for the elimination of toxic levels of free fatty acids.
- ☑ Fatty acid oxidation is regulated by the delivery of substrate to the oxidation enzymes. This reflects a balance between hormonal signals, such as insulin and glucagon, designed to control energy storage and energy production, respectively.
- ☑ Glucose and fatty acids reciprocally regulate the utilization of each other in energy generation pathways through substrate-product interactions termed the glucose-fatty acid cycle.
- ☑ Ketogenesis represents the pathway carried out in the liver to divert acetyl-CoA into carbon sources of energy, the ketone bodies, for use by the brain and other peripheral tissues primarily during periods of fasting and starvation. In type 1 diabetes, the unregulated release of glucagon leads to excess adipose tissue release of fatty acids which are converted to ketone bodies by the liver in excess of peripheral tissue utilization resulting in the condition referred to as diabetic ketoacidosis, DKA.
- ☑ Defects in enzymes of fatty acid oxidation can lead to potentially the life-threatening conditions of hypoglycemia and fatty deposition in organs such as the liver resulting in cirrhosis. Additionally, peroxisomal fatty acid oxidation defects manifest with symptoms similar to the more classical peroxisomal biogenesis disorders such as Zellweger syndrome.

REVIEW QUESTIONS

1. A 12-year-old boy is brought to the emergency department after a day of training for his school cross-country track team with complaints of intense pain in his legs and that he felt almost too weak to walk. Serum studies show hypoketotic hypoglycemia and hyperammonemia. Urinalysis finds myoglobinuria. Histopathology of muscle biopsy tissue is positive for Sudan black staining. Given the findings in this patient, which of the following enzymes is most likely to be defective?
(A) Carnitine palmitoyltransferase-2
(B) Glucose-6-phosphatase
(C) Glycogen phosphorylase
(D) Medium-chain acyl-CoA dehydrogenase
(E) Mitochondrial trifunctional protein

2. A 1-year-old girl is brought to the emergency department by her parents due to their inability to rouse her to eat. Physical examination finds hypotonia and hepatomegaly. Blood laboratory studies find hypoglycemia, hyperammonemia, and free carnitine level of less than 5 mM (normal 25 mM–50 mM). Liver function enzymes (AST and ALT) are variably elevated. This infant is most likely suffering from which of the following disorders?
(A) Carnitine deficiency, systemic primary
(B) Maple syrup urine disease (MSUD)
(C) Medium-chain acyl-CoA dehydrogenase deficiency (MCADD)
(D) Multiple acyl-CoA dehydrogenase deficiency (MADD)
(E) von Gierke disease

3. Following a minor respiratory illness, a seemingly healthy, developmentally normal 15-month-old boy exhibited repeated episodes of severe lethargy and vomiting following periods of fasting, such as during the middle of the night. The parents brought the infant to the emergency department following a seizure. The child was hypoglycemic and was administered 10% dextrose but remained lethargic. Blood ammonia was high, liver function tests were slightly elevated, and his serum contained an accumulation of dicarboxylic acids. Which of the following disorders most likely corresponds to the symptoms observed in this infant?
(A) Andersen disease
(B) Maple syrup urine disease (MSUD)
(C) Medium-chain acyl-CoA dehydrogenase deficiency (MCADD)
(D) Multiple acyl-CoA dehydrogenase deficiency (MADD)
(E) von Gierke disease
(F) Zellweger syndrome

4. A 1-year-old boy is brought to the emergency department by his anguished parents following a seizure. The parents report that their child has not eaten well during the past 3 days because of an upper respiratory tract infection. Physical examination shows lethargy and mild hepatomegaly. Blood work indicates he is hypoglycemic and hypoketotic. Urinalysis finds increased levels of octanoylcarnitine, octanedioic acid, and hexanedioic acid. Which of the following is the most likely cause of the findings in this patient?
(A) Carnitine palmitoyltransferase-1 deficiency
(B) Fructose-1,6-bisphosphatase deficiency

(C) Glucose-6-phosphatase deficiency
(D) Medium-chain acyl-CoA dehydrogenase deficiency
(E) Mitochondrial trifunctional protein deficiency

5. A 14-year-old girl is brought to the emergency department unresponsive. History reveals that the patient is a type 1 diabetic. Physical examination shows dehydration. Serum studies show hyperglycemia, metabolic acidosis, ketonemia, and hypertriglyceridemia. Urinalysis shows glucosuria and ketonuria. Which of the following is most likely contributing to the hypertriglyceridemia in this patient?
(A) Decreased clearance of VLDL-cholesterol
(B) Decreased LDL receptor activity
(C) Decreased lipoprotein lipase activity
(D) Increased hepatic influx of free fatty acids from adipose tissue
(E) Increased hepatic lipase activity
(F) Increased lecithin:cholesterol acyltransferase activity

6. Experiments are being carried out to determine the function of a novel compound. Results of the experiments find that the compound inhibits the conversion of riboflavin to its active coenzyme. Under these conditions, which of the following metabolic processes is most likely to be directly impaired if this compound was administered to humans?
(A) Synthesis of malonyl-CoA
(B) Peroxisomal oxidation of phytanoyl-CoA
(C) Mitochondrial β-oxidation of palmitate
(D) Peroxisomal ω-oxidation of butyric acid
(E) Synthesis of palmitate

7. Experiments are being conducted on the metabolic profile of a cell line derived from a breast cancer compared to normal epithelial cells. Results from these experiments show the rate of malonyl-CoA biosynthesis is five times higher in the tumor-derived cell line than in the normal epithelial cells. Given these results, the rate of biosynthesis of which of the following classes of compounds is most likely higher in the cancer cells compared with normal epithelial cells?
(A) Cholesterol
(B) Fatty acids
(C) Glycosphingolipids
(D) Phospholipids
(E) Prostaglandins

8. A 37-year-old female patient is being examined by her physician. Her chief complaint is that her stools are very foul smelling and float on the surface of the toilet water. An MRI of her abdomen reveals no apparent abnormalities in the gallbladder or pancreas. Biopsy of the main pancreatic duct also shows no overt pathology. Pancreatic secretions from this patient would most likely be found to be deficient is which of the following?
(A) Carboxyl ester lipase (CEL)
(B) Carboxypeptidase A
(C) Chymotrypsinogen
(D) Lipase
(E) Phospholipase A_2 (PLA_2)

9. A 12-year-old boy is brought to the emergency department after a day of training for his school cross-country track team with complaints of intense pain in his legs and that he felt almost too weak to walk. Serum studies show hypoketotic hypoglycemia and hyperammonemia. Urinalysis finds myoglobinuria. Histopathology of muscle biopsy tissue is positive for Sudan black staining. A defect in which of the following processes is most likely to be the cause of the patient's symptoms?
(A) Amino acid metabolism
(B) Glycogen metabolism
(C) Mitochondrial function
(D) Peroxisomal biogenesis
(E) Protein *N*-glycosylation

10. A 5-month-old male child is brought into the ER by his parents following a seizure. On examination it is found that the child has hypoplastic supraorbital ridges, epicanthal folds, a small nose with anteverted nares, a broad nasal bridge, full forehead, and large anterior fontanelle. Suspecting chromosomal abnormality as the cause of the physical signs in this patient a karyotype analysis is ordered but finds no anomalies. A defect in which of the following processes is most likely associated with the observed symptoms in this child?
(A) Genomic imprinting
(B) Glycogen metabolism
(C) Mitochondrial function
(D) Peroxisomal biogenesis
(E) Protein *N*-glycosylation

11. A 22-year-old man is being examined by his physician because he is concerned about growths on his eyelids. He is 180 cm (5 ft 11 in) tall and weighs 85 kg (188 lb); BMI is 26 kg/m^2. Physical examination shows no other abnormalities except for the xanthelasmas. Serum studies show a total cholesterol concentration of 300 mg/dL, HDL-cholesterol concentration of 37 mg/dL, and triglyceride concentration of 1500 mg/dL. A deficiency in which of the following is the most likely cause of these findings?
(A) Cortisol
(B) Essential fatty acids
(C) Hepatic lipase
(D) HDL receptor
(E) Lipoprotein lipase

12. During an episode of gastroenteritis that significantly compromises food intake, a 13-month-old girl develops progressive vomiting followed by coma. She is hypoglycemic and no ketone bodies are detected in the urine. A specific defect in the metabolism of which of the following is the most likely cause of these findings?
(A) Acetoacetate
(B) Glycogen
(C) Lactate
(D) Leucine
(E) Palmitate

13. A 3-month-old infant is brought to the emergency department by distraught parents, frightened by the extreme lethargy and near comatose state of their child. Serum analysis shows glucose 57 md/dL (N: 70–140 mg/dL) and elevated octanoylcarnitine. Suspecting a specific enzyme deficiency, the child's physician requests an additional serum assay. An assay for which of the following would be most useful from a diagnostic perspective?
(A) Acetone
(B) Bilirubin
(C) Dicarboxylic acids
(D) Glucocerebrosidase
(E) Methylmalonic acid
(F) Sphingomyelin

14. A 6-year-old boy with progressive muscle weakness is found to have a systemic defect in the production of carnitine. Which of the following is the most likely outcome, within skeletal muscle, in this patient as a result of the identified defect?
(A) Decreased utilization of glucose
(B) Decreased cholesterol stores
(C) Decreased glucose oxidation
(D) Increased lactate production
(E) Increased triglyceride stores
(F) Increased utilization of acetoacetate

15. An 8-month-old girl is brought to the emergency department because her parents have been unable to fully rouse her for 3 hours. She had repeated episodes of vomiting and diarrhea the previous day, and she has not eaten for the past 12 hours. Physical examination shows lethargy and mild hepatomegaly. Serum analysis determines no detectable ketones and urinalysis finds elevated acylcarnitines. A deficiency in which of the following processes is the most likely contributing to the pathology in this patient?
(A) Amino acid metabolism
(B) Fatty acid metabolism
(C) Glucose metabolism
(D) Glycogen metabolism
(E) Lysosomal glycosphingolipid metabolism

16. A 2-year-old boy is admitted to the hospital because of generalized weakness, repeated episodes of vomiting, and coma after several days of reduced food intake because of a minor febrile illness. He is treated successfully with intravenous glucose. After 13 hours of fasting when the child is well, his serum glucose and β-hydroxybutyrate levels are low while free carnitine concentrations are increased. Triglycerides containing only medium-chain fatty acids are fed, and the serum β-hydroxybutyrate concentration increases to the reference range. Which of the following is most likely to be defective in this child?
(A) Carnitine palmitoyltransferase-1
(B) Carnitine synthesis
(C) Fatty acyl-CoA synthetases
(D) Medium-chain acyl-CoA dehydrogenase
(E) Peroxisomal fat oxidation

17. A 3-month-old infant is brought to the emergency department by distraught parents, frightened by the extreme lethargy and near comatose state of their child. Serum analysis shows glucose 57 md/dL (N: 70–140 mg/dL) and little detectable β-hydroxybutyrate. A work-up of the infant finds no known mutations associated with defects in fatty acid oxidation that are typically associated with these symptoms. Functional studies on adipose tissue from the infants finds that glucagon and epinephrine bind and activate their respective receptors and associated G-proteins but there is no increase in triglyceride metabolism. A defect in which of the following would most likely account for the observations in this infant?
(A) Adipose triglyceride lipase
(B) Monoglyceride lipase
(C) Phosphodiesterase
(D) Protein kinase A
(E) Protein kinase B

18. A 12-year-old boy is being examined by his pediatrician with complaints of decreased ability to see at night as well as experiencing numbness in his hands and feet. Ophthalmoscopic examination finds clear signs of retinitis pigmentosum. A defect in which of the following processes is most likely to account for the signs and symptoms in this patient?
(A) Bile acid metabolism
(B) Branched-chain amino acid metabolism
(C) Lysosomal glycosphingolipid metabolism
(D) Mitochondrial fatty acid oxidation
(E) Peroxisomal fatty acid oxidation

19. Experiments are being conducted on fatty acid oxidation using cells in culture following their treatment with the carcinogen, ethylnitrosourea. Results from the experiments find that ATP consumption and overall levels of $FADH_2$ production are reduced compared to normal cells. Which of the following enzyme activities is the most likely to be deficient accounting for the observed results?
(A) Acyl-CoA synthetase
(B) Carnitine palmitoyltransferase-1
(C) Carnitine palmitoyltransferase-2
(D) Medium-chain acyl-CoA dehydrogenases
(E) Mitochondrial trifunctional protein

20. Experiments are being conducted on the oxidation of hexacosanoic acid (C26:0) using cells in culture. Results of the experiments find that very little of the lipid is metabolized. A defect in which of the following processes is most likely to account for these observations?
(A) Lysosomal glycolipid metabolism
(B) Microsomal fatty acid ω-oxidation
(C) Mitochondrial fatty acid β-oxidation
(D) Peroxisomal fatty acid α-oxidation
(E) Peroxisomal fatty acid β-oxidation

21. Excess uptake and metabolism of fatty acids by the pancreas significantly contributes to the progressive loss of β-cell function in overweight and obese individuals. Which of the following best explains this effect of fatty acids?
(A) Deficiency in peroxisomal oxidative capacity resulting in increased fat droplet production which results in apoptosis
(B) Excess accumulation of triglycerides derived from the fatty acids causing steatosis
(C) Increase in endoplasmic reticulum stress due to incorporation of the fats into membrane lipids triggering apoptosis
(D) Increased fat oxidation in the peroxisomes results in release of cytochrome *c* triggering apoptosis
(E) Low levels of β-cell catalase leads to reactive oxygen species excess resulting in mitochondrial dysfunction

22. A 54-year-old man of Asian ethnicity is undergoing molecular studies to determine the cause of his hypertension. A particular polymorphism was identified in his *CYP4A11* gene. Based on his genetic makeup, which of the following processes is most likely to be altered, contributing to his pathology?
(A) Lysosomal glycolipid metabolism
(B) Microsomal fatty acid ω-oxidation
(C) Mitochondrial fatty acid β-oxidation
(D) Peroxisomal fatty acid α-oxidation
(E) Peroxisomal fatty acid β-oxidation

23. A 10-year-old boy is taken to the emergency department after a day of riding his bike with his friends. He is complaining of intense pain in his legs. Urinalysis finds myoglobinuria. Which of the following would most likely aid in the correct diagnosis in this patient?

(A) Histopathology of muscle using periodic acid-Schiff (PAS)
(B) Histopathology of muscle using Sudan black
(C) Liver biopsy staining using periodic acid-Schiff (PAS)
(D) Liver biopsy staining using Sudan black
(E) Serum analysis of dicarboxylic acid levels
(F) Urinalysis for medium-chain acylcarnitines

24. An individual suffers from a defect in one of the enzymes required for the synthesis of carnitine. If this individual does not have an adequate intake of carnitine in the diet and is fasting, which of the following would be the most likely observation in this person compared to conditions of normal carnitine intake?

(A) Elevated levels of dicarboxylic acids in the blood
(B) Elevated long-chain fatty acid levels in the blood
(C) Hyperglycemia
(D) Increased levels of fatty acid oxidation
(E) Hyperketonuria

25. Experiments are being conducted on a hepatocyte cell line derived from a patient with hepatocellular carcinoma. Results of these experiments demonstrate that β-hydroxybutyrate is effectively metabolized to acetyl-CoA in these cells but does not occur in normal hepatocytes. Expression of which of the following activities, in the tumor-derived hepatocytes, would best explain the experimental results?

(A) β-Hydroxybutyrate dehydrogenase
(B) Hydroxymethylglutaryl-CoA-lyase
(C) Hydroxymethylglutaryl-CoA-synthetase
(D) Medium-chain acyl-CoA dehydrogenase
(E) Succinyl-CoA: 3-oxoacid-CoA-transferase

26. A 1-year-old boy is brought to the emergency department by his parents following a seizure. The parents report that their child has not eaten well during the past 3 days because of an upper respiratory tract infection. Physical examination shows lethargy and mild hepatomegaly. Urinalysis finds increased levels of octanoylcarnitine, octanedioic acid, and hexanedioic acid. Which of the following signs and symptoms would most likely also be found in this child due to the 3-day period of reduced food intake?

(A) Bone and joint pain from thrombocytopenia
(B) Hyperammonemia and hyperketonemia
(C) Hyperuricemia
(D) Hypoglycemia and metabolic acidosis
(E) Metabolic alkalosis and decreased serum bicarbonate

27. A 53-year-old woman diagnosed with Crohn disease has her terminal ileum resected. Five years later, she comes to the physician because of weakness and fatigue. Physical examination shows skin pallor. Laboratory studies show a hemoglobin concentration of 9 g/dL N = 12–15 g/L), a mean corpuscular volume (MCV) of 110 fL (N = 82–98 fL), and a hematocrit of 33% (N = 36%–44%). Which of the following processes is most likely to be deficient in this patient?

(A) Microsomal fatty acid ω-oxidation
(B) Mitochondrial oxidation of even-chain fatty acids
(C) Mitochondrial oxidation of odd-chain fatty acids
(D) Peroxisomal fatty acid α-oxidation
(E) Peroxisomal fatty acid β-oxidation

28. A 15-year-old boy has been diagnosed with retinitis pigmentosa, peripheral polyneuropathy, and cerebellar ataxia. Analysis of his cerebrospinal fluid indicated a high protein content but no elevation of cell number. Serum studies found phytanic acid levels above normal. Which of the following processes is most likely defective in this patient?

(A) Lysosomal glycolipid metabolism
(B) Microsomal fatty acid ω-oxidation
(C) Mitochondrial fatty acid β-oxidation
(D) Peroxisomal fatty acid α-oxidation
(E) Peroxisomal fatty acid β-oxidation

29. The product of the mitochondrial β-oxidation of fatty acids with odd numbers of carbon atoms is further oxidized in the TCA cycle. Which of the following would most likely be found elevated in the serum of a person with a deficiency that negatively impacts this process?

(A) Alanine
(B) Glucose
(C) Lactate
(D) Methylmalonic acid
(E) Palmitate

30. Which of the following best explains why the carbons of palmitic acid cannot be utilized for the direct synthesis of glucose via the pathway of gluconeogenesis?

(A) Fat oxidation occurs in mitochondria and gluconeogenesis occurs in the cytosol
(B) States of catabolism and anabolism are never concurrently active
(C) Storage of fats occurs in adipose tissue and gluconeogenesis occurs in liver and kidney
(D) The carbons of acetyl-CoA from fat oxidation are lost as CO_2 in the TCA cycle
(E) The carbons of acetyl-CoA from fat oxidation inhibit conversion of pyruvate to oxaloacetate

31. Experiments are being carried out to study the rate of fatty acid metabolism using a cell line derived from the treatment of normal cells with a carcinogen. Results of these experiments find that palmitic acid synthesis and oxidation occur at equivalent rates in response to treatment of the cells with insulin. Which of the following proteins most likely possesses an abnormal activity accounting for the observed results?

(A) Acyl-CoA synthetase
(B) Carnitine palmitoyltransferase-1
(C) Carnitine palmitoyltransferase-2
(D) Medium-chain acyl-CoA dehydrogenases
(E) Mitochondrial trifunctional protein

32. A 2-month-old male infant has been brought to the emergency department by his parents due to their failure to rouse him to eat. Physical examination of the infant finds dysmorphic facial features and the presence of hypospadias, a condition in which the opening of the penis is on the underside rather than the tip. Blood work shows severe metabolic acidosis, nonketotic hypoglycemia, and hyperammonemia. Which of the following disorders most likely corresponds to the signs and symptoms observed in this infant?

(A) Andersen disease
(B) Maple syrup urine disease (MSUD)
(C) Medium-chain acyl-CoA dehydrogenase deficiency (MCADD)

(D) Multiple acyl-CoA dehydrogenase deficiency (MADD)
(E) von Gierke disease
(F) Zellweger syndrome

33. A 15-year-old boy has been diagnosed with retinitis pigmentosa, peripheral polyneuropathy, and cerebellar ataxia. Analysis of his cerebrospinal fluid indicated a high protein content but no elevation of cell number. Serum studies found phytanic acid levels above normal. Which of the following is the most likely disorder causing this patient's symptoms?
(A) Carnitine deficiency, systemic primary
(B) Medium-chain acyl-CoA dehydrogenase deficiency
(C) Mitochondrial trifunctional protein deficiency
(D) Refsum disease
(E) Zellweger syndrome

34. A 4-month-old girl is being examined by her pediatrician because her parents are concerned that she is difficult to rouse in the mornings and seems irritable when they try to feed her. The parents report that their daughter seems to have had more frequent episodes of vomiting in the past few weeks. There is no significant family history. The patient was born vaginally at 39 weeks gestation following an uncomplicated pregnancy. Physical examination finds that the infant is at the 10th percentile for length and weight and at the 25th percentile for head circumference. Serum studies reveal a glucose concentration of 42 mg/dL (N = 70–150 mg/dL) and a bicarbonate concentration of 14 mEq/L (N = 16–24 mEq/L). Urinalysis is negative for both glucose and β-hydroxybutyrate. Measurement for which of the following would be most useful in the determination of the cause of the patient's symptoms?
(A) Acetoacetate
(B) Dicarboxylic acids
(C) Long-chain acylcarnitines
(D) Phytanoyl-CoA
(E) Propionyl-CoA

35. A 9-month-old male infant is brought to the Emergency Department by his parents due to their inability to rouse him to eat. Physical examination finds hypotonia and hepatomegaly. Blood laboratory studies find hypoglycemia, hyperammonemia, and free carnitine level of less than 5 mM (normal 25 mM–50 mM). Liver function enzymes (AST and ALT) are variably elevated. Which of the following processes is most likely impaired by this patient's underlying disorder?
(A) Fatty acid synthesis
(B) Gluconeogenesis
(C) Glycogen catabolism
(D) Glycolysis
(E) Ketone body synthesis
(F) Peroxisomal fatty acid oxidation

ANSWERS

1. Correct answer is **A.** The patient most likely suffers from a disorder known as adult myopathic CPT deficiency. This disorder is caused by mutations in the gene (*CPT2*) encoding the enzyme, carnitine palmitoyltransferase 2 (CPT-2). The myopathic form of CPT-2 deficiency is the most common inherited disorder of lipid metabolism that affects skeletal muscle as well as the most common cause of inherited myoglobinuria. This form of CPT-2 deficiency is characterized by recurrent episodes of muscle pain, rhabdomyolysis, and myoglobinuria that is triggered by prolonged exercise. Deficiency in glucose-6-phosphatase (choice B) results in the glycogen storage disease known as von Gierke. Deficiency in glycogen phosphorylase (choice C) results in the disorder referred to as McArdle disease. The symptoms of McArdle disease are very similar to the symptoms associated with adult myopathic CPT deficiency except in the case of McArdle disease the accumulating substance in skeletal muscle cells is carbohydrate as opposed to lipid. Deficiency in medium-chain acyl-CoA dehydrogenase (choice D) results in the disorder known as MCAD deficiency. MCAD deficiency is associated with severe hypoglycemia along with hypoketonemia in the early neonatal stages. Mitochondrial trifunctional protein (choice E) is a complex composed of α-subunits and β-subunits encoded by the *HADHA* and *HADHB* genes, respectively. The major form of MTP deficiency results from mutations in that *HADHA* gene. The clinical symptoms associated with MTP deficiency include hypoketotic hypoglycemia, metabolic acidosis, metabolic encephalopathy, liver dysfunction, cardiomyopathy, exercise-induced myoglobinuria, and rhabdomyolysis.

2. Correct answer is **A.** The low levels of carnitine present in this patient suggest that the patient has a defect in the ability to properly obtain carnitine. This indicates that the patient is most likely suffering from primary carnitine deficiency, more commonly referred to as carnitine deficiency, systemic primary. The typical metabolic presentation in patients with primary carnitine deficiency occurs most frequently before 2 years of age. Infants with primary carnitine deficiency exhibit poor feeding and can become lethargic and minimally responsive. The presentation of primary carnitine deficiency is quite variable with respect to the age of onset, the severity of the symptoms, and the involved organs. Maple syrup urine disease (choice B) results from mutations in the gene encoding branched-chain ketoacid dehydrogenase (BCKD). Classic MSUD is defined by neonatal onset of encephalopathy and is the most severe form of the disorder. Medium chain acyl-CoA dehydrogenase deficiency (choice C) results from mutations in the gene encoding medium chain acyl-CoA dehydrogenase. The most common symptom of MCAD deficiency is episodic hypoketotic hypoglycemia brought on by fasting. Symptoms appear within the first 2 years of life. Clinical crisis is characterized by an infant presenting with episodes of vomiting and lethargy that may progress to seizures and ultimately coma. Multiple acyl-CoA dehydrogenase deficiency (choice D) is a form of lipid storage myopathy (LSM). MADD results from mutations in either of the two genes that encode the protein components of the heterodimeric complex identified as electron transfer flavoprotein (ETF) or the gene encoding electron transfer flavoprotein dehydrogenase (encoded by the *ETFDH* gene). There are three different classifications of MADD based upon the timing and severity of symptoms and are referred to as the neonatal-onset with congenital anomalies (MADD type I), neonatal-onset without congenital anomalies (MADD type II), and the mild- and/or later-onset form (MADD type III). von Gierke disease (choice E) results from mutations in the gene encoding glucose-6-phosphatase. von Gierke disease can present during the neonatal period with lactic acidosis and hypoglycemia. More commonly though, infants of 3–4 months of age will manifest with hepatomegaly and hypoglycemic seizures. The hallmark features of this disease are hypoglycemia, lactic acidosis, hyperuricemia, and hyperlipidemia. The severity of the hypoglycemia and lactic acidosis can be such that in the past affected individuals died in infancy.

3. Correct answer is **C.** The infant is exhibiting all the signs and symptoms of medium chain acyl-CoA dehydrogenase (MCAD) deficiency. Deficiency in MCAD is the most common inherited defect in the pathways of mitochondrial fatty acid β-oxidation. The most common presentation of infants with this disorder is episodic hypoketotic hypoglycemia following periods of fasting. Although the first episode may be fatal, and incorrectly ascribed to sudden infant death syndrome, patients with MCAD deficiency are normal between episodes and are treated by avoidance of fasting and treatment of acute episodes with intravenous glucose. Accumulation of medium-chain acylcarnitines and dicarboxylic acids is diagnostic, in particular octanoylcarnitine. Andersen disease (choice A) is a glycogen storage disease that results from mutations in the glycogen-branching enzyme. Classic Andersen disease is a rapidly progressive disorder that will result in early lethality as a result of liver failure. Maple syrup urine disease (choice B) results from mutations in the gene encoding branched-chain ketoacid dehydrogenase. Classic MSUD is defined by neonatal onset of encephalopathy and is the most severe form of the disorder. The levels of the BCAAs, especially leucine, and their α-keto acids, are dramatically elevated in the blood, urine, and cerebrospinal fluid of afflicted infants. Multiple acyl-CoA dehydrogenase deficiency (choice D) is a form of lipid storage myopathy (LSM). MADD results from mutations in either of the two genes that encode the protein components of the heterodimeric complex identified as electron transfer flavoprotein (ETF) or the gene encoding electron transfer flavoprotein dehydrogenase (encoded by the *ETFDH* gene). There are three different classifications of MADD based upon the timing and severity of symptoms and are referred to as the neonatal-onset with congenital anomalies (MADD type I), neonatal-onset without congenital anomalies (MADD type II), and the mild- and/or later-onset form (MADD type III). von Gierke disease (choice E) results from mutations in the gene encoding glucose-6-phosphatase. von Gierke disease can present during the neonatal period with lactic acidosis and hypoglycemia. More commonly though, infants of 3–4 months of age will manifest with hepatomegaly and hypoglycemic seizures. The hallmark features of this disease are hypoglycemia, lactic acidosis, hyperuricemia, and hyperlipidemia. Zellweger syndrome (choice F) represents a constellation of disorders due to defects in the biogenesis and function of the peroxisomes. Zellweger syndrome is a lethal disorder usually before infants reach the age of 2 years.

4. Correct answer is **D.** The patient is most likely experiencing the signs and symptoms of medium chain acyl-CoA dehydrogenase deficiency (MCADD). Deficiency in MCAD is the most common inherited defect in the pathways of mitochondrial fatty acid oxidation. The most common presentation of infants with this disorder is episodic hypoketotic hypoglycemia following periods of fasting. Although the first episode may be fatal, and incorrectly ascribed to sudden infant death syndrome, patients with MCAD deficiency are normal between episodes and are treated by avoidance of fasting and treatment of acute episodes with intravenous glucose. Accumulation of medium-chain acylcarnitines, in particular octanoylcarnitine, and dicarboxylic acids is diagnostic of MCAD deficiency. Carnitine palmitoyltransferase-1 deficiency (choice A) affects primarily the liver and leads to reduced fatty acid oxidation and ketogenesis. The most common symptom associated with CPT-1 deficiency is hypoketotic hypoglycemia associated with hepatic pathology. Fructose-1,6-bisphosphatase deficiency (choice B), resulting from mutations in the *FBP1* gene which encodes the liver form of the enzyme, results in severely impaired hepatic gluconeogenesis and leads to episodes of hypoglycemia, apnea, hyperventilation, ketosis, and lactic acidosis. These symptoms can take on a lethal course in neonates. Glucose-6-phosphate dehydrogenase deficiency (choice C) results in the glycogen storage disorder known as von Gierke disease. von Gierke disease can present during the neonatal period with lactic acidosis and hypoglycemia. More commonly though, infants of 3–4 months of age will manifest with hepatomegaly and hypoglycemic seizures. Mitochondrial trifunctional protein (choice E) is a complex composed of α-subunits and β-subunits encoded by the *HADHA* and *HADHB* genes, respectively. The major form of MTP deficiency results from mutations in that *HADHA* gene. The clinical symptoms associated with MTP deficiency include hypoketotic hypoglycemia, metabolic acidosis, metabolic encephalopathy, liver dysfunction, cardiomyopathy, exercise-induced myoglobinuria, and rhabdomyolysis.

5. Correct answer is **C.** Even with injected insulin, the normal processes that are regulated by insulin are poorly controlled in type 1 diabetics. The poorly regulated insulin function leads to inappropriate and ineffective regulation of the expression of lipoprotein lipase in the endothelium of cardiac muscle, skeletal muscle, and adipose tissue. The lack of appropriate levels of lipoprotein lipase activity result in the inability to remove fatty acids from circulating triglycerides present in chylomicrons and VLDL. The absence of sufficient lipoprotein lipase activity results in the hypertriglyceridemia common in type 1 diabetics. Clearance of VLDL cholesterol (choice A) is not significantly affected in type 1 diabetics. LDL receptor activity (choice B) is not significantly affected in type 1 diabetics. The poorly regulated release of glucagon from the pancreas in type 1 diabetics results in increased delivery of free fatty acids to the liver from adipose tissue (choice D); however, this is not a contributor to the hypertriglyceridemia as is typical in type 1 diabetes. Hepatic lipase activity (choice E) is not significantly altered or abnormal in type 1 diabetics. The activity of lecithin:cholesterol acetyltransferase (choice F) is not significantly altered in type 1 diabetics.

6. Correct answer is **C.** Riboflavin serves as a precursor for the coenzyme form of the vitamin, flavin adenine dinucleotide (FAD). Mitochondrial β-oxidation of fatty acids, such as palmitate, requires several dehydrogenases, the first being the acyl-CoA dehydrogenases that require FAD as a cofactor for their reaction. Therefore, reduced ability to generate FAD would have a negative impact on the abilities of mitochondrial fatty acid β-oxidation to take place. Synthesis of the malonyl-CoA (choice A) requires the enzyme acetyl-CoA carboxylase which is a biotin-dependent enzyme and therefore would not be affected by reduced riboflavin. Peroxisomal oxidation of phytanoyl-CoA (choice B) involves the α-oxidation pathway which requires the nicotinic acid-derived cofactor, NAD^+. Peroxisomal omega oxidation (choice D) involves enzymes of the alcohol dehydrogenase and aldehyde dehydrogenase family which require NAD^+ as cofactor, not FAD. Synthesis of palmitate (choice E) involves the enzyme fatty acid synthase which requires the reduced cofactor, NADPH, and therefore does not involve the use of riboflavin-derived coenzyme.

7. Correct answer is **B.** Malonyl-CoA is the product of the acetyl-CoA carboxylase (ACC) reaction. Acetyl-CoA carboxylase is the rate-limiting enzyme in fatty acid biosynthesis, therefore, increased production of malonyl-CoA from ACC would result in increased fatty acid biosynthesis. Synthesis of none of the other lipids (choices A, C, D, and E) involves the intermediate, malonyl-CoA.

8. Correct answer is **D.** Pancreatic lipase is the primary lipase that hydrolyzes dietary triglycerides in the small intestines. The action of alkaline pancreatic juice results in inhibition of the activity of the acid lipases (lingual and gastric) that begin the process of triglyceride hydrolysis in the stomach. Although a normal diet contains phospholipids and cholesterol, the predominant lipids are triglycerides. Loss of pancreatic lipase secretion would, therefore, result in incomplete digestion of dietary triglycerides preventing their absorption and leading to increased fat content of the feces. Carboxyl ester lipase (choice A) is involved in the hydrolysis of the fatty acid esterified to the carbon-3 position of cholesterol. Carboxypeptidase A (choice B) and chymotrypsinogen (choice C) are pancreatic proteases involved in protein digestion, not lipid digestion. Phospholipase A_2 (choice E) is a pancreatic enzyme involved in hydrolysis of dietary phospholipids not triglycerides.

9. Correct answer is **C.** The patient is most likely suffering the consequences of the disorder known as adult myopathic CPT deficiency. Myopathic CPT deficiency results from mutations in the gene encoding carnitine palmitoyltransferase 2 (CPT-2). CPT-2 is an enzyme present on the inner mitochondrial membrane involved in the transport of fatty acylcarnitines into the matrix of the mitochondria for oxidation. The adult form of CPT-2 deficiency, the myopathic form, is the most common form of CPT-2 deficiency. The myopathic form of CPT-2 deficiency is also the most common disorder of lipid metabolism that affects skeletal muscle as well as the most common cause of inherited myoglobinuria. This form of CPT-2 deficiency is characterized by recurrent episodes of muscle pain, rhabdomyolysis, and myoglobinuria that is triggered by prolonged exercise. Defects in this none of the other processes (choices A, B, D, and E) would account for the signs and symptoms in this patient.

10. Correct answer is **D.** The patient is manifesting the hallmarks of Zellweger syndrome (ZWS). Zellweger syndrome is not a single disorder but a family of pathologically related disorders that result from mutations in several genes involved in the biogenesis of the peroxisomes. Classic Zellweger syndrome is a neonatal presenting severe disorder. The most common clinical manifestations of ZWS include a series of characteristic craniofacial abnormalities that can lead to a diagnosis of Down syndrome. Due to the lack of proper peroxisomal lipid metabolism very long-chain fatty acids and various branched-chain fatty acids accumulate in the tissues impairing their functions. Since the peroxisomes are also important in ether phospholipid and plasmalogen synthesis, which are critical lipids in brain function, there is progressive impairment of neuronal migration and neuronal positioning as well as decreased myelin production. Definitive diagnosis of ZWS is commonly accomplished through measurement of the levels of plasma very long-chain fatty acids. Most common observations are increased levels of C26:0 (hexacosanoic acid; also called cerotic acid) and C26:1 (cis-17-hexacosenoic acid). Defects in this none of the other processes (choices A, B, C, and E) would account for the signs and symptoms in this patient.

11. Correct answer is **E.** Patients manifesting symptoms of hyperlipidemia, that include severely elevated triglyceride levels, as in this patient, are most likely deficient in lipoprotein lipase or its necessary cofactor apoC-II. Deficiency in either LPL or apoC-II is a cause of a family of related monogenic disorders collectively identified as familial chylomicronemia syndrome (FCS) (see Clinical Box 16–1). A predominant and characteristic feature of FCS is that affected individuals have highly elevated levels of triglycerides. Additional symptoms include episodes of abdominal pain, recurrent acute pancreatitis, eruptive xanthomas, and hepatosplenomegaly. Deficiencies in none of the other options (choices A, B, C, and D) would properly account for the signs and symptoms in this patient.

12. Correct answer is **E.** The infant is most likely suffering from the signs and symptoms of a deficiency in medium chain acyl-CoA dehydrogenase, MCAD. Mitochondrial β-oxidation of long-chain fatty acids, such as palmitate, cease when these fats become medium-chain length. Therefore, in patients with MCAD deficiency, oxidation of palmitate would be deficient. Metabolism of none of the other substrates (choices A, B, C, and D) would be defective in patients with MCAD deficiency.

13. Correct answer is **C.** The patient is most likely exhibiting the symptoms of medium chain acyl-CoA dehydrogenase, MCAD deficiency (MCADD). In infants, the supply of glycogen lasts less than 6 hours and gluconeogenesis is not sufficient to maintain adequate blood glucose levels. Normally, during periods of fasting (in particular during the night) the oxidation of fatty acids provides the necessary ATP to fuel hepatic gluconeogenesis as well as ketone bodies for non-hepatic tissue energy production. Normally, hypoglycemia is accompanied by an increase in ketone formation from the increased oxidation of fatty acids. In MCAD deficiency there is a reduced level of fatty acid oxidation, hence near normal, or low levels of ketones are detected in the serum. Accumulation of medium-chain acylcarnitines, in particular octanoylcarnitine, and dicarboxylic acids is diagnostic of MCAD deficiency. Acetone (choice A) is the nonenzymatic product of acetoacetate, a ketone body, whose levels would be low in MCAD deficiency. Bilirubin (choice B) would be elevated in any patient where there is increased hemolysis. Glucocerebrosidase (choice D) is found at elevated levels in patients suffering from Gaucher disease. The predominant form of Gaucher disease manifests in adults, not infants. Increased levels of methylmalonic acid (choice E) are found in patients with a vitamin B_{12} deficiency or a deficiency in the methylmalonyl-CoA mutase enzyme that requires B_{12} for its activity. Increased accumulation of sphingomyelin (choice F) occurs in patients suffering from the lysosomal storage disease identified as Niemann-Pick disease.

14. Correct answer is **E.** Skeletal muscle prefers to oxidize fatty acids for the production of energy. Oxidation of the predominant forms of fatty acids in the human body, long-chain fatty acids, requires prior attachment to carnitine in order to be transferred into the mitochondrial matrix for oxidation. A reduced capacity to carry out mitochondrial fatty acid oxidation in the absence of sufficient carnitine production would result in the accumulation of triglycerides within skeletal muscle cells. None of the other options (choices A, B, C, D,

and F) would be associated with the consequences of a deficiency in carnitine production.

15. Correct answer is **B.** The infant is most likely exhibiting the symptoms of MCAD deficiency (MCADD). In infants, the supply of glycogen lasts less than 6 hours and gluconeogenesis is not sufficient to maintain adequate blood glucose levels. Normally, during periods of fasting (in particular during the night) the oxidation of fatty acids provides the necessary ATP to fuel hepatic gluconeogenesis as well as ketone bodies for nonhepatic tissue energy production. Normally, hypoglycemia is accompanied by an increase in ketone formation from the increased oxidation of fatty acids. In MCAD deficiency there is a reduced level of fatty acid oxidation, hence near normal, or low levels of ketones are detected in the serum. Accumulation of medium-chain acylcarnitines, in particular octanoylcarnitine, and dicarboxylic acids is diagnostic of MCAD deficiency. Defects in amino acid metabolism (choice A) would be associated with disorders such as phenylketonuria and Maple syrup urine disease. The most likely disorder of glucose metabolism (choice C) would be erythrocyte pyruvate kinase deficiency. Defects in glycogen metabolism (choice D) are associated with multiple forms of glycogen storage disease such as von Gierke disease. Numerous lysosomal storage diseases are the result of defects in glycosphingolipid metabolism (choice E) such as in the case of Tay-Sachs disease.

16. Correct answer is **A.** Deficiencies in the activity of the carnitine palmitoyltransferases lead to impaired energy production from fatty acid oxidation. Deficiencies in CPT-1 are relatively rare and affect primarily the liver and lead to reduced fatty acid oxidation and ketogenesis. The most common symptom associated with CPT-1 deficiency is hepatic encephalopathy presenting with hypoketotic hypoglycemia and sudden onset of liver failure. There is also an elevation in blood levels of carnitine. The liver involvement results in hepatomegaly and in muscles results in weakness. A high carbohydrate, low-fat diet composed of primarily short- and medium-chain triglycerides is required. Medium- and short-chain fatty acids can enter the mitochondria without the need for the carnitine shuttle. A defect in carnitine synthesis (choice B) would not allow for free carnitine concentration to be increased in the patient. Defects in fatty acyl-CoA synthetases (choice C) have not been identified associated with any significant pathology. Medium-chain acyl-CoA dehydrogenase deficiency (choice D) results from mutations in the gene encoding medium chain acyl-CoA dehydrogenase. The most common symptom of MCAD deficiency is episodic hypoketotic hypoglycemia brought on by fasting. Disorders of peroxisomal fat oxidation (choice E) predominantly include disorders such as Refsum disease and Zellweger syndrome.

17. Correct answer is **D.** The signs and symptoms in the infant are most likely indicative of a defect in fatty acid oxidation. The most common causes of hypoketotic hypoglycemia in an infant are medium-chain acyl-CoA dehydrogenase deficiency or defects in carnitine uptake or synthesis. Since these possibilities were ruled out, the infant must harbor a defect at some other level of the regulation of fatty acid oxidation. The results of the adipose tissue assays indicated that glucagon and epinephrine cannot stimulate the release of fatty acids from triglycerides thereby preventing adequate fatty acid oxidation in the liver to support gluconeogenesis. Since both hormones bind their receptors and activate the associated G-protein the defect lies downstream and interferes with activated release of fatty acids. Both glucagon and epinephrine signaling activates PKA which in turn phosphorylates and activates hormone-sensitive lipase resulting in increased fatty acid release from adipose tissue. Adipose triglyceride lipase (choice A) is responsible for the removal of a fatty acid from adipose tissue triglycerides which generates the substrate for hormone-sensitive lipase. This enzyme is not regulated by glucagon or epinephrine. Monoglyceride lipase (choice B) hydrolyzes the last fatty acid from the monoglycerides generated by hormone-sensitive lipase. This enzyme is not regulated by glucagon or epinephrine. Phosphodiesterase (choice C) and PKB (choice E) are both activated by insulin in adipose tissue to prevent the breakdown of triglycerides. Defects in both would most likely be associated with increased, not decreased, fatty acid release from adipose tissue.

18. Correct answer is **E.** The patient is most likely experiencing the signs and symptoms of Refsum disease. Refsum disease is the result of deficiencies in the peroxisomal enzyme responsible for one of the initial steps in the oxidation of phytanic acid, a 3-methyl substituted fatty acid derived from the chlorophyll, phytol, specifically phytanoyl-CoA hydroxylase (also called phytanoyl-CoA dioxygenase). Phytanoyl-CoA hydroxylase carries out an initial α-oxidation reaction in the pathway resulting in the generation of the 19-carbon fatty acid, pristanic acid. The cardinal clinical features of Refsum disease are retinitis pigmentosa, chronic polyneuropathy, cerebellar ataxia, and elevated protein levels in cerebrospinal fluid. Most Refsum patients have electrocardiographic changes, and some have sensorineural hearing loss and/or ichthyosis. Multiple epiphyseal dysplasia (skeletal malformations) is a conspicuous feature in some cases. Refsum disease is a slowly developing, progressive peripheral neuropathy. Progression of the disease results in severe motor weakness and muscle wasting, particularly in the lower extremities. Defects in bile acid metabolism (choice A) are most often discovered in the neonatal period and associated with progressive hepatic involvement. Defects in branched-chain amino acid metabolism (choice B) result in the potentially neonatal lethal disorder called maple syrup urine disease. The most likely disorder of lysosomal glycosphingolipid metabolism (choice C) is Tay-Sachs disease which is a lethal disorder resulting in death by 2–3 years of age. The most common disorder of mitochondrial fatty acid β-oxidation (choice D) is medium-chain acyl-CoA dehydrogenase deficiency (MCADD). The symptoms of MCADD manifest in the neonatal period and include severe hypoglycemia associated with hypoketonemia.

19. Correct answer is **A.** Mitochondrial fatty acid β-oxidation requires that these fats be activated by attachment to CoA. Activation is catalyzed by a family of fatty acyl-CoA synthetases (also called acyl-CoA ligases or thiokinases). The net result of this activation process is the consumption of two molar equivalents of ATP. The process of mitochondrial fatty acid β-oxidation involves two different classes of dehydrogenases. The first group of dehydrogenases utilize FAD as a cofactor and in the course of oxidizing their substrate generate $FADH_2$. A defect in fatty acid activation would, consequently, result in decreased ATP consumption associated with their activation and a decrease in $FADH_2$ production via their oxidation. Defects in none of the other enzymes (choices B, C, D, and E) would be associated with reduced ATP consumption and reduction in $FADH_2$ production.

20. Correct answer is **E.** Oxidation of fatty acids occurs in the mitochondria and the peroxisomes via similar enzymatic pathways referred to as β-oxidation. Fatty acids of between 4 to 8 and between 6 to 12 carbon atoms in length, referred to as short- and medium-chain fatty acids (SCFA and MCFA, respectively), are oxidized exclusively in the mitochondria. Long-chain fatty acids (LCFA: 10–16 carbons long) are oxidized in both the mitochondria and the peroxisomes with the peroxisomes exhibiting preference for 14-carbon and longer LCFAs. Very-long-chain fatty acids (VLCFA: C17–C26) undergo oxidation initiated exclusively in the peroxisomes. Lysosomal glycolipid metabolism (choice A) is not associated with the metabolism of very long-chain saturated fatty acids. Microsomal fatty acid ω-oxidation (choice B) is a pathway by which a carboxylic acid group is added to the ω-end of fatty acids. Mitochondrial fatty acid β-oxidation (choice C) does not include the oxidation of very long-chain fatty acids. Peroxisomal fatty acid α-oxidation (choice D) involves the oxidation of methyl substituted fatty acids such as phytanic acid.

21. Correct answer is **E.** Peroxisomes oxidize long-chain fatty acid via a β-oxidation pathway where the first reaction generates H_2O_2 (a reactive oxygen species, ROS) instead of $FADH_2$ as for mitochondrial β-oxidation. A diet high in fatty acids results in higher levels of peroxisomal fatty acid oxidation resulting in increased levels of H_2O_2 production. Within the β-cells of the pancreas this increased ROS production cannot be tolerated due to low, to no, catalase production in these cells. The net result is β-cell dysfunction and the triggering mitochondrially-induced apoptosis (see Chapter 34). None of the other options (choices A, B, C, and D) reflect contributions to the destruction of pancreatic insulin secreting cells on a high-fat diet as is typical of overweight and obese individuals.

22. Correct answer is **B.** The microsomal (endoplasmic reticulum, ER) pathway of fatty acid ω-oxidation represents a minor pathway of overall fatty acid oxidation. Human ω-hydroxylases are all members of the cytochrome P450 family (CYP) of enzymes. These enzymes are abundant in the liver and kidneys. Specifically, it is members of the CYP4A and CYP4F families that preferentially hydroxylate the terminal methyl group of C10–C26 length fatty acids. The ω-hydroxylated form of arachidonic acid, 20-hydroxyeicosatetraenoic acid (20-HETE) is produced through the action of CYP4A11. 20-HETE has been shown to be involved in the activation of pro-inflammatory pathways, and the signaling pathways leading to hypertension, both of which contribute to the development of obesity, type 2 diabetes, and cardiovascular disease. None of the other pathways (choice A, C, D, and E) are associated with the function of CYP4A11.

23. Correct answer is **B.** The patient most likely suffers from a disorder known as adult myopathic CPT deficiency. This disorder is caused by mutations in the gene (CPT2) encoding the enzyme, carnitine palmitoyltransferase 2. The myopathic form of CPT-2 deficiency is the most common inherited disorder of lipid metabolism that affects skeletal muscle as well as the most common cause of inherited myoglobinuria. This form of CPT-2 deficiency is characterized by recurrent episodes of muscle pain, rhabdomyolysis, and myoglobinuria that is triggered by prolonged exercise. Myopathic CPT deficiency can be diagnosed by performing histopathology of skeletal muscle biopsy using the lipophilic stain, Sudan black. Histopathology using PAS stain (choice A and C) is used to assay for the accumulation of carbohydrate, not lipids. None of the other assays (choice D, E, and F) would be useful in the correct diagnosis of myopathic CPT deficiency.

24. Correct answer is **B.** Carnitine is required for the transport of long-chain fatty acids from the outer mitochondrial membrane into the mitochondria matrix for oxidation. Limiting levels of carnitine would, therefore, result in reduced rates of mitochondrial β-oxidation of fatty acids. A reduced capacity for mitochondrial β-oxidation would ultimately result in a reduced capacity for cells to take fatty acids from the blood ultimately leading to hyperlipidemia. Since fatty acid oxidation would be impaired there would be reduced ketogenesis (choice E) occurring and less energy production would restrict gluconeogenesis (choice C). Increased levels of dicarboxylic acids (choice A) are diagnostic for medium chain acyl-CoA dehydrogenase deficiency. Reduced levels of carnitine would result in decreased, not increased (choice D), levels of fatty acid oxidation.

25. Correct answer is **E.** Ketogenesis occurs in the liver from acetyl-CoA during high rates of fatty acid oxidation such as would be occurring during early starvation or on high-fat diets. The principal ketone bodies are acetoacetate and β-hydroxybutyrate, which are reversibly synthesized in a reaction catalyzed by β-hydroxybutyrate dehydrogenase. The liver delivers acetoacetate and β-hydroxybutyrate to the circulation where they are taken up by nonhepatic tissue for use as an oxidizable fuel. The brain will derive much of its energy from ketone body oxidation during prolonged fasting and starvation. Within extrahepatic tissues, β-hydroxybutyrate is converted to acetoacetate by β-hydroxybutyrate dehydrogenase. Acetoacetate is reactivated to acetoacetyl-CoA in a reaction catalyzed by succinyl-CoA: 3-oxoacid-CoA-transferase (also called succinyl-CoA-acetoacetate-CoA-transferase or acetoacetate: succinyl-CoA-CoA transferase), which uses succinyl-CoA as the source of CoA. This enzyme is not expressed in hepatocytes. Therefore, the ability to utilize β-hydroxybutyrate in the hepatoma cells indicates that expression of the succinyl-CoA: 3-oxoacid-CoA-transferase gene has been activated. All of the other enzyme options (choices A, B, C, and D) are normally expressed in hepatocytes.

26. Correct answer is **D.** The patient is most likely experiencing the signs and symptoms of medium-chain acyl-CoA dehydrogenase deficiency (MCADD). Deficiency in MCAD is the most common inherited defect in the pathways of mitochondrial fatty acid β-oxidation. The most common presentation of infants with this disorder is episodic hypoketotic hypoglycemia following periods of fasting. With MCAD deficiency there is a reduced level of fatty acid oxidation, hence near normal, or low levels of ketones are detected in the serum. Accumulation of medium-chain acylcarnitines, in particular octanoylcarnitine, and dicarboxylic acids is diagnostic of MCAD deficiency. The reduced capacity to generate sufficient ATP via fatty acid oxidation in MCAD deficiency patients results in an inability to carry out hepatic gluconeogenesis. The reduced hepatic gluconeogenesis leads to severe hypoglycemia and an increased accumulation of red blood cell-derived lactate in the blood. This lactic acidemia is the basis for the metabolic acidosis that is common in MCAD deficiency patients. Hyperammonemia (choice B) is commonly found in MCAD deficient patients, but never associated with hyperketonemia. None of the other signs and symptoms (choices A, C, and E) are associated with the overall pathology of MCAD deficiency.

27. Correct answer is **C.** As a result of the patient's surgery, she lacks the distal ileum of her small intestine necessary for the absorption of vitamin B_{12} resulting in her macrocytic anemia. Vitamin B_{12} is a required cofactor for methylmalonyl-CoA mutase. Methyl malonyl-CoA mutase catalyzes the last reaction in the conversion of propionyl-CoA to succinyl-CoA. The mitochondrial oxidation of fatty acids with an odd number of carbon atoms, as well as the oxidation of several amino acids (methionine, isoleucine, threonine, and valine), produces propionyl-CoA. Therefore, a deficiency in vitamin B_{12} is associated with a lack of ability to metabolize fatty acids with an odd number of carbon atoms. None of the other processes (choices A, B, D, and E) would be affected in this patient with a vitamin B_{12} deficiency.

28. Correct answer is **D.** The signs and symptoms in this patient are most likely indicative of Refsum disease. Refsum disease is an autosomal recessive disorder that results from defects in peroxisomal fatty acid metabolism. Specifically, the disorder is due to deficiencies in the peroxisomal enzyme, phytanoyl-CoA hydroxylase, responsible for one of the initial steps in the oxidation of phytanic acid, a 3-methyl substituted fatty acid derived from the chlorophyll, phytol. The cardinal clinical features of Refsum disease are retinitis pigmentosa, chronic polyneuropathy, cerebellar ataxia, and elevated protein levels in cerebrospinal fluid. Most Refsum patients have electrocardiographic changes, and some have sensorineural hearing loss and/or ichthyosis. Multiple epiphyseal dysplasia (skeletal malformations) is a conspicuous feature in some cases. Refsum disease is a slowly developing, progressive peripheral neuropathy. Progression of the disease results in severe motor weakness and muscle wasting, particularly in the lower extremities. Defects in none of the other processes (choices A, B, C, and E) result in the characteristic signs and symptoms of Refsum disease seen in this patient.

29. Correct answer is **D.** Propionyl-CoA is converted to succinyl-CoA in a series of reactions using three different enzymes. It is first carboxylated in an ATP-dependent reaction catalyzed by propionyl-CoA carboxylase, an enzyme that requires biotin as a cofactor. The product of the first reaction, D-methylmalonyl-CoA is then converted to L-methylmalonyl-CoA by methylmalonyl-CoA racemase. Finally, methylmalonyl-CoA is converted to succinyl-CoA by the vitamin B_{12}-requiring enzyme, methylmalonyl-CoA mutase. A defect in this pathway would result in the accumulation of the substrate of whichever enzyme was defective. Most commonly mutations are found in propionyl-CoA carboxylase or methylmalonyl-CoA mutase. Mutations in methylmalonyl-CoA mutase or deficiency of vitamin B_{12} will result in increased serum and urine concentrations of methylmalonic acid. None of the other substances (choices A, B, C, and E) are associated with the metabolism of fatty acids with an odd number of carbon atoms.

30. Correct answer is **D.** When the carbons of fatty acids are oxidized for energy production, the by-product of that process is the two-carbon compound, acetyl-CoA. Acetyl-CoA can then enter the TCA cycle for complete oxidation. Although, several compounds of the TCA cycle can be directed into the gluconeogenic pathway of glucose synthesis, the carbons of acetyl-CoA cannot provide a net source of carbon in that latter pathway. This is due to the fact that, following entry of the two carbons of acetyl-CoA into the TCA cycle, two carbons are lost as CO_2 during the subsequent reactions of the cycle, one by the reaction catalyzed by isocitrate dehydrogenase and the other by the reaction catalyzed by 2-oxoglutarate dehydrogenase (α-ketoglutarate dehydrogenase). None of the other options (choices A, B, C, and E) correctly explains the biochemical mechanism that prevents the carbons of fatty acids contributing to net glucose synthesis.

31. Correct answer is **B.** Insulin stimulates fatty acid synthesis through its activation of the activity of the rate-limiting enzyme, acetyl-CoA carboxylase (ACC). The product of the ACC reaction is malonyl-CoA. Malonyl-CoA binds to the outer mitochondrial membrane-associated enzyme, carnitine palmitoyltransferase 1 (CPT1), inhibiting its ability to exchange the CoA on an activated fatty acid for carnitine. The inhibition of CPT1 prevents the newly synthesized palmitic acid from being oxidized. Since fat oxidation is occurring in the cells in this study the binding site for malonyl-CoA must be defective. The loss of inhibition of CPT1 allows palmitoyl-CoA to be converted to palmitoyl-carnitine and transported into the matrix of the mitochondria for oxidation. Although an abnormal activity of each of the other enzymes (choices A, C, D, and E) might result in fatty acid oxidation under insulin-stimulation, the most direct effect of insulin is at the level of CPT1.

32. Correct answer is **D.** The infant is most likely exhibiting the signs and symptoms of multiple acyl-CoA dehydrogenase deficiency (MADD) which is a form of lipid storage myopathy (LSM). MADD results from mutations in either of the two genes that encode the protein components of the heterodimeric complex identified as electron transfer flavoprotein (ETF) or the gene encoding electron transfer flavoprotein dehydrogenase (encoded by the *ETFDH* gene). There are three different classifications of MADD based upon the timing and severity of symptoms and are referred to as the neonatal-onset with congenital anomalies (MADD type I), neonatal-onset without congenital anomalies (MADD type II), and the mild- and/or later-onset form (MADD type III). Onset of type I or II MADD is usually in the neonatal period and symptoms include severe metabolic acidosis, nonketotic hypoglycemia, and hyperammonemia. Many of these affected patients will die in the neonatal period despite metabolic treatment. Infants who survive the neonatal period will suffer from recurrent episodes of metabolic decompensation resembling Reye syndrome. Very often these infants will also develop hypertrophic cardiomyopathy. In type I MADD the congenital anomalies may include dysmorphic facial features and large cystic kidneys. In males, the type I disease is associated with hypospadias. Andersen disease (choice A) is a glycogen storage disease that results from mutations in the glycogen branching enzyme. Classic Andersen disease is a rapidly progressive disorder that will result in early lethality as a result of liver failure. Maple syrup urine disease (choice B) results from mutations in the gene encoding branched-chain ketoacid dehydrogenase. Classic MSUD is defined by neonatal onset of encephalopathy and is the most severe form of the disorder. The levels of the BCAAs, especially leucine, and their α-keto acids, are dramatically elevated in the blood, urine and cerebrospinal fluid of afflicted infants. Medium-chain acyl-CoA dehydrogenase deficiency (choice C) is the most common inherited defect in the pathways of mitochondrial fatty acid oxidation. The most common presentation of infants with this disorder is episodic hypoketotic hypoglycemia following periods of fasting. Although the patient in this case exhibits similar symptoms to those of MCAD deficiency, there is no associated hypospadias with MCAD deficiency. von Gierke disease (choice E) results from mutations in the gene encoding glucose-6-phosphatase. von Gierke disease can present during the neonatal period with lactic acidosis and hypoglycemia. More commonly though, infants of 3–4 months of age will manifest with hepatomegaly and hypoglycemic seizures. The hallmark features of this disease are hypoglycemia, lactic acidosis, hyperuricemia, and hyperlipidemia. Zellweger syndrome (choice F) represents a constellation of disorders due to defects in the biogenesis and function of the peroxisomes. Zellweger syndrome is a lethal disorder usually before infants reach the age of 2 years.

33. Correct answer is **D.** The patient is most likely experiencing the signs and symptoms of Refsum disease. Refsum disease is the result of deficiencies in the peroxisomal enzyme responsible for one of the initial steps in the oxidation of phytanic acid, a 3-methyl substituted fatty acid derived from the chlorophyll, phytol, specifically phytanoyl-CoA hydroxylase (also called phytanoyl-CoA dioxygenase). Phytanoyl-CoA hydroxylase carries out an initial α-oxidation reaction in the pathway resulting in the generation of the 19-carbon fatty acid, pristanic acid. The cardinal clinical features of Refsum disease are retinitis pigmentosa, chronic polyneuropathy, cerebellar ataxia, and elevated protein levels in cerebrospinal fluid. Most Refsum patients have electrocardiographic changes, and some have sensorineural hearing loss and/or ichthyosis. Multiple epiphyseal dysplasia (skeletal malformations) is a conspicuous feature in some cases. Refsum disease is a slowly developing, progressive peripheral neuropathy. Progression of the disease results in severe motor weakness and muscle wasting, particularly in the lower extremities. Carnitine deficiency, systemic primary (choice A) typically presents in patients before 2 years of age. Infants with primary carnitine deficiency exhibit poor feeding and can become lethargic and minimally responsive. The presentation of primary carnitine deficiency is quite variable with respect to the age of onset, the severity of the symptoms, and the involved organs. Medium chain acyl-CoA dehydrogenase deficiency (choice B) results in the disorder known as MCAD deficiency. MCAD deficiency is associated with severe hypoglycemia along with hypoketonemia in the early neonatal stages. Mitochondrial trifunctional protein (choice C) is a complex composed of α-subunits and β-subunits encoded by the *HADHA* and *HADHB* genes, respectively. The major form of MTP deficiency results from mutations in that *HADHA* gene. The clinical symptoms associated with MTP deficiency include hypoketotic hypoglycemia, metabolic acidosis, metabolic encephalopathy, liver dysfunction, cardiomyopathy, exercise-induced myoglobinuria, and rhabdomyolysis. Zellweger syndrome (choice E) represents a constellation of disorders due to defects in the biogenesis and function of the peroxisomes. Zellweger syndrome is a lethal disorder usually before infants reach the age of 2 years.

34. Correct answer is **B.** The infant is exhibiting all the signs and symptoms of medium-chain acyl-CoA dehydrogenase (MCAD) deficiency. Deficiency in MCAD is the most common inherited defect in the pathways of mitochondrial fatty acid β-oxidation. The most common presentation of infants with this disorder is episodic hypoketotic hypoglycemia following periods of fasting. Although the first episode may be fatal, and incorrectly ascribed to sudden infant death syndrome, patients with MCAD deficiency are normal between episodes and are treated by avoidance of fasting and treatment of acute episodes with intravenous glucose. Accumulation of medium-chain acylcarnitines and dicarboxylic acids is diagnostic, in particular octanoylcarnitine. Since MCAD deficiency impairs fatty acid oxidation and, thus ketogenesis, the measurement of acetoacetate (choice A) would not aid in a diagnosis in this patient. Accumulation of long-chain acylcarnitines (choice C) would be indicative of a defect in mitochondrial fatty acid oxidation and, thus, reduced production of ketones. However, a deficiency in mitochondrial very long-chain acyl-CoA dehydrogenase (VLCAD), which is responsible for oxidation of long-chain fatty acids, is not as common as MCAD deficiency, and this disorder is also associated with early onset cardiac and multiorgan failure that does not appear to be the situation with this patient. Measurement for phytanoyl-CoA levels (choice D) would be useful for aiding a diagnosis of Refsum disease. Refsum disease is a slowly developing, progressive peripheral neuropathy but is not associated with disturbances in glucose or mitochondrial fatty acid metabolism. Measurement for propionyl-CoA levels (choice E) would be useful for aiding a diagnosis of propionic acidemia. Metabolic disturbances that are common to the neonatal form of propionic acidemia include ketonuria, hypoglycemia, hyperammonemia, and high anion gap metabolic acidosis.

35. Correct answer is **E.** The low levels of carnitine present in this patient suggest that the patient has a defect in the ability to properly obtain carnitine. This indicates that the patient is most likely suffering from primary carnitine deficiency, more commonly referred to as carnitine deficiency, systemic primary. The typical metabolic presentation in patients with primary carnitine deficiency occurs most frequently before 2 years of age. Infants with primary carnitine deficiency exhibit poor feeding and can become lethargic and minimally responsive. The presentation of primary carnitine deficiency is quite variable with respect to the age of onset, the severity of the symptoms, and the involved organs. The lack of adequate carnitine results in impaired ability of the mitochondria to oxidize long-chain fatty acids which in turn impairs the process of ketogenesis. The inability to oxidize fatty acids in patients with primary carnitine deficiency would lead to decreased hepatic ATP production and, as a result, a reduced capacity to carry out gluconeogenesis (choice B), but it would not be the most likely impaired process in the patient. Impairment in none of the other processes (choices A, C, D, and F) would be significantly affected in a patient with primary carnitine deficiency.

CHAPTER

14

Ethanol Metabolism

High-Yield Terms

Alcohol dehydrogenase (ADH)	Any of a family of enzymes that catalyze the interconversion of alcohols and aldehydes or ketones; humans express multiple forms of ADH from at least seven distinct genes
Aldehyde dehydrogenase (ALDH)	Any of a family of enzymes that catalyze the oxidation of aldehydes; two primary enzymes, ALDH1A1 and ALDH2, involved in metabolizing acetaldehyde generated during ethanol oxidation
Microsomal ethanol oxidizing system, MEOS	Inducible ethanol metabolizing system employing a cytochrome P450 enzyme (CYP2E1)
Hepatic steatosis	Condition of fatty liver that can result from excess alcohol consumption
Nonalcoholic fatty liver disease (NAFLD)	One cause of a fatty liver (steatosis) not due to excessive alcohol use; most common form of chronic liver disease; obesity and activation of CYP2E1 are major contributors to development of NAFLD and NASH
Nonalcoholic steatohepatitis, NASH	Progression of NAFLD to state of inflammation and fibrosis; the major feature in NASH is fat in the liver; along with inflammation and cellular damage, obesity and activation of CYP2E1 are major contributors to development of NAFLD and NASH
NAPQI	*N*-acetyl-p-benzoquinone imine (NAPQI) is a toxic metabolite of acetaminophen (paracetamol) whose levels are enhanced by ethanol consumption

ETHANOL METABOLIZING PATHWAYS

The bulk of ingested alcohol is metabolized in the liver. The process of ethanol oxidation can proceed via several pathways but two are prevalent and clinically the most significant.

The primary pathway of hepatic ethanol metabolism is that initiated by class I alcohol dehydrogenases (ADH). These enzymes require NAD^+ and are expressed at high concentrations in the cytosol of hepatocytes. ADH oxidizes ethanol to acetaldehyde while simultaneously reducing NAD^+ to NADH (Figure 14–1). The acetaldehyde then enters the mitochondria where it is oxidized to acetate by one of the aldehyde dehydrogenases (ALDH) while simultaneously reducing NAD^+ to NADH.

The second major pathway for ethanol metabolism is the microsomal ethanol oxidizing system (MEOS) which involves the NADPH-dependent cytochrome P450 enzyme, CYP2E1 (see Figure 14–2). The MEOS pathway is induced in individuals who chronically consume alcohol.

HIGH-YIELD CONCEPT

Humans evolved to express multiple ADH genes and isoforms, not for metabolism of ethanol, but to metabolize naturally occurring alcohols found in foods as well as those produced by intestinal bacteria. As an example, one form of ADH is responsible for the metabolism of not only ethanol but also retinol to retinaldehyde which is the form of vitamin A necessary for vision.

HIGH-YIELD CONCEPT

Due to the negative physiologic effects of one of the alleles of the *ALDH2* gene (identified as ALDH2*2 allele), even heterozygous individuals are strongly protected against alcohol dependence.

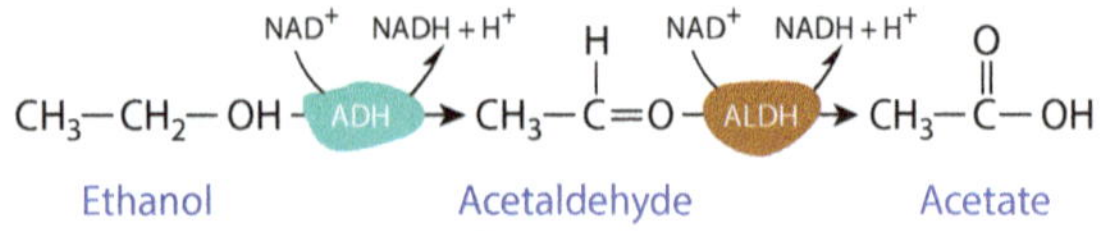

FIGURE 14–1 Reactions of ethanol metabolism. (Reproduced with permission from themedicalbiochemistrypage, LLC.)

HIGH-YIELD CONCEPT

Increased activity of CYP2E1 results in accelerated production of lipid hydroperoxides and is a significant contributor to the development of nonalcoholic fatty liver disease (NAFLD) and nonalcoholic steatohepatitis (NASH). Both NAFLD and NASH are commonly associated with obesity, type 2 diabetes, and hyperlipidemia.

There are two primary ALDH genes in humans that are responsible for the oxidation of acetaldehyde generated during the oxidation of ethanol. The ALDH1 protein is a cytosolic enzyme while the ALDH2 protein resides in the mitochondria. The bulk of acetaldehyde oxidation occurs in the mitochondria via ALDH2.

MICROSOMAL ETHANOL OXIDATION SYSTEM

Under conditions of chronic alcohol ingestion, the increased level of ethanol metabolism cannot be accounted for solely via the ADH and ALDH catalyzed reactions. Induction of an alternative ethanol metabolism pathway in the microsomes occurs. This ethanol-induced metabolic system is, therefore, referred to as the microsomal ethanol oxidation system, MEOS (Figure 14–2). The MEOS contains a cytochrome P450 activity that is distinct from ADH and is designated as CYP2E1. Induction of CYP2E1 mRNA and enzyme activity ranges from 4- to 10-fold in the liver following alcohol intake.

ACUTE AND CHRONIC EFFECTS OF ETHANOL METABOLISM

The primary acute metabolic effects of ethanol consumption are the result of the altered NADH/NAD$^+$ ratio that is the consequence of both the ADH- and ALDH-catalyzed reactions (Figure 14–3). Acute effects of acetaldehyde are also evident with ethanol consumption. Acetaldehyde forms adducts with proteins, nucleic acids, and other compounds resulting in impaired activity of the affected compounds.

The NADH produced in the cytosol by ADH must be reduced back to NAD$^+$ via mitochondrial electron transport. However, mitochondrial TCA cycle activity and oxidative phosphorylation are impaired due to the high levels of NADH resulting from the ALDH reaction. Reduced cytosolic NAD$^+$ impairs the flux of glucose through glycolysis at the glyceraldehyde-3-phosphate dehydrogenase reaction. Additionally, there is an increased rate of hepatic lactate production due to the effect of increased NADH on the direction of the hepatic lactate dehydrogenase (LDH) reaction. This reversal of the LDH reaction diverts pyruvate (also alanine)

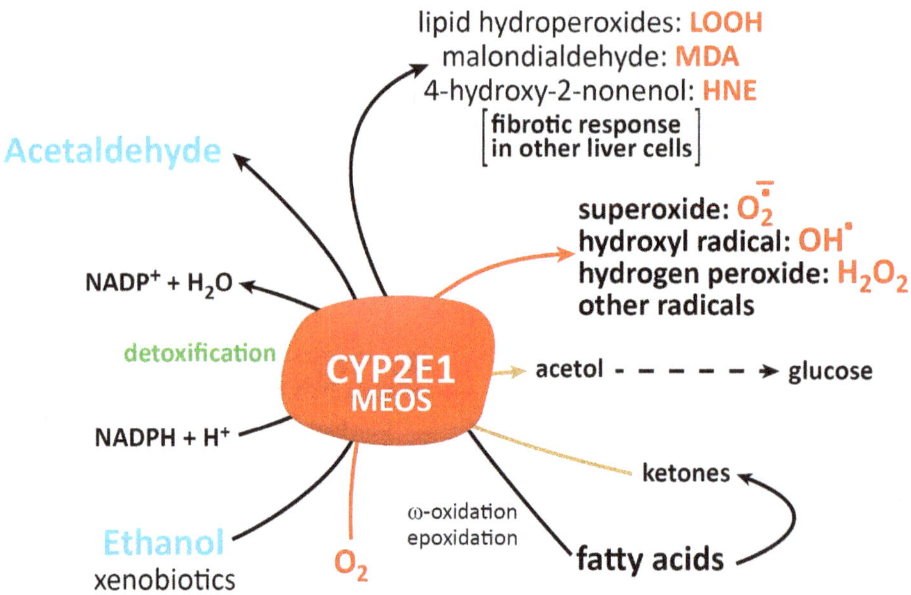

FIGURE 14–2 Physiologic and toxic activities associated with hepatic CYP2E1. (Reproduced with permission from themedicalbiochemistrypage, LLC.)

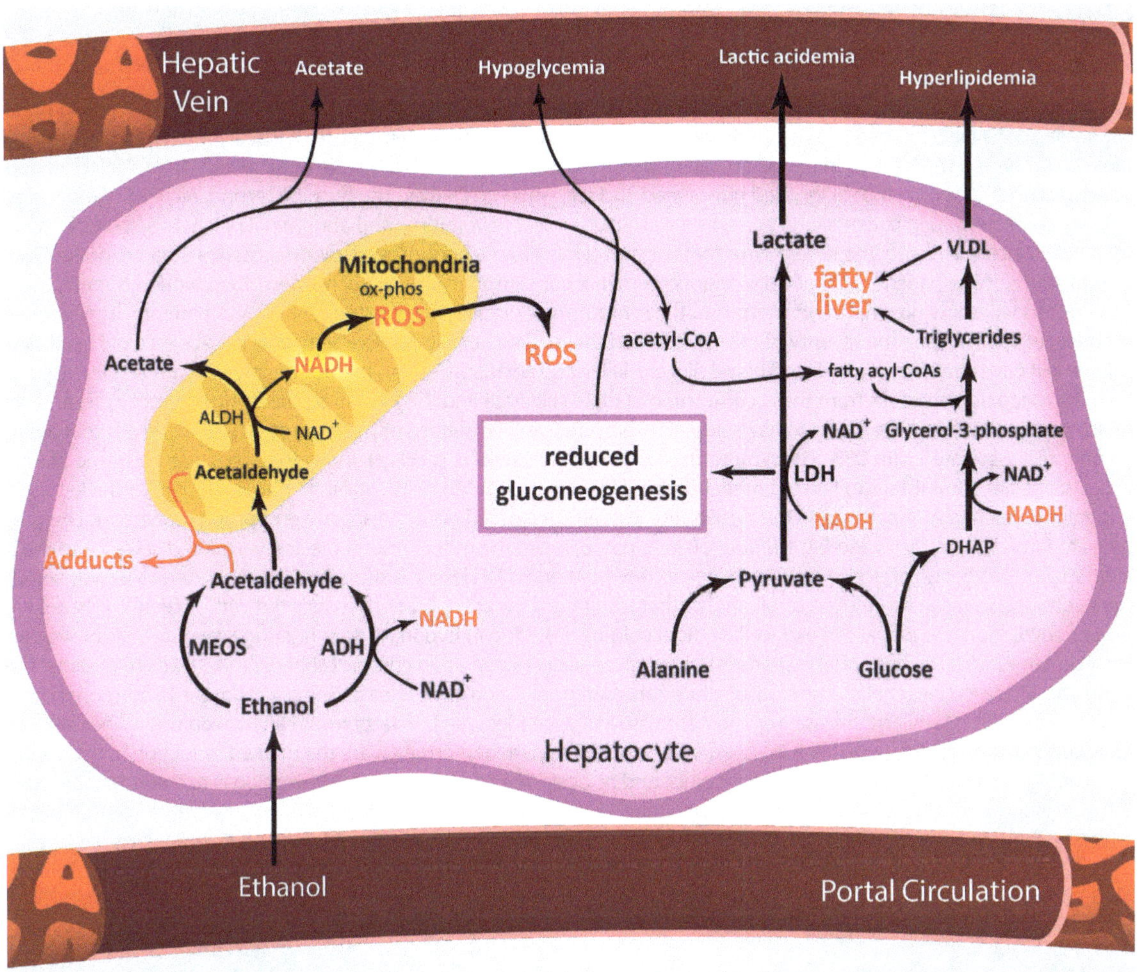

FIGURE 14–3 Metabolic disruptions in liver due to ethanol metabolism. Hepatic metabolism of ethanol results in the generation of large quantities of cytosolic and mitochondrial NADH leading to disruptions in the normal metabolic processes in the liver. Acute and chronic ethanol metabolism results in impaired gluconeogenesis leading to potentially severe hypoglycemia. The elevated cytosolic NADH levels lead to diversion of pyruvate into lactate, as well as an inability to convert lactate to pyruvate which represents the major disruption in normal hepatic gluconeogenesis. The increased lactate production in turn results in excessive lactate delivery to the blood and a consequent lactic acidemia. The excess acetate, derived from the mitochondrial oxidation of acetaldehyde, is converted to acetyl-CoA via the action of mitochondrial and cytoplasmic acetyl-CoA synthetases. The acetyl-CoA is then diverted into fatty acid synthesis. In addition, chronic ethanol metabolism leads to impaired fatty acid oxidation and the diversion of carbons into fats results in increased triglyceride and VLDL production causing fatty infiltration and ultimately liver damage and failure. Contributing to the progression to liver damage and failure is the increased production of reactive oxygen species (ROS) within the mitochondria as a consequence of the increased levels of mitochondrial NADH. The ROS cause mitochondrial stress leading to the triggering of the mitochondrial apoptosis pathway and hepatocyte death. (Reproduced with permission from themedicalbiochemistrypage, LLC.)

from gluconeogenesis leading to a reduction in the capacity of the liver to deliver glucose to the blood resulting in hypoglycemia.

In addition to the negative effects of the altered $NADH/NAD^+$ ratio on hepatic gluconeogenesis, fatty acid oxidation is also reduced as this process requires NAD^+ as a cofactor. Concomitant with reduced fatty acid oxidation is enhanced fatty acid synthesis and increased triglyceride production by the liver. The source of the carbons for fatty acid synthesis is the acetyl-CoA made from the acetate end-product of ethanol metabolism. The altered cytosolic $NADH/NAD^+$ ratio leads to glycerol-3-phosphate dehydrogenase generating more glycerol-3-phosphate, the backbone for the synthesis of the triglycerides. Increased fatty acid and triglyceride synthesis results in the fatty liver syndrome and hyperlipidemia typical in chronic alcohol consumption.

Ethanol consumption and metabolism negatively affects many other metabolic pathways, thereby contributing to the spectrum of metabolic disorders frequently found in alcoholics such as alcoholic ketoacidosis (Clinical Box 14–1). The induction of the MEOS in chronic ethanol consumption will also lead to altered hepatic metabolism of xenobiotics and drugs. Particularly significant is the effect of the MEOS on acetaminophen (paracetamol) metabolism (Clinical Box 14–2).

CLINICAL BOX 14–1 ALCOHOLIC KETOACIDOSIS

Alcoholic ketoacidosis (AKA) represents a pathology that is often associated with prolonged and excessive ethanol consumption. Alcoholic ketoacidosis (also referred to as alcoholic ketosis or alcoholic acidosis) manifests with nausea, intractable vomiting, and abdominal pain. These symptoms overlap with manifestations of crises in individuals who are addicted to ethanol (alcohol dependence) and as such AKA is often not diagnosed nor treated and managed properly in the hospital setting. Alcoholic ketoacidosis was originally characterized in patients who presented with nausea, severe vomiting, and abdominal pain whose history includes prolonged heavy alcohol misuse. The severe symptoms occurred following a bout of particularly excessive ethanol intake. Due to the onset of symptoms, these patients will have discontinued ethanol consumption, and as such when blood work is done in the hospital setting the results will show no ethanol. In contrast to the symptoms of diabetic ketoacidosis (DKA), AKA patients usually present in an alert and lucid state despite the severity of the acidosis and the marked ketonemia. In addition to the absence of blood alcohol, AKA patients will have a normal or a reduced blood glucose level, and a variably severe metabolic acidosis with an increased anion gap. The metabolic acidosis results from the accumulation of plasma lactate and the ketone bodies, β-hydroxybutyrate, and acetoacetate. Often patients with AKA are found to have extremely elevated concentrations of plasma free fatty acids, levels that are much higher than those associated with DKA. The symptoms of AKA normally resolve quickly if intravenous glucose and large amounts of intravenous saline are administered. Elevated mitochondrial NADH is thought to be pivotal in the development of the ketoacidosis and lactic acidosis seen in AKA patients. In the cytosol, the acetyl-CoA derived from the acetate end-product of ethanol metabolism, contributes to fatty acid synthesis and fatty infiltration in hepatocytes. In the mitochondria the acetyl-CoA is diverted into the ketone synthesis pathway producing acetoacetate which, due to the elevated NADH levels, is preferentially converted to β-hydroxybutyrate. The severe vomiting that can be induced by alcohol or that result from the complications associated with excessive ethanol ingestion lead to dehydration and decreased extracellular fluid volume, resulting in hypotension triggering a sympathetic nervous system response. Combined with the hormonal responses to hypoglycemia and starvation chronic ethanol intake leads to reduced insulin production and increased catecholamine, cortisol, glucagon, and growth hormone release. The effects of these hormonal disturbances include increased fatty acid release from adipose tissue triglycerides. The free fatty acids can be oxidized in the liver contributing to the potential for increased ketogenesis. The greatest threats to patients with AKA are the marked reduction in extracellular fluid volume (resulting in shock), hypokalemia, hypoglycemia, and acidosis. The recommended intervention is to institute rapid isotonic saline infusion along with glucose, and if necessary, potassium. The addition of glucose results in progressively increased pH, reductions in lactate, β-hydroxybutyrate, plasma free fatty acid, growth hormone, and cortisol levels, and an increased insulin level.

CLINICAL BOX 14–2 ACETAMINOPHEN-INDUCED HEPATOTOXICITY

Acetaminophen (*N*-acetyl-*p*-aminophenol [APAP]), also commonly called paracetamol, is a widely used over-the-counter medication for its analgesic and antipyretic properties in both adults and children. The maximum recommended therapeutic dose of acetaminophen/paracetamol is 4 g/day in adults and 50–75 mg/kg/day in children. Consumption of a single dose greater than 7 g in an adult and 150 mg/kg in a child is considered potentially toxic to the liver and kidneys. The toxicity of acetaminophen is due to its metabolism to the highly active metabolite, *N*-acetyl-*p*-benzoquinone imine (NAPQI). Indeed, acetaminophen overdose is one of the most common drug-related toxicities. The metabolism of acetaminophen occurs primarily in the liver (Figure 14–4) and, to a lesser extent, the kidneys and intestines. At normal therapeutic dosing, only a minor fraction of acetaminophen is oxidized to NAPQI. The glucuronidation of acetaminophen is catalyzed by at least four different UDP-glucuronyltransferase (UGT) enzymes. The sulfation of acetaminophen is catalyzed by a number of different sulfotransferase enzyme family members. Following glucuronidation or sulfation the modified acetaminophen is transported out of hepatocytes into the blood or the bile canaliculi via ATP-binding cassette (ABC) family transporters. NAPQI is highly reactive and is primarily responsible for acetaminophen-induced hepatotoxicity. Metabolism of acetaminophen to NAPQI is carried out by various cytochrome P450 (CYP) enzymes including CYP2E1. Of particular significance to ethanol metabolism and acetaminophen toxicity is the role of CYP2E1 in the generation of NAPQI. Chronic consumption of ethanol results in the induction of the *CYP2E1* gene and this can result in severe toxicity to acetaminophen due to enhanced conversion to NAPQI. The normal route for the detoxification of NAPQI is through its binding to the sulfhydryl group of glutathione (GSH). Following glutathione conjugation NAPQI is ultimately excreted in the urine as cysteine and mercapturic acid conjugates. Although most of the NAPQI is formed in the liver, the kidney also metabolizes acetaminophen to the toxic metabolite and releases the cysteine conjugate into the bile as well as the blood for further elimination in urine. At doses of acetaminophen that exceed 4 g/day the normal sulfation pathway becomes saturated, whereas glucuronidation and oxidation to NAPQI increase. This situation is demonstrably exacerbated in the context of ethanol consumption and the induction of CYP2E1. The glucuronidation pathway can also become saturated leading to even more acetaminophen oxidation to NAPQI, especially during ethanol consumption and metabolism. In the context of excessive NAPQI production there is an eventual depletion of GSH stores. Under these conditions NAPQI will form adducts with proteins through the sulfhydryl side chains of cysteines. In this protein adduct pathway, NAPQI primarily targets mitochondrial proteins and ion channels, leading to the loss of energy production, disturbances in ionic balance, and ultimately cell death. In conditions of acetaminophen toxicity, the administration of *N*-acetylcysteine (NAC) has been shown to replenish GSH stores, to scavenge reactive oxygen species (ROS) in the mitochondria, and to enhance the metabolism of acetaminophen via the sulfation pathway. If NAC is administered within 8–10 hours after an acute acetaminophen overdose, there is a reduced risk for hepatotoxicity and protection from renal failure.

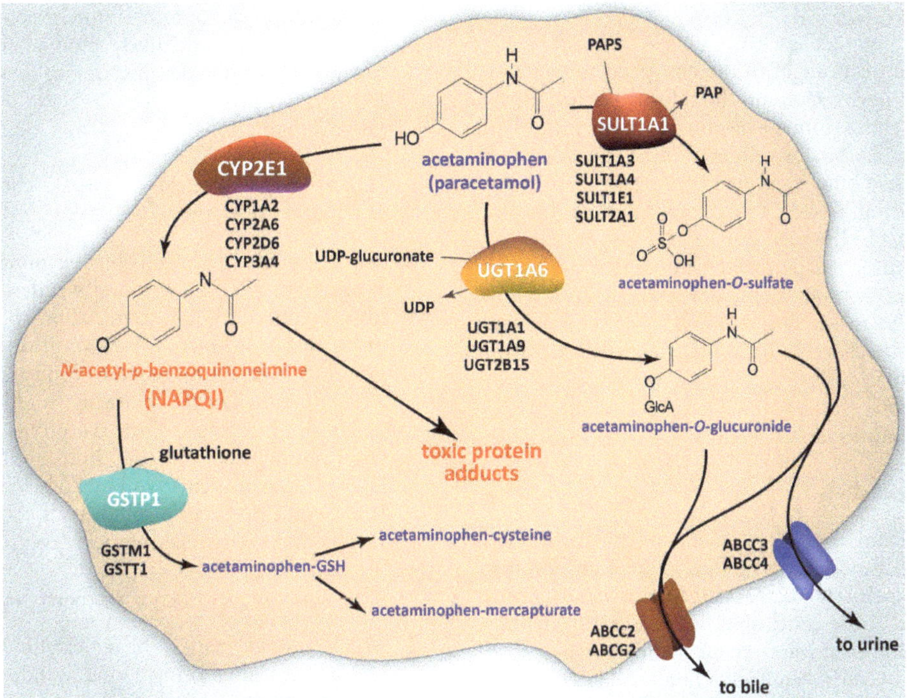

FIGURE 14–4 Pathways of acetaminophen metabolism. The normal pathway for elimination of acetaminophen (paracetamol), when taken at the recommended normal dosages, is either via glucuronidation or via sulfation. These two pathways are catalyzed by a variety of UDP-glucuronosyltransferases (UGT) and sulfotransferases (SULT). The primary hepatic UGT enzyme catalyzing the metabolism of acetaminophen is encoded by the *UGT1A6* gene and the primary sulfotransferase is encoded by the *SULT1A1* gene. The excretion of acetaminophen-*O*-sulfate (APAP-sulfate) and acetaminophen-*O*-glucuronide (APAP-glucuronide) is via the urine or in the bile. The hepatic transporters that transport the sulfated and glucuronidated APAP to the blood are ATP-binding cassette family members, ABCC3 and ABCC4. The transporters for bile excretion are ABCC2 and ABCG2. Very little acetaminophen is normally oxidized to the toxic metabolite, NAPQI. However, at high dosages, or especially in the context of ethanol-induced increases in CYP2E1 activity, oxidation of acetaminophen to NAPQI increases dramatically. NAPQI can be metabolized and excreted by glutathione-*S*-transferase (GST) enzymes utilizing glutathione (GSH), but this pathway becomes limiting at high levels of NAPQI due to depletion of GSH. The major NAPQI metabolizing GST enzymes are encoded by the *GSTP1*, *GSTM1*, and *GSTT1* genes, with the GSTP1-encoded enzyme being the most significant. The product of the GST reaction is acetaminophen-GSH which is further metabolized to either acetaminophen-cysteine or to acetaminophen-mercapturic acid. (Reproduced with permission from themedicalbiochemistrypage, LLC.)

CHECKLIST

- ☑ The primary pathway for ethanol metabolism occurs within the liver and involves oxidation by alcohol dehydrogenases and aldehyde dehydrogenases.
- ☑ Alcohol dehydrogenase (ADH) catalyzes a cytosolic oxidation reaction converting ethanol to acetaldehyde.
- ☑ The major aldehyde dehydrogenase (ALDH) is a mitochondrial enzyme catalyzing the oxidation of acetaldehyde to acetate; a cytosolic ALDH exists in humans but is a minor contributor to overall ethanol metabolism.
- ☑ Metabolism of ethanol disrupts the NADH/NAD$^+$ ratio within the hepatocyte resulting in the inhibition of gluconeogenesis, fatty acid oxidation, and TCA cycle activity.
- ☑ Excess acetate from ethanol metabolism is converted to acetyl-CoA and diverted into fatty acid biosynthesis.
- ☑ A second major alcohol metabolizing pathway involves the microsomal cytochrome P450 enzyme, CYP2E1 referred to as the microsomal ethanol oxidizing system, MEOS.
- ☑ Chronic alcohol consumption results in induction of the CYP2E1-mediated MEOS pathway which is a major contributor to liver cell damage due to high rates of reactive oxygen species (ROS) production.
- ☑ Increased ROS production during chronic ethanol metabolism is associated with cancer, atherosclerosis, diabetes, inflammation, aging, and other harmful metabolic processes.
- ☑ Chronic alcohol consumption leads to excess deposition of fat resulting in hepatic steatosis (fatty liver).
- ☑ Various alleles of ADH and ALDH are associated with variable rates of ethanol metabolism. ADH and ALDH are most frequently seen in high rates of alcoholism.

REVIEW QUESTIONS

1. A 62-year-old man is brought to the emergency department after being found unconscious on the side of the road. Physical examination shows him to be unclean with filthy hair, wearing dirty torn clothing, smelling of urine and alcohol. In an attempt to revive him, he is given a dose of naloxone via nasal spray and administered an IV containing 10% dextrose. History reveals that he has been seen in the emergency department four times over the past year with similar symptoms. The patient never regained consciousness and died within hours of admission to the hospital. Which of the following is the most likely biochemical reason for the patient's death?
   (A) Diabetic ketoacidosis
   (B) Hyperlipidemia
   (C) Protein Malnutrition
   (D) Sepsis
   (E) Severe lactic acidosis

2. Experiments are being conducted on ethanol metabolism in a mammalian animal model system. Test animals are administered ethanol via their water chronically for 3 weeks. Genomic studies performed at the conclusion of this experiment show increased expression of at least one metabolic enzyme encoding gene, relative to control animals. The altered level of activity of this enzyme is most likely to contribute to which of the following?
   (A) Decreased rate of acetaldehyde production
   (B) Decreased rate of acetyl-CoA production
   (C) Decreased rate of ethanol clearance from blood
   (D) Increased level of ethanol tolerance
   (E) Increased protection from alcohol-induced hepatic steatosis
   (F) Increased protection from effects of reactive oxygen species

3. Experiments are being conducted on ethanol metabolism in a mammalian animal model system. Test animals are chronically administered ethanol via their water for 3 weeks. Genomic studies performed at the conclusion of this experiment show induced expression of at least one metabolic enzyme encoding gene, relative to control animals. Which of the following classes of enzymes are most likely to represent the product of the induced gene?
   (A) Alcohol dehydrogenases
   (B) Aldehyde dehydrogenases
   (C) Catalases
   (D) Cytochrome P450 (CYP)
   (E) Peroxidases

4. A study is being conducted on chronic ethanol consumption in humans. There are 12 volunteers in this study, all of whom have been identified with the onset of steatohepatitis. Which of the following enzymes would most likely be found to have altered activity in the liver of these patients, thus contributing to their liver pathology?
   (A) Alcohol dehydrogenase
   (B) Glucose-6-phosphate dehydrogenase
   (C) Glycerol-3-phosphate dehydrogenase
   (D) Lactate dehydrogenase
   (E) Medium-chain Acyl-CoA dehydrogenase

5. Experiments are being conducted on ethanol metabolism using a hepatocyte cell line. Addition of ethanol leads to the identification of abnormal protein complexes. Which of the following is the most likely product of ethanol metabolism accounting for the identification of these complexes?
   (A) Acetaldehyde
   (B) Acetate
   (C) Formaldehyde
   (D) Hydrogen peroxide
   (E) Superoxide anion

6. A 57-year-old man is being examined in the emergency department after being found wandering in the middle of a busy avenue. Physical examination shows the patient to be disheveled, smelling of urine, vomit, and ethanol. The patient is found to have an unsteady gait and vertical nystagmus. Assay for which of the following would be most useful in the diagnosis of the cause of the symptoms in this patient?
   (A) Iron deficiency by total iron-binding capacity, TIBC
   (B) Mean corpuscular volume, MCV
   (C) Serum indirect bilirubin levels
   (D) Serum methylmalonic acid level to confirm vitamin B_{12} deficiency
   (E) Thiamine levels by erythrocyte transketolase activity

7. A 57-year-old man is being examined in the Emergency Department after being found wandering in the middle of a busy avenue. Physical examination shows the patient to be disheveled, smelling of urine, vomit, and ethanol. The patient is found to have an unsteady gait and vertical nystagmus. Given the findings in this patient, which of the following hepatic enzymes would be most likely to exhibit reduced activity?
   (A) Acetyl-CoA carboxylase
   (B) Glycogen phosphorylase
   (C) α-Ketoglutarate dehydrogenase
   (D) Lactate dehydrogenase
   (E) Medium-chain acyl-CoA dehydrogenase

8. The consumption of ethanol while taking acetaminophen, also commonly called paracetamol, can lead to severe pathologic consequences in the liver. This pathology is related to an acetaminophen metabolite interfering with the functions of glutathione. Which of the following would provide the best metabolic explanation for this consequence?
   (A) Alcohol dehydrogenase converts acetaminophen to acetaminophen-*O*-sulfate
   (B) Alcohol dehydrogenase converts acetaminophen to *N*-acetyl-*p*-benzoquinone imine (NAPQI)
   (C) Aldehyde dehydrogenase converts acetaminophen to acetaminophen-*O*-glucuronide
   (D) Aldehyde dehydrogenase converts acetaminophen to *N*-acetyl-*p*-benzoquinone imine (NAPQI)
   (E) CYP2E1 converts acetaminophen to acetaminophen-*O*-sulfate
   (F) CYP2E1 converts acetaminophen to acetaminophen-*O*-glucuronide
   (G) CYP2E1 converts acetaminophen to *N*-acetyl-*p*-benzoquinone imine (NAPQI)

9. A 37-year-old female alcoholic has been told by her physician that she has the onset of steatohepatitis. If this patient were to dramatically change to a healthy lifestyle, which of the following chronic effects of her addiction is most likely to be irreversible?
   (A) Enhanced triglyceride synthesis
   (B) Hepatic fibrosis

(C) Inhibition of fatty acid oxidation
(D) Ketoacidosis
(E) Lactic acidosis

10. Chronic ethanol consumption and its metabolism contributes to elevations in cellular and serum levels of acetate. Which of the following represents the most likely fate of this organic acid?
(A) It directly enters the TCA cycle and is oxidized
(B) It is oxidized by alcohol dehydrogenase generating NADH
(C) It is taken up by nonhepatic tissues and converted to acetyl-CoA
(D) It is transported to the bile canaliculi and excreted in the bile
(E) Its toxicity contributes to liver necrosis

11. Experiments are being conducted on ethanol metabolism in a mammalian animal model system. Test animals are chronically administered ethanol via their water for 3 weeks. Which of the following metabolic changes would be most likely to be observed in the test animals?
(A) Activation of fatty acid oxidation
(B) Increased rate of gluconeogenesis
(C) Increased ratio of NAD^+ to NADH
(D) Inhibition of ketogenesis
(E) Lactic acidosis

12. A 63-year-old man has been released from jail following his arrest for fourth offense of driving while intoxicated. As a condition of his release, he has been ordered to take a particular medication every day to help prevent alcohol consumption. Which of the following represents the most likely mechanism by which the prescribed medication deters the consumption of alcohol?
(A) Activating the excessive metabolism of ethanol to acetate resulting in rapid inebriation with limited alcohol consumption
(B) Blocking the conversion of acetaldehyde to acetate resulting in rapid accumulation of toxic acetaldehyde adducts
(C) Inhibiting ethanol absorption so that an individual cannot become intoxicated
(D) Inhibiting the conversion of ethanol to acetaldehyde, thereby, causing ethanol to be excreted before it can be metabolized
(E) Preventing the excretion of acetate resulting in severe nausea and vomiting

13. Experiments are being conducted on ethanol metabolism in a mammalian animal model system. Test animals are chronically administered ethanol via their water for 3 weeks. One of the findings of these experiments is a dramatic increase in the NADH to NAD^+ ratio. Which of the following is the most likely outcome of this observed alteration?
(A) Altered membrane fluidity resulting in decreased hepatocyte function
(B) Hyperglycemia due to increased rates of hepatic gluconeogenesis
(C) Increased production of glycerol-3-phosphate contributing to triglyceride production
(D) Increased TCA cycle activity resulting in increased carbon dioxide output
(E) Potentiation of central nervous system activity

14. Experiments are being conducted on ethanol metabolism in a mammalian animal model system. Test animals are chronically administered ethanol via their water for 3 weeks. Histopathological studies on liver sections from these animals shows the appearance of numerous lipid droplets. An alteration in the activity of which of the following enzymes is most likely responsible for the histopathological results?
(A) Fatty acid synthase
(B) Fatty acyl-CoA synthetase
(C) Glucose-6-phosphate dehydrogenase
(D) Glycerol-3-phosphate dehydrogenase
(E) Medium-chain acyl-CoA dehydrogenase

15. A 57-year-old man is being examined in the emergency department after being found wandering in the middle of a busy avenue. Physical examination shows the patient to be disheveled, smelling of urine, vomit, and ethanol. The patient is found to have an unsteady gait and vertical nystagmus. The attending physician orders tests to assist in the assessment of the level of pathology in this patient. Which of the following is the most likely finding of the assay the physician requested?
(A) Decreased level of serum AST
(B) Decreased prothrombin time (PT)
(C) Decreased urine urate
(D) Elevated serum ammonia
(E) Elevated serum ketones
(F) Elevated urine glucose

ANSWER

1. Correct answer is **E.** The patient is presumed to be an alcoholic and does not consume a normal healthy diet which most likely resulted in thiamine deficiency. Consumption of alcohol reduces the ability of the liver to carry out gluconeogenesis because the alcohol dehydrogenase reaction generates large amounts of cytosolic NADH. This NADH drives the lactate dehydrogenase reaction in the direction of pyruvate reduction to lactate, thereby reducing pyruvate incorporation into gluconeogenesis. Providing IV dextrose without supplemen tal thiamine further increases the concentration of pyruvate, via glycolysis, which is then also reduced to lactate instead of being oxidized to acetyl-CoA because the pyruvate dehydrogenase complex (PDHc) requires thiamine pyrophosphate to function. In addition to the lack of thiamine, exerting a negative impact on the PDHc, the mitochondrial NADH level is very high as a result of the aldehyde dehydrogenase reaction of ethanol metabolism, and this NADH allosterically activates PDHc kinases that then phosphorylate and inhibit the PDHc. The overall consequence of ethanol metabolism is lactic acidosis which is then further enhanced by the administration of the dextrose resulting in lethal metabolic acidosis. The naloxone treatment is an opioid receptor antagonist for treatment of opioid overdose which is a differential diagnosis for acute ethanol intoxication. There is no indication that the patient was a type 1 diabetic and thus, diabetic ketoacidosis (choice A) is not a likely contributor to his death. Chronic alcohol consumption results in hyperlipidemia (choice B) but this would not have been significantly enhanced, to a lethal condition, by the administration of dextrose. Chronic alcohol consumption is often associated with nutritional deficit, including protein (choice C), but this is unlikely to have contributed to the patient's death following administration of dextrose. There were no indications that the patient was experiencing symptoms of sepsis (choice D).

2. Correct answer is **D.** Chronic consumption of ethanol results in the induction of the gene encoding the metabolic enzyme, CYP2E1. This enzyme comprises what is referred to as the microsomal ethanol oxidizing system (MEOS). The MEOS operates primarily in the liver to metabolize ethanol when the concentration is chronically high. CYP2E1 is the primary P450 enzyme responsible for converting ethanol to acetaldehyde. Because CYP2E1-encoding gene is induced the metabolism of ethanol is increased, relative to controls, resulting in a potential for increased ethanol tolerance as well as increased, not decreased, ethanol clearance (choice C). Ethanol induction of the MEOS increases, not decreases, acetaldehyde production (choice A). Acetyl-CoA production will be increased, not decrease (choice B), in ethanol metabolism through the action of acetyl-CoA synthetases. These enzymes produce acetyl-CoA from acetate which is the end-product of ethanol metabolism. The acetyl-CoA produced from ethanol-derived acetate contributes to increased fatty acid synthesis resulting in fatty infiltration (steatosis) of the liver as opposed to providing protection from steatosis (choice E). Activation of the MEOS system and the metabolism of ethanol via this system results in dramatic increases in reactive oxygen species (ROS) production. As opposed to protecting from the effects of ROS (choice F), this effect of the MEOS exacerbates ROS damage of hepatocytes.

3. Correct answer is **D.** Chronic consumption of ethanol results in the induction of the gene encoding the metabolic enzyme, CYP2E1 which is a member of the large cytochrome P540 family of enzymes. This enzyme comprises what is referred to as the microsomal ethanol oxidizing system (MEOS). The MEOS operates primarily in the liver to metabolize ethanol when the concentration is chronically high. CYP2E1 is the primary P450 enzyme responsible for converting ethanol to acetaldehyde. Alcohol dehydrogenases (choice A) and aldehyde dehydrogenases (choice B) are not significantly induced by chronic ethanol metabolism. Due to the increased production of reactive oxygen species (ROS) by the MEOS it is possible that there will be induction of enzymes involved in detoxification of ROS such as catalase (choice C) and peroxidases (choice E), but these would be indirect responses where induction of CYP2E1 is direct.

4. Correct answer is **C.** The metabolism of ethanol results in dramatic elevation of both cytosolic and mitochondrial NADH. Glycerol-3-phosphate dehydrogenase reduces the glycolytic intermediate, dihydroxyacetone phosphate, to glycerol-3-phosphate (G3P) while also oxidizing NADH to NAD^+. As a result of the elevated cytosolic NADH, from the alcohol dehydrogenase catalyzed reaction, there is excess production of G3P. Glycerol-3-phosphate is the initial acceptor of fatty acids for the synthesis of triglycerides. The acetate byproduct of ethanol metabolism is converted to acetyl-CoA via acetyl-CoA synthetases, and this excess acetyl-CoA can serve as a precursor for the synthesis of fatty acids which contributes to triglyceride synthesis. The triglycerides are packaged into very low-density lipoproteins (VLDL) which, when transported to the blood, contribute to hyperlipidemia. Although some VLDL is exported from hepatocytes, the ethanol in the cells interferes with effective transport which, together with increased fatty acid and triglyceride synthesis, results in the steatohepatitis associated with chronic ethanol consumption. None of the other enzymes (choices A, B, D, and E) are contributory in any direct or significant way to the development of steatohepatitis.

5. Correct answer is **A.** Acetaldehyde is the product of the alcohol dehydrogenase catalyzed reaction. Acetaldehyde enters the mitochondria and is oxidized to acetate by aldehyde dehydrogenase. Acetaldehyde is highly reactive and can interact with proteins and other biomolecules in the cell to form both stable and unstable adducts. Acetaldehyde preferably interacts with certain amino acids in proteins but not all amino acids are equally susceptible to adduct formation with acetaldehyde. Lysine, cysteine, and aromatic amino acids are commonly altered via acetaldehyde interaction. In addition, certain proteins are particularly susceptible to forming adducts with acetaldehyde. These include proteins found in red blood cell membranes, lipoproteins, hemoglobin, albumin, collagen, tubulin, and several cytochromes including CYP2E1. Acetate (choice B) is either released to the blood and picked up by other tissues and converted to acetyl-CoA or converted to acetyl-CoA in hepatocytes. Formaldehyde (choice C) is a product of methanol oxidation but not ethanol metabolism. Hydrogen peroxide (choice D) and superoxide anion (choice E) levels increase as a result of the metabolism of ethanol, especially when CYP2E1 of the microsomal ethanol oxidizing system (MEOS) is induced. However, these are not direct products of ethanol oxidation.

6. Correct answer is **E.** The patient is most likely a chronic alcohol consumer who also has a poor diet resulting in deficiencies in several nutrients. Deficiency in water soluble vitamins is common in alcoholics due to their poor diet, with deficiency in thiamine and folate being particularly problematic due to ethanol-mediated inhibition of absorption from the intestines. Deficiency in thiamine affects important dehydrogenases of metabolism such as pyruvate dehydrogenase (PDHc), 2-oxoglutarate dehydrogenase (α-ketoglutarate dehydrogenase), and branched-chain keto acid dehydrogenase. Impaired PDHc activity is the major contributor to the signs and symptoms in this patient. The transketolase enzyme of the pentose phosphate pathway also requires thiamine for its activity. Assay for erythrocyte transketolase activity is a rapid and relatively noninvasive test for the diagnosis of thiamine deficiency. Deficiency in iron (choice A) is not associated with the signs and symptoms in this patient. Macrocytic or microcytic anemias, detectable with MCV determination (choice B), can result from vitamin deficiencies but are not often associated with the complications of chronic ethanol consumption. The chronic consumption of ethanol will result in steatohepatitis leading to impaired liver function which will result in elevation in unconjugated bilirubin (choice C) but this measurement would not be useful in diagnosis of the cause of the patients symptoms. Deficiency in most vitamins, such as B_{12} (choice D), could be apparent in an alcoholic with a poor diet but the measurement of methylmalonic acid would not be useful in the diagnosis of the symptoms in this patient.

7. Correct answer is **C.** The patient is most likely a chronic alcohol consumer who also has a poor diet resulting in deficiencies in several nutrients. Deficiency in water-soluble vitamins is common in alcoholics due to their poor diet, with deficiency in thiamine and folate being particularly problematic due to ethanol-mediated inhibition of absorption from the intestines. Deficiency in thiamine affects important dehydrogenases of metabolism such as pyruvate dehydrogenase (PDHc),

2-oxoglutarate dehydrogenase (α-ketoglutarate dehydrogenase), and branched-chain keto acid dehydrogenase. Deficiency in most vitamins, such as biotin, B_6, niacin, and riboflavin, could be apparent in an alcoholic with a poor diet resulting in reduced activity of the biotin-dependent enzyme, acetyl-CoA carboxylase (choice A), the B_6-dependent enzyme, glycogen phosphorylase (choice B), the NAD^+-dependent enzyme, lactate dehydrogenase (choice D), and the FAD-dependent enzyme, medium-chain acyl dehydrogenase (choice E), but reduced activity of these enzymes do not correlate to the symptoms in this patient.

8. Correct answer is **G.** In the absence of ethanol metabolism acetaminophen is normally metabolized to acetaminophen-*O*-sulfate and acetaminophen-*O*-glucuronide, both of which are transported out of hepatocytes to the blood and excreted in the urine and the bile. Consumption of ethanol results in the induction of the microsomal ethanol metabolizing system (MEOS) which constitutes the cytochrome P450 enzyme, CYP2E1. CYP2E1, along with several other CYP enzymes, catalyzes the conversion of acetaminophen to *N*-acetyl-*p*-benzoquinone imine (NAPQI), with CYP2E1 activity being the most significant relative to the toxic effects of combining ethanol consumption with acetaminophen. NAPQI rapidly depletes hepatocytes of glutathione, thereby rendering the cells highly susceptible to damage by reactive oxygen species. None of the other option (A, B, C, D, E, and F) correctly defines the metabolism of acetaminophen in the liver either in the presence or absence of ethanol.

9. Correct answer is **B.** Chronic ethanol consumption and alcohol metabolism contributes to the spectrum of metabolic disorders frequently found in alcoholics. These disorders include fatty liver syndromes such as the patient's steatohepatitis, as well as hyperlipidemia, lactic acidosis, ketoacidosis, and hyperuricemia. The first stage of liver damage following chronic alcohol consumption is the appearance of fatty liver, which is followed by inflammation, apoptosis, fibrosis, and finally cirrhosis. These negative and toxic changes within the liver are irreversible even when alcohol consumption is terminated. All of the other consequences of ethanol metabolism (choices A, C, D, and E) will resolve upon the cessation of ethanol intake.

10. Correct answer is **C.** Acetate, from whatever source, is converted to acetyl-CoA by ATP-dependent acetyl-CoA synthetases (AceCS). Following the consumption of ethanol, acetate levels can be elevated by as much as 20-fold. The primary causes of fatty liver syndrome (hepatic steatosis), induced by excess alcohol consumption are the altered $NADH/NAD^+$ levels that in turn inhibit gluconeogenesis, inhibit fatty acid oxidation, and inhibit the activity of the TCA cycle. Each of these inhibited pathways results in the diversion of acetyl-CoA into *de novo* fatty acid synthesis in nonhepatic tissues as well as in the liver. Acetate cannot be directly oxidized via the TCA cycle (choice A), it must first be activated to acetyl-CoA. Acetate is not a substrate for alcohol dehydrogenases (choice B) and is not transported to the bile canaliculi (choice D). Acetate itself does not directly contribute to liver necrosis (choice E), but does so only after conversion to acetyl-CoA and its subsequent use as a substrate for fatty acid synthesis.

11. Correct answer is **E.** The majority of the aberrant metabolic effects of chronic ethanol consumption stem from the altered NADH to NAD^+ ratio as a result of the actions of alcohol dehydrogenase and aldehyde dehydrogenase. The increased levels of cytosolic NADH drive the lactate dehydrogenase (LDH) reaction in the direction of pyruvate reduction to lactate. Any blood lactate, that would normally be oxidized to pyruvate by LDH in the normal process of the Cori cycle, which involves incorporation of lactate into glucose production via gluconeogenesis, remains as lactate. The consequences of the shift in the LDH reaction and inhibited gluconeogenesis (choice B) are lactic acidosis. Ethanol metabolism yields acetate which is converted to acetyl-CoA both in the cytosol, leading to increased fatty acid synthesis, not oxidation (choice A), and in the mitochondria where it contributes to ketone body synthesis as opposed to inhibiting the process (choice D). The effects of alcohol dehydrogenase and aldehyde dehydrogenase are increased NADH and reduced NAD^+ (choice C).

12. Correct answer is **B.** The most likely medication being mandated is disulfiram. Disulfiram blocks the processing of alcohol in the body by inhibiting aldehyde dehydrogenase which results in a rapid rise in the level of acetaldehyde derived from the action of alcohol dehydrogenase. Acetaldehyde is highly reactive and can interact with proteins and other biomolecules in the cell to form both stable and unstable adducts. Acetaldehyde preferably interacts with certain amino acids in proteins but not all amino acids are equally susceptible to adduct formation with acetaldehyde. Lysine, cysteine, and aromatic amino acids are commonly altered via acetaldehyde interaction. In addition, certain proteins are particularly susceptible to forming adducts with acetaldehyde. These include proteins found in red blood cell membranes, lipoproteins, hemoglobin, albumin, collagen, tubulin, and several cytochromes including CYP2E1. These toxic effects of acetaldehyde result in promoting a highly negative response to ethanol consumption. None of the other options (choices A, C, D, and E) correspond to the actions of disulfiram.

13. Correct answer is **C.** The dramatic increases in both cytosolic and mitochondrial NADH, that occurs due to the metabolism of ethanol, results in the inhibition of gluconeogenesis, fatty acid oxidation, and the activity of the TCA cycle. The reduction in NAD^+ impairs the flux of glucose through glycolysis at the glyceraldehyde-3-phosphate dehydrogenase reaction, thereby limiting energy production. The increase in cytosolic NADH drives the glycerol-3-phosphate dehydrogenase in the direction of reducing the glycolytic intermediate, dihydroxyacetone phosphate (DHAP) to glycerol-3-phosphate which is the backbone for the synthesis of the triglycerides. One of the major outcomes of the altered $NADH/NAD^+$ ratio is fatty acid deposition in the liver leading to fatty liver syndrome and hyperlipidemia as a result of increased hepatic VLDL production. The $NADH/NAD^+$ ratio does not alter membrane fluidity (choice A), inhibits hepatic gluconeogenesis resulting in hypoglycemia (choice B), and reduces the activity of the TCA cycle dehydrogenase (choice D). Ethanol itself alters membrane fluidity and action potential propagation in the central nervous system resulting in inhibition of nervous activity (choice E).

14. Correct answer is **D.** The metabolism of ethanol by the liver leads to a large increase in both cytosolic and mitochondrial NADH. This increase in NADH disrupts the normal processes of metabolic regulation such as hepatic gluconeogenesis, TCA cycle function, and fatty acid oxidation. Concomitant with reduced fatty acid oxidation is enhanced fatty acid synthesis and increased triglyceride production by the liver. In the mitochondria, the production of acetate from acetaldehyde leads to increased levels of acetyl-CoA. Since the increased generation

of NADH also reduces the activity of the TCA cycle, the acetyl-CoA is diverted to fatty acid synthesis. The increase in cytosolic NADH drives the glycerol-3-phosphate dehydrogenase in the direction of reducing the glycolytic intermediate, dihydroxyacetone phosphate (DHAP) to glycerol 3-phosphate which is the backbone for the synthesis of the triglycerides. The increased fatty acid synthesis and the increased levels of triglyceride production result in fatty acid deposition in the liver leading to fatty liver syndrome and excessive levels of lipids in the blood as a result of increased VLDL production and release by the liver. Although fatty acid and triglyceride synthesis is enhanced in the liver in response to ethanol metabolism, the activity of fatty acid synthase (choice A) and fatty acyl-CoA synthetases (choice B) is less significant to triglyceride infiltration in the liver and VLDL production than the increased activity of glycerol-3-phosphate dehydrogenase. Glucose-6-phosphate dehydrogenase (choice C) activity will provide some of the NADPH required for fatty acid synthesis, but the increased activity of glycerol-3-phosphate dehydrogenase is more significant to overall triglyceride and VLDL production. Medium-chain acyl-CoA dehydrogenase (choice E) is a fatty acid oxidizing enzyme and fat oxidation is impaired due to the reduced levels of NAD^+ required by mitochondrial trifunctional protein (MTP) which carries out the last three steps of fat oxidation.

15. Correct answer is **D.** Chronic ethanol metabolism, as is most likely in this patient, results in progressive damage to the liver beginning with fatty infiltration and the ultimate development of cirrhotic lesions. The damage to the liver reduces its capacity to detoxify xenobiotics, conjugate bilirubin, synthesize blood coagulation factors, and synthesize urea from waste nitrogen, etc. The compromised ability of the liver to synthesize urea will lead to drastically elevated ammonium ion in the blood. This is a medical emergency because it can cross the blood-brain barrier and cause neurologic dysfunction and even death. Damage to the liver will result in increased levels of AST (choice A) and ALT being found in the blood; however, these are not as diagnostic to the level of pathology that is likely in this patient. The decreased ability to produce coagulation factors, such as prothrombin (choice B) can contribute to bleeding dysfunction, but not serve as a useful diagnostic tool to the level of pathology that is likely in this patient as does the measurement of plasma ammonium levels. The progressive liver damage resulting from chronic ethanol consumption will lead to increased purine nucleotide catabolism and increased, not reduced (choice C), urine levels of uric acid. Both ketone production (choice E) and glucose (choice F) delivery to the blood (via gluconeogenesis and glycogenolysis) will be reduced in this patient due to progressive liver failure.

C H A P T E R

15

Cholesterol and Bile Metabolism

High-Yield Terms

Cholesterol ester	Product of fatty acid esterification of the 3-OH catalyzed by ACAT or LCAT
SREBP2	Sterol-regulated element-binding protein 2, controls the expression of genes involved in hepatic cholesterol biosynthesis
Isoprenoid	Any compound containing the 5-carbon organic molecule isoprene (also called terpene) with the formula: CH_2=C-(CH_3)-CH=CH_2
Prenylation	Process of attaching isoprenoid intermediates of the cholesterol biosynthetic pathway (farnesyl pyrophosphate and geranylgeranyl pyrophosphate) to proteins
Classic (neutral) pathway	Major pathway for bile acid synthesis, initiated from cholesterol via the action of CYP7A1; both cholic and chenodeoxycholic acid synthesized via the classic pathway
Acidic pathway	Alternative, minor pathway for bile acid synthesis initiated via the action of sterol 27-hydroxylase (CYP27A1); only chenodeoxycholic acid synthesized via the acidic pathway
CYP7A1	7α-hydroxylase, rate-limiting enzyme in the classic pathway of bile acid synthesis
Primary bile acids	The end-products of hepatic bile acid synthesis and includes cholic acid and chenodeoxycholic acid
Secondary bile acids	Products of the actions of intestinal bacteria on the primary bile acids generating deoxycholate (from cholate) and lithocholate (from chenodeoxycholate)
Enterohepatic circulation	The circulation of bile acids, or other substances, from the liver to the gallbladder, followed by secretion into the small intestine, absorption by intestinal enterocytes and transport back to the liver

CHOLESTEROL BIOSYNTHESIS

Cholesterol is an extremely important biological molecule that has roles in membrane structure as well as being a precursor for the synthesis of the steroid hormones (see Chapter 32) and the bile acids. In addition, the cholesterol biosynthesis pathway is required for endogenous synthesis of vitamin D (see Chapter 3). Both dietary cholesterol, and that synthesized *de novo*, are transported through the circulation in lipoprotein particles (see Chapter 16). The same is true of cholesterol esters, the form in which cholesterol is stored in cells. Due to its important role in membrane function, all cells express the enzymes of cholesterol biosynthesis.

The synthesis and utilization of cholesterol must be tightly regulated in order to prevent overaccumulation and abnormal deposition within the body. Of particular clinical importance is the abnormal deposition of cholesterol and cholesterol-rich lipoproteins in the coronary arteries. Such deposition, eventually leading to atherosclerosis, is the leading contributory factor in diseases of the coronary arteries. Because of the pathology associated with excess serum cholesterol, measurement of total serum cholesterol, as well as cholesterol content of lipoprotein particles (Clinical Box 15–1), is routine practice.

Cholesterol synthesis (Figure 15–1) originates from the 2-carbon acetate group of acetyl-CoA which can be derived from glucose oxidation (see Chapter 5), amino acid oxidation (see Chapter 18), and lipid oxidation (see Chapter 13). The major metabolic origin of acetyl-CoA is the mitochondria and since cholesterol synthesis occurs in the cytosol, the acetyl-CoA must be transported out of the mitochondria. Acetyl-CoA transport to the cytoplasm occurs via the mechanism depicted in Figure 11–3.

HIGH-YIELD CONCEPT

Production of acetyl-CoA from ethanol metabolism is one reason that excess alcohol consumption is a significant contributor to elevated serum cholesterol and lipid levels.

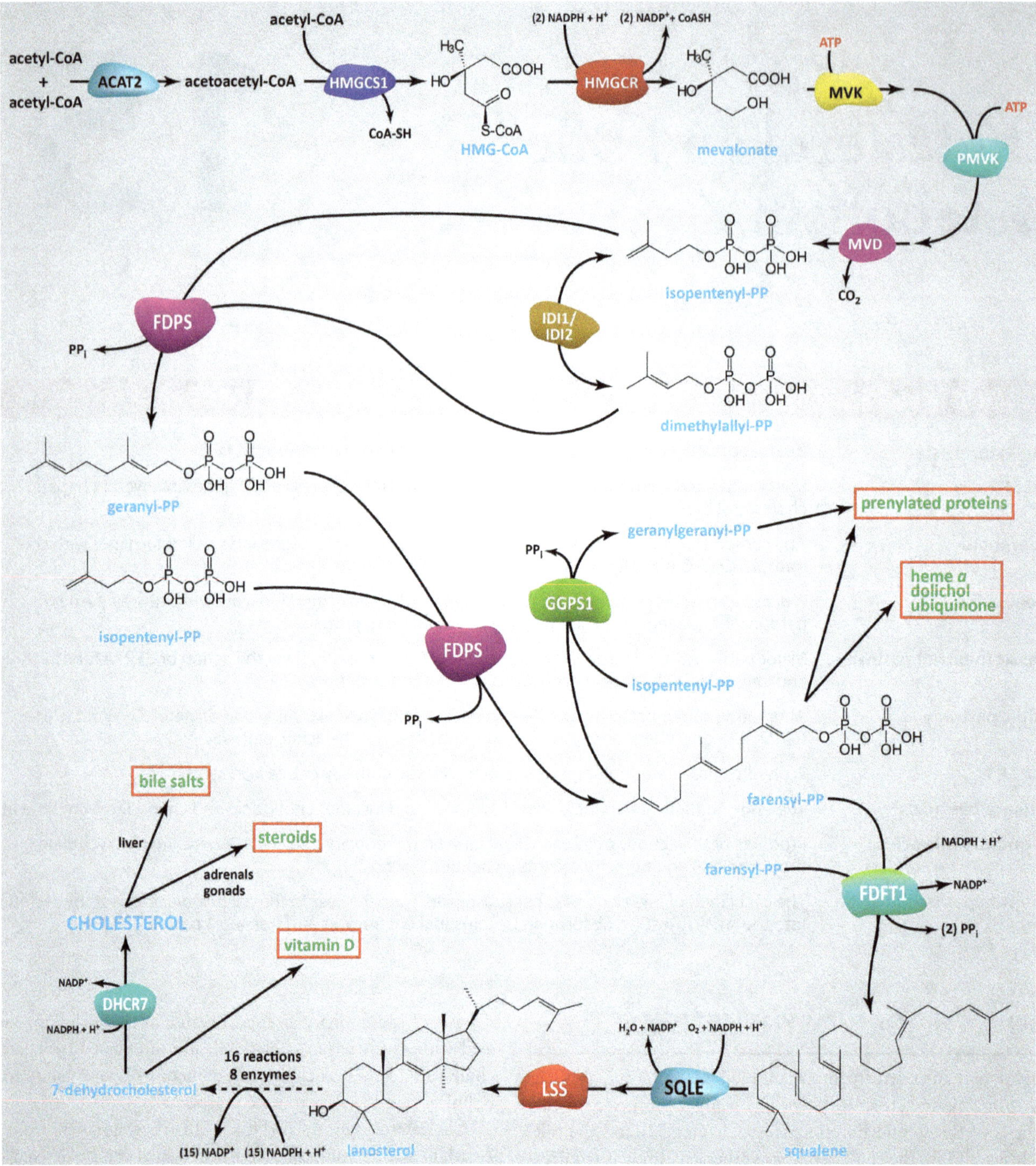

FIGURE 15–1 Pathway of cholesterol biosynthesis. Synthesis of cholesterol begins with the transport of acetyl-CoA from within the mitochondria to the cytosol. The rate-limiting step in cholesterol synthesis occurs at the 3-hydroxy-3-methylglutaryl-CoA (HMG-CoA) reductase, HMGR, catalyzed step. The phosphorylation reactions are required to solubilize the isoprenoid intermediates in the pathway. Intermediates in the mevalonate pathway are used for the synthesis of prenylated proteins, dolichol, coenzyme Q, and the side chain of heme *a*. The abbreviation "PP" (eg, isopentenyl-PP) stands for pyrophosphate. ACAT2: acetyl-CoA acetyltransferase 2. DHCR7: 7-dehydrocholesterol reductase. FDPS: farnesyl diphosphate synthase. FDFT1: farnesyl-diphosphate farnesyltransferase 1 (more commonly called squalene synthase). GGPS1: geranylgeranyl diphosphate synthase 1. HMGCS1: HMG-CoA synthase 1 (cytosolic). HMGCR: HMG-CoA reductase. LSS: lanosterol synthase (2,3-oxidosqualene-lanosterol cyclase). MVD: diphosphomevalonate decarboxylase. MVK: mevalonate kinase. PMVK: phosphomevalonate kinase. SQLE: squalene epoxidase (also called squalene monooxygenase). (Reproduced with permission from themedicalbiochemistrypage, LLC.)

CLINICAL BOX 15–1 CHOLESTEROL VALUES

Standard fasting blood tests for cholesterol will include values for total cholesterol, HDL cholesterol (so-called "good" cholesterol), and LDL cholesterol (so-called "bad" cholesterol). Family history and lifestyle, including factors such as blood pressure and whether or not one smokes, affect what would be considered ideal versus nonideal values for fasting blood-lipid profiles.

Total Serum Cholesterol

<200 mg/dL = desired values
200–239 mg/dL = borderline to high risk
240 mg/dL and above = high risk

HDL Cholesterol

With HDL cholesterol the higher the better.
<40 mg/dL for men and <50 mg/dL for women = higher risk
40–50 mg/dL for men and 50–60 mg/dL for woman = normal values
>60 mg/dL is associated with some level of protection against heart disease

LDL Cholesterol

With LDL cholesterol the lower the better.
<100 mg/dL = optimal values
100 mg/dL–129 mg/dL = optimal to near optimal
130 mg/dL–159 mg/dL = borderline high risk
160 mg/dL–189 mg/dL = high risk
190 mg/dL and higher = very high risk

The process of cholesterol synthesis can be considered to be composed of five major steps where the reactions that culminate in the synthesis of isopentenyl pyrophosphate and its isomeric form, dimethylallyl pyrophosphate, are commonly referred to as the mevalonate pathway:

1. Acetyl-CoA is converted to 3-hydroxy-3-methylglutaryl-CoA (HMG-CoA).
2. HMG-CoA is converted to mevalonate.
3. Mevalonate is converted to the isoprene-based molecule, isopentenyl pyrophosphate (IPP).
4. IPP molecules are converted to squalene.
5. Squalene is converted to cholesterol.

Synthesis of HMG-CoA is the rate-limiting and highly regulated step of cholesterol biosynthesis. This reaction is catalyzed by the NADPH-dependent enzyme, HMG-CoA reductase, HMGR. The terminal reaction of cholesterol biosynthesis involves the enzyme, 7-dehydrocholesterol reductase. Defects in the gene (*DHCR7*) encoding this latter enzyme results in Smith-Lemli-Opitz syndrome (SLOS, Clinical Box 15–2)

CLINICAL BOX 15–2 SMITH-LEMLI-OPITZ SYNDROME

Smith-Lemli-Opitz syndrome (SLOS) is an autosomal recessive disorder that was first described in 1964 by three doctors whose last names constitute the name of this syndrome. SLOS results in multiple malformations and behavioral problems as a consequence of a defect in cholesterol synthesis. The defect resides in the terminal enzyme of the cholesterol biosynthesis pathway, 7-dehydrocholesterol reductase. Defects in this gene result in increased levels of 7-dehydrocholesterol and reduced levels (15–27% of normal) of cholesterol in SLOS patients. The highest frequency of SLOS appears in Caucasians of northern European descent with a frequency of around 1 in 20,000 to 1 in 70,000. Over 130 different mutations in the *DHCR7* gene have been identified in SLOS patients including missense, nonsense, and splice site mutations. Six mutations have been shown to account for greater than 60% of all SLOS mutations. These mutations include a cysteine for arginine substitution at amino acid 404 (identified as the R404C mutation), a methionine for threonine substitution at amino acid 93 (identified as the T93M mutation), a leucine for valine substitution at amino acid 362 (identified as the V362L mutation), a nonsense mutation at amino acid 151 resulting in termination of translation (identified as the W151X mutation), and a splice site mutation in intron 8 of the *DHCR7* gene. The splice site mutation is the most frequently observed mutation in the *DHCR7* gene accounting for one-third of all mutations in SLOS. One of the most important development regulating proteins of early embryos, sonic hedgehog (Shh), is modified by cholesterol addition. Shh is necessary for patterning events that take place in the central nervous system, during limb development, and in the formation of facial structures. The involvement of cholesterol in normal Shh function explains many of the abnormalities that are observed in SLOS patients. The clinical spectrum of SLOS is very broad, ranging from the most severe form manifesting as a lethal malformation syndrome, to a relatively mild disorder that encompasses behavioral and learning disabilities. Frequent observations in SLOS infants is poor feeding and postnatal growth failure. The growth failure may necessitate the insertion of a gastronomy tube to ensure adequate nutritional support. There are distinct craniofacial

CLINICAL BOX 15–2 (CONTINUED)

anomalies associated with SLOS. These include microcephaly (head size smaller than normal), micrognathia (abnormally small lower jaw), ptosis (drooping eyelids), a small upturned nose, and cleft palate or bifid uvula. Male infants with SLOS exhibit genital abnormalities that range from a small penis to ambiguous genitalia or gender reversal. Abnormalities in limb development are common in SLOS patients and include short thumbs, postaxial polydactyly, and single palmar creases. In addition, the most common clinical finding in SLOS patients is syndactyly (fusion of digits) of the second and third toes. This latter limb deformity is found in over 95% of SLOS patients.

REGULATION OF HMGR ACTIVITY

Regulation of HMGR activity is the primary means for controlling the level of cholesterol biosynthesis. The level of enzyme activity is regulated by four distinct mechanisms: (1) feedback inhibition, (2) control of gene expression, (3) rate of enzyme degradation, and (4) phosphorylation-dephosphorylation.

The first three control mechanisms are exerted by cholesterol itself. Cholesterol acts as a feedback inhibitor of preexisting HMGR as well as an inducer of rapid ubiquitin-mediated degradation of the enzyme. When cholesterol is in excess the amount of mRNA for HMGR is reduced as a result of decreased expression of the gene. The mechanism by which cholesterol (and other sterols) affects the transcription of the *HMGR* gene is via control of the activity of a member of the sterol-regulated element-binding protein (SREBP) family of transcription factors.

Regulation of HMGR through covalent modification occurs as a result of phosphorylation and dephosphorylation (Figure 15–2). The enzyme is most active in the unphosphorylated state. Phosphorylation of the enzyme decreases its activity. HMGR is phosphorylated by AMP-activated protein kinase (AMPK) and dephosphorylated by HMGR phosphatase.

The activity of HMGR is additionally controlled by the cAMP signaling pathway via the regulation of PKA activity. Since the

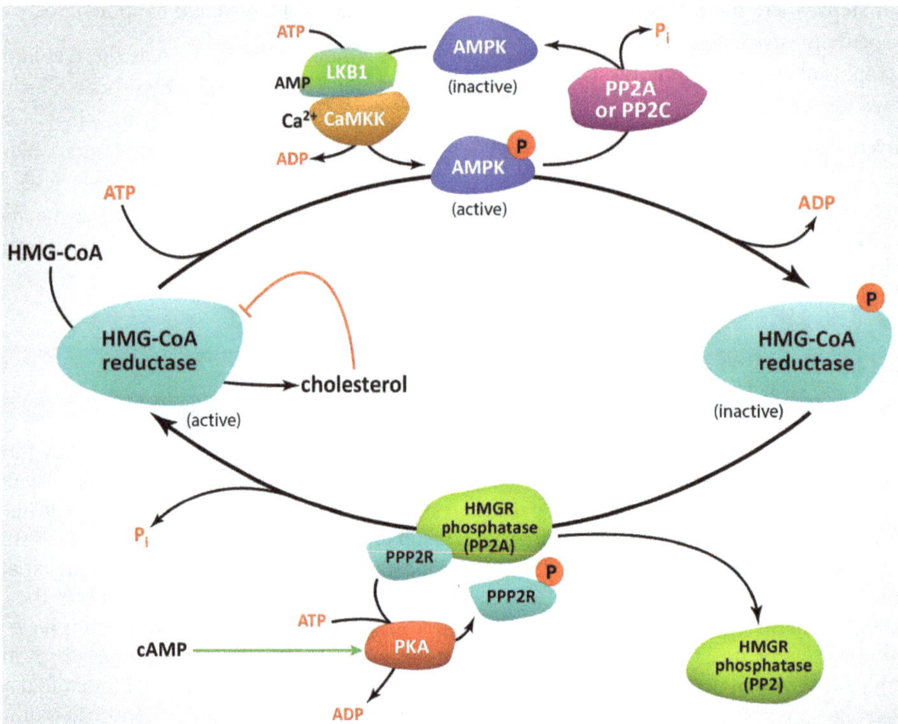

FIGURE 15–2 Regulation of HMGR by covalent modification. HMGR is most active in the dephosphorylated state. Phosphorylation is catalyzed by AMP-activated protein kinase (AMPK) an enzyme whose activity is also regulated by phosphorylation. Phosphorylation of AMPK is catalyzed by at least two enzymes: LKB1 and CaMKKβ. Dephosphorylation of HMGR, returning it to the more active state, is a consequence of the activity of protein phosphatases of the 2A family (PP2A). The PP2A core enzyme interacts with a variable regulatory subunit to assemble into a holoenzyme. The major function of the PP2A regulatory subunits is to target phosphorylated substrate proteins to the phosphatase activity of the PP2A catalytic subunits. PPP2R represents one of the 15 different PP2A regulatory subunits. Hormones such as glucagon and epinephrine negatively affect cholesterol biosynthesis by increasing the activity of the specific regulatory subunits of the PP2A family enzymes. PKA-mediated phosphorylation of PPP2 results in release of PP2A from HMGR preventing it from being dephosphorylated. Opposing the effects of glucagon and epinephrine, insulin stimulates the removal of phosphates and, thereby, activates HMGR activity. (Reproduced with permission from themedicalbiochemistrypage, LLC.)

intracellular level of cAMP is regulated by hormonal stimuli, regulation of cholesterol biosynthesis is, therefore, under hormonal control. Insulin decreases cAMP which in turn activates cholesterol synthesis. Alternatively, glucagon and epinephrine, which increase the level of cAMP, inhibit cholesterol synthesis.

HIGH-YIELD CONCEPT

AMPK is a master metabolic regulator whose activity increases the rate of ATP production and inhibits ATP consumption. AMPK activity is itself regulated via phosphorylation. In addition to regulating the activity of HMGR, AMPK activity influences the transcriptional regulation of numerous metabolic genes.

THE UTILIZATION OF CHOLESTEROL

Cholesterol is transported in the plasma predominantly as cholesteryl esters associated with lipoproteins (see Chapter 16). Dietary cholesterol is transported from the small intestine to the liver within chylomicrons. Cholesterol synthesized by the liver, as well as any dietary cholesterol in the liver that exceeds hepatic needs, is transported in the serum within very-low-density lipoproteins (VLDL). VLDL are converted to low-density lipoproteins (LDL) through the action of endothelial cell-associated lipoprotein lipase (LPL) present exclusively in the vasculature of skeletal muscle, cardiac muscle, and adipose tissue. The inability to properly utilize and dispose of serum cholesterol due to inherited mutations in several genes results in the autosomal dominant familial hypercholesterolemias (Clinical Box 15–3).

CLINICAL BOX 15–3 THE FAMILIAL HYPERCHOLESTEROLEMIAS

Classic familial hypercholesterolemia, FH (type 2a hyperlipidemia) is an autosomal dominant disorder that results from mutations affecting the structure and function of the cell-surface receptor that binds plasma LDL (low-density lipoproteins) removing them from the circulation. The defects in LDL-LDL receptor (LDLR) interaction result in lifelong elevation of LDL-cholesterol (LDL-C) in the blood. The resultant hypercholesterolemia leads to premature coronary artery disease and atherosclerotic plaque formation in the coronary arteries and the aorta. Although the primary causes of FH are mutations in the *LDLR* gene (representing 60–80% of FH patients), mutations in the apolipoprotein B (*APOB*) gene that cause familial ligand-defective apoB (often referred to as familial hypercholesterolemia type 2) and gain-of-function mutations in the proprotein convertase subtilisin/kexin type 9 (*PCSK9*) gene are also associated with autosomal dominant forms of familial hypercholesterolemia. Mutations in the *APOB* gene represent about 1–5% of FH cases, whereas mutations in the *PCSK9* gene represent no more than 3% of identified cases of FH. Although classic FH is inherited in an autosomal dominant manner, the disease exhibits a gene dosage effect. Homozygous individuals are more severely affected than are heterozygotes. Heterozygotes for FH occur with a frequency of 1 in 500 which makes this disease one of the most common inherited disorders in metabolism. Six different classes of receptor mutation have been identified in FH with each class having multiple alleles. More than 700 different mutations in the *LDLR* gene have been found in FH. The class 1 mutations are null mutations because these result in a failure to make any detectable LDLR protein. Class 2 mutations are the most common and represent intracellular transport defects. The LDLR does not move between the endoplasmic reticulum (ER) and the Golgi membranes. Class 3 mutations represent LDLRs that are delivered to the cell surface but fail in their ability to bind LDL. Class 4 mutations are the rarest and result in LDLR protein that will bind LDL but the LDLR-LDL complexes cannot be internalized. Class 5 mutations result in receptors that bind and internalize the LDL particle but cannot release the particles in the endosomes so the receptors cannot recycle back to the cell surface. Class 6 mutations are in the cytoplasmic tail of the protein which leads to failure to reach the hepatocyte plasma membrane. The clinical characteristics of FH include elevated concentrations of plasma LDL and deposition of LDL-cholesterol in the arteries, tendons, and skin. Fat deposits in the arteries are called atheromas and in the skin and tendons they are called xanthomas. In heterozygotes, hypercholesterolemia is the earliest clinical manifestation in FH and remains the only clinical finding during the first decade of life. Xanthomas and the characteristic arcus cornea (whitish ring on the peripheral cornea) begin to appear in the second decade. The symptoms of coronary heart disease present in the fourth decade. At the time of death 80% of heterozygotes will have xanthomas. The clinical picture is more uniform and severe in homozygotes. Homozygotes present with marked hypercholesterolemia at birth and it will persist throughout life. Xanthomas, arcus cornea, and atherosclerosis will develop during childhood in homozygotes. Death from myocardial infarction usually will occur before the age of 30 in homozygotes. The pathology associated with *APOB* gene mutations in familial ligand-defective apoB is similar to the pathology of LDLR mutations, namely severe elevations in serum LDL cholesterol and early onset coronary atherosclerosis. However, familial ligand-defective apoB patients usually have less severe hypercholesterolemia, reduced incidence of xanthomas, and slightly lower incidence of coronary artery disease. Familial ligand-defective apoB results from four different mutations in the *APOB* gene. The most common mutation in the *APOB* gene found in this disorder results in the substitution of a glutamine (Gln; Q) for arginine (Arg; R) at amino acid 3500, identified as the R3500Q mutation. Another mutation at the same codon results in substitution of the Arg for tryptophan (Trp; W), identified as the R3500W mutation. The other two identified mutations alter codon 3531 resulting in substitution of cysteine (Cys; C) for Arg, identified as the C3531R mutation, and codon 3480 where Trp is substituted for Arg, identified as the R3480W mutation. The normal function of PCSK9 is to degrade some of the LDL receptors that are endocytosed following binding of LDL. PCSK9 is a secreted protein that associates with the extracellular domain of the LDL receptor, predominantly on hepatocytes, and is co-internalized

CLINICAL BOX 15–3 (CONTINUED)

with LDL-LDL receptor complexes. The action of PCSK9 on LDL receptor protein in the endosomal compartment following internalization results in less than 100% of the LDL receptors being recycled to the plasma membrane. Therefore, PCSK9 mutations that enhance the activity of the enzyme will result in even greater level of LDL receptor degradation and dramatically less LDL receptor recycling. This will result in significant reduction in the capacity for LDL binding with a consequent elevation in serum LDL levels, typical of familial hypercholesterolemia.

PHARMACOLOGIC INTERVENTION IN HYPERCHOLESTEROLEMIA

Reductions in circulating cholesterol levels can have profound positive impacts on cardiovascular disease, particularly on atherosclerosis, as well as other metabolic disruptions of the vasculature. Numerous therapies have been developed for intervention in conditions of hypercholesterolemia and hyperlipoproteinemia.

A. Alirocumab (Praluent), Evolocumab (Repatha)

These drugs are the newest type of anti-hypercholesterolemia drugs recently approved by the FDA for use in the United States. Both drugs are injectable antibodies that block the function of proprotein convertase subtilisin/kexin type 9, PCSK9. PCSK9 is serine protease of the subtilisin-like proprotein convertase-2 family whose major function is the endosomal degradation of the LDL receptor (LDLR), thereby reducing the recycling of the LDLR to the plasma membrane. Hypercholesterolemic patients taking another cholesterol-lowering drug while simultaneously utilizing either of these new PCSK9 inhibitors saw further reductions in serum LDL levels between 55% and 77%.

B. Atorvastatin (Lipitor), Simvastatin (Zocor), Lovastatin (Mevacor)

These drugs are fungal HMG-CoA reductase (HMGR) inhibitors and are members of the family of drugs referred to as the statins. The net result of treatment with statins is an increased cellular uptake of LDL, since the intracellular synthesis of cholesterol is inhibited and cells are therefore dependent on extracellular sources of cholesterol.

C. Nicotinic acid (Niacor and Niaspan)

Nicotinic acid reduces the plasma levels of both VLDL and LDL by inhibiting hepatic VLDL secretion, as well as suppressing the flux of free fatty acid release from adipose tissue by inhibiting lipolysis. In addition, nicotinic acid administration strongly increases the circulating levels of HDL.

D. Gemfibrozil (Lopid), Fenofibrate (TriCor)

These compounds (called fibrates) are derivatives of fibric acid. The fibrates acts as activators of the peroxisome proliferator-activated receptor-α (PPARα) class of proteins that are members of the nuclear receptor coactivator family. Activation of PPARα results in modulation of the expression of genes involved in lipid metabolism, carbohydrate metabolism, and adipose tissue differentiation. Fibrates result in the activation of PPARα in liver and muscle. In the liver this leads to increased peroxisomal β-oxidation of fatty acids, thereby decreasing the liver's secretion of triacylglycerol- and cholesterol-rich VLDL, as well as increased clearance of chylomicron remnants, increased levels of HDL, and increased lipoprotein lipase activity which in turn promotes rapid VLDL turnover.

E. Cholestyramine or colestipol (resins)

These compounds are nonabsorbable resins that bind bile acids in the intestines preventing their reentry via the enterohepatic circulation. The drop in bile acid return to the liver reduces the bile acid-mediated inhibition of bile acid synthesis. As a result, a greater amount of cholesterol is converted to bile acids to maintain a steady level in circulation. Additionally, the synthesis of LDL receptors increases to allow increased cholesterol uptake for bile acid synthesis, and the overall effect is a reduction in plasma cholesterol.

F. Ezetimibe

This drug is sold under the trade names Zetia or Ezetrol and is also combined with the statin drug simvastatin and sold as Vytorin or Inegy. Ezetimibe functions to reduce intestinal absorption of cholesterol by blocking the intestinal cholesterol uptake transporter known as Niemann-Pick type C1-like 1 (NPC1L1). The combination drug of ezetimibe and simvastatin has shown efficacy equal to or slightly greater than atorvastatin (Lipitor) alone at reducing circulating cholesterol levels.

G. Lomitapide

Certain patient populations, especially individuals that are homozygous for mutations in the LDL receptor are not effectively treated with drugs such as alirocumab and statins. Two recent drugs, that were designed to target liver lipoprotein homeostasis, have been approved for use in humans. One drug, lomitapide (Juxtapid), is a small molecule inhibitor of the microsomal triglyceride transfer protein (MTTP; also referred to as MTP). MTTP is a heterodimeric complex that is required for the incorporation of apoB-48 into chylomicrons in the intestines and apoB-100 into VLDL by the liver. Lomitapide has been shown to reduce circulating LDL in homozygous FH patients by up to 50%.

H. Mipomersen

The drug mipomersen (Kynamro) is an antisense oligonucleotide (ASO) that targets the apoB mRNA in the liver, thereby resulting in reduced synthesis of the apoB-100 protein. Since apoB-100 is required for VLDL assembly in the liver, there is reduced VLDL secretion by the liver.

I. Bempedoic Acid

Bempedoic acid is a dicarboxylic acid that was demonstrated to inhibit fatty acid and cholesterol synthesis that correlated to reductions in plasma triglyceride and lipoprotein levels. Bempedoic acid is a prodrug that is converted exclusively in the liver to its active CoA-derivative, bempedoyl-CoA. The conversion of bempedoic acid to its CoA derivative is required for its ability to suppress lipid synthesis and to also stimulate mitochondrial fatty acid β-oxidation. One advantage of bempedoic acid over statins in the treatment of hypercholesterolemia is that the lack of expression of the enzyme that attaches CoA to the drug in skeletal muscle prevents any adverse side effects in that tissue. The US FDA approved the use of orally administered bempedoic acid alone (Nexletol) or in combination with ezetimibe (Nexlizet) in February of 2020.

CHECKLIST

- ☑ Cholesterol is required for synthesis of the bile acids required for lipid digestion and absorption, synthesis of the steroid hormones, and incorporation into membranes and lipoprotein particles.
- ☑ Cholesterol synthesis occurs in the cytosol and mitochondrially derived acetyl-CoA must first be transported to the cytosol as citrate.
- ☑ Cholesterol synthesis requires many reactions, some of which generate byproducts that are utilized in other important biological processes.
- ☑ Cholesterol synthesis is tightly regulated at the level of HMGR activity and level.
- ☑ The master metabolic regulator, AMPK, is a critical enzyme in the control of HMGR activity.
- ☑ Transcriptional regulation of genes involved in cholesterol biosynthesis (eg, HMGR) occurs via regulated activity of SREBP.
- ☑ Defects in the terminal enzyme of cholesterol biosynthesis, 7-dehydrocholesterol reductase (DHCR7) result in SLOS.
- ☑ FH is one of the most common genetic causes of hypercholesterolemia.
- ☑ Treatment of hypercholesterolemia can be affected by several approaches with the statin drugs being the most prescribed class.

BILE ACID SYNTHESIS PATHWAYS

Although several of the enzymes involved in bile acid synthesis are active in many cell types, the liver is the only organ where their complete biosynthesis can occur. The major pathway for the synthesis of the bile acids is referred to as the "classic" or "neutral" pathway (Figure 15–3). This pathway is initiated via

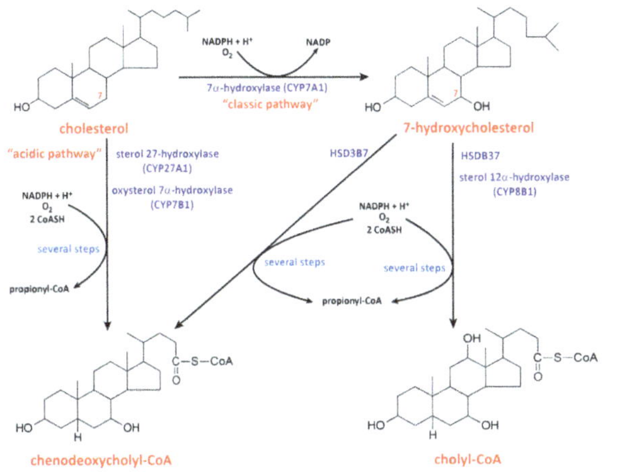

FIGURE 15–3 Synthesis of the two primary bile acids, cholic acid (CA) and chenodeoxycholic acid (CDCA). The reaction catalyzed by the 7α-hydroxylase (CYP7A1) is the rate-limiting step in bile acid synthesis. Expression of CYP7A1 occurs only in the liver. Conversion of 7α-hydroxycholesterol to the bile acids requires several steps not shown in detail in this image. Only the relevant cofactors needed for the synthesis steps are shown. Sterol 12α-hydroxylase (CYB8B1) controls the synthesis of cholic acid and as such is under tight transcriptional control. (Reproduced with permission from themedicalbiochemistrypage, LLC.)

hydroxylation of cholesterol at the 7 position via the action of cholesterol 7α-hydroxylase (CYP7A1).

There is an alternative pathway that involves hydroxylation of cholesterol at the 27 position by the mitochondrial enzyme sterol 27-hydroxylase (CYP27A1). This alternative pathway is referred to as the "acidic" pathway of bile acid synthesis. In humans this alternative bile acid synthesis pathway accounts for no more than 6% of total bile acid production.

The end-products of hepatic bile acid synthesis are chenodeoxycholic acid (CDCA) and cholic acid (CA) and are referred to as the primary bile acids. Chenodeoxycholic acid represents around 45% and cholic acid around 30% of the bile acids in human bile excretions from the gallbladder. Before the CDCA and CA are secreted into the canalicular lumen, they are conjugated via an amide bond at the terminal carboxyl group with either of the two amino acids glycine or taurine. This conjugation process increases the amphipathic nature of the bile acids making them more water soluble as well as less cytotoxic.

ENTEROHEPATIC CIRCULATION AND BILE ACID MODIFICATION

Following secretion by the liver the bile acids enter the bile canaliculi which join with the bile ductules which then form the bile ducts. Bile acids are carried from the liver through these ducts to the gallbladder, where they are stored for future use. In the gallbladder bile acids are concentrated up to 1000-fold. Following stimulation by food intake the gallbladder releases the bile into the duodenum, via the action of the gut hormone cholecystokinin,

CCK (see Chapter 31), where they aid in the emulsification of dietary lipids.

Within the intestines the primary bile acids are acted upon by bacteria and undergo a deconjugation process that removes the glycine and taurine residues. The deconjugated bile acids are either excreted or reabsorbed by the gut and returned to the liver. Anaerobic bacteria modify the primary bile acids converting them to the secondary bile acids, identified as deoxycholate (from cholate) and lithocholate (from chenodeoxycholate). As much as 95% of total bile acid synthesized by the liver is absorbed by the distal ileum and returned to the liver. This process of secretion from the liver to the gallbladder and then to the intestines and finally reabsorption is termed the enterohepatic circulation.

REGULATION OF BILE ACID SYNTHESIS

Bile acids regulate the expression of genes involved in their synthesis, thereby creating a feedback loop. This regulatory mechanism involves the receptors called the farnesoid X receptors, FXR. The FXR belong to the superfamily of nuclear receptors that includes the steroid/thyroid hormone receptor family as well as the retinoid X receptors (RXR) and the peroxisome proliferator-activated receptors (PPAR). FXR forms a heterodimer with members of the RXR family. One major target of FXR is the small heterodimer partner (*SHP*) gene. Activation of SHP expression by FXR results in inhibition of transcription of the cholesterol 7α-hydroxylase gene (CYP7A1) (Clinical Box 15–4).

CLINICAL BOX 15–4 GALLSTONES

Gallstones are hard, pebble-like deposits that form inside the gallbladder. The clinical term for this condition is cholelithiasis. Gallstones may be as small as a grain of sand or as large as a golf ball. Gallstones are more common in women, Native Americans, and other ethnic groups, and people older than 40 years. Gallstones may also run in families. There are a variety of causes for the formation of gallstones. There are two main types of gallstones, those composed primarily of cholesterol and those composed of bilirubin. Gallstones formed from cholesterol are the most common type. Gallstones formed from too much bilirubin in the bile are called pigment stones. Gallstones can remain asymptomatic for many years. Migration of the stones into the ductal system of the gallbladder can result in obstruction of bile flow resulting in inflammation. If a large stone blocks either the cystic duct or the common bile duct (called choledocholithiasis), symptoms will include a cramping pain in the middle to right upper abdomen. This is known as biliary colic. The pain goes away if the stone passes into the duodenum via the common bile duct. Once gallstones become symptomatic, definitive surgical intervention with excision of the gallbladder (cholecystectomy) is usually indicated. Cholecystectomy is among the most frequently performed abdominal surgical procedures.

CHECKLIST

- ☑ Bile acids represent the major pathway for the metabolism of cholesterol.
- ☑ Bile acids are synthesized in the liver, stored within the gallbladder, and secreted into the intestines, via the actions of cholecystokinin (CCK), in response to food intake in order to aid in the solubilization of lipids and lipid-soluble vitamins.
- ☑ The most abundant bile acids in human bile are chenodeoxycholic acid (45%) and cholic acid (31%) which are referred to as the primary bile acids.
- ☑ Bile acids are modified, prior to secretion into the bile canaliculi, by amino acid addition which increases their amphipathic nature making them more easily secretable as well as less cytotoxic.
- ☑ Within the intestines the primary bile acids are acted upon by bacteria and undergo a deconjugation process that removes the glycine and taurine residues. Anaerobic bacteria present in the colon modify the primary bile acids converting them to the secondary bile acids, identified as deoxycholate (from cholate) and lithocholate (from chenodeoxycholate).
- ☑ Both primary and secondary bile acids are reabsorbed by the intestines and delivered back to the liver via the portal circulation which results in as much as 95% of total bile acid synthesized by the liver being returned to the liver. This process of secretion from the liver to the gallbladder, to the intestines, and finally reabsorption is termed the enterohepatic circulation.
- ☑ Bile acids and bile acid metabolites are bioactive lipids that bind to transcription factors of the nuclear receptor family leading to a wide range of biological effects.
- ☑ Defects in enzymes of bile acid metabolism and membrane transport of bile acids can result in liver dysfunction, cholestatic liver disease, cirrhosis, progressive jaundice, and fatty diarrhea (steatorrhea).

REVIEW QUESTIONS

1. Experiments are being conducted on the effects of a novel compound designed to inhibit the synthesis of intestinal fibroblast growth factor 19 (FGF19). Given the compound elicits the expected effect, which of the following is the most likely response that would be observed in experimental animals to whom the compound is administered?
(A) Enhanced expression of SREBP
(B) Enhanced expression of the rate-limiting enzyme in bile acid synthesis
(C) Enhanced secretion of bile acids onto the bile canaliculi
(D) Inhibited expression of SREBP
(E) Inhibited expression of the rate-limiting enzyme of bile acid synthesis
(F) Inhibition of secretion of bile acids onto the bile canaliculi

2. Physical examination of a neonate shows microcephaly (small head), micrognathia (small jaw), ptosis (drooping eyelids), cleft palate, and syndactyly of the second and third toes. These findings are most likely the result of a defect in which of the following metabolic processes?
(A) Bile acid synthesis
(B) Cholesterol esterification of protein
(C) Cholesterol synthesis
(D) Dolichol synthesis
(E) Protein acetylation

3. A physician has been treating a 57-year-old male patient who had a myocardial infarction 6 months previously. The prescribed treatment was the use of a high dose of a statin-type drug. The outcome from this therapy was a reduction in the patient's total serum cholesterol from 345 mg/dL to 250 mg/dL. Which of the following processes most likely accounts for the drug-induced reduction in the patient's total cholesterol?
(A) Increased cleavage of SREBP in the Golgi
(B) Increased transcription of the *CETP* gene
(C) Reduced transcription of the LDL receptor gene
(D) Retention of SCAP/SREBP in the endoplasmic reticulum by INSIG
(E) Targeting of the ubiquitin ligase machinery to HMG-CoA reductase

4. A 53-year-old male patient who had a myocardial infarction 6 months ago has been taking a high-dose statin therapy. This therapy resulted in a reduction of his total cholesterol from 325 mg/dL to 240 mg/dL. In order to obtain a further reduction in his serum cholesterol levels, his cardiologist adds evolocumab (a PCSK9 inhibitor) to his therapy. Which of the following best describes the common effect of these two distinct therapies?
(A) Activation of cholesterol ester transfer protein (CETP)
(B) Decrease in the level of HMG-CoA reductase activity
(C) Decrease in the recycling of bile acids from the intestines
(D) Increasing the quantity of plasma membrane-associated HDL receptors
(E) Increasing the quantity of plasma membrane-associated LDL receptors
(F) Inhibition of the synthesis of HMG-CoA reductase

5. A 39-year-old man is being examined by his physician with complaints of recurrent bouts of abdominal pain for the past 6 months. Physical examination finds the presence of numerous xanthomas on his feet, hands, knees, and buttocks. Abdominal palpation finds hepatomegaly. Serum studies show triglyceride levels of 1540 mg/dL (N = <150 mg/dL) along with below normal levels of both LDL and HDL. A deficiency in which of the following would most likely account for the signs and symptoms in this patient?
(A) ApoA-I
(B) ApoB-100
(C) ApoB-48
(D) ApoC-II
(E) HDL receptors (SR-B1)
(F) LDL receptors

6. During an examination in the emergency department following a suspected heart attack it is found that a 39-year-old woman has a total serum cholesterol level of 385 mg/dL (N = <200 mg/dL). A mutation in the gene encoding which of the following proteins would most likely explain the pathology in this patient?
(A) ApoA-I
(B) ApoB-100
(C) ApoC-II
(D) Cholesterol ester transfer protein (CETP)
(E) Lipoprotein lipase

7. A 6-month-old infant presents with progressive neurologic dysfunction, cholestasis, bilateral cataracts, and chronic diarrhea. A diagnosis is made of a bile acid metabolism defect due to deficiency in the sterol 27-hydroxylase gene. Which of the following would most likely be an additional finding in this infant?
(A) Decreased overall levels of chenodeoxycholic acid
(B) Decreased overall levels of cholic acid
(C) Decreased overall levels of 7-dehydrocholesterol
(D) Elevated cholesterol ester levels in the gallbladder
(E) Elevated taurocholic acid levels in the biliary canaliculi
(F) Elevated deoxycholic acid levels in the gallbladder

8. A 67-year-old woman is being examined in the emergency department with complaints of chest pain radiating to her left arm. Blood work reveals her total cholesterol to be 290 mg/dL (N = <200 mg/dL). The attending physician prescribes a statin. Which of the following best describes the benefit of the prescribed therapy for this patient?
(A) Decrease of the serum level of LDL by promoting catabolism
(B) Increase in the serum level of HDL thereby promoting increased reverse cholesterol transport
(C) Inhibition of the synthesis of LDL receptors
(D) Inhibition of the formation of LDL from VLDL
(E) Inhibition of the rate-limiting step in cholesterol biosynthesis

9. A 39-year-old woman is being examined in the emergency department with complaints of chest pain radiating to her left arm. Her serum cholesterol level is 430 mg/dL (N = <200 mg/dL). History reveals that her father died at the age of 37 from a heart attack and that her brother also died of a heart attack at the age of 32. Given the patients pathology and family history, it is most likely that she inherited a mutation resulting in which of the following?
(A) Abnormal LDL receptors
(B) Decreased activity of HMG-CoA reductase
(C) Increased conversion of VLDL to LDL

(D) Decreased activity of 7-dehydrocholesterol reductase
(E) Reduced plasma concentration of HDL

10. Physical examination of a neonate shows microcephaly (small head), micrognathia (small jaw), ptosis (drooping eyelids), cleft palate, and syndactyly of the second and third toes. These findings are most likely the result of a defect in which of the following enzymes?
(A) 7-Dehydrocholesterol reductase
(B) 3-Hydroxy-3-methylglutaryl-CoA (HMG-CoA) reductase
(C) 3-Hydroxy-3-methylglutaryl-CoA (HMG-CoA) synthase
(D) Lanosterol synthase
(E) Mevalonate kinase

11. Physical examination of a neonate shows microcephaly (small head), micrognathia (small jaw), ptosis (drooping eyelids), cleft palate, and syndactyly of the second and third toes. Measurement of the blood levels of which of the following compounds would be most useful for a correct diagnosis in this infant?
(A) 7-Dehydrocholesterol
(B) Farnesylpyrophosphate
(C) Geranylpyrophosphate
(D) Lanosterol
(E) Mevalonate
(F) Squalene

12. A 5-month-old infant is taken to her pediatrician because her parents are concerned about her general failure to thrive and a progressive yellowing of her eyes and skin. Physical examination finds that the infant has slight bowing of the legs, indicative of rickets. Additional physical findings include hepatomegaly and steatorrhea. The pediatrician suspects the infant has an inherited defect in bile acid metabolism. Which of the following enzymes is most likely to be defective in this infant?
(A) Bile salt export protein (BSEP)
(B) 3β-Hydroxy Δ^5 C_{27}-steroid oxidoreductase (HSD3B7)
(C) 7α-Hydroxylase (CYP7A1)
(D) Multidrug resistance associated protein 2 (MRP2)
(E) Sterol 27-hydroxylase (CYP27A1)

13. A 27-year-old man who has suffered a heart attack has a serum total cholesterol concentration of 480 mg/dL (N = <200 mg/dL). Despite changing his lifestyle and diet, the patient seems incapable of attaining optimal total serum cholesterol levels. The patient's cardiologist prescribed a drug that promotes LDL receptor recycling to the plasma membrane, particularly in hepatocytes. Which of the following is the most likely target of this drug?
(A) HMG-CoA reductase (HMGR)
(B) Lecithin:cholesterol acyltransferase (LCAT)
(C) Lipoprotein lipase (LPL)
(D) Microsomal triglyceride transfer protein (MTTP)
(E) Proprotein convertase subtilisin/kexin type 9 (PCSK9)

14. Experiments are being performed with a novel compound that has been shown to alter the processes of bile acid synthesis. The effects of this compound are very nearly identical to those exerted on this process by chenodeoxycholic acid. Given these results, which of the following represents the most likely target of this novel compound?
(A) Carbohydrate response element-binding protein (ChREBP)
(B) Farnesoid X receptor (FXR)
(C) 7α-Hydroxylase (CYP7A1)
(D) HMG-CoA reductase
(E) Sterol response element-binding protein (SREBP)

15. A 67-year-old man is undergoing tests following a heart attack. Blood work reveals his total cholesterol to be 290 mg/dL (N = <200 mg/dL) and his LDL cholesterol is 132 mg/dL (N = <100 mg/dL). Studies performed on hepatocytes from a liver biopsy determine the number of LDL receptors are equivalent to controls. Which of the following could best explain the observations in this patient?
(A) Hepatocytes from the patient are defective in the selective removal of cholesterol from the LDL complex
(B) Hepatocytes from the patient have decreased levels of acyl-CoA:cholesterol acyltransferase, ACAT
(C) The patient has a mutated form of apoB-100
(D) The patient's hepatic vascular endothelial cells lack functional lipoprotein lipase
(E) The patient's LDL receptor is likely to be abnormally phosphorylated

16. A 9-year-old girl presents with low red blood cell count, corneal opacities, and renal insufficiency. She is diagnosed with lecithin:cholesterol acyltransferase (LCAT) deficiency. Given these findings, which of the following is most likely to be defective in this patient?
(A) Fatty acid esterification of cholesterol
(B) Conversion of 7-dehydrocholesterol to cholesterol
(C) Hepatic removal of cholesterol from HDL
(D) Transfer of cholesterol esters from HDL to LDL
(E) Receptor-mediated hepatic LDL uptake

17. An autopsy is conducted on a stillborn female fetus exhibiting multiple lethal congenital malformations and osteosclerosis. Analysis of lipids accumulated in tissues showed high levels of desmosterol and extremely low levels of cholesterol. Which of the following enzymes was most likely defective in this fetus resulting in the lethality?
(A) 7-Dehydrocholesterol reductase
(B) 24-Dehydrocholesterol reductase
(C) HMG-CoA reductase
(D) Mevalonate kinase
(E) Squalene monooxygenase

18. A line of transgenic mice has been generated in which the gene encoding the transcription factor, small heterodimer partner (SHP) has been disabled specifically in hepatocytes. Which of the following processes associated with bile acid metabolism, would most likely be altered in the livers of these mice?
(A) Activation of bile acid synthesis
(B) Bile acid conjugation
(C) Bile acid export to bile canaliculi
(D) Bile acid reuptake from the intestine
(E) Synthesis of chenodeoxycholate

19. A 35-year-old man who has suffered a heart attack has a serum total cholesterol concentration of 480 mg/dL (N = <200 mg/dL). His father died at 41 years of age from a massive heart attack. One of his two siblings had recently had his fasting plasma lipid levels tested and was found to have a serum total cholesterol level of 375 mg/dL. The best explanation for the clinical findings in this patient and his family is a reduced level of which of the following?
(A) Acyl-CoA:cholesterol acyltransferase (ACAT)
(B) HMG-CoA reductase (HMGR)
(C) Lecithin:cholesterol acyltransferase

(D) Low-density lipoprotein (LDL) receptor
(E) Lipoprotein lipase

20. A 22-year-old man is being examined by his physician with complaints of abdominal pain and because he is concerned about growths on his eyelids. He is 180 cm (5ft 11 in) tall and weighs 85 kg (188 lb); BMI is 26 kg/m^2. Physical examination shows no other abnormalities except for xanthelasmas. Serum studies show a total cholesterol concentration of 250 mg/dL (N = <200 mg/dL), HDL-cholesterol concentration of 37 mg/dL (N = >50 mg/dL), and triglyceride concentration of 3500 mg/dL (N = <150 mg/dL). A deficiency in which of the following would best explain the findings in this patient?
(A) 7-Dehydrocholesterol reductase
(B) Hepatic lipase
(C) HMG-CoA reductase
(D) Hormone-sensitive lipase
(E) Lipoprotein lipase

21. Experiments are being conducted on hepatocytes in culture to study the effects of a novel compound structurally related to atorvastatin. When added to the cultures it is found that the level of plasma membrane-associated glycoproteins is significantly reduced when compared to untreated cells. Given these results, measurement for which of the following would most likely show reduced levels in the treated cells?
(A) Acetoacetyl-CoA
(B) Chenodeoxycholic acid
(C) Cholic acid
(D) Dolichol phosphate
(E) HMG-CoA

22. Experiments are being carried out to assess the function of the cholesterol biosynthesis pathway in a cell line derived from a hepatoma. Protein localization studies find that functional sterol regulated element binding protein (SREBP) is not associated with membranes of the endoplasmic reticulum, as is the case in normal hepatocytes. Given these results, which of the following activities would most likely be enhanced in the cancer cells relative to normal hepatocytes?
(A) 7-Dehydrocholesterol reductase
(B) HMG-CoA reductase
(C) HMG-CoA synthase
(D) Mevalonate kinase
(E) SCAP

23. Experiments are being conducted on the pathway of cholesterol biosynthesis using a cell line derived from a human hepatoma. Results from these experiments find that the addition of 25-hydroxycholesterol to the cells does not lead to a reduction in measurable amounts of newly synthesized cholesterol. These observations are the opposite of what is determined when 25-hydroxycholesterol is added to normal hepatocytes in culture. These results indicate that normal regulation of which of the following enzymes is defective in these hepatoma cells?
(A) 7-Dehydrocholesterol reductase (DHCR7)
(B) HMG-CoA reductase (HMGR)
(C) HMG-CoA synthase
(D) Mevalonate kinase
(E) Squalene monoxygenase

24. Experiments are being carried out on cells in culture with a novel compound that represses mitochondrial ATP production. Addition of the compound results in a dramatic decrease in the production of farnesylated proteins. Which of the following proteins exhibits reduced activity in the presence of the compound accounting for the observed reduction in modified proteins?
(A) AMP-activated kinase (AMPK)
(B) HMG-CoA reductase phosphatase
(C) HMG-CoA reductase (HMGR)
(D) Protein phosphatase-1 (PP1)
(E) Protein kinase A (PKA)

25. Experiments are being conducted on a newly identified plasma membrane G-protein coupled receptor (GPCR). Characterization of the receptor shows that it is coupled to a G_s-type G-protein. Activation of this receptor is most likely to affect the rate of cholesterol biosynthesis because of which of the following?
(A) cAMP activates AMP-regulated kinase (AMPK) which then phosphorylates and activates HMG-CoA reductase
(B) cAMP-dependent protein kinase (PKA) is activated leading to inhibition of HMGR phosphatase
(C) cAMP-dependent protein kinase (PKA) is activated which then phosphorylates and inhibits HMGR
(D) cAMP-dependent protein kinase (PKA) is activated which phosphorylates and inhibits AMPK allowing HMGR to remain active
(E) The resultant increased cAMP directly inhibits HMGR via allosteric interaction

26. Experiments are being conducted on a cell line derived from a human hepatoma. Results of these studies find that even though the cells have no detectable expression of ATP-citrate lyase (ACL), the rate of cholesterol synthesis is observed to be approximately 60% of that occurring in control hepatocytes. The most likely explanation for this observation is an enhanced activity of which of the following enzymes?
(A) Acetyl-CoA synthetase
(B) Acetoacetyl-CoA synthetase
(C) HMG-CoA reductase
(D) HMG-CoA synthase
(E) Mevalonate kinase

27. In familial hypercholesterolemia the elevated plasma LDL cholesterol is highly susceptible to oxidation forming oxidized LDL (oxLDL). oxLDL are taken up by macrophages, which become engorged to form foam cells. Which of the following best explains the oxLDL-induced formation of foam cells?
(A) Cholesterol cannot be extracted from macrophages by HDL
(B) Expression of the receptors for oxLDL is increased in the macrophages
(C) LDL enters by pinocytosis to form foam cells
(D) LDL receptors on peripheral cells are upregulated
(E) There is increased synthesis of cholesterol in macrophages as a result

28. Experiments are being conducted on the pathway of cholesterol biosynthesis using a cell line derived from a liver biopsy. Results from these experiments find that the addition of 25-hydroxycholesterol to the cells results in a measurable reduction in newly synthesized cholesterol. Which of the following most closely reflects the mechanism by which this compound exerts its effect?
(A) Condensation of acetyl-CoA and acetoacetyl-CoA to form hydroxymethyl glutaryl-CoA
(B) Cyclizing of squalene to form lanosterol

(C) Formation of mevalonate from HMG-CoA
(D) Induces phosphorylation of HMG-CoA reductase
(E) Reduction of 7-dehydrocholesterol to form cholesterol

29. A 58-year-old man, who suffered a heart attack, is undergoing a follow-up examination. Immediately after his heart attack his physician prescribed a statin. The patient now indicates that the drug has caused severe leg cramping and pain. His physician recommends a switch to a vitamin-based therapy. Which of the following processes is most likely to be affected by this new therapeutic protocol?
(A) Adipocyte fatty acid release
(B) Adipocyte triglyceride synthesis
(C) HDL-mediated reverse cholesterol transport
(D) Hepatic LDL receptor synthesis
(E) HMG-CoA synthesis

30. A 2-year-old girl who is exhibiting a failure to thrive is diagnosed with hepatic failure and cholestasis. Her pediatrician suspects the girl is suffering from a form of familial intrahepatic cholestasis. Which of the following processes is most likely to be defective in this patient?
(A) Bile acid synthesis
(B) Cholesterol synthesis
(C) Gallbladder excretion into the intestines
(D) Hepatic bile acid export
(E) Mevalonate synthesis

31. Experiments are being conducted on the processes of bile acid metabolism using a cell line derived from a hepatoma. Mass spec and gas chromatographic studies indicate that the cell line produces chenodeoxycholic acid and related metabolites but does not produce cholic acid nor any metabolites of this compound. Which of the following is the most likely enzyme missing or defective in these cells?
(A) Bile acid-CoA synthetase
(B) 7-Dehydrocholesterol reductase (DHC7R)
(C) HMG-CoA reductase
(D) 7 α-Hydroxylase (CYP7A1)
(E) Sterol 27-hydroxylase (CYP27A1)

32. An 11-year-old boy is being evaluated for progressive neuropathy. Physical examination shows the boy to be short for his age, he exhibits a spastic gait, his deep tendon reflexes are decreased, and his proprioception is impaired. Ophthalmoscopic examination finds pigmentary retinal degeneration. History reveals that in addition to frequent diarrhea he has steatorrhea. Laboratory studies on his serum lipids find that the total cholesterol is 33 mg/dL (N = <170 mg/dL), triglycerides are undetectable (N = <150 mg/dL), and HDL cholesterol is 28 mg/dL (N = >45 mg/dL). The identification of a mutation in the gene encoding which of the following would most likely account for the signs and symptoms in this patient?
(A) ApoC-II
(B) 7-Dehydrocholesterol reductase
(C) Lecithin acyl cholesterol transferase (LCAT)
(D) LDL receptor
(E) Microsomal triglyceride transfer protein (MTTP)

33. A 27-year-old man is being examined by his physician because he is concerned about fatty-looking growths on his eyelids. The patient also states that he has been having abdominal pain of varying intensity for the past week. He is 180 cm (5ft 11 in) tall and weighs 85 kg (188 lb); BMI is 26 kg/m^2. Serum studies show a total cholesterol concentration of 675 mg/dL (N = < 200 mg/dL), LDL-cholesterol concentration of 240 mg/dL (N = < 100 mg/dL), HDL-cholesterol concentration of 43 mg/dL (N = > 50 mg/dL), and triglyceride concentration of 152 mg/dL (N = < 150 mg/dL). Which of the following processes is the most likely cause of this patient's signs and symptoms?
(A) A mutation in a gene encoding a microsomal lipid transfer protein
(B) A mutation in a gene encoding a protein receptor
(C) A mutation in a gene encoding an endoplasmic reticulum-localized enzyme
(D) Reduced bile duct function
(E) Reduced enterohepatic circulation
(F) Reduced peroxisomal fatty acid oxidation

34. A 58-year-old man, who suffered a heart attack, is undergoing a follow-up examination. Immediately after his heart attack, his physician prescribed a statin. The patient now indicates that the drug has caused severe leg cramping and pain. His physician recommends a switch to a vitamin-based therapy. Which of the following is most likely to be a complication of this new therapeutic approach?
(A) Easy bruising
(B) Facial flushing
(C) Gastrointestinal pain
(D) Myoglobinuria
(E) Tachycardia

35. A 47-year-old man arrives in the Emergency Department complaining of severe chest pain, shortness of breath, and nausea. Physical examination shows the patient is diphoretic, is exhibiting labored breathing, and has visible xanthelasmas and xanthomas. Blood work finds the patient's total cholesterol is 478 mg/dL (N = < 200 mg/dL), LDL cholesterol is 194 mg/dL (N = < 100 mg/dL), and triglycerides are 165 mg/dL (N = < 150 mg/dL). The attending physician suspects the patient may be experiencing a myocardial infarction and initiates appropriate therapeutic intervention. Following an overnight stay for treatment and observation, the patient is released. It is recommended that he contact his personal physician for follow-up and further investigation. In the course of a follow-up examination, it is found that the patient's LDL receptor gene contains no mutations. Mutation in the gene encoding which of the following proteins is most likely to account for the signs and symptoms in this patient?
(A) ApoB-100
(B) ApoC-II
(C) 7-Dehydrocholesterol reductase
(D) HMG-CoA reductase
(E) Lipoprotein lipase

ANSWERS

1. Correct answer is **B.** When bile acids are secreted by the gallbladder, these compounds can be absorbed by ileal enterocytes. Within the enterocytes the bile acids bind to, and activate, the nuclear receptor FXR. Bile acid activation of FXR leads to the enhanced expression of numerous genes in the enterocytes, with the *FGF19* gene being one of these FXR targets. Activation of the *FGF19* gene results in the protein being secreted into the enterohepatic circulation. When the hormone reaches the liver, it interacts with the βKlotho/FGFR4 complex and triggers activation of a signal transduction cascade. The net result, in the liver, is transcriptional repression of the *CYP7A1* gene, which encodes the rate-limiting enzyme in the "classic pathway" of bile acid synthesis. Therefore, the inhibition of FGF19 production in the intestines would result in enhanced bile acid synthesis in the liver. None of the other options (choices A, C, D, E, and F) reflect significant effects that would be observed in response to the inhibition of FGF19 synthesis in the intestine.

2. Correct answer is **C.** The neonate is most likely manifesting the developmental abnormalities associated with Smith-Lemli-Opitz syndrome (SLOS). SLOS results in multiple malformations and behavioral problems as a consequence of a defect in cholesterol synthesis. The defect resides in the terminal enzyme of the cholesterol biosynthesis pathway, namely 7-dehydrocholesterol reductase. Mutations in the gene (*DHCR7*) encoding this enzyme result in increased levels of 7-dehydrocholesterol and reduced levels (15–27% of normal) of cholesterol in SLOS patients. One of the most important development regulating proteins of early embryos is modified by cholesterol addition. This protein is called sonic hedgehog (abbreviated Shh). Shh is necessary for patterning events that take place in the central nervous system, during limb development, and in the formation of facial structures. Shh function requires that the amino terminal end of the protein be modified by attachment of cholesterol. The involvement of cholesterol in normal Shh function explains many of the abnormalities that are observed in SLOS patients. Defects in none of the other processes (choices A, B, D, and E) result in the developmental abnormalities observed in this neonate.

3. Correct answer is **A.** Control of cholesterol homeostasis is exerted by a number of mechanisms, with transcriptional control of genes encoding key regulatory enzymes is the most significant. Sterols themselves, such as cholesterol are at the heart of this transcriptional regulatory network. Sterol-regulated transcription of key rate-limiting enzymes and by the regulated degradation of HMGR. Activation of transcrip tional control occurs through the regulated cleavage of the membrane-bound transcription factor, sterol-regulated element binding protein, SREBP. SREBP is proteolytically activated, and the proteolysis is controlled by the level of sterols in the cell. Full-length SREBP is embedded in the membrane of the endoplasmic reticulum (ER). Release of the transcription factor domain of SREBP from the ER is controlled by its interaction with a protein called SREBP cleavage-activating protein (SCAP). When cells have sufficient sterol content SREBP and SCAP are retained in the ER preventing SREBP from being released and activating transcription of genes including the gene encoding the rate-limiting step of cholesterol synthesis, 3-hydroxy-3-methylglutaryl-CoA reductase (HMGR). The statin drugs inhibit HMGR which will lower overall cholesterol synthesis resulting in SREBP being released from SCAP, as opposed to being retained in the ER (choice D), allowing it to migrate to the Golgi where it is proteolyzed releasing the transcription factor domain. In addition to the *HMGR* gene, SREBP activates transcription of the gene encoding the LDL receptor so its level of transcription will increase, not decrease (choice C). Neither of the other options (choices B and E) reflect changes resulting from stain-mediated suppression of HMGR.

4. Correct answer is **E.** PCSK9 is secreted by the liver, and it binds to LDL-LDL receptor complexes on hepatocytes which, following endocytosis, stimulates the lysosomal degradation of the LDL receptor (LDLR), thereby reducing the recycling of the LDLR to the plasma membrane. This effect of PCSK9 leads to a reduced ability of the liver to remove IDL and LDL from the blood contributing to the potential for hypercholesterolemia. Therefore, drugs designed to inhibit the function of PCSK9 exert their benefits by allowing for more LDL receptor to be recycled to the plasma membrane enabling more serum LDL to be bound and internalized, thus lowering overall serum levels. None of the other options (choices A, B, C, D, and F) reflect the effects of PCSK9 inhibition.

5. Correct answer is **D.** Significantly elevated levels of serum triglycerides, such as in this patient, most likely reflect defects in one of the two proteins critical to the removal of fatty acids from the triglycerides contained in circulating lipoprotein particles such as chylomicrons and very-low-density lipoprotein (VLDL) particles. These two proteins are the lipoprotein-associated apolipoprotein C-II (apoC-II) and the endothelial cell-associated enzyme, lipoprotein lipase, LPL. LPL is expressed only in the vasculature of skeletal and cardiac muscle and adipose tissue. The activity of LPL requires interaction with apoC-II for its activity. Chylomicrons and VLDL acquire apoC-II through interactions with high-density lipoprotein (HDL) particles. Defects in each of the other proteins (choices A, B, C, E, and F) are associated with pathologies but are distinct from the severe hypertriglyceridemia found in this patient.

6. Correct answer is **B.** High serum total cholesterol levels can result from a number of different causes, with one of the most likely being a defect in the ability of LDL receptors to bind LDL. The LDL receptor requires the presence of apolipoprotein B-100 (apoB-100) in intermediate density (IDL) and LDL particles in order for them to bind. Deficiencies in either apoC-II (choice C) or lipoprotein lipase (choice E) are associated with relatively normal levels of serum cholesterol but significantly elevated levels of triglycerides. Mutations in the gene (*APOA1*) encoding apoA I (choice A) are extremely rare and are the cause of familial HDL deficiency, a disorder associated with corneal opacities, xanthomas, xanthelasmas, and premature coronary artery disease but patients have normal levels of VLDL and LDL cholesterol. Mutation in CETP (choice D) is associated with a positive phenotype of dramatic elevation in the level of high-density lipoprotein (HDL) particles conferring protection from coronary artery disease.

7. Correct answer is **A.** The infant is most likely manifesting the symptoms associated with a defect in the synthesis of bile acids. The alternative bile acid synthesis pathway involves hydroxylation of cholesterol at the carbon 27 position by the mitochondrial enzyme sterol 27-hydroxylase (CYP27A1). This alternative pathway is referred to as the "acidic" pathway of bile acid synthesis. The product of this pathway is chenodeoxycholic acid, the same as for the classic pathway initiated by CYP7A1. However, the acidic pathway does not lead to the synthesis of cholic acid so this bile acid and its metabolites would not be reduced in individuals with a deficiency in CYP27A1. Although the acidic pathway accounts for no more than 6% of total bile acid production, it is an important pathway of bile synthesis as evidenced by the symptoms seen in infants harboring mutations in genes encoding enzymes of the acidic pathway. None of the other options (choices B, C,

D, E, and F) correlate to effects associated with mutation in the *CYP27A1* gene.

8. Correct answer is **E.** The statin drugs inhibit the rate-limiting enzyme in *de novo* cholesterol biosynthesis, 3-hydroxy-3-methylglutaryl-CoA reductase (HMGR). Thus, inhibition of cholesterol synthesis with the use of statin drugs reduces the amount of total cholesterol, such as LDL- and HDL-associated, in the plasma. The statin-mediated reduction in the level of LDL is due to reduced hepatic VLDL production and increased LDL receptor expression, not increased, due to LDL catabolism (choice A). The level of HDL (choice B) does not increase significantly with statin therapy. The statin drugs, by virtue of inhibiting cholesterol synthesis result in increased synthesis of LDL receptors as opposed to inhibition of their synthesis (choice C). The conversion of VLDL to LDL is the result of the action of lipoprotein lipase removing fatty acids from the triglycerides in the VLDL particles and this process is not inhibited (choice D) by statin drugs.

9. Correct answer is **A.** Given the signs and symptoms in this patient, combined with her family history, she is most likely suffering from the most common inherited form of familial hypercholesterolemia, FH. FH is an autosomal dominant disorder that predominantly results from mutations affecting the structure and function of the LDL receptor. The defects in LDL receptor impair binding and uptake of LDL from the blood resulting in lifelong elevation of LDL-cholesterol in the blood. The resultant hypercholesterolemia leads to premature coronary artery disease and atherosclerotic plaque formation. Decreased activity of HMG-CoA reductase (choice B) would result in lower levels of total cholesterol not elevated as in this patient. An increased rate of VLDL conversion to LDL (choice C) would not, in and of itself, result in elevated total serum cholesterol. The enzyme, 7-dehydrocholesterol reductase (choice D) is the terminal enzyme in cholesterol biosynthesis and so a decrease in its activity would result in reduced overall levels of total cholesterol. Genetic causes of reduced plasma HDL levels (choice E) are associated with mutations in the gene encoding the cholesterol transporter, ABCA1, or the gene encoding apoA-I. These mutations are associated with corneal opacities, xanthomas, xanthelasmas, and premature coronary artery disease but patients have normal levels of VLDL and LDL cholesterol.

10. Correct answer is **A.** The neonate is most likely manifesting the developmental abnormalities associated with Smith-Lemli-Opitz syndrome (SLOS). SLOS results in multiple malformations and behavioral problems as a consequence of a defect in cholesterol synthesis. The defect resides in the terminal enzyme of the cholesterol biosynthesis pathway, namely 7-dehydrocholesterol reductase. Mutations in the gene encoding this enzyme result in increased levels of 7-dehydrocholesterol and reduced levels (15–27% of normal) of cholesterol in SLOS patients. One of the most important development regulating proteins of early embryos is modified by cholesterol addition. This protein is called sonic hedgehog (abbreviated Shh). Shh is necessary for patterning events that take place in the central nervous system, during limb development, and in the formation of facial structures. Shh function requires that the amino terminal end of the protein be modified by attachment of cholesterol. Defects in HMG-CoA reductase (choice B) have not been described in humans. Defects in HMG-CoA synthase (choice C) are characterized by episodes of severe hypoketotic hypoglycemia, accompanied by vomiting, hepatomegaly, and lethargy, and which can progress to life-threatening coma. Defects in lanosterol synthase (choice D) are characterized by hypotrichosis and intellectual disability or developmental delay, frequently associated with early-onset epilepsy and other dermatologic features. Defects in mevalonate kinase (choice E) is the cause of a rare genetic autoinflammatory disorder characterized by recurrent episodes of fever which typically begin during infancy.

11. Correct answer is **A.** The neonate is most likely manifesting the developmental abnormalities associated with Smith-Lemli-Opitz syndrome (SLOS). SLOS results in multiple malformations and behavioral problems as a consequence of a defect in cholesterol synthesis. The defect resides in the terminal enzyme of the cholesterol biosynthesis pathway, namely 7-dehydrocholesterol reductase. Mutations in the gene encoding this enzyme result in increased levels of 7-dehydrocholesterol and reduced levels (15–27% of normal) of cholesterol in SLOS patients. Whereas, the loss of function of the terminal enzyme in cholesterol synthesis is likely to result in increased levels of other intermediates (choices B, C, D, E, and F) in the pathway, elevation in 7-dehydrocholesterol levels is the most useful diagnostically for SLOS.

12. Correct answer is **B.** The infant is most likely manifesting the symptoms associated with a defect in the synthesis of bile acids. Defects in 3β-hydroxy Δ^5 C_{27}-steroid oxidoreductase (HSD3B7) are the most commonly reported inborn errors in bile acid synthesis. The disorder is characterized by neonatal onset of progressive liver disease with cholestatic jaundice and malabsorption of lipids and lipid-soluble vitamins from the gastrointestinal tract resulting from a primary failure to synthesize bile acids. Affected infants also show failure to thrive, secondary coagulopathy, progressive jaundice, hepatomegaly, and malabsorption with resultant steatorrhea (fatty diarrhea). Inherited defects in the gene (*ABCB11*) encoding BSEP (choice A) are the cause of progressive familial intrahepatic cholestasis type 2 (PFIC2) which is associated with severe jaundice, pruritus, and intrahepatic cholestasis, followed by liver failure and juvenile hepatobiliary carcinoma. Defects in CYP7A1 (choice C) are associated with decreased bile acid production resulting in increased intracellular cholesterol accumulation leading to downregulation of LDL receptors and consequent hypercholesterolemia. Mutations in the *ABCC2* gene that encodes MRP2 (choice D) are the cause of Dubin-Johnson syndrome, which is associated with mild, predominantly conjugated hyperbilirubinemia. Loss of function of the *CYP27A1* gene (choice E) is associated with nodule formation in tendons and brain (preferentially in the cerebellum) which are rich in cholesterol and cholestanol.

13. Correct answer is **E.** PCSK9 is secreted by the liver, and it binds to LDL-LDL receptor complexes on hepatocytes which, following endocytosis, stimulates the lysosomal degradation of the LDL receptor (LDLR), thereby reducing the recycling of the LDLR to the plasma membrane. This effect of PCSK9 leads to a reduced ability of the liver to remove IDL and LDL from the blood contributing to the potential for hypercholesterolemia. Therefore, drugs designed to inhibit the function of PCSK9 exert their benefits by allowing for more LDL receptor to be recycled to the plasma membrane enabling more serum LDL to be bound and internalized, thus lowering overall serum levels. None of the other enzymes (choices A, B, C, and D) contribute to LDL receptor recycling to the plasma membrane.

14. Correct answer is **B.** Bile acids, in particular chenodeoxycholic acid (CDCA) and cholic acid (CA), can regulate the expression of genes involved in their synthesis, thereby, creating a feedback loop. When bile acids are secreted by the gallbladder, these compounds can be absorbed by ileal enterocytes. Within the enterocytes the bile acids bind to, and activate, the nuclear receptor FXR. Bile acid activation of FXR leads to the enhanced expression of numerous genes in the enterocytes, with the *FGF19* gene being one of these FXR targets. Activation of the *FGF19* gene results in the protein being secreted into the enterohepatic circulation. When the hormone reaches the liver, it interacts with the βKlotho/FGFR4 complex and triggers activation of a signal transduction cascade. The net result, in the liver, is transcriptional repression of the *CYP7A1* gene, which encodes the rate-limiting enzyme in the "classic pathway" of bile acid synthesis. None of the other options (choices A, C, D, and E) represent the target for activation by bile acids such as chenodeoxycholate.

15. Correct answer is **C.** LDL particles are removed from the blood through their binding to the LDL receptor. Following binding the LDL-LDL receptor complexes are internalized through receptor-mediated endocytosis. In order for LDL receptors to recognize and bind LDL, the LDL particles must contain functional apoB-100. Therefore, in this patient with elevated serum LDL in the presence of normal levels of hepatic LDL receptors, the most likely possible cause is a defective apoB-100 protein associated with the circulating LDL. Mutations that affect the LDL receptor binding domain of apoB-100 result in a form of familial hypercholesterolemia referred to as familial ligand-defective apoB. None of the other options (choices A, B, D, and E) correlate to the findings in this patient.

16. Correct answer is **A.** The primary mechanism by which HDL acquires peripheral tissue cholesterol is via an interaction with the ABCA1 cholesterol transporter on macrophages within the subendothelial spaces of the tissues. The free cholesterol transferred from macrophages to HDL is esterified by HDL-associated lecithin:cholesterol acyltransferase (LCAT). LCAT is synthesized in the liver and so named because it transfers a fatty acid from the *sn*2 position of a phosphatidylcholine (a lecithin) to the hydroxyl (–OH) on carbon 3 (A ring) of cholesterol. The action of LCAT thus generates a cholesteryl ester and lysolecithin. None of the other options (choices B, C, D, and E) refer to the function of LCAT.

17. Correct answer is **B.** The findings in the stillborn female are most likely indicative of the disorder called desmosterolosis. Desmosterolosis is an extremely rare disorder, but the presentations are useful for an understanding of the role of cholesterol in early neonatal developments. Skeletal abnormalities found in desmosterolosis are similar to, but more severe than, those presenting in Smith-Lemli-Opitz syndrome (SLOS) which is caused by mutations in the gene encoding 7-dehydrocholesterol reductase (choice A). Desmosterolosis results from a defect in the gene encoding 3-β-hydroxysterol Δ^{24}-reductase (DHCR24) which catalyzes the reduction of the Δ^{24} double bond of sterol intermediates during cholesterol biosynthesis. Loss of DHCR4, therefore, causes a loss of cholesterol production with accumulation of the intermediate, desmosterol. Defects in HMG-CoA reductase (choice C) or squalene monooxygenase (choice E) have not been described in humans. Defects in mevalonate kinase (choice D) are the cause of a rare genetic autoinflammatory disorder characterized by recurrent episodes of fever which typically begin during infancy.

18. Correct answer is **A.** Small heterodimer partner (SHP) is a transcriptional repressor. Activation of SHP expression by FXR results in inhibition of transcription of SHP target genes. Of significance to bile acid metabolism, SHP represses the expression of the cholesterol 7α-hydroxylase gene (*CYP7A1*). CYP7A1 is the rate-limiting enzyme in the synthesis of bile acids from cholesterol via the classic pathway. Loss of SHP expression would, therefore, result in unregulated CYP7A1 expression. Chenodeoxycholate synthesis (choice E) occurs via the classic, and the acidic pathways, of bile acid synthesis, therefore, unregulated synthesis of the CYP7A1 enzyme would increase its synthesis but the more correct answer is activation of all of bile acid synthesis, not just chenodeoxycholate. SHP regulates the expression of several additional genes involved in overall bile acid homeostasis but does not directly influence bile acid conjugation (choice B), export (choice C), or reuptake from the intestines (choice D).

19. Correct answer is **D.** Given the signs and symptoms in this patient, combined with his family history, he is most likely suffering from the most common inherited form of familial hypercholesterolemia, FH. FH is an autosomal dominant disorder that predominantly results from mutations affecting the structure and function of the LDL receptor. The defects in LDL receptor impair binding and uptake of LDL from the blood resulting in lifelong elevation of LDL-cholesterol in the blood. The resultant hypercholesterolemia leads to premature coronary artery disease and atherosclerotic plaque formation. Reduction in hepatic ACAT (choice A), which is encoded by the sterol-*O*-acyltransferase 2 (*SOAT2*) gene, is associated accumulation of free cholesterol. Deficiencies in HMGR (choice B) have not been described in humans. Deficiency in LCAT (choice C) results in the disorder associated with characteristic abnormalities in blood lipid profiles that includes low HDL (<10 mg/dL), low apoA-I (20–30 mg/dL), low cholesteryl esters, and low LDL. Mutations in lipoprotein lipase (choice E) are associated with dramatic elevation in serum triglycerides with mild to moderate levels of LDL cholesterol.

20. Correct answer is **E.** Significantly elevated levels of serum triglycerides, such as in this patient, most likely reflect defects in one of the two proteins critical to the removal of fatty acids from the triglycerides contained in circulating lipoprotein particles such as chylomicrons and very-low-density lipoprotein (VLDL) particles. These two proteins are the lipoprotein-associated apolipoprotein C-II (apoC-II) and the endothelial cell-associated enzyme, lipoprotein lipase, LPL. LPL is expressed only in the vasculature of skeletal and cardiac muscle and adipose tissue. The activity of LPL requires interaction apoC-II for its activity. Chylomicrons and VLDL acquire apoC-II through interactions with high-density lipoprotein (HDL) particles. Defects in none of the other enzymes (choices A, B, C, and D) are associated with severe hypertriglyceridemia.

21. Correct answer is **D.** Inhibition of *de novo* cholesterol biosynthesis, through inhibition of the rate-limiting enzyme, HMG-CoA reductase, with the use of statin drugs such as atorvastatin, leads to reduction in the synthesis of several isoprenoid compounds such as dolichol phosphate. The reduction in dolichol production leads to the inhibition of the ability to effectively carry out *N*-linked glycosylation of many cellular proteins. Inhibition of HMG-CoA reductase could increase, not decrease, concentrations of substrates upstream of the enzyme such as acetoacetyl-CoA (choice A) and HMG-CoA (choice E). Chenodeoxycholate (choice B) and cholate (choice C) are bile acids, and their levels could decrease as a result of reduced hepatic cholesterol synthesis in the presence of a statin drug. However, these substances are not involved in glycoprotein synthesis.

22. Correct answer is **B.** Sterol-regulated transcription of the key rate-limiting enzyme of cholesterol biosynthesis, HMG-CoA reductase, occurs through the regulated cleavage of the membrane-bound transcription factor, sterol-regulated element-binding protein, SREBP. SREBP is proteolytically activated and the proteolysis is controlled by the level of sterols in the cell. Full-length SREBP is embedded in the membrane of the endoplasmic reticulum (ER). Release of the transcription factor domain of SREBP from the ER is controlled by its interaction with a protein called SREBP cleavage-activating protein (SCAP). When cells have sufficient sterol content SREBP and SCAP are retained in the ER preventing SREBP from being released and activating transcription of genes. If SREBP is not associated with the ER it is likely going to be unregulated by cellular sterol concentration because it will not be bound to SCAP. This would lead to unregulated activation of the gene encoding HMG-CoA reductase. None of the other enzymes (choices A, C, D, and E) is transcriptionally controlled by SREBP.

23. Correct answer is **B.** Sterols, such as oxysterols and cholesterol, regulate overall cholesterol synthesis by controlling the activity of transcription factor, sterol-regulated element-binding protein, SREBP. SREBP is proteolytically activated and the proteolysis is controlled by the level of sterols in the cell. Full-length SREBP is embedded in the membrane of the endoplasmic reticulum (ER). Release of the transcription factor domain of SREBP from the ER is controlled by its interaction with a protein called SREBP cleavage-activating protein (SCAP). When cells have sufficient sterol content SREBP and SCAP are retained in the ER preventing SREBP from being released and activating transcription of genes. Normal oxysterol regulation of SREB would lead to reduced cholesterol synthesis due, in part, to reduced expression of HMGR. Thus, continued transcriptional activation of target genes by SREBP, even in the presence of oxysterols, would be measurable with continued cholesterol synthesis due to unregulated transcription of HMGR. None of the other enzymes (choices A, C, D, and E) is transcriptionally controlled by SREBP.

24. Correct answer is **C.** The only enzyme listed whose activity is directly affected by the level of ATP synthesis is AMPK (choice A). However, when ATP levels fall, AMP levels will rise, and AMPK becomes fully activated, not reduced. One of the important cholesterol biosynthetic enzymes that is a target of AMPK is HMGR. Phosphorylation of HMGR by AMPK results in reduced activity of the enzyme and therefore, reduced synthesis of the isoprenoid intermediates in the cholesterol biosynthesis pathway, such as farnesyl pyrophosphate and geranyl pyrophosphate. Therefore, an aberrant increase in AMPK activity will result in reduced synthesis of the isoprenoid intermediates of the pathway resulting in reduced farnesylation of proteins. None of the other enzymes (choices B, D, and E) is a target for AMPK or is not directly involved in cholesterol synthesis.

25. Correct answer is **B.** G_s-coupled GPCRs activate adenylate cyclase upon receptor activation. Adenylate cyclase then produces cAMP which, in turn, activates cAMP-dependent protein kinase, PKA. Activation of PKA in hepatocytes will lead to increased phosphorylation of the regulatory subunit of HMGR phosphatase which can then no longer activate the phosphatase. The reduced level of phosphate removal from HMGR will keep this enzyme in a less active state. The net effect will be a reduction in cholesterol biosynthesis which will preserve ATP for use in gluconeogenesis which is a primary response of liver to glucagon stimulation. Activated PKA does not result in any of the other changes (choices A, C, D, and E).

26. Correct answer is **B.** Cholesterol biosynthesis occurs in the cytosol and begins with acetyl-CoA which is almost exclusively generated in the mitochondria. Mitochondrial acetyl-CoA is transported to the cytosol in the form of citrate. In the cytosol citrate is hydrolyzed to acetyl-CoA and oxaloacetate by the ATP-dependent enzyme, ATP-citrate lyase. During ketogenesis mitochondrial acetoacetate can diffuse to the cytosol where it is converted to acetoacetyl-CoA via the cytosolic enzyme, acetoacetyl-CoA synthetase. The resulting acetoacetyl-CoA could then serve as a direct substrate for incorporation into cholesterol. It is important to understand, however, that although this reaction process can occur, under conditions where ketogenesis is occurring in the liver the level of active cytosolic HMG-CoA reductase would be significantly reduced. Acetyl-CoA synthetases (choice A) generate acetyl-CoA from CoASH and acetate where the amount of acetate in the hepatocytes is insufficient to account for 60% of normal cholesterol synthesis. Hepatic acetate only rises significantly during the metabolism of ethanol. The other three enzymes (choices C, D, and E) all function downstream of acetyl-CoA entry into cholesterol synthesis and thus require the presence of acetyl-CoA from either ATP-citrate lyase or acetoacetyl-CoA synthetase.

27. Correct answer is **B.** There are a number of cell surface receptors that bind lipoproteins of the LDL family such as the classic LDL receptor but also includes members of the LDL receptor-related proteins. Modified LDL, such as oxidized LDL (oxLDL), do not bind to the LDL receptor. Instead, these lipoprotein particles are taken up into macrophages via the scavenger receptor, FAT/CD36. Presentation of this receptor on macrophage plasma membranes is not downregulated in response to oxLDL uptake as is the case for the LDL receptor in response to LDL uptake by hepatocytes, adrenal tissues, and gonads. Conversely, uptake of oxLDL by macrophages actually results in increased density of FAT/CD36 on these cells. None of the other options (choices A, C, D, and E) correspond to the role of oxLDL and the generation of foam cells.

28. Correct answer is **C.** Sterols, such as oxysterols, like 25-hydroxycholesterol, regulate overall cholesterol synthesis by controlling the activity of transcription factor, sterol-regulated element-binding protein, SREBP. SREBP is proteolytically activated and the proteolysis is controlled by the level of sterols in the cell. Full-length SREBP is embedded in the membrane of the endoplasmic reticulum (ER). Release of the transcription factor domain of SREBP from the ER is controlled by its interaction with a protein called SREBP cleavage-activating protein (SCAP). When cells have sufficient sterol content SREBP and SCAP are retained in the ER preventing SREBP from being released and activating transcription of genes. Normal oxysterol regulation of SREBP would lead to reduced cholesterol synthesis due, in large part, to reduced expression of the gene encoding HMG-CoA reductase. HMG-CoA reductase catalyzes the conversion of 3-hydroxy-3-methylglutaryl-CoA (HMG-CoA) to mevalonate. Therefore, reduced expression of the HMG-CoA reductase gene will lead to reduced formation of mevalonate. None of the other options (choices A, B, D, and E) reflect processes that would be affected by addition of 25-hydroycholesterol to cells.

29. Correct answer is **A.** Numerous medications have been developed for the control and treatment of serum cholesterol levels, such as the statins. However, because the statins block HMG-CoA reductase activity, the resultant mevalonate-derived isoprenoid compounds, that are utilized in numerous other pathways and processes, decline. One important isoprenoid from this pathway is farnesyl pyrophosphate which is required for the synthesis of ubiquinone. Ubiquinone is required for electron transport and the synthesis of ATP. Tissues, like skeletal muscle, that need large quantities of ATP are particularly susceptible to the side-effects of statin therapy. Another option for the treatment of hypercholesterolemia is nicotinic acid (but not nicotinamide). Use of nicotinic acid as a therapeutic stems from the fact that it binds to and activates the hydroxycarboxylic acid receptor 2 (HCA2) in adipocytes. Activation of this receptor inhibits fatty acid release from stored triglycerides which subsequently reduces fatty acid uptake by the liver, thereby reducing the plasma levels of both VLDL and LDL. In addition, nicotinic acid administration strongly increases the circulating levels of HDL. Patient compliance with nicotinic acid administration is sometimes compromised because of the unpleasant side effect of cutaneous vasodilation resulting in flushing of the face. None of the other options (choices B, C, D, and E) correspond to effects of a vitamin-based therapeutic for hypercholesterolemia.

30. Correct answer is **D.** Progressive familial intrahepatic cholestasis type 2 (PFIC2) is caused by mutations in the *ABCB11* gene encoding the bile transporter identified as bile salt export protein (BSEP). BSEP is involved in the process of exporting bile acids out of hepatocytes into the bile canaliculi thus reducing their toxicity to these cells. None of the other options (choices A, B, C, and E) relate to processes associated with familial intrahepatic cholestasis.

31. Correct answer is **D.** The major pathway for the synthesis of the bile acids is initiated via hydroxylation of cholesterol at the carbon 7 position via the action of cholesterol 7α-hydroxylase (CYP7A1). The pathway initiated by CYP7A1 is referred to as the "classic" or "neutral" pathway of bile acid synthesis. The hydroxyl group on cholesterol at the 3 position is in the β-orientation and must be epimerized to the α-orientation during the synthesis of the bile acids. This epimerization is initiated by conversion of the 3β-hydroxyl to a 3-oxo group catalyzed by 3β-hydroxy-Δ^5-C_{27}-steroid oxidoreductase (HSD3B7). Following the action of HSD3B7 the bile acid intermediates can proceed via two pathways whose end products are chenodeoxycholic acid (CDCA) and cholic acid (CA). The alternative bile acid synthesis pathway, referred to as the acidic pathway, is initiated by sterol 27-hydroxylase (CYP27A1). This pathway yields only chenodeoxycholic acid. Defects in none of the other enzymes (choices A, B, C, and E) would lead to the synthesis of chenodeoxycholate in the absence of cholate.

32. Correct answer is **E.** The patient is most likely suffering from the effects of the disorder known as abetalipoproteinemia. Abetalipoproteinemia is a rare autosomal recessive disorder characterized by very low levels of serum cholesterol and triglyceride and the absence of apoB-containing lipoproteins (chylomicrons, VLDL, and LDL). ApoB-48 (chylomicrons) and apoB-100 (VLDL and LDL) are encoded by the same gene. Absence of chylomicron formation produces a deficiency of essential fatty acids (linolenic and linoleic acids) and the fat-soluble vitamins. Symptoms include malabsorption, spinocerebellar dysfunction, retinopathy that causes impaired night and color vision, and acanthocytosis (thorny-appearing red cells). Abetalipoproteinemia results from mutations in the gene (*MTTP*) encoding microsomal triglyceride transfer protein. There are three essential functions associated with MTTP including lipid transfer, apoB binding, and membrane association. The characterization of the dramatically reduced plasma levels of LDL cholesterol in patients with abetalipoproteinemia prompted investigations aimed at targeting MTTP inhibition in the treatment of various hypercholesterolemias. Indeed, lomitapide, a small molecule inhibitor of microsomal triglyceride transfer protein has been approved for use in the treatment of familial hypercholesterolemia. Deficiency of apoC-II (choice A) produces hypertriglyceridemia because apoC-II is an activator of lipoprotein lipase, LPL. LPL is required for metabolism of VLDL and chylomicrons in the capillaries of adipose and muscle. Symptoms include pancreatitis, pain after a fatty meal, and xanthomas. Deficiency in 7-dehydrocholesterol reductase (choice B) results in the disorder called Smith-Lemli-Opitz syndrome, SLOS. SLOS results in multiple malformations and behavioral problems as a consequence of a defect in cholesterol synthesis. Deficiency in LCAT (choice C) results in the disorder associated with characteristic abnormalities in blood lipid profiles that includes low HDL (<10 mg/dL), low apoA-I (20–30 mg/dL), low cholesteryl esters, and low LDL. Deficiency of the LDL receptor (choice D) results in hypercholesterolemia associated with high levels of LDL cholesterol.

33. Correct answer is **B.** The patient is most likely suffering from the consequences of familial hypercholesterolemia (FH). The clinical characteristics of FH include dramatically elevated concentrations of total plasma cholesterol, LDL-cholesterol, and deposition of LDL-cholesterol in the arteries, tendons, and skin. Fat deposits in the arteries are called atheromas, in the skin and tendons they are called xanthomas, and on the eyelids they are termed xanthelasmas. The most common form of FH results from mutations in the gene encoding the LDL receptor. Mutations in the gene (*MTTP*) encoding microsomal triglyceride transfer protein (choice A) are the cause of abetalipoproteinemia (ABL) which is a rare autosomal recessive disease that is characterized by very low plasma concentrations of triglyceride and total cholesterol (<30 mg/dL) and is also associated with undetectable levels of LDL and apoB. Many of the enzymes of cholesterol biosynthesis are localized to the endoplasmic reticulum (choice C) but mutations in the genes encoding these enzymes would result in defective cholesterol synthesis, not significantly elevated levels of plasma cholesterol. None of the other effects (choices D, E, and F) would lead to the significant increase in serum cholesterol seen in this patient.

34. Correct answer is **B.** The patient was most likely prescribed nicotinic acid therapy as a means to help reduce his serum cholesterol. Nicotinic acid reduces the plasma levels of both VLDL and LDL by inhibiting hepatic VLDL secretion, as well as suppressing the flux of free fatty acid release from adipose tissue by inhibiting lipolysis. In addition, nicotinic acid administration strongly increases the circulating levels of HDL. Patient compliance with nicotinic acid administration is sometimes compromised because of the unpleasant side-effect of facial flushing (strong cutaneous vasodilation). None of the other adverse side effects (choices A, C, D, and E) are associated with therapeutic intervention of hypercholesterolemia.

35. Correct answer is **A.** The patient is most likely suffering from the consequences of a form of familial hypercholesterolemia (FH). The clinical characteristics of FH include dramatically elevated concentrations of total plasma cholesterol, LDL-cholesterol, and deposition of LDL cholesterol in the arteries, tendons, and skin. Fat deposits in the arteries are called atheromas and in the skin and tendons they are called xanthomas. The most common form of FH results from mutations in the gene encoding the LDL receptor. There are three other causes of FH including mutations in the *APOB* gene (commonly referred to as familial ligand-defective apoB) which encodes apoB-100 and apoB-48. Mutations in none of the other genes (choices B, C, D, and E) would result in the characteristic elevations in total cholesterol and LDL cholesterol observed in this patient. Mutations in the gene encoding apoC-II (choice B) and lipoprotein lipase (choice E) are associated with significant elevations in serum triglycerides and chylomicrons and represent two of the causes of familial chylomicronemia. Mutations in the *DHCR7* gene, encoding 7-dehydrocholesterol reductase (choice C) are the cause of Smith-Lemli-Opitz syndrome whose symptoms are observable at birth.

CHAPTER

16

Lipoproteins and Blood Lipids

High-Yield Terms

Lipoprotein	Complex of variable protein and lipid composition responsible for transport of fats throughout the body
Apolipoprotein	Lipid-binding proteins of lipoprotein complexes
Chylomicron	Lipoprotein complex generated from dietary lipids within the enterocytes of the intestines
VLDL	Lipoprotein complex generated from endogenous (or dietary) lipids within the liver; circulation in the vasculature leads to progressive loss of fatty acids converting these lipoproteins to IDL and finally LDL
HDL	High-density lipoprotein involved in the removal of cholesterol from peripheral tissue for return to the liver; the process is referred to as reverse cholesterol transport, RCT
Acyl-CoA-cholesterol acyltransferase, ACAT	Key intracellular enzyme for esterifying cholesterol
Lecithin:cholesterol acyltransferase, LCAT	Key HDL-associated enzyme involved in the esterification of cholesterol, removed from peripheral tissue, prior to exchange for triglyceride with VLDL and LDL
Cholesterol ester transfer protein, CETP	HDL-associated protein that transfers cholesterol esters from HDLs to VLDL and LDL in exchange of triglycerides from the VLDL/LDL to HDL
Lipoprotein(a), Lp(a)	Clinically significant apolipoprotein disulfide bonded to apoB-100 in LDL, easily oxidized and phagocytosed by macrophages enhancing proinflammatory responses; inhibits the process of fibrin clot dissolution

Lipoprotein complexes consist of various proteins and lipids. The lipid portion of lipoproteins consists of cholesterol, cholesterol esters, triglycerides, and/or phospholipids. Lipoproteins can be derived from dietary lipids via synthesis in enterocytes of the intestine or from endogenous lipids via synthesis in the liver. The generalization of lipoprotein types is defined by the amount of protein and lipid as depicted in Table 16–1.

The proteins associated with lipoproteins are referred to as apolipoproteins. Different apolipoprotein classes, defined by the use of letters (eg, apoA), are found in functionally distinct lipoprotein complex types. The clinically significant apolipoproteins are members of the apoA, apoB, apoC, and apoE families (Table 16–2).

LIPOPROTEIN LIPASE

In the capillaries of adipose tissue, skeletal muscle, and the heart, the fatty acids of chylomicrons and VLDL/IDL/LDL are removed from the triglycerides by the action of lipoprotein lipase (LPL), which is found on the surface of the endothelial cells of the capillaries. Lipoprotein lipase is encoded by the *LPL* gene.

Synthesis of LPL occurs on the rough endoplasmic reticulum (ER) within parenchymal cells of adipose tissue (adipocytes) and of cardiac and skeletal muscle (cardiomyocytes and myocytes, respectively). As LPL is being synthesized, the activity of lipase maturation factor 1 (LMF1) is required for the maturation of LPL and its migration through the secretory pathway. LPL is then subsequently exocytosed from the parenchymal cell, where it binds to **heparin sulfated proteoglycans (HSPG)** present on the surface of the cell facing the subendothelial spaces. The enzyme is then picked up and transported from the subendothelial spaces of the capillaries to the capillary endothelial cells via the action of glycosylphosphatidylinositol-anchored HDL-binding protein 1 which is encoded by the *GPIHBP1* gene. Functional LPL is a homodimer which remains associated with the apical (lumen) surface of the endothelial cells through its interactions with GPIHBP1.

ApoC-II and apoA-V present in the chylomicrons and VLDL activate LPL in the presence of phospholipid. In addition to apoC-II and apoA-V, several angiopoietin-like proteins (discussed later) are critical to the regulation of LPL activity. During the removal of fatty acids from lipoprotein-associated triglycerides,

TABLE 16–1 Composition of the lipoproteins in plasma of humans.

		Composition					
Lipoprotein	Source	Diameter (nm)	Density (g/mL)	Protein (%)	Lipid (%)	Main Lipid Components	Apolipoproteins
Chylomicrons	Intestine	90–1000	<0.95	1–2	98–99	Triacylglycerol	A-I, A-II, A-IV,[1] B-48, C-I, C-II, C-III, E
Chylomicron remnants	Chylomicrons	45–150	<1.006	6–8	92–94	Triacylglycerol, phospholipids, cholesterol	B-48, E
VLDL	Liver (intestine)	30–90	0.95–1.006	7–10	90–93	Triacylglycerol	B-100, C-I, C-II, C-III
IDL	VLDL	25–35	1.006–1.019	11	89	Triacylglycerol, cholesterol	B-100, E
LDL	VLDL	20–25	1.019–1.063	21	79	Cholesterol	B-100
HDL	Liver, intestine, VLDL, chylomicrons					Phospholipids, cholesterol	A-I, A-II, A-IV, C-I, CII, C-III, D,[2] E
HDL_1		20–25	1.019–1.063	32	68		
HDL_2		10–20	1.063–1.125	33	67		
HDL_3		5–10	1.125–1.210	57	43		
Pre²-HDL[3]		<5	>1.210				A-I
Albumin/free fatty acids	Adipose tissue		>1.281	99	1	Free fatty acids	

[1]Secreted with chylomicrons but transfers to HDL.

[2]Associated with HDL2 and HDL3 subfractions.

[3]Part of a minor fraction known as very-high-density lipoproteins (VHDL).

Abbreviations: HDL, high-density lipoproteins; IDL, intermediate-density lipoproteins; LDL, low-density lipoproteins; VLDL, very-low-density lipoproteins.

Reproduced with permission from Rodwell VW, Bender DA, Botham KM, et al: *Harper's Illustrated Biochemistry*, 31st ed. New York, NY: McGraw Hill; 2018.

a substantial portion of phospholipid, apoA-V and apoC-II is transferred to HDL. The loss of apoC-II and apoA-V prevents LPL from further degrading the chylomicron remnants.

Mutations in the *LPL*, *GPIHBP1*, *LMF1*, *APOC2*, and *APOAV* genes are all causes of familial chylomicronemia syndrome, FCS (see Clinical Box 16–1). Mutations in several of these genes were originally identified as causes of the type 1 hyperlipoproteinemias.

Chylomicronemia syndrome refers to a disorder that is caused by minor genetic variants that collectively result in polygenic hypertriglyceridemia. In this context, it is appropriate to term the disorder multifactorial chylomicronemia syndrome. Originally, the polygenic form of chylomicronemia syndrome was identified as hyperlipidemia, type 5.

In addition to mutations in the *LPL* gene, mutations in genes that encode regulators of LPL function also result in familial chylomicronemia syndrome. These LPL regulators are encoded by the *APOC2*, *APOA5*, *LMF1*, and *GPIHBP1* genes which encode apoC-II (apoC-2), apoA-V (apoA-5), lipase maturation factor 1, and glycosylphosphatidylinositol-anchored HDL binding protein 1, respectively. The *LMF1* and *GPIHBP1* encoded proteins are involved in the synthesis and maturation of LPL, while the *APOC2* and *APOA5* encoded proteins (apolipoproteins) are found in **chylomicrons and VLDL** and serve to activate LPL in the presence of phospholipid.

Most individuals manifesting with chylomicronemia have the multifactorial (polygenic) form of the disorder. When FCS is caused by mutations in the *LPL* gene, the disorder is referred to as classic FCS. The characteristic feature of familial chylomicronemia syndrome, which is also characteristic of multifactorial chylomicronemia syndrome, is intermittent or persistent fasting chylomicronemia. The chylomicronemia, in turn, results in hypertriglyceridemia. The hypertriglyceridemia is defined as a serum triglyceride level in excess of 1000 mg/dL (normal is <150 mg/dL). The disorder also predisposes affected individuals to acute pancreatitis. Additional clinical findings in FCS patients are eruptive xanthomas, episodic abdominal pain, hepatosplenomegaly, and lipemia retinalis (creamy white appearance in peripheral retinal vessels).

In the course of the correct diagnosis of FCS, it is important to exclude any secondary causes of polygenic hyperchylomicronemia as well as secondary hypertriglyceridemia. These other

TABLE 16–2 Major apolipoprotein classifications.

Apolipoprotein	Lipoprotein Association	Function and Comments
apoA-I	Chylomicrons, HDL	Major protein of HDL, binds ABCA1 on macrophages, critical antioxidant protein of HDL, activates lecithin:cholesterol acyltransferase, LCAT
apoA-II	Chylomicrons, HDL	Near exclusive to HDL, represents the second most abundant protein in HDL, enhances hepatic lipase activity, extrahepatic expression as well as misfolding of proprotein contribute to senile amyloidosis
apoB-48	Chylomicrons	Exclusively found in chylomicrons, derived from *apoB*-gene by RNA editing in intestinal enterocytes; lacks the LDL receptor-binding domain of apoB-100; the designation of apoB-48 refers to the fact that this protein contains 48% of the full-length apoB-100 protein
apoB-100	VLDL, IDL, and LDL	Major protein of LDL, binds to LDL receptor; one of the longest known proteins in humans; the designation of apoB-100 refers to the fact that this protein contains 100% of the coding capacity of the apoB mRNA
apoC-II	Chylomicrons, VLDL, IDL, and HDL	Activates lipoprotein lipase; clustered with *APOC1* and *APOE* genes on chromosome 19
apoC-III	Chylomicrons, VLDL, IDL, and HDL	Predominantly synthesized in the liver; inhibits lipoprotein lipase and hepatic lipase, interferes with hepatic uptake and catabolism of apoB-containing lipoproteins, appears to enhance the catabolism of HDL particles, enhances monocyte adhesion to vascular endothelial cells, activates inflammatory signaling pathways; loss-of-function mutations associated with reduced serum triglycerides and decreased incidence of cardiovascular disease; RNA interference technique to reduce levels of apoC-III has shown promise in treatment of familial chylomicronemia syndrome and in patients with severe high triglycerides
Cholesterol ester transfer protein, CETP	HDL	Plasma glycoprotein secreted primarily from the liver and is associated with cholesteryl ester transfer from HDL to LDL and VLDL in exchange for triglycerides
apoE	Chylomicron remnants, VLDL, IDL, and HDL	At least 3 alleles E2, E3, E4; the apoE2 allele has Cys at amino acids 112(TGC) and 158(TGC); apoE3 has Cys(TGC) and Arg(CGC) at these two positions, respectively; apoE4 has Arg(both codons CGC) at both positions; binds to LDL receptor; the apoE3 allele is the most common; apoE4 allele amplification associated with an inherited form of late-onset Alzheimer disease
apo(a)	LDL	Protein ranges in size from 300,000–800,000 as a result of from 2–43 copies of the Kringle-type domain; Kringle domains contain around 80 amino acids which form the domain via three intrachain disulfide bonds; disulfide bonded to apoB-100, forms a complex with LDL identified as lipoprotein(a), Lp(a); functions as a serine protease that inhibits tissue-type plasminogen activator 1 (tPA); strongly resembles plasminogen; may deliver cholesterol to sites of vascular injury, high-risk association with premature coronary artery disease and stroke

clinical situations can include poorly controlled **type 2 diabetes**, **obesity**, severe hypothyroidism, **metabolic syndrome** and its associated insulin resistance, systemic lupus erythematosus, and alcoholism.

CLINICAL BOX 16–1 FAMILIAL CHYLOMICRONEMIA SYNDROME

Familial chylomicronemia syndrome (FCS) represents a family of related monogenic disorders that manifest with symptoms typical of the related, polygenic disorder simply termed chylomicronemia syndrome. FCS is primarily caused by autosomal recessive inheritance of mutations in the *LPL* gene which encodes the enzyme **lipoprotein lipase (LPL)**. When the disorder results from mutations in the *LPL* gene it is also known as hyperlipoproteinemia, type 1a.

Management of FCS focuses primarily on treating the pancreatitis due to the high morbidity and mortality associated with this condition. Patients with FCS need to adopt a very low-fat diet where the total intake of fats represents less than 10% to 15% of total calories. The lipids in FCS patients diets should be enriched in medium-chain triglycerides (MCT) since these do not require pancreatic lipase or bile acids for digestion, and the fatty acids that are released are delivered from intestinal enterocytes to the blood and are not packaged into chylomicrons. Two drugs that have been approved by the US FDA for use in the treatment of various hyperlipidemias have been shown to provide benefit in classic FCS patients. The drug **lomitapide**, which is an inhibitor of **microsomal triglyceride transfer protein** (MTP; also abbreviated MTTP) has been used to treat classic FCS patients but with limited success. The drug volanesorsen, which is an antisense oligonucleotide to the mRNA encoding apoC-III, has been found to reduce triglyceride levels in classic FCS patients on the order of 50% to 80%. Although approved for use by the European Union, the US FDA has rejected approval of volanesorsen due to a high (25%) levels of trial participants developing thrombocytopenia (low platelet count associated with abnormal bleeding).

MICROSOMAL TRIGLYCERIDE TRANSFER PROTEIN

Incorporation of apoB proteins into lipoprotein particles requires the activity of the endoplasmic reticulum (ER) chaperone identified as microsomal triglyceride transfer protein (MTP; also identified as MTTP). The critical role of MTP in lipoprotein assembly and maturation is evidenced in a form of abetalipoproteinemia that is associated with mutations in the gene (MTTP) that encodes MTP. Abetalipoproteinemia is characterized by fat malabsorption, steatorrhea, acanthocytosis (thorny looking cells), and hypocholesterolemia in infancy. Later in life, deficiency of fat-soluble vitamins is associated with development of atypical retinitis pigmentosa, coagulopathy, posterior column neuropathy, and myopathy.

The drug lomitapide, is a small molecule inhibitor of MTP that has been approved for the treatment of certain patient populations, especially individuals that are homozygous for mutations in the LDL receptor and are not effectively treated with drugs such as alirocumab and statins.

ANGIOPOIETIN-LIKE PROTEINS AND SERUM TRIGLYCERIDES

Lipoprotein lipase is the rate-limiting enzyme for the removal of fatty acids present in the triglycerides in circulating lipoproteins, particularly chylomicrons. Three of the angiopoietin-like proteins (ANGPTL3, ANGPTL4, and ANGPTL8) play crucial roles in the posttranslational regulation of LPL activity. ANGPTL3 is involved in the regulation of overall lipoprotein metabolism through its ability to inhibit the activity of LPL, as well as to inhibit the activity of endothelial lipase, EL. ANGPTL4 also inhibits LPL activity. The role of ANGPTL8 is to activate ANGPTL3.

The clinical significance of the ANGPTL proteins is demonstrated in patients harboring mutations in the *ANGPTL3* gene. These individuals have what is called familial combined hypolipidemia. This has also been called familial hypobetalipoproteinemia type 2. Because of the associated hypobetalipoproteinemia, familial combined hypolipidemia actually belongs to the family of hypolipidemic disorders identified as familial hypobetalipoproteinemia syndrome, FHBL.

The most commonly detected ANGPTL3 mutation in familial combined hypolipidemia is a double nonsense mutation affecting codon 17 such that the normal Ser (S) codon at that position (TCC) is mutated to a stop codon, TGA. This mutation is referred to as the S17X mutation. Individuals homozygous for the S17X mutation have on average a 48% reduction in LDL, a 62% reduction in triglyceride, a 46% reduction in HDL, a 44% reduction in apoB, and a 48% reduction in apoA-I.

A monoclonal antibody against ANGPTL3 (evinacumab) has shown promise at lowering circulating levels of LDL in homozygous familial hypercholesterolemia patients. Patients administered the monoclonal antibody over a period of 24 weeks showed an average reduction in LDL cholesterol (LDL-c) of 49%.

CHYLOMICRONS

Chylomicrons (Figure 16–1) are assembled in intestinal enterocytes as a means to transport dietary cholesterol, triglycerides, phospholipids, and fat-soluble vitamins to the rest of the body. Chylomicrons are, therefore, the molecules formed to mobilize dietary (exogenous) lipids. The predominant lipids of chylomicrons are triglycerides (see Table 16–1). The apolipoprotein, apoB-48, is exclusive to chylomicrons.

Chylomicrons leave the intestine via the lymphatic system and enter the circulation at the left subclavian vein. In the bloodstream, important apolipoproteins acquired from HDL are apoC-II and apoE. In the capillaries of adipose tissue, skeletal muscle, and cardiac muscle, the fatty acids of chylomicrons are removed from the triglycerides by the action of lipoprotein lipase (LPL), which is found on the surface of the endothelial cells of the capillaries (Figure 16–2).

Chylomicron remnants, containing primarily cholesterol esters, apoE and apoB-48, are then taken up by hepatocytes via interaction with various lipoprotein receptors including the LDL receptor (LDLR), the chylomicron remnant receptor, which is a member of the LDL receptor-related protein (LRP) family, and heparan sulfate proteoglycans (HSPG).

VLDL, IDL, AND LDL

Very-low-density lipoproteins (VLDL) are the complexes involved in the transport of lipid (primarily triglyceride) from the liver to the extrahepatic tissues. In addition to triglycerides, VLDL contain some cholesterol and cholesterol esters, and phospholipids. The apolipoprotein that is exclusive to VLDL is apoB-100. Like nascent chylomicrons, newly released VLDL obtain apoC and apoE from circulating HDL. The fatty acid portion of triglycerides in VLDL is released to adipose tissue, skeletal muscle, and cardiac muscle in the same way as for chylomicrons, through the action of LPL (Figure 16–3).

The action of LPL, coupled with the transfer of apoC to HDL, converts VLDL to intermediate density lipoproteins (IDL), also termed VLDL remnants. Further loss of triglycerides and transfer of apoE back to HDL converts IDL to LDL. The interaction of VLDL, IDL, and LDL with HDL is the major means for the return of extrahepatic cholesterol to the liver.

LDL are taken up by cells via LDL receptor-mediated endocytosis. LDL receptor recognition of LDL requires the presence of

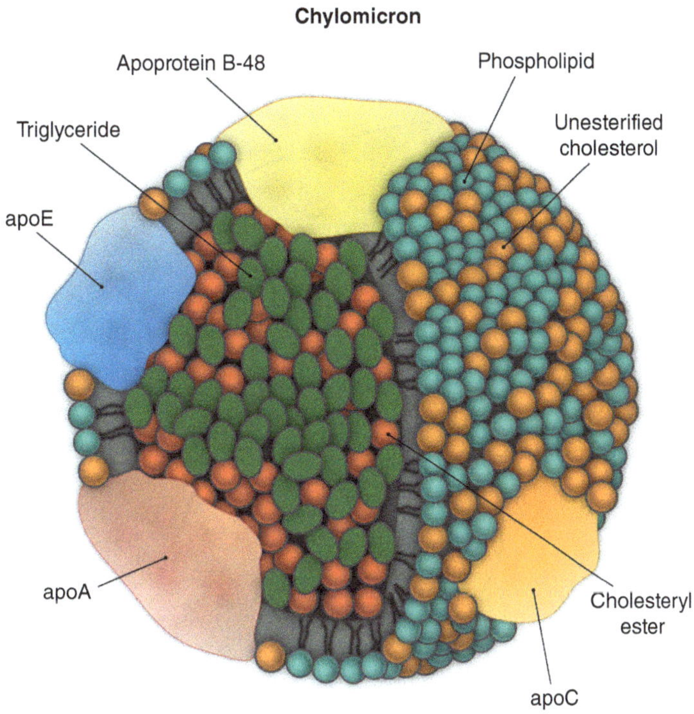

FIGURE 16–1 Structure of a chylomicron as a representative structure of a typical lipoprotein particle. Image demonstrates the outer layer of phospholipid and free cholesterol with primarily triglycerides and cholesteryl esters internally. Included in chylomicrons and other lipoprotein cores but not shown are triglycerides (TG). Each lipoprotein type, chylomicron, LDL, and HDL, contains apolipoproteins. Apolipoprotein B-48 (apoB-48) is specific for chylomicrons just as apoB-100 is specific for LDL. (Reproduced with permission from themedicalbiochemistrypage, LLC.)

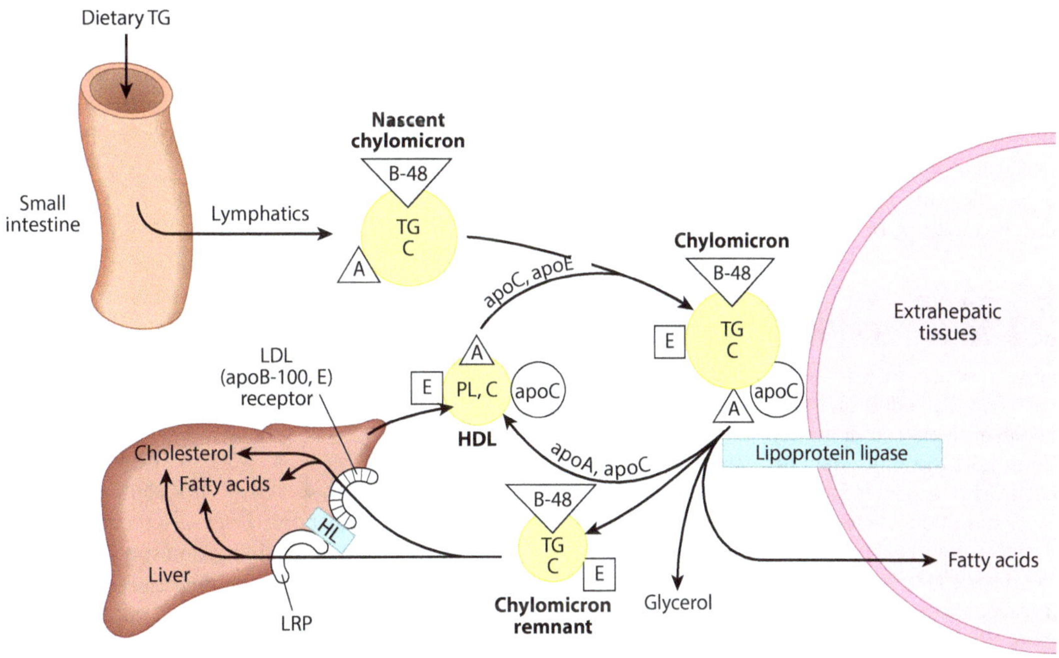

FIGURE 16–2 Metabolic fate of chylomicrons. (A, apolipoprotein A; B-48, apolipoprotein B-48; C, cholesterol and cholesteryl ester; E, apolipoprotein E; HDL, high-density lipoprotein; HL, hepatic lipase; LRP, LDL-receptor-related protein; PL, phospholipid; TG, triacylglycerol.) Only the predominant lipids are shown. (Reproduced with permission from Rodwell VW, Bender DA, Botham KM, et al: *Harper's Illustrated Biochemistry*, 31st ed. New York, NY: McGraw Hill; 2018.)

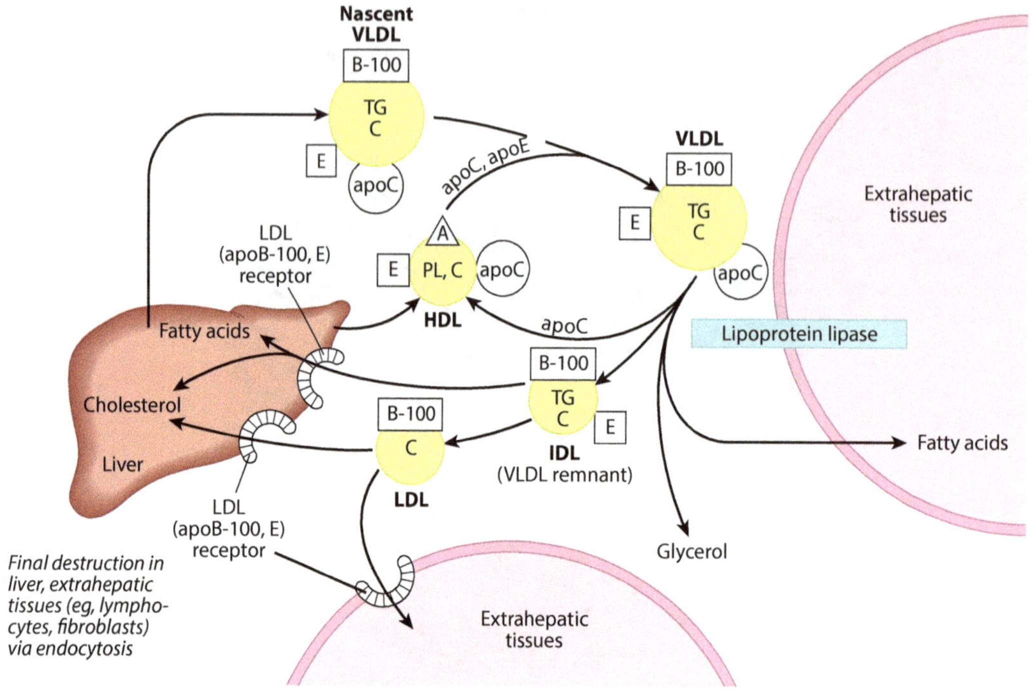

FIGURE 16–3 Metabolic fate of very-low-density lipoproteins (VLDL) and production of low-density lipoproteins (LDL). (A, apolipoprotein A; B-100, apolipoprotein B-100; C, cholesterol and cholesteryl ester; E, apolipoprotein E; HDL, high-density lipoprotein; IDL, intermediate-density lipoprotein; PL, phospholipid; TG, triacylglycerol.) Only the predominant lipids are shown. It is possible that some IDL is also metabolized via the low-density lipoprotein receptor–related protein (LRP). (Reproduced with permission from Rodwell VW, Bender DA, Botham KM, et al: *Harper's Illustrated Biochemistry*, 31st ed. New York, NY: McGraw Hill; 2018.)

both apoB-100 and, with respect to IDL, is enhanced by the presence of apoE. The uptake of LDL occurs predominantly in liver (75%), adrenal glands, gonads, and adipose tissue.

On binding of LDL to the LDLR the complexes are internalized by a receptor-mediated endocytotic process. The endocytosed membrane vesicles (endosomes) fuse with lysosomes, in which the apolipoproteins are degraded, and the cholesterol esters are hydrolyzed to yield free cholesterol. The cholesterol can then be utilized for hepatic bile acid synthesis, steroid hormone synthesis, incorporated into membranes, or stored.

HIGH-YIELD CONCEPT

The consumption of alcohol is associated with either a protective or a negative effect on the level of circulating LDL. Low-level alcohol consumption, particularly red wines which contain the antioxidant resveratrol, appear to be beneficial with respect to cardiovascular health. Resveratrol consumption is associated with a reduced risk of cardiovascular, cerebrovascular, and peripheral vascular disease. One major effect of resveratrol in the blood is the prevention of oxidation of LDL, (forming oxLDL). Oxidized LDL contribute significantly to the development of atherosclerosis. Conversely excess alcohol consumption is associated with the development of fatty liver which in turn impairs the ability of the liver to take up LDL via the LDLR resulting in increased LDL in the circulation.

HIGH-DENSITY LIPOPROTEINS

HDL represent a heterogeneous population of lipoproteins in that they exist as functionally distinct particles possessing different sizes, protein content, and lipid composition. One of the major functions of HDL is to acquire cholesterol from peripheral tissues and transport this cholesterol back to the liver where it can ultimately be excreted following conversion to bile acids. This function is referred to as reverse cholesterol transport (RCT). The role of HDL in RCT represents the major atheroprotective (prevention of the development of atherosclerotic lesions in the vasculature) function of this class of lipoprotein. In addition to RCT, HDL exert anti-inflammatory, antioxidant, and vasodilatory effects that together represent additional atheroprotective functions of HDL. HDL also possess anti-apoptotic, anti-thrombotic, and anti-infectious properties.

HDL begin as the single protein, apolipoprotein A-I (apoA-I), which is synthesized *de novo* in the liver and small intestine. Nascent HDL are devoid of any cholesterol, cholesterol esters, lipids, and any other proteins. Cells, predominantly macrophages, bind nascent HDL containing almost exclusively apoA-I, through interaction with the ATP-binding cassette transport protein A1, ABCA1 (Figure 16–4). The interaction of apoA-I with ABCA1 facilitates transport of free cholesterol from membranes to HDL. The free cholesterol is then esterified by HDL-associated lecithin:cholesterol-acyltransferase, LCAT, a liver synthesized enzyme. The activity of LCAT requires interaction with apoA-I. The importance of ABCA1 in RCT is evident in individuals

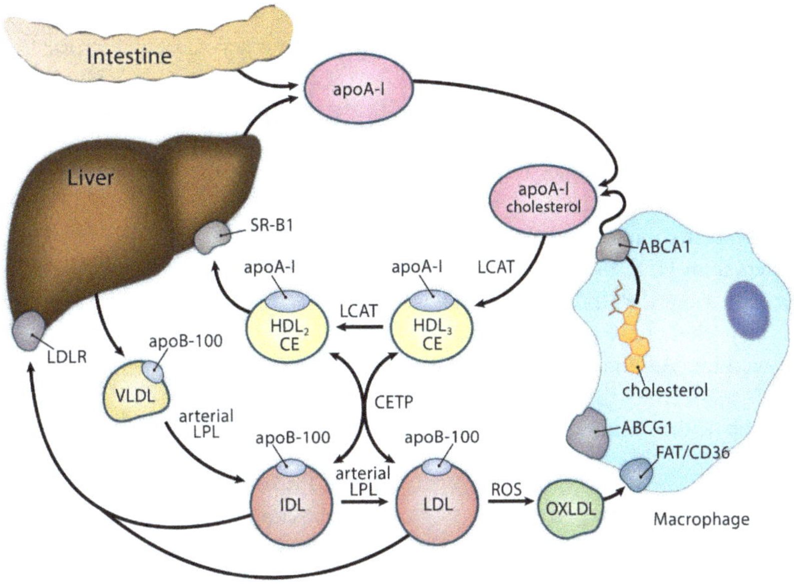

FIGURE 16–4 Details of the interactions between HDL and LDL within the vasculature. As indicated in the text, HDL begins as protein-rich discoidal structures, composed primarily of apoA-I, produced by the liver and intestines. Within the vasculature, apoA-I interacts with the ATP-binding cassette transporter, ABCA1 (such as is diagrammed for interaction with macrophages) and extracts cholesterol from cells. Through the action of LCAT, the apoA-I–associated cholesterol is esterified forming cholesterol esters. This process results in the generation of HDL3 particles. As the HDL3 particles continue through the circulation, they pick up more cholesterol and through the action of LCAT, generate more cholesterol esters. As HDL migrates through the vasculature, there is an interaction between them and IDL and LDL. This interaction occurs through the action of CETP, which exchanges the cholesterol esters in the HDL for triglycerides from LDL. This interaction results in the conversion of HDL3 particles to HDL2. The differences between these two types of HDL particle are detailed in Table 28–1. HDL can also remove cholesterol from cells via interaction with the ATP-binding cassette transporter ABCG1. Approximately 20% of HDL uptake of cellular cholesterol occurs via ABCG1. HDL is then removed from the circulation by the liver through binding of the HDL to hepatic scavenger receptor SR-B1. Cholesterol ester–rich IDL and LDL can return to the liver and be taken up through interaction with the LDL receptor (LDLR). Within the vasculature, the generation of ROS results in oxidation of lipid components of LDL, generating oxidized LDL (oxLDL) that is taken up by the macrophages via the scavenger receptor, FAT/CD36. (Reproduced with permission from themedicalbiochemistrypage, LLC.)

harboring defects in *ABCA1* gene. These individuals suffer from a disorder called Tangier disease (Clinical Box 16–2).

As HDL circulate and acquire more cholesterol, they also accu mulate numerous additional apolipoproteins as well as hundreds of other proteins. Indeed, a fully formed HDL contains more than 300 different proteins, many of which have no known role in lipid transport but are critical to the antioxidant, anti-inflammatory, and anti thrombotic functions of HDL.

Cholesterol-rich HDL return to the liver, where they bind to a receptor that is a member of the scavenger receptor family,

CLINICAL BOX 16–2 TANGIER DISEASE

Tangier disease (TD) is an autosomal recessive disorder resulting from defects in the ATP-binding cassette (ABC) transporter family gene encoding ABCA1. The disease is so named because it was originally identified in two individuals living on Tangier Island, Virginia. TD is a rare disease with only around 50 cases identified worldwide. Although a rare disease, the identification of the gene defective in the disease and an analysis of the function of the encoded transporter protein have provided insight into overall cellular cholesterol homeostasis. Expression of the *ABCA1* gene is highest in placenta, liver, lung, and adrenal glands. Numerous pathways of transcriptional regulation of ABCA1 have been identified including cAMP, nuclear receptors (such as LXRs, RXRs, and PPARs), hormones, and cytokines. The involvement of cytokines in the regulation of ABCA1 expression demonstrates the crosstalk between cellular cholesterol management and inflammatory responses. Pro-inflammatory cytokines such as tumor necrosis factor-α (TNF-α) and interleukin-1β (IL-1β) interfere with the transcriptional enhancement of ABCA1 exerted by LXRs. The predominant site of ABCA1 protein localization is the plasma membrane. In nonhepatic tissue the role of ABCA1 is to promote the efflux of cholesterol principally to the HDL class of lipoprotein particles which in turn transport the cholesterol back to the liver for catabolism. The clinical hallmarks of TD are a lack of HDL and apoA-I. The clinical manifestations of TD are related to an accumulation of cholesterol esters in reticuloendothelial tissues (eg, tonsils, lymph nodes, spleen, thymus, and bone marrow). The first symptom seen in almost all TD patients is enlarged tonsils that appear orange in color. Additional typical clinical findings include splenomegaly, a variable incidence of cardiovascular disease, and peripheral neuropathy.

specifically the scavenger receptor BI, SR-BI. HDL binding to SR-BI does not result in internalization as in the case of LDL receptor-mediated endocytosis. The cholesterol esters of HDL are taken up by the hepatocytes through caveolae while the HDL and SR-BI remain on the plasma membrane.

RCT also involves the transfer of cholesterol esters from HDL to VLDL, IDL, and LDL. This transfer requires the activity of the plasma glycoprotein cholesterol ester transfer protein (CETP). The transfer of cholesterol esters from HDL to VLDL involves a reciprocal exchange of triglycerides from the VLDL to the HDL. This action allows excess cellular cholesterol to be returned to the liver through the LDL receptor. Additionally, when HDL particles become enriched with triglycerides they are better substrates for the action of hepatic lipase that in turn facilitates HDL interaction with SR-B1

LIPOPROTEIN RECEPTORS

LDL Receptors

The LDL receptor spans the plasma membrane and it is the extracellular domain that is responsible for apoB-100/apoE binding. The intracellular domain is responsible for the clustering of LDL receptors into regions of the plasma membrane termed clathrin-coated pits. Associated with the extracellular domain of the LDL receptor is the enzyme proprotein convertase subtilisin/kexin type 9 (PCSK9).

Once LDL binds the receptor, the LDL-PCSK9-LDLR complexes are rapidly internalized (endocytosed). ATP-dependent proton pumps lower the pH in the endosomes, which results in dissociation of the LDL from the receptor. The portion of the endosomal membranes harboring the LDL receptor are then recycled to the plasma membrane and the LDL-containing endosomes fuse with lysosomes. However, within the endosome some of the LDL receptor protein is degraded via the action of PCSK9 resulting in less than 100% recycling of the LDL receptor to the plasma membrane.

Storage of any free cholesterol released from the LDLR involves re-esterification catalyzed by sterol-*O*-acyltransferase 2 (SOAT2), for intracellular storage. The original name given to SOAT2 was acyl-CoA-cholesterol acyltransferase, ACAT.

LDL Receptor–Related Proteins

The LDL receptor–related protein (LRP) family represents a group of structurally related transmembrane proteins involved in a diverse range of biological activities including lipid metabolism, nutrient transport, protection against atherosclerosis, as well as numerous developmental processes. The LRP includes LRP1, LRP1b, LRP2, LRP4, LRP5/6, LRP8, the VLDL receptor (VLDLR), and LR11/SorLA1. LRP1 (also known as CD91 or α_2-macroglobulin receptor) is expressed in numerous tissues and is known to be involved in diverse activities that include lipoprotein transport, modulation of platelet-derived growth factor receptor-β (PDGFRβ) signaling, regulation of cell-surface protease activity, and the control of cellular entry of bacteria and viruses. LRP1 has been shown to bind more than 40 different ligand.

Scavenger Receptors

The scavenger receptor family was identified in studies that were attempting to determine the mechanism by which LDL accumulated in macrophages in atherosclerotic plaques. The scavenger receptor family proteins are identified as class A receptors, class B receptors, mucin-like receptors, and endothelial receptors. The class B receptors include CD36 and scavenger receptor class B type I (SR-BI). The CD36 receptor is also known as fatty acid translocase (designated FAT/CD36) and it is one of the receptors responsible for the cellular uptake of fatty acids (see Chapter 13). The SR-BI is the hepatic receptor for HDL.

Abnormal Lipoprotein Homeostasis and Disease

Inherited mutations in genes encoding the proteins of lipoprotein metabolism are associated with the hyper- and hypolipoproteinemias (see Tables 16–3 and 16–4). In addition, people suffering from

TABLE 16–3 The high-yield hyperlipoproteinemias.

Disorder	Defect	Comments
Familial chylomicronemia syndrome (see Clinical Box 16–1)	Mutations in one of five genes; *LPL*, *GPIHBP1*, *LMF1*, *APOA5*, *APOC2*	Represents the type 1 hyperlipoproteinemias; deficiency in LPL is type 1a, deficiency in apoC-II is type 1b, deficiency in GPIHBP1 is type 1d; slow chylomicron clearance, reduced LDL and HDL levels; characterized by very severe hypertriglyceridemia, episodes of abdominal pain, recurrent acute pancreatitis, eruptive xanthomas, hepatosplenomegaly; treated by low fat/complex carbohydrate diet; no increased risk of coronary artery disease
Familial hypercholesterolemias, FH, (type 2a hyperlipidemia); see Clinical Box 15–3	Six classes of LDL receptor defect; loss-of-function mutations in the *APOB* gene; gain-of-function mutations in the *PCSK9* gene	Reduced LDL clearance leads to hypercholesterolemia (dramatic elevation in LDL cholesterol), resulting in early onset atherosclerosis and coronary artery disease; disorder originally referred to as familial ligand-defective apoB is now classified as one of the autosomal dominant forms of FH; *APOB* mutations that result in FH affect the LDL receptor-binding domain where the Gln for Arg mutation at amino acid 3500 (R3500Q) or Cys for Arg mutation at amino acid 3531 (R3531C) are the most commonly identified mutations

(*Continued*)

TABLE 16–3 The high-yield hyperlipoproteinemias. (*Continued*)

Disorder	Defect	Comments
Familial dysbetalipoproteinemia (type 3 hyperlipidemia; remnant removal disease, broad beta disease, apolipoprotein E deficiency)	*APOE* gene mutations; patients only express the apoE2 isoform	apoE binds to several lipoprotein receptors including the LDL receptor, VLDL receptor, lipoprotein receptor-related protein 1 (LRP1; also called APOER), and LRP8 (also called apoE receptor 2, APOER2); apoE2 isoform interacts poorly with these receptors; results in severely reduced hepatic remnant clearance; causes tendon xanthomas, hypercholesterolemia and atherosclerosis in peripheral and coronary arteries due to elevated levels of chylomicrons and VLDL
Familial LCAT deficiency (Norum disease); Fish-eye disease	Complete (familial LCAT deficiency) or partial (Fish-eye disease) loss of LCAT	Complete or partial absence of LCAT leads to inability of HDL to take cholesterol from cells due to loss of esterification capability; decreased levels of plasma cholesteryl esters and lysolecithin; abnormal LDL (Lp-X) and VLDL; diffuse corneal opacities, swelling of optic nerve, accumulation of fat under the skin around the eyes (xanthelasma), target cell hemolytic anemia, and proteinuria with renal failure
Wolman disease and cholesteryl ester storage disease (CESD)	Mutations in lysosomal acid lipase (*LIPA*) gene	Lysosomal acid lipase is also called cholesteryl ester hydrolase; Wolman disease is severe form of LIPA deficiency (no enzyme activity), CESD mild form (some residual enzyme activity); Wolman disease associated with massive infiltration of organs with macrophages filled with triglycerides and cholesteryl esters, death occurs early in life; CESD is slowly progressing disease that primarily affects the liver

TABLE 16–4 The high-yield hypolipoproteinemias.

Disorder	Defect	Comments
Abetalipoproteinemia: ABL (acanthocytosis, Bassen-Kornzweig syndrome)	Mutations in the *MTTP* gene	MTTP encodes microsomal triglyceride transfer protein; loss of function results similar pathology to familial hypobetalipoproteinemia (FHBL); intestine and liver accumulate VLDL and chylomicrons, respectively; results in malabsorption of fat, steatorrhea, deficiency in fat-soluble vitamins, retinitis pigmentosa, acanthocytosis (erythrocytes with a thorny appearance), and ataxic neuropathic disease
Familial hypobetalipoproteinemia syndromes: FHBL	Truncating mutations in the *APOB* gene; also due to loss-of-function mutations in *PCSK9* gene	Inherited as an autosomal dominant condition; serum LDL concentrations 10–20% of normal; hepatic steatosis
Familial combined hypolipidemia	Mutations in *ANGPTL3* gene	Angiopoietin-like protein 3 inhibits lipoprotein lipase and endothelial lipase activities; therefore loss of activity results in enhanced fatty acid removal from circulating triglycerides; associated with reduced levels of both apoB (VLDL/LDL) and apoA-I (HDL) containing lipoproteins; primary cause in most patients thus far characterized is a double mutation (TCC → TGA) converting the Ser at codon 17 to a stop codon (designated the S17X mutation)
Tangier disease (see Clinical Box 16–2)	Mutations in the *ABCA1* gene	Reduced HDL concentrations, no effect on chylomicron or VLDL production; tendency to hypertriglyceridemia; some elevation in VLDL; hypertrophic tonsils with orange appearance

type 2 diabetes, hypothyroidism, cholestatic liver disease, and kidney disease, as examples, often exhibit abnormal lipoprotein metabolism as a result of secondary effects of their primary disorders.

Lipoprotein(a)

Lipoprotein(a), Lp(a) is composed of a common LDL nucleus linked to a molecule of apolipoprotein(a) [apo(a)] by disulfide bonds to apoB-100. Elevated plasma levels of Lp(a) are a significant risk factor for the development of atherosclerotic disease. Apo(a) contains numerous secondary structures called Kringle domains. The Kringle domains of apo(a) exhibit 75 to 85% similarity to the Kringle domains of plasminogen which is involved in the process of blood coagulation (see Chapter 33).

Lp(a) competitively inhibits the binding of plasminogen to its receptor on endothelial cells as well as to its binding sites on fibrinogen and fibrin. Lp(a)-mediated interference of plasminogen binding leads to reduced surface-dependent activation of plasminogen to plasmin preventing fibrin clots from being degraded (Figure 16–5).

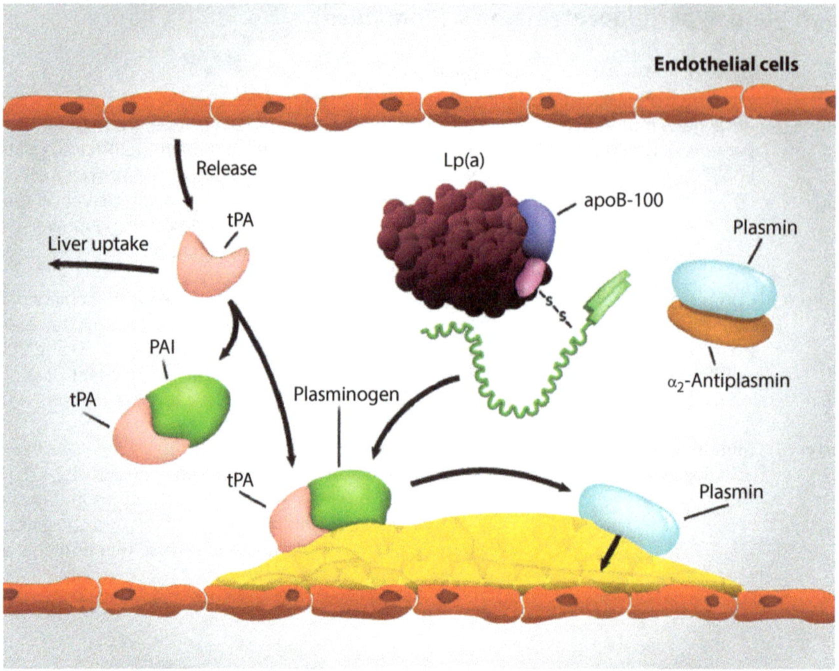

FIGURE 16–5 Mechanism of Lp(a) interference with normal fibrinolysis. The apo(a) protein disulfide bonded to apoB-100 in LDL contains Kringle domains that interfere with plasminogen binding to fibrin clots and also interfere with the ability of tPA to hydrolyze plasminogen to active plasmin, thereby, interfering with the normal course of fibrin clot dissolution. (Reproduced with permission from themedicalbiochemistrypage, LLC.)

CHECKLIST

- ☑ Lipid transport, both dietary lipids and endogenous lipids, are transported in the blood associated with proteins in complexes referred to as lipoproteins.
- ☑ Dietary lipoproteins are called chylomicrons and endogenous lipoproteins are either very-low-density lipoproteins (VLDL) or high-density lipoproteins (HDL).
- ☑ Chylomicrons are synthesized in intestinal enterocytes and are composed primarily of triglyceride and apolipoproteins. These lipoproteins are delivered to the circulation through the subclavian vein via the lymphatic system.
- ☑ VLDL are synthesized in the liver to deliver fatty acid (triglyceride) and cholesterol to peripheral tissues. As they circulate and lose lipid they become progressively more dense becoming low-density lipoproteins (LDL). HDL begin as apolipoprotein A-I and acquire cholesterol via interactions with peripheral tissues and macrophages and acquire triglycerides from VLDL and LDL.
- ☑ LDL are highly susceptible to oxidation (oxLDL) and are then preferentially phagocytosed by macrophages inducing proinflammatory responses from these cells; this phenomenon is a major reason LDL are referred to as "bad cholesterol."
- ☑ HDL play a critical role in the removal of cholesterol from macrophages and other peripheral tissues and return the cholesterol to the liver either directly or through exchange to VLDL and LDL, this process is referred to as reverse cholesterol transport (RCT) and is the reason HDL are often referred to as "good cholesterol."
- ☑ Numerous HDL-associated proteins are critical for the antioxidant and anti-inflammatory properties of these lipoproteins. Pharmacological elevation in plasma levels of HDL are beneficial in the prevention of atherosclerosis and coronary heart disease (CHD); inhibition of CETP has demonstrated efficacy in increasing circulating HDL levels.
- ☑ Lipoproteins, chylomicrons, LDL, and HDL bind to specific cell-surface receptors and are either internalized or deliver constituents such as cholesterol to cell to which they bind. LDL receptors require the presence of both apoB-100 and apoE for maximal binding. Chylomicron remnants can bind to the LDL receptor, LDL receptor-related protein (LRP), or to heparin sulfate proteoglycans (HSPG) in the space of Disse in the liver. HDL bind to the scavenger receptor SR-B1 on hepatocytes to deliver cholesterol to this tissue.
- ☑ Defects in overall lipoprotein synthesis and metabolism can lead to severe clinical outcomes associated with hypercholesterolemia and resulting in atherosclerosis and CHD. Familial hypercholesterolemia (FH) results from defects in LDL receptor-mediated hepatic LDL uptake and is the most common inherited disorder of lipoprotein metabolism.

REVIEW QUESTIONS

1. A 23-year-old man presents in the emergency department with complaints of severe epigastric pain. Physical examination reveals extensive xanthomas and palpable hepatosplenomegaly. Blood is drawn for routine tests, and it is noted to have a somewhat milky appearance. Which of the following processes is most likely abnormal accounting for the observations in this patient?
   (A) Adipose tissue triglyceride metabolism
   (B) Hepatic LDL receptor endocytosis
   (C) Hepatic VLDL synthesis
   (D) Intestinal chylomicron synthesis
   (E) Vascular chylomicron metabolism

2. A 15-year-old girl with type 1 diabetes is undergoing a routine physical examination. Laboratory results indicate her serum triglyceride level is 520 mg/dL (N = <150 mg/dL). Which of the following best explains the findings in this patient?
   (A) Decreased activity of hormone-sensitive lipase
   (B) Decreased activity of lipoprotein lipase
   (C) Defective LDL receptors
   (D) Deficiency in apoA-I
   (E) Increased hepatic triglyceride synthesis

3. A 23-year-old woman presents with low red blood cell count, corneal opacities, and renal insufficiency. Her physician makes a diagnosis of lecithin:cholesterol acyltransferase (LCAT) deficiency. Given this diagnosis, which of the following processes is most likely to be defective in this patient?
   (A) Adipose tissue triglyceride metabolism
   (B) Hepatic uptake of HDL cholesterol
   (C) Hepatic uptake of LDL cholesterol
   (D) Transfer of cholesterol esters from HDL to VLDL
   (E) Vascular chylomicron metabolism

4. A 22-year-old man is undergoing an investigation to determine the cause of his moderate hypertriglyceridemia. Serum studies revealed the presence of abnormal lipid and lipoprotein profiles. Both HDL and LDL were less dense than normal and showed significant elevations in triglyceride content with the mass of triglycerides approximately the same as that of cholesterol. A deficiency in which of the following is the most likely cause of the observed lipid abnormalities?
   (A) ApoB-100
   (B) Cholesterol ester transfer protein, CETP
   (C) Hepatic triglyceride lipase
   (D) Lecithin:cholesterol acyltransferase, LCAT
   (E) Lipoprotein lipase

5. Clinical trials are being undertaken of an investigational drug for the treatment of hypercholesterolemia. Results of these experiments indicate that in test subjects who consume the drug there is a statistically significant elevation in circulating HDL when compared to control subjects. Given these results, which of the following proteins is most likely the target of the investigational drug?
   (A) ApoB-100
   (B) ApoC-II
   (C) Cholesterol ester transfer protein, CETP
   (D) Hepatic triglyceride lipase, HTGL
   (E) Lecithin:cholesterol acyltransferase, LCAT

6. A 13-year-old girl presents with extensive eruptive xanthomas. Physical examination shows a palpable liver lateral to the rectus abdominus. History reveals that the girls' stools are oily and odorous. Additional history reveals that the girl does not have type 1 or type 2 diabetes and an analysis of circulating insulin and glucose levels indicates they are within normal ranges and responses. Examination of plasma indicates that it is quite milky indicating a lipemia. Analysis of the lipid content of the plasma shows a significant accumulation of chylomicrons and triglycerides. The child is placed on a fat-free diet which reduces the lipemia and all of the other clinical manifestations. Given the findings in this patient, which of the following processes is most likely defective?
   (A) Adipose tissue triglyceride synthesis
   (B) Hepatic bile acid synthesis
   (C) Intestinal lipid digestion
   (D) Skeletal muscle glycogen storage
   (E) Vascular lipoprotein hydrolysis

7. A patient presents with very high levels of serum cholesterol. After a series of tests, it is concluded that the patient has high circulating levels of LDL cholesterol but has normal levels of the hepatic LDL receptor. Which of the following would best explain the observations in this patient?
   (A) Hepatocytes from the patient are defective in the selective removal of cholesterol from the LDL complex
   (B) Hepatocytes from the patient have decreased levels of ACAT
   (C) The absence of the enzyme lipoprotein lipase in the endothelial cells of the liver
   (D) The patient has a mutated form of apoB-100
   (E) There is an altered level of phosphorylation of the LDL receptor

8. A 47-year-old man is being examined by his cardiologist as a follow-up of his myocardial infarct that he suffered 6 weeks ago. The patient has been taking atorvastatin and lisinopril for his hypercholesterolemia and hypertension, respectively. Physical examination finds the presence of corneal arcus and nodules were noted on both Achilles tendons and the right leg was warm, mildly erythematous, and painful to palpation. His latest fasting lipid profile shows total cholesterol of 355 mg/dL (N = < 200 mg/dL), LDL of 300 mg/dL (N = 130–160 mg/dL), and HDL of 34 mg/dL (N = 40–50 mg/dL). Which of the following is the most likely contributor to this patient's clinical status?
   (A) Abnormally elevated production of lipoprotein lipase
   (B) Abnormally elevated production of VLDL by the liver
   (C) Abnormally reduced production of HDL, resulting in a diminished capacity of reverse cholesterol transport
   (D) Defective LDL receptors leading to reduced uptake of plasma LDL and IDL
   (E) Defective lipoprotein lipase activity

9. Experiments are being conducted on a novel compound developed with the aim of enhancing the process of reverse cholesterol transport. Which of the following proteins would be the most likely target of such a compound?
   (A) ApoB-48
   (B) ApoB-100
   (C) ApoE
   (D) Cholesteryl ester transfer protein (CETP)
   (E) Lipoprotein lipase

10. A 47-year-old man is being examined by his cardiologist as a follow-up of his myocardial infarct that he suffered

6 weeks ago. The patient has been taking atorvastatin and lisinopril for his hypercholesterolemia and hypertension, respectively. Recently analyzed serum samples show that the patient has significantly elevated levels of lipoprotein-associated phospholipase A_2 (Lp-PLA_2). Which of the following represents the most likely role of the patient's Lp-PLA_2 levels in his cardiovascular pathology?
(A) Binding to the LDL receptor on hepatocytes
(B) Disulfide bonding to apoB-100 in LDL
(C) Hydrolysis of oxidized phospholipids
(D) Inactivation of platelet-activating factor
(E) Interaction with tissue plasminogen activator (tPA)

11. Experiments are being conducted on a novel molecule designed to mimic the observations observed in patients with the disorder known as familial combined hypolipidemia. Observations in these patients show that on average they have a 48% reduction in LDL, a 62% reduction in triglyceride, a 46% reduction in HDL, a 44% reduction in apoB, and a 48% reduction in apoA-I. Which of the following proteins would be the expected target of this novel molecule?
(A) Angiopoietin-like protein 3 (ANGPTL3)
(B) ApoB-100
(C) ApoC-II
(D) Cholesterol ester transfer protein
(E) Lipoprotein lipase

12. During periods of fasting changes in gene expression in the heart result in an increased efficiency of access to fatty acids. A deficiency in which of the following would most likely result in loss of this normal cardiac response to fasting?
(A) Angiopoietin-like protein 3 (ANGPTL3)
(B) ApoB-100
(C) Hormone-sensitive lipase
(D) LDL receptor
(E) Lipoprotein lipase

13. During a routine clinical trial of a new drug designed to lower serum cholesterol levels, a trial participant was discovered who had only 20% of normal circulating LDL cholesterol, even in the absence of the test drug. Which of the following would most likely account for the observations in this trial participant?
(A) Gain-of-function mutations in angiopoietin-like protein 3 gene
(B) Gain-of-function mutations in HDL receptor gene
(C) Gain-of-function mutations in HMG-CoA reductase gene
(D) Loss-of-function mutations in LDL receptor gene
(E) Loss-of-function mutations in lipoprotein lipase gene
(F) Loss-of-function mutations in *PCSK9* gene

14. A 47-year-old man is being examined by his cardiologist as a follow-up of his myocardial infarct that he suffered 6 weeks ago. The patient has been taking atorvastatin and lisinopril for his hypercholesterolemia and hypertension. Physical examination finds the presence of corneal arcus and nodules were noted on both Achilles tendons and the right leg was warm, mildly erythematous, and painful to palpation. His latest fasting lipid profile shows total cholesterol of 355 mg/dL (N = < 200 mg/dl), LDL of 300 mg/dL (N = 130–160 mg/dL), and HDL of 34 mg/dL (N = 40–50 mg/dL). Which of the following medications would be most beneficial for use in this patient?
(A) Colestipol
(B) Evolocumab
(C) Ezetimibe
(D) Gemfibrozil
(E) Niacin

15. A 28-year-old man is being examined by his physician with complaints of fatigue and loss of visual acuity. Ophthalmoscopic examination finds diffuse grayish corneal opacities. Serum and urine analyses find anemia, hyperlipemia, and proteinuria. Plasma triglycerides and unesterified cholesterol levels are elevated, as are levels of phosphatidylcholine. A defect in which of the following would most likely account for the signs and symptoms in this patient?
(A) Cholesterol ester transfer protein (CETP)
(B) 7-Dehydrocholesterol reductase
(C) Hepatic triglyceride lipase
(D) Lecithin:cholesterol acyltransferase (LCAT)
(E) Lipoprotein lipase

16. Elevated plasma levels of the lipoprotein particle identified as lipoprotein(a) [Lp(a)] are a primary risk factor for coronary heart disease and stroke. The glycoprotein apolipoprotein(a) [apo(a)] is most likely to contribute to the formation of Lp(a) due to covalent attachment to which of the following?
(A) ApoB-100
(B) ApoC-II
(C) Cholesterol ester transfer protein
(D) HDL
(E) Lipoprotein lipase

17. Experiments are being carried out with the use of a compound designed to reduce the antioxidant functions of HDL. Administration of this compound to experimental animals results in elevated plasma concentration of oxidized LDL (oxLDL). Given these results this compound is most likely targeting the function of which of the following?
(A) ApoA-I
(B) ApoC-II
(C) Cholesterol ester transfer protein, CETP
(D) Glutathione peroxidase 1
(E) Lecithin:cholesterol acyltransferase, LCAT
(F) Sphingosine-1-phosphate

18. A 24-year-old man is being seen by his physician with complaints of smelly and oily stools and frequent diarrhea. Biochemical studies determine that the patient has a dramatically reduced capacity to produce chylomicrons. Given these findings, which of the following is most likely to be an additional consequence of this patient's clinical status?
(A) Fasting hyperglycemia
(B) Increased risk of hypertriglyceridemia
(C) Lactic acidosis
(D) Prolonged prothrombin time
(E) Reduced circulating HDL concentration

19. A strain of mice has been developed that have normal levels of lipoprotein lipase enzyme but significantly reduced levels of lipoprotein lipase hydrolytic activity. These mice are most likely harboring a defective gene encoding which of the following?
(A) ApoA-IV
(B) ApoB-48
(C) ApoC-II
(D) Hepatic LDL receptor
(E) Hormone-sensitive lipase

20. A 2-month-old male infant is being examined to determine the cause of his physical abnormalities which includes microcephaly, micrognathia, ptosis, and cleft palate. A defect in which of the following processes would most likely account for the signs and symptoms in this infant?
(A) Branched-chain amino acid metabolism
(B) Cholesterol synthesis
(C) Mannose phosphorylation of lysosomal enzymes
(D) Mitochondrial fatty acid oxidation
(E) Peroxisomal fatty acid metabolism

21. A 46-year-old man is being treated in the emergency department following an apparent heart attack. Physical examination shows that the patient is of optimal weight for his height. Measurement of his serum cholesterol level indicates it is 460 mg/dL. History reveals that his father died at 39 years of age from a massive heart attack, and one of his two younger siblings also was found to have significant elevation in serum total cholesterol. Given the pathology in this patient and his family history, which of the following additional symptoms would be most likely?
(A) Corneal arcus
(B) Hyperammonemia
(C) Hypoglycemia
(D) Lactic acidosis
(E) Nonalcoholic fatty liver

22. A 23-year-old man is found to harbor a mutation in the gene that encodes the enzyme, cytidine deaminase, responsible for editing of C to U in mRNA. With respect to this patient and the observed mutation, which of the following would be the most likely consequence?
(A) Fat-soluble vitamin deficiency
(B) Hyperammonemia
(C) Hypercholesterolemia
(D) Hypertriglyceridemia
(E) Hyperuricemia
(F) Unconjugated hyperbilirubinemia

23. A 22-year-old man is being examined by his physician because he is concerned about growths on his eyelids. He is 180 cm (5 ft 11 in) tall and weighs 85 kg (188 lb); BMI is 26 kg/m^2. Physical examination shows no other abnormalities. Serum studies show a total cholesterol concentration of 300 mg/dL (N = <200 mg/dL), HDL-cholesterol concentration of 37 mg/dL (N = >40 mg/dL), and triglyceride concentration of 3500 mg/dL (N = <150 mg/dL). A deficiency in which of the following is the most likely cause of these findings?
(A) Cortisol
(B) Glucagon
(C) Hepatic lipase
(D) Insulin
(E) Lipoprotein lipase
(F) Pancreatic lipase

24. A 41-year-old man is being examined by his physician with complaints of recurrent abdominal pain for the past several years. Physical examination shows the patient has hepatomegaly and the presence of numerous xanthomas. Plasma triglycerides and chylomicrons were markedly elevated, whereas LDL and HDL were decreased. A deficiency in which of the following is the most likely cause of this patient's condition?
(A) ApoA-I
(B) ApoB-100
(C) ApoC-II
(D) Chylomicron receptors
(E) HDL receptors
(F) LDL receptors

25. A 17-year-old boy is being examined by his physician with complaints of reddish-orange-colored bumps under the skin on his elbows, back of his legs, and buttocks. Additional physical signs include a palpable liver. Laboratory studies show normal insulin and glucose levels. Plasma lipid analysis shows a triglyceride concentration of 775 mg/dL (N = <150 mg/dL), 95% of which is associated with chylomicrons. In addition to being counseled to reduce fat intake in his diet, which of the following therapeutic interventions is most appropriate in this patient?
(A) HMG-CoA reductase inhibitor
(B) Intestinal cholesterol uptake inhibitor
(C) PCSK9 inhibitor
(D) PPARα activator
(E) PPARγ activator

26. A 28-year-old man has come to his physician with complaints of blurry vision. Physical examination shows diffuse grayish corneal opacities. Serum and blood analysis indicate the patient has anemia, proteinuria, and hyperlipemia. Renal function is compromised, and serum albumin level is elevated. Plasma triglycerides and unesterified cholesterol levels are elevated, as are levels of phosphatidylcholine. These symptoms are most likely to be indicative of which of the following disorders?
(A) Familial apoC-II deficiency
(B) Familial hypercholesterolemia
(C) Familial hypertriglyceridemia
(D) Familial lecithin:cholesterol acyltransferase deficiency
(E) Familial ligand defective apoB

27. Experiments are being conducted with an investigational compound designed for the treatment of hypercholesterolemia. The results of clinical trials in 300 individuals indicate that consumption of the drug causes a clear elevation in the circulating levels of HDL in 87% of the test subjects. Given these results, which of the following proteins is most likely the target of the investigational drug?
(A) ApoB-100
(B) ApoC-II
(C) Cholesterol ester transfer protein, CETP
(D) Hepatic triglyceride lipase, HTGL
(E) Lecithin:cholesterol acyltransferase, LCAT

28. A 23-year-old man is found to harbor a mutation in the gene that encodes the enzyme responsible for editing the intestinal apoB mRNA. The mutation results in a significant loss in the ability to produce intestinal lipoproteins. Which of the following is the most likely consequence in this individual?
(A) Fasting hyperglycemia
(B) Impaired absorption of dietary lipids
(C) Increased risk of hypertriglyceridemia
(D) Increased risk of lactic acidosis
(E) Increased serum urea nitrogen concentration

29. A 37-year-old man comes to his physician because of a 2-month history of a rash on his arms. He also says that he has had moderate to severe upper abdominal pain for the past 24 hours and that these abdominal symptoms have been coming and going during the preceding 12–18 months. Physical examination

shows yellow papules on the extensor surfaces of the upper extremities. Palpation of the epigastric region causes sharp pain. Laboratory studies show a serum amylase concentration of 187U/L. If this patient has inherited a mutation in a gene from the *APOC* family, which of the following would most likely be an additional expected finding?
(A) Hyperbilirubinemia
(B) Hypertriglyceridemia
(C) Hypervolemia
(D) Hypoglycemia
(E) Reduced levels of HDL
(F) Reduced levels of serum insulin

30. A 39-year-old man is being examined by his physician during a follow-up to discuss a fasting lipid profile result that showed elevated total cholesterol and elevated LDL cholesterol. History reveals that the patient had a similar lipid panel result the previous year. The patient is otherwise healthy and has no other medical conditions or complaints. His father had a history of hypercholesterolemia and died as a result of an acute myocardial infarction at the age of 48 years. The patient reports that he has smoked one pack of cigarettes daily for the past 15 years. Despite attempts to change his lifestyle with respect to diet and exercise, there has been no significant change in his serum cholesterol values. His physician explains that his serum cholesterol and lifestyle, along with family history indicate that his risk for cardiovascular disease is elevated. The physician prescribes lovastatin and strongly encourages his patient to work on his diet and exercise. Given the function of the prescribed medication, which of the following is most likely to be decreased in the plasma of this patient?
(A) ApoA-I
(B) ApoB-48
(C) ApoB-100
(D) Cholesterol ester transfer protein (CETP)
(E) Lecithin-cholesterol ester transferase (LCAT)

31. A 43-year-old man is undergoing a routine examination required for the purchase of life insurance. History reveals that the patient has not seen a doctor in over 5 years, and there is hypertension, hypercholesterolemia, and cardiovascular disease in his family. The patient reports that he has smoked one pack of cigarettes daily for the past 12 years. A fasting lipid profile is ordered, and the results show that the patient's total cholesterol is 227 mg/dL (N = < 200 mg/dL), LDL-cholesterol is 163 mg/dL (N = < 100 mg/dL), and triglycerides are 172 mg/dL (N = < 150 mg/dL). The physician prescribes bempedoic acid. Given the function of the prescribed medication, the activity of which of the following is most likely to be decreased in this patient?
(A) Acetyl-CoA carboxylase
(B) Angiopoietin-like protein 3
(C) ApoB-100
(D) ATP citrate lyase
(E) HMG-CoA reductase
(F) Lipoprotein lipase
(G) Microsomal triglyceride transfer protein

32. A 63-year-old woman is undergoing a routine examination required by her new employer. History reveals that the patient has not seen a doctor in over 5 years, and there is hypertension, hypercholesterolemia, and cardiovascular disease in her family, with her father having succumbed to a myocardial infarction at the age of 61 years. A fasting lipid profile is ordered, and the results show that the patient's total cholesterol is 257 mg/dL (N = < 200 mg/dL), LDL-cholesterol is 153 mg/dL (N = < 100 mg/dL), and triglycerides are 172 mg/dL (N = < 150 mg/dL). Given the family history and recent blood work from this patient, the physician prescribes cholestyramine. Which of the following is the most likely effect of this medication on the patient's lipid profile?

	LDL	HDL	Triglyceride
A.	↓	↑↑	↓
B.	↓↓	↑	↑
C.	↓↓↓	↑↑	↓
D.	↑	↑	↓↓
E.	↑↑	↑	↓↓↓
F.	↑↑↑	↓↓↓	↓↓↓

(A)
(B)
(C)
(D)
(E)
(F)

33. A 43-year-old man is undergoing a routine examination required by his new employer. History reveals that there is hypertension, hypercholesterolemia, and cardiovascular disease in his family. A fasting lipid profile is ordered, and the results show that the patient's total cholesterol is 227 mg/dL (N = < 200 mg/dL), LDL-cholesterol is 133 mg/dL (N = < 100 mg/dL), and triglycerides are 478 mg/dL (N = < 150 mg/dL). Based on the results of the lipid screening the patient's physician prescribes the most appropriate medication for reducing serum triglyceride levels. Given the function of the prescribed medication, this patient will most likely be at an increased risk for which of the following adverse effects?
(A) Cholelithiasis
(B) Hyperuricemia
(C) Muscle weakness and pain
(D) Myoglobinuria
(E) Steatorrhea

34. A 59-year-old man is being examined by his physician during a follow-up to discuss a fasting glucose and lipid profile result that showed total cholesterol of 245 mg/dL (N = < 200 mg/dL), HDL-cholesterol 30 mg/dL (N = > 40 mg/dL), LDL cholesterol 170 mg/dL (N = < 100mg/dL), triglycerides 250 mg/dL (N = < 150 mg/dL), and glucose 112 mg/dL (N = 70–100 mg/dL). The patient is otherwise healthy and has no other medical conditions or complaints. His father had a history of hypercholesterolemia and died as a result of an acute myocardial infarction at the age of 63 years. His physician explains that his serum cholesterol and lifestyle, along with family history, indicate that his risk for cardiovascular disease is elevated, and therefore, he is going to prescribe the most appropriate medication to help lower his serum lipids. Which of the following most likely represents the class of drug that was prescribed to this patient?
(A) ATP-citrate lyase inhibitor
(B) Fibrate
(C) Microsomal triglyceride transfer protein inhibitor
(D) PCSK9 inhibitor
(E) Statin

35. A 43-year-old man is undergoing a routine examination required for the purchase of life insurance. History reveals that the patient has not seen a doctor in over 5 years, and there is hypertension, hypercholesterolemia, and cardiovascular disease in his family. The patient reports that he has smoked one pack of cigarettes daily for the past 12 years. A fasting lipid profile is ordered, and the results show that the patient's total cholesterol is 227 mg/dL (N = < 200 mg/dL), LDL-cholesterol is 163 mg/dL (N = < 100 mg/dL), and triglycerides are 172 mg/dL (N = < 150 mg/dL). Given the family history and recent blood work from this patient, which of the following is most likely to be increased in the plasma of this patient?
(A) ApoA-I
(B) ApoB-48
(C) ApoB-100
(D) Cholesterol ester transfer protein (CETP)
(E) Lecithin-cholesterol ester transferase (LCAT)

36. A 29-year-old man is meeting with his physician to discuss a recommended treatment plan. During a previous wellness check he was diagnosed with elevated levels of serum lipids, particularly total cholesterol, and he was placed on a statin class drug. However, the patient developed severe muscle pain and indicated to his physician that he could not tolerate the side effects of the drug. The patient has a significant family history of hyperlipidemia with his father suffering from several myocardial infarctions between the ages of 43 and 58 years. The patient's paternal grandfather died following an acute myocardial infarction when he was 52 years of age. Other than the elevated hyperlipidemia, the patient reports no other medical issues. He states that following the initial diagnosis of elevated serum lipids, he switched to a strictly vegan diet. He states that he does not smoke, use illicit drugs, or drink alcohol. At this most recent examination his fasting lipid profile shows a total serum cholesterol level of 322 mg/dL (N = < 200 mg/dL), an LDL-cholesterol level of 154 mg/dL (N = < 100 mg/dL)), an HDL-cholesterol level of 35 mg/dL (N = > 40 mg/dL), and a triglyceride level of 135 mg/dL (N = < 150 mg/dL). Given the patient's prior adverse response to statin therapy, combined with the family history and the patient's current level of hyperlipidemia, the doctor is most likely to prescribe a class of drug whose mechanism of action is best described by which of the following?
(A) Activates PPARα resulting in increased hepatic apoA-I synthesis
(B) Activates PPARγ resulting in suppression of expression of the *APOB* gene
(C) Increases the binding of LDL to hepatic LDL receptors
(D) Increases the synthesis and processing of lipoprotein lipase
(E) Interferes with intestinal cholesterol uptake
(F) Interferes with LDL receptor degradation

37. A 40-year-old man is undergoing a routine examination as a part of his annual physical. The patient has no medical concerns and has an unremarkable medical history. He does not smoke nor drink alcohol to excess and is currently taking no medication. As a part of his physical examination, he has had fasting blood work done. The results of this blood work show that his complete blood count and basic metabolic panel are within expected ranges for his age but the lipid profile finds that his total cholesterol is 215 mg/dL (N = < 200 mg/dL), LDL cholesterol is 107 mg/dL (N = < 100 mg/dL), HDL cholesterol is 41 mg/dL (N = > 40 mg/dL), and triglycerides are 678 mg/dL (N = < 150 mg/dL). Based on the results of the lipid screening, which of the following classes of medication is most likely to be of the highest benefit to this patient?
(A) ATP-citrate lyase inhibitor
(B) Fibrate
(C) Microsomal triglyceride transfer protein inhibitor
(D) PCSK9 inhibitor
(E) Statin

38. An 11-year-old girl is brought to her pediatrician by her mother because she has been complaining of abdominal pain and nausea for the past 2 days. Physical examination finds hepatosplenomegaly, lipemia retinalis, and the presence of numerous reddish-yellow papules on her lower back, buttocks, and the extensor surfaces of her extremities. The pediatrician orders blood work which finds the patient's plasma is milky. Given the most likely diagnosis, which of the following is the most likely near-term medical complication that will affect this patient?
(A) Achilles tendon xanthomas
(B) Acute pancreatitis
(C) Myocardial infarction
(D) Nephrolithiasis
(E) Steatorrhea

39. A 26-year-old man is being examined by his physician with a primary complaint of yellowish growths on the back of his hands and near the corners of his eyes. The patient has a significant family history of cardiovascular disease with his father suffering from several myocardial infarctions between the ages of 43 and 58 years. The patient's paternal grandfather died following an acute myocardial infarction when he was 52 years of age. His physician orders a fasting lipid profile and the results show a total serum cholesterol level of 342 mg/dL (N = < 200 mg/dL), an LDL-cholesterol level of 154 mg/dL (N = < 100 mg/dL)), an HDL-cholesterol level of 35 mg/dL (N = > 40 mg/dL), and a triglyceride level of 115 mg/dL (N = < 150 mg/dL). A deficiency in which of the following is the most likely contributing factor to the signs and symptoms in this patient?
(A) ApoA-I
(B) Glycosylphosphatidylinositol-anchored HDL binding protein 1, GPIHBP1
(C) Hepatic lipase
(D) LDL receptor
(E) Lecithin-cholesterol acyltransferase, LCAT

40. An 11-year-old has been taken to the Emergency Department by his adoptive father because he has been complaining of nausea and severe abdominal pain that is radiating to his back for the past several hours. Physical examination finds the patient's abdomen is tender to palpation and there is demonstrable hepatosplenomegaly. Several yellowish papules are noted on the patient's lower back, buttocks, and the extensor surfaces of his extremities. The attending physician orders blood work, and the technician finds that the patient's blood is quite milky. Given the most likely diagnosis in this patient, which of the following proteins is most likely defective?
(A) ApoC-II
(B) Lysosomal acid lipase
(C) ApoB-100
(D) LDL receptor
(E) Lecithin-cholesterol ester transferase, LCAT

ANSWERS

1. Correct answer is **E.** Chylomicrons are assembled in the intestinal mucosa as a means to transport dietary triglycerides, phospholipids, and cholesterol to the rest of the body. Following the digestive process, the absorbed fatty acids, monoacylglycerides, phosphatidic acid, and cholesterol are reassembled into triglycerides, phospholipids, and cholesterol esters and packaged into chylomicrons. Chylomicrons leave the intestine via the lymphatic system and enter the circulation at the left subclavian vein. High levels of chylomicrons in the blood can give it a milky appearance and can be indicative of defects in the processes of lipoprotein lipase-mediated triglyceride metabolism and subsequent tissue uptake of the released fatty acids. The term "chylo" refers to the milky fluid consisting of lymph and emulsified fats or free fatty acids which is how the term chylomicron was derived. None of the other options (choices A, B, C, and D) reflect processes, that, when abnormal, would result in a milky appearance to the plasma.

2. Correct answer is **B.** The triglyceride components of VLDL and chylomicron are hydrolyzed to free fatty acids and glycerol in the capillaries of tissues such as cardiac muscle, skeletal muscle, and adipose tissue by the actions of lipoprotein lipase (LPL) and in the liver by the actions of hepatic triglyceride lipase (HTGL, also called hepatic lipase, HL). Insulin exerts numerous effects on overall metabolic homeostasis. One of the effects of insulin, that relate to the symptoms in this patient, is the regulation of the expression of LPL on the surface of endothelial cells. Since type 1 diabetics do not synthesize insulin, they do not properly regulate the level of LPL which contributes to hypertriglyceridemia in these individuals. Decreased activity of hormone-sensitive lipase (choice A) would result in reduced ability to release free fatty acid from adipose tissue triglycerides and would have no direct correlation to elevated serum triglycerides in type 1 diabetics. If LDL receptors were defective (choice C) the level of triglycerides would be normal, but LDL cholesterol levels would be dramatically elevated as is typical in familial hypercholesterolemia. A deficiency in apoA-I (choice D) is a rare disorder called familial HDL deficiency and is associated with extremely low plasma high-density lipoprotein (HDL) cholesterol, corneal opacities, xanthomas, and premature coronary heart disease (CHD). Increased hepatic triglyceride synthesis (choice E) would most likely result in increased levels of VLDL secretion from the liver but the action of LPL would lead to the formation of LDL and thus, triglyceride levels would be normal, but LDL cholesterol levels would be increased.

3. Correct answer is **D.** The primary mechanism by which HDL acquires peripheral tissue cholesterol is via an interaction with macrophages in the subendothelial spaces of the tissues. The free cholesterol that is transferred from macrophages to HDL is esterified by HDL-associated LCAT. LCAT is synthesized in the liver and so named because it transfers a fatty acid from the *sn*2 position of a phosphatidylcholine (lecithin) to the free hydroxyl group on carbon-3 of cholesterol, generating a cholesterol ester and a lysolecithin. The cholesterol esters in these HDL are then transferred to VLDL, IDL, and LDL via the actions of the HDL-associated enzyme, cholesterol ester transfer protein (CETP). None of the other options (choices A, B, C, and E) are associated with the function of LCAT.

4. Correct answer is **C.** Hepatic triglyceride lipase (HTGL, also called hepatic lipase, HL) is an enzyme that is made primarily by hepatocytes, hence the name of the enzyme. Hepatic lipase hydrolyzes phospholipids and triglycerides present in chylomicron remnants, LDL, and HDL. The apoB-48 present in chylomicrons directly binds to hepatic lipase on the surface of hepatocytes. The binding of LDL to the LDL receptor and the binding of triglyceride-rich HDL to the HDL receptor (SR-BI) on the surface of hepatocytes allows for the action of hepatic lipase to hydrolyze the triglycerides in these lipoprotein particles. The potential significance of the HTGL pathway is that it is predominant in the conversion of intermediate-density lipoproteins to LDL and the conversion of postprandial triglyceride-rich HDL into the postabsorptive triglyceride-poor HDL. HTGL plays a secondary role in the clearance of chylomicron remnants by the liver. A prominent feature of HTGL deficiency is the increase in HDL cholesterol and an approximately 10-fold increase in HDL triglyceride. Deficiency in apoB-100 (choice A) occurs in familial hypobetalipoproteinemia (FHBL) which is most commonly due to truncating mutations in the *APOB* gene. The characteristic features of FHBL, caused by these APOB truncating mutations, are low plasma concentrations of total cholesterol, LDL cholesterol (LDL-C), and apoB-100. Deficiency in CETP (choice B) is associated with increased HDL cholesterol levels. The HDL particles are enriched in cholesterol esters and depleted of triglycerides. Individuals with CETP deficiency have a reduced risk for coronary heart disease (CHD). Familial LCAT deficiency (choice D) patients have an abnormal lipoprotein particle in their blood called lipoprotein-X (Lp-X). Lp-X is characterized by the very low protein content of the particle (around 5%) and its predominant phospholipid (>65%) content. The protein in Lp-X is almost exclusively albumin in the inner core and apoC on the surface. Deficiency in lipoprotein lipase (choice E) is associated with severe increases in serum triglycerides on the order of 10 times the normal.

5. Correct answer is **C.** Cholesterol ester transfer protein (CETP) is plasma glycoprotein secreted primarily from the liver and plays a critical role in HDL metabolism by facilitating the exchange of cholesterol esters (CE) from HDL for triglycerides (TG) in apoB containing lipoproteins, such as VLDL, IDL, and LDL. The activity of CETP directly lowers the cholesterol levels of HDL and enhances HDL catabolism by providing HDL with the triglyceride substrate of hepatic lipase. Thus, CETP plays a critical role in the regulation of circulating levels of HDL, LDL, and apoA-I. Deficiency in CETP is associated with increased HDL cholesterol levels. The HDL particles are enriched in cholesterol esters and depleted of triglycerides. Individuals with CETP deficiency have a reduced risk for coronary heart disease (CHD). Pharmacologic targeting of none of the other proteins (choices A, B, D, and E) would lead to significant elevations in HDL.

6. Correct answer is **E.** The triglyceride components of VLDL and chylomicron are hydrolyzed to free fatty acids and glycerol in the capillaries of cardiac muscle, skeletal muscle, and adipose tissue by the actions of lipoprotein lipase (LPL) and in the liver by the actions of hepatic triglyceride lipase (HTGL, also called hepatic lipase, HL). Insulin exerts numerous effects on overall metabolic homeostasis. One of the effects of insulin, that relate to the symptoms in this patient, is the regulation of the expression of LPL on the surface of endothelial cells. The loss of peripheral insulin sensitivity in type 2 diabetes and the poorly regulated function of insulin in

type 1 diabetics will lead to hyperlipidemia. Therefore, assessing whether either form of diabetes is present in a patient can help identify the causes of hyperlipidemia. Since the patient had neither type 1 nor type 2 diabetes, the cause of her hyperlipidemia must be mediated by another mechanisms. The role of chylomicrons and triglycerides in producing milky plasma was confirmed. Therefore, the most likely cause of the symptoms in the patient is the inability to hydrolyze fatty acids from the circulating lipoprotein particles. None of the other options (choices A, B, C, and D) would account for the observations in this patient.

7. Correct answer is **D.** The presence of normal levels of hepatic LDL receptor in a patient with hypercholesterolemia is suggestive of a defect in LDL binding to the receptor or the inability of the receptor to internalize in response to LDL binding. The inability of the LDL receptor to bind LDL could be the result of a mutation in the LDL binding site of the receptor or a mutation in the LDL receptor binding site in the apoB-100 proteins of VLDL, IDL, and LDL. The inability to remove LDL from the receptor (choice A) when internalized would lead to reduced LDL receptor returned to the plasma membrane. The function of ACAT (choice B) is to esterify cholesterol once it is released from LDL receptor within the cell. Endothelial cells of the vasculature of the liver do not express lipoprotein lipase (choice C). The LDL receptor is not a substrate for phosphorylation (choice E).

8. Correct answer is **D.** The most common cause of familial hypercholesterolemia, FH (type II hyperlipoproteinemia) is an autosomal dominant disorder that results from mutations affecting the structure and function of the LDL receptor. The defects in LDL receptor presentation or function result in lifelong elevation of LDL-cholesterol in the blood. The resultant hypercholesterolemia leads to premature coronary artery disease and atherosclerotic plaque formation. Elevation in lipoprotein lipase expression (choice A) would result in a higher level of fatty acid removal from circulating chylomicrons and VLDL but would not lead to significant increases in LDL and total cholesterol. Elevated production in VLDL (choice B) could lead to increased levels of IDL and LDL but their subsequent uptake by the LDL receptor pathway would most likely reduce overall levels in the blood or at least only lead to moderate elevation of their levels, not the severe elevations observed in this patient. Reduced HDL levels (choice C), as is seen in familial HDL deficiency (FHD) is associated with extremely low plasma HDL cholesterol, corneal opacities, xanthomas, and premature coronary heart disease (CHD). Defective lipoprotein lipase activity (choice E) is associated with severe hypertriglyceridemia with relatively normal levels of total cholesterol.

9. Correct answer is **D.** Cholesterol ester transfer protein (CETP) is a plasma glycoprotein secreted primarily from the liver and plays a critical role in HDL metabolism by facilitating the exchange of cholesterol esters (CE) from HDL for triglycerides (TG) in apoB containing lipoproteins, such as VLDL, IDL, and LDL. The activity of CETP directly lowers the cholesterol levels of HDL and enhances HDL catabolism by providing HDL with the triglyceride substrate of hepatic lipase. Thus, CETP plays a critical role in the regulation of circulating levels of HDL, LDL, and apoA-I. It has also been shown that in mice naturally lacking CETP most of their cholesterol is found in HDL and these mice are relatively resistant to atherosclerosis. ApoB-48 (choice A) is found exclusively in chylomicrons which do not participate in reverse cholesterol transport. ApoB-100 (choice B) and apoE (choice C) are both components of VLDL and IDL which accept cholesterol esters from HDL. As such they participate secondarily in reverse cholesterol transport but require that function CETP be present in HDL to accept the esters. Lipoprotein lipase (choice E) removes fatty acids from circulating triglycerides and, therefore, does not participate in the process of reverse cholesterol transport.

10. Correct answer is **C.** The enzymatic activity of Lp-PLA_2 is specific for short-chain acyl groups (up to 9 methylene groups) at the *sn*2 position of phospholipids. When PAF is the substrate for Lp-PLA_2 the products are lyso-PAF and acetate. When phospholipids of the phosphatidylcholine (PC) family are oxidized by free radical activity (referred to as oxPL), they can be a substrate for Lp-PLA_2 even if the unsaturated fatty acid at the *sn*2 position is longer than 9 carbon atoms. The ability of Lp-PLA_2 to recognize oxPL as substrates is due to the presence of aldehydic or carboxylic moieties at the omega (ω) end of the peroxidized fatty acyl residues at the *sn2* position. The products of Lp-PLA_2 activity on oxPL are oxidized free fatty acids (oxFFA) and lysophosphatidylcholine. Numerous types of oxPL have been identified in oxidized LDL (oxLDL) particles and many of them exhibit biological activity that promote atherogenesis and the development of coronary heart disease (CHD). None of the other options (choices A, B, D, and E) relate to the functions of Lp-PLA_2.

11. Correct answer is **A.** Familial combined hypolipidemia results from mutations in the gene (*ANGPTL3*) encoding the angiopoietin-like protein 3 protein. Familial combined hypolipidemia is associated with reduced circulating levels of VLDL, LDL, and HDL due to increased activities of both lipoprotein lipase (LPL) and endothelial lipase (EL). Three of the angiopoietin-like proteins (ANGPTL3, ANGPTL4, and ANGPTL8) play crucial roles in the posttranslational regulation of LPL activity. Angiopoietin-like protein 3 is produced exclusively by the liver and secreted into the circulation. Prior to its release from hepatocytes, a portion of the ANGPTL3 proprotein is cleaved into N-terminal and C-terminal fragments. Both full-length and the cleaved fragments of ANGPTL3 are secreted into the circulation. The N-terminal portion of ANGPTL3 is involved in the regulation of overall lipoprotein metabolism through its ability to inhibit the activity of LPL, as well as to inhibit the activity of endothelial lipase, EL. As a result of deciphering the cause of familial combined hypolipidemia, drugs have been developed to inhibit the action of ANGPTL3 as a means to lower total serum cholesterol and triglycerides. Inhibition of none of the other proteins (choices B, C, D, and E) would result in the observed beneficial changes in serum lipoprotein levels.

12. Correct answer is **E.** Lipoprotein lipase (LPL) is expressed exclusively in the vasculature of cardiac muscle, skeletal muscle, and adipose tissue. The level of LPL present in the vasculature of these tissues changes in response to tissue demands for energy during periods of fasting and following feeding. During fasting the level of LPL activity decreases in adipose tissue but increases in cardiac and skeletal muscle. This increase in LPL activity allows these muscle tissues to maximally access circulating fatty acids in the triglycerides of lipoprotein particles. Deficiency in none of the other proteins (choices A, B, C, and D) results in reduced cardiac tissue access to fatty acids during periods of fasting.

13. Correct answer is **F.** The enzyme, proprotein convertase subtilisin/kexin type 9 (PCSK9), plays a role in the metabolism of LDL receptors. PCSK9 normally functions to degrade some of the LDL receptors within the endosome thereby, reducing the overall level of LDL receptor recycling to the plasma membrane. A loss-of-function mutation in the *PCSK9* gene would result in reduced degradation of LDL receptors within the endosome resulting in an increased number of LDL receptors being returned to the plasma membrane. This increased LDL receptor recycling would allow for increased LDL removal from the blood. Indeed, naturally occurring loss-of-function mutations in the *PCSK9* gene were the basis for the development of drugs to inhibit the activity of PCSK9 for the treatment of hypercholesterolemia as is typical in familial hypercholesterolemia. The product of the *ANGPTL3* gene (choice A) is responsible for reducing the concentration of lipoprotein lipase present on the surface of the endothelium. Gain-of-function mutations in the *ANGPTL3* gene would, therefore, result in hypertriglyceridemia. Gain-of-function mutations in the HDL receptor gene (choice B) could result in reductions in serum HDL but would not contribute to reductions in LDL cholesterol. Gain-of-function mutations in the HMG-CoA reductase gene (choice C) would result in increased synthesis of cholesterol which would result in increased circulating levels of LDL. Loss-of-function mutations in the LDL receptor (choice D) would result in lack of ability to remove the LDL from the blood resulting in hypercholesterolemia. Loss-of-function mutations in the lipoprotein lipase gene (choice E) would lead to the inability of plasma triglycerides to be hydrolyzed resulting in hypertriglyceridemia.

14. Correct answer is **B.** The patient most likely has a form of familial hypercholesterolemia, FH. FH is most often the result of defects in the processing and/or function of the LDL receptor. Common treatments for FH include the use of the statin class of drugs. Quite often these drugs are ineffective at reducing total serum cholesterol levels to nonpathologic levels in FH patients. Recent approvals by the FDA include drugs like evolocumab which is an inhibitor of the function of the enzyme proprotein convertase subtilisin/kexin type 9 (PCSK9). PCSK9 normally functions to degrade some of the LDL receptors within the endosome thereby, reducing the overall level of LDL receptor recycling to the plasma membrane. The inhibition of PCSK9 allows for a higher level of LDL receptor recycling which enhances the ability to remove LDL cholesterol from the blood. Colestipol (choice A) is a type of bile acid chelating resin used to enhance bile acid excretion in the feces, thereby inducing the liver to drive more cholesterol into bile acid synthesis. Although useful for treating high cholesterol, cholestipol is not as effective as is the inhibition of PCSK9. Ezetimibe (choice C) is a drug that inhibits the cholesterol uptake transporter in the small intestine. Inhibition of cholesterol absorption from the diet leads to reduction in overall circulating cholesterol. Although useful for treating high cholesterol, ezetimibe is not as effective as is the inhibition of PCSK9. Gemfibrozil (choice D) is a member of the fibrate class of drugs whose effects are exerted by the induction of the activity of peroxisome proliferator activated receptor alpha (PPARα). Fibrates are useful for treating hypertriglyceridemia but are not as useful for treating hypercholesterolemia. Niacin (choice E), specifically nicotinic acid, is used to interfere with fatty acid release from adipose tissue, thereby reducing overall VLDL production by the liver. Although useful for treating high cholesterol, nicotinic acid is not as effective as is the inhibition of PCSK9. In addition, side effects of nicotinic acid lead to noncompliance by patients.

15. Correct answer is **D.** The patient is most likely suffering from the effects of a disorder referred to as familial LCAT deficiency, FLD. FLD is also called fish-eye disease or Norum disease. Individuals with FLD have characteristic abnormalities in blood lipid profiles that includes low HDL (<10 mg/dL), low apo A-I (20–30 mg/dL), low cholesterol esters, and low LDL. The HDL particles in FLD patients, in addition to being lower than normal, are also small and resemble immature HDL. FLD patients may also experience hypertriglyceridemia, but this blood lipid abnormality does not appear in all patients. FLD patients always develop corneal opacities that give their eyes the appearance of fish eyes, hence the association with the name fish-eye disease. FLD patients will also have an abnormal lipoprotein particle in their blood called lipoprotein-X (Lp-X). Lp-X is characterized by the very low protein content of the particle (around 5%) and its predominant phospholipid (>65%) content. The protein in Lp-X is almost exclusively albumin in the inner core and apoC on the surface. Patients with FLD also develop normochromic anemia as a result of the enrichment of cholesterol in the plasma membranes of erythrocytes. Eventually, FLD patients develop proteinuria and end-stage renal disease. Defects in cholesteryl ester transfer protein (choice A) are associated with increased circulating levels of HDL cholesterol providing protection from coronary heart disease. Defects in 7-dehydrocholesterol reductase (choice B) are associated with the disorder known as Smith-Lemli-Opitz syndrome, SLOS. SLOS is associated with a characteristic set of developmental abnormalities apparent at birth. Defects in hepatic triglyceride lipase (choice C) are associated with hypertriglyceridemia, increased levels of HDL cholesterol, and decreased levels of LDL cholesterol. Deficiency in lipoprotein lipase (choice E) is associated with severe hypertriglyceridemia.

16. Correct answer is **A.** Lipoprotein(a) [Lp(a)] is composed of a common LDL nucleus linked to a molecule of apolipoprotein(a) [apo(a); encoded by the *LPA* gene] by disulfide bonds between a cysteine residue in a Kringle-IV (KIV) type 9 domain in apo(a) and a cysteine residue in apolipoprotein B-100 (apoB-100). When attached to apoB-100 the apo(a) protein surrounds the LDL molecule. Synthesis of Lp(a) occurs in the liver. The half-life of Lp(a) in the circulation is approximately 3–4 days. Numerous epidemiologic studies have demonstrated that elevated plasma levels of Lp(a) are a significant risk factor for the development of atherosclerotic disease. Apolipoprotein(a) does not form complexes with any of the other proteins or lipoprotein particles (choices B, C, D, and E).

17. Correct answer is **A.** Numerous lines of evidence demonstrate that apoA-I is a major anti-atherogenic and antioxidant factor in HDL due to its critical role in the HDL-mediated process of reverse cholesterol transport. In addition to reverse cholesterol transport, apoA-I can remove oxidized phospholipids from oxidized LDL (oxLDL) directly contributing to a reduced level of oxLDL in the circulation. Specific methionine residues (Met112 and Met148) of apoA-I have been shown to directly reduce cholesterol ester hydroperoxides and phosphatidylcholine hydroperoxides. oxLDL are taken up by macrophages which stimulates a proinflammatory response in these cells. Therefore, a reduction in oxLDL concentration will lead to reduced intravascular inflammation. ApoC-II (choice B) is involved in the removal of fatty acids from circulating triglycerides and plays no role in antioxidant activity in the vasculature. Cholesteryl ester transfer protein (choice C) is involved in the transfer of cholesterol esters from HDL to IDL and LDL, but plays no direct role in antioxidant activity in the vasculature. Both glutathione peroxidase-1 (choice D) and sphingosine-1-phosphate (choice F) are antioxidant proteins that are found associated with HDL but have limited direct roles in preventing oxidation of LDL. Lecithin:cholesterol ester transferase (choice E) is responsible for esterifying cholesterol within HDL but plays no role in the vasculature.

18. Correct answer is **D.** Chylomicrons are assembled in the intestinal mucosa as a means to transport dietary cholesterol and triglycerides to the rest of the body. Chylomicrons are, therefore, the molecules formed to mobilize dietary (exogenous) lipids. In addition to the delivery of dietary fatty acids and cholesterol to the vasculature, chylomicrons are required for the uptake and delivery of fat-soluble vitamins, such as vitamin K, to the body. Failure to produce chylomicrons would, therefore, lead to impaired absorption of dietary lipids, including fat-soluble vitamins. Vitamin K is required to produce the active forms of several coagulation factors including prothrombin, factor VII, factor IX, factor X, protein C, and protein S. The net effect of reduced uptake of vitamin K will be a prolonged prothrombin time in patients with fat malabsorption as in this patient. None of the other options (choices A, B, C, and E) would be expected to be observed in this patient whose primary defect is in the synthesis of chylomicrons.

19. Correct answer is **C.** The activity of lipoprotein lipase requires the cofactor protein, apolipoprotein C-II (apoC-II). Loss, or defective activity, of apoC-II would result in loss of lipoprotein lipase activity with the consequences being circulating lipoproteins of all types enriched in triglyceride leading to hypertriglyceridemia. None of the other proteins (choices A, B, D, and E) are required for or associated with the activity of lipoprotein lipase.

20. Correct answer is **B.** The signs and symptoms present in this infant are most indicative of the developmental abnormality identified as Smith-Lemli-Opitz syndrome, SLOS. SLOS is an autosomal recessive disorder resulting from a defect in cholesterol synthesis. The defect resides in the terminal enzyme of the cholesterol biosynthesis pathway, namely 7-dehydrocholesterol reductase. Defects in this gene result in increased levels of 7-dehydrocholesterol and reduced levels (15–27% of normal) of cholesterol in SLOS patients. The clinical spectrum of SLOS is very broad, ranging from the most severe form manifesting as a lethal malformation syndrome, to a relatively mild disorder that encompasses behavioral and learning disabilities. There are distinct craniofacial anomalies associated with SLOS which includes microcephaly (head size smaller than normal), micrognathia (abnormally small lower jaw), ptosis (drooping eyelids), a small, upturned nose, and cleft palate or bifid uvula. Defects in branched-chain amino acid metabolism (choice A) are the cause of maple syrup urine disease. Defects in mannose phosphorylation of lysosomal enzymes (choice C) result in the disorder known as I-cell disease. Numerous disorders of mitochondrial fatty acid oxidation (choice D) are known with medium chain acyl-CoA dehydrogenase deficiency being the most common and most severe. Defects in peroxisomal fatty acid metabolism (choice E) encompass numerous disorders such as Refsum disease and the lethal spectrum of disorders termed Zellweger syndrome.

21. Correct answer is **A.** This patient most likely has a form of familial hypercholesterolemia (FH) resulting from defects in the function of the LDL receptor. The clinical characteristics of FH include elevated concentrations of plasma LDL and deposition of LDL-cholesterol in the arteries, tendons, skin, and numerous other tissues. Fat deposits in the arteries are called atheromas and those in the skin and tendons are called xanthomas. When fat begins to deposit withing the eye there is a characteristic bilateral gray, white, or yellowish circumferential deposition in the peripheral cornea, referred to as corneal arcus. None of the other symptoms (choices B, C, D, and E) are common in patients with familial hypercholesterolemia.

22. Correct answer is **A.** The editing of C residues to U residues in mRNA occurs in several different mRNAs but of particular significance is the editing of the APOB mRNA in the small intestine. When this mRNA is edited, the change introduces a stop codon resulting in the translation of a shorter protein identified as apoB-48. The function of apoB-48 is to allow for the formation of functional chylomicrons in intestinal enterocytes. The lack of intestinal chylomicron production will lead to fat malabsorption and, consequently, deficiencies in the fat-soluble vitamins. None of the other options (choices B, C, D, E, and F) would be associated with an inability to edit the APOB mRNA.

23. Correct answer is **E.** The most telling finding in this patient is the massively elevated levels of triglycerides. The removal of fatty acids from circulating lipoprotein particles, such as chylomicrons and VLDL, requires the converted actions of lipoprotein lipase (LPL) and apoC-II. The activity of the endothelial cell-associated LPL requires apoC-II which is associated with chylomicron and VLDL. Loss of, or reduced, activity of LPL would, therefore, lead to a decreased capacity to remove fatty acids from the triglycerides resulting in significant increase in serum triglyceride levels as seen in this patient. A deficiency in cortisol (choice A) or glucagon (choice B) would result in reduced fatty acid release from adipose tissue and reduced hepatic gluconeogenesis, collectively resulting in reduced substrate availability for endogenous VLDL production by the liver. Hepatic lipase (choice C) predominantly removes fatty acids from triglyceride-rich HDL and so would not contribute to hypertriglyceridemia associated with decreased chylomicron and VLDL triglyceride metabolism. Deficiency in insulin (choice D) would result in reduced levels of lipoprotein lipase in the vasculature but would also lead to significant reduction in VLDL production by the liver such that serum triglycerides would not be elevated to the extent seen in this patient. Pancreatic lipase (choice F) is secreted into the small intestine via the pancreas where it serves the function of dietary lipid digestion.

24. Correct answer is **C.** The most telling finding in this patient is the massively elevated levels of triglycerides. The removal of fatty acids from circulating lipoprotein particles, such as chylomicrons and VLDL, requires the converted actions of lipoprotein lipase (LPL) and apoC-II. The activity of the endothelial cell-associated LPL requires apoC-II which is associated with chylomicron and VLDL. Loss of, or reduced, activity of LPL would, therefore, lead to a decreased capacity to remove fatty acids from the triglycerides resulting in significant increase in serum triglyceride levels as seen in this patient. A deficiency in apoA-I (choice A) would result in the lack of HDL production as this protein is the precursor of these lipoprotein particles. Symptoms of apoA-I deficiency include corneal opacities, xanthomas, and premature coronary heart disease (CHD). Deficiency in apoB-100 (choice B) would result in loss in production of VLDL by the liver and thus, would reduce the likelihood of hypertriglyceridemia. Deficiency in chylomicron receptors (choice D) have not been identified in humans. Deficiency in HDL receptors (choice E) which are one of the scavenger receptors (SR-BI) have not been identified in humans. Deficiency in LDL receptors (choice F) is the cause of the most common form of familial hypercholesterolemia (FH), a disease associated with dramatic elevation in LDL cholesterol leading to early onset atherosclerosis and coronary heart disease (CHD).

25. Correct answer is **D.** Treatment of patients with hypertriglyceridemia includes the use of drugs in the fibrate class, such as gemfibrozil. The fibrates activate peroxisome proliferator-activated receptor alpha (PPARα) in the liver and muscle which results in modulation of the expression of genes involved in lipid metabolism. In the liver, the activation of PPARα leads to increased mitochondrial β-oxidation of fatty acids, thereby decreasing the liver's secretion of triglyceride- and cholesterol-rich VLDL, as well as increased clearance of chylomicron remnants, increased levels of HDL. Activation of PPARα in skeletal muscle contributes to increased lipoprotein lipase activity which in turn promotes rapid VLDL turnover. The statin class of drugs are HMG-CoA reductase inhibitors (choice A) which are used to reduce the synthesis of cholesterol leading to increased LDL receptor expression and increased cellular uptake of LDL cholesterol. The drug ezetimibe inhibits the intestinal cholesterol transporter, thereby reducing intestinal cholesterol uptake (choice B) leading to reductions in total plasma cholesterol levels. PCSK9 inhibitors (choice C) lead to increased levels of LDL receptor recycling to the plasma membrane of cells allowing for increased LDL cholesterol removal from the blood. The thiazolidinedione drugs (see Chapter 30) are peroxisome proliferator-activated receptor gamma (PPARγ) inhibitors (choice E) used in the treatment of the hyperglycemia associated with type 2 diabetes.

26. Correct answer is **D.** The patient is most likely exhibiting the signs and symptoms typical of familial lecithin:cholesterol acyltransferase deficiency (FLD), also referred to as fish-eye disease. Individuals with FLD have characteristic abnormalities in blood lipid profiles that include low HDL (<10 mg/dL), low apo A-I (20–30 mg/dL), low cholesteryl esters, and low LDL. The HDL particles in FLD patients, in addition to being lower than normal, are also small and resemble immature HDL. FLD patients may also experience hypertriglyceridemia, but this blood lipid abnormality does not appear in all patients. FLD patients always develop corneal opacities that give their eyes the appearance of fish eyes, hence the association with the name fish-eye disease. Familial apoC-II deficiency (choice A) is associated with severe hypertriglyceridemia. Familial hypercholesterolemia (choice B) is most commonly caused be defects in the LDL receptors and as such, is associated with significant elevation in plasma LDL levels resulting in atherosclerosis and early coronary heart disease (CHD). Familial hypertriglyceridemia (choice C) results from mutations in the gene encoding apoC-II or in the gene encoding lipoprotein lipase. Familial ligand defective apoB (choice E) is associated with mutant forms of apoB-100 that lack the function of the domain required to bind the LDL receptor. This results in one of the less common forms of familial hypercholesterolemia.

27. Correct answer is **C.** Cholesterol ester transfer protein (CETP) is a plasma glycoprotein secreted primarily from the liver, and it plays a critical role in HDL metabolism by facilitating the exchange of cholesterol esters (CE) from HDL for triglycerides (TG) in apoB containing lipoproteins, such as VLDL, IDL, and LDL. The potential for the therapeutic use of CETP inhibitors in humans was first suggested when it was discovered that a small population of Japanese had an inborn error in the *CETP* gene leading to hyperalphalipoproteinemia associated with very high HDL levels and protection from atherosclerosis and coronary heart disease (CHD). Although numerous clinical trials of several different potential CETP inhibitors have been undertaken, none has proven to be as efficacious as predicted. Pharmacologic targeting of none of the other proteins (choices A, B, D, and E) would result in significant increases in HDL levels.

28. Correct answer is **B.** When the apoB gene is expressed in intestinal enterocytes the mature mRNA is identical to the mRNA found in hepatocytes. However, following the processing of the mRNA in the intestine it is a substrate for a cytidine deaminase that edits a particular C residue, in a CAA codon, to a U resulting in the generation of a UAA stop codon. The effect of this mRNA editing is the synthesis of a shorter protein (apoB-48) in intestines relative to the liver (apoB-100). Chylomicrons are assembled in the intestinal enterocytes as a means to transport dietary cholesterol and triglycerides to the rest of the body. In order to assemble functional chylomicrons, the enterocytes need to incorporate apoB-48 into the lipoprotein particles. Failure to produce chylomicrons would, therefore, lead to impaired absorption of dietary lipids. None of the other options (choices A, C, D, and E) would be associated with an inability to edit the apoB mRNA.

29. Correct answer is **B.** There are several apolipoproteins of the apoC family with the protein encoded by the *APOC2* gene being involved in the regulation of fatty acid removal from circulating triglycerides. A mutation in the *APOC2* gene would most likely result in the mutant apoC family member protein that was identified in this patient. Functional apoC-II is required to activate lipoprotein lipase, LPL. The activity of LPL is required to hydrolyze fatty acids from the triglycerides of chylomicrons and VLDL. A mutant form of apoC-II would, therefore, be associated with hypertriglyceridemia. None of the other options (choices A, C, D, E, and F) would be associated with defects in members of the *APOC* gene family.

30. Correct answer is **C.** The patient has a lifestyle and family history indicative of hypercholesterolemia and recent fasting lipid profile results confirm his medical condition. The use of the statin class of drugs is common for the treatment of hypercholesterolemia. These drugs lower overall circulating and cellular levels of cholesterol by inhibiting the rate-limiting enzyme of *de novo* cholesterol biosynthesis, HMG-CoA reductase. When intracellular levels of cholesterol fall due to reduced synthesis, there is a consequent increase in the transcription of the gene encoding the LDL receptor. The presentation of more LDL receptor proteins on the surface of cells, such as hepatocytes, will result in increased rates of LDL receptor-mediated endocytosis following LDL interaction with the receptor. Since the apolipoprotein, apoB-100, is unique to VLDL, IDL, and LDL, the endocytosis of more LDL particles is most likely going to be associated with a reduction in the plasma levels of LDL and consequently the levels of apoB-100. ApoA-I (choice A) is the precursor protein for the formation of HDL particles, while CETP (choice D) and LCAT (choice E) are proteins associated with HDL, and reducing plasma LDL-cholesterol would more likely lead to increased levels of HDL and the associated proteins, not a decrease. ApoB-48 (choice B) is unique to chylomicrons whose synthesis is tied to dietary lipid intake, not endogenous lipid and lipoprotein production. Thus, reducing *de novo* cholesterol synthesis will not lead to reduced levels of chylomicrons.

31. Correct answer is **D.** Bempedoic acid is a dicarboxylic acid that inhibits fatty acid and cholesterol synthesis, leading to a correlated reduction in plasma triglyceride and lipoprotein levels. Bempedoic acid is a pro-drug that is converted exclusively in the liver to its active CoA-derivative, bempedoyl-CoA. The CoA addition to bempedoic acid is catalyzed by very long-chain acyl-CoA synthetase-1 which is highly expressed in the liver but is not expressed in adipose tissue, the intestines, or in skeletal muscle. The conversion of bempedoic acid to its CoA derivative is required for its ability to suppress fatty acid and cholesterol synthesis and to also stimulate mitochondrial fatty acid β-oxidation. One of the targets of bempedoyl-CoA is the enzyme ATP-citrate lyase (ACL) that hydrolyzes cytosolic citrate to acetyl-CoA and oxaloacetic acid. The acetyl-CoA can then be utilized in *de novo* fatty acid and cholesterol synthesis. None of the other proteins (choices A, B, C, E, and F) are targets for the actions of bempedoic acid. Current hyperlipidemia targeting medications include ARO-ANG3 which is an RNA interference-based complex that reduces the level of the mRNA encoding angiopoietin-like protein 3 (choice B). The drug mipomersen is an antisense oligonucleotide (ASO) that targets the apoB mRNA in the liver, thereby resulting in reduced synthesis of the apoB-100 protein (choice C). Since apoB-100 is required for VLDL assembly in the liver there is reduced VLDL secretion by the liver. The statin class of drugs target HMG-CoA reductase (choice E) activity. Lomitapide is a small molecule inhibitor of the microsomal triglyceride transfer protein (choice G).

32. Correct answer is **B.** The physician prescribed cholestyramine which is a drug in the bile acid binding resin family. These drugs work by binding bile acids in the intestines preventing their reabsorption via the enterohepatic circulation. The reduced return of bile acids to the liver leads to increased diversion of hepatic cholesterol into bile acids, thereby lowering intracellular cholesterol levels. Reduced intracellular cholesterol results in increased expression of the LDL receptor gene leading to an increased capacity to remove LDL from the blood. One consequence of increased bile acid synthesis is increased VLDL production by hepatocytes which can lead to increased triglyceride concentrations in the blood. All of the other options (choices A, C, D, E, and F) indicate reduced triglycerides and thus are not the most likely outcomes with the use of cholestyramine.

33. Correct answer is **A.** The physician most likely prescribed a drug in the fibrate class, such as gemfibrozil and fenofibrate. The fibrates are the drugs of choice for patients with hypertriglyceridemia and either normal or mildly elevated total cholesterol. The fibrates result in the activation of PPARα in liver and muscle. In the liver, this leads to increased peroxisomal β-oxidation of fatty acids, thereby decreasing the liver's secretion of triglyceride- and cholesterol-rich VLDL, as well as increased clearance of chylomicron remnants, increased levels of HDL, and increased lipoprotein lipase activity which in turn promotes rapid VLDL turnover. Fibrate use is associated with increased cholesterol content of bile, which can elevate the risk of developing gallstones, referred to as cholelithiasis. Although there is a slight risk of muscle pain and weakness (choice C) and myoglobinuria (choice D) with the use of fibrates, especially when used in combination with a statin drug, these side effects are not the most likely consequences of fibrate therapy. Hyperuricemia (choice B) and steatorrhea (choice E) are not commonly associated side effects of the fibrates.

34. Correct answer is **E.** The physician most likely prescribed a statin class drug as these are generally considered the ideal drugs for lowering moderately elevated levels of total cholesterol and LDL cholesterol. The statin drugs work to lower total cholesterol as a result of their inhibition of the rate-limiting enzyme of *de novo* cholesterol biosynthesis, HMG-CoA-reductase. The ATP-citrate lyase (choice A) inhibitor, bempedoic acid, has been shown to be effective at lowering plasma LDL levels but is most often administered with a statin. The fibrate class of drugs (choice B) are primarily used for the treatment of hypertriglyceridemia in the context of normal to mildly elevated total cholesterol and LDL cholesterol. Microsomal triglyceride transfer protein (choice C) inhibitors and PCSK9 (choice D) inhibitors are generally only prescribed in conjunction with other cholesterol-lowering drugs, such as the statins, for individuals who have familial hypercholesterolemia.

35. Correct answer is **C.** The patient most likely has reduced capacity to endocytose LDL-receptor complexes, accounting for the elevated levels of total cholesterol and LDL cholesterol found in the patient's blood test. ApoB-100 is exclusive to VLDL, IDL, and LDL, and thus, an increased plasma level of LDL, as evidenced in this patient, will be associated with elevated levels of apoB-100 in the blood. ApoA-I (choice A), CETP (choice D), and LCAT (choice E) are all HDL-associated proteins and are not likely to be elevated in the blood of this patient. Indeed, individuals with a family history of hypercholesterolemia are more likely to have HDL levels that are below the suggested minimum level of 40 mg/dL. ApoB-48 (choice B) is unique to chylomicrons which are produced in intestinal enterocytes from dietary lipids. The level of chylomicrons is generally not elevated in patients with a deficiency in LDL receptor binding and endocytosis.

36. Correct answer is **F.** The family history and current level of total cholesterol in this relatively young patient strongly indicates that he is most likely heterozygous for a mutation in the LDL receptor gene. Since statin therapy was not tolerated the most likely drug to be prescribed is a PCSK9 inhibitor such as evolocumab. PCSK9 (proprotein convertase subtilisin/kexin type 9) function in the endosomal degradation of the LDL receptor (LDLR), thereby reducing the recycling of the LDLR to the plasma membrane. This effect of PCSK9 leads to a reduced ability of the liver to remove IDL and LDL from the blood contributing to the potential for hypercholesterolemia.

None of the other processes (choices A, B, C, D, and E) relate to the function of the PCSK9 inhibitors.

37. Correct answer is **B.** The most useful medication class for patients with dramatically elevated triglycerides is the fibrate class. The fibrates are activators of peroxisome proliferator-activated receptor-α (PPARα). Activation of PPARα results in modulation of the expression of genes involved in lipid metabolism. In addition, PPARα modulates carbohydrate metabolism and adipose tissue differentiation. Fibrates result in the activation of PPARα in the liver and muscle. In the liver, this leads to increased peroxisomal β-oxidation of fatty acids, thereby decreasing the liver's secretion of triacylglycerol- and cholesterol-rich VLDL, as well as increased clearance of chylomicron remnants, increased levels of HDL, and increased lipoprotein lipase activity which in turn promotes rapid VLDL turnover. There are many drug classes currently utilized to treat patients with hypercholesterolemia and other hyperlipidemias, however, none of these (choices A, C, D, and E) are useful for specifically targeting the treatment of hypertriglyceridemia.

38. Correct answer is **B.** The patient is most likely manifesting the signs and symptoms of familial chylomicronemia syndrome (FCS). FCS is caused by mutations in one of the five genes that are responsible for the synthesis, processing, and regulation of lipoprotein lipase (LPL). The characteristic feature of familial chylomicronemia syndrome, which is also characteristic of multifactorial chylomicronemia syndrome, is intermittent or persistent fasting chylomicronemia. Chylomicronemia, in turn, results in hypertriglyceridemia. The hypertriglyceridemia is defined as a serum triglyceride level in excess of 1000 mg/dL (normal is <150 mg/dL). The disorder also predisposes affected individuals to acute pancreatitis. Additional clinical findings in FCS patients are eruptive xanthomas, episodic abdominal pain, hepatosplenomegaly, and lipemia retinalis (creamy white appearance in peripheral retinal vessels). While several of the other symptoms (choices A, C, D, and E) can be consequences of diseases associated with hyperlipidemia, they are not the characteristic near-term complications in FCS.

39. Correct answer is **D.** The patient is most likely experiencing the signs and symptoms of the most common form of familial hypercholesterolemia (FH). Classic familial hypercholesterolemia is an autosomal dominant disorder that results from mutations affecting the structure and function of the cell-surface receptor that binds plasma LDL (low-density lipoproteins) removing them from the circulation. The defects in LDL-receptor (LDLR) interaction result in lifelong elevation of LDL-cholesterol (LDL) in the blood. The resultant hypercholesterolemia leads to premature coronary artery disease and atherosclerotic plaque formation in the coronary arteries and the aorta. The clinical characteristics of FH include elevated concentrations of plasma LDL and deposition of LDL-cholesterol in the arteries, tendons, and skin. Fat deposits in the arteries are called atheromas, in the skin and tendons they are called xanthomas, and in the skin around the eyes they are referred to as xanthelasmas. Deficiencies in none of the other proteins (choices A, B, C, and E) are associated with early onset and severe hypercholesterolemia as evidenced in this patient.

40. Correct answer is **A.** The patient is most likely manifesting the signs and symptoms of familial chylomicronemia syndrome (FCS). FCS is caused by mutations in one of the five genes that are responsible for the synthesis, processing, and regulation of lipoprotein lipase (LPL). The genes that, when mutated, contribute to the development of FCS include the lipoprotein lipase gene, and the genes, *APOC2*, *APOA5*, *LMF1*, and *GPIHBP1* that encode proteins required for LPL processing and regulation. These genes encode apoC-II (apoC-2), apoA-V (apoA-5), lipase maturation factor 1, and glycosylphosphatidylinositol-anchored HDL-binding protein 1, respectively. The characteristic feature of familial chylomicronemia syndrome, which is also characteristic of multifactorial chylomicronemia syndrome, is intermittent or persistent fasting chylomicronemia. The chylomicronemia, in turn, results in hypertriglyceridemia. The hypertriglyceridemia is defined as a serum triglyceride level in excess of 1000 mg/dL (normal is <150 mg/dL). The disorder also predisposes affected individuals to acute pancreatitis. Additional clinical findings in FCS patients are eruptive xanthomas, episodic abdominal pain, hepatosplenomegaly, and lipemia retinalis (creamy white appearance in peripheral retinal vessels). Deficiencies in none of the other proteins (choices B, C, D, and E) are associated with the development of FCS.

CHAPTER

17

Nitrogen Metabolism

High-Yield Terms

Aminotransferase	Any of a family of enzymes that catalyze the transfer of an amino group between an α-amino acid and an α-keto acid
AST and ALT	Aspartate aminotransferase, AST (also called serum glutamate-oxaloacetate-aminotransferase, SGOT) and alanine transaminase, ALT (also called serum glutamate-pyruvate aminotransferase, SGPT) prevalent liver enzymes whose elevations in the blood have been used as clinical markers of tissue damage
Glucose-alanine cycle	Mechanism for skeletal muscle to eliminate nitrogen while replenishing its glucose supply. Glucose oxidation produces pyruvate which can undergo transamination to alanine; the alanine then enters the blood stream and is transported to the liver where it is converted back to pyruvate which is then a source of carbon atoms for gluconeogenesis.
Urea	Nitrogen compound composed of two amino groups (–NH_2) joined by a carbonyl (–C=O) functional group, is the main nitrogen-containing substance in human urine
kwashiorkor	An acute form of childhood protein-energy malnutrition with adequate caloric intake, characterized by edema, irritability, anorexia, ulcerating dermatoses, and an enlarged liver with fatty infiltrates

TRANSAMINASES (AMINOTRANSFERASES)

Nitrogen enters the human body as dietary free amino acids, protein, nucleotides, and the ammonia (as ammonium ion, NH_4^+) produced by intestinal bacteria. A pair of principal enzymes, glutamate dehydrogenase and glutamine synthetase, incorporates this ammonia into carbon skeletons generating the amino acids glutamate and glutamine, respectively. Amino and amide groups from these latter two amino acids are then freely transferred to other carbon skeletons by transamination (Figure 17–1) and transamidation reactions. Transaminases (also called aminotransferases) exist for all amino acids except threonine and lysine.

HIGH-YIELD CONCEPT

Serum transaminases, such as aspartate transaminase, AST (also called serum glutamate-oxaloacetate-aminotransferase, SGOT) and alanine transaminase, ALT (also called serum glutamate-pyruvate aminotransferase, SGPT) have been used as clinical markers of tissue damage, with increasing serum levels indicating an increased extent of damage.

Alanine transaminase has an important function in the delivery of skeletal muscle nitrogen (in the form of alanine) to the liver. In the liver, alanine transaminase transfers the ammonia, from alanine to α-ketoglutarate (2-oxoglutarate) regenerating pyruvate which can then be diverted into gluconeogenesis (see Chapter 6). This process is referred to as the glucose-alanine cycle. The nitrogen is eventually incorporated into urea for excretion.

Three critical enzymes contribute most significantly to overall nitrogen homeostasis. These enzymes are glutamate dehydrogenase, glutamine synthetase, and glutaminase.

THE GLUTAMATE DEHYDROGENASE REACTION

Glutamate dehydrogenase (Figure 17–2) utilizes NAD^+ in the direction of nitrogen liberation from glutamate and NADPH for nitrogen incorporation into α-ketoglutarate (2-oxoglutarate). In the forward reaction glutamate dehydrogenase is important in converting free ammonia and 2-oxoglutarate to glutamate, forming one of the 20 amino acids required for protein synthesis. On the other hand, the reverse reaction is a key anapleurotic process linking amino acid metabolism with TCA cycle activity while simultaneously providing the reduced electron carrier, NADH, that can be used for ATP synthesis.

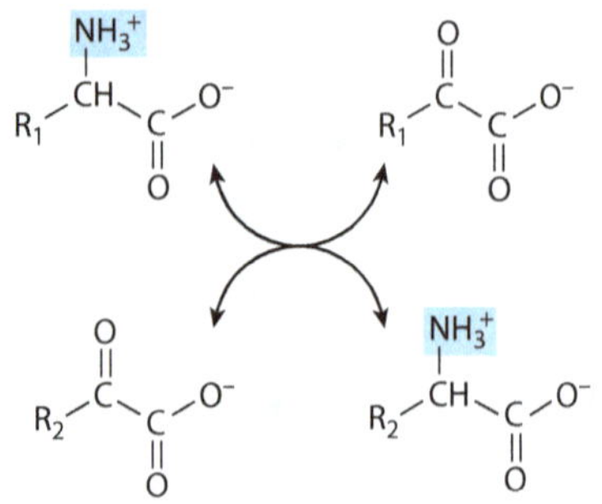

FIGURE 17–1 Transamination. The reaction is freely reversible with an equilibrium constant close to unity. (Reproduced with permission from Rodwell VW, Bender DA, Botham KM, et al: *Harper's Illustrated Biochemistry*, 31st ed. New York, NY: McGraw Hill; 2018.)

HIGH-YIELD CONCEPT

The multiple roles of glutamate in nitrogen homeostasis make it a gateway between free ammonia and the amino groups of most amino acids.

THE GLUTAMINE SYNTHETASE AND GLUTAMINASE REACTIONS

The glutamine synthetase reaction (Figure 17–3) produces glutamine, one of the 20 major amino acids, and a major plasma carrier of ammonia in a nontoxic form. Of physiologic significance is the removal of nitrogen from glutamine in the kidney through the concerted actions of glutaminase (Figure 17–4) and glutamate dehydrogenase, a mechanism utilized by the kidney to maintain acid-base balance in the blood.

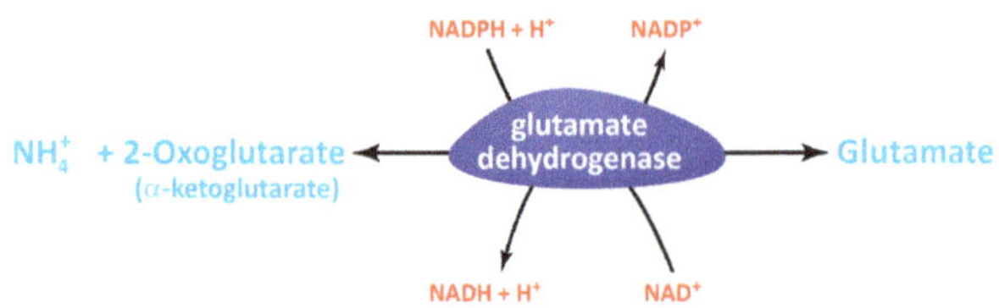

FIGURE 17–2 Reactions catalyzed by glutamate dehydrogenase (GDH). Glutamate dehydrogenase represents an important "gateway" enzyme in that it can catalyze reactions in two different directions dependent on overall cellular energy and metabolic needs. When energy and carbon levels are high, glutamate can incorporate nitrogen (from NH_4^+) into 2-oxoglutarate (α-ketoglutarate) which is driven by the increased levels of NADPH generated from the oxidation of glucose in the pentose phosphate pathway. Conversely, when energy levels are reduced glutamate can be oxidatively deaminated in the opposite direction allowing 2-oxoglutarate (α-ketoglutarate) to be utilized in the TCA cycle for production of energy. Important to the reaction in this direction is that glutamine, which is the major circulating amino acid, effectively serves as the "carrier" of the carbons of 2-oxoglutarate (α-ketoglutarate). (Reproduced with permission from themedicalbiochemistrypage, LLC.)

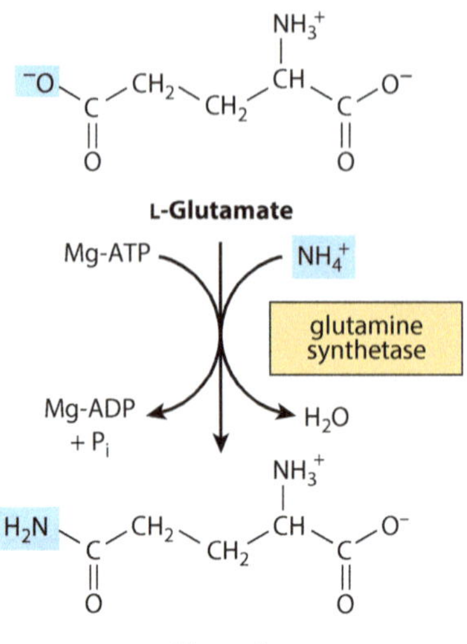

FIGURE 17–3 The glutamine synthetase reaction strongly favors glutamine synthesis. (Reproduced with permission from Rodwell VW, Bender DA, Botham KM, et al: *Harper's Illustrated Biochemistry*, 31st ed. New York, NY: McGraw Hill; 2018.)

HIGH-YIELD CONCEPT

During periods of metabolic acidosis, the body will divert more glutamine from the liver to the kidney. This allows for the conservation of bicarbonate ion since the incorporation of ammonia into urea requires bicarbonate. When glutamine enters the kidney, glutaminase releases one mole of ammonia generating glutamate and then glutamate dehydrogenase releases another mole of ammonia generating α-ketoglutarate (2-oxoglutarate). The ammonia will ionize to ammonium ion (NH_4^+) which is excreted. The net effect is a reduction in the concentration of hydrogen ion, [H^+], and thus an increase in the pH of the blood.

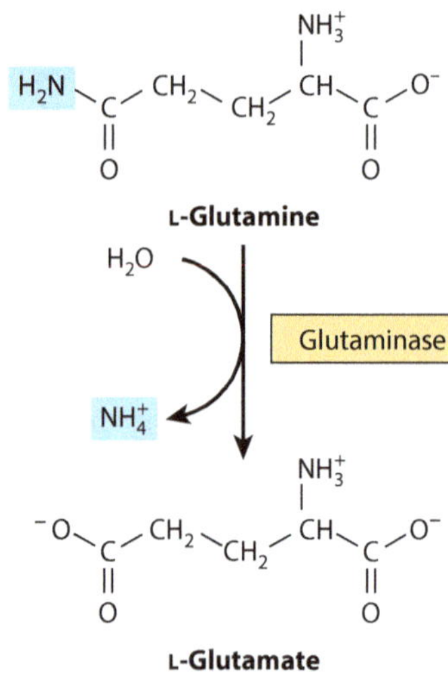

FIGURE 17–4 The glutaminase reaction proceeds essentially irreversibly in the direction of glutamate and NH_4^+ formation. Note that the amide nitrogen, not the α-amino nitrogen, is removed. (Reproduced with permission from Rodwell VW, Bender DA, Botham KM, et al: *Harper's Illustrated Biochemistry*, 31st ed. New York, NY: McGraw Hill; 2018.)

NITROGEN BALANCE

Unlike fats and carbohydrates, nitrogen has no designated storage depots in the body. Since the half-life of many proteins is short (on the order of hours), insufficient dietary quantities of even one amino acid can quickly limit the synthesis, and lower the body levels, of many essential proteins. The result of limited synthesis and normal rates of protein degradation is that the balance of nitrogen intake and nitrogen excretion is rapidly and significantly altered.

HIGH-YIELD CONCEPT

Normal, healthy adults are generally in nitrogen balance, with intake and excretion being very well matched. Young growing children, adults recovering from major illness, and pregnant women are often in positive nitrogen balance. Their intake of nitrogen exceeds their loss as net protein synthesis proceeds. When more nitrogen is excreted than is incorporated into the body, an individual is in negative nitrogen balance. Insufficient quantities of even one essential amino acid are adequate to turn an otherwise normal individual into one with a negative nitrogen balance.

Diets deficient in protein, but sufficient in fat and carbohydrate, lead to an inability to synthesize protein (because of missing essential amino acids) and ultimately to a syndrome known as kwashiorkor, common among children in underdeveloped and poor countries. The edema characteristic of kwashiorkor results from the lack of ability to synthesize sufficient albumin, a major osmolyte in the blood.

THE UREA CYCLE

Although glutamine transport to the kidneys and the concerted actions of glutaminase and glutamate dehydrogenase can support a pathway for the elimination of waste nitrogen, about 80% of the excreted nitrogen is in the form of urea. The formation of urea takes place exclusively in the liver, in a series of reactions that are distributed between the mitochondrial matrix and the cytosol. The series of reactions that form urea is known as the urea cycle or the Krebs-Henseleit Cycle (Figure 17–5).

Carbamoyl phosphate is synthesized from bicarbonate (HCO_3^-) and ammonium ion (NH_4^+) via the action of carbamoyl phosphate synthetase 1 (CPS1). This reaction is energetically expensive, consuming two molar equivalents of ATP. Humans express two

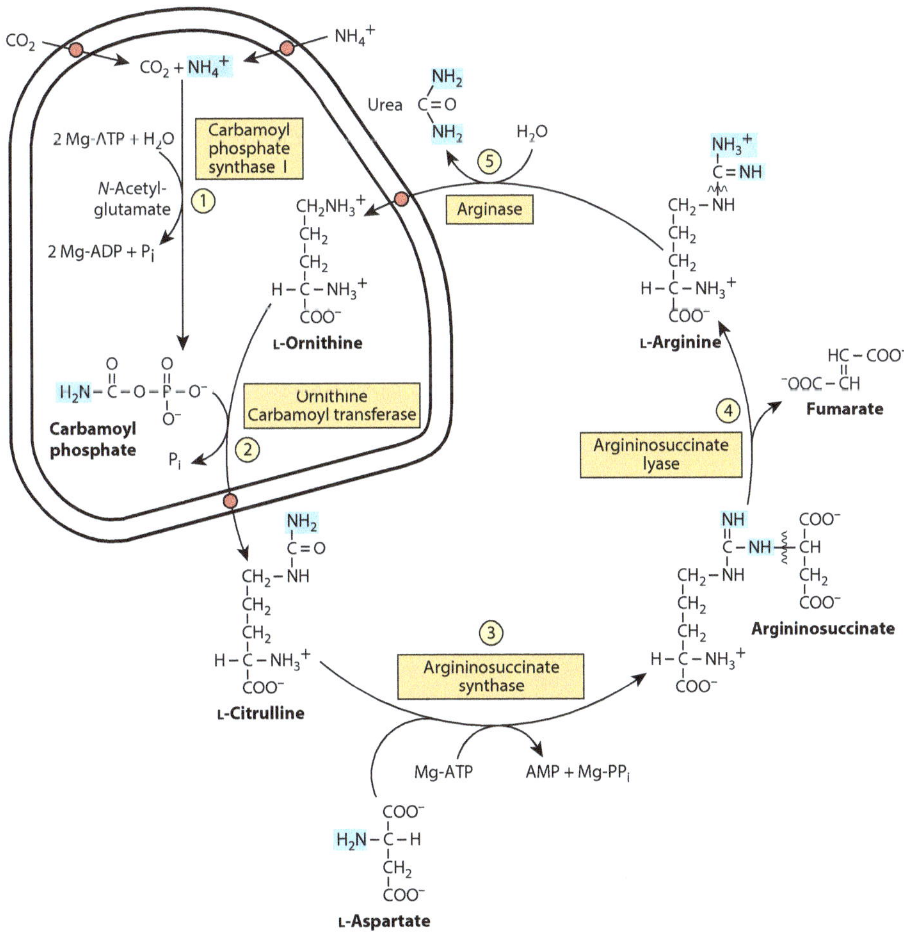

FIGURE 17–5 Reactions and intermediates of urea biosynthesis. The nitrogen-containing groups that contribute to the formation of urea are shaded. Reactions 1 and 2 occur in the matrix of liver mitochondria and reactions 3, 4, and 5 in liver cytosol. CO_2 (as bicarbonate), ammonium ion, ornithine, and citrulline enter the mitochondrial matrix via specific carriers (see red dots) present in the inner membrane of liver mitochondria. (Reproduced with permission from Rodwell VW, Bender DA, Botham KM, et al: *Harper's Illustrated Biochemistry*, 31st ed. New York, NY: McGraw Hill; 2018.)

CLINICAL BOX 17–1 CITRULLINEMIA TYPE II (CTLN2)

The major form of citrullinemia (CTLN1) is the result of defects in the urea cycle enzyme argininosuccinate synthetase (Table 17–1). Another form of citrullinemia, with sudden onset between the ages of 11 and 79 years, is called citrullinemia type II (CTLN2). Manifestations of CTLN2 are recurrent hyperammonemia with neuropsychiatric symptoms including nocturnal delirium, aggression, irritability, hyperactivity, delusions, disorientation, restlessness, drowsiness, loss of memory, flapping tremor, convulsive seizures, and coma. The symptoms of CTLN2 are often provoked by alcohol and sugar intake, as well as by certain medications, and/or surgery. CTLN2 is caused by deficiency in the gene encoding citrin. Citrin is a mitochondrial solute carrier protein (SLC25A13) involved in the mitochondrial uptake of glutamate and export of aspartate and as such functions in the malate-aspartate shuttle. Deficiencies in SLC25A13 result in mild hyperammonemia and citrullinemia. The clinical course in adults with citrullinemia type II is milder than that of CTLN1, possibly distinguishing it from milder late-onset citrullinemia type I. It is not known why CTLN2 is milder and later in onset than CTLN1 and distinguishing between the two forms of citrullinemia is difficult. Citrin deficiency can manifest in newborns as neonatal intrahepatic cholestasis caused by citrin deficiency (NICCD) and in older children as failure to thrive and dyslipidemia caused by citrin deficiency (FTTDCD). One of the most common characteristics of citrin deficiency is a fondness for protein-rich and/or lipid-rich foods and aversion to carbohydrate-rich foods. In NICCD children younger than age 1 year exhibit growth retardation with transient intrahepatic cholestasis, hepatomegaly, diffuse fatty liver, and parenchymal cellular infiltration associated with hepatic fibrosis, variable liver dysfunction, hypoproteinemia, decreased coagulation factors, hemolytic anemia, and/or hypoglycemia. NICCD is generally not severe and symptoms may often resolve by 1 year of age provided appropriate treatment is given. However, some infants will die due to infection and liver cirrhosis. FTTDCD is usually observed in children around 1–2 years of age with the aforementioned food preferences being apparent. Some FTTDCD patients have growth retardation, hypoglycemia, hyperlipidemia, pancreatitis, fatty liver, hepatoma, and fatigue. In some cases of FTTDCD, the affected individual will manifest with characteristic CTLN2 symptoms later in life.

carbamoyl phosphate synthetases. The CPS2 activity is associated with the cytosolic trifunctional enzyme that initiates pyrimidine biosynthesis (see Chapter 20).

Ornithine, arising in the cytosol, is transported to the mitochondrial matrix via the action of ornithine translocase encoded by the *ORNT1* gene. In the mitochondria ornithine transcarbamylase (OTC) catalyzes the condensation of ornithine with carbamoyl phosphate, producing citrulline. Concomitant with ornithine transport into the mitochondria is the export of citrulline to the cytosol where the remaining reactions of the urea cycle take place.

In addition to the ORNT1-encoded transporter, the mitochondrial transporter called citrin is critical to urea cycle function. Citrin is involved in the mitochondrial uptake of glutamate and export of aspartate and as such functions in the malate-aspartate shuttle. Deficiencies in citrin are the causes of citrullinemia type II, CTLN2 (Clinical Box 17–1).

TABLE 17–1 Urea Cycle Disorders.

UCD	Enzyme Deficiency	Symptoms/Comments
Type I Hyperammonemia, CPSD (Clinical Box 17–2)	Carbamoyl phosphate synthetase 1	Within 24–72 h after birth infant becomes lethargic, needs stimulation to feed, vomiting, increasing lethargy, hypothermia and hyperventilation; without measurement of serum ammonia levels and appropriate intervention infant will die: treatment with arginine which activates *N*-acetylglutamate synthetase
N-acetylglutamate synthetase deficiency	*N*-acetylglutamate synthetase	Severe hyperammonemia, mild hyperammonemia associated with deep coma, acidosis, recurrent diarrhea, ataxia, hypoglycemia, hyperornithinemia: treatment includes administration of carbamoyl glutamate to activate CPS-1
Type 2 hyperammonemia, OTCD (Clinical Box 17–3)	Ornithine transcarbamylase	Most commonly occurring UCD, only X-linked UCD, ammonia and amino acids elevated in serum, increased serum orotic acid due to mitochondrial carbamoyl phosphate entering cytosol and being incorporated into pyrimidine nucleotides which leads to excess production and consequently excess catabolic products: treat with high-carbohydrate, low-protein diet, ammonia detoxification with sodium phenylacetate or sodium benzoate
Classic (type I) Citrullinemia (CTLN1), ASD	Argininosuccinate synthetase	Episodic hyperammonemia, vomiting, lethargy, ataxia, seizures, eventual coma: treat with arginine administration to enhance citrulline excretion, also with sodium benzoate for ammonia detoxification
Argininosuccinic aciduria, ALD	Argininosuccinate lyase (argininosuccinase)	Episodic symptoms similar to classic citrullinemia, elevated plasma and cerebral spinal fluid argininosuccinate: treat with arginine and sodium benzoate
Hyperargininemia, AD	Arginase	Rare UCD, progressive spastic quadriplegia and intellectual impairment, ammonia and arginine high in cerebral spinal fluid and serum, arginine, lysine and ornithine high in urine: treatment includes diet of essential amino acids excluding arginine, low-protein diet

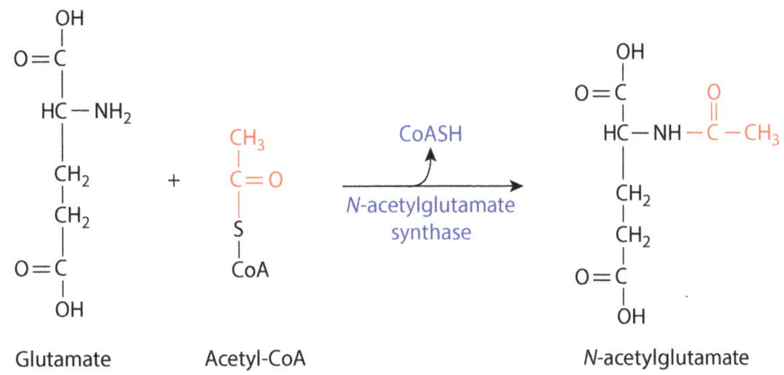

FIGURE 17–6 *N*-acetylglutamate synthetase reaction. (Reproduced with permission from themedicalbiochemistrypage, LLC.)

Argininosuccinate synthetase catalyzes the formation of argininosuccinate from citrulline and aspartate. This reaction, like the CPS1 catalyzed reaction, is energetically expensive, consuming two molar equivalents of ATP.

Arginine and fumarate are produced from argininosuccinate by argininosuccinate lyase (also called argininosuccinase).

Arginase hydrolyzes urea from arginine, regenerating cytosolic ornithine, which can then be transported to the mitochondrial matrix for another round of urea synthesis.

REGULATION OF THE UREA CYCLE

With long-term changes in the quantity of dietary protein, changes of 20-fold or greater in the concentration of urea cycle enzymes are observed. When dietary proteins increase significantly, enzyme concentrations rise. On return to a balanced diet, enzyme levels decline. Under conditions of starvation, enzyme levels rise as proteins are degraded and amino acid carbon skeletons are used to provide energy, thus increasing the quantity of nitrogen that must be excreted.

Short-term regulation of the urea cycle occurs principally at CPS1, which is essentially inactive in the absence of its obligate activator *N*-acetylglutamate. The synthesis of *N*-acetylglutamate is catalyzed by *N*-acetylglutamate synthetase, NAGS (Figure 17–6). NAGS is allosterically activated by arginine, a required intermediate of the urea cycle.

UREA CYCLE DISORDERS

Deficiencies in each of the enzymes of the urea cycle, including NAGS, have been identified. These disorders are referred to as urea cycle disorders, UCD. A common thread to most UCD is hyperammonemia leading to ammonia intoxication. Blood chemistry will also show elevations in glutamine. In addition to hyperammonemia, UCD also present with encephalopathy and respiratory alkalosis. The most dramatic presentation of UCD symptoms occurs in neonates between 24 and 48 hours after birth. Afflicted infants exhibit progressively deteriorating symptoms due to the elevated ammonium levels. Clinical symptoms are most severe when the UCD is at the level of CPS1 (Clinical Box 17–2).

CLINICAL BOX 17–2 CARBAMOYL PHOSPHATE SYNTHETASE 1 DEFICIENCY

Carbamoyl phosphate synthetase 1 deficiency is an autosomal recessive disorder that, as the name implies, is due to mutations in the carbamoyl phosphate synthetase 1 (*CPS1*) gene. There are at least 25 known mutations in the *CPS1* gene that result in carbamoyl phosphate synthetase deficiency (CPSD). Mutations in the *CPS1* gene that cause CPSD include missense, nonsense, and exon deletions. The frequency of CPSD is approximately 1 per 62,000 live births. Because CPS1 is responsible for the first reaction of the urea cycle, defects in this gene manifest with the most severe symptoms of all UCDs. CPSD is, like the other neonatal onset forms of UCD, most severe when presenting in newborn infants. As with each of the four neonatal onset UCD, CPSD is characterized by the accumulation of ammonium ion and glutamine with clinical manifestations appearing in full-term infants with no prior obstetric risk factors. The classic symptoms appear between 24 and 48 hours after birth (but not prior to 24 hours) and include convulsions, hyperventilation, ataxia, hypothermia, lethargy, vomiting, and poor feeding. If left untreated, the hyperammonemia will result in coma and death. The severe effects of hyperammonemia are described in the section on Neurotoxicity Associated with Ammonia. Even though sepsis is a rare event in a normal term infant with no prior obstetric complications, this disorder is misdiagnosed in almost half of neonatal UCD cases. Initial laboratory findings will include respiratory alkalosis which is the earliest objective indication of encephalopathy. The encephalopathy will progress to the point where mechanical ventilation is required. Another routine laboratory finding is reduced serum (blood) urea nitrogen (BUN) which may be as low as 1 mg/dL (normal for newborns is 3–12 mg/dL). If plasma ammonia levels are not measured the infants' death will be attributed to sepsis, intracranial hemorrhage, or some other disorder that would normally be associated with a preterm delivery. CPSD patients are treated in much the same ways as for other neonatal UCDs in that protein intake must be highly regulated and the hyperammonemia must be controlled. Hemodialysis is the only effective means to rapidly lower serum ammonia levels in

CLINICAL BOX 17–2 (CONTINUED)

these patients. Acute episodes of hyperammonemia can be treated with intravenous administration of Ammunol and with oral Buphenyl for chronic adjunctive therapy of hyperammonemia. Additionally, CPSD patients are treated with a strict dietary regimen that includes 0.7 g/kg/day of protein and 0.7 g/kg/day of an essential amino acid mixture. The diet is also supplemented with citrulline to serve as a source of arginine. As development proceeds and the need for protein declines, it is necessary to adjust the dietary intake of protein accordingly.

When making a diagnosis of a neonatal UCD, based on presenting symptoms and observed hyperammonemia, it is possible to perform a differential diagnosis by analyzing for plasma levels of citrulline as well as for levels of urinary orotic acid. High urinary orotic acid is indicative of OTC deficiency, whereas, high plasma citrulline is indicative of defects in argininosuccinate synthetase or argininosuccinate lyase.

TREATMENT OF UREA CYCLE DISORDERS

Hemodialysis is the only effective means to rapidly reduce the level of circulating ammonia in UCD patients, particularly during an initial presentation in the emergency department. Overall treatment of UCD involves the reduction of protein in the diet, removal of excess ammonia and replacement of intermediates missing from the urea cycle. Administration of levulose reduces ammonia through its action of acidifying the colon. Antibiotics can be administered to kill intestinal ammonia producing bacteria. Sodium benzoate and sodium phenylacetate can be administered to covalently bind glycine (forming hippurate) and glutamine (forming phenylacetylglutamine), respectively. Ammunol is an FDA-approved intravenous solution of 10% sodium benzoate and 10% sodium phenylacetate for management of hyperammonemia in UCD. Buphenyl is an FDA-approved oral medication for chronic adjunctive therapy of hyperammonemia in UCD patients.

Dietary supplementation with arginine or citrulline can increase the rate of urea production and/or waste nitrogen excretion in certain UCD. Arginine supplementation activates NAGS which in turn generates the activator of CPS-1.

NEUROTOXICITY ASSOCIATED WITH AMMONIA

Ammonium ion in the blood can be quite neurotoxic. Aside from its effect on blood pH, ammonium ion readily traverses the brain-blood barrier and in the brain it is converted to glutamate via glutamate dehydrogenase, depleting the brain of α-ketoglutarate (2-oxoglutarate). As the 2-oxoglutarate is depleted, oxaloacetate falls correspondingly, and ultimately TCA cycle activity is severely reduced.

The increased glutamate leads to glutamine formation within glial cells resulting in depletion of glutamate required as a neurotransmitter and as a precursor for the synthesis of γ-aminobutyrate: GABA, another neurotransmitter.

Glial cell volume is controlled by intracellular glutamine. As glutamine levels rise in the brain the volume of fluid increases resulting in the associated cerebral edema seen in infants with hyperammonemia caused by urea cycle defects.

Elevated glutamine also exerts an adverse effect on mitochondrial function because of the action of mitochondrial glutaminase. The action of mitochondrial glutaminase in the astrocytes leads to further increases in intramitochondrial ammonia levels negatively affecting the H^+ gradients required for ATP synthesis.

CLINICAL BOX 17–3 ORNITHINE TRANSCARBAMYLASE DEFICIENCY

Deficiency in ornithine transcarbamylase (OTC) is the most commonly occurring UCD with a frequency of approximately 1 case in every 14,000 live births. OTC is encoded by the *OTC* gene which is located on the X chromosome and the disorder is inherited as an X-linked recessive disorder. There have been over 158 different mutant alleles of the *OTC* gene identified in OTC deficiency. In males, 98% receive a mutant allele from their mothers, whereas, in females, 9–10% of mutant OTC carriers acquired their mutation sporadically. OTC deficiency is, like the other neonatal onset forms of UCDs, most severe when presenting in newborn infants. As with each of the four neonatal onset UCDs, OTCD is characterized by the accumulation of ammonia and glutamine with clinical manifestations appearing in full-term infants with no prior obstetric risk factors. The classic symptoms appear between 24 and 48 hours after birth (but not prior to 24 hours) and include convulsions, hyperventilation, ataxia, hypothermia, lethargy, vomiting, and poor feeding. If left untreated, the hyperammonemia will result in coma and death. The severe effects of hyperammonemia are described in the section on Neurotoxicity Associated with Ammonia. Even though sepsis is a rare event in a normal term infant with no prior obstetric complications, this disorder is misdiagnosed in almost half of neonatal UCD cases. Initial laboratory findings will include respiratory alkalosis which is the earliest objective indication of encephalopathy. The encephalopathy will progress to the point where mechanical ventilation is required. Another routine laboratory finding is reduced serum (blood) urea nitrogen (BUN) which may be as low as 1 mg/dL (normal for newborns is 3–12 mg/dL). If plasma

CLINICAL BOX 17–3 (CONTINUED)

ammonia levels are not measured the infants' death will be attributed to sepsis, intracranial hemorrhage, or some other disorder that would normally be associated with a preterm delivery. OTC deficiency patients are treated in much the same ways as for other neonatal UCDs in that protein intake must be highly regulated and the hyperammonemia must be controlled. Hemodialysis is the only effective means to rapidly lower serum ammonia levels in these patients. Acute episodes of hyperammonemia can be treated with intravenous administration of Ammunol and with oral Buphenyl for chronic adjunctive therapy of hyperammonemia. OTCD patients are treated with a strict dietary regimen that includes 0.7 g/kg/day of protein and 0.7 g/kg/day of an essential amino acid mixture. The diet is also supplemented with citrulline to serve as a source of arginine. As development proceeds and the need for protein declines it is necessary to adjust the dietary intake of protein accordingly.

CHECKLIST

- ☑ Nitrogen from the biosphere enters the human body as dietary free amino acids, protein, and the ammonia produced by intestinal tract bacteria. Glutamate dehydrogenase and glutamine synthetase effect the conversion of ammonia into the amino acids glutamate and glutamine, respectively. Amino and amide groups from these two substances are freely transferred to other carbon skeletons by transamination and transamidation reactions.
- ☑ Glutamate dehydrogenase and glutamine synthetase represent the major nitrogen mobilizing enzymes in the body. Glutamate dehydrogenase is considered a gateway enzyme serving to regulate energy production and waste removal during amino acid metabolism.
- ☑ Glutamine is the major form of nontoxic nitrogen in the circulation. In this capacity it plays a major role in delivering waste nitrogen to the kidneys for excretion and also the release of the nitrogen allows the kidneys to balance fluid pH.
- ☑ Nitrogen homeostasis in the brain is critical for maintaining adequate levels of the neurotransmitter glutamate and to prevent nitrogen toxicity. Within the CNS there is an interaction between the cerebral blood flow, neurons, and the protective astrocytes that regulates the metabolism of glutamate, glutamine, and ammonia.
- ☑ The urea cycle represents the primary pathway for converting waste nitrogen from amino acid catabolism into a soluble nontoxic substance that is easily excreted. The cycle takes place both in the cytosol and the mitochondria of hepatocytes.
- ☑ Defects in enzymes of the urea cycle are the primary cause of potentially severe and fatal hyperammonemia. The earlier in the cycle that a defect is encountered the higher the potential for more severe hyperammonemia.
- ☑ Treatment of urea cycle disorders is principally aimed at controlling the level of free ammonia. This includes the reduction of protein in the diet, removal of excess ammonia, and replacement of intermediates missing from the urea cycle.

REVIEW QUESTIONS

1. A 3-day-old infant is being examined in the emergency department following a seizure. The infant was born at home following an uneventful and complete term. He was examined following his birth, and no issues or abnormalities were noted. While being tended to in the ED, the infant lapsed into a coma and died. Serum and urine analyses postmortem found severe hyperammonemia and urinary orotic acid that was well above normal. Plasma concentrations of citrulline and argininosuccinate were in the low-normal range. Which of the following enzyme activities was most likely deficient in this infant?

(A) Argininosuccinate lyase
(B) Argininosuccinate synthetase
(C) Carbamoyl phosphate synthetase 1
(D) *N*-Acetylglutamate synthetase
(E) Ornithine transcarbamylase

2. An infant, who was born at home, developed seizures 2 days after birth. On examination in the emergency department, it was found that the infant had elevated serum NH_4^+, glutamate, and alanine. The attending physician suspected that the child was suffering from a defect in nitrogen homeostasis and ordered a test for confirmation of his diagnosis. To make a definitive differential diagnosis in this case, which of the following, if elevated in the blood, would be the most useful?

(A) Alanine
(B) Lactate
(C) Homocysteine
(D) Methionine
(E) Orotic acid

3. During periods of prolonged fasting skeletal muscle acquires some required energy from amino acid catabolism. Which of the following is most likely released from skeletal muscle under these conditions?

(A) Alanine
(B) Asparagine
(C) Aspartate
(D) Glutamate
(E) Glutamine

4. Experiments are being conducted in a primate model system to study the metabolic responses to conditions of induced systemic acidosis. Under these experimental conditions which of the following is most likely to constitute the primary hepatic response to these induced conditions?
(A) Glutamine conversion to glutamate releasing ammonia
(B) Incorporation of ammonia into glutamate forming glutamine
(C) Incorporation of ammonia into α-ketoglutarate (2-oxoglutarate) forming glutamate
(D) Incorporation of ammonia into pyruvate forming alanine
(E) Increased production of urea to dispose of ammonia

5. Experiments are being conducted on the activity of glutamate dehydrogenase using a cell line derived from a human hepatoma. Results of these experiments have shown that the enzyme does not respond to positive allosteric regulation during the liberation of ammonia from glutamate as is the case for wild-type enzyme. This result suggests that the enzyme from the hepatoma cells most likely acquired a mutation in the binding site for which of the following?
(A) ADP
(B) ATP
(C) Citrate
(D) Glutamine
(E) GTP

6. During periods of prolonged fasting, skeletal muscle acquires some required energy from amino acid catabolism. As a result of these catabolic processes, there is increased nitrogen metabolism in the liver. Which of the following is most likely to increase in the blood under these conditions?
(A) Alanine
(B) Asparagine
(C) Aspartate
(D) Glutamate
(E) Glutamine

7. A 3-day-old infant is being examined in the emergency department following a seizure. The infant was born at home following an uneventful and complete term. He was examined following his birth and no issues or abnormalities were noted. While being tended to in the ED the infant lapsed into a coma. Serum analyses found severe hyperammonemia and concentrations of citrulline and argininosuccinate that were in the low-normal range. Assay for which of the following would be most useful to make a diagnosis in this infant?
(A) Alloisoleucine
(B) Lactate
(C) Orotic acid
(D) Phenylacetate
(E) Suberic acid

8. A novel mutation has been identified in the alanine transaminase gene that allows the enzyme to function even in the absence of its required cofactor. This mutation has most likely eliminated the necessary binding site for which of the following?
(A) Ascorbate
(B) Biotin
(C) NAD^+
(D) Pyridoxal phosphate
(E) Thiamine pyrophosphate

9. A newborn who developed seizures 2 days after birth was diagnosed with elevated serum NH_4^+, glutamate, and alanine and elevated levels of orotic acid in the urine. A defect in which of the following metabolic processes is most consistent with the findings in the infant?
(A) Hepatic ammonium ion metabolism
(B) Mitochondrial fatty acid β-oxidation
(C) Peroxisomal amino acid oxidation
(D) Purine nucleotide catabolism
(E) Pyrimidine nucleotide biosynthesis

10. A 3-day-old infant is being examined in the emergency department following a seizure. The infant was born at home following an uneventful and complete term. He was examined following his birth and no issues or abnormalities were noted. While being tended to in the ED, the infant lapsed into a coma and died. Serum and urine analyses postmortem found severe hyperammonemia and urinary orotic acid well above normal. Plasma concentrations of citrulline and argininosuccinate are in the low-normal range. Administration of which of the following would have been the most successful course of action in treating this infant prior to his death?
(A) Ammunol
(B) Bicarbonate
(C) Hemodialysis
(D) Iron chelation
(E) Phenobarbital

11. A 2-day-old infant is brought to the emergency department suffering a seizure. Analysis of serum NH_4^+ reveals it to be quite high. Suspecting a urea cycle impairment, the attending physician infuses the infant with arginine. Which of the following most likely explains the utility of this therapeutic intervention?
(A) Allosteric activation of carbamoyl phosphate synthetase 1
(B) Allosteric activation of ornithine transcarbamylase
(C) Enhanced synthesis of an activator of carbamoyl phosphate synthetase 1
(D) Enhanced synthesis of an activator of ornithine transcarbamylase
(E) Inhibition of ammonia release by glutamate dehydrogenase
(F) Inhibition of ammonia release by glutaminase

12. A child was born at home and developed seizures 2 days after birth. On examination in the emergency department, it was found that the infant had elevated serum NH_4^+, glutamate, and alanine. Urinary orotic acid levels were found to be above normal and serum citrulline was barely detectable. A defect in which of the following would most likely account for the signs and symptoms observed in this infant?
(A) Argininosuccinate synthetase
(B) Carbamoyl phosphate synthetase 1
(C) Glutamate dehydrogenase
(D) Ornithine transcarbamylase
(E) Pyruvate carboxylase
(F) UMP synthase

13. A 3-day-old infant is being examined in the emergency department following a seizure. The infant was born at home following an uneventful and complete term. He was examined following his birth and no issues or abnormalities were noted. While being tended to in the ED the infant lapsed into a coma and died. Serum and urine analyses postmortem found severe hyperammonemia. The levels of citrulline and

argininosuccinate were in the low-normal range and urinary orotic acid was not detected. Which of the following enzyme activities was most likely deficient in this infant?
(A) Argininosuccinate lyase
(B) Argininosuccinate synthetase
(C) Carbamoyl phosphate synthetase 1
(D) *N*-acetylglutamate synthetase
(E) Ornithine transcarbamylase

14. An infant, born at home, developed seizures 2 days after birth. On examination in the emergency department, it was found that the infant had elevated serum NH_4^+, glutamate, and alanine. Molecular studies identified a small deletion in the coding region of the ornithine transcarbamylase gene. Given this finding, which of the following measurable abnormalities would most likely also be present in this infant?
(A) Citrullinemia
(B) Elevated urinary excretion of argininosuccinic acid
(C) Elevation in blood orotic acid
(D) Hyperuremia
(E) Uric acid deposition in the joints

15. A 2-day-old boy, delivered at full term, has become lethargic and requires stimulation for feeding. When vomiting and hyperventilation ensued, routine laboratory results showed blood urea nitrogen (BUN) of 1.2 mg/dL (N = 3–12 mg/dL). Bulging of the fontanel suggested an intracranial hemorrhage, but a CT scan revealed only cerebral edema. Blood samples taken at admission show dramatically elevated serum ammonium ion and citrulline levels that are 100 times normal. A deficiency in which of the following enzymes would most likely account for the signs and symptoms in this infant?
(A) Argininosuccinate synthetase
(B) Carbamoyl phosphate synthetase 1
(C) 3-Hydroxy-3-methylglutaryl-CoA (HMG-CoA) reductase
(D) Medium-chain acyl-CoA dehydrogenase
(E) Ornithine transcarbamylase
(F) Pyruvate carboxylase

16. A 3-day-old infant is being examined in the emergency department following a seizure. The infant was born at home following an uneventful and complete term. He was examined following his birth and no issues or abnormalities were noted. While being tended to the infant experienced another seizure and required mechanical ventilation. Analysis of serum found citrulline and argininosuccinate levels were in the low to normal range. Assessment for which of the following would be most significant to ensure that proper interventions were instituted to ensure the survival of this infant?
(A) Level of ammonium ion in the blood
(B) Level of urea in the blood
(C) Level of citrulline in the blood
(D) Level of orotic acid in the urine
(E) Odor of acetone on the breath

17. An unconscious 37-year-old man is brought to the emergency department. His wife reports that they were at home having dinner celebrating his birthday. She states that normally he does not drink but they were having champagne for the celebration and that shortly after they finished the bottle he became disorientated and irritable and then he began experiencing delusions. When he began to have a seizure, she called 911. By the time the ambulance arrived he was unconscious. Blood tests taken when he was admitted show significantly elevated serum ammonium ion. A deficiency in which of the following activities is most likely the cause of this patient's symptoms?
(A) Carbamoyl phosphate synthetase 1
(B) Citrin
(C) Glucocerebrosidase
(D) Glutamate dehydrogenase
(E) Ornithine transcarbamylase

18. The release of ammonia from glutamine, in the proximal tubule of the nephron in the kidney, represents a vital role of nitrogen homeostasis in overall acid-base balance. Which of the following enzymes is most likely to be an additional critical component of this process?
(A) Alanine transaminase
(B) Asparagine synthetase
(C) Glutamine synthetase
(D) α-Ketoglutarate dehydrogenase (2-Oxoglutarate dehydrogenase)
(E) Pyruvate dehydrogenase

19. A 37-year-old man is brought to the emergency department by his wife as she is concerned about his rapid onset of aggression, hyperactivity, and disorientation. The wife reports that they were at home having dinner celebrating his birthday. She states that normally he does not drink but they were having champagne for the celebration and that shortly after they finished the bottle, he became disorientated and irritable. Blood tests show significantly elevated levels of citrulline. A defect in which of the following processes would most likely explain the signs and symptoms in this patient?
(A) Mitochondrial glutamate and aspartate transport
(B) Mitochondrial urea synthesis
(C) Protein *N*-glycosylation
(D) Protein *O*-glycosylation
(E) Peroxisomal dicarboxylic acid metabolism

20. A 2-month-old infant has been experiencing poor feeding and episodic vomiting began. Additional abnormal behavior includes episodes of screaming, agitation, and hyperventilation followed by periods of extreme lethargy. Physical examination shows the infant has a distended abdomen. Serum studies identify below normal levels of citrulline and above normal levels of ornithine. Given the signs and symptoms in this patient, which of the following additional symptoms would most likely be present?
(A) Elevated serum alloisoleucine and ketoacidosis
(B) Elevated urine orotic acid and serum glutamine
(C) Ketoacidosis and needle-shaped urinary crystals
(D) Megaloblastic anemia and metabolic acidosis
(E) Methylmalonic acidemia and anemia

21. A 53-year-old woman is admitted to the emergency department experiencing lethargy, confusion, nausea, and vomiting following completion of a marathon. Examination of the patient shows elevated respiration rate. Blood pH was found to be 7.15 (N = 7.35–7.45). Given these results, which of the following is most likely to be found elevated in the patient's blood?
(A) Ammonium ion
(B) Alanine
(C) Asparagine
(D) Glutamate
(E) Glutamine
(F) Urea

22. A 3-day-old infant is being examined in the emergency department following a seizure. The infant was born, at full term, at home. The mother reports that there were no obstetric complications during the pregnancy. He was examined following his birth and no issues or abnormalities were noted. The attending physician requests a comprehensive metabolic panel with addition of serum ammonium ion assessment. Results of the blood work show ammonia 105 μmol/L (N = <50 μmol/L). Assessment of above normal levels of which of the following would be most useful in determining if the cause of the hyperammonemia in this patient was the result of a defect in a cytoplasmic urea cycle enzyme?
(A) Asparagine
(B) Carbamoyl phosphate
(C) Citrulline
(D) Ornithine
(E) Orotic acid

23. A 4-month-old infant is being examined by her pediatrician due to her poor feeding, vomiting, and extreme lethargy. Blood work shows ammonia level of 105 μmol/L (N = <50 μmol/L) and a citrulline level of 130 μmol/L (N = <40 μmol/L). Molecular testing found no definitive mutation in any of the genes encoding urea cycle enzymes nor in the gene encoding *N*-acetylglutamate synthetase. Which of the following is the most likely abnormal protein causing the symptoms in this patient?
(A) Branched-chain keto acid dehydrogenase
(B) Citrin
(C) Glycogen-branching enzyme
(D) Medium-chain acyl-CoA dehydrogenase
(E) Phytanoyl-CoA hydroxylase

24. A 3-day-old infant is being examined in the emergency department following a seizure. The infant was born, at full term, at home. The mother reports that there were no obstetric complications during the pregnancy. He was examined following his birth and no issues or abnormalities were noted. The attending physician requests a comprehensive metabolic panel with addition of serum ammonium ion assessment. Results of the blood work shows an ammonia level of 105 μmol/L (N = <50 μmol/L). Which of the following would be most useful for the long-term control of the symptoms in this patient?
(A) Dietary addition of lactulose
(B) High-protein diet
(C) Lactose-free diet
(D) Phenylalanine restriction
(E) Protein-free diet

25. A child who was born at home developed seizures 2 days after birth. On examination in the emergency department, it was found that the infant had elevated serum NH_4^+ and glutamine. Blood work indicates that citrulline and lactate levels were within normal ranges. Urine analysis shows normal levels of ketones. Supplementation with which of the following would be most useful in treating the symptoms observed in this infant?
(A) Asparagine
(B) Bicarbonate
(C) Phenobarbital
(D) Red blood cell transfusion
(E) Sodium phenylacetate

ANSWERS

1. Correct answer is **E.** The infant is most likely manifesting the symptoms of a deficiency in the urea cycle enzyme, ornithine transcarbamylase. Ornithine transcarbamylase deficiency (OTCD) is also referred to as type 2 hyperammonemia. The presentation of hyperammonemia between 24 and 48 hours after birth (but not before 24 hours after birth) would most likely indicate a urea cycle disorder. This diagnosis can be confirmed by the absence of acidosis or ketosis. Severe deficiency or total absence of activity of any of the first four enzymes in the urea cycle, or the enzyme that produces the required cofactor for carbamoyl phosphate synthetase 1, results in the accumulation of ammonium ion and other precursor metabolites during the first few days of life. Infants with a severe urea cycle disorder are normal at birth but rapidly develop cerebral edema and the related signs of lethargy, anorexia, hyper- or hypoventilation, hypothermia, seizures, neurologic posturing, and coma. In milder (or partial) deficiencies of these enzymes and in arginase (ARG) deficiency, ammonium ion accumulation may be triggered by illness or stress at almost any time of life. In these disorders the elevations of plasma ammonium ion concentration and symptoms are often subtle, and the first recognized clinical episode may not occur for months or decades. Due to the similarity in symptoms of several of the urea cycle disorders the use of a differential diagnosis allows for accurate determination of which enzyme is deficient in the pathway resulting in the observed pathology. The first diagnostic test is to assay for plasma levels of citrulline. Moderately high levels of citrulline are indicative of argininosuccinate lyase deficiency, ALD (choice A) and extremely high levels are indicative of argininosuccinate synthetase deficiency, ASD (choice B). If no, or trace, citrulline is detected then analysis of urine orotic acid can be used to distinguish between carbamoyl synthetase 1 (CPS1) deficiency, CPSD (choice C) and ornithine transcarbamylase (OTC) deficiency (OTCD). The presence of elevated levels of urinary orotic acid in OTCD results from the mitochondrial carbamoyl phosphate, synthesized by a CPS1, spilling into the cytoplasm, and serving as a substrate for the first enzyme in the pathway of pyrimidine nucleotide biosynthesis. A deficiency in *N*-acetyl glutamate synthetase, NAGS (choice D) would mimic the effects of CPS1 due to the fact that *N*-acetylglutamate is required to activate CPS1. Given that the postmortem examination found significantly elevated levels of urinary orotic acid the most likely enzyme deficiency in this patient was OTC.

2. Correct answer is **E.** The presentation of hyperammonemia between 24 and 48 hours after birth (but not before 24 hours after birth) would most likely indicate a urea cycle disorder. This diagnosis can be confirmed by the absence of acidosis or ketosis. Severe deficiency or total absence of activity of any of the first four enzymes in the urea cycle, or the enzyme that produces the required cofactor for carbamoyl phosphate synthetase 1, results in the accumulation of ammonium ion and other precursor metabolites during the first few days of life. Infants with a severe urea cycle disorder are normal at birth but rapidly develop cerebral edema and the related signs of lethargy, anorexia, hyper- or hypoventilation, hypothermia, seizures, neurologic posturing, and coma. Due to the similarity in symptoms of several of the urea cycle disorders the use of a differential diagnosis allows for accurate determination of which enzyme is deficient in the pathway resulting in the observed pathology. The first diagnostic test is to assay for plasma levels of citrulline. Moderately high levels of citrulline are indicative of argininosuccinate lyase deficiency, ALD and extremely high levels are indicative of argininosuccinate synthetase deficiency, ASD. If no, or trace, citrulline is detected then analysis of urine orotic acid can be used to distinguish between carbamoyl synthetase 1 (CPS1) deficiency, CPSD and ornithine transcarbamylase (OTC) deficiency (OTCD). The presence of elevated levels of urinary orotic acid in ornithine transcarbamylase deficiency results from the mitochondrial carbamoyl phosphate, synthesized by a CPS1, spilling into the cytoplasm, and serving as a substrate for the first enzyme in the pathway of pyrimidine nucleotide biosynthesis. Measurement of the serum levels of none of the other substances (choices A, B, C, and D) would allow for a differential diagnosis in the urea cycle disorders.

3. Correct answer is **A.** During periods of prolonged fasting, skeletal muscle protein is broken down to provide the amino acids for oxidation allowing for energy production. During this process the waste nitrogen needs to be released from skeletal muscle in a nontoxic form. The primary mechanism for the release of waste nitrogen from skeletal muscle amino acid catabolism is through incorporation of the ammonia into pyruvate generating alanine catalyzed by alanine transaminase. The alanine is then transported to the blood where it is delivered to the liver. In the liver, alanine transaminase transfers the ammonia to α-ketoglutarate (2-oxoglutarate) which regenerates pyruvate. The pyruvate can then be diverted into gluconeogenesis. This process is referred to as the glucose-alanine cycle. In most other tissues waste nitrogen from amino acid catabolism is used to generate glutamine (choice E) through the concerted actions of glutamate dehydrogenase, generating glutamate from 2-oxoglutarate and NH_4^+, and glutamine synthetase, generating glutamine from glutamate and NH_4^+. None of the other amino acids (choices B, C, and D) represent the amino acid release from skeletal muscle during periods of prolonged fasting.

4. Correct answer is **B.** Major reactions that involve the regulation of plasma pH as well as the level of circulating ammonium ion (NH_4^+) involve the hepatic and renal enzymes glutamate dehydrogenase (GDH), glutamine synthetase (GS), and glutaminase. The liver compartmentalizes GS and glutaminase in order to control the flow of ammonia into glutamine or urea. Under acidotic conditions the liver incorporates NH_4^+ into glutamine via the GS reaction. The glutamine then enters the circulation. In fact, glutamine is the major amino acid of the circulation, and its role is to ferry NH_4^+ to and from various tissues in a nontoxic form. In the epithelial cells of the proximal tubule of the nephron in the kidneys, glutamine is hydrolyzed by glutaminase (yielding glutamate) releasing the ammonia. Another mole of ammonia is released through the action of glutamate dehydrogenase acting on the glutamate derived from the glutaminase reaction. Within the proximal tubule cells, the ammonia ionizes with a hydrogen ion (H^+) yielding ammonium ion, NH_4^+. The net effect is that a single mole of glutamine, taken up by the proximal tubule, generates two moles of NH_4^+ effectively reducing the circulating concentration of H^+ by two moles resulting in an increase in the pH. This process of coordination between the liver and kidney is crucial to overall regulation of acid-base balance. Within the proximal tubule of the kidney, the release of ammonia from glutamine and the generation of NH_4^+ is referred to as renal ammoniagenesis. None of the other processes (choices A, C, D, and E) correctly represent the response of the liver to the induced systemic acidosis in these experimental animals.

5. Correct answer is **A.** Glutamate dehydrogenase (GDH) represents an important "gateway" enzyme in that it can catalyze reactions in two different directions dependent upon overall cellular energy and metabolic needs. When energy and carbon levels are high glutamate can incorporate nitrogen (from NH_4^+) into α-ketoglutarate (2-oxoglutarate) which is driven by the increased levels of NADPH generated from oxidation of glucose in the pentose phosphate pathway. Conversely, when energy levels are reduced glutamate can be oxidatively deaminated in the opposite direction allowing α-ketoglutarate (2-oxoglutarate) to be utilized in the TCA cycle for production of energy. Given its critical gateway function, it is easy to understand that glutamate dehydrogenase is regulated by the cell energy charge. ATP (choice B) and GTP (choice E) are positive allosteric effectors of the formation of glutamate, and conversely, ATP and GTP exert potent negative allosteric effects on the formation of 2-oxoglutarate. Given that low energy charge would be expected to increase the conversion of glutamate to α-ketoglutarate, it is not surprising that ADP is a positive allosteric effector of the GDH reaction in this direction. Thus, when the level of ATP is high, conversion of glutamate to α-ketoglutarate and other TCA cycle intermediates is limited and when the cellular energy charge is low, glutamate is converted to ammonia and oxidizable TCA cycle intermediates. The lack of an expected positive allosteric response of GDH in the direction of ammonia liberation from glutamate would most likely reflect a loss of the ADP-binding site in the enzyme from the hepatoma cells. Citrate (choices C) and glutamine (choice D) do not exert any allosteric effects on the activity of GDH.

6. Correct answer is **E.** During periods of prolonged fasting, skeletal muscle protein is broken down to provide the amino acids for oxidation allowing for energy production. During this process, the waste nitrogen needs to be released from skeletal muscle in a nontoxic form. The primary mechanism for the release of waste nitrogen from skeletal muscle amino acid catabolism is through incorporation of the ammonia into pyruvate generating alanine catalyzed by alanine transaminase. The alanine is then transported to the blood where it is picked up by the liver. In the liver, alanine transaminase transfers the ammonia from alanine to α-ketoglutarate which regenerates pyruvate. The pyruvate can then be diverted into gluconeogenesis. This process is referred to as the glucose-alanine cycle. Other tissues that are utilizing the carbon skeletons of amino acids for energy production transfer the waste nitrogen to 2-oxoglutarate ultimately generating glutamine. The glutamine is then delivered, via the blood, to either the liver or the kidneys. Within the liver the waste nitrogen that was derived from amino acid oxidation in the peripheral tissues has two primary states. Through the action of various aminotransferases, including alanine transaminase and aspartate transaminase, the liver can divert the waste nitrogen, as ammonium ion (NH_4^+) into the production of urea. In addition to generating urea, the liver, via the action of glutamate dehydrogenase and glutamine synthetase, can divert the waste nitrogen into α-ketoglutarate (2-oxoglutarate) generating glutamine. Just as the glutamine generated in tissues other than

the liver can be delivered to the kidney, the glutamine generated in the liver is a critical metabolic pathway for eventual excretion of the waste nitrogen as NH_4^+ in the urine. Alanine (choice A) is not released from the liver but instead is deaminated by alanine transaminase to yield the pyruvate which is then used in the pathway of gluconeogenesis. Asparagine (choice B), aspartate (choice C), and glutamate (choice D) are not released from the liver to the blood in the context of hepatic nitrogen metabolism.

7. Correct answer is **C.** The presentation of hyperammonemia between 24 and 48 hours after birth (but not before 24 hours after birth) would likely indicate a urea cycle disorder. This diagnosis can be confirmed by the absence of acidosis or ketosis. Severe deficiency or total absence of activity of any of the first four enzymes in the urea cycle, or the enzyme that produces the required cofactor for carbamoyl phosphate synthetase 1, results in the accumulation of ammonium ion and other precursor metabolites during the first few days of life. Infants with a severe urea cycle disorder are normal at birth but rapidly develop cerebral edema and the related signs of lethargy, anorexia, hyper- or hypoventilation, hypothermia, seizures, neurologic posturing, and coma. Due to the similarity in symptoms of several of the urea cycle disorders the use of a differential diagnosis allows for accurate determination of which enzyme is deficient in the pathway resulting in the observed pathology. The first diagnostic test is to assay for plasma levels of citrulline. Moderately high levels of citrulline are indicative of argininosuccinate lyase deficiency, ALD and extremely high levels are indicative of argininosuccinate synthetase deficiency, ASD. If no, or trace, citrulline is detected then analysis of urine orotic acid can be used to distinguish between carbamoyl synthetase 1 (CPS1) deficiency, CPSD and ornithine transcarbamylase (OTC) deficiency (OTCD). The presence of elevated levels of urinary orotic acid in ornithine transcarbamylase deficiency results from the mitochondrial carbamoyl phosphate, synthesized by a CPS1, spilling into the cytoplasm, and serving as a substrate for the first enzyme in the pathway of pyrimidine nucleotide biosynthesis. Measurement of the serum alloisoleucine (choice A) is diagnostic for the disorder resulting from deficiency of branched-chain amino acid dehydrogenase known as maple syrup urine disease. Measurement of serum of lactate (choice B) would be useful for identifying one of the specific causes of metabolic acidosis. Measurement of serum phenylacetate (choice D) is diagnostic for phenylketonuria, PKU. Measurement of serum suberic acid (choice E), a dicarboxylic acid, is diagnostic for medium-chain acyl-CoA dehydrogenase deficiency.

8. Correct answer is **D.** All transaminases (aminotransferases) require pyridoxal phosphate as a cofactor for carrying out the transfer of ammonia from an α-amino acid to an acceptor α-keto acid. None of the other vitamin derived cofactors (choices A, B, C, and E) are required for the activity of transaminases such as alanine transaminase.

9. Correct answer is **E.** There are two unrelated metabolic pathways that, when defective, can present with elevated levels of urinary orotic acid. One pathway is the urea cycle where deficiency in ornithine transcarbamylase (OTC) is associated with severe hyperammonemia as well as orotic aciduria. OTC deficiency is apparent by 24 to 48 hours after birth and will be lethal if not correctly diagnosed. The other pathway is the *de novo* pyrimidine nucleotide biosynthesis pathway. Deficiencies in UMP synthase, a bifunctional enzyme that catalyzes the conversion of orotic acid to orotate monophosphate (OMP) and then OMP to UMP, result in orotic aciduria as well as megaloblastic anemia. The characteristic feature of this megaloblastic anemia is that it is nonresponsive to supplementation with folate and cobalamin, both of which the history reveals are being provided to the infant. Given the age of this patient and the physical findings, particularly the crystals produced in the infant's urine upon exposure to the air, the most likely defective metabolic process is the pyrimidine nucleotide biosynthesis pathway. Defects in none of the other metabolic processes (choices A, B, C, and D) would lead to the signs and symptoms manifesting in this patient.

10. Correct answer is **C.** The presentation of hyperammonemia between 24 and 48 hours after birth (but not before 24 hours after birth) would most likely indicate a urea cycle disorder, UCD. This diagnosis can be confirmed by the absence of acidosis or ketosis. Severe deficiency or total absence of activity of any of the first four enzymes in the urea cycle, or the enzyme that produces the required cofactor for carbamoyl phosphate synthetase 1, results in the accumulation of ammonium ion and other precursor metabolites during the first few days of life. Infants with a severe urea cycle disorder are normal at birth but rapidly develop cerebral edema and the related signs of lethargy, anorexia, hyper- or hypoventilation, hypothermia, seizures, neurologic posturing, and coma. In general, the treatment of the neonatal urea cycle disorders has as common elements the reduction of protein in the diet, removal of excess ammonium ion, and replacement of intermediates missing from the urea cycle. However, upon initial diagnosis hemodialysis is the only effective means to rapidly reduce the level of circulating ammonium ion in UCD patients. Ammunol (choice A) is an FDA-approved intravenous solution of 10% sodium benzoate and 10% sodium phenylacetate used in the treatment of the acute hyperammonemia in UCD patients. However, it is not effective at dealing with the severe hyperammonemia, in an undiagnosed UCD patient, that has led to seizures. Administration of none of the other interventions (choices B, D, and E) would have provided any benefit to this patient.

11. Correct answer is **A.** The primary control mechanism regulating the rate of the urea cycle is the availability of intermediates in the pathway. However, short-term regulation of the urea cycle does occur at the level of the carbamoyl phosphate synthetase 1 (CPS1) catalyzed step. CPS1 is essentially inactive in the absence of its obligate activator *N*-acetylglutamate. The steady-state concentration of *N*-acetylglutamate is determined by the level of activity of the enzyme, *N*-glutamate synthetase (NAGS), that synthesizes this activator. The activity of NAGS is allosterically regulated by the amino acid arginine. The allosteric regulation of NAGS explains the utility of supplementation of urea cycle disorder (UCD) patients with arginine. Even in UCD patients whose primary defect is in CPS1, administration of arginine allows for maximal activation of any residual CPS1 activity, thereby providing some benefit. None of the other options (choices B, C, D, E, and F) correctly explain the utility of arginine infusion in a patient suspected of harboring a defect in the urea cycle.

12. Correct answer is **D.** The presentation of hyperammonemia between 24 and 48 hours after birth (but not before 24 hours after birth) would most likely indicate a urea cycle disorder. This diagnosis can be confirmed by the absence of acidosis or ketosis. Severe deficiency or total absence of activity of any of

the first four enzymes in the urea cycle, or the enzyme that produces the required cofactor for carbamoyl phosphate synthetase 1, results in the accumulation of ammonium ion and other precursor metabolites during the first few days of life. Infants with a severe urea cycle disorder are normal at birth but rapidly develop cerebral edema and the related signs of lethargy, anorexia, hyper- or hypoventilation, hypothermia, seizures, neurologic posturing, and coma. Due to the similarity in symptoms of several of the urea cycle disorders the use of a differential diagnosis allows for accurate determination of which enzyme is deficient in the pathway resulting in the observed pathology. The first diagnostic test is to assay for plasma levels of citrulline. Moderately high levels of citrulline are indicative of argininosuccinate lyase deficiency, ALD and extremely high levels are indicative of argininosuccinate synthetase deficiency, ASD. If no, or trace, citrulline is detected then analysis of urine orotic acid can be used to distinguish between carbamoyl synthetase 1 (CPS1) deficiency, CPSD and ornithine transcarbamylase (OTC) deficiency (OTCD). Given the hyperammonemia and orotic aciduria in this patient the most likely defective enzyme is OTC. Hyperammonemia in the presence of orotic aciduria eliminates CPS1 (choice B) as the likely defective enzyme. Defects in none of the other enzymes (choices A, C, E, and F) would result in hyperammonemia and orotic aciduria as evidenced in this patient.

13. Correct answer is **C.** The presentation of hyperammonemia between 24 and 48 hours after birth (but not before 24 hours after birth) would most likely indicate a urea cycle disorder. This diagnosis can be confirmed by the absence of acidosis or ketosis. Severe deficiency or total absence of activity of any of the first four enzymes in the urea cycle, or the enzyme that produces the required cofactor for carbamoyl phosphate synthetase 1, results in the accumulation of ammonium ion and other precursor metabolites during the first few days of life. Infants with a severe urea cycle disorder are normal at birth but rapidly develop cerebral edema and the related signs of lethargy, anorexia, hyper- or hypoventilation, hypothermia, seizures, neurologic posturing, and coma. Due to the similarity in symptoms of several of the urea cycle disorders the use of a differential diagnosis allows for accurate determination of which enzyme is deficient in the pathway resulting in the observed pathology. The first diagnostic test is to assay for plasma levels of citrulline. Moderately high levels of citrulline are indicative of argininosuccinate lyase deficiency, ALD and extremely high levels are indicative of argininosuccinate synthetase deficiency, ASD. If no, or trace, citrulline is detected then analysis of urine orotic acid can be used to distinguish between carbamoyl phosphate synthetase 1 (CPS1) deficiency (CPSD) and ornithine transcarbamylase (OTC) deficiency (OTCD). Given the hyperammonemia and the lack of detectable orotic aciduria, the most likely defective enzyme in this patient is CPS1. Whereas a deficiency in *N*-acetylglutamate synthetase, NAGS (choice D) would result in symptoms essentially identical to those of CPSD and would be differentiated from OTCD similarly, the frequency of NAGS deficiency is the least of all the urea cycle disorders and, therefore, not as likely to be the cause of this patient's disease. Hyperammonemia in the absence of orotic aciduria eliminates OTC (choice E) as the likely defective enzyme. The low to normal levels of citrulline and argininosuccinate eliminate deficiencies in the other enzymes (choices A and B) as being the cause of the patient's death.

14. Correct answer is **C.** The presentation of hyperammonemia between 24 and 48 hours after birth (but not before 24 hours after birth) would most likely indicate a urea cycle disorder. Ornithine transcarbamylase (OTC) is one of the enzymes of the urea cycle. Deficiency in OTC is the cause of one of the urea cycle disorders that are the major causes of hyperammonemia in the newborn. Differentiation of which urea cycle enzyme is defective and causing the hyperammonemia can be accomplished by analysis of the levels of the various intermediates in the cycle. Since a defect in OTC prevents the incorporation of carbamoyl phosphate into ornithine, the carbamoyl phosphate will leave the mitochondria and serve as a precursor for the synthesis of the pyrimidine nucleotides. The excess synthesis of the intermediates in pyrimidine synthesis, such as orotic acid as a result of deficiency in OTC, can be detected in the blood and urine. None of the other options (choices A, B, D, and E) would correspond to an abnormality associated with mutations in the gene encoding ornithine transcarbamylase.

15. Correct answer is **A.** The presentation of hyperammonemia between 24 and 48 hours after birth (but not before 24 hours after birth) would most likely indicate a urea cycle disorder. This diagnosis can be confirmed by the absence of acidosis or ketosis. Severe deficiency or total absence of activity of any of the first four enzymes in the urea cycle, or the enzyme that produces the required cofactor for carbamoyl phosphate synthetase 1, results in the accumulation of ammonium ion and other precursor metabolites during the first few days of life. Infants with a severe urea cycle disorder are normal at birth but rapidly develop cerebral edema and the related signs of lethargy, anorexia, hyper- or hypoventilation, hypothermia, seizures, neurologic posturing, and coma. Due to the similarity in symptoms of several of the urea cycle disorders the use of a differential diagnosis allows for accurate determination of which enzyme is deficient in the pathway resulting in the observed pathology. The first diagnostic test is to assay for plasma levels of citrulline. Moderately high levels of citrulline are indicative of argininosuccinate lyase deficiency, ALD and extremely high levels are indicative of argininosuccinate synthetase deficiency, ASD. If no, or trace, citrulline is detected then analysis of urine orotic acid can be used to distinguish between carbamoyl synthetase 1 (CPS1) deficiency, CPSD and ornithine transcarbamylase (OTC) deficiency (OTCD). The clinical presentation of patients with defects in several enzymes of urea synthesis are virtually identical. These enzymes are CPS1, ornithine transcarbamylase (OTC), argininosuccinate synthetase (AS), and argininosuccinase. Given that the level of citrulline in this patient was 100 times normal it is most likely that the deficiency causing the symptoms was in argininosuccinate synthetase. Deficiency in carbamoyl phosphate synthetase 1 (choice B) and ornithine transcarbamylase (choice E) are both associated with low to no detectable citrulline. Deficiency in HMG-CoA reductase (choice C) has not been identified in humans. Deficiency in medium-chain acyl-CoA dehydrogenase deficiency (choice D) is a disorder of mitochondrial fatty acid β-oxidation that does not manifest with significant hyperammonemia. Deficiency in pyruvate carboxylase (choice F) is associated with severe hypoglycemia but not hyperammonemia.

16. Correct answer is **A.** The presentation of hyperammonemia between 24 and 48 hours after birth (but not before 24 hours after birth) would most likely indicate a urea cycle disorder.

This diagnosis can be confirmed by the absence of acidosis or ketosis. Severe deficiency or total absence of activity of any of the first four enzymes in the urea cycle, or the enzyme that produces the required cofactor for carbamoyl phosphate synthetase 1, results in the accumulation of ammonium ion and other precursor metabolites during the first few days of life. Infants with a severe urea cycle disorder are normal at birth but rapidly develop cerebral edema and the related signs of lethargy, anorexia, hyper- or hypoventilation, hypothermia, seizures, neurologic posturing, and coma. Serum analytes allow for differential diagnosis of which enzyme in the urea cycle is deficient resulting in the hyperammonemia and other symptoms associated with urea cycle disorders. However, given that hyperammonemia can be fatal, in particular in the neonate, it is essential that the level of serum ammonium ion be assessed whenever a urea cycle disorder is suspected. Rapid intervention with hemodialysis is necessary to ensure survival of infants presenting with the level of severity of the symptoms in this patient. Measurement of serum levels of urea (choice A) and citrulline (choice B) and the level of orotic acid in the urine (choice D) are useful in the confirmation of, and differential diagnosis of, urea cycle disorders but do not represent the critically important measurements to ensure the proper therapeutic intervention is instituted in this patient. An odor of acetone on the breath (choice E) would most likely be indicative of diabetic ketoacidosis in a patient with type 1 diabetes. However, this is not likely to be observed in a 3-day-old infant.

17. Correct answer is **B.** The patient is most likely exhibiting the symptoms of citrullinemia type II. Citrullinemia type II (CTLN2) commonly presents with sudden onset between the ages of 11 and 79 years. Manifestations of CTLN2 are recurrent hyperammonemia with neuropsychiatric symptoms including nocturnal delirium, aggression, irritability, hyperactivity, delusions, disorientation, restlessness, drowsiness, loss of memory, flapping tremor, convulsive seizures, and coma. The symptoms of CTLN2 are often provoked by alcohol and sugar intake, as well as by certain medications, and/or surgery. CTLN2 is caused by deficiency in the gene encoding citrin. Citrin is a mitochondrial solute carrier protein (SLC25A13) involved in the mitochondrial uptake of glutamate and export of aspartate and as such functions in the malate-aspartate shuttle. Deficiency in carbamoyl phosphate synthetase 1 (choice A) and ornithine transcarbamylase (choice E) would be associated with little to no detectable citrulline. Deficiency in glucocerebrosidase (choice C) is the cause of Gaucher disease. Deficiency in glutamate dehydrogenase (choice D) has not been observed in humans.

18. Correct answer is **D.** With respect to the role of the kidney in acid-base balance, the function of the proximal tubule is the generation of ammonia (NH_3) which is in equilibrium with ammonium ion (NH_4^+). The production of ammonia is referred to as ammoniagenesis. Although ammonia and ammonium ion excretion in the urine constitutes a portion of the total waste nitrogen excretion, ammoniagenesis in the kidney is critically important in acid-base regulation. The production, secretion, and reabsorption of bicarbonate (HCO_3^-), by the kidney, is a major contributor to the renal responsibility to regulate acid-base balance. However, on its own renal bicarbonate production is not sufficient, thus the need for ammonia generation. The ionization of NH_3 to NH_4^+ is an effective means to reduce the overall H^+ load, and thus raise the pH of the blood during periods of acidosis. In addition to releasing two moles of NH_4^+, the benefits of renal glutamine metabolism are that bicarbonate (HCO_3^-) is also generated. The HCO_3^- is derived from the α-ketoglutarate (2-oxoglutarate) dehydrogenase-mediated oxidation of the α-ketoglutarate (2-oxoglutarate) in the TCA cycle. The source of the α-ketoglutarate being generated from the concerted glutaminase and glutamate dehydrogenase reactions. The HCO_3^- is then transported to the blood from the proximal tubule cells via the basolateral membrane Na^+-coupled bicarbonate transporter identified as NBC1 which is encoded by the *SLC4A4* gene. Mutations in the *SLC4A4* gene result in type 2 (proximal) renal tubular acidosis (type 2 RTA). The HCO_3^- produced by the proximal tubule via glutamine metabolism represents new HCO_3^- being added to the pool already in the blood, thereby enhancing the buffering capacity of the blood. None of the other enzymes (choices A, B, C, and E) contribute to the process of acid-base balance at the level of renal ammoniagenesis.

19. Correct answer is **A.** The patient is most likely exhibiting the symptoms of citrullinemia type II. Citrullinemia type II (CTLN2) commonly presents with sudden onset between the ages of 11 and 79 years. Manifestations of CTLN2 are recurrent hyperammonemia with neuropsychiatric symptoms including nocturnal delirium, aggression, irritability, hyperactivity, delusions, disorientation, restlessness, drowsiness, loss of memory, flapping tremor, convulsive seizures, and coma. The symptoms of CTLN2 are often provoked by alcohol and sugar intake, as well as by certain medications, and/or surgery. CTLN2 is caused by deficiency in the gene encoding citrin. Citrin is a mitochondrial solute carrier protein (SLC25A13) involved in the mitochondrial uptake of glutamate and export of aspartate and as such functions in the malate-aspartate shuttle. Deficiencies in none of the other processes (choices B, C, D, and E) would account for the signs and symptoms in this patient.

20. Correct answer is **B.** The infant is most likely manifesting the signs and symptoms of a neonatal urea cycle disorder. The normal levels of citrulline and elevated levels of ornithine strongly suggest that the infant has a deficiency in the urea cycle enzyme, ornithine transcarbamylase. Deficiency in ornithine transcarbamylase results in mitochondrial carbamoyl phosphate spilling into the cytosol where it contributes to *de novo* pyrimidine nucleotide biosynthesis. The increase in pyrimidine nucleotide biosynthesis results in elevated levels of urinary orotic acid. The impaired urea cycle results in the liver diverting waste nitrogen into α-ketoglutarate (2-oxoglutarate) via the glutamate dehydrogenase reaction and into glutamate via the glutamine synthetase reaction. This increased production of glutamine by the liver will lead to an elevation of glutamine in the blood. Elevated alloisoleucine and ketoacidosis (choice A) are characteristic findings in maple syrup urine disease, a disorder resulting from deficiency in branched-chain keto acid dehydrogenase. Orotic aciduria resulting from a deficiency in the pyrimidine nucleotide biosynthetic enzyme, UMP synthase, would be associated with the potential for ketoacidosis and crystals forming in the urine (choice C) as well as megaloblastic anemia (choice D). Methylmalonic acidemia and anemia (choice E) are hallmarks of a vitamin B_{12} deficiency.

21. Correct answer is **E.** The patient is most likely experiencing symptoms of severe metabolic acidosis which is confirmed

by the blood pH value of 7.15. The most likely cause of the patient's metabolic acidosis is the lactate produced by her skeletal muscles in the course of her running the marathon. During periods of metabolic acidosis numerous physiological changes take place to respond to elevated level of acid in body fluids. The role of the liver in the response to metabolic acidosis is to shift from the production of urea to incorporating ammonia into α-ketoglutarate (2-oxoglutarate) and then glutamate yielding glutamine. As a result, the level of blood glutamine increases in response to metabolic acidosis. Within the proximal tubules epithelial cells of the nephron in the kidney the ammonia is released from glutamine allowing hydrogen ion to interact with ammonia forming ammonium ion (NH_4^+) which is then eliminated in the urine effectively removing acid (H^+) from the blood. This metabolic interrelationship between the liver and kidney is a critical mechanism ensuring overall acid-base balance. None of the other substances (choices A, B, C, D, and F) would be elevated in the blood under the conditions of metabolic acidosis.

22. Correct answer is **C.** The infant is most likely manifesting the signs and symptoms of a neonatal urea cycle disorder. The urea cycle begins in the mitochondria with the condensation of ammonium ion and bicarbonate through the action of carbamoyl phosphate synthetase 1 (CPS1) and finishes in the cytosol with the release of urea and ornithine via the action of arginase. The ornithine is then transported into the mitochondria where it is complexed with the carbamoyl phosphate generated by CPS1 via the action of ornithine transcarbamylase (OTC) forming citrulline. The citrulline is then transported to the cytosol. A defect in either of the mitochondrial enzymes of the urea cycle will result in little to no detectable citrulline. Conversely, if the defect in the urea cycle was in a cytoplasmic enzyme, which would most likely be argininosuccinate synthetase (AS) or argininosuccinate lyase (AL), there would be elevation in the detectable level of citrulline. Asparagine levels (choice A) would not be affected by a defect in any urea cycle enzyme. A defect in the CPS1 would result in little to no detectable carbamoyl phosphate (choice B). A defect in ornithine transcarbamylase would result in reduced levels of detectable ornithine (choice D). Elevated levels of orotic acid (choice E) are indicative of a defect in ornithine transcarbamylase.

23. Correct answer is **B.** Given the absence of apparent mutations in any urea cycle enzyme, the infant is most likely exhibiting the symptoms of type II citrullinemia. Mutations in two genes are the known causes of citrullinemia. One gene encodes the urea cycle enzyme argininosuccinate synthetase. Mutations in argininosuccinate synthetase are the cause of type I citrullinemia, also known as classic citrullinemia. However, since the molecular analyses showed no definitive mutation in any gene encoding a urea cycle enzyme this cannot be the cause of the infants hyperammonemia and citrullinemia. The other gene associated with citrullinemia is the *SLC25A13* gene which encodes the transporter identified as citrin. Mutations in the *SLC25A13* gene are the cause of type II citrullinemia. Citrin deficiency can manifest in newborns as neonatal intrahepatic cholestasis caused by citrin deficiency (NICCD) and in older children as failure to thrive and dyslipidemia caused by citrin deficiency (FTTDCD). One of the most common characteristics of citrin deficiency is a fondness for protein-rich and/or lipid-rich foods and aversion to carbohydrate-rich foods. In NICCD children younger than age 1 year exhibit growth retardation with transient intrahepatic cholestasis, hepatomegaly, diffuse fatty liver, and parenchymal cellular infiltration associated with hepatic fibrosis, variable liver dysfunction, hypoproteinemia, decreased coagulation factors, hemolytic anemia, and/or hypoglycemia. NICCD is generally not severe, and symptoms may often resolve by 1 year of age provided appropriate treatment is given. However, some infants will die due to infection and liver cirrhosis. FTTDCD is usually observed in children around 1–2 years of age with the aforementioned food preferences being apparent. Some FTTDCD patients have growth retardation, hypoglycemia, hyperlipidemia, pancreatitis, fatty liver, hepatoma, and fatigue. Mutations in the gene encoding branched-chain ketoacid dehydrogenase (choice A) are the cause of maple syrup urine disease. Mutations in the gene encoding glycogen branching enzyme (choice C) are the cause of the glycogen storage disease identified as Andersen disease. Mutations in the gene encoding medium-chain acyl-CoA dehydrogenase, MCAD (choice D) result in the fatty acid β-oxidation disorder identified as MCAD deficiency. Mutations in the gene encoding phytanoyl-CoA hydroxylase (choice E) are the cause of Refsum disease.

24. Correct answer is **A.** The infant is most likely exhibiting the symptoms of a neonatal urea cycle disorder, UCD. In general, the treatment of UCD has as common elements the reduction of protein in the diet, removal of excess ammonia, and replacement of intermediates missing from the urea cycle. Administration of lactulose (a nonabsorbable disaccharide) results in reduced ammonia production in the gut and, therefore, less ammonium ion is delivered to the portal circulation from the intestines. Bacteria metabolize lactulose to acidic byproducts which then promotes excretion of ammonia in the feces as ammonium ion (NH_4^+) and interferes with the production of ammonia through reduced catabolism of other nitrogenous compounds. A high-protein diet (choice B) is strongly contraindicated in patients with UCD since this would dramatically increase NH_4^+ levels in these patients. A lactose-free diet (choice C) is the recommended diet for patients suffering from classic galactosemia. Phenylalanine restriction (choice D) is required of patients with phenylketonuria, PKU. A protein-free diet (choice E) would reduce the level of waste nitrogen production; however, it would not allow for normal growth and development in the infant.

25. Correct answer is **E.** The infant is most likely manifesting the signs and symptoms of a neonatal urea cycle disorder, UCD. In general, the treatment of UCD has as common elements the reduction of protein in the diet, removal of excess ammonia, and replacement of intermediates missing from the urea cycle. Sodium benzoate and sodium phenylacetate can be administered to covalently bind glycine (forming hippurate) and glutamine (forming phenylacetylglutamine), respectively. These latter compounds, which contain the ammonia nitrogen, are excreted in the feces. Supplementation with none of the other options (choices A, B, C, and D) is of therapeutic benefit in the treatment of patients with urea cycle disorders.

C H A P T E R

18

Amino Acid Metabolism

High-Yield Terms

Glucogenic	Relating to amino acids whose catabolic products can be used for net glucose synthesis during gluconeogenesis
Ketogenic	Relating to amino acids whose catabolic products enter the TCA cycle but cannot be used for net glucose synthesis during gluconeogenesis
Essential amino acid	Any amino acid that cannot be formed *de novo* or from other precursor compounds within mammalian cells
Asparaginase	Enzyme catalyzing the deamination of asparagine to aspartate; enzyme is used clinically as a chemotherapeutic treatment for certain leukemias
Cystathionine β-synthase	Enzyme involved in cysteine biosynthesis; deficiencies are most common cause of homocysteinemias/homocystinurias
Phenylketonuria, PKU	A particular form of hyperphenylalaninemia resulting from defects in the phenylalanine hydroxylase gene
Maple syrup urine disease	In the catabolic enzyme, branched-chain α-keto acid dehydrogenase (BCKD) result in Maple syrup urine disease, MSUD
Alkaptonuria	First inherited error in metabolism to be characterized; benign disease caused by defects in the tyrosine catabolizing enzyme homogentisate oxidase, urine of afflicted patients turns brown on exposure to air

AMINO ACID UPTAKE

The process of protein digestion followed by peptide and amino acid uptake by the gut is reviewed in Chapter 28. Briefly, proteins are degraded to free amino acids, di- and tri-peptides by gut and pancreatic peptidases. Intestinal uptake of amino acids involves numerous transporter proteins that collectively are divided into three broad categories: acidic, basic, and neutral amino acid transporters. The inability to effectively absorb amino acids from the gut can lead to serious developmental and physiologic consequences such as in the case of Hartnup disorder (Clinical Box 18–1).

METABOLIC CLASSIFICATIONS OF AMINO ACIDS

Amino acids fall into three categories: glucogenic, ketogenic, or glucogenic and ketogenic. Glucogenic amino acids are those that give rise to a net production of pyruvate or TCA cycle intermediates, such as α-ketoglutarate (2-oxoglutarate) or oxaloacetate, all of which are precursors to glucose via gluconeogenesis. All amino acids except lysine and leucine are at least partly glucogenic. Lysine and leucine are the only amino acids that are solely ketogenic, giving rise only to acetyl-CoA or acetoacetyl-CoA, neither of which can bring about net glucose production.

Amino acids that cannot be made at all or in sufficient amounts in human cells are classified as essential amino acids (Table 18–1). Those amino acids, that humans can synthesize are, classified as nonessential. The amino acids arginine, methionine, and phenylalanine are considered conditionally essential for reasons not directly related to lack of synthesis. Arginine is synthesized by mammalian cells but at a rate that is insufficient to meet the growth needs of the body and the majority that is synthesized is cleaved to form urea. Methionine is required in large amounts to produce cysteine if the latter amino acid is not adequately supplied in the diet. Similarly, phenylalanine is needed in large amounts to form tyrosine if the latter is not adequately supplied in the diet.

GLUTAMATE AND GLUTAMINE METABOLISM

The relationships between 2-oxoglutarate (α-ketoglutarate), glutamate, and glutamine are reviewed in Chapter 17.

CLINICAL BOX 18–1 HARTNUP DISORDER

Hartnup disorder is an autosomal recessive disorder that was first described in 1956 in the Hartnup family in London. The originally characterized patients exhibited a renal aminoaciduria of neutral amino acids associated with a pellagra-like skin rash and episodes of cerebellar ataxia. Indeed, in the original publication documenting this disorder the authors described the clinical features as: "hereditary pellagra-like skin rash with temporary cerebellar ataxia, constant renal aminoaciduria, and other bizarre biochemical features." Since its initial characterization, Hartnup disorder has been found to have a frequency of occurrence on the order of 1:30,000 in European populations. However, although the original patient presented with the symptoms described, many individuals with the disorder remain nearly asymptomatic with skin rashes and diarrhea in infancy being the most severe manifestations. Regardless of the broad range of symptom presentation the hallmark of Hartnup disorder is aminoaciduria. Almost all affected individuals are correctly diagnosed through urine analysis. Hartnup disorder is caused by a defect in neutral amino acid transport in the apical brush border membranes of the small intestine and in kidney proximal tubules, the latter accounting for the aminoaciduria in Hartnup disorder patients. The transporter is a member of the solute carrier family, specifically the SLC6A19 transporter. SLC6A19 is also known as the system B(0) [also written as B^0] neutral amino acid transporter 1 [B(0)AT1 or B0AT1]. The B refers to a broad specificity transporter, the 0 denotes the transporter as one for neutral amino acids, and the superscripting of the 0 denotes that the transporter is a Na^+-dependent transporter. The SLC6A19 transporter prefers large aliphatic neutral amino acids. Of significance to overall amino acid homeostasis is the fact that the SCL6A19 encoded transporter transports eight of the ten essential amino acids, namely leucine, isoleucine, valine, methionine, phenylalanine, tryptophan, threonine, and histidine. Of significance, specifically to Hartnup disorder is that SLC6A19 is the major transporter of tryptophan in the intestines and its lack, in Hartnup disorder, is key to the pathology of the disorder. To date a total of 21 different mutations have been identified with missense mutations representing the bulk of the identified mutations. Within Europeans the most frequent mutation is a missense mutation converting an Asp codon at amino acid 173 to an Asn, designated as the D173N mutation. Symptoms of Hartnup disorder may begin in infancy or early childhood, but sometimes they begin as late as early adulthood. Symptoms may be triggered by sunlight, fever, drugs, or emotional or physical stress. Most symptoms occur sporadically and are caused by a deficiency of the enzyme cofactors, NAD^+ and $NADP^+$. These cofactors become sporadically deficient due to the fact that tryptophan serves as an endogenous precursor for quinolinic acid which can be converted, via several reactions, to NAD^+. The significance of tryptophan to the overall NAD^+ and $NADP^+$ pool can be clearly demonstrated in Hartnup disorder given that the symptoms of skin rash in these patients resolve on niacin (vitamin B_3) supplementation. When Hartnup disorder manifests during infancy the symptoms can be variable in clinical presentation. These symptoms include failure to thrive, photosensitivity, intermittent ataxia, nystagmus, and tremor. Since tryptophan is also required for the synthesis of melatonin, it is believed that skin sensitivity to sunlight is exerted, in part, by a lack or reduction in melatonin synthesis. In addition to the regulation of circadian rhythm melatonin has been shown to exert protective effects in the skin as well as being a regulator of skin structure and function. The cerebellar ataxia associated with Hartnup disorder is likely due to reduced synthesis of serotonin which is derived from tryptophan. The lack of intestinal tryptophan transport is responsible for most, if not all, clinical phenotypes of Hartnup disorder. The pellagra-like skin rash seen on sun-exposed areas of skin in Hartnup disorder patients is most likely the result of NAD^+ and $NADP^+$ deficiency. Variability in presentation of Hartnup disorder symptoms arises due to both dietary influences and the fact that other proteins associate with, and affect the activity of, SLC6A19. As to dietary effects, persons who consume a high-protein diet tend to be the most asymptomatic due to the contribution of intestinal peptide transport to the overall absorption of tryptophan. Indeed, most patients with Hartnup disorder can remain asymptomatic on a high-protein diet due to intestinal peptide absorption via the actions of the peptide transporter, PepT1. In comparison, individuals who consume high-carbohydrate, low-protein diets are more likely to exhibit the most severe manifestations of Hartnup disorder.

ROLE OF GLUTAMINE METABOLISM IN CANCER

Glutamine represents the most abundant amino acid in the blood. By circulating in the plasma, glutamine represents a major contributor to the energy needs of cells, particularly cancer cells (see Chapter 34). Glutamine metabolism contributes to the generation of numerous other amino acids, contributes to the pool of acetyl-CoA required for fatty acid and cholesterol synthesis, participates in the generation of NADPH required for lipid and nucleic acid synthesis, serves as a precursor for the antioxidant, glutathione, and as a precursor for the hexosamine, UDP-*N*-acetylglucosamine (UDP-GlcNAc). All of these pathways are required for the generation of the biomass that is necessary for cancer cell proliferation and for the regulation of transcription programs in cancer cells that promote the proliferative state.

ASPARTATE AND ASPARAGINE METABOLISM

Aspartate is synthesized by a simple one-step transamination reaction catalyzed by aspartate aminotransferase, AST (Figure 18–1). The transfer of nitrogen to oxaloacetate is an important component of substrate generation (aspartate) for the production of ornithine in the urea cycle (see Chapter 17). Aspartate can also be formed by deamination of asparagine catalyzed by asparaginase (Figure 18–2). Asparaginase has utility as a chemotherapeutic in the treatment of certain leukemias (Clinical Box 18–2).

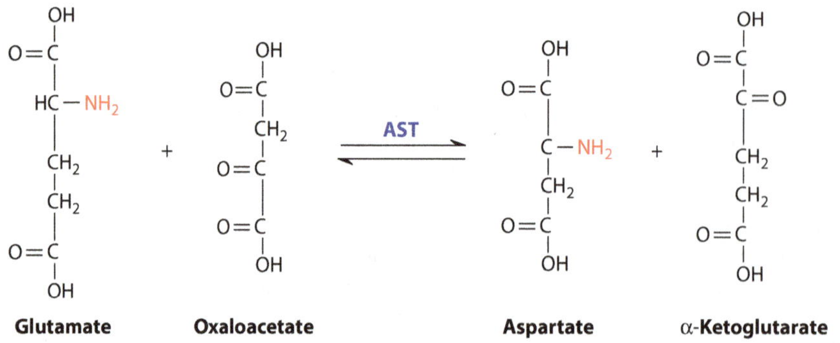

FIGURE 18–1 Aspartate aminotransferase (AST) reaction. (Reproduced with permission from themedicalbiochemistrypage, LLC.)

TABLE 18–1 Essential vs nonessential amino acids.

Nonessential	Essential
Alanine	Arginine
Asparagine	Histidine
Aspartate	Isoleucine
Cysteine	Leucine
Glutamate	Lysine
Glutamine	Methionine
Glycine	Phenylalanine
Proline	Threonine
Serine	Tryptophan
Tyrosine	Valine

Reproduced with permission from King MW: *Integrative Medical Biochemistry Examination and Board Review*. New York, NY: McGraw Hill; 2014.

CLINICAL BOX 18-2 ASPARAGINASE AS ANTI-CANCER DRUG

Asparaginase is used as a chemotherapeutic drug in the treatment of acute lymphocytic leukemias, ALL. The rationale for the use of asparaginase in this capacity stems from the fact that ALL cells are unable to synthesize asparagine, whereas normal cells are able to make their own asparagine. Therefore, leukemic cells require high amounts of circulating asparagine for protein synthesis and growth. Since asparaginase catalyzes the conversion of asparagine to aspartic acid and ammonia the leukemic cells are deprived of circulating asparagine. The inability to acquire sufficient asparagine leads to the activation of amino acid deprivation responses in the leukemic cells which culminates with the triggering of programmed cell death pathways in these cells.

Asparagine is synthesized from aspartate via the action of asparagine synthetase (Figure 18–3), an ATP-dependent amidotransferase reaction.

ALANINE AND THE GLUCOSE-ALANINE CYCLE

Alanine is second only to glutamine in prominence as a circulating amino acid. In this capacity it serves a unique role in the transfer of nitrogen from peripheral tissues, primarily skeletal muscle, to the liver. Alanine is formed from pyruvate at a rate proportional to intracellular pyruvate levels. Liver accumulates plasma alanine, reverses the transamination that occurs in muscle, and proportionately increases urea production. When alanine transfer from muscle to liver is coupled with glucose transport from liver back to muscle, the process is known as the glucose-alanine cycle.

CYSTEINE AND METHIONINE METABOLISM

Cysteine and methionine metabolism are interrelated as the sulfur for cysteine synthesis comes from methionine (Figure 18–4). Two enzymes of this pathway, cystathionine β-synthase (CBS) and cystathionase (cystathionine γ-lyase), use pyridoxal phosphate (vitamin B_6) as a cofactor. The intermediate in this pathway, homocysteine can undergo oxidation with itself to form the disulfide-bonded homodimer, homocystine.

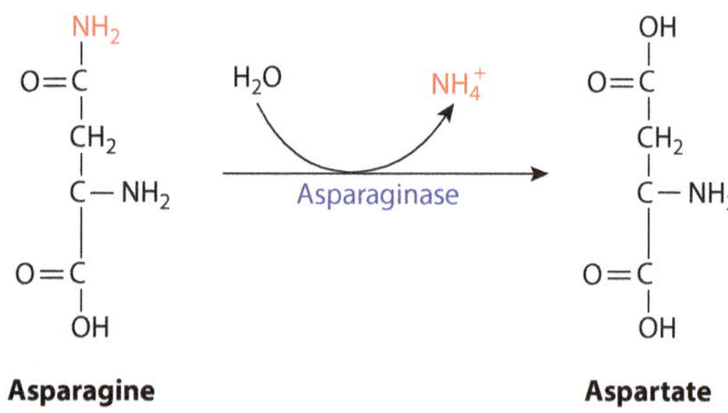

FIGURE 18–2 Asparagine synthetase reaction. (Reproduced with permission from themedicalbiochemistrypage, LLC.)

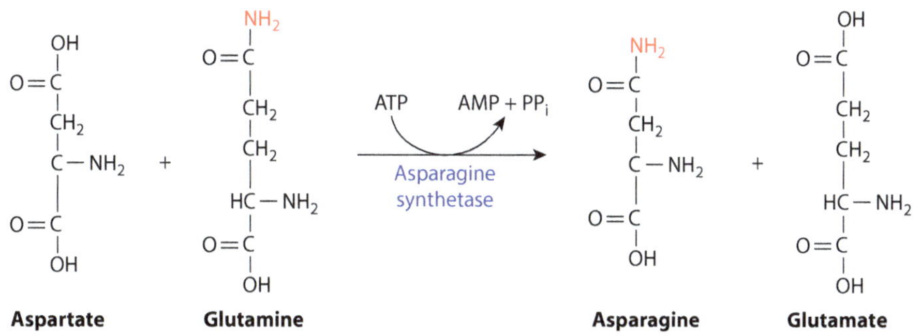

FIGURE 18–3 Asparaginase reaction. (Reproduced with permission from themedicalbiochemistrypage, LLC.)

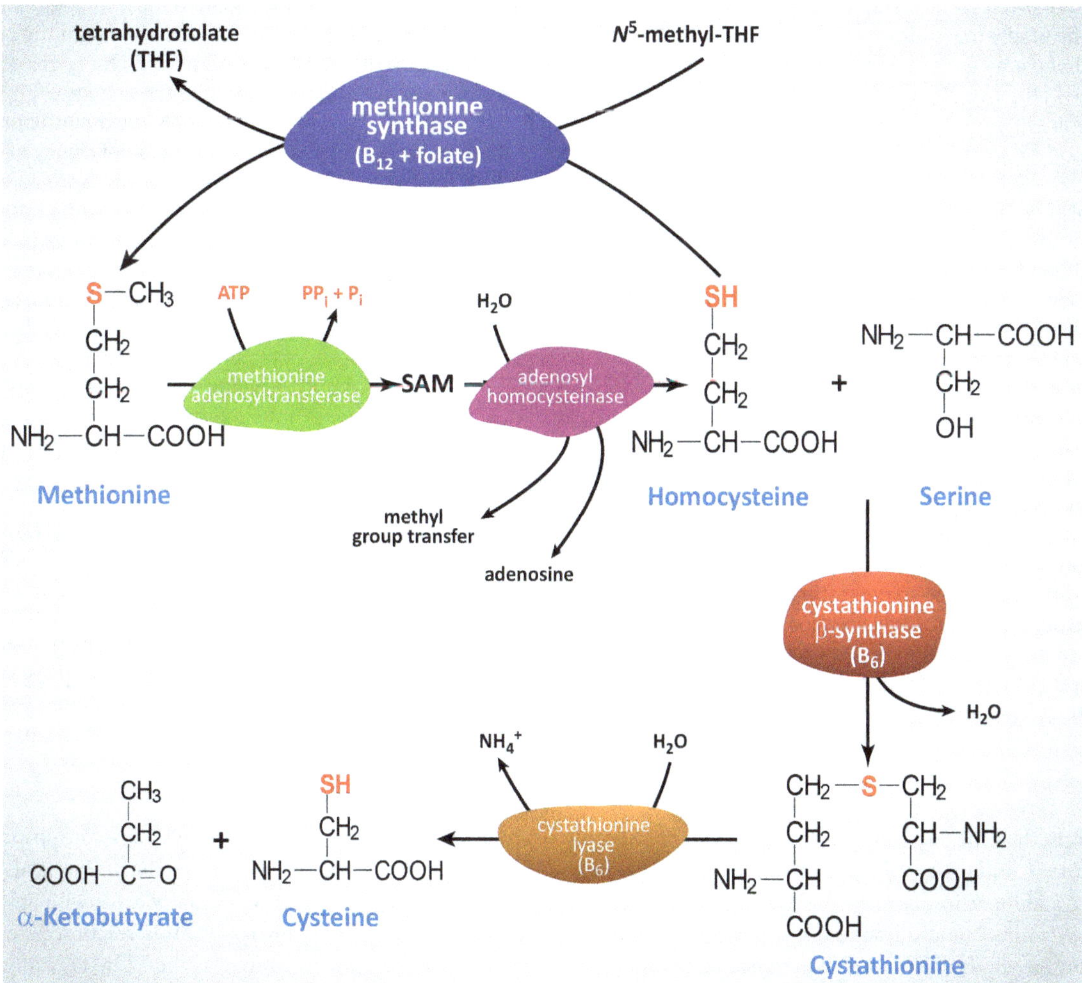

FIGURE 18–4 Utilization of methionine in the synthesis of cysteine. The sulfur from the essential amino acid, methionine, is required for the synthesis of cysteine. The synthesis of cysteine represents an extremely important and clinically relevant biochemical pathway. Several vitamins are required for this metabolic pathway to proceed emphasizing the nutritional impact. Folate, pyridoxal phosphate (PLP, B_6), and B_{12} are all necessary for cysteine synthesis. The enzyme methionine synthase (homocysteine methyltransferase) requires both folate and B_{12} for activity. Deficiency in either of these vitamins contributes to homocysteinemia/homocystinuria and also to the development of macrocytic (megaloblastic) anemias. Cystathionine β-synthase is a PLP requiring enzyme demonstrating why vitamin B_6 deficiency is also associated with the development of homocysteinemia/homocystinuria. SAM: *S*-adenosylmethionine. Adenosylhomocysteinase is also known as *S*-adenosylhomocysteine hydrolase. The release of adenosine from SAM in this pathway represents a major mechanism for the intracellular production of this important cardiovascular and immune regulatory molecule. (Reproduced with permission from themedicalbiochemistrypage, LLC.)

CLINICAL BOX 18–3 HOMOCYSTEINEMIA/HOMOCYSTINURIA

Homocysteinemias (also termed homocystinurias) represent a family of inherited disorders resulting from defects in several of the genes involved in the conversion of methionine to cysteine. As the name implies, these disorders result in elevated levels of homocysteine and homocystine in the blood, where the elevated urine output of the metabolite is referred to as homocysteinurina or homocystinuria. Homocystine is a disulfide-bonded homodimer of two homocysteines. This is similar to the formation of cystine from two cysteines. In addition to homocystinuria, patients excrete elevated levels of methionine and metabolites of homocysteine. The most common causes of homocystinuria (classic homocystinuria) are defects in the gene (*CBS*) encoding cystathionine β-synthase. Homocystinuria is often associated with intellectual impairment, although the complete syndrome is multifaceted and many individuals with this disease are mentally normal, while others experience variable levels of developmental delay along with learning problems. Common symptoms of homocystinuria are dislocated optic lenses (*ectopia lentis*), osteoporosis, lengthening and thinning of the long bones, and an increased risk of abnormal blood clotting (thromboembolism). The nature of the lens dislocation (subluxation), evident in homocysteinemia patients, can serve as a differential diagnostic tool. Lens dislocation is also found in patients suffering from Marfan syndrome, which is a connective tissue disorder caused by defects in the fibrillin gene (*FBN1*). In homocystinuria the lens subluxation occurs in a downward and inward (inferonasally) direction, whereas in Marfan syndrome the lens subluxation occurs upward and outward. Some instances of genetic homocysteinemia respond favorably to pyridoxine therapy suggesting that in these cases the defect in CBS is a decreased affinity for the cofactor, pyridoxal phosphate. Homocysteinemia can also result from vitamin deficiencies due to the role of the cofactor forms of B_6, B_{12}, and folate in the overall metabolism of methionine. Vitamin B_6 (as pyridoxal phosphate) is required for the activity of CBS and cystathionine γ-lyase, and the homocysteinemia that results with B_6 deficiency is also associated with elevated methionine levels in the blood. Vitamin B_{12} and folate (as methyl-THF) are required for the methionine synthase reaction so a deficiency of either vitamin can result in homocysteinemia presenting with reduced levels of plasma methionine. The enzyme methylmalonyl-CoA mutase also requires B_{12} and so a homocystinuria resulting from a deficiency in this vitamin is also associated with methylmalonic academia. Indeed, the measurement of serum methionine and methylmalonic acid in cases of homocysteinemia (homocystinuria) allows for a differential diagnosis of the nutritional (nongenetic) cause. Another related disorder, sometimes referred to as hyperhomocysteinemia, is most often associated with manifestation of symptoms much later in life. The characteristic pathology of hyperhomocysteinemia is coronary artery disease (CAD) and an increased risk for deep vein thromboses, DVT. In addition, there is an increased risk for mild cognitive impairment and dementia. An inherited form of hyperhomocysteinemia results from mutations in the methylene tetrahydrofolate reductase (*MTHFR*) gene. The most common mutation in this gene that results in hyperhomocysteinemia is a C to T change at nucleotide position 677 (C677T). Mutations in the methionine synthase (*MTR*) gene are also associated with inherited hyperhomocysteinemia. In the case of the *MTR* gene the most common mutation is a change of an A for a G at nucleotide position 2756 (A2756G). Elevated levels of homocysteine in the blood have been shown to correlate with cardiovascular dysfunction. The role of homocysteine in cardiovascular disease is related to its ability to induce a state of inflammation. Homocysteine inhibits the extracellular collagen processing enzyme, lysyl oxidase leading to impaired collagen. In addition, homocysteine is highly reactive with proteins in the blood and on the surface of the endothelial cells. Together with the disturbed collagen processing these events trigger inappropriate activation of neutrophils contributing to the induced inflammatory state. Homocysteine also serves as a negatively charged surface that attracts the contact phase of the intrinsic pathway of blood coagulation (see Chapter 33). Activation of the intrinsic coagulation cascade leads to inappropriate thrombolytic events as well as resulting in increases in inflammatory cytokine release from leukocytes that are activated as a result of the procoagulant state.

Mutations in the gene encoding CBS are the primary causes of homocystinuria (Clinical Box 18–3). Due to the roles of the vitamins, B_6, B_{12}, and folate in this metabolic pathway, deficiencies in any of these vitamins can also lead to accumulation of homocysteine/homocystine in the blood and homocysteine/homocystine in the urine.

The catabolism of methionine involves the pathway to cysteine synthesis which also yields α-ketobutyrate (2-ketobutyrate) which is then converted to propionyl-CoA. The propionyl-CoA is converted to succinyl-CoA which then enters the TCA cycle for further oxidation. The enzymes required for this conversion are propionyl-CoA carboxylase, methylmalonyl-CoA epimerase, and methylmalonyl-CoA mutase, respectively. The clinical significance of methylmalonyl-CoA mutase in this pathway is that it is one of only two enzymes that require a vitamin B_{12}-derived cofactor for activity. This propionyl-CoA conversion pathway is also required for the metabolism of the amino acids, valine, isoleucine, and threonine as well as fatty acids with an odd number of carbon atoms. For this reason, this reaction pathway is often remembered by the mnemonic as the VOMIT pathway, where V stands for valine, O for odd-chain fatty acids, M for methionine, I for isoleucine, and T for threonine.

The major cysteine catabolic pathway in humans generates the intermediate cysteine sulfinate (Figure 18–5). Cysteine sulfinate can serve as a biosynthetic intermediate in the production of taurine used in bile acid metabolism (see Chapter 15) or as the precursor of the sulfate used in the synthesis of 3′-phosphoadenosine-5′-phosphosulfate, (PAPS). PAPS is used for the transfer of sulfate to biological molecules such as the sugars of the glycosphingolipids (see Chapter 12).

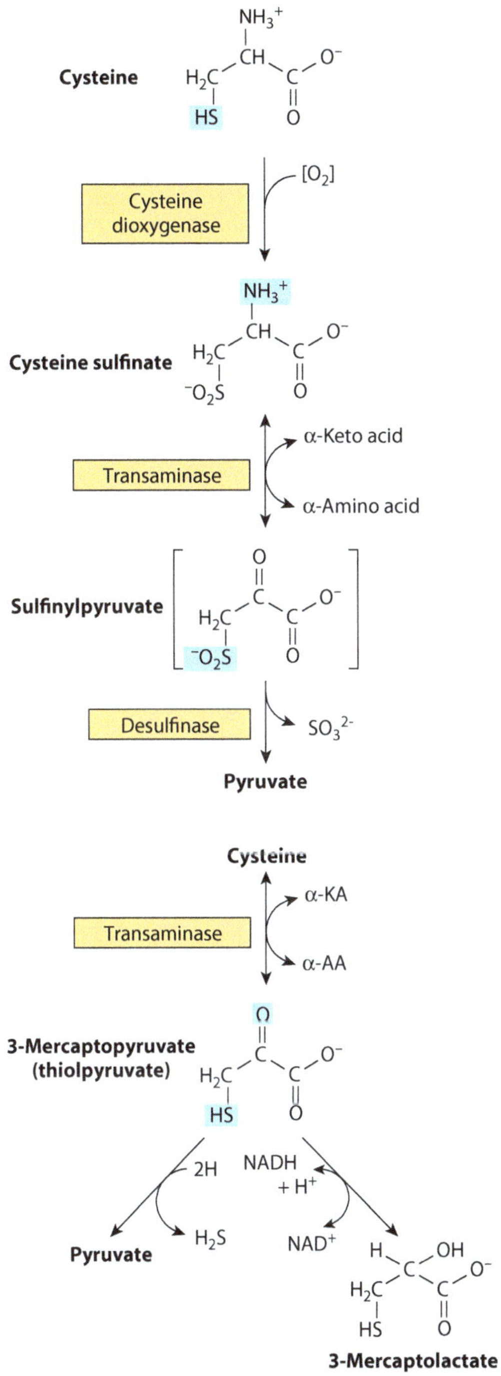

FIGURE 18–5 Two pathways catabolize L-cysteine: the cysteine sulfinate pathway (top) and the 3-mercaptopyruvate pathway (bottom). (Reproduced with permission from Rodwell VW, Bender DA, Botham KM, et al: *Harper's Illustrated Biochemistry*, 31st ed. New York, NY: McGraw Hill; 2018.)

Methionine serves as the methyl donor in the synthesis of *S*-adenosylmethionine, SAM (also abbreviated as AdoMet). SAM is critical in numerous methyl transfer reactions involving those in the synthesis or modification of nucleic acids, lipids, proteins (particularly histones), neurotransmitters, and small molecules.

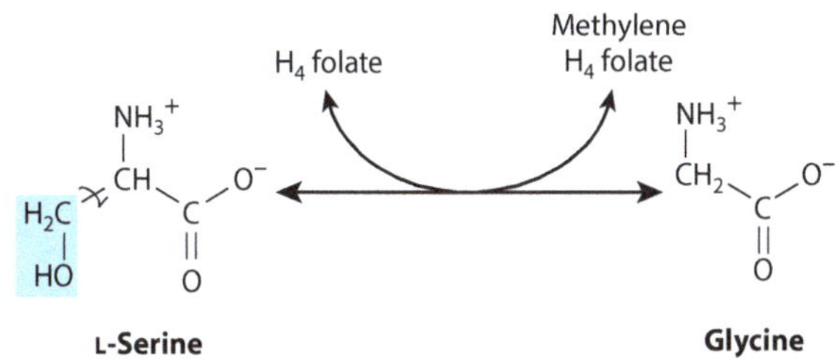

FIGURE 18–6 Interconversion of serine and glycine by serine hydroxymethyltransferase. (H4 folate, tetrahydrofolate). (Reproduced with permission from Rodwell VW, Bender DA, Botham KM, et al: *Harper's Illustrated Biochemistry*, 31st ed. New York, NY: McGraw Hill; 2018.)

GLYCINE AND SERINE METABOLISM

Glycine and serine are interchangeable through the action of the cytosolic form of serine hydroxymethyltransferase (SHMT1). This enzyme is a member of the family of 1-carbon transferases and is also known as glycine hydroxymethyltransferase (Figure 18–6) or serine/glycine hydroxymethyltransferase. This reaction involves the transfer of the hydroxymethyl group from serine to tetrahydrofolate (THF), producing glycine and N^5,N^{10}-methylene-THF.

The main pathway to *de novo* biosynthesis of serine utilizes the glycolytic intermediate 3-phosphoglycerate (Figure 18–7). As indicated in Figure 18–6, serine can also be derived from glycine.

The catabolism of serine occurs via its conversion first to glycine. Glycine can then be oxidized by glycine decarboxylase (also referred to as the glycine cleavage complex, GCC) to yield ammonia, CO_2, and a second equivalent of N^5,N^{10}-methylene-THF (Figure 18–8). Glycine decarboxylase is a mitochondrial enzyme complex composed of four distinct proteins identified as H, L, P, and T. The H protein is a lipoic acid-containing protein. The L protein is a dihydrolipoamide dehydrogenase (DLD) similar to the DLD subunit of the pyruvate dehydrogenase and α-ketoglutarate (2-oxoglutarate) dehydrogenase complexes. The P protein is a pyridoxal phosphate-dependent glycine decarboxylase. The T protein is a tetrahydrofolate-requiring aminotransferase. Mutations in the genes encoding the H, P, or T proteins results in nonketotic hyperglycinemia (glycine encephalopathy, Clinical Box 18–4).

HIGH-YIELD CONCEPT

In addition to its role in protein synthesis and the formation of serine, glycine functions in the central nervous system as a major inhibitory neurotransmitter. In this capacity glycine participates in regulating signals that process motor and sensory information that permit movement, vision, and audition. Glycine also functions as an excitatory neurotransmitter in conjunction with glutamate binding to the *N*-methyl-D-aspartate (NMDA) family of glutamate receptors.

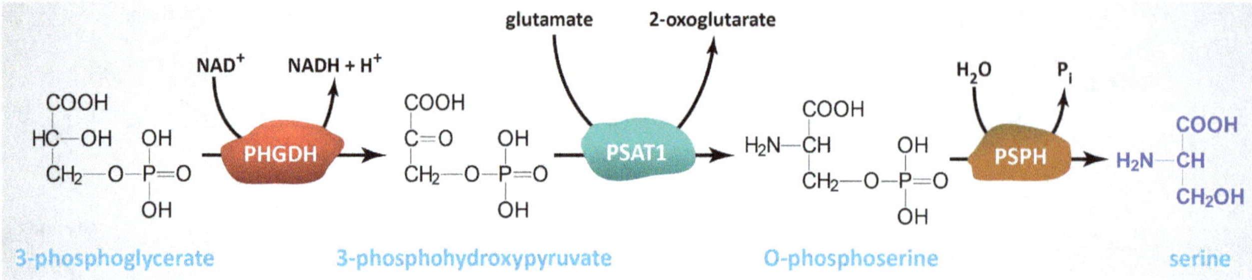

FIGURE 18–7 Reactions of serine biosynthesis. Serine can be derived from the glycolytic intermediate, 3-phosphoglycerate, in a three-step reaction pathway. The first reaction is catalyzed by phosphoglycerate dehydrogenase (PHGDH). The second reaction is a simple transamination catalyzed by phosphoserine aminotransferase 1 (PSAT1) which utilizes glutamate as the amino donor and releases 2-oxoglutarate (α-ketoglutarate). The last step in the reaction pathway is catalyzed by phosphoserine phosphatase (PSPH). (Reproduced with permission from themedicalbiochemistrypage, LLC.)

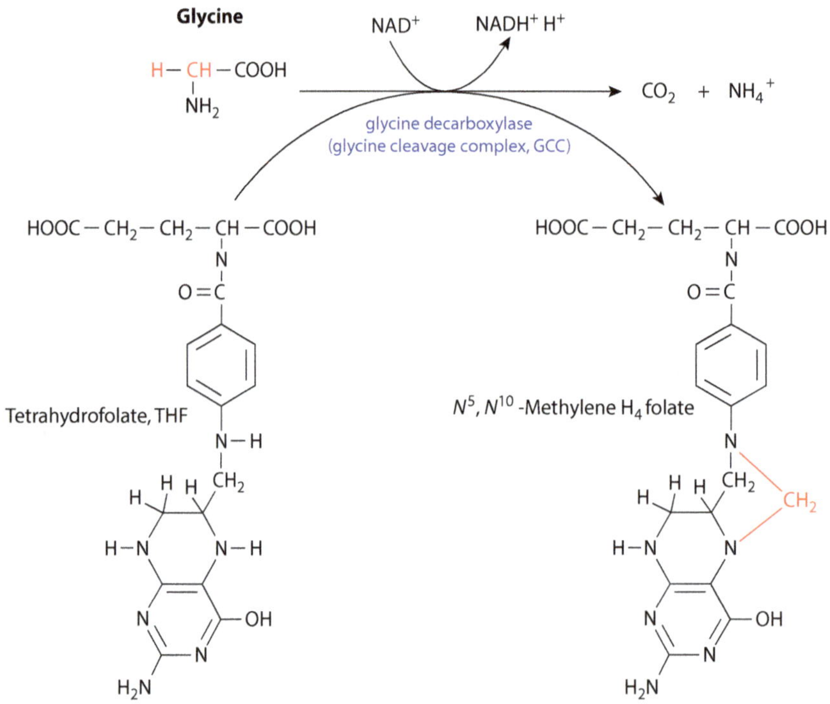

FIGURE 18–8 Reaction catalyzed by glycine decarboxylase. (Reproduced with permission from themedicalbiochemistrypage, LLC.)

CLINICAL BOX 18–4 NONKETOTIC HYPERGLYCINEMIA

Nonketotic hyperglycinemia (NKH) is an autosomal recessive inborn error of glycine metabolism due to deficiencies in the H, P, or T proteins of the glycine decarboxylase complex. Mutations in the P protein are the most common. NKH, also known as glycine encephalopathy, is characterized by severe mental retardation that is due to highly elevated levels of glycine in the CNS. Infants generally present with severe lethargy, seizures, and respiratory depression requiring mechanical ventilation. A diagnosis of NKH associated with these symptoms is made secondary to elevated plasma and cerebrospinal fluid glycine concentrations. The prognosis for infants with NKH is poor, with severe neurologic impairment, intractable seizures, and death common before 5 years of age.

ARGININE METABOLISM

The synthesis and catabolism of arginine in mammals takes place within the context of the urea cycle (see Chapter 17).

PROLINE AND ORNITHINE METABOLISM

Glutamate is the precursor of both proline and ornithine (Figure 18–9), with glutamate semialdehyde being a branch point intermediate leading to one or the other of these two amino acids. While ornithine is not one of the 20 amino acids used in protein synthesis, it plays a significant role as the acceptor of carbamoyl phosphate in the urea cycle. Ornithine serves an additional important role as the precursor for the synthesis of the polyamines. Because proline can be converted to ornithine, the catabolism of both proline and ornithine involves the entry of ornithine into the urea cycle.

PHENYLALANINE AND TYROSINE METABOLISM

Phenylalanine serves as the precursor for tyrosine via the tetrahydrobiopterin-requiring enzyme, phenylalanine hydroxylase, PAH (Figure 18–10). Thus, phenylalanine catabolism initiates with its conversion to tyrosine and then the pathway of tyrosine catabolism. During the course of the PAH-catalyzed reaction, tetrahydrobiopterin (BH_4) is converted to an intermediate identified as pterin 4α-carbinolamine (also called 4α-hydroxypterin or

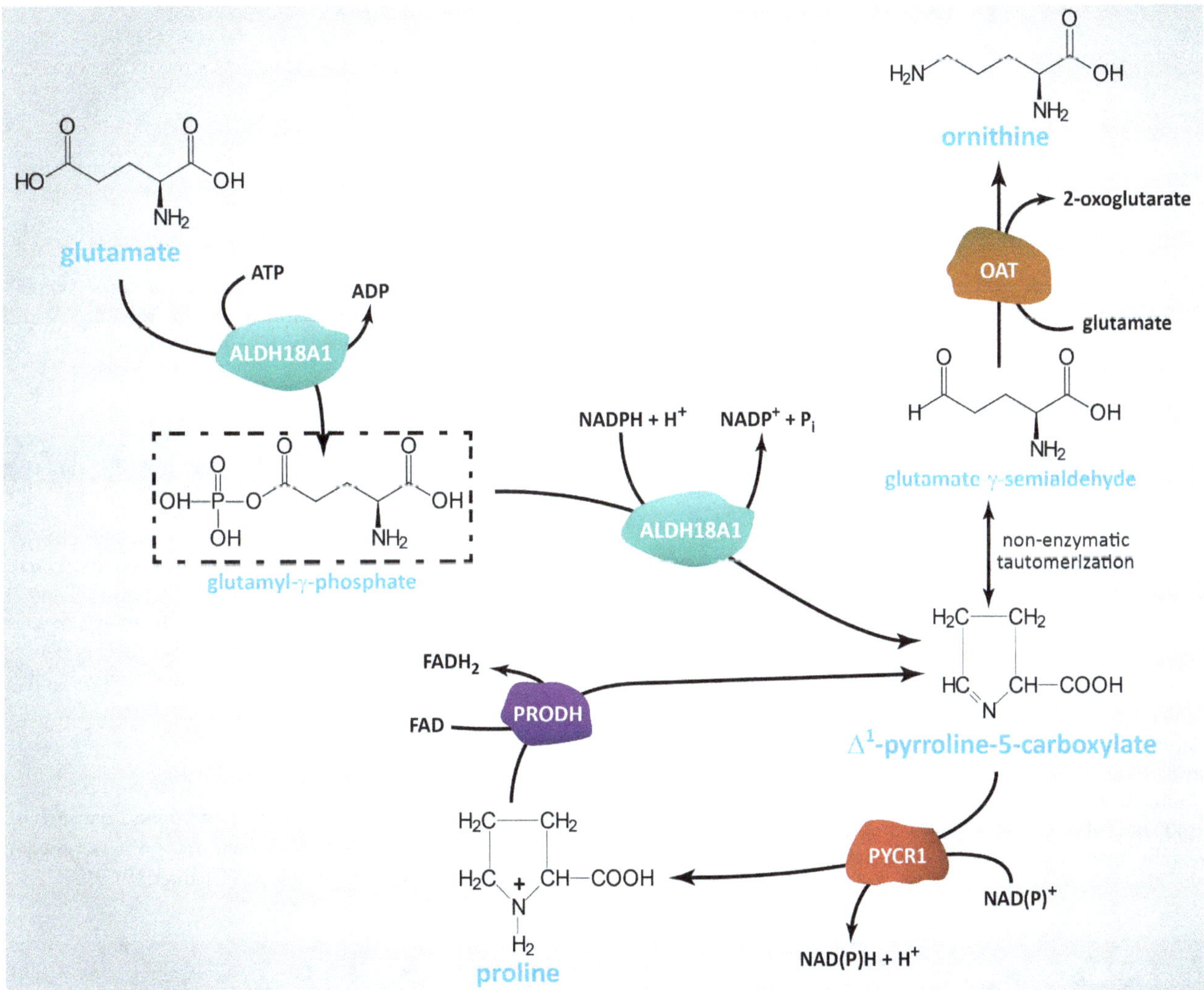

FIGURE 18–9 Synthesis of ornithine and proline. Glutamate serves as the precursor for the synthesis of both ornithine and proline which are derived from the Δ^1-pyrroline-5-carboxylate intermediate in the pathway. Formation of Δ^1-pyrroline-5-carboxylate occurs via the action of the bifunctional enzyme, aldehyde dehydrogenase 18 family, member A1 (also known as delta-1-pyrroline-5-carboxylate synthase). The transamination of the tautomeric form of Δ^1-pyrroline-5-carboxylate (glutamate γ-semialdehyde) results in the generation of ornithine. The reduction of Δ^1-pyrroline-5-carboxylate to proline occurs via the action of pyrroline-5-carboxylate reductase 1 (PYCR1). PRODH is proline dehydrogenase, the first enzyme in the pathway of proline catabolism which converts proline back to Δ^1-pyrroline-5-carboxylate. (Reproduced with permission from themedicalbiochemistrypage, LLC.)

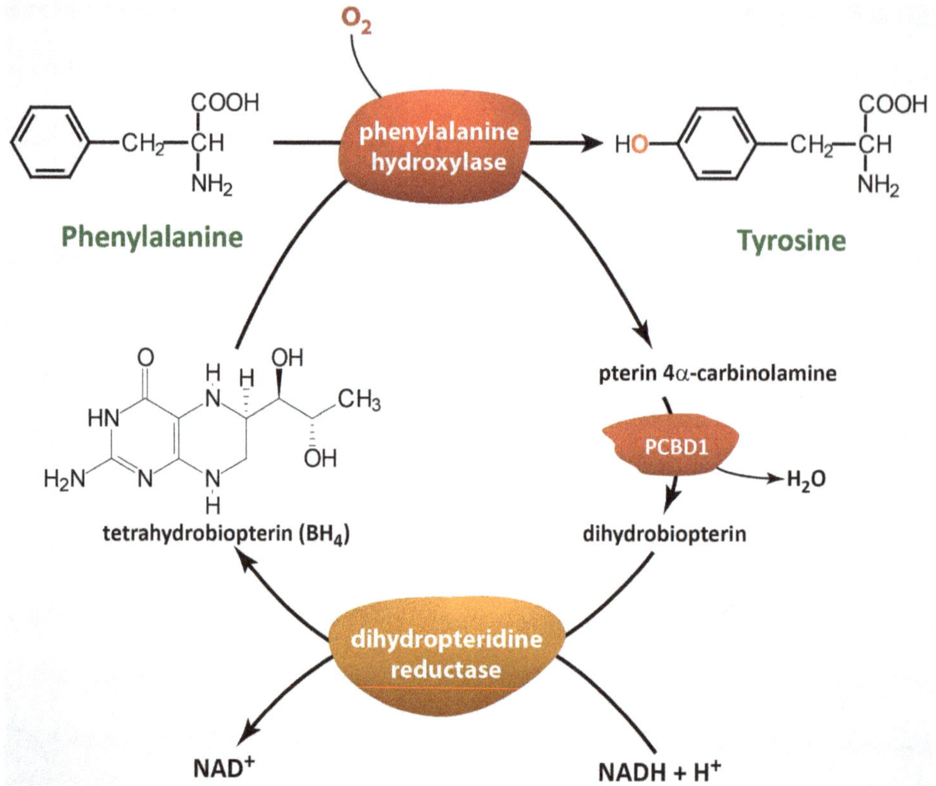

FIGURE 18–10 Biosynthesis of tyrosine from phenylalanine. Phenylalanine serves as the precursor for tyrosine. The conversion of phenylalanine to tyrosine can also be considered the first step in the catabolism of phenylalanine as this conversion reaction is necessary to catabolize phenylalanine. PCBD1 is pterin 4α-carbinolamine dehydratase. (Reproduced with permission from themedicalbiochemistrypage, LLC.)

4α-hydroxydihydrobiopterin). The regeneration of BH_4 involves the enzymes pterin 4α-carbinolamine dehydratase 1 and dihydropteridine reductase (DHPR).

HIGH-YIELD CONCEPT

Missing or deficient PAH results in hyperphenylalaninemia. Hyperphenylalaninemia is defined as a plasma phenylalanine concentration greater than 2 mg/dL (120 μM). The most widely recognized hyperphenylalaninemia (and most severe) is the genetic disease known as phenylketonuria, PKU (Clinical Box 18–5). Patients suffering from PKU have plasma phenylalanine levels more than 1000 μM, whereas the non-PKU hyperphenylalaninemias exhibit levels of plasma phenylalanine less than 1000 μM.

HIGH-YIELD CONCEPT

Because of the requirement for BH_4 in the function of PAH, deficiencies in DHPR can manifest with hyperphenylalaninemia. However, since BH_4 is a cofactor in several other enzyme-catalyzed reactions (eg, the tyrosine- and tryptophan-derived neurotransmitters), the effects of missing or defective DHPR cause even more severe neurologic difficulties than those usually associated with PKU caused by deficient PAH activity.

In addition to its role in protein synthesis, tyrosine is the precursor for the catecholamine neurotransmitters, dopamine, norepinephrine, and epinephrine (see Chapter 19).

CLINICAL BOX 18–5 PHENYLKETONURIA: PKU

Phenylketonuria (PKU) is an autosomal recessive disorder associated with hyperphenylalaninemia that results from defects in the metabolism of phenylalanine. PKU represents the most severe form of the hyperphenylalaninemias. There are several hyperphenylalaninemias that are not PKU and are called non-PKU hyperphenylalaninemias (HPA). Hyperphenylalaninemia is defined as a plasma phenylalanine concentration more than 120 μM. PKU is characterized by plasma phenylalanine more than 1000 μM and non-PKU hyperphenylalaninemias have plasma phenylalanine amounts that are less than 1000 μM. PKU is caused by muta catalyzed by PAH involves tetrahydrobiopterin (BH_4) as a cofactor, the HPAs can result from defects in any of the several genes

CLINICAL BOX 18–5 (CONTINUED)

required for synthesis and recycling of BH_4. Removal of excess phenylalanine normally proceeds via the tyrosine biosynthesis reaction and then via tyrosine catabolism. The first reaction in this process is the PAH catalyzed hydroxylation of phenylalanine. Several hundred disease-causing mutations have been identified in the *PAH* gene. The non-PKU HPAs can result from any defect in phenylalanine hydroxylation. Many are the result of defects in the metabolism of the BH_4 cofactor of PAH. During the PAH catalyzed reaction BH_4 is converted to 4α-hydroxytetrahydrobiopterin. The regeneration of BH_4 is catalyzed by reactions that involve 4α-carbinolamine dehydratase and dihydropteridine reductase (DHPR). In addition to these latter two enzymes, BH_4 can be synthesized in a pathway that requires guanosine triphosphate cyclohydrolase, 6-pyruvoyltetrahydrobiopterin synthase, and sepiapterin reductase. A deficiency in any of the five enzymes will lead to defects in phenylalanine hydroxylation and consequently hyperphenylalaninemia. Because BH_4 is involved in additional hydroxylation reactions, notably tryptophan and tyrosine in the brain in the formation of serotonin and the catecholamines, respectively, it is important to correctly diagnose any HPA as being the result of abnormal BH_4 homeostasis or defects in PAH. The major clinical manifestation associated with PKU and many HPAs is impaired cognitive development and function. The precise mechanism for the intellectual impairment associated with PKU has not been worked out but is thought to be the result of the accumulation of phenylalanine in the brain, which becomes a major donor of amino groups in aminotransferase activity and depletes neural tissue of α-ketoglutarate (2-oxoglutarate). The absence of α-ketoglutarate in the brain shuts down the TCA cycle and the associated production of aerobic energy, which is essential to normal brain development. Another hypothesis proposed to explain the severe intellectual impairment that can result in untreated PKU patients is that the accumulating phenylalanine impairs the transport of tyrosine into the brain. The reduction in brain tyrosine levels would then negatively impact the synthesis of the neurotransmitters, dopamine and norepinephrine. The product of phenylalanine transamination, phenylpyruvic acid, is reduced to phenylacetate and phenyllactate, and all three compounds appear in the urine (Figure 18–11). The presence of phenylacetate in the urine and sweat imparts a "mousy" odor. Currently in this country (and many others as well), newborns are routinely screened for PKU by measurement of serum phenylalanine levels. All HPAs, including PKU, occur with a frequency of 5–350 cases/million live births. In order to classify the phenotype of PKU into severe and less severe forms, as well as to exclude BH_4-deficient HPAs, it is necessary to measure the plasma, urine, and cerebrospinal fluid levels of phenylalanine, pterins, and the derivatives of the neurotransmitters derived from tryptophan and tyrosine. The mainstay in treatment of PKU is the low-phenylalanine diet. Optimal treatment requires both early-onset (hence the utility of the postnatal assessments in this country) and continuous treatment throughout adolescence and possibly for life. Because of the necessity for phenylalanine in protein synthesis and neurotransmitter synthesis (via conversion to tyrosine) it is important to carefully control the intake of the amino acid. Too little and developmental impairment will occur, too much and severe neurologic dysfunction will result.

The catabolism of tyrosine (and phenylalanine) yields fumarate and acetoacetate. Mutations in genes encoding three of the enzymes of phenylalanine and tyrosine catabolism result in a family of disorders referred to as the tyrosinemias, also called hypertyrosinemias (Clinical Box 18–6).

HIGH-YIELD CONCEPT

The first inborn error in metabolism ever recognized, alkaptonuria, was demonstrated to be the result of a defect in phenylalanine and tyrosine catabolism. Alkaptonuria is caused by defective homogentisic acid oxidase. Homogentisic acid accumulation is relatively innocuous, causing urine to darken on exposure to air, but no life-threatening effects accompany the disease. The only untoward consequence of alkaptonuria is ochronosis (bluish-black discoloration of the tissues) and arthritis.

TRYPTOPHAN METABOLISM

Aside from its role as an amino acid in protein biosynthesis, tryptophan also serves as a precursor for the synthesis of the neurotransmitters, serotonin and melatonin (see Chapter 19) and as the precursor for the synthesis of NAD^+.

During the catabolism of tryptophan (Figure 18–12) the non-protein amino acid, kynurenine is produced. Kynurenine yields kynurenic acid by transamination of α-ketoglutarate (2-oxoglutarate). Kynurenic acid and its metabolites act as antiexcitotoxics and anticonvulsives. High levels of kynurenic acid are found in the urine of individuals suffering from schizophrenia.

Catabolism of kynurenine yields α-amino-β-carboxymuconate-ε-semialdehyde (ACMS) which can undergo complete oxidation to acetoacetyl-CoA or it can spontaneously cyclize to quinolinic acid. Quinolinic acid serves as the precursor for NAD^+ synthesis.

Figure 18-12 Catabolism of tryptophan

THREONINE METABOLISM

There are at least three pathways for threonine catabolism that have been identified in mammals. The principal threonine catabolizing pathway in humans involves a glycine-independent serine/threonine dehydratase (also known as serine dehydratase/threonine deaminase) yielding α-ketobutyrate (2-ketobutyrate) which is further catabolized to propionyl-CoA. The resulting propionyl-CoA is converted to succinyl-CoA via the same VOMIT pathway that is a part of the catabolism of methionine, isoleucine, and valine. The succinyl-CoA can then enter the TCA cycle for further oxidation.

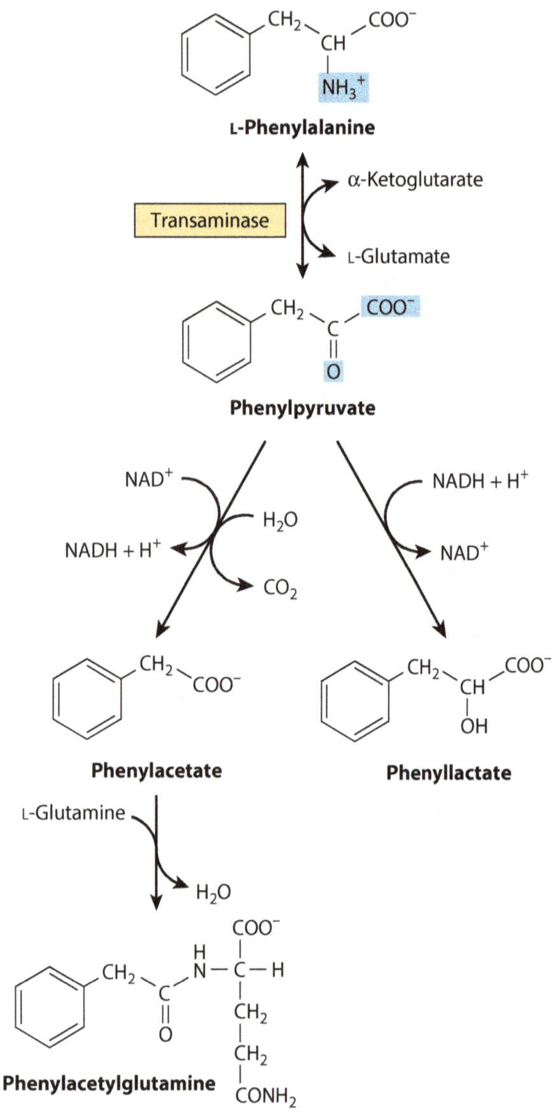

FIGURE 18–11 Alternative pathways of phenylalanine catabolism in phenylketonuria. The reactions also occur in normal liver tissue but are of minor significance. (Reproduced with permission from Rodwell VW, Bender DA, Botham KM, et al: *Harper's Illustrated Biochemistry*, 31st ed. New York, NY: McGraw Hill; 2018.)

LYSINE METABOLISM

Although at least three pathways for lysine catabolism have been identified, the primary pathway utilized in humans occurs within the liver and is called saccharopine pathway (Figure 18–13). The ultimate end product of lysine catabolism, via this pathway, is acetoacetyl-CoA.

Lysine is also important as a precursor for the synthesis of carnitine, required for the transport of fatty acids into the mitochondria for oxidation. Free lysine does not serve as the precursor for this reaction, rather the trimethyllysine found in proteins, particularly the histones.

CLINICAL BOX 18–6 TYROSINEMIAS

Defects in three of the enzymes of tyrosine catabolism result in increased concentrations of tyrosine and metabolites in the blood and urine. These disorders are referred to as the tyrosinemias and are also often referred to as the hypertyrosinemias. Because of the involvement of mutations in three distinct genes in the etiology of tyrosinemia, there are three distinct forms identified as tyrosinemia type 1, type 2, and type 3. Mutations in the *FAH* gene result in life-threatening disorder, tyrosinemia type 1 (TYRSN1). TYRSN1 is an autosomal recessive disorder characterized by hypertyrosinemia and progressive liver disease. This disorder also leads to a secondary renal tubular dysfunction resulting in hypophosphatemic rickets. Defects in the *FAH* gene result in the accumulation of the upstream tyrosine metabolites, maleylacetoacetate and fumarylacetoacetate, as well as their metabolic by-products succinylacetone and succinylacetoacetate. The compounds are toxic to cells, particularly liver and kidney, explaining the pathology associated with this disease. Succinylacetone is also a potent inhibitor of δ-aminolevulinic acid dehydratase (also called porphobilinogen synthase) leading to accumulation of δ-aminolevulinic acid (ALA). ALA is neurotoxic and thought to be the cause of the acute porphyria-like pathology in this TYRSN1. Inherited mutations in the *TAT* gene lead to tyrosinemia type 2 (TYRSN2; also called Richner-Hanhart syndrome) which, as the name implies, is associated with elevated tyrosine levels in the blood and, consequently the urine. This form of tyrosinemia is associated with intellectual impairment, painful corneal eruptions, photophobia, keratitis, and painful palmoplantar hyperkeratosis. Mutations in the *HPD* gene result in tyrosinemia type 3 (TYRSN3). TYRSN3 is an autosomal recessive disease that, in addition to hypertyrosinemia, is associated with mild intellectual impairment and/or convulsions but these patients do not display hepatic damage as is characteristic of tyrosinemia type 1.

HISTIDINE METABOLISM

In addition to serving in protein synthesis, histidine is the precursor for the biogenic amine, histamine (Figure 18–14). Catabolism of histidine is an important pathway for the generation of the tetrahydrofolate (THF) derivative, N^5-formimino-THF catalyzed by formimidoyltransferase cyclodeaminase (FTCD). The end product of histidine catabolism is glutamate.

Inherited defects in the *FTCD* gene represent the second most common cause of inborn errors in folate metabolism. Potential for severe intellectual impairment is the main clinical feature associated with FTCD deficiency. Patients with FTCD defects will also present with megaloblastic anemia due to the role of folate derivatives in the synthesis of purine and thymine nucleotides.

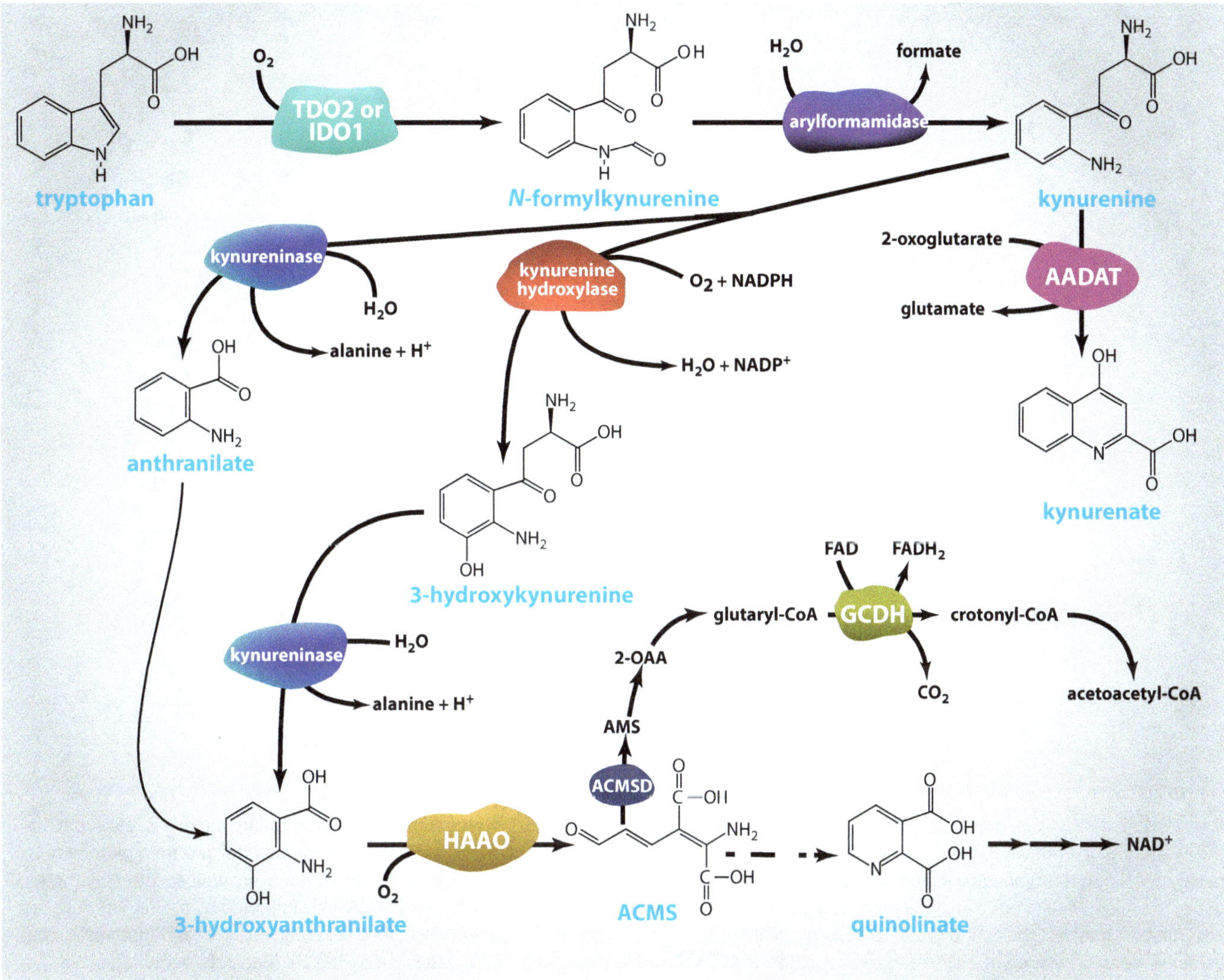

FIGURE 18–12 Tryptophan catabolism to acetoacetate also involves functional metabolism to several important bioactive compounds. These compounds include the nicotinamide adenine dinucleotide co-factors, NAD^+ and $NADP^+$, kynurenic acid, and quinolinic acid. TDO2: tryptophan 2,3-dioxygenase; IDO1: indoleamine 2,3-dioxygenase 1; AADAT: aminoadipate aminotransferase. Kynurenine hydroxylase is also identified as kynurenine 3-monooxygenase. HAAO: 3-hydroxyanthranilate 3,4-dioxygenase; ACMSD: α-amino-β-carboxymuconate-ε-semialdehyde decarboxylase; ACMS: α-amino-β-carboxymuconate-ε-semialdehyde; AMS: α-aminomuconate-ε-semialdehyde; 2-OAA: 2-oxoadipic acid (also called α-ketoadipic acid or 2-ketoadipic acid); GCDH: glutaryl-CoA dehydrogenase. ACMS spontaneously cyclizes into quinolinic acid (quinolinate). (Reproduced with permission from themedicalbiochemistrypage, LLC.)

LEUCINE, ISOLEUCINE, AND VALINE: BRANCHED-CHAIN AMINO ACID METABOLISM

Leucine, isoleucine, and valine are the branched-chain amino acids, BCAA. The catabolism of all three amino acids occurs in most cells but the highest rates of catabolism take place in skeletal muscle. BCAA catabolism yields both NADH and $FADH_2$ which can be utilized for ATP generation which is a primary reason for their high rates of catabolism in skeletal muscle. The catabolism of all three of these amino acids uses the same enzymes in the first two steps (Figure 18–15).

The principal products of leucine catabolism are acetyl-CoA and acetoacetyl-CoA. The end product of valine is propionyl-CoA which is converted to succinyl-CoA in the VOMIT pathway. Isoleucine catabolism terminates with production of acetyl-CoA and propionyl-CoA.

There are a number of genetic diseases associated with faulty catabolism of the BCAA. These disorders include isovaleric

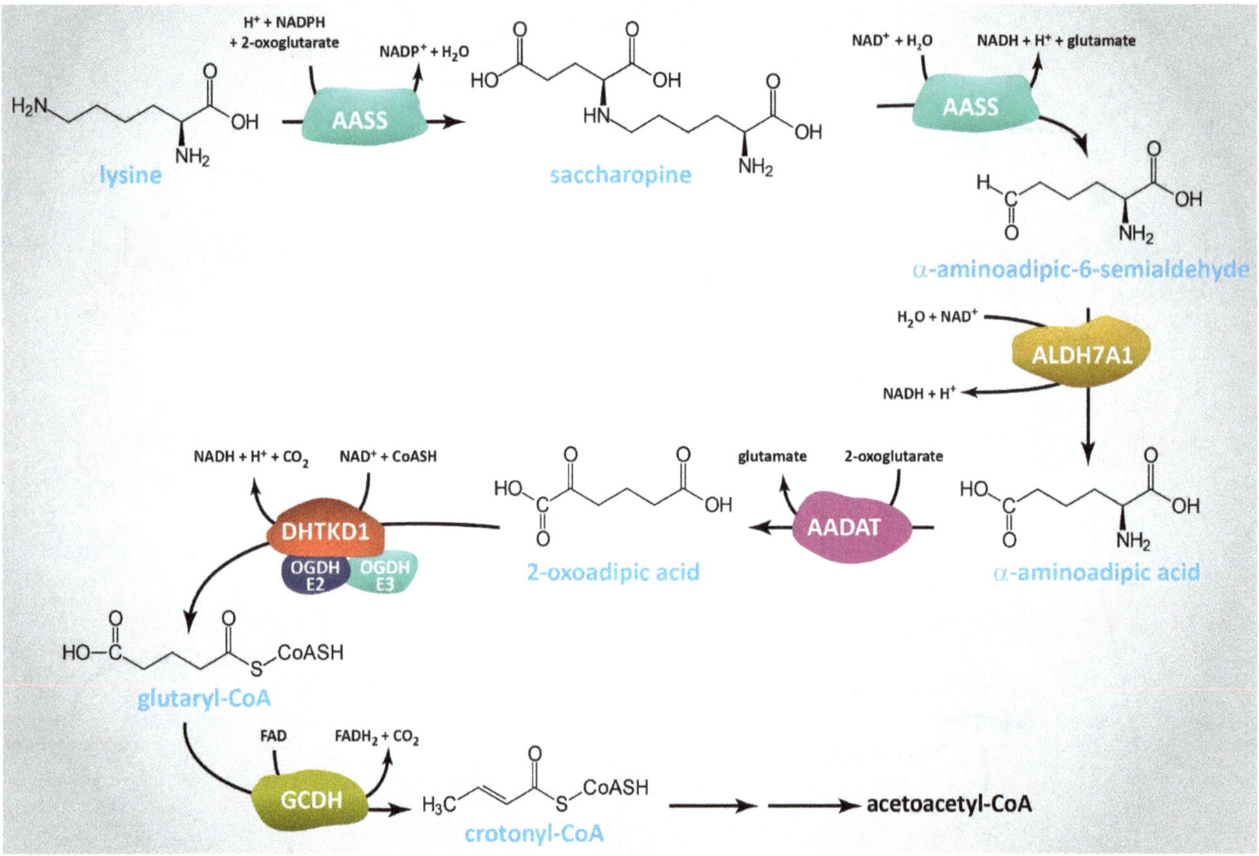

FIGURE 18–13 Catabolism of lysine via the major hepatic pathway. The major pathway for lysine catabolism in humans is referred to as the saccharopine pathway. Lysine is converted to saccharopine by condensation with 2-oxoglutarate (α-ketoglutarate) and then glutamate is released yielding α-aminoadipic-6-semialdehyde (2-AMAS). These two reactions are catalyzed by the bifunctional enzyme encoded by the *AASS* gene. The ALDH7A1 encoded enzyme then reduces 2-AMAS to α-aminoadipic acid (2-AMA). The 2-AMA is deaminated by the AADAT encoded enzyme that transfers the amino group to 2-oxoglutarate yielding 2-oxoadipic acid (2-OAA; also called α-ketoadipic acid) and glutamate. The oxidative decarboxylation of 2-OAA and condensation with CoASH to form glutaryl-CoA is catalyzed by the 2-oxoadipate dehydrogenase complex whose E1 subunits are encoded by the *DHTKD1* gene. The E2 and E3 subunits of this complex are shared with the 2-oxoglutarate dehydrogenase (α-ketoglutarate dehydrogenase) complex of the TCA cycle. Glutaryl-CoA is oxidatively decarboxylated to crotonyl-CoA via glutaryl-CoA dehydrogenase (GCDH). The crotonyl-CoA is converted to β-hydroxybutyryl-CoA and β-hydroxybutyryl-CoA is converted to acetoacetyl-CoA, the end product of lysine catabolism. (Reproduced with permission from themedicalbiochemistrypage, LLC.)

acidemia, 3-methylcrotonylglycinuria, 3-hydroxy-3-methylglutaric aciduria, isobutyrylglycinuria, short/branched-chain acyl-CoA dehydrogenase deficiency, and beta-ketothiolase deficiency. This latter disease results from mutations in the *ACAT1* (acetyl-CoA acetyltransferase 1) gene which is somewhat inappropriately identified as β-ketothiolase (3-ketothiolase) deficiency.

The most common defect in the catabolism of the BCAA is in the branched-chain α-keto acid dehydrogenase, BCKD. Since there is only one dehydrogenase enzyme for all three amino acids, all three α-keto acids accumulate and are excreted in the urine. The disease is known as maple syrup urine disease, MSUD, (Clinical Box 18–7) because of the characteristic odor of the urine in afflicted individuals.

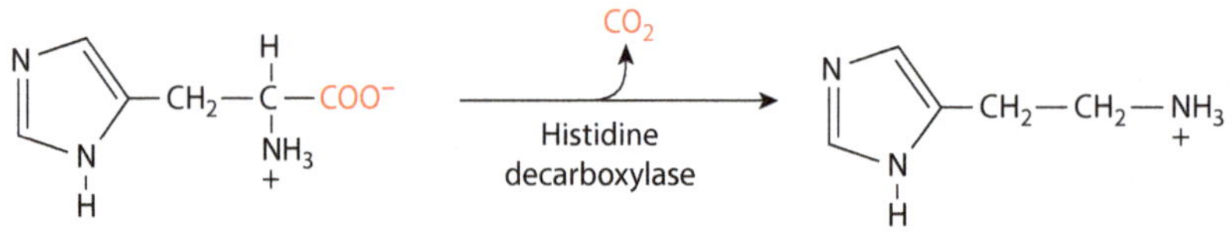

FIGURE 18–14 Synthesis of histamine. (Reproduced with permission from themedicalbiochemistrypage, LLC.)

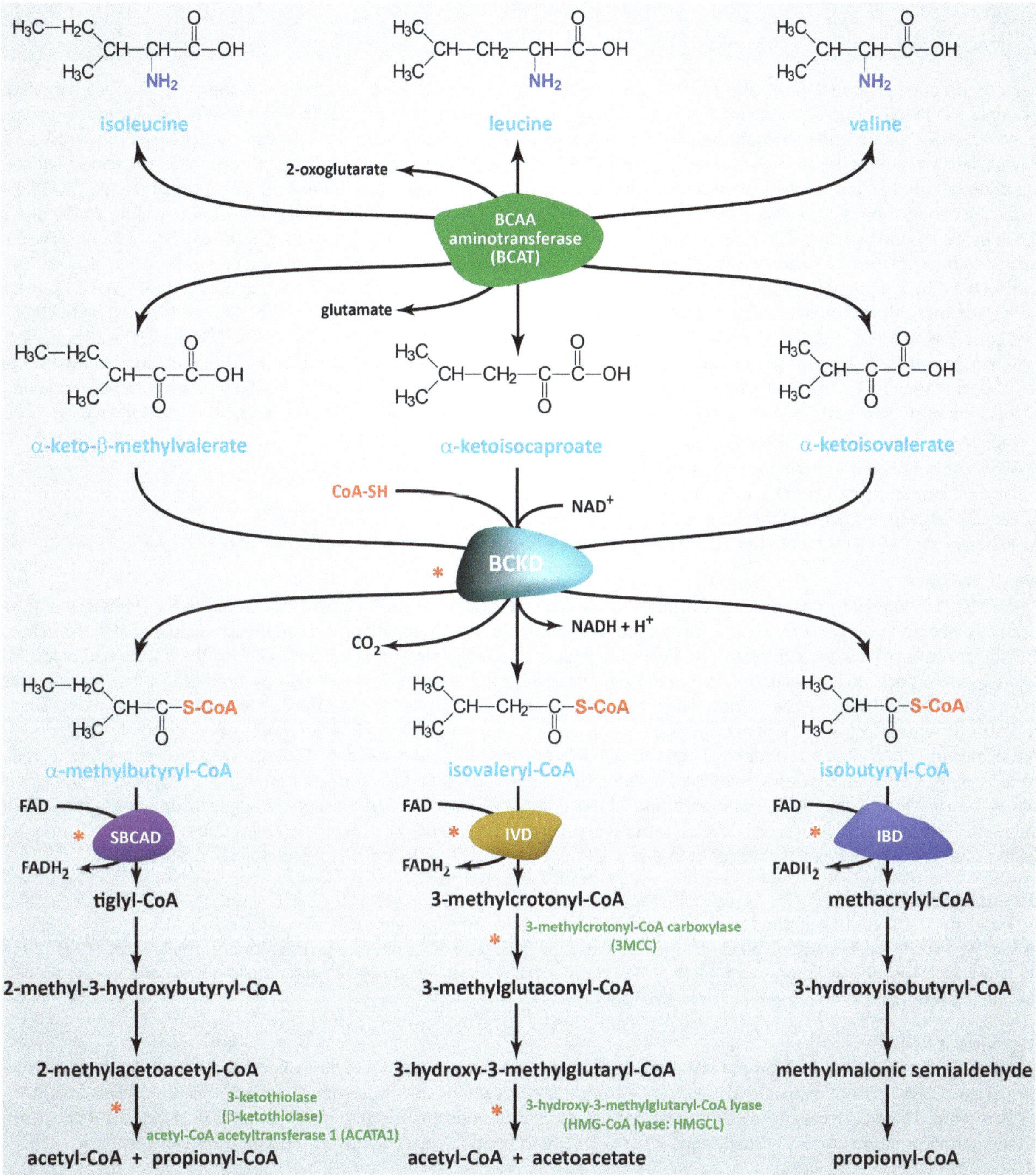

FIGURE 18–15 Catabolism of the branched-chain amino acids. The three branched-chain amino acids, isoleucine, leucine, and valine enter the catabolic pathway via the action of the same two enzymes. The initial deamination of all three amino acids is catalyzed by one of two branched-chain amino acid transaminases (BCATc or BCATm). The resulting α-ketoacids are then oxidatively decarboxylated via the action of the enzyme complex, branched-chain α-keto acid dehydrogenase (BCKD). The BCKD reaction generates the CoA derivatives of the decarboxylated ketoacids while also generating the reduced electron carrier, NADH. After these first two reactions the remainder of the catabolic pathways for the three amino acids diverges. The third reaction of branched-chain amino acid catabolism involves a dehydrogenation step that involves three distinct enzymes, one for each of the CoA derivatives generated via the BCKD reaction. This latter dehydrogenation step also yields additional reduced electron carrier as $FADH_2$. The third reaction of isoleucine catabolism involves the enzyme short/branched-chain acyl-CoA dehydrogenase (SBCAD). The SBCAD enzyme is encoded by the *ACADSB* gene. The third reaction of leucine catabolism involves the enzyme isovaleryl-CoA dehydrogenase (IVD). The third reaction of valine catabolism involves the enzyme isobutyryl-CoA dehydrogenase (IBD). The IBD enzyme is encoded by the acyl-CoA dehydrogenase family, member 8 (*ACAD8*) gene. These CoA dehydrogenases belong to the same family of dehydrogenases involved in the process of mitochondrial fatty acid oxidation. Red asterisks denote enzymes whose deficiencies are associated with known disorders. (Reproduced with permission from themedicalbiochemistrypage, LLC.)

CLINICAL BOX 18–7 MAPLE SYRUP URINE DISEASE

Maple syrup urine disease (MSUD), also called branched-chain aminoaciduria, is so called because the urine of affected individuals smells like maple syrup or burnt sugar. MSUD is an autosomal recessive disorder that results from a deficiency in the enzyme, branched-chain α-keto acid dehydrogenase (BCKD), that is involved in the catabolism of the branched-chain amino acids (BCAAs) leucine, isoleucine, and valine. A deficiency in BCKD leads to an accumulation of those three amino acids and their corresponding branched-chain α-keto acids (BCKA). MSUD is associated with a worldwide frequency of approximately 1 in 185,000 people. In certain inbred populations such as the Old Order Mennonites the incidence of MSUD is extremely high, on the order of 1 in every 175 births. The BCKD complex is a multimeric mitochondrial enzyme composed of three catalytic subunits. The E1 portion of the complex is a thiamine pyrophosphate (TPP)-dependent decarboxylase with a subunit structure of $\alpha_2\beta_2$. The E2 portion is a dihydrolipoamide branched-chain transacylase composed of 24 lipoic acid-containing polypeptides. The E3 portion is a homodimeric flavoprotein identified as dihydrolipoamide dehydrogenase, DLD. The E1α subunits are encoded by the *BCKDHA* gene. The E1β subunits are encoded by the *BCKDHB* gene. The E2 subunits are encoded by the *DBT* gene. The E3 subunits are encoded by the *DLD* gene, the same gene that encodes the dihydrolipoamide dehydrogenase subunits found in the PDH and the 2-oxoglutarate (α-ketoglutarate) dehydrogenase complexes. The genetic heterogeneity in MSUD patients can be explained by the complexity in the structure of BCKD. There are four molecular phenotypes of MSUD based on the affected locus:

Type IA is due to mutations in the E1α gene.
Type IB is due to mutations in the E1β gene.
Type II is due to mutations in the E2 gene.
Type III is due to mutations in the E3 gene.
To date, a total of 63 mutations have been identified in the four genes of the catalytic portion of BCKD.

Classic MSUD

Classic MSUD is defined by neonatal onset of encephalopathy and is the most severe form of the disorder. The levels of the BCAAs, especially leucine, and their α-keto acids, are dramatically elevated in the blood, urine, and cerebrospinal fluid of afflicted infants. The primary cause of the encephalopathy and neurodegeneration in MSUD infants is the high levels of the α-keto acid of leucine, α-ketoisocaproic acid, in the brain. This compound triggers apoptosis in neurons and glial cells by interfering with mitochondrial energy metabolism. The presence of alloisoleucine in the fluids is highly diagnostic of MSUD. The level of BCKD activity in classic MSUD patients is less than 2% of normal. Affected infants appear normal at birth but symptoms develop rapidly appearing by 4–7 days after birth. The first distinctive signs are lethargy and little interest in feeding. As the disease progresses, infants will exhibit weight loss and progressive neurologic deterioration. Neurologic signs will alternate from hypo- to hypertonia and extension of the arms resembling decerebrate posturing. At this time the characteristic burnt sugar or maple syrup odor to the urine is apparent. If left untreated infants will develop seizures, lapse into a coma, and die. The prognosis for untreated infants is poor with death occurring within several months of birth due to complications of metabolic crisis and neurologic deterioration.

Intermediate MSUD

Intermediate MSUD is distinguished from classic in that patients do not experience the severity of classic MSUD in the neonatal period. Infants will have persistent elevation in BCAAs in body fluids as well as neurologic impairment. The level of BCKD in intermediate MSUD individuals ranges from 3% to 30% of normal. Many intermediate MSUD patients do not experience the acute metabolic decompensation present in classic MSUD.

Intermittent MSUD

In patients with the intermittent form of MSUD the activity of BCKD ranges from 5% to 50% of normal. These individuals will show normal early development with normal intelligence. During periods when patients are asymptomatic their fluid levels of BCAAs will be normal. These patients are however, at risk for acute metabolic decompensation during periods of stress. Initial symptoms of the intermittent form of MSUD usually appear between 5 months and 2 years of age in association with an infection.

Thiamine-responsive MSUD

There is a similar course of progress in the symptoms of thiamine-responsive MSUD patients to that seen in intermediate MSUD patients. Plasma BCAA levels are around five times normal and alloisoleucine is characteristically detectable in these patients. Administration of thiamine and consumption of a low-protein diet results in a reduction of BCAA levels to normal. Withdrawal of thiamine treatment results in a rapid rebound in the elevation of plasma BCAA concentration. These responses to thiamine are the reason for this classification of MSUD. There is a wide range of heterogeneity in thiamine-responsive MSUD patients and thiamine treatment alone is insufficient to result in lower levels of BCAAs.

Dihydrolipoyl dehydrogenase (E3)-deficient MSUD

As the name of this classification implies, this form of MSUD is due to a deficiency in the E3 component of the BCKD complex. This form of MSUD is very rare with only 20 reported cases. The symptoms of the E3-deficient form are similar to those of intermediate MSUD, but there is an accompanying severe lactic acidosis. Infants with the E3-deficient form of MSUD are relatively normal for the first few months of life. Persistent lactic acidosis will be seen to develop between 2 and 6 months of age.

CHECKLIST

- ☑ Amino acids serve at least two critically important functions in cells. They are precursors for protein synthesis and conversely, they can be oxidized to yield energy for ATP synthesis. Many amino acids serve additional functions in the body such as the neurotransmitter amino acids and amino acid derivatives.
- ☑ Dietary amino acids are absorbed via the action of specific intestinal enterocyte transporter proteins. Deficiency in the neutral amino acid transporter, found in the intestines and the kidneys, is the cause of Hartnup disorder.
- ☑ Amino acids are classified as essential if they cannot be synthesized by cells of the body or derived from precursor compounds.
- ☑ Oxidation of amino acids yields carbon compounds that can serve as precursors for glucose synthesis via gluconeogenesis or compounds that can only be delivered to the TCA cycle for further oxidation. The former are referred to as glucogenic amino acids, the latter as ketogenic.
- ☑ Glutamate and glutamine are two of the most important metabolic amino acids in the body; they serve as reservoirs of nitrogen and as the carbon skeletons for the TCA cycle intermediate, α-ketoglutarate. Glutamine is the major nitrogen containing compound in the blood.
- ☑ Glutamate serves as the precursor for the synthesis of the neurotransmitter, GABA.
- ☑ Alanine plays a critical role in the delivery of waste nitrogen, primarily from skeletal muscle, to the liver. The carbon skeleton of alanine is pyruvate which can be used for glucose synthesis; this process is termed the glucose-alanine cycle.
- ☑ Methionine serves as the precursor for the synthesis of cysteine; deficiency in cystathione β-synthase is the major cause of homocystinurias. Methionine is also the precursor for *S*-adenosylmethionine which is the principal methyl donor for the synthesis of the catecholamines and polyamines.
- ☑ Glycine and serine are interconverted via the action of serine-hydroxymethyltransferase. Serine can be synthesized from a glycolytic intermediate. Glycine is a neurotransmitter and also serves as a precursor in the synthesis of heme, creatine, and purine nucleotides.
- ☑ Tyrosine is derived from the hydroxylation of phenylalanine. Deficiency in the enzyme catalyzing this reaction results in the hyperphenylalaninemia called PKU. Tyrosine also serves as the precursor for the synthesis of the catecholamines.
- ☑ Tryptophan serves an important role as the precursor for the synthesis of serotonin and melatonin.
- ☑ Lysine serves as the precursor for the synthesis of carnitine which is required for mitochondrial uptake of fatty acids.
- ☑ Histidine serves as the precursor for the neurotransmitter histamine.
- ☑ Leucine, isoleucine, and valine are the branched-chain amino acids. Catabolism of these amino acids initially involves the same two enzymes. Deficiency in one of these enzymes, branched-chain α-keto-acid decarboxylase (BCKD) is the cause of maple syrup urine disease.

REVIEW QUESTIONS

1. A 7-year-old girl with mild intellectual impairment was healthy at birth but presented during the first week of life with vomiting, lethargy, seizures, and hypertonia. During this early period blood work showed ketoacidosis with elevated levels of α-ketoisocaproic acid. Based upon these findings, the patient was placed on an amino acid restrictive diet which relieved many of the symptoms and allowed for relatively normal physical development. Which of the following enzymes is most likely deficient in this child?
(A) Branched chain α-keto acid dehydrogenase
(B) Cystathionine β-synthase
(C) Glycine decarboxylase (glycine cleavage complex)
(D) Phenylalanine hydroxylase
(E) Propionyl-CoA carboxylase

2. An 11-month-old boy has been brought to the physician because of lethargy and irritability for the past 3 days. These symptoms appeared following the diagnosis of acute otitis media for which the pediatrician prescribed amoxicillin. At the time of examination, laboratory studies indicated the serum was pH 7.29 (N = 7.35–7.45) and bicarbonate was 14 mEq/L (N = 22–26 mEq/L). In addition, there was a measurable increase in serum valine concentration. Given the most likely metabolic disorder associated with these signs and symptoms, which of the following would also most likely be elevated in the serum of this patient?
(A) Arginine and lysine
(B) Asparagine and glutamine
(C) Homocysteine and cysteine
(D) Leucine and isoleucine
(E) Phenylalanine and tyrosine

3. A 10-day-old girl is being examined by her pediatrician due to concerns raised by her parents about the odd shape of her eyes. Physical examination shows no other overt abnormalities. Serum studies show a methionine concentration

of 1175 μM (N <50 μM). Based upon the findings in this infant, which of the following enzymes is most likely to be deficient?
(A) Branched-chain α-keto acid dehydrogenase
(B) Cystathionine β-synthase
(C) Methionine synthase
(D) Phenylalanine hydroxylase
(E) Tyrosine aminotransferase

4. A 2-year-old boy is brought to the physician's office for evaluation of severe developmental delay. The parents say that his urine has always had a strange musty odor. Physical examination shows the boy has fair colored hair, pale skin, and pale blue irises. Which of the following processes is most likely deficient in this patient?
(A) Glycine conversion to serine
(B) Homocysteine conversion to cystathionine
(C) Phenylalanine conversion to tyrosine
(D) Tryptophan conversion to serotonin
(E) Tyrosine conversion to melanin

5. A physician is examining a pediatric patient brought in by his parents because they are disturbed by his progressive mood changes and apparent heightened anxiety. In addition, the parents report that the child appears to have a high degree of sensitivity to sunlight, with a rash forming with only a few minutes of exposure. Physical examination shows signs of cerebellar ataxia that include unsteady gait and uncoordinated eye movements. Additional findings include a reddish rash on the child's face, arms, and hands. Serum and urinalysis show significant aminoacidemia and aciduria. Measurement of urine levels of which of the following would be most informative for a correct diagnosis?
(A) Alanine
(B) Alloisoleucine
(C) Glutamine
(D) β-Hydroxybutyrate
(E) Tryptophan

6. A 23-year-old woman is brought to the ER because of a 1-hour history of severe pain and coldness of her left leg. History shows that she dropped out of high school in the 10th grade due to difficulty with comprehension. Intelligence testing demonstrated her IQ to be 80 at that time. Her parents and two older siblings have normal intelligence and have no history of these symptoms. Physical examination shows mottling and loss of pulses in the left lower extremity and foot. Arteriography of the left lower extremity shows thrombosis of the femoral artery. This patient most likely has a metabolic disorder involving which of the following amino acids?
(A) Glycine
(B) Leucine
(C) Methionine
(D) Phenylalanine
(E) Tyrosine

7. A 3-year-old boy with severe intellectual impairment is brought to the physician because of a 4-week history of progressively frequent generalized tonic-clonic seizures. There is no available record of newborn screening. He has blond hair and blue eyes. Physical examination shows patches of dry thickened skin on the face, neck, and inner creases of the elbows and knees. Serum studies for amino acid concentrations are pending. Urine studies show increased concentrations of phenylpyruvate. Given these findings, which of the following is most likely to be disrupted in this patient?
(A) Amino acid metabolism
(B) Catecholamine synthesis
(C) Glycosphingolipid metabolism
(D) Odd-chain number fatty acid metabolism
(E) Vitamin B_{12} absorption

8. A 5-day-old infant is rushed to the emergency department suffering from a seizure. History reveals that the infant has not fed well since birth and has been vomiting for the past 3 days. Physical examination finds that the infant is extremely lethargic. Blood work finds ketonuria, hypoglycemia, hyperammonemia, and high anion gap metabolic acidosis. Based on the signs and symptoms in this infant, which of the following is the most likely disorder?
(A) Alkaptonuria
(B) Homocystinuria
(C) Isovaleric acidemia
(D) Maple syrup urine disease
(E) Propionic acidemia

9. A physician is examining a pediatric patient brought in by his parents because they are disturbed by his progressive mood changes and apparent heightened anxiety. Physical examination shows pellegra-like skin eruptions and signs of cerebellar ataxia that include unsteady gait and uncoordinated eye movements. Serum and urinalysis show significant aminoacidemia and aciduria. Measurement of urine levels of which of the following would be most informative for a correct diagnosis?
(A) Alanine
(B) Alloisoleucine
(C) Glutamine
(D) β-Hydroxybutyrate
(E) Tryptophan

10. A 4-year-old boy is being examined by his pediatrician because his parents are disturbed by his progressive mood changes and apparent hightened anxiety. Physical examination shows peeling, redness, and scaling of sun-exposed areas of his skin. The patient also exhibits an unsteady gait and uncoordinated eye movements. Urinalysis finds elevated levels of citrulline, glutamine, phenylalanine, tyrosine, leucine, and tryptophan. Analysis of serum finds normal levels of amino acids. These signs and symptoms are most likely due to which of the following disorders?
(A) Alkaptonuria
(B) Glycine decarboxylase deficiency
(C) Hartnup disorder
(D) Maple syrup urine disease
(E) Phenylketonuria (PKU)

11. A 6-month-old female infant is undergoing examination in the emergency department following a seizure. Shortly after admission to the hospital the infant experiences severe respiratory depression necessitating mechanical ventillation. The parents report that their child appeared normal at birth and continued to develop at what was an apparently normal pace until about 1 month earlier when they noticed changes in her behavior. These changes included sleepiness, poor feeding behavior, and a general "floppiness" when they held their infant. Fluid chemistry reveals aminoacidemia, aminoaciduria, and increased amino acid in the CSF. Suspecting an inborn error in metabolism, the attending physician orders a specific molecular test to be performed, the results of which

demonstrate a mutation in a pyridoxal phosphate-dependent dehydrogenase gene. Given the results of these tests, measurement for increased serum levels of which of the following specific amino acids would be most useful in aiding in an acurate diagnosis in this infant?
(A) Arginine
(B) Glutamine
(C) Glycine
(D) Leucine
(E) Phenylalanine

12. A 29-month-old boy has been hospitalized due to chronic diarrhea. He exhibits considerable weight loss such that he is only about 70% of expected weight for age. Physical examination shows areas of scaly peeling skin, significant atrophy of muscle tissue in his limbs, and the presence of a protuberant abdomen. He appears to have a normal amount of subcutaneous adipose tissue. These findings are most consistent with which of the following conditions?
(A) Infectious hepatitis
(B) Kwashiorkor
(C) Marasmus
(D) Type 1 diabetes
(E) von Gierke disease

13. A 3-month-old female infant is being examined by her pediatrician because her mother is concerned about her difficulty in being roused, poor suckling behavior, and that she seems uninterested in eating. In addition, the mother notes that the baby's diapers often smell like burnt sugar. This infant most likely has a defect in which of the following enzymes?
(A) Branched-chain α-keto acid dehydrogenase
(B) Cystathionine β-synthase
(C) Glycine cleavage complex (GCC)
(D) Homogentisate oxidase
(E) Phenylalanine hydroxylase

14. A 5-year-old boy with severe intellectual impairment is brought to the physician because of a 4-week history of progressively frequent generalized tonic-clonic seizures. There is no available record of newborn screening. He has blond hair and blue eyes. Physical examination shows patches of dry, thickened skin on his neck and inner creases of the elbows and knees. Serum studies for amino acid concentrations are pending. Urine studies show increased concentrations of phenylpyruvic and phenyllactic acids. The activity of which of the following enzymes is most likely defective in this patient?
(A) Branched-chain α-keto acid dehydrogenase
(B) Dihydropteridine reductase
(C) Homogentisate oxidase
(D) Phenylalanine hydroxylase
(E) Tyrosine aminotransferase

15. A 13-year-old girl with moderate intellectual impairment is brought to the physician by her mother who is concerned that her daughter has been having difficulty with her vision for the past several weeks. Physical examination shows a fair complexion, malar erythema, and she has long, slender hands and fingers. Ophthalmologic examination shows ectopia lentis bilaterally and inferonasally. Blood tests reveal her cystathionine concentration is below normal. This patient is most likely to have an increased urine concentration of which of the following amino acids?
(A) Cysteine
(B) Leucine
(C) Methionine
(D) Phenylalanine
(E) Tryptophan

16. A 29-year-old man is being examined by his physician with complains of severe pain in his lower right back, nausea, vomiting, and intense sweating. The physician makes a diagnosis of nephrolithiasis. This patient most likely has an increased urine concentration of which of the following?
(A) Arginine and citrulline
(B) Glycine and alanine
(C) Lysine and cystine
(D) Methionine and homocysteine
(E) Phenylalanine and tyrosine

17. A 3-month-old infant is being examined in the emergency department following a seizure. Blood work indicates the child has a serum phenylalanine concentration of 650 μM (N = 30–60 μM). The attending physician places the infant on a low-phenylalanine diet. Upon follow-up 3-days later the level of serum phenylalanine is found to be reduced to 250 μM. However, while at home the infant developed progressive movement disorders, difficulty swallowing, seizures, and a fever. A defect in which of the following enzymes would best explain the lack of a positive outcome on the low phenylalanine diet?
(A) Branched-chain α-keto acid dehydrogenase
(B) Dihydropteridine reductase
(C) Phenylalanine hydroxylase
(D) Tryptophan hydroxylase
(E) Tyrosine hydroxylase

18. A 4-month-old male infant is being examined in the emergency department for behavior that appears to be decerebrate posturing. The infant was examined by a pediatrician 1-month earlier to ascertain the cause of his poor suckling behavior and general lack of interest in feeding. History reveals that the mother notes that in the past few days the infant's urine has taken on an odd odor somewhat like caramelized sugar. Given all the signs and symptoms presenting in this infant it is most likely that he suffers from which of the following conditions?
(A) Alkaptonuria
(B) Homocystinuria
(C) Isovaleric acidemia
(D) Maple syrup urine disease
(E) Phenylketonuria (PKU)
(F) Propionic acidemia

19. A 1-year-old female is being treating in the Emergency Department following a seizure. History indicates that the child was born at home and did not undergo screening for known congenital disorders. Blood work indicates phenylalanine concentration to be 3.7 mg/dL (N = <2 mg/dL) and tyrosine to be 0.6 mg/dL (N = 0.8 ± 0.4 mg/dL). Measurement of serum serotonin level shows it to be abnormally low. A deficiency in which of the following would most likely explain the observations in this patient?
(A) Branched-chain α-keto acid dehydrogenase
(B) Dihydropteridine reductase
(C) Phenylalanine hydroxylase
(D) Propionyl-CoA carboxylase
(E) Tyrosine aminotransferase

20. A 10-year-old girl is undergoing a routine examination by her pediatrician. Physical examination indicates that the child

is thin and has long fingers and toes. Physical examination finds ectopia lentis bilaterally and inferonasally. Psychological profile indicates that the girl is cognitively impaired. Given the observations in this patient, which of the following would most likely have been elevated in her serum shortly after birth?
(A) Leucine
(B) Methionine
(C) Phenylalanine
(D) Serine
(E) Tyrosine

21. A physician is examining a pediatric patient brought in by his parents because they are disturbed by his progressive mood changes and apparent heightened anxiety. In addition, the parents report that the child appears to have a high degree of sensitivity to sunlight, with a rash forming with only a few minutes of exposure. Physical examination shows signs of cerebellar ataxia that include unsteady gait and uncoordinated eye movements. Additional findings include a reddish rash on the child's face, arms, and hands. Which of the following would be the most useful dietary supplement in the treatment of this patient?
(A) High carbohydrate
(B) High fat
(C) High protein
(D) Phenylalanine
(E) Tryptophan
(F) Tyrosine

22. A 5-month-old infant who has been experiencing lethargy, recurrent vomiting, respiratory distress, and muscular hypotonia is brought to the emergency room in a near comatose state. Lab studies show serum pH of 7.27 (N = 7.35–7.45) and bicarbonate of 12 mEq/L (N = 22–26 mEq/L). Further analysis finds elevated levels of methylmalonic acid in both serum and urine. A deficiency in which of the following enzymes would most likely allow for elimination of cobalamin deficiency as the cause of the observations in this patient?
(A) Malonyl-CoA decarboxylase
(B) Methionine synthase
(C) Methylmalonyl-CoA mutase
(D) Methylmalonyl-CoA racemase
(E) Propionyl-CoA carboxylase

23. Arginine is classified as an essential amino acid. Which of the following processes is most likely to be able to provide some of the required daily amount of arginine, even when it may be limiting in the diet?
(A) Catecholamine synthesis
(B) Heme biosynthesis
(C) Peroxisomal fatty acid α-oxidation
(D) Phenylalanine catabolism
(E) Urea cycle

24. A 3-month-old female infant is being examined by her pediatrician because her mother is concerned about her difficulty in being roused, poor suckling behavior, and that she seems uninterested in eating. In addition, the mother notes that the baby's diapers often smell like burnt sugar. This infant most likely has a defect in which of the following metabolic processes?
(A) Amino acid catabolism
(B) Hepatic glycogen synthesis
(C) Mitochondrial fatty acid β-oxidation
(D) Peroxisomal fatty acid α-oxidation
(E) Synthesis of eicosanoids

25. A 3-year-old boy is brought to the emergency department after suffering frequent generalized tonic-clonic seizures. Physical examination shows the boy has blonde hair and blue eyes. History reveals that there is no available record of newborn screening. Given the signs and symptoms in this patient, which of the following is most likely necessary to add as a supplement to his diet?
(A) Citrulline
(B) Linolenic acid
(C) Methionine
(D) Niacin
(E) Tyrosine

26. A 67-year-old woman is being examined by her physician with complaints of chronic back, hip, and knee pain. Physical examination finds bluish-grey macules over the cartilaginous portions of her ears and on the sclera of her eyes. Past medical history included an aortic stenosis. The patient reported that when she sweats it seems to permanently stain her clothing. She also stated that her urine seems to get darker if she does not flush the toilet. These signs and symptoms are most likely indicative of a defect in which of the following processes?
(A) Aromatic amino acid catabolism
(B) Bilirubin conjugation
(C) Branched-chain amino acid catabolism
(D) Peroxisomal fatty acid α-oxidation
(E) Purine nucleotide catabolism

27. A 5-month-old infant who has been experiencing lethargy, recurrent vomiting, respiratory distress, and muscular hypotonia is brought to the emergency room in a near comatose state. Serum studies show elevated levels of methylmalonic acid in both serum and urine. Given the signs and symptoms, which of the following is most likely to also be apparent in this infant?
(A) Homocystinuria
(B) Hyperammonemia
(C) Hypoglycemia
(D) Metabolic acidosis
(E) Metabolic alkalosis

28. A 3-year-old boy with severe intellectual impairment is brought to the physician because of a 4-week history of progressively frequent generalized seizures. There is no available record of newborn screening. He has blond hair and blue eyes. Physical examination shows patches of dry thickened skin on the face, neck, and inner creases of the elbows and knees. Serum studies for amino acid concentrations are pending. Urine studies show increased concentrations of phenylpyruvate. Given the symptoms and findings in this infant, which is the most likely mode with which his disease was inherited?
(A) Autosomal dominant
(B) Autosomal recessive
(C) Mitochondrial
(D) X-linked dominant
(E) X-linked recessive

29. A 7-day-old male neonate, who has been breast-fed since birth, is brought to the emergency department because of a 2-day history of poor feeding associated with frequent vomiting. Physical examination shows lethargy, dehydration, hypertonicity, and rigidity of the extremities. Laboratory studies

show metabolic acidosis, ketosis, and hypoglycemia. Following treatment of this patient's acute condition, long-term therapy is begun. This therapy is most likely to limit which of the following substances in the infant's diet?
(A) Galactose, fructose, and lactose
(B) Leucine, isoleucine, and valine
(C) Methionine, homocysteine, and cystathionine
(D) Medium-chain fatty acids
(E) Ornithine, citrulline, and arginine
(F) Phenylalanine and tyrosine

30. A 1-month-old male infant is brought to the physician for a routine examination. Physical examination shows hypopigmentation of the skin, light blonde hair, and translucent irises. His parents both have olive-colored skin, dark hair, and dark eyes. This infant most likely has a defect in the metabolism of which of the following?
(A) Epinephrine
(B) Homocysteine
(C) Serotonin
(D) Tryptophan
(E) Tyrosine

31. A 10-day-old newborn is being examined in the emergency department due to an inability to feed, vomiting, and extreme lethargy. Blood work finds massive metabolic acidosis accompanied by hyperammonemia. Physical examination finds that the infant exudes an odor of sweaty feet. A deficiency in the metabolism of which of the following is most likely to account for the symptoms in this infant?
(A) Glycine
(B) Leucine
(C) Methionine
(D) Phenylalanine
(E) Tyrosine

32. A 7-month-old boy has failed to gain weight normally. His diet consists of a dilute milk formula. His weight and length are below normal for his age, and he appears emaciated. His temperature is below normal, and his pulse is slow. Which of the following is the most likely cause of the infant's condition?
(A) Chronic renal failure
(B) Growth hormone deficiency
(C) Hypothyroidism
(D) Kwashiorkor
(E) Marasmus

33. A 67-year-old woman is being examined by her physician with complaints of chronic back, hip, and knee pain. Physical examination finds bluish-grey macules over the cartilaginous portions of her ears and on the sclera of her eyes. Past medical history included an aortic stenosis. The patient reported that when she sweats it seems to permanently stain her clothing. She also stated that her urine seems to get darker if she does not flush the toilet. These signs and symptoms are most likely indicative of which of the following?
(A) Alkaptonuria
(B) Homocystinuria
(C) Hyperbilirubinemia
(D) Maple syrup urine disease
(E) Phenylketonuria

34. A 1-year-old boy has recently been diagnosed with hepatocellular carcinoma following a period of progressive liver failure. Of significance to the progression of the infant's disease was the measurement of elevated levels of tyrosine and succinylacetone in the plasma. Given these findings, which of the following disorders is most likely to be the root cause of the liver cancer in this infant?
(A) Isovaleric acidemia
(B) Maple syrup urine disease
(C) Phenylketonuria (PKU)
(D) Propionic acidemia
(E) Tyrosinemia type 1

35. A 10-day-old neonate is being examined in the emergency department due to an inability to feed, vomiting, and extreme lethargy. Blood work finds massive metabolic acidosis accompanied by hyperammonemia. Physical examination finds that the infant exudes an odor of sweaty feet. Which of the following most likely accounts for the signs and symptoms in this infant?
(A) 3-Hydroxy-3-methylglutaric aciduria
(B) Isovaleric acidemia
(C) 3-Methylcrotonylglycinuria
(D) Phenylketonuria (PKU)
(E) Propionic acidemia

36. A 24-year-old man is being examined in the Emergency Department with severe anxiety resulting from the rapid onset of a crushing chest pain. The attending physician orders an EKG, the results of which show classic ST-elevation myocardial infarction (STEMI) with elevation of the ST-segment in leads V1, V2, and V3. Physical examination shows a patient who is tall with thin extremities and with arachnodactyly. Examination of the patient's eyes shows ectopia lentis bilaterally and inferonasally. Given these signs and symptoms, this patient is most likely to have elevated levels of which of the following in their blood?
(A) Cysteine
(B) Leucine
(C) Methionine
(D) Phenylalanine
(E) Tyrosine

37. A 47-year-old man is being examined by his physician with complaints of chronic and worsening pain in both hips, both knees, and his lower back. He reports that the pain has been persistent and increasing in intensity over the past year. He states that the pain was originally managed with over-the-counter NSAID medication, but lately he is getting little relief. Physical examination shows an otherwise healthy patient with the only untoward physical sign being the presence of ochronotic pigmentation of his ears. Given the signs and symptoms presented, which of the following enzymes is most likely deficient in this patient?
(A) Branched-chain α-keto acid dehydrogenase
(B) Ferrochelatase
(C) Homogentisic acid oxidase
(D) Phenylalanine hydroxylase
(E) Porphobilinogen deaminase
(F) Uroporphyrinogen decarboxylase

38. A 7-day-old girl has been rushed to the Emergency Department by her parents following two seizures. The infant was born at home to a 29-year-old Gravida 2, parity 1 mother and has not undergone the Recommended Uniform Screening Panel (RUSP). The mother and father are healthy, and they are unaware of any family history of disease. The patient

has been breast fed, but the mother reports that over the past 48 hours she has had difficulty getting her daughter to feed. Physical examination finds that the infant is hypotonic and lethargic. The attending physician notes that the patient has a distinctive, but faint, odor of sugar to her skin. These signs and symptoms are most likely the result of a deficiency in which of the following processes?
(A) Catecholamine biosynthesis
(B) Glycine catabolism
(C) Intestinal tryptophan uptake
(D) Leucine catabolism
(E) Lysosomal glycoprotein degradation

39. A 2-week-old boy is undergoing a routine post-natal examination by his pediatrician. There is no available record of the newborn undergoing the Recommended Uniform Screening Panel (RUSP) at birth. Physical examination shows the infant has fair skin, blue eyes, blonde hair, and patches of dry thickened skin on the face, neck, and inner creases of the elbows and knees. The pediatrician notes that the patient's breath has a distinctive odor. Given the most likely diagnosis in this patient, which of the following compounds is most likely to be detected at levels well above normal?
(A) Alloisoleucine
(B) Glycine
(C) Homogentisate
(D) Lysine
(E) Phenylacetate
(F) Tyrosine

40. A physician is examining a 9-year-old girl who was brought in by her parents because they are disturbed by her progressive mood changes and apparent heightened anxiety. In addition, the parents report that the child appears to have a high degree of sensitivity to sunlight, with a rash forming on sun-exposed surfaces of skin with only a few minutes of exposure. Physical examination shows signs of cerebellar ataxia that include unsteady gait and uncoordinated eye movements. Given the most likely diagnosis in this patient, which of the following would be the most beneficial supplement provided in her diet?
(A) Niacin
(B) Phenylalanine
(C) Riboflavin
(D) Thiamine
(E) Tyrosine
(F) Tryptophan

ANSWERS

1. Correct answer is **A.** The patient is most likely experiencing the signs and symptoms of maple syrup urine disease (MSUD) which is the result of mutations in the gene encoding branched-chain α-keto acid dehydrogenase. Classic MSUD is defined by neonatal onset of encephalopathy and is the most severe form of the disorder. The levels of the branched-chain amino acids (BCAA), especially leucine, and their α-keto acids, are dramatically elevated in the blood, urine, and cerebrospinal fluid of afflicted infants. Deficiency in the cystathionine β-synthase (choice B) which is associated with homocysteinemia, ectopia lentis, high risk for atherosclerosis and deep vein thrombosis, and intellectual impairment. Deficiency in glycine decarboxylase (choice C) results in glycine encephalopathy (GCE) which is characterized by nonketotic hyperglycinemia (NKH). Several forms of GCE have been characterized with the neonatal phenotype being the most common. Deficiency in phenylalanine hydroxylase (choice D) results in phenylketonuria, PKU. Deficiency in propionyl-CoA carboxylase (choice E) results in propionic acidemia. This disorder is associated with episodic ketoacidosis following consumption of protein. The accumulation of propionyl-CoA within the cell leads to inhibition of mitochondrial metabolism, thereby resulting in reduced production of ATP, GTP, and citrate.

2. Correct answer is **D.** The patient is most likely experiencing the signs and symptoms of maple syrup urine disease (MSUD) which is the result of mutations in the gene encoding branched-chain α-keto acid dehydrogenase. Classic MSUD is defined by neonatal onset of encephalopathy and is the most severe form of the disorder. The levels of the branched-chain amino acids (BCAA), especially leucine, and their α-keto acids, are dramatically elevated in the blood, urine, and cerebrospinal fluid of afflicted infants. There are no metabolic disorders associated with increased serum levels of arginine and lysine (choice A) or asparagine and glutamine (choice B). Elevation in serum homocysteine (choice C), but not cysteine, occurs with mutations in the cystathionine β-synthase gene, as well as in conditions of vitamin B_6, B_{12}, and folate deficiency. Increased serum levels of phenylalanine (choice E), but not tyrosine, are significant in phenylketonuria, PKU.

3. Correct answer is **B.** The patient is most likely exhibiting the signs and symptoms associated with deficiency in cystathionine β-synthase (CBS) activity. Cystathionine β-synthase catalyzes the reaction converting homocysteine and serine to cystathionine in the pathway from methionine to cysteine. Mutations in the CBS gene are the most common causes of homocysteinemia (commonly referred to as homocystinuria). The inability to convert homocysteine to cystathionine results in increased availability for the methionine synthase reaction resulting in increased methionine production as well as the homocysteinemia. Therefore, an increase in methionine and homocysteine is indicative of mutations in, or inhibition of, the cystathionine β-synthase reaction. Deficiency in branched-chain α-keto acid dehydrogenase (choice A) would lead to accumulation of the branched-chain amino acids as well as their α-ketoacid forms as is the case in maple syrup urine disease. Deficiencies in methionine synthase (choice C) would result in homocysteinemia, such as in this patient, however there would not be a consequent increase in methionine. Deficiency in phenylalanine hydroxylase (choice D) is the cause of phenylketonuria, PKU, which is associated with highly elevated levels of phenylalanine and the metabolic byproducts, phenyllactate, phenylpyruvate, and phenylacetate. Deficiency in tyrosine aminotransferase (choice E) is the cause of tyrosinemia type 2 (TYRSN2) which is an autosomal recessive disease characterized as an oculocutaneous syndrome. Tyrosinemia type 2 is also known as Richner-Hanhart syndrome. Tyrosinemia type 2 presents with hyperkeratotic plaques on the hands and soles of the feet and photophobia due to deposition of tyrosine crystals within the cornea.

4. Correct answer is **C.** The patient is most likely exhibiting signs and symptoms associated with deficiency in phenylalanine hydroxylase which results in the disorder known as phenylketonuria, PKU. Mutation in phenylalanine hydroxylase decreases the ability to generate tyrosine from phenylalanine. Reduced production of tyrosine leads to decreased melanin production resulting in the pale skin, fair colored hair, and pale blue eyes typical of PKU patients. The lack of melanin production from tyrosine (choice E) would account for the fair hair and blue eyes of this patient but would not result in severe developmental delay. None of the other amino acid conversions (choices A, B, and D) would correlate with the findings in this patient.

5. Correct answer is **E.** The patient is most likely suffering from Hartnup disorder. This disease is caused by a defect in neutral amino acid transport in the apical brush-border membranes of the small intestine and in kidney proximal tubules. The lack of intestinal tryptophan transport is responsible for most, if not all, clinical phenotypes of Hartnup disorder. The pellagra-like skin rash seen on sun-exposed areas of skin in Hartnup disorder patients is the result of mild NAD^+ deficiency due to a lack of tryptophan absorption. Tryptophan is utilized by the body to contribute to the total pool of NAD^+. Symptoms of Hartnup disorder may begin in infancy or early childhood, but sometimes they begin as late as early adulthood. Symptoms may be triggered by sunlight, fever, drugs, or emotional or physical stress. Most symptoms occur sporadically and are caused by a deficiency in the production of NAD^+. Accumulation of alanine (choice A) in the blood is most likely to occur during periods of fasting when skeletal muscle protein is degraded for energy production from the amino acids. Accumulation of alloisolecine (choice B), derived from isoleucine, in the blood and urine is indicative of a deficiency in the branched-chain α-keto acid dehydrogenase (BCKD) responsible for the catabolism of the branched-chain amino acids. The disorder associated with defects in BCKD is known as maple syrup urine disease. Glutamine (choice C) is the major amino acid found in the blood. Changes in the level of this amino acid correlate very well to changes in overall acid-base balance. Indeed, during periods of metabolic acidosis the level of glutamine in the blood increases since the liver diverts waste nitrogen, which would normally enter the urea cycle, to glutamine synthesis. This allows glutamine to be mobilized to the kidneys where removal of the nitrogen results in the generation of ammonium ion (NH_4^+) resulting in removal of H^+ in the urine. Accumulation of β-hydroxybutyrate (choice D) in the blood would signify an increase in fatty acid oxidation and the resultant diversion of the acetyl-CoA byproduct into ketone synthesis.

6. Correct answer is **C.** The patient is exhibiting the signs and symptoms associated with deficiency in cystathionine β-synthase (CBS) which results in a disorder referred to as homocystinuria. Common symptoms of homocystinuria are dislocated optic lenses (ectopia lentis; also termed lens subluxation), osteoporosis, lengthening and thinning of the long bones, and an increased risk of abnormal blood clotting (thromboembolism). In addition to homocysteinuria, patients excrete elevated levels of methionine and metabolites of homocysteine. The most common causes of homocystinuria (classic homocystinuria) are defects in the cystathionine β-synthase (*CBS*) gene. Homocystinuria is often associated with intellectual impairment, although the complete syndrome is multifaceted and many individuals with this disease are mentally normal, while others experience variable levels of developmental delay along with learning problems. A metabolic defect in glycine metabolism (choice A) is the cause of glycine encephalopathy, also known as noketotic hyperglycinemia (NKH). Deficiency in leucine metabolism (choice B) is associated with defects in branched-chain α-keto acid dehydrogenase (BCKD) and results in the disorder known as maple syrup urine disease (MSUD). Deficiency in the phenylalanine metabolism (choice D) results in the disorder known as phenylketonuria, PKU. Deficiency in metabolism of tyrosine (choice E) is most likely to be associated with the tyrosinemias, of which there are three distinct types dependent upon which tyrosine metabolizing enzyme is affected.

7. Correct answer is **A.** The patient is most likely exhibiting the signs and symptoms of phenylketonuria, PKU. Phenylalanine metabolizing enzyme, phenylalanine hydroxylase. The major clinical manifestation associated with PKU is impaired cognitive development and function. A disturbance in catecholamine synthesis (choice B) would be associated with neurologic dysfunction due to reduced synthesis of dopamine and norepinephrine. Disturbances in glycosphingolipid metabolism (choice C) are seen in several of the lysosomal storage diseases. A disruption in the metabolism of fatty acids with an odd number of carbon atoms (choice D) would result in propionic acidemia or methylmalonic acidemia. A defect in vitamin B_{12} absorption (choice E) would result in megaloblastic anemia.

8. Correct answer is **E.** The infant is most likely exhibiting the signs and symptoms of neonatal onset propionic acidemia. Propionic acidemia results from mutations in either of the two genes encoding the subunits of propionyl-CoA carboxylase. Measurement of propionyl-CoA levels in humans is difficult so the assay that is used is to measure for the carnitine ester (propionyl-carnitine) in blood and urine. Additional metabolites that are elevated in propionic acidemia, and can be assayed in the urine, include methylcitrate and 3-hydroxypropionate. Methylcitrate is formed by conjugation of propionyl-CoA with oxaloacetic acid from the TCA cycle. The accumulation of propionyl-CoA, within the cell, leads to inhibition of mitochondrial metabolism thereby resulting in reduced production of ATP, GTP, and citrate. Propionyl-CoA also directly inhibits carbamoyl phosphate synthase 1 (CPS-1) of the urea cycle. Methylcitrate has been shown to inhibit the function of isocitrate dehydrogenase (encoded by the *IDH3* gene) and citrate synthase. Alkaptonuria (choice A) is a relatively benign disorder associated with ochronotic arthritis resulting from mutations in homogentisate oxidase. Homocystinuria (choice B), also referred to as homocysteinemia, is most commonly caused by mutations in the gene encoding cystathionine β-synthase. Common symptoms of homocystinuria are dislocated optic lenses (ectopia lentis; also termed lens subluxation), osteoporosis, lengthening and thinning of the long bones, and an increased risk of abnormal blood clotting (thromboembolism). Symptoms of homocystinuria do not manifest within the first few days after birth. Isovaleric acidemia (choice C) results from mutations in the gene (*IVD*) encoding isovaleryl-CoA dehydrogenase. In the severe neonatal lethal form infants suffer from massive metabolic acidosis within a few days of birth accompanied by hyperammonemia, encephalopathy, lethargy, poor feeding, vomiting, and the characteristic "sweaty foot" odor. Maple syrup urine disease (choice D) results from deficiencies in branched-chain α-keto acid dehydrogenase leading to an accumulation of leucine, isoleucine, and lysine and their corresponding branched-chain α-keto acids (BCKA). Classic MSUD is defined by neonatal onset of encephalopathy and is the most severe form of the disorder. Affected infants appear normal at birth but symptoms develop rapidly appearing by 4–7 days after birth. As the disease progresses, infants will exhibit weight loss and progressive neurologic deterioration. Neurologic signs will alternate from hypo- to hypertonia and extension of the arms resembling decerebrate posturing. At this time the characteristic burnt sugar or maple syrup odor to the urine is apparent. Phenylketonuria, PKU (choice E) results from mutations in the phenylalanine hydroxylase gene. The major clinical manifestations associated with PKU are impaired cognitive development and function, but these symptoms do not appear within days of birth.

9. Correct answer is **E.** The patient is most likely suffering from Hartnup disorder. This disease is caused by a defect in neutral amino acid transport in the apical brush-border membranes of the small intestine and in kidney proximal tubules. The lack of intestinal tryptophan transport is responsible for most, if not all, clinical phenotypes of Hartnup disorder. The inability to reabsorb neutral amino acids, including tryptophan, in the proximal tubule of the kidney is the cause of the aminoaciduria. Increased levels of urinary alanine (choice A) would most likely be associated with increased skeletal muscle protein breakdown during periods of prolonged fasting. Increased levels of alloisoleucine (choice B) in the urine is associated with defects in branched-chain α-keto acid dehydrogenase (BCKD), a disorder called maple syrup urine disease. Increased levels of glutamine (choice C) in the urine would most likely be associated with metabolic acidosis. Increased levels of β-hydroxybutyrate (choice D) in the urine are indicative of ketoacidosis due to disorders such as type 1 diabetes or increased fatty acid oxidation.

10. Correct answer is **C.** The patient is most likely suffering from Hartnup disorder. This disease is caused by a defect in neutral amino acid transport in the apical brush-border membranes of the small intestine and in kidney proximal tubules. The lack of intestinal tryptophan transport is responsible for most, if not all, clinical phenotypes of Hartnup disorder. The pellagra-like skin rash seen on sun-exposed areas of skin in Hartnup disorder patients is the result of mild NAD^+ deficiency due to a lack of tryptophan absorption. Tryptophan is utilized by the body to contribute to the total pool of NAD^+. Symptoms of Hartnup disorder may begin in infancy or early childhood, but sometimes they begin as late as early adulthood. Symptoms may be triggered by sunlight, fever, drugs, or emotional or physical stress. Most symptoms occur sporadically and are caused by a deficiency in the production of NAD^+. When Hartnup disorder manifests during infancy the symptoms can be variable in clinical presentation. These symptoms include failure to thrive, photosensitivity, intermittent ataxia, nystagmus, and tremor. Alkaptonuria (choice A) is a relatively benign disorder associated with mutations in homogentisate oxidase. The only significant symptom of alkaptonuria is referred to as ochronotic arthritis which only manifest in adulthood. Glycine decarboxylase deficiency (choice B) result in glycine encephalopathy (GCE) which is characterized by nonketotic hyperglycinemia (NKH). Several forms of GCE have been characterized with the neonatal phenotype being the most common. Hartnup disorder (choice C) results from mutations in the intestinal and renal neutral amino acid transporter. Common symptoms of Hartnup disorder are very similar to pellagra. Maple syrup urine disease (choice D) results due to mutations in branched-chain α-keto acid dehydrogenase (BCKD). Phenylketonuria, PKU (choice E) results from mutations in phenylalanine hydroxylase. The major clinical manifestation associated with PKU and many HPA is impaired cognitive development and function.

11. Correct answer is **C.** The infant is most likely suffering from glycine encephalopathy (nonketotic hyperglycinemia, NKH) which is an autosomal recessive inborn error of glycine metabolism due to deficiencies in proteins of the glycine decarboxylase complex. Glycine encephalopathy, is characterized by the development of severe intellectual impairment, following a relatively normal early postnatal period. The intellectual impairment results from the highly elevated levels of glycine in the CNS. Infants generally present with severe lethargy, seizures, and respiratory depression requiring mechanical ventilation. A diagnosis of NKH associated with these symptoms is made secondary to elevated plasma and cerebrospinal fluid glycine concentrations. The prognosis for infants with NKH is poor, with severe neurologic impairment and intractable seizures progressing ultimately to death before 5 years of age. Measurement for increased serum levels of arginine (choice A) or glutamine (choice B) would not be useful in diagnosis of disease. Measurement for increased serum levels of leucine (choice D) would be useful in a diagnosis of maple syrup urine disease. Measurement of increased serum levels of phenylalanine (choice E) would be indicative of phenylketonuria, PKU.

12. Correct answer is **B.** The patient is most likely exhibiting the signs and symptoms of malnutrition, specifically the disorder referred to as kwashiorkor. Kwashiorkor is a condition resulting from inadequate protein intake. Early symptoms include fatigue, irritability, and lethargy. As protein deprivation continues, one sees growth failure, loss of muscle mass, generalized swelling (edema), and decreased immunity. A large, protuberant belly, due to ascites, is common in children suffering from this disorder. Marasmus (choice C) is another disorder associated with malnutrition resulting from inadequate intake of carbohydrate, protein, and fat. Muscle wasting and loss of subcutaneous fat are the main clinical signs of marasmus. None of the other conditions (choices A, D, and E) are reflective of the signs and symptoms in this patient.

13. Correct answer is **A.** The symptoms exhibited by the infant are most indicative of maple syrup urine disease (MSUD). This disease is caused by defects in branched-chain α-keto acid dehydrogenase, one of the enzymes used in the catabolism of the branched-chain amino acids (BCAAs) and the associated branched-chain α-keto acids (BCKAs). The classical symptom of this disease is the odor of burnt sugar in the diapers of afflicted infants. Left untreated, infants will die in the first few months of life from recurrent metabolic crises and neurological deterioration. Deficiency in cystathionine β-synthase (choice B) results in homocystinuria. Mutations in several of the components of the glycine cleavage complex (choice C) result in the disorder referred to as glycine encephalopathy, also known as nonketotic hyperglycinemia (NKH). Mutations in homogentisate oxidase (choice D) result in the relatively benign disorder called alkaptonuria. Mutations in phenylalanine hydroxylase (choice E) are the cause of the hyperphenylalaninemia known as phenylketonuria, PKU.

14. Correct answer is **D.** The patient is most likely exhibiting the signs and symptoms of phenylketonuria, PKU. PKU results from mutations in phenylalanine hydroxylase.

The major clinical manifestation associated with PKU is impaired cognitive development and function. The product of phenylalanine transamination, phenylpyruvic acid, is reduced to phenyllactate and metabolized to phenylacetate, and all three compounds appear in the urine. Deficiency in branched-chain α-keto acid dehydrogenase (choice A) results in the disorder known as maple syrup urine disease, MSUD. Typical findings in MSUD are elevated levels of the branched-chain amino acids and their α-keto acid metabolites. Deficiency in dihydropteridine reductase (choice B) is associated with hyperphenylalaninemia, similar to PKU but at much lower levels, due to its role in the regeneration of tetrahydrobiopterin, required by phenylalanine hydroxylase. The regeneration of tetrahydrobiopterin by dihydropteridine reductase is also required by tyrosine hydroxylase and tryptophan hydroxylase and therefore, mutations in this enzyme result in deficiencies in the production of catecholamines and reduced serotonin, respectively. Deficiency in homogentisate oxidase (choice C) results in the relatively benign disorder known as alkaptonuria. Deficiency in tyrosine aminotransferase (choice E) is the cause of tyrosinemia type 2 (TYRSN2) is an autosomal recessive disease characterized as an oculocutaneous syndrome. Tyrosinemia type 2 is also known as Richner-Hanhart syndrome. Tyrosinemia type 2 presents with hyperkeratotic plaques on the hands and soles of the feet and photophobia due to deposition of tyrosine crystals within the cornea.

15. Correct answer is **C.** The patient is most likely exhibiting the signs and symptoms associated with deficiency in cystathionine β-synthase (CBS) activity. Cystathionine β-synthase catalyzes the reaction converting homocysteine and serine to cystathionine in the pathway from methionine to cysteine. Mutations in the CBS gene are the most common causes of homocysteinemia (also referred to as homocystinuria). The inability to convert homocysteine to cystathionine results in increased availability for the methionine synthase reaction resulting in increased methionine production as well as the homocysteinemia. None of the other amino acids (choices A, B, D, and E) would be found elevated in this patient.

16. Correct answer is **C.** Nephrolithiasis, commonly referred to as kidney stones, is most commonly caused by dehydration and the presence of calcium oxalate crystals. Cystine is the oxidized disulfide homodimer of two cysteines. Type I cystinuria is an autosomal recessive disorder that results from a failure of the renal proximal tubules to reabsorb cystine that was filtered by the glomerulus. The accumulation of cystine and its formation of crystals within the distal tubules results in the formation of cystine stones in the kidneys. Cystinuria results from defects in either of the two protein subunits of the cystine transporter which is distinct from the renal cysteine transporter. The same cystine transporter is expressed within the small intestine but a defect in its function in this tissue does not contribute to pathology. In addition to excess cystine in the urine, the disorder is associated with increased urinary excretion of the dibasic amino acids, arginine, lysine, and ornithine. Increased urinary excretion of none of the other amino acids (choices A, B, D, and E) are associated with cystinuria.

17. Correct answer is **B.** The serum phenylalanine concentration in this patient indicates that there is a form of hyperphenylalaninemia (HPA). There are several hyperphenylalaninemias that are not phenylketonuria (PKU) and are called non-PKU hyperphenylalaninemias. Hyperphenylalaninemia is defined as a plasma phenylalanine concentration greater than 120 μM. PKU is characterized by plasma phenylalanine greater than 1000 μM and non-PKU HPA have plasma phenylalanine amounts that are less than 1000 μM. Dihydropteridine reductase (DHPR) catalyzes the conversion of dihydrobiopterin to tetrahydrobiopterin. Dihydrobiopterin is generated in the course of the phenylalanine hydroxylase reaction as well as the reactions catalyzed by tyrosine hydroxylase and phenylalanine hydroxylase. Dihydropteridine reductase deficiency leads to neurologic signs appearing around 4 or 5 months of age, although clinical signs are often obvious from birth. The principal symptoms include psychomotor retardation, tonicity disorders, drowsiness, irritability, abnormal movements, hyperthermia, hypersalivation, and difficult swallowing. Deficiency in branched-chain α-keto acid dehydrogenase (choice A) is the cause of maple syrup urine disease, MSUD. Deficiency in phenylalanine hydroxylase (choice C) is the cause of the severe hyperphenylalaninemia referred to as phenylketonuria, PKU. Deficiency in tryptophan hydroxylase (choice D) is associated with hypoxia-induced pulmonary arterial hypertension. Deficiency in tyrosine hydroxylase (choice E) is characterized by a wide spectrum of disease whose symptoms can vary widely, even among members of the same family. Common symptoms include an uncoordinated or clumsy manner of walking and dystonia.

18. Correct answer is **D.** The infant is most likely exhibiting the signs and symptoms of maple syrup urine disease (MSUD), also called branched-chain aminoaciduria. The name of this disorder is derived from the fact that the urine of affected individuals smells like maple syrup or burnt sugar. MSUD results from deficiencies in branched-chain α-keto acid dehydrogenase leading to an accumulation of leucine, isoleucine, and lysine and their corresponding branched-chain α-keto acids (BCKA). Classic MSUD is defined by neonatal onset of encephalopathy and is the most severe form of the disorder. The levels of the BCAA, especially leucine, are dramatically elevated in the blood, urine, and cerebrospinal fluid of afflicted infants. Affected infants appear normal at birth but symptoms develop rapidly appearing by 4–7 days after birth. The first distinctive signs are lethargy and little interest in feeding. As the disease progresses, infants will exhibit weight loss and progressive neurologic deterioration. Neurologic signs will alternate from hypo- to hypertonia and extension of the arms resembling decerebrate posturing. At this time the characteristic burnt sugar or maple syrup odor to the urine is apparent. Alkaptonuria (choice A) is a relatively benign disorder associated with ochronotic arthritis resulting from mutations in homogentisate oxidase. Homocystinuria (choice B), also referred to as homocysteinemia, is most commonly caused by mutations in the gene encoding cystathionine β-synthase. Common symptoms of homocystinuria are dislocated optic lenses (ectopia lentis; also termed lens subluxation), osteoporosis, lengthening and thinning of the long bones, and an increased risk of abnormal blood clotting (thromboembolism). Isovaleric acidemia (choice C) results from mutations in the gene (IVD) encoding isovaleryl-CoA dehydrogenase. Isovaleric acidemia is divided into two distinct symptomatic forms, a severe lethal form and a chronic intermittent form. The severe lethal form of IVA is the most common. In the severe neonatal lethal form infants suffer from massive metabolic acidosis within a few days of birth accompanied by hyperammonemia, encephalopathy, lethargy,

poor feeding, vomiting, and the characteristic "sweaty foot" odor. Phenylketonuria (choice E) results from mutations in the phenylalanine hydroxylase gene. Propionic acidemia (choice F) results from mutations in either of the two genes encoding the subunits of propionyl-CoA carboxylase. The accumulation of propionyl-CoA, within the cell, leads to inhibition of mitochondrial metabolism thereby resulting in reduced production of ATP, GTP, and citrate. Propionyl-CoA also directly inhibits carbamoyl phosphate synthase 1 (CPS-1) of the urea cycle.

19. Correct answer is **B.** The serum phenylalanine concentration in this patient indicates that there is a form of hyperphenylalaninemia (HPA). There are several hyperphenylalaninemias that are not phenylketonuria (PKU) and are called non-PKU hyperphenylalaninemias. Hyperphenylalaninemia is defined as a plasma phenylalanine concentration greater than 120 μM. PKU is characterized by plasma phenylalanine greater than 1000 μM and non-PKU HPA have plasma phenylalanine amounts that are less than 1000 μM. Dihydropteridine reductase (DHPR) catalyzes the conversion of dihydrobiopterin to tetrahydrobiopterin. Dihydrobiopterin is generated in the course of the phenylalanine hydroxylase reaction as well as the reactions catalyzed by tyrosine hydroxylase and phenylalanine hydroxylase. Dihydropteridine reductase deficiency leads to neurologic signs appearing around 4 or 5 months of age, although clinical signs are often obvious from birth. The principal symptoms include psychomotor retardation, tonicity disorders, drowsiness, irritability, abnormal movements, hyperthermia, hypersalivation, and difficult swallowing. Deficiency in branched-chain α-keto acid dehydrogenase (choice A) is the cause of maple syrup urine disease, MSUD. Deficiency in phenylalanine hydroxylase (choice C) results in the more common hyperphenylalaninemia referred to as phenylketonuria, PKU. Mutations in either of the two genes encoding the subunits of propionyl-CoA carboxylase (choice D) result in propionic acidemia. Deficiency in tyrosine aminotransferase (choice E) is the cause of tyrosinemia type 2 (TYRSN2) which is an autosomal recessive disease characterized as an oculocutaneous syndrome. Tyrosinemia type 2 is also known as Richner-Hanhart syndrome. Tyrosinemia type 2 presents with hyperkeratotic plaques on the hands and soles of the feet and photophobia due to deposition of tyrosine crystals within the cornea.

20. Correct answer is **B.** The patient is most likely exhibiting the signs and symptoms associated with deficiency in cystathionine β-synthase (CBS) which results in a disorder referred to as homocystinuria. Common symptoms of homocystinuria are dislocated optic lenses (ectopia lentis; also termed lens subluxation), osteoporosis, lengthening and thinning of the long bones, and an increased risk of abnormal blood clotting (thromboembolism). In addition to homocysteinuria, patients excrete elevated levels of methionine and metabolites of homocysteine. Homocystinuria is often associated with intellectual impairment, although the complete syndrome is multifaceted and many individuals with this disease are mentally normal, while others experience variable levels of developmental delay along with learning problems. Measurement of serum methionine levels at birth would be most useful in making a correct diagnosis in this patient. None of the other amino acids (choices A, C, D, and E) would be elevated in this patient at birth.

21. Correct answer is **C.** The patient is most likely suffering from Hartnup disorder. This disease is caused by a defect in neutral amino acid transport in the apical brush-border membranes of the small intestine and in kidney proximal tubules. The lack of intestinal tryptophan transport is responsible for most, if not all, clinical phenotypes of Hartnup disorder. As a result of the inability to absorb tryptophan from the diet supplementing the diet of a Hartnup disease patient with tryptophan alone (choice E) is ineffective. Due to the transport of small peptides, derived from protein digestion, into the intestinal enterocytes, supplementation of Hartnup disease patients with a high-protein diet can supply the necessary tryptophan through the absorption of di-, tri-, and tetrapeptides. None of the other supplements (choices A, B, D, and F) would provide therapeutic benefit to Hartnup disease patients.

22. Correct answer is **C.** There are only two enzymes in the human body that require vitamin B_{12} (cobalamin) as a cofactor. These two enzymes are methionine synthase (also known as homocysteine methyltransferase) and methyl malonyl-CoA mutase. The oxidation of fatty acids with an odd number of carbon atoms, and the oxidation of the amino acids, methionine, threonine, isoleucine, and valine all yield propionyl-Co. Propionyl-CoA is converted to succinyl-CoA via a series of three reactions, where the last one is the vitamin B_{12}-requiring methylmalonyl-CoA mutase. Mutations in methylmalonyl-CoA mutase, and deficiency of vitamin B_{12} both result in increased levels of methylmalonic acid. The most common physical symptoms seen in patients with defective methylmalonyl-CoA mutase activity are failure to thrive, lethargy, vomiting, muscular hypotonia, and respiratory distress. Characteristic laboratory findings will be methylmalonic acidemia. Deficiency in the malonyl-CoA decarboxylase (choice A) would be associated with the inability to regulate fatty acid oxidation level of carnitine palmitoyltransferase 1. Signs and symptoms of malonyl-CoA decarboxylase deficiency can include hypoglycemia, hypotonia, seizures, diarrhea, vomiting, and cardiomyopathy. Deficiency in methionine synthase (choice B) is associated with homocysteinemia and megaloblastic anemia. Deficiency in methylmalonyl-CoA racemase (choice D) has not been identified in humans. Deficiency in propionyl-CoA carboxylase (are choice E) is the cause of propionic acidemia.

23. Correct answer is **E.** The amino acids arginine, methionine, and phenylalanine are considered essential for reasons not directly related to lack of synthesis. Arginine is synthesized by mammalian cells but at a rate that is insufficient to meet the growth needs of the body and the majority that is synthesized is cleaved to form urea. None of the other processes (choices A, B, C, and D) could provide for the synthesis of arginine in the absence of dietary intake.

24. Correct answer is **A.** The patient is most likely experiencing the signs and symptoms of maple syrup urine disease (MSUD) which is the result of mutations in the gene encoding branched-chain α-keto acid dehydrogenase. Classic MSUD is defined by neonatal onset of encephalopathy and is the most severe form of the disorder. The levels of the branched-chain amino acids (BCAA), especially leucine, and their α-keto acids, are dramatically elevated in the blood, urine, and cerebrospinal fluid of afflicted infants. Left untreated, infants will die in the first few months of life from recurrent metabolic crisis and neurologic deterioration. Defects in hepatic glycogen synthesis (choice B) are most likely associated with the glycogen storage disease known as Anderson disease. Anderson disease results from deficiency in the glycogen-branching enzyme and usually results in death by 2 years of age due to liver failure. Defects in mitochondrial fatty acid β-oxidation (choice C) encompass several disorders, the most common being medium-chain acyl-CoA dehydrogenase deficiency, MCADD. MCADD is associated with potentially lethal hypoglycemia accompanied by hypoketonemia. Defective peroxisomal fatty acid α-oxidation (choice D) results in the disorder known as Refsum disease. Defective synthesis of eicosanoids (choice E) can result in numerous abnormalities associated with multiple different tissue types.

25. Correct answer is **E.** The patient is most likely exhibiting the signs and symptoms of phenylketonuria, PKU. PKU results from mutations in phenylalanine hydroxylase. The major clinical manifestation associated with PKU is impaired cognitive development and function. The product of phenylalanine transamination, phenylpyruvic acid, is reduced to phenyllactate and metabolized to phenylacetate, and all three compounds appear in the urine. Deficiency in phenylalanine hydroxylase results in the inhibition of tyrosine synthesis. Indeed, half of the phenylalanine required in the diet goes into the production of tyrosine. If the diet is enriched in tyrosine, the requirements for phenylalanine are reduced by about 50%. Supplementation with none of the other compounds (choices A, B, C, and D) would be beneficial in the treatment of PKU.

26. Correct answer is **A.** The patient is most likely exhibiting the signs and symptoms of a deficiency in the enzyme homogentisate oxidase which results in the disorder referred to as alkaptonuria. A deficiency of homogentisate oxidase results in the accumulation of homogentistatic acid, which when in the urine can cause the urine to darken to a blackish color upon standing. Homogentistate can also cause the cartilage to darken in a process called ochronosis. Alkaptonuria is relatively benign, with ochronotic arthritis being the most severe complication. Hyperbilirubinemia (choice B) can be the result of many problems including hemolytic anemia or blockage of the bile duct as well as the inability of the liver to effectively conjugate bilirubin. Elevated direct bilirubin would cause the urine to be a dark brown color. A defect in branched-chain amino acid catabolism (choice C) manifests as the disease known as maple syrup urine disease, MSUD. MSUD is caused by a defect in branched chain α-keto acid dehydrogenase. A defect in the process of peroxisomal fatty acid α-oxidation (choice D) is the cause of the disorder called Refsum disease. Disorders in purine nucleotide catabolism (choice E) represent multiple disorders with the most severe being adenosine deaminase (ADA) deficient SCID.

27. Correct answer is **D.** The infant is most likely exhibiting signs and symptoms associated with defective methylmalonyl-CoA mutase. Defects in methylmalonyl-CoA mutase activity comprise four distinct genotypes whose clinical symptoms are remarkably similar. Characteristic findings in methylmalonyl-CoA mutase deficiency include failure to thrive leading to developmental abnormalities, recurrent vomiting, respiratory distress, hepatomegaly, and muscular hypotonia. In addition, patients have severely elevated levels of methylmalonic acid in the blood and urine. Unaffected individuals have near undetectable levels of methylmalonate in their plasma, whereas, affected individuals have been found to have levels ranging from 3 to 40 mg/dL in their blood. Methylmalonic acid, being an organic acid, would contribute to metabolic acidosis when elevated, such as would be the case in this patient. None of the other abnormalities (choices A, B, C, and E) would be present in an infant suffering from methylmalonyl-CoA mutase deficiency.

28. Correct answer is **B.** The patient is most exhibiting the signs and symptoms of phenylketonuria, PKU. Phenylalanine metabolizing enzyme, phenylalanine hydroxylase. The major clinical manifestation associated with PKU is impaired cognitive development and function. Phenylketonuria is inherited as an autosomal recessive disorder. None of the other modes of inheritance (choices A, C, D, and E) are related to the inheritance of phenylketonuria.

29. Correct answer is **B.** The patient is most likely experiencing the signs and symptoms of maple syrup urine disease (MSUD) which is the result of mutations in the gene encoding branched-chain α-keto acid dehydrogenase (BCKD) that is involved in the catabolism of the branched-chain amino acids (BCAAs), leucine, isoleucine, and valine. Classic MSUD is defined by neonatal onset of encephalopathy and is the most severe form of the disorder. The levels of the branched-chain amino acids (BCAA), especially leucine, and their α-keto acids, are dramatically elevated in the blood, urine, and cerebrospinal fluid of afflicted infants. Maple syrup urine disease (MSUD), also called branched-chain aminoaciduria, is so called because the urine of affected individuals smells like maple syrup or burnt sugar. Due to the deficiency in BCKD, infants need to be placed on a carefully controlled diet that provides sufficient branched-chain amino acids for growth and development but that does not promote their metabolism which would contribute to manifestation of pathology. Dietary restriction of none of the other compounds (choices A, C, D, and E) would be beneficial in a patient suffering from MSUD.

30. Correct answer is **E.** The infant is most likely manifesting the signs and symptoms of albinism. Albinism is a congenital disorder characterized by the complete or partial absence of pigment in the skin, hair, and eyes due to absence or defect of tyrosinase. Tyrosinase is expressed in melanocytes, which are specialized cells that produce a pigment called melanin from the amino acid tyrosine. Melanin is the substance that gives skin, hair, and eyes their color. Melanin is also found in the light-sensitive tissue at the back of the eye (the retina), where it plays a role in normal vision. A defect in the metabolism of none of the other substances (choices A, B, C, and D) would be associated with the signs and symptoms in this infant.

31. Correct answer is **B.** The infant is most likely manifesting all of the signs and symptoms of isovaleric acidemia. Isovaleric acidemia results from mutations in the gene (*IVD*) encoding isovaleryl-CoA dehydrogenase. Isovaleryl-CoA dehydrogenase catalyzes the oxidation of isovaleryl-CoA to 3-methylcrotonyl-CoA. Isovaleryl-CoA is the product of the branched-chain α-keto acid dehydrogenase metabolism of the α-keto acid of leucine. Isovaleric acidemia is divided into two distinct symptomatic forms, a severe lethal form and a chronic intermittent form. The severe lethal form of IVA is the most common. In the severe neonatal lethal form infants suffer from massive metabolic acidosis within a few days of birth accompanied by hyperammonemia, encephalopathy, lethargy, poor feeding, vomiting, and the characteristic "sweaty foot" odor. Metabolic ketoacidosis with an unexplained anion gap is typical in infants suffering from the severe lethal form of IVA. Early neonatal presentation is highly associated with mortality. Defects in the metabolism of none of the other amino acids (choices A, C, D, and E) would account for the signs and symptoms presenting in this infant.

32. Correct answer is **E.** The infant is most likely exhibiting the signs and symptoms associated with the nutritional deficit disorder identified as marasmus. Marasmus is generally known as the gradual wasting away of the body due to severe malnutrition or inadequate absorption of food. It is a severe form of malnutrition caused by inadequate intake of total calories from protein, carbohydrate, and fat. A child with marasmus looks emaciated and exhibits a body weight that is reduced to less than 60% of the normal body weight for the age. Marasmus can be distinguished from kwashiorkor (choice D) in that kwashiorkor results from protein malnutrition but with adequate energy intake, whereas marasmus is inadequate energy intake in all forms, including protein. None of the other options (choices A, B, and C) would account for the signs and symptoms in this infant.

33. Correct answer is **A.** The patient is most likely exhibiting the signs and symptoms of a deficiency in the enzyme homogentisate oxidase which results in the disorder referred to as alkaptonuria. A deficiency of homogentisate oxidase results in the accumulation of homogentistatic acid, which when in the urine can cause the urine to darken to a blackish color upon standing. Homogentistate can also cause the cartilage to darken in a process called ochronosis. Alkaptonuria is relatively benign, with ochronotic arthritis being the most severe complication. Causes of homocystinuria (choice B), also referred to as homocysteinemia, include mutations in the gene encoding the enzyme cystathionine β-synthase. Hyperbilirubinemia (choice C) can be the result of many problems including hemolytic anemia or blockage of the bile duct. Elevated direct bilirubin would cause the urine to be a dark brown color. Maple syrup urine disease (choice D) is caused by defects in branched chain α-keto acid dehydrogenase. A defect in the enzyme would cause intellectual impairment, abnormal muscle tone, and a caramel-colored urine. Phenylketonuria, PKU (choice E) is due to a defect in phenylalanine hydroxylase or its coenzyme tetrahydrobiopterin. Besides intellectual impairment and microcephaly, another characteristic is musty odor of urine.

34. Correct answer is **E.** The symptoms and plasma analytes in this infant are highly indicative of tyrosinemia type I. Tyrosinemia type 1 (TYRSN1) is an autosomal recessive disease and represents the most severe form of the tyrosinemias. Tyrosinemia type 1, is a potentially fatal childhood disorder associated with liver failure, painful neurologic crises, rickets, and hepatocarcinoma. This disorder is caused by a deficiency of fumarylacetoacetate hydrolase which catalyzes the final reaction of tyrosine catabolism. If untreated, death typically occurs at less than 2 years of age. Urine organic acids in TYRSN1 show elevated, tyrosine, 4-hydroxyphenyl organic acids, and succinylacetone, the latter being a particularly toxic metabolite. Isovaleric acidemia (choice A) results from mutations in the gene (*IVD*) encoding isovaleryl-CoA dehydrogenase. In the severe neonatal lethal form of this disease infants suffer from massive metabolic acidosis within a few days of birth accompanied by hyperammonemia, encephalopathy, lethargy, poor feeding, vomiting, and the characteristic "sweaty foot" odor. Maple syrup urine disease, MSUD (choice B) results from mutations in branched-chain α-keto acid dehydrogenase. Classic MSUD is defined by neonatal onset of encephalopathy and is the most severe form of the disorder. The levels of the branched-chain amino acids and their α-keto acids are dramatically elevated in the blood, urine, and cerebrospinal fluid of afflicted infants. Phenylketonuria (choice C) results from deficiency in phenylalanine hydroxylase. PKU is associated with highly elevated levels of phenylalanine and the metabolic byproducts, phenyllactate, phenylpyruvate, and phenylacetate. Propionic acidemia (choice D) results from mutations in either of the two genes encoding the subunits of propionyl-CoA carboxylase. This disorder is associated with episodic ketoacidosis following consumption of protein. The accumulation of propionyl-CoA within the cell leads to inhibition of mitochondrial metabolism, thereby resulting in reduced production of ATP, GTP, and citrate.

35. Correct answer is **B.** The infant is most likely manifesting all of the signs and symptoms of isovaleric acidemia. Isovaleric acidemia results from mutations in the gene (*IVD*) encoding isovaleryl-CoA dehydrogenase. Isovaleryl-CoA dehydrogenase catalyzes the oxidation of isovaleryl-CoA to 3-methylcrotonyl-CoA. Isovaleryl-CoA is the product of the branched-chain α-keto acid dehydrogenase metabolism of the α-keto acid of leucine. Isovaleric acidemia is divided into two distinct symptomatic forms, a severe lethal form and a chronic intermittent form. The severe lethal form of IVA is the most common. In the severe neonatal lethal form infants suffer from massive metabolic acidosis within a few days of birth accompanied by hyperammonemia, encephalopathy, lethargy, poor feeding, vomiting, and the characteristic "sweaty foot" odor. Metabolic ketoacidosis with an unexplained anion gap is typical in infants suffering from the severe lethal form of IVA. Early neonatal presentation is highly associated with mortality. Deficiency in 3-hydroxy-3methylglutaryl-CoA lyase (HMG-CoA lyase), results in a disorder referred to as 3-hydroxy-3-methylglutaric aciduria (choice A). Characteristic findings in patients with this disorder are accumulation of leucine metabolites, 3-hydroxy-3-methylglutaric acid, 3-methylglutaconic acid, 3-methylglutaric acid, and 3-hydroxyisovaleric acid. Since the enzyme is also involved in ketone body synthesis, mutations in the gene result in defects in ketone synthesis. 3-Methylcrotonylglycinuria (choice C) results from defects in either of the two subunits of the biotin-requiring enzyme, 3-methylcrotonyl-CoA carboxylase (3MCC), another enzyme involved in the catabolism of leucine. The characteristic features of the severe forms of 3MCC deficiency include difficulty feeding, recurrent episodes of vomiting and diarrhea, lethargy, and hypotonia. Phenylketonuria (choice D) results from deficiency in phenylalanine hydroxylase. PKU is associated with highly elevated levels of phenylalanine and the metabolic byproducts, phenyllactate, phenylpyruvate, and phenylacetate. Propionic acidemia (choice E) results from mutations in either of the two genes encoding the subunits of propionyl-CoA carboxylase. This disorder is associated with episodic ketoacidosis following consumption of protein. The accumulation of propionyl-CoA, within the cell, leads to inhibition of mitochondrial metabolism, thereby resulting in reduced production of ATP, GTP, and citrate.

36. Correct answer is **C.** The patient most likely has a deficiency in cystathionine β-synthase (CBS) resulting in homocysteinemia/homocystinuria. Classic homocystinuria is often associated with intellectual impairment, although the complete syndrome is multifaceted and many individuals with this disease are mentally normal, while others experience variable levels of developmental delay along with learning problems. Common symptoms of homocystinuria are dislocated optic lenses (ectopia lentis), osteoporosis, and lengthening and thinning of the long bones. Elevated levels of homocysteine in the blood induce a state of inflammation. Homocysteine serves as a negatively charged surface that attracts the contact phase of the intrinsic pathway of blood coagulation. Activation of the intrinsic coagulation cascade leads to inappropriate thrombolytic events. Abnormal blood clotting is associated with a risk for deep vein thrombotic (DVT) episodes as well as for myocardial infarction (MI). The MI is associated with characteristic features on an EKG that are visible by ST-segment elevation seen in leads V1, V2, and V3, as is the case for this patient. Cystathionine β-synthase converts homocysteine and serine to cystathionine. The elevated levels of homocysteine, that result from CBS deficiency, lead to increased conversion of homocysteine to methionine resulting in an associated methioninemia. Elevated blood levels of none of the other amino acids (choices A, B, D, and E) would be found in a patient with homocysteinemia/homocystinuria.

37. Correct answer is **C.** The patient is most likely exhibiting the signs and symptoms of ochronotic arthritis which is associated with a deficiency in the activity of the phenylalanine and tyrosine catabolic enzyme, homogentisate oxidase. Deficiency in homogentisate oxidase causes the disorder referred to as alkaptonuria. Alkaptonuria is characterized by homogentisic aciduria, ochronosis (a bluish-black discoloration of tissues), and arthritis (termed ochronotic arthritis). In some alkaptonuria patients, there is skin pigmentation in splotches around the mouth and in the cartilage of the ears. Homogentisic acid accumulation in the heart can lead to valve damage. Deficiency in branched-chain α-keto acid dehydrogenase (choice A) is the cause of maple syrup urine disease, a disease that, in the classic form, manifests with neonatal-onset encephalopathy. Deficiency in ferrochelatase (choice B) is the cause of erythropoietic protoporphyria (EPP). Light-sensitive dermatitis commencing in childhood, usually before 10 years of age, is the primary clinical finding in EPP. Common symptoms are itching, swelling, and painful erythema (skin redness due to capillary congestion) which can develop within minutes on sun-exposed areas of the skin. Deficiency in phenylalanine hydroxylase (choice D) is the cause of the severe form of hyperphenylalaninemia called phenylketonuria (PKU). The major clinical manifestation associated with PKU is impaired cognitive development and function. The product of phenylalanine transamination, phenylpyruvic acid, is reduced to phenylacetate and phenyllactate, and all three compounds appear in the urine. The presence of phenylacetate in the urine and sweat imparts a "mousy" odor. Deficiency in porphobilinogen deaminse (choice E) causes the late-onset disorder identified as acute intermittent porphyria (AIP). The clinical manifestations of AIP are related to the visceral, autonomic, peripheral, and central nervous system involvement of the disease. In fact, almost all of the symptoms of AIP result from neurologic dysfunction. Deficiency in uroporphyrinogen decarboxylase (UROD) (choice F) is the cause of porphyria cutanea tarda (PCT). The symptoms of PCT are characterized by blistering skin lesions on sun-exposed areas of the skin. In addition to blistering skin lesions, the typical sign of PCT is dark red or purple coloration of the urine, which is the origin of the term porphyria used to describe all disorders of heme biosynthesis.

38. Correct answer is **D.** The infant is most likely manifesting the signs and symptoms of maple syrup urine disease (MSUD) which gets its name from the fact that the urine of affected individuals smells like maple syrup or burnt sugar. MSUD results from a deficiency in the enzyme, branched-chain α-keto acid dehydrogenase (BCKD), that is involved in the catabolism of the branched-chain amino acids (BCAA), leucine, isoleucine, and valine. Classic MSUD is defined by neonatal onset of encephalopathy and is the most severe form of the disorder. The levels of the BCAA, especially leucine, and their α-keto acids, are dramatically elevated in the blood, urine, and cerebrospinal fluid of afflicted infants. Deficiency in catecholamine biosynthesis (choice A) is a common consequence of mutations in genes encoding enzymes responsible for the synthesis of tetrahydrobiopterin or in the gene encoding dihydropteridin reductase (DHPR). DHPR is required of tyrosine hydroxylase, the rate-limiting enzyme in catecholamine synthesis. Deficieny in glycine catabolism (choice B) results from mutations in any of the three genes encoding subunits of glycine decarboxylase (also known as glycine cleavage complex, GCC) resulting in glycine encephalopathy (GCE). The most common form of GCE is the neonatal form and symptoms appear in the first few days of life and include lethargy, hypotonia, myoclonic jerks, and often death. Deficiency in intestinal tryptophan uptake (choice C) is the cause of Hartnup disorder. Symptoms of Hartnup disorder may begin in infancy or early childhood, but sometimes they begin as late as early adulthood. Symptoms may be triggered by sunlight, fever, drugs, or emotional or physical stress. When Hartnup disorder manifests during infancy, the symptoms can be variable in clinical presentation. These symptoms include failure to thrive, photosensitivity, intermittent ataxia, nystagmus, and tremor. Deficiency in lysosomal glycoprotein degradation (choice E) is associated with several disorders such as Sandhoff disease, aspartylglucosaminuria, and sialidosis. None of these diseases is associated with the typical odor seen in this patient.

39. Correct answer is **E.** The infant is most likely suffering from the signs and symptoms of phenylketonuria (PKU). The major clinical manifestation associated with PKU, and many HPA, is impaired cognitive development and function. The product of phenylalanine transamination, phenylpyruvic acid, is reduced to phenylacetate and phenyllactate, and all three compounds appear in the urine. The presence of phenylacetate in the urine and sweat imparts a "mousy" odor. Elevated levels of none of the substances (choices A, B, C, D, and F) would be associated with PKU. Elevations in alloisoleucine (choice A) are characteristic of maple syrup urine disease which results from deficiency in brached-chain keto acid dehydrogenase (BCKD). Elevated levels of homogentisic acid (choice C) is characteristic of the relatively benign disorder of phenylalanoine and tyrosine catabolism termed alkaptonuria, a disorder caused by deficieny in homogentisate oxidase.

40. Correct answer is **A.** The patient is most likely experiencing the signs and symptoms of Hartnup disorder which is caused by a defect in a neutral amino acid transporter (SLC6A19) in the apical brush border membranes of the small intestine and in kidney proximal tubules. This transporter transports eight of the ten essential amino acids, namely leucine, isoleucine, valine, methionine, phenylalanine, tryptophan, threonine, and histidine. Of significance, specifically to Hartnup disorder, is that SLC6A19 is the major transporter of tryptophan in the intestines and its lack, in Hartnup disorder, is key to the pathology of the disorder. Symptoms of

Hartnup disorder may begin in infancy or early childhood, but sometimes they begin as late as early adulthood. Symptoms may be triggered by sunlight, fever, drugs, or emotional or physical stress. Most symptoms occur sporadically and are caused by reduced levels of the niacin (vitamin B_3) derived enzyme cofactors, NAD^+ and $NADP^+$. When Hartnup disorder manifests during infancy the symptoms can be variable in clinical presentation. These symptoms include failure to thrive, photosensitivity, intermittent ataxia, nystagmus, and tremor. Since tryptophan is also required for the synthesis of melatonin, it is believed that skin sensitivity to sunlight is exerted, in part, by a lack or reduction in melatonin synthesis. In addition to the regulation of circadian rhythm, melatonin has been shown to exert protective effects in the skin as well as being a regulator of skin structure and function. The cerebellar ataxia associated with Hartnup disorder is likely due to reduced synthesis of serotonin which is derived from tryptophan. Since tryptophan conversion to NAD^+ is significantly reduced, dietary supplementation with niacin is essential. Supplementation with none of the other substances (choices B, C, D, E, and F) would be beneficial in a patient with Hartnup disorder.

CHAPTER

19

Amino Acid–Derived Biomolecules

High-Yield Terms

Nitric oxide (NO)	Produced and released by vascular endothelium to promote smooth muscle relaxation
Catecholamines	Neurotransmitter family derived from tyrosine including dopamine, norepinephrine, and epinephrine; a catechol is an organic compound composed of a benzene ring and at least two hydroxyl groups attached, hence the derivation of the name of these compounds
Glutamate	Major excitatory neurotransmitter in the central nervous system, CNS
GABA	γ-aminobutyric acid, synthesized from glutamate, major inhibitory neurotransmitter in the CNS
Glycine	Inhibitory neurotransmitter
Creatine phosphate	Energy storage molecule in skeletal muscle, nonenzymatic breakdown generates creatinine
Glutathione	A tripeptide composed of glutamate, cysteine, and glycine that serves as a critical biological reductant; it is also conjugated to drugs to make them more water soluble and is involved in amino acid transport across cell membranes

Amino acids are required for protein synthesis and are important sources of energy during periods of fasting. Aside from these critical functions, amino acids function as neurotransmitters or as precursors for neurotransmitter synthesis. They help to control the levels of reactive oxygen species (ROS), contribute to energy stores in skeletal muscle, and serve many additional nonprotein functions.

NITRIC OXIDE SYNTHESIS AND FUNCTION

Vasodilators, such as acetylcholine, bradykinin, and adenosine exert their effects upon the vascular smooth muscle cell by activating signal transduction pathways in the overlying endothelium. The receptors to which these vasodilators bind on the endothelial cell are all members of the G-protein coupled receptor (GPCR) family (see Chapter 26). Acetylcholine binds the M3 (muscarinic) receptor, bradykinin binds the B2 bradykinin receptor, and adenosine binds the adenosine A_{2a} receptor. The G-protein to which these receptors are coupled is a G_q-type G-protein. G_q-type G-proteins activate phospholipase C-β (PLCβ) which hydrolyzes membrane phosphatidylinositol-4,5-bisphosphate (PIP_2) into diacylglycerol (DAG) and inositol-1,4,5-trisphosphate (IP_3). IP_3 binds to receptors on the endoplasmic reticulum (ER) that act as ligand-gated calcium channels. Activation of the IP_3 receptors results in release of Ca^{2+} from the ER which then binds to the calmodulin subunit of nitric oxide synthase (NOS) activating the enzyme. NOS synthesizes nitric oxide (NO) from the amino acid arginine (Figure 19–1).

HIGH-YIELD CONCEPT

There are three isozymes of NOS in mammalian cells: neuronal NOS (nNOS), also called NOS-1; inducible or macrophage NOS (iNOS), also called NOS-2, and endothelial NOS (eNOS), also called NOS-3. Nitric oxide synthases are very complex enzymes, employing five redox cofactors: NADPH, FAD, FMN, heme, and tetrahydrobiopterin (BH_4 also sometimes written H_4B). In addition, NOS enzymes form a complex with the Ca^{2+}-binding protein, calmodulin.

Both eNOS and nNOS are constitutively expressed and regulated by Ca^{2+} binding to their calmodulin subunits. Although iNOS contains calmodulin subunits, its activity is unaffected by changes in Ca^{2+} concentration. iNOS is transcriptionally activated in macrophages, neutrophils, and smooth muscle cells in response to inflammatory signals.

The NO produced by endothelial cells passes into the underlying smooth muscle cells to exert its effects. Within smooth muscle cells, NO reacts with the heme moiety of a soluble guanylyl

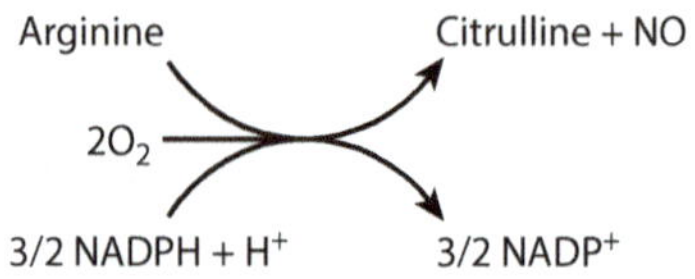

FIGURE 19–1 The reaction catalyzed by nitric oxide synthase. (Reproduced with permission from Rodwell VW, Bender DA, Botham KM, et al: *Harper's Illustrated Biochemistry*, 31st ed. New York, NY: McGraw Hill; 2018.)

HIGH-YIELD CONCEPT

Nitric oxide is involved in a number of other important cellular processes in addition to its impact on vascular smooth muscle cells. Events initiated by NO that are important for blood coagulation include inhibition of platelet aggregation and adhesion and inhibition of neutrophil adhesion to platelets and to the vascular endothelium.

cyclase, resulting in its activation which leads to elevation of intracellular levels of cGMP. The cGMP directly inhibits the plasma membrane localized L-type Ca^{2+} channels resulting in decreasing overall intracellular Ca^{2+} that would normally serve to activate myosin light-chain kinase (MLCK) and lead to vasoconstriction. The same L-type Ca^{2+} channels can be directly inhibited by NO via *S*-nitrosylation. The cGMP also activates protein kinase G (PKG) resulting in the phosphorylation and activation of myosin light-chain phosphatase resulting in phosphate removal from myosin light chains resulting in vasodilation. The cGMP also activates K^+ channels inducing hyperpolarization of the smooth muscle resulting in relaxation.

Drugs that are used clinically to mimic the actions of naturally occurring NO include organic nitrates (nitroglycerin, amyl nitrate, and isosorbide dinitrate) and sodium nitroprusside.

TYROSINE-DERIVED NEUROTRANSMITTERS

Tyrosine is the precursor for the synthesis of the catecholamines. The catecholamine neurotransmitters are dopamine, norepinephrine, and epinephrine (Figure 19–2).

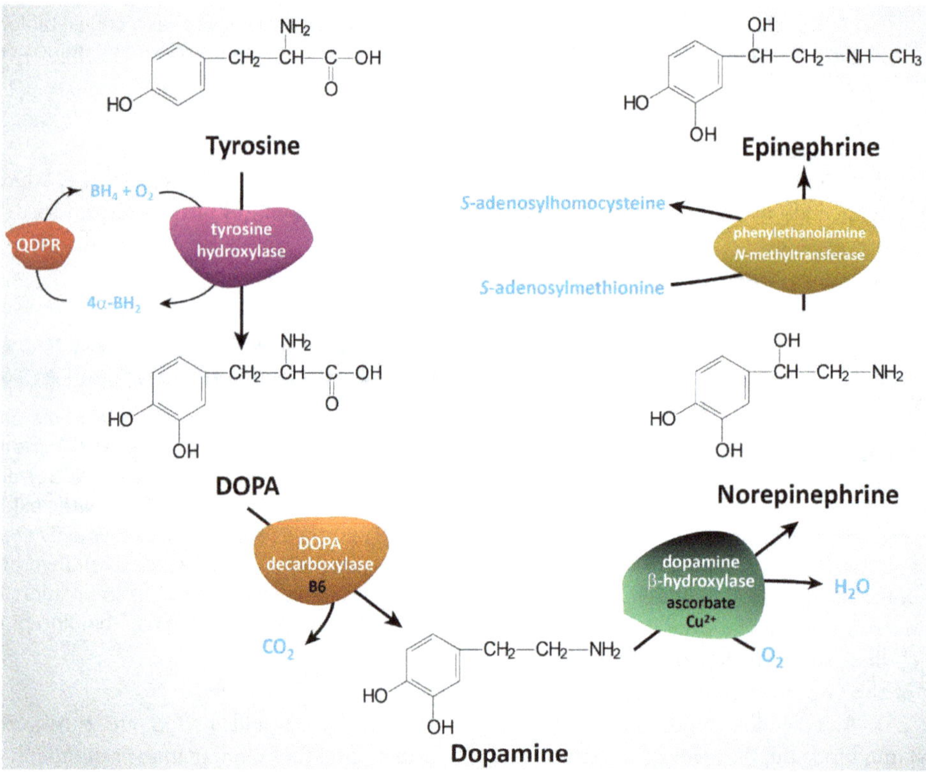

FIGURE 19–2 Synthesis of the catecholamine neurotransmitters from tyrosine. Tyrosine is converted to each of the three catecholamines through a series of four reactions. The tissue from which the neurotransmitter/hormone is derived expresses a specific set, or all, of these enzymes such that only dopamine (substantia nigra) is the result, or only norepinephrine (locus coeruleus), or both norepinephrine and epinephrine (adrenal medulla). DOPA decarboxylase, a vitamin B_6-dependent enzyme also known as aromatic L-amino acid decarboxylase, is encoded by the *DDC* gene. Dopamine β-hydroxylase is a critical vitamin C (ascorbate) and copper (Cu^{2+})-dependent enzyme. QDPR is quinoid dihydropteridine reductase which is more commonly just called dihydropteridine reductase. BH_4 and 4α-BH_2 are tetrahydrobiopterin and 4α-dihydrobiopterin, respectively. (Reproduced with permission from themedicalbiochemistrypage, LLC.)

HIGH-YIELD CONCEPT

Both epinephrine and norepinephrine actions underlie the fight-or-flight response which encompasses increased heart rate, increased blood flow to skeletal muscle, and increased glucose mobilization from glycogen.

The first step in catecholamine synthesis involves tyrosine hydroxylase, which like phenylalanine hydroxylase (see Figure 18–10) requires tetrahydrobiopterin (BH_4) as cofactor and generates 3,4-dihydrophenylalanine (L-DOPA). DOPA decarboxylase converts DOPA to dopamine, dopamine β-hydroxylase converts dopamine to norepinephrine, and phenylethanolamine *N*-methyltransferase converts norepinephrine to epinephrine. Once synthesized, dopamine, norepinephrine, and epinephrine are packaged in granulated vesicles.

The actions of the catecholamines are exerted via interaction with GPCR. There are three distinct types of adrenergic receptors: α_1, α_2, and β (Table 19–1). Within each class of adrenergic receptor there are several subclasses. The α_1 receptor class is coupled to G_q-type G-proteins that activate PLCβ resulting in increases in IP_3 and DAG release from membrane PIP_2. The α_2 receptor class is coupled to G_i-type G-proteins that inhibit the activation of adenylate cyclase. The β class of receptors is composed of three subtypes: β_1, β_2, and β_3, each of which couple to G_s-type G-proteins resulting in activation of adenylate cyclase and increases in cAMP with concomitant activation of PKA.

Dopamine binds to dopaminergic receptors identified as D-type receptors and there are five subclasses identified as D_1, D_2, D_3, D_4, and D_5. The D_1 and D_5 receptors are coupled to G_s-type G-proteins that activate adenylate cyclase and the D_2, D_3, and D_4 receptors are coupled to G_i-type G-proteins that inhibit adenylate cyclase.

TRYPTOPHAN-DERIVED NEUROTRANSMITTERS

Tryptophan serves as the precursor for the synthesis of serotonin (5-hydroxytryptamine, 5-HT) and melatonin (*N*-acetyl-5-methoxytryptamine). Serotonin synthesis initiates with the action of the enzyme tryptophan hydroxylase, which like phenylalanine hydroxylase (see Figure 18–10) and tyrosine hydroxylase (Figure 19–3) requires tetrahydrobiopterin (BH_4) as cofactor.

Serotonin is present at the highest concentrations in platelets and in the gastrointestinal tract. Lesser amounts are found in the brain and the retina. After release from serotonergic neurons, most of the released serotonin is recaptured by an active reuptake mechanism. The function of the selective serotonin reuptake inhibitors (SSRI) is to inhibit this reuptake process, thereby resulting

TABLE 19–1 Adrenergic pharmacology.

Drug Class	Target(s)	Effects/Comments
Nonselective α blockers	Both classes of α receptor; primary responses at α_1 receptors	Reduce vasoconstriction caused by both norepinephrine and epinephrine acting at α_1 receptors; inhibition of α_2 receptors exerted within sympathetic nervous system; phenoxybenzamine is most well-known in this class, was once also used to treat benign prostatic hyperplasia (BPH)
Selective α blockers	α_1 Receptors	All drugs in this class end with the suffix **'osin'** (eg, prazosin); drugs in this class can induce orthostatic hypotension
α_1 Agonists	α_1 Receptors	Function systemically to increase blood pressure; methoxamine and phenylephrine increase peripheral vascular resistance resulting in increased blood pressure; these drugs are used in the treatment of hypotension and shock
α_2 Agonists	α_2 Receptors	Function centrally (ie, within the CNS) to lower blood pressure; methyldopa is longest used drug in this class, although not used often any longer it is still the drug of choice (DOC) for the treatment of hypertension in pregnancy; cause vasodilation and reduction in blood pressure; also used to treat BPH; although classified as a nonselective agonist, clonidine is widely used drug for the treatment of hypertension and hot flashes in menopausal females; clonidine is also approved for the treatment of attention deficit hyperactivity disorder (ADHD)
Nonselective β blockers	β_1 and β_2 receptors	Some nonselective β blocker drugs have the **'olol'** suffix (eg, propranolol) like the β_1-selective blockers; because of their non-selectivity these drugs affect the heart, kidneys, lungs, gastro-intestinal tract, liver, uterus, vascular smooth muscle (VSM), and skeletal muscle
β_1 Blockers	β_1 Receptors	β_1 blocker drugs (eg, metoprolol) all have a name with the suffix **'olol'**; β_1-specific blockers function to decrease heart rate (chronotropic effects) and contractility (inotropic effects) leading to decreased blood pressure; β blockers are also sometimes prescribed for the treatment of glaucoma, migraine headaches, and anxiety
β_2 Agonists	β_2 Receptors	β_2 Agonists are principally used to induce bronchodilation in asthmatics and others with pulmonary dysfunction; these drugs are divided into the short-acting and long-acting subtypes; salbutamol is the most common of the prescribed short-acting drugs; all of the long-acting drugs have a name with the suffix **'terol'** (eg, formoterol)

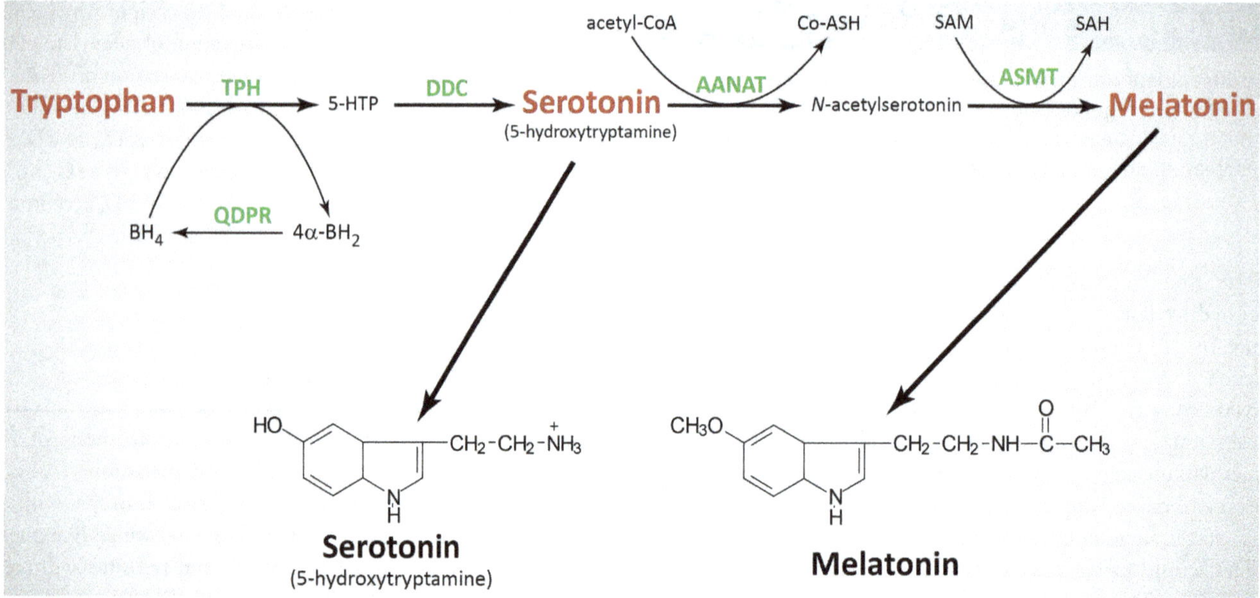

FIGURE 19–3 Pathway for serotonin and melatonin synthesis from tryptophan. Abbreviations: THP: tryptophan hydroxylase; QDPR: quinoid dihydropteridine reductase (more commonly called dihydropteridine reductase); 4α-BH_2: 4α-dihydrobiopterin; BH_4: tetrahydrobiopterin, 5-HTP: 5-hydroxytryptophan; DDC: DOPA decarboxylase; AANAT: aralkylamine *N*-acetyltransferase; ASMT: acetylserotonin-*O*-methyltransferase. SAM is *S*-adenosylmethionine. SAH is *S*-adenosylhomocysteine. (Reproduced with permission from themedicalbiochemistrypage, LLC.)

in prolonged serotonin presence in the synaptic cleft. The SSRI drugs are used in the treatment of depression, generalized anxiety disorder, post-traumatic stress disorder, and certain phobias.

The function of serotonin is exerted upon its interaction with specific receptors. Several serotonin receptor groups have been characterized and are identified as $5HT_1$, $5HT_2$, $5HT_3$, $5HT_4$, $5HT_5$, $5HT_6$, and $5HT_7$. Within the $5HT_1$ group, there are subtypes $5HT_{1A}$, $5HT_{1B}$, $5HT_{1D}$, $5HT_{1E}$, and $5HT_{1F}$. There are three $5HT_2$ subtypes, $5HT_{2A}$, $5HT_{2B}$, and $5HT_{2C}$ as well as two $5HT_5$ subtypes, $5HT_{5A}$ and $5HT_{5B}$. Most of these receptors are coupled to G-proteins that affect the activities of either adenylate cyclase or PLCβ. The $5HT_3$ receptors are ion channels (ionotropic receptors).

Synthesis and secretion of melatonin increases during the dark period of the day and is maintained at a low level during daylight hours. The primary effect of melatonin is the regulation of circadian rhythms such as sleep-wake cycles and in the regulation of blood pressure. Melatonin functions by inhibiting the synthesis and secretion of other neurotransmitters such as dopamine and γ-aminobutyric acid, GABA.

GLUTAMATE

Within the central nervous system (CNS) glutamate is the main excitatory neurotransmitter. Glutamate exerts its neurotransmitter effects through binding to four distinct classes of ion channel (ionotropic) receptors. Three of these glutamate receptor classes have been identified on the basis of their binding affinities for certain substrates and are, thus, referred to as the kainate, AMPA (2-amino-3-hydroxy-5-methyl-4-isoxazolepropionic acid), and NMDA (*N*-methyl-D-aspartate) receptors. The fourth class of ionotropic glutamate receptor is termed the delta (δ) receptors. Glutamate also binds to a family of GPCR identified as mGluR, where the "m" refers to metabotropic.

Within the CNS glutamatergic neurons are responsible for the mediation of many vital processes such as the encoding of information, the formation and retrieval of memories, spatial recognition, and the maintenance of consciousness. Excessive excitation of glutamate receptors has been associated with the pathophysiology of hypoxic injury, hypoglycemia, strokes, and epilepsy.

GLYCINE

Within the CNS glycine functions as an inhibitory neurotransmitter through binding to specific receptors identified as GlyR. The GlyR are members of the ionotropic family of ligand-gated ion channels. As a neurotransmitter, glycine mediates fast inhibitory neurotransmission within the spinal cord, brain stem, and caudal brain. The effects of glycine exert control over a variety of motor and sensory functions, including vision and audition. Glycine can also exert excitatory neurotransmission through co-binding with glutamate to the NMDA class of glutamate receptors.

GABA: INHIBITORY NEUROTRANSMITTER

The inhibitory neurotransmitter, γ-aminobutyric acid (GABA) is derived from glutamate. GABA is a major inhibitor of presynaptic transmission in the CNS, and also in the retina. Neurons that secrete GABA are termed GABAergic neurons.

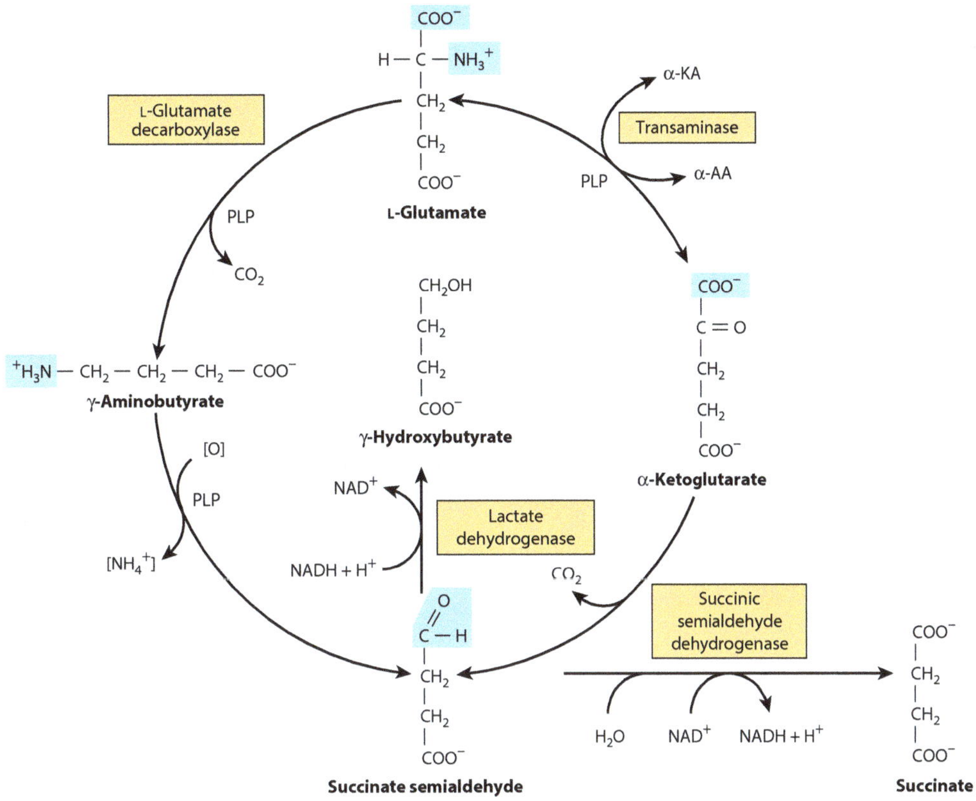

FIGURE 19–4 Metabolism of γ-aminobutyrate. (α-KA, α-keto acids; α-AA, α-amino acids; PLP, pyridoxal phosphate.) (Reproduced with permission from Rodwell VW, Bender DA, Botham KM, et al: *Harper's Illustrated Biochemistry*, 31st ed. New York, NY: McGraw Hill; 2018.)

The formation of GABA occurs via a metabolic pathway referred to as the GABA shunt (Figure 19–4). The pyridoxal phosphate-dependent enzyme, glutamic acid decarboxylase (GAD), catalyzes the decarboxylation of glutamate to form GABA. There are two GAD genes in humans identified as *GAD1* and *GAD2*. The GAD isoforms produced by these two genes are identified as GAD_{67} (*GAD1* gene: GAD67) and GAD_{65} (*GAD2* gene: GAD65), which is reflective of their molecular weights. Both the *GAD1* and *GAD2* genes are expressed in the brain, and GAD2 expression also occurs in the pancreas.

HIGH-YIELD CONCEPT

The presence of anti-GAD antibodies (both anti-GAD65 and anti-GAD67) is a strong predictor of the future development of type 1 diabetes in high-risk populations.

GABA exerts its effects by binding to two distinct receptors, GABA-A and GABA-B. The GABA-A receptors are heteropentameric (most commonly: $\alpha_2\beta_2\gamma$) ionotropic receptors that form a Cl^- channel. The binding of GABA to GABA-A receptors increases the Cl^- conductance of presynaptic neurons. The GABA-B receptors are GPCR that are coupled to a G_i-type G-protein. On postsynaptic membranes the GABA-B associated G-protein increases the conductance of G-protein-coupled inwardly rectifying potassium channels (GIRK). On presynaptic membranes binding of GABA to GABA-B receptors decreases neurotransmitter release by inhibiting voltage-activated Ca^{2+} channels.

GABA PHARMACOLOGY

The anxiolytic/sedative effects of the barbiturates and benzodiazepines are exerted via their binding to subunits of the GABA-A receptors. Benzodiazepines potentiate the effects of GABA binding to GABA-A receptors by binding to a site on the receptor created by the association of the gamma (γ) subunit and one of the alpha (α) subunits. There are two distinct subtypes of benzodiazepine receptors termed BZ1 and BZ2. The BZ1 receptor is formed by the interaction of γ and α_1 subunits, whereas the BZ2 receptors are formed by the interaction of the γ and α_2, α_3, or α_5 subunits. The BZ1 receptor is involved in mediating the induction of sleep. This fact has led to the development of several classes of drug that specifically target this GABA-A receptor isoform. The nonbenzodiazepine drug, zolpidem (Ambien), exerts its hypnotic sleep-inducing effects due to near selective binding to the BZ1 site.

The receptor for the barbiturates is the beta (β) subunit of the GABA-A receptor. Barbiturates can induce GABA-A channel opening in the absence of GABA and for this reason they can induce a lethal level of CNS suppression.

CREATINE AND CREATININE BIOSYNTHESIS

Creatine is synthesized (Figure 19–5) in the liver by methylation of guanidoacetate. Guanidoacetate itself is formed in the kidney from the amino acids, arginine and glycine.

HIGH-YIELD CONCEPT

Both creatine and creatine phosphate are found in muscle, brain, and blood. Creatinine is formed in muscle from creatine phosphate by a nonenzymatic dehydration and loss of phosphate. The amount of creatinine produced is related to muscle mass and remains remarkably constant from day to day. Creatinine is excreted by the kidneys and the level of excretion (creatinine clearance rate) is a measure of renal function.

GLUTATHIONE

Glutathione (abbreviated GSH) is a tripeptide composed of glutamate, cysteine, and glycine and it is synthesized in the cytosol of all mammalian cells (Figure 19–6). Glutathione serves as a potent reductant eliminating hydroxy radicals, peroxynitrites, and hydroperoxides; it is conjugated to drugs to make them more water soluble; it is involved in amino acid transport across cell membranes (the γ-glutamyl cycle); it is a substrate for the synthesis of the peptidoleukotrienes (Chapter 12); it serves as a cofactor for some enzymatic reactions; and it serves as an aid in the rearrangement of protein disulfide bonds.

HIGH-YIELD CONCEPT

The role of GSH as a reductant is extremely important particularly in the highly oxidizing environment of the erythrocyte. In this capacity GSH serves as a cofactor in the reduction of hydrogen peroxide (H_2O_2) to H_2O catalyzed by glutathione peroxidase, GPx (see Figure 8–3).

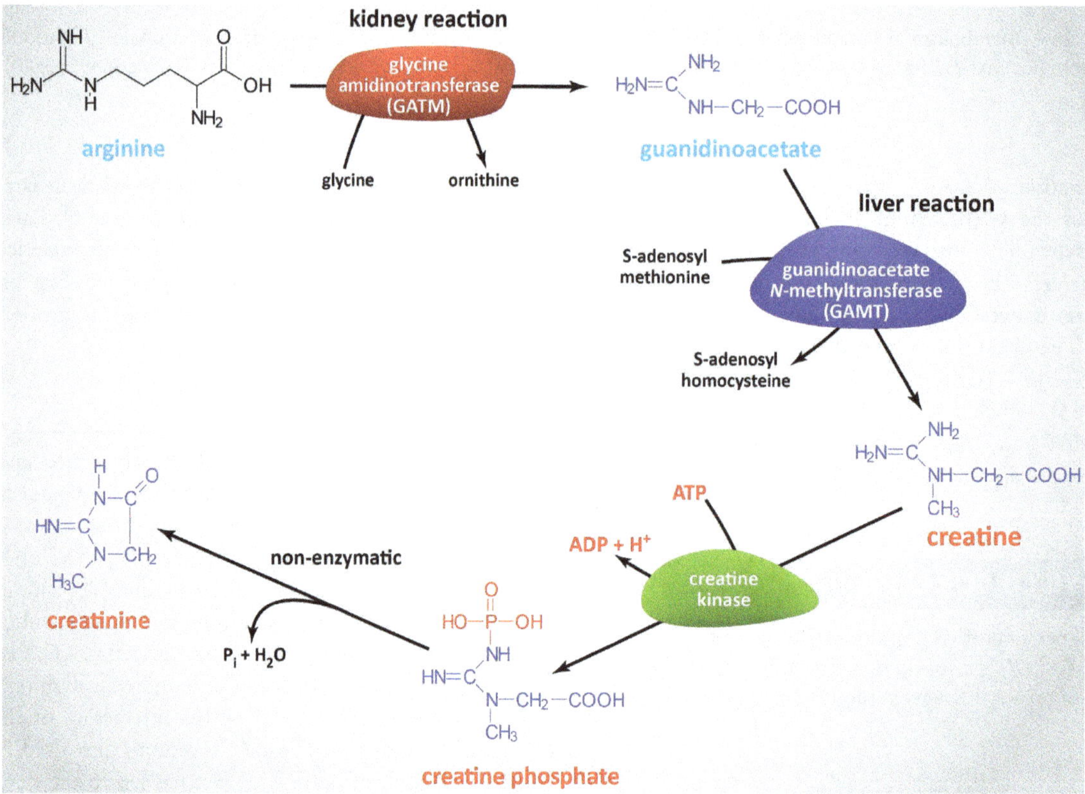

FIGURE 19–5 Synthesis of creatine and creatinine. The synthesis of creatine begins from arginine and glycine via the renal enzyme glycine amidinotransferase (GATM). The product, guanidinoacetate, is transported to the liver where it is methylated via the action of guanidinoacetate N-methyltransferase (GAMT) forming creatine. The methyl group is donated from S-adenosylmethionine (SAM). Creatine is released to the blood and picked up by the brain and skeletal muscle cells via the action of the SLC6A8 transporter. Creatine kinase (creatine phosphokinase) transfers a phosphate from ATP generating the high-energy intermediate, creatine phosphate. (Reproduced with permission from themedicalbiochemistrypage, LLC.)

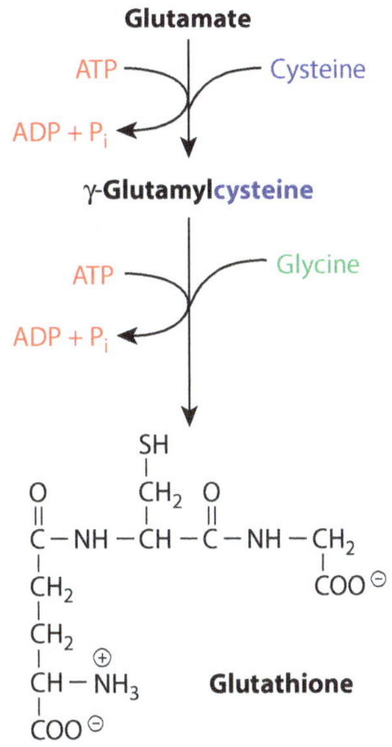

FIGURE 19–6 Synthesis of glutathione. The synthesis of glutathione, which occurs in the cytosol of all cells, proceeds via a two-step reaction involving the ATP-requiring enzymes glutamate-cysteine ligase (GCL) and glutathione synthetase (GSS). The common designation for reduced glutathione (monomeric) is GSH. When glutathione reduces reactive oxygen or nitrogen species, or upon its involvement in many other reduction reactions, it becomes oxidized to the dimeric form which is abbreviated as GSSG. (Reproduced with permission from themedicalbiochemistrypage, LLC.)

The oxidized form of GSH consists of two molecules that are disulfide bonded together (abbreviated GSSG). The enzyme, glutathione reductase, utilizes NADPH as a cofactor to reduce GSSG back to two moles of GSH. Hence, the pentose phosphate pathway is an extremely important pathway of erythrocytes for the continuing production of the NADPH needed by glutathione reductase.

Detoxification of xenobiotics or their metabolites is another major function of GSH. These compounds form conjugates with GSH either spontaneously or enzymatically in reactions catalyzed by GSH *S*-transferase. The conjugates formed are usually excreted from the cell and, in the case of the liver they are excreted in the bile.

CHECKLIST

- ☑ Nitric oxide is a major regulator of blood pressure, vascular homeostasis, coagulation, and immune functions. It is synthesized from the amino acid arginine via the action of three different nitric oxide synthases, NOS.
- ☑ The catecholamines are a family of neurotransmitters and hormones derived from the amino acid tyrosine. This family includes norepinephrine, epinephrine, and dopamine. Norepinephrine and epinephrine regulate cardiac, vascular, and metabolic processes of the periphery, whereas dopamine functions primarily within the CNS regulating reward circuitry.
- ☑ Serotonin and melatonin are neurotransmitters derived from the amino acid tryptophan. Serotonin (5-hydroxytryptamine, 5-HT) functions within the periphery, primarily the GI tract, and in the CNS. Within the CNS serotonin is a crucial regulator of affect, and drugs that increase its life time at nerve endings promotes increase in mood and behavior. Melatonin is diurnally synthesized and primarily regulates sleep-wake cycles.
- ☑ GABA is the major inhibitory neurotransmitter in the CNS. It is synthesized from the amino acid glutamate.
- ☑ Creatine phosphate is a major intramyocellular energy storage molecule, readily capable of donating its high-energy phosphate to ADP generating ATP via the action of creatine kinase (creatine phosphokinase). Creatine phosphate spontaneously dephosphorylates to creatinine which is excreted in the urine at a constant rate. The creatinine clearance rate is a measure of renal function.
- ☑ Glutathione is a major biological reductant important for detoxification of reactive oxygen species and oxidized macromolecules particularly membrane lipids. Glutathione is a tripeptide composed of glutamate, cysteine, and glycine.

REVIEW QUESTIONS

1. A 32-year-old woman who is at 32 weeks of gestation with her first child is being examined in the emergency department following a seizure. Additional symptoms found in this patient are swollen hands and feet, blood pressure of 165/125, right quadrant belly pain, and significant proteinuria. Additional blood work finds that her plasma zinc concentration is 0.3 μg/mL (N = 0.67–1.10 μg/mL). Given the results of the blood tests, which of the following is most likely deficient in this patient accounting for the neurologic pathology?
   (A) Acetylcholine
   (B) γ-Amino butyric acid (GABA)
   (C) Anandamide
   (D) Dopamine
   (E) Epinephrine
   (F) Tryptamine

2. Experiments are being carried out to examine the processes of DNA replication using a cell line derived from prostate cancer tissue. Results of these experiments find that the DNA in these cells fragments easily and does not replicate well. Additional results find that the level of spermidine is significantly reduced when compared to normal cells. It is most likely that these cancer cells are deficient in which of the following?
   (A) Adenosylhomocysteinase
   (B) Glutamate dehydrogenase
   (C) Methionine adenosyltransferase
   (D) Ornithine decarboxylase
   (E) Pyrroline-5-carboxylate reductase 1

3. Experiments are being conducted in an animal model system on a novel compound developed to act as a vasodilator via activation of an endothelial cell G_q-coupled receptor. Initial results find that the compound does indeed activate the receptor as evidenced by enhanced phospholipase Cβ (PLCβ) activity. However, there is no measurable decrease in vascular tone. The activity of which of the following is most likely impaired in the test animals?
   (A) Adenylate cyclase
   (B) Calmodulin
   (C) cGMP phosphodiesterase
   (D) Endothelial nitric oxide synthase
   (E) Guanylate cyclase

4. A 45-year-old man visits his physician with the complaint that he has an inability to perform sexually. History reveals that he experiences full nocturnal erections but during sex, although he is capable of erections, they do not last as long and that they are of lesser strength than 6 months ago. Which of the following is most likely associated with the reported symptoms in this patient?
   (A) Decreased cGMP phosphodiesterase activity
   (B) Decreased nitric oxide synthase activity
   (C) Decreased protein kinase C (PKC) activity
   (D) Increased protein kinase C (PKC) activity
   (E) Increased cAMP phosphodiesterase activity
   (F) Increased phospholipase Cβ (PLCβ) activity

5. A 61-year-old woman is being examined by her physician because of a 5-month history of progressive memory loss and cognitive difficulties. History reveals that she has been extremely forgetful, often misplaces her keys, and frequently does not remember where she parked the car. Physical examination and laboratory studies show no abnormalities. Her physician makes a tentative diagnosis of Alzheimer-type dementia. Which of the following neurotransmitters would be the ideal pharmacologic target of antagonism for treatment with this diagnosis?
   (A) Acetylcholine
   (B) γ-Aminobutyrate (GABA)
   (C) Dopamine
   (D) Glutamate
   (E) Norepinephrine

6. A 57-year-old man is undergoing examination by his physician for treatment of his hypertension. History indicates that the patient has experienced episodic severe hypertension for the past 18 months. Results of a CT scan show a large tumor of the adrenal gland on his right kidney with evidence that the cancer has metastasized to his liver. Blood work finds elevated levels of both norepinephrine and epinephrine. The physician prescribes a drug therapy to reduce adrenal medullary hormone production. Which of the following would represent the most likely target of this therapy?
   (A) Catecholamine-*O*-methyltransferase
   (B) Dopamine β-hydroxylase
   (C) DOPA decarboxylase
   (D) Monoamine oxidase
   (E) Phenylethanolamine-*N*-methyltransferase
   (F) Tyrosine hydroxylase

7. A 58-year-old man is seeing his physician with a complaint of impotence. History reveals that the patient is capable of attaining an erection but that they are not as turgid as he would like and that they do not last very long. This patient is most likely experiencing a reduction in the effects of which of the following?
   (A) Acetylcholine
   (B) γ-Aminobutyric acid (GABA)
   (C) Epinephrine
   (D) Nitric oxide
   (E) Serotonin

8. Experiments are being conducted on the process of creatine phosphate synthesis using cells derived from a human hepatoma. Results of these experiments show that creatine levels are reduced in these cells compared to normal hepatocytes. When an amino acid mixture is added to the culture system there is observed an increase in creatine level. Which of the following is the most likely amino acid in the added mixture accounting for the observed result?
   (A) Arginine
   (B) Asparagine
   (C) Aspartate
   (D) Glutamate
   (E) Glutamine

9. Experiments are being conducted on the process of creatine phosphate synthesis using cells derived from a human hepatoma. Results of these experiments show that creatine levels are reduced in these cells compared to normal hepatocytes. Which of the following is most likely defective in these cells?
   (A) Dihydropteridine reductase
   (B) Glutamate decarboxylase
   (C) Glycine amidinotransferase
   (D) Ornithine decarboxylase
   (E) Phenylethanolamine-*N*-methyltransferase

10. A 50-year-old man is being examined by his physician because of difficulty sleeping. History reveals that his insomnia is most likely caused by work-related stress. As a first approach to treatment, the physician suggests drinking a glass of warm whole milk before bedtime. Which of the following processes is most likely to be stimulated by this therapeutic approach?
(A) Catabolism of dopamine
(B) Catabolism of melatonin
(C) Catabolism of serotonin
(D) Synthesis of dopamine
(E) Synthesis of melatonin
(F) Synthesis of serotonin

11. A 29-year-old woman is being examined by her physician with complaints of having no energy, a lack of ability to concentrate with apparent attention deficit. In addition, the patient reports that she has been moody and feeling somewhat depressed. Following a complete physical, including a complete blood count and a comprehensive metabolic panel, it is discovered that the patient's level of copper is extremely low. Given the symptoms and findings in this patient which of the following processes is most likely impaired and accounts for her symptoms?
(A) Catecholamine catabolism
(B) Catecholamine synthesis
(C) GABA catabolism
(D) GABA synthesis
(E) Serotonin catabolism
(F) Serotonin synthesis

12. Experiments are being conducted on erythrocytes from a patient who suffers from recurrent episodes of mild hemolytic anemia. Analysis of these cells shows that they are highly sensitive to oxidative stress, likely due to the fact that they contain significantly less glutathione than normal erythrocytes. A deficiency in which of the following enzymes is most likely in these erythrocytes?
(A) Cystathionine β-synthase
(B) Glutamate-cysteine ligase
(C) Glutamate dehydrogenase
(D) Methionine synthase
(E) Ornithine decarboxylase

13. A 57-year-old man was seen by his physician with complaints of difficulty with starting and stopping urination, frequent urgency, and having to urinate frequently at night. His physician prescribed an appropriate medication and indicated that the patient return in 3 weeks to report results. At his follow-up visit the patient reports that he has observed no changes in urinary difficulties. Given these results, which of the following proteins is most likely to be impaired resulting in the negative pharmacologic effects?
(A) A G_i-type G-protein
(B) A G_s-type G-protein
(C) A G_q-type G-protein
(D) cAMP-dependent protein kinase, PKA
(E) cGMP-dependent protein kinase, PKG
(F) Phosphodiesterase 5, PDE5

14. Clinical trials are being performed to examine the efficacy of a novel monoamine oxidase inhibitor in the treatment of certain forms of major depressive disorder. The concentration of which of the following compounds is most likely to be increased in trial participants receiving this novel drug?
(A) γ-Aminobutyric acid, GABA
(B) Dihydroxyphenylalanine
(C) Epinephrine
(D) Melatonin
(E) Phenyllactate

15. Experiments are being conducted on a cell line derived from an adrenal medullary tumor. Assay of culture media shows high levels of vanillylmandelic acid? Given these results it is most likely that these cells have an enhanced level of which of the following processes?
(A) Acetylcholine synthesis
(B) γ-Aminobutyric acid (GABA) catabolism
(C) Catecholamine catabolism
(D) Creatine synthesis
(E) Tryptamine catabolism

ANSWERS

1. Correct answer is **B.** The patient is most likely exhibiting the signs and symptoms of pre-eclampsia that are exacerbated by a co-existent deficiency in zinc. The glutamate derivative, γ-aminobutyrate (GABA; also called 4-aminobutyrate) is a major inhibitor of presynaptic transmission in the central nervous system (CNS). Glutamic acid decarboxylase (GAD) catalyzes the decarboxylation of glutamic acid to form GABA. The activity of GAD requires pyridoxal phosphate (PLP) as a cofactor. PLP is generated through the action of pyridoxal kinase. Pyridoxal kinase itself requires zinc for activation. A deficiency in zinc or defects in pyridoxal kinase can lead to seizure disorders, particularly as seen in this pre-eclamptic patient. A deficiency in zinc would have little to no effect on any of the synthesis and/or function of the other neurotransmitters (choices A, C, D, E, and F).

2. Correct answer is **D.** Spermine and spermidine are polyamines whose functions include stabilization of DNA during the processes of replication. The initial step in polyamine synthesis is catalyzed by ornithine decarboxylase (ODC) which decarboxylates the amino acid ornithine producing putrescine. One of the earliest signals that cells have entered their replication cycle is the appearance of elevated levels of mRNA for ornithine decarboxylase 1 (ODC1). Adenosylhomocysteinase (choice A) is an enzyme in the methionine cycle that catalyzes the conversion of *S*-adenosylhomocysteine to homocysteine. Glutamate dehydrogenase (choice B) is a key enzyme in overall nitrogen homeostasis and catalyzes the formation of glutamate from ammonium ion and 2-oxoglutarate or in the reverse direction generates 2-oxoglutarate and ammonium ion from glutamate. Methionine adenosyltransferase (choice C) synthesizes *S*-adenosylmethionine from methionine and ATP. Pyrroline-5-carboxylate reductase 1 (choice E) is involved in the pathway of proline synthesis from glutamate.

3. Correct answer is **B.** The ability of G_q-coupled receptors in endothelial cells to exert vasodilatory effects is directly attributable to the release of calcium ions from the endoplasmic reticulum, ER. The activation of PLCβ by G_q-type G proteins leads to production of DAG and IP_3 from membrane-associated PIP_2. The IP_3 binds to receptors in the ER stimulating release of stored calcium. Both endothelial nitric oxide synthase (eNOS) and neuronal NOS (nNOS) are constitutively expressed and regulated by Ca^{2+}. The calcium regulation is imparted through the associated calmodulin subunits of NOS. Once activated NOS generates nitric oxide (NO) which then diffuses to the underlying smooth muscle cells where it initiates a cascade of event resulting in relaxation of the cells and consequent vasodilation. A defect in calmodulin would, therefore, lead to reduced calcium binding and consequent reduction in NOS activation. Adenylate cyclase (choice A) does not contribute to the effects of G_q-type G proteins. A defect in cGMP phosphodiesterase (choice C) or guanylate cyclase (choice E) in smooth muscle cells would affect expected changes in vascular tone since NO in smooth muscle activates guanylate cyclase and the production of cGMP. However, the defect associated with the activation of PLCβ would most likely be associated with the endothelium and not the smooth muscle. Although NOS deficiency (choice D) could account for lack of change in vascular tone in response to the novel compound, the association of a lack of response to activation of PLCb is more likely due to a defect in the function of calmodulin.

4. Correct answer is **B.** Penile erection involves the relaxation of smooth muscle in the corpus cavernosum. The key mediator of smooth muscle relaxation is nitric oxide (NO), which acts by increasing level of cGMP within smooth muscle cells. The production of NO occurs in the endothelial cells of the vasculature through activation of nitric oxide synthase (NOS). The production of cGMP results in activation of cGMP-dependent protein kinase (PKG; specifically, the PKGI isoforms) and the phosphorylation of various protein substrates. Significant targets and the effects of PKGI in SMC are activation of myosin light chain phosphatase, inhibition of PLCβ, inhibition of the IP_3 receptor, inhibition of plasma membrane localized L-type Ca^{2+} channels, and activation of plasma membrane localized calcium-activated K^+ channels (commonly called the big potassium, BK, channels). The net effect of all these phosphorylation events is smooth muscle cell relaxation. In addition to activating PKGI, cGMP itself contributes to smooth muscle relaxation through direct inhibition of the plasma membrane localized L-type Ca^{2+} channels. Therefore, a decrease in NOS activity would contribute to a decrease in smooth muscle relaxation in the corpus cavernosum and erectile dysfunction. A decrease in cGMP phosphodiesterase activity (choice A) would result in enhanced smooth muscle relaxation due to reduced degradation of any generated cGMP. This would enhance erectile function as opposed to the decrease present in this patient. Protein kinase C (choices C and D) does not contribute to the signaling processes directly controlling erectile function. Although cAMP does play a role in smooth muscle relaxation (choice E), it is not as significant as cGMP. An increase in PLCβ activity (choice F) would increase smooth muscle contraction preventing erection; however, in the presence of active NO production by the endothelium and its actions in smooth muscle this would not be the most likely contributor to a patient's erectile dysfunction.

5. Correct answer is **D.** The patient is most likely exhibiting the early symptoms of Alzheimer disease. Within the central nervous system (CNS) glutamate is the main excitatory neurotransmitter. Glutamatergic neurons possess four distinct classes of ionotropic (ion channel) receptors that bind glutamate released from presynaptic neurons. Three of these receptor classes were identified on the basis of their binding affinities for certain substrates and are thus, referred to as the kainate, 2-amino-3-hydroxy-5-methyl-4-isoxazolepropionic acid (AMPA), and *N*-methyl-D-aspartate (NMDA) receptors. The fourth class of ionotropic glutamate receptor is termed the delta (δ) receptors. Neurons that respond to glutamine (glutamatergic neurons) are responsible for the mediation of many vital processes such as the encoding of information, the formation and retrieval of memories, spatial recognition, and the maintenance of consciousness. Dysfunction in glutamatergic neurotransmission is believed to play a role in the etiology of Alzheimer disease. Targeting glutamatergic neurotransmission, specifically via the NMDA receptors, has shown efficacy in treating Alzheimer disease. Memantidine, approved for use in treating Alzheimer disease, is an antagonist of the NMDA receptor. Antagonism of the other neurotransmitters (choices A, B, C, and E) is not associated with efficacy in the treatment of Alzheimer disease.

6. Correct answer is **F.** The medullary tumor identified in this patient is most likely contributing to his symptoms due to excess medullary catecholamine synthesis. Tyrosine is transported into catecholamine-secreting neurons and adrenal medullary chromaffin cells where catecholamine synthesis takes place. The first step in the process involves the enzyme tyrosine hydroxylase which represents the rate-limiting reaction of catecholamine biosynthesis. Therefore, inhibition of tyrosine hydroxylase would represent an effective mechanism for reducing the adrenal medullary synthesis of epinephrine and norepinephrine. Catecholamine-*O*-methyltransferase (choice A) and monoamine oxidase (choice D) are enzymes of catecholamine catabolism, therefore, inhibiting these enzymes would most likely result in increased levels of epinephrine and norepinephrine. The other three enzymes (choices B, C, and E) are involved in catecholamine synthesis downstream of the tyrosine hydroxylase reaction. Since phenylethanolamine *N*-methyltransferase (choice E) synthesizes epinephrine from norepinephrine, inhibition of this enzyme would only reduce epinephrine levels in the patient.

7. Correct answer is **D.** Penile erection involves the relaxation of smooth muscle in the corpus cavernosum. The key mediator of smooth muscle relaxation is nitric oxide (NO), which acts by increasing the level of cGMP within smooth muscle cells. The production of NO occurs in the endothelial cells of the vasculature through activation of nitric oxide synthase (NOS). The endothelial cell NO then diffuses into the underlying smooth muscle cells where it binds to the heme moiety of a soluble guanylyl cyclase (also identified as guanylate cyclase), thereby activating the enzyme. The activated guanylate cyclase converts GTP to cGMP which then exerts effects in the smooth muscle cell leading to relaxation and consequent vasodilation. None of the other neurotransmitters (choices A, B, C, and E) play a direct role in the processes of penile erection.

8. Correct answer is **A.** Creatine synthesis occurs predominantly in the kidneys and the liver. The synthesis of creatine begins in the kidneys using the amino acids arginine and glycine. The formation of guanidinoacetate (GAA) from these two amino acids is catalyzed by the enzyme glycine amidinotransferase, also called L-arginine:glycine amidinotransferase (AGAT). None of the other amino acids (choices B, C, D, and E) are involved in the synthesis of creatine.

9. Correct answer is **C.** Creatine synthesis occurs predominantly in the kidneys and the liver. The synthesis of creatine begins in the kidneys using the amino acids arginine and glycine. The formation of guanidinoacetate (GAA) from these two amino acids is catalyzed by the enzyme glycine amidinotransferase,

also called L-arginine:glycine amidinotransferase (AGAT). Dihydropteridine reductase (choice A) is involved in the reactions catalyzed by phenylalanine hydroxylase, tyrosine hydroxylase, and tryptophan hydroxylase. Glutamate decarboxylase (choice B) synthesizes γ-aminobutyric acid (GABA) from glutamate. Ornithine decarboxylase (choice D) catalyzes the rate-limiting reaction in the synthesis of the polyamines. Phenylethanolamine-*N*-methyltransferase (choice E) converts norepinephrine to epinephrine.

10. Correct answer is **F.** Whole milk is one of the largest sources of tryptophan. Serotonin is synthesized from the amino acid tryptophan. Low serotonin levels result in sleep disruption and sleep disorders, including insomnia. Stress is a common cause of low serotonin levels, resulting in a snowballing feedback cycle of disrupted sleep, depression, anxiety, and fatigue during the day. None of the other options (choices A, B, C, D, and E) correlate to the sleep-inducing effect of milk consumption.

11. Correct answer is **B.** The signs and symptoms in this patient are most closely reflective of a deficiency in norepinephrine, one of the three catecholamine neurotransmitters. Low levels of norepinephrine can cause lethargy, lack of concentration, attention deficit hyperactivity disorder (ADHD), and possibly depression. Norepinephrine is derived from the amino acid tyrosine and involves the enzyme, dopamine β-hydroxylase. Dopamine β-hydroxylase is an ascorbate- and copper-dependent enzyme, therefore, deficiency in copper would result in reduced levels of norepinephrine. None of the other processes (choices A, C, D, E, and F) would be significantly affected by a copper deficiency.

12. Correct answer is **B.** Glutathione (GSH) is synthesized in the cytosol of all mammalian cells via a two-step reaction. The rate of GSH synthesis is dependent upon the availability of cysteine and the activity of the rate-limiting enzyme, glutamate-cysteine ligase (GCL). The second reaction of GSH synthesis involves the enzyme, glutathione synthetase, which condenses γ-glutamylcysteine with glycine. Cystathionine β-synthase (choice A) is an enzyme involved in the synthesis of cysteine from methionine. Glutamate dehydrogenase (choice C) catalyzes a reaction that can proceed in either direction, dependent on energy needs and nitrogen levels. This reaction condenses ammonium ion with 2-oxoglutarate, forming glutamate, or carries out the reverse reaction. Methionine synthase (choice D), which is also known as homocysteine methyltransferase, produces methionine from homocysteine and N^5-methyltetrahydrofolate. Ornithine decarboxylase (choice E) catalyzes the rate-limiting reaction in the synthesis of the polyamines.

13. Correct answer is **C.** The patient is most likely experiencing the effects of benign prostatic hyperplasia (BPH). BPH is a common condition occurring in males as they age. An enlarged prostate gland can cause uncomfortable urinary symptoms, such as blocking the flow of urine out of the bladder. One of the most common therapeutic interventions in BPH is the use of α_1-adrenergic receptor blockers. The α_1-adrenergic receptor is coupled to a G_q-type G protein. When the receptor is activated by epinephrine (or norepinephrine), the activation of the associated G protein leads to activation of phospholipase Cβ (PLCβ). PLCβ hydrolyzes diacylglycerol (DAG) and inositol-1,4,5-trisphosphate (IP_3) from membrane-localized phosphatidylinositol-4,5-bisphosphate (PIP_2). IP_3 binds to receptors in the sarcoplasmic reticulum of smooth muscle cells stimulating release of stored calcium to the cytosol. The calcium will bind to the calmodulin subunit of myosin light-chain kinase (MLCK) activating the kinase. MLCK then phosphorylates myosin light chains causing smooth muscle contraction. Therefore, the antagonism of α_1-adrenergic receptors should lead to the relaxation of the smooth muscles of the prostate and bladder neck to improve urine flow and reduce bladder blockage. The fact that the medication does not work as expected is most likely due to a defect in the signaling of α_1-adrenergic receptors in these tissues, such as the associated G_q-type G protein. Although phosphodiesterase 5 (choice F) inhibitors do show positive effects in patient with BPH, these drugs are primarily used to treat erectile dysfunction. None of the other options (choices A, B, D, E, and F) are related to drug targets in the treatment of BPH.

14. Correct answer is **C.** Epinephrine and norepinephrine are catabolized to inactive compounds through the sequential actions of catecholamine-*O*-methyltransferase (COMT) and monoamine oxidase (MAO). Compounds that inhibit the action of MAO have been shown to have beneficial effects in the treatment of clinical depression and anxiety disorders. The inhibition of MAO would, therefore, result in increasing levels of both epinephrine and norepinephrine. The action of MAO is not involved in the catabolism of the other options (choices A, B, D, and E).

15. Correct answer is **C.** Epinephrine and norepinephrine are catabolized to inactive compounds through the sequential actions of catecholamine-*O*-methyltransferase (COMT) and monoamine oxidase (MAO). The terminal catabolic product of the actions of these two enzymes, with respect to norepinephrine catabolism, is vanillylmandelic acid. None of the other options (choices A, B, D, and E) correspond to substances whose synthesis or catabolism involves vanillylmandelic acid as an intermediate or end product.

C H A P T E R

20

Nucleotide Metabolism

High-Yield Terms	
5-phosphoribosyl-1-pyrophosphate, PRPP	Activated form of ribose used in *de novo* synthesis of purine and pyrimidine nucleotides
Gout	A disorder that is related to excess production and deposition of uric acid crystals, does not occur in the absence of hyperuricemia
Severe-combined immunodeficiency, SCID	A disorder related to defects in the activity of the purine nucleotide catabolism enzyme, adenosine deaminase (ADA)
Tumor lysis syndrome, TLS	Potentially fatal condition characterized by acute urate nephropathy resulting from significant increases in purine nucleotide degradation from dying cancer cells

PURINE NUCLEOTIDE BIOSYNTHESIS

The *de novo* synthesis pathways of both purines and pyrimidines, as well as the pathway of purine salvage utilize the activated sugar intermediate, 5-phosphoribosyl-1-pyrophosphate (PRPP). PRPP is synthesized from ribose-5-phosphate via the action of PRPP synthetase (Figure 20–1).

Synthesis of the purine nucleotides begins with PRPP and leads to the first fully formed nucleotide, inosine 5′-monophosphate (IMP) (Figure 20–2).

IMP represents a branch point for purine biosynthesis, because it can be converted into either AMP or GMP through two distinct reaction pathways (Figure 20–3). The pathway leading to AMP requires energy in the form of GTP; the pathway leading to GMP requires energy in the form of ATP.

REGULATION OF PURINE NUCLEOTIDE SYNTHESIS

Control over purine nucleotide synthesis is exerted at the first two reactions of the pathway, PRPP synthetase and glutamine phosphoribosylpyrophosphate amidotransferase, commonly referred to simply as amidotransferase (Figure 20–4). The activity of PRPP synthetase is enhanced by increased levels of ribose-5-phosphate. This fact explains the hyperuricemia associated with the glycogen storage disease, von Gierke disease (see Clinical Box 7–4). Conversely, PRPP synthetase is feedback inhibited by purine-5′-nucleotides (predominantly AMP and GMP). The amidotransferase is feedback inhibited by binding ATP, ADP, and AMP at one inhibitory site and GTP, GDP, and GMP at another. Conversely, the activity of the enzyme is stimulated by PRPP. Additionally, purine biosynthesis is regulated in the branch pathways from IMP to AMP and GMP (Figure 20–5). The accumulation of excess ATP leads to enhanced synthesis of GMP, and excess GTP leads to enhanced synthesis of AMP.

CATABOLISM AND SALVAGE OF PURINE NUCLEOTIDES

Catabolism of the purine nucleotides leads ultimately to the production of uric acid (Figure 20–6), which is insoluble and is excreted in the urine. Uric acid excretion and reabsorption occurs within the proximal tubules of the kidney. Elevation in uric acid levels can result in precipitation of urate crystals, with monosodium urate crystals being the most commonly occurring, in the synovial fluids of the joints. The accumulation of urate crystals in the joints is the hallmark of gout (Clinical Box 20–1).

In the treatment of numerous cancers, particularly the treatment of leukemias and lymphomas, the increased uric acid produced by the dying cells contributes to the potentially fatal condition termed, tumor lysis syndrome (Clinical Box 20–2).

Purine nucleotide salvage (Figure 20–7) is highly efficient; thus, the need for *de novo* synthesis is generally minimal. Deficiencies in several of the enzymes of purine salvage are known with hypoxanthine-guanine phosphoribosyltransferase (Clinical Box 20–3) and adenosine deaminase (Clinical Box 20–4) deficiencies resulting in severe disorders.

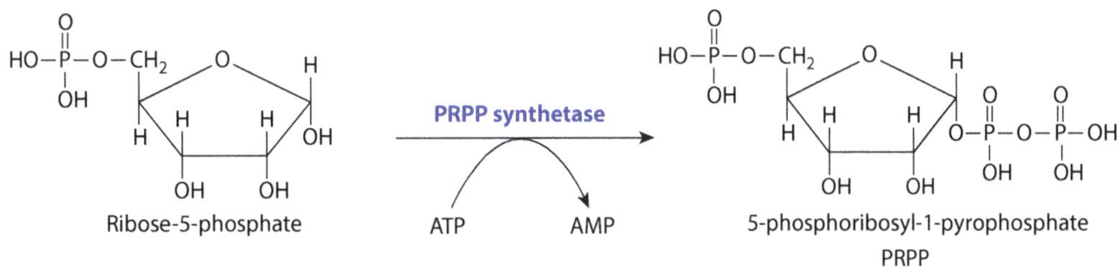

FIGURE 20–1 PRPP synthetase reaction. (Reproduced with permission from themedicalbiochemistrypage, LLC.)

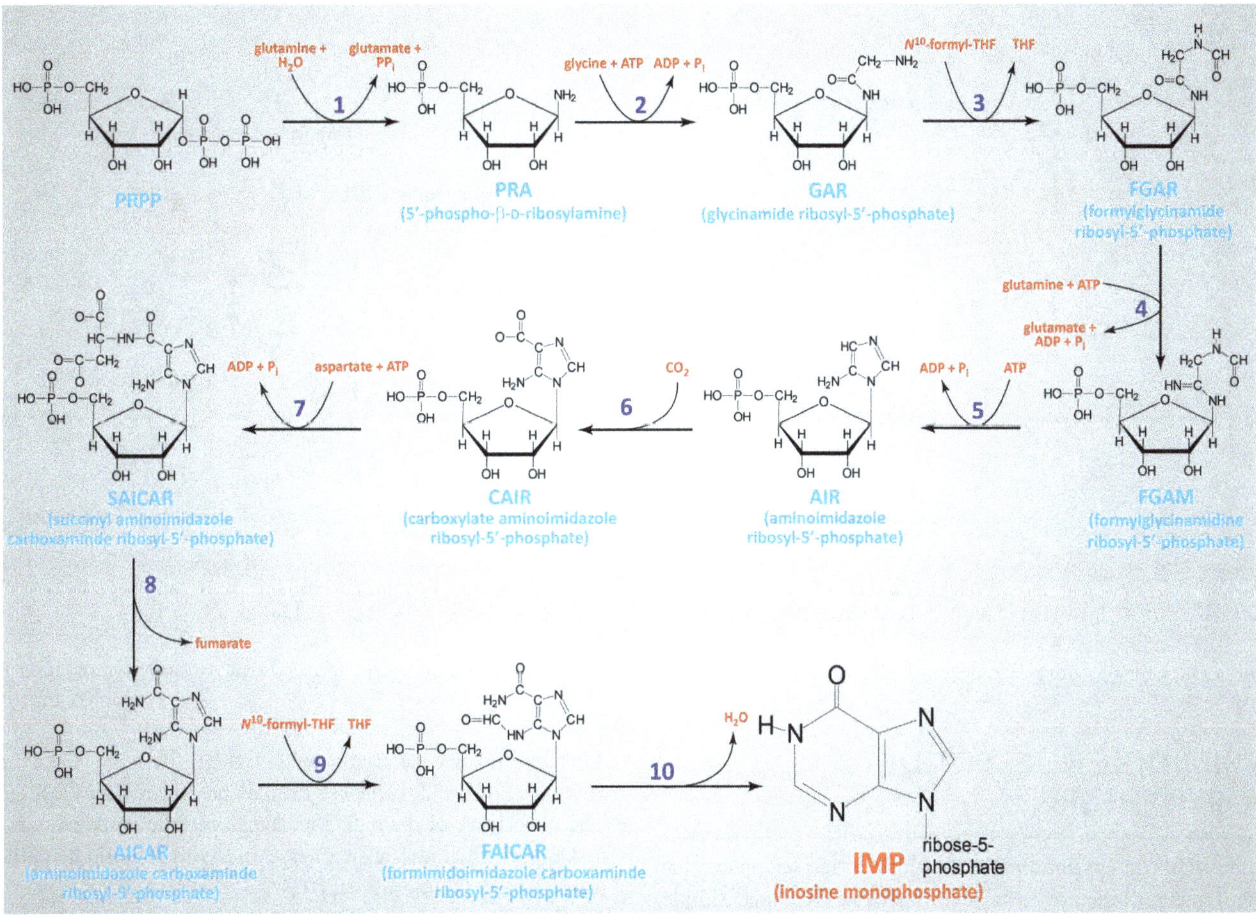

FIGURE 20–2 De novo purine nucleotide synthesis pathway. Synthesis of the first fully formed purine nucleotide, inosine monophosphate, IMP begins with PRPP. Through a series of reactions utilizing ATP, tetrahydrofolate (THF) derivatives, glutamine, glycine, and aspartate, this pathway yields IMP. The rate-limiting reaction is catalyzed by glutamine PRPP amidotransferase, the enzyme indicated by 1 in the figure. The numbers in the figure correspond to the following enzyme activity names:

1. glutamine phosphoribosylpyrophosphate amidotransferase (GPAT activity of the *PPAT* gene)
2. glycinamide ribonucleotide synthetase (GARS activity of the *GART* gene)
3. glycinamide ribonucleotide formyltransferase (GART activity of the *GART* gene)
4. phosphoribosylformylglycinamide synthase (PFAS activity of the *PFAS* gene)
5. aminoimidazole ribonucleotide synthetase (AIRS activity of the *GART* gene)
6. aminoimidazole ribonucleotide carboxylase (AIRC activity of the *PAICS* gene)
7. succinylaminoimidazolecarboxamide ribonucleotide synthetase (SAICAR activity of the *PAICS* gene)
8. adenylosuccinate lyase (ADSL activity of the *ADSL* gene)
9. 5-aminoimidazole-4-carboxamide ribonucleotide formyltransferase (AICARFT activity of the *ATIC* gene)
10. IMP cyclohydrolase (IMPCH activity of the *ATIC* gene) (Reproduced with permission from themedicalbiochemistrypage, LLC.)

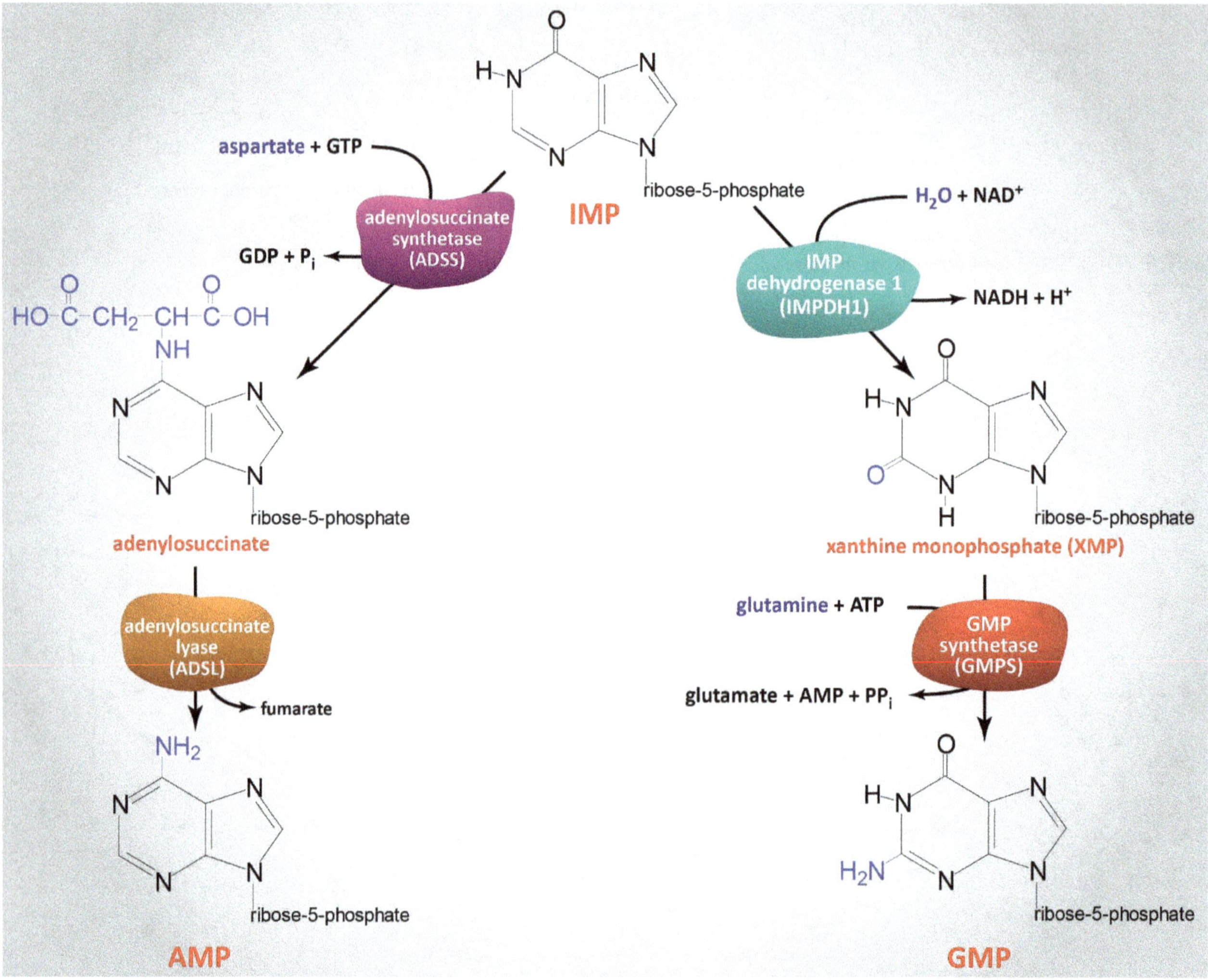

FIGURE 20–3 Synthesis of AMP and GMP from IMP. (Reproduced with permission from themedicalbiochemistrypage, LLC.)

PYRIMIDINE NUCLEOTIDE BIOSYNTHESIS

Synthesis of the pyrimidine nucleotides is less complex than that of the purines since the base is chemically much simpler (Figure 20–8). The first completed pyrimidine base is orotate monophosphate (OMP). OMP is subsequently decarboxylated to UMP. UMP is phosphorylated twice to yield UTP. CTP is synthesized from UTP via the action of CTP synthase (Figure 20–9).

THYMIDINE NUCLEOTIDE SYNTHESIS

The *de novo* pathway to thymidine nucleotide (dTTP) synthesis first requires the use of dUMP. The dUMP is converted to dTMP (5-methyl-dUMP) by the action of thymidylate synthetase (Figure 20–10). This reaction requires the cofactor, N^5-N^{10}-methylene-THF (methyleneTHF), which is oxidatively demethylated to dihydrofolate (DHF). The DHF is reduced to THF by dihydrofolate reductase (DHFR), the same enzyme that generates DHF and then THF from dietary folates (see Chapter 3). The critical role of thymidine nucleotides in the synthesis of DNA makes both thymidylate synthetase and DHFR ideal chemotherapeutic targets (Clinical Box 20–5).

The salvage pathway to dTTP synthesis involves the enzyme thymidine kinase which can use either thymidine or deoxyuridine as substrate. The activity of the cytoplasmic version of thymidine kinase (TK1) is regulated in a cyclic manner with peak expression of the *TK1* gene occurring during S-phase of the cell cycle.

REGULATION OF PYRIMIDINE BIOSYNTHESIS

The regulation of pyrimidine synthesis occurs mainly at the first step catalyzed by the trifunctional enzyme encoded by the *CAD* gene. The CPS2 domain of the CAD enzyme is activated by ATP and inhibited by UDP, UTP, dUTP, and CTP. Pyrimidine

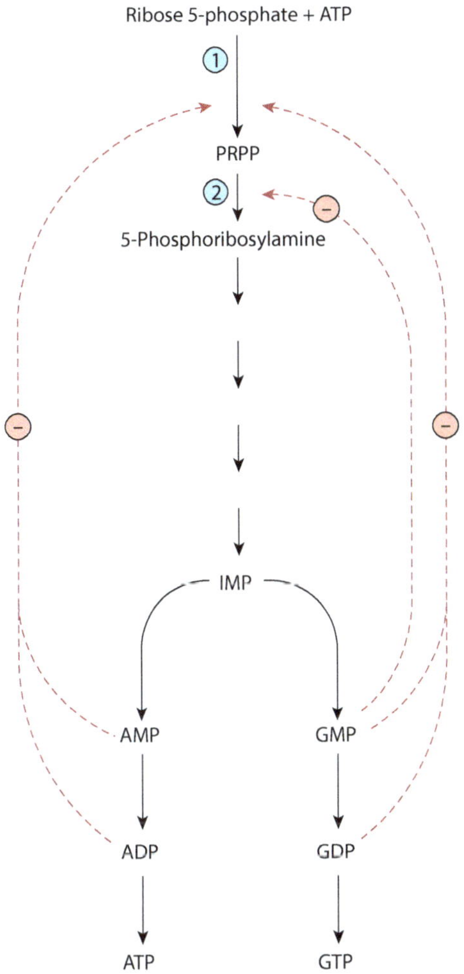

FIGURE 20–4 Control of the rate of *de novo* purine nucleotide biosynthesis. Reactions 1 and 2 are catalyzed by PRPP synthase and by PRPP glutamyl amidotransferase, respectively. Solid lines represent chemical flow. Broken red lines represent feedback inhibition by intermediates of the pathway. (Reproduced with permission from Rodwell VW, Bender DA, Botham KM, et al: *Harper's Illustrated Biochemistry*, 31st ed. New York, NY: McGraw Hill; 2018.)

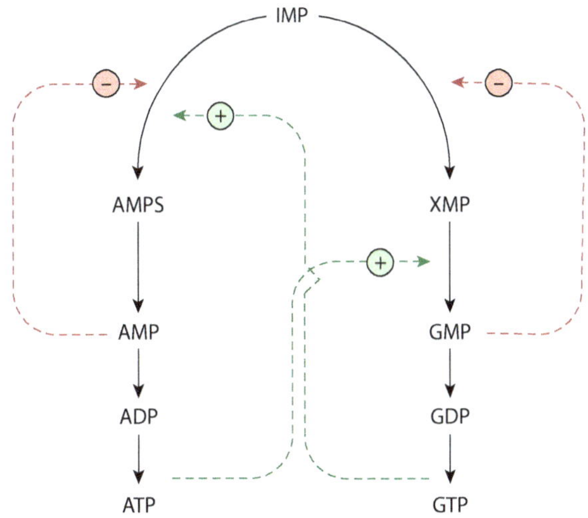

FIGURE 20–5 Regulation of the conversion of IMP to adenosine nucleotides and guanosine nucleotides. Solid lines represent chemical flow. Broken green lines represent positive feedback loops +, and broken red lines represent negative feedback loops ⊖. Abbreviations include AMPS (adenylosuccinate) and XMP (xanthosine monophosphate). (Reproduced with permission from Rodwell VW, Bender DA, Botham KM, et al: *Harper's Illustrated Biochemistry*, 31st ed. New York, NY: McGraw Hill; 2018.)

synthesis is also regulated by the level of PRPP. The OMP decarboxylase activity of the bifunctional enzyme, UMP synthase, is competitively inhibited by UMP and, to a lesser degree, by CMP. Finally, CTP synthase is feedback-inhibited by CTP and activated by GTP.

CATABOLISM OF PYRIMIDINE NUCLEOTIDES

Catabolism of the pyrimidine nucleotides leads ultimately to β-alanine (when CMP and UMP are degraded) or β-aminoisobutyrate (when dTMP is degraded) and NH_3 and CO_2. Because the products of pyrimidine catabolism are water soluble there are few clinical signs or symptoms due to increased pyrimidine catabolism.

Two rare inherited disorders affecting pyrimidine biosynthesis are the result of deficiencies in the bifunctional, UMP synthase. These deficiencies result in a megaloblastic anemia, impaired growth, and severe orotic aciduria. The megaloblastic anemia cannot be treated by addition of vitamin B_{12} or folate to the diet. These disorders can be treated with uridine and/or cytidine, which increase UMP production and consequently thymidine nucleotides. The UMP will also inhibit the CPS2 activity of the CAD enzyme, the result of which is attenuated orotic acid production.

FORMATION OF DEOXYRIBONUCLEOTIDES

The deoxynucleotides are generated from the corresponding nucleotide diphosphates (NDP) via the action of ribonucleotide reductase (RR). Ribonucleotide reductase is the only enzyme used in the generation of all the deoxyribonucleotides, therefore, its activity and substrate specificity must be tightly regulated (Figure 20–11). The allosteric regulatory sites of RR bind ATP, dATP, dGTP, or dTTP with high affinity. The binding of ATP at activity sites leads to increased enzyme activity, while the binding of dATP inhibits the enzyme.

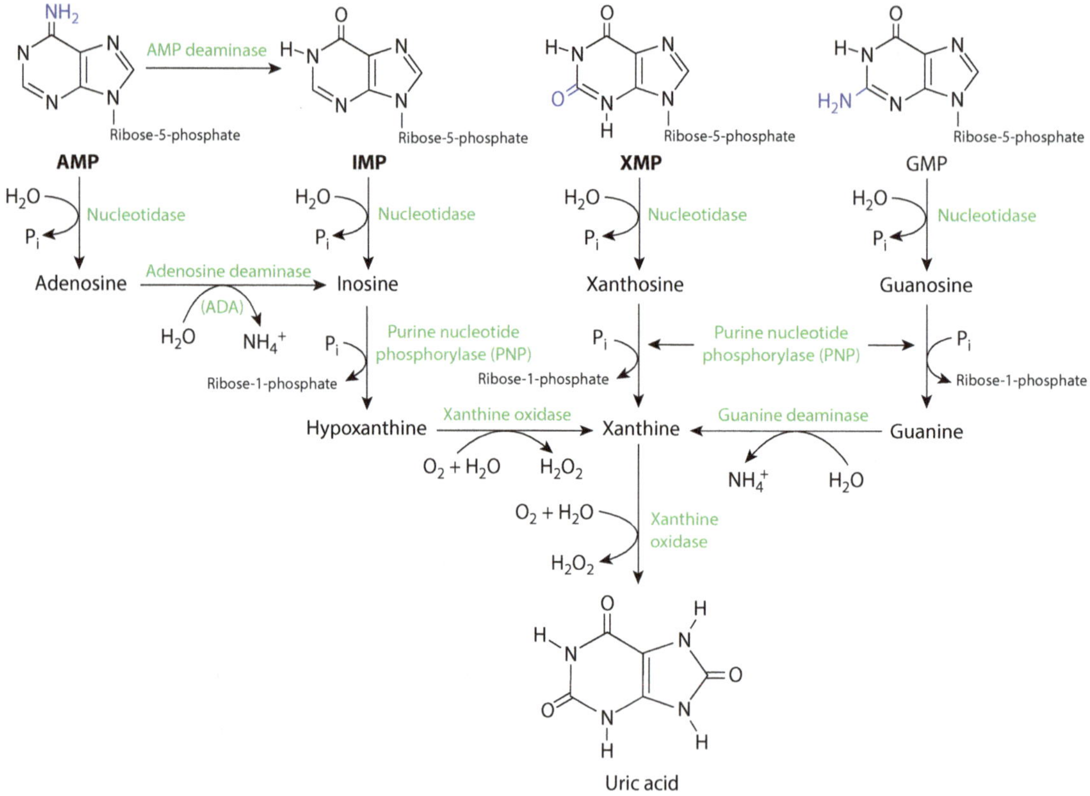

FIGURE 20–6 Pathways of purine nucleotide catabolism. The purine mononucleotides, (d)AMP, (d)GMP, IMP, and XMP (where the lower case "d" refers to the deoxyribonucleotide forms) are all catabolized to uric acid. Each mononucleotide is first converted to the phosphate free nucleoside form through the actions of one of several cytosolic 5′-nucleotidases. The nitrogen is removed from dAMP and AMP by AMP deaminase generating IMP. Alternatively, adenosine is deaminated to inosine by the critical enzyme, adenosine deaminase, ADA. The ribose is removed from the nucleotides by purine nucleoside phosphorylase (PNP) yielding the nucleobases, hypoxanthine, xanthine, and guanine. The nitrogen is removed from guanine by guanine deaminase yielding xanthine. Hypoxanthine and xanthine are then converted to the terminal product of purine catabolism, uric acid, by the enzyme xanthine oxidase. (Reproduced with permission from themedicalbiochemistrypage, LLC.)

CLINICAL BOX 20–1 HYPERURICEMIA AND GOUT

Gout is a disorder that is related to excess production and deposition of uric acid crystals. Uric acid is the byproduct of purine nucleotide catabolism. The root cause of gout is hyperuricemia and it is characterized by recurrent attacks of acute inflammatory arthritis. The formation of urate crystals leads to the formation of tophaceous deposits (sandy, gritty, nodular masses of urate crystals), particularly in the joints which precipitates the episodes of gouty arthritis. Gouty arthritis is the most painful manifestation of gout and is caused when urate crystals interact with neutrophils triggering an inflammatory response. Gout does not occur in the absence of hyperuricemia. Hyperuricemia is defined as a serum urate concentration exceeding 6.8 mg/dL in both men and women. However, it should be noted that serum urate concentrations vary markedly among different populations and the values are influenced by such things as age, sex, ethnicity, body weight, and the surface area of the body. Hyperuricemia can result from either excess uric acid production or reduced excretion or a combination of both mechanisms. Primary gout is a biochemically and genetically heterogeneous disorder resulting from inborn metabolic errors that alter uric acid homeostasis. There are at least three different inherited defects that lead to early development of severe hyperuricemia and gout: glucose-6-phosphatase (gene symbol: G6PT) deficiency; severe and partial hypoxanthine-guanine phosphoribosyltransferase (HGPRT, gene symbol: HPRT) deficiency; and elevated 5′-phosphoribosyl-1′-pyrophosphate synthetase (PRPP synthetase) activity. At least three different enzymes with PRPP synthetase activity have been identified which are encoded by three distinct genes. These genes are identified as *PRPS1, PRPS2*, and *PRPS1L1*. Mutations in the *PRPS1* gene are those that are associated with PRPP synthetase superactivity. In addition, mutations in the *PRPS1* gene are associated with Arts syndrome and Charcot-Marie-Tooth disease X-linked recessive type 5. A complete or virtually complete loss of HGPRT activity results in the severe disorder, Lesch-Nyhan syndrome (see Clinical Box 20–3). Although Lesch-Nyhan syndrome is known more for the associated bizarre emotional behaviors, there is also overproduction and excretion of uric acid and gouty manifestation. Less dramatic reductions in HGPRT activity do cause

CLINICAL BOX 20–1 (CONTINUED)

hyperuricemia and gout due to the reduced salvage of hypoxanthine and guanine leading to increased uric acid production. Deficiencies in glucose-6-phosphatase result in type I glycogen storage disease (von Gierke disease, Clinical Box 7–4). However, associated with this defect is increased uric acid production and symptoms of gout. The inability to dephosphorylate glucose-6-phosphate leads to an increase in the diversion of this sugar into the pentose phosphate pathway (PPP). One major product of the PPP is ribose-5-phosphate. An increase in the production of ribose-5-phosphate results in substrate-level activation of PRPP synthetase. Hyperuricemia does not always lead to the typical clinical manifestations of gout. These symptoms usually only appear in a person suffering with hyperuricemia for 20–30 years. The normal course of untreated hyperuricemia, leading to progressive urate crystal deposition, begins with uric acid urolithiasis (urate kidney stones) and progresses to acute gouty arthritis, then intercritical gout and chronic tophaceous gout. Intercritical gout refers to the period between gouty attacks. Diagnosis of gout during these periods is difficult, but analysis for urate crystals in the synovial fluids of a previously affected joint can establish a correct diagnosis. Numerous circumstances can precipitate gouty attacks such as trauma, surgery, excessive alcohol consumption, administration of certain drugs, and the ingestion of purine-rich foods. Acute gouty arthritis consists of painful episodes of inflammatory arthritis and represents the most common manifestation of gout. Typical descriptions of this symptom include a patient who goes to bed and awakens by severe pain in the big toe but may also be experienced in the heel, instep or ankle. The pain is described as that of a dislocated joint and is often accompanied or preceded by chills and a slight fever. The pain progresses and is often described as if a dog were gnawing on the limb. The pain can become so severe that the simple act of cloth touching the area is unbearable. Gouty arthritis attacks usually dissipate within several hours but can also last for several weeks. The inflammatory processes initiated in gouty arthritis are the result of neutrophil ingestion (phagocytosis) of urate crystals and the subsequent release of numerous inflammatory mediators. Gouty arthritis usually develops in males in the fourth to sixth decade of life and in the sixth to eight decade in women. Episodes of gouty arthritis that occur in childhood, in early adults or in premenopausal women should suggest an underlying inherited enzyme defect or the ingestion of some agent that interferes with uric acid metabolism. Chronic tophaceous gout results after a number of years in an untreated individual. Episodes of acute gouty arthritis become more frequent and severe and the intercritical period may disappear completely. This stage of the disease is characterized by the deposition of solid urate (tophi) in the articular (cartilage covering the bony ends of the articulating joints) and other connective tissues. The continued development of tophi results in destructive arthropathy (disease of a joint). Aside from gouty arthritis and tophus formation, renal disease is the most frequent complication of hyperuricemia. Kidney disease in patients with gout is of numerous types. Urate nephropathy is the result of the deposition of monosodium urate crystals in the renal interstitial tissue. Uric acid nephropathy is caused by the deposition of uric acid crystals in the collecting tubules, renal pelvis or the ureter and results in impaired urine flow. Calcium oxalate urolithiasis also occurs in hyperuricemic patients. Uric acid urolithiasis (uric acid kidney stones) accounts for approximately 10% of all urinary calculi (stones) in the United States. Additional renal effects of hyperuricemia include metabolic acidosis caused by defective lactic acid excretion which in turn exacerbates the hyperuricemia due to reduced urate excretion. The major renal urate-anion exchanger is encoded by the solute carrier gene, *SLC22A12* (originally identified as the urate transporter 1, URAT1 protein). Expression of SLC22A12 is very high in the epithelial cells of the proximal tubule of the renal cortex but is not expressed in the distal tubules. The SLC22A12 transporter cotransports urate along with chloride and iodine anions. Transport of urate via SLC22A12 is selectively inhibited by lactate, succinate, β-hydroxybutyrate, and acetoacetate. Urate reabsorption is coupled to renal lactate reabsorption at the apical membrane of the proximal tubule cell via interactions between SLC22A12 and the lactate transporters SLC5A8 and SCL5A12. Due to this interaction lactic acidemia impairs urate reabsorption and excretion while hyperuricemia results in impaired lactate excretion and reabsorption. Treatments aimed at lowering serum urate levels in hyperuricemic patients are usually only a consideration in the context of gout. Because acute gouty arthritis is an inflammatory event, treatment with anti-inflammatory drugs is often successful in reducing the symptoms. The inflammation caused by acute attacks of hyperuricemia can be treated with the use of colchicine. Colchicine is a microtubule polymerization inhibitor that functions by binding to tubulin. Failure to form functional microtubule filaments results in inhibition of immune cell (B and T cell) division as well as inhibition of phagocytosis of urate crystals by monocytes/macrophages. The overall effect of colchicine is a reduction in inflammatory processes. Treatments for chronic hyperuricemia and the resultant gout include the use of uricosuric drugs and drugs that inhibit the production of uric acid. The commonly prescribed uricosuric drug in the United States is probenecid. The use of two additional uricosurics, sulfinpyrazone and lesinurad, has been discontinued in the United States. These uricosuric drugs function, at high doses, by competing for urate reuptake from the glomerular filtrate via SLC22A12 and, therefore, reduce renal reabsorption of uric acid allowing for increased excretion in the urine. However, it is important to be careful with the initial dosing of probenecid (and was also the case for sulfinpyrazone) due to the fact that at the initial low circulating levels of the drug it actually acts to inhibit urate excretion resulting in transient increases in serum urate. The most commonly prescribed drug for reducing the production of uric acid is the xanthine oxidase inhibitor, allopurinol. Allopurinol is a purine analog that is a structural isomer of hypoxanthine. A more recent xanthine oxidase inhibitor is febuxostat, approved in the United States in 2009. Febuxostat is a non-purine analog that functions as a selective noncompetitive inhibitor of the active site of xanthine oxidase. Febuxostat is generally only prescribed for patients who do not tolerate allopurinol.

CLINICAL BOX 20–2 TUMOR LYSIS SYNDROME

Chemotherapeutic treatment of leukemias, non-Hodgkin lymphomas, and Burkitt lymphomas often results in tumor lysis syndrome (TLS). TLS is caused by massive tumor cell lysis with the release of large amounts of potassium, phosphate, and nucleic acids into the systemic circulation. Catabolism of the purine nucleic acids to uric acid leads to hyperuricemia. The dramatic increase in uric acid excretion can result in the precipitation of uric acid in the renal tubules and can also induce renal vasoconstriction, impaired autoregulation, decreased renal blood flow, and inflammation, referred to as acute urate nephropathy. Hyperphosphatemia with calcium phosphate deposition in the renal tubules can also cause acute kidney injury. Treatment of TLS includes aggressive hydration and diuresis, monitoring of electrolyte abnormalities, and control of hyperuricemia with allopurinol and rasburicase (recombinant urate oxidase).

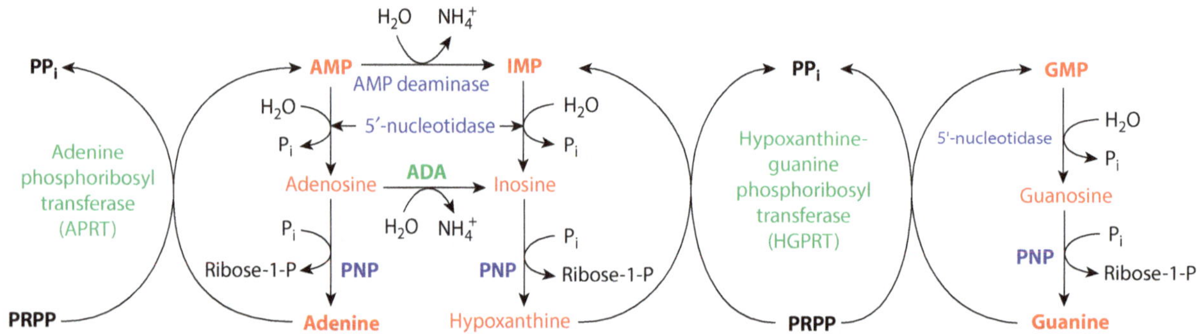

FIGURE 20–7 Pathways of purine nucleotide salvage. ADA, adenosine deaminase; PNP, purine nucleotide phosphorylase. (Reproduced with permission from themedicalbiochemistrypage, LLC.)

CLINICAL BOX 20–3 LESCH-NYHAN SYNDROME

Lesch-Nyhan syndrome (LNS) is an X-linked recessive disorder resulting from the near complete lack of activity of the purine nucleotide salvage enzyme, hypoxanthine-guanine phosphoribosyltransferase, HGPRT (encoded by the *HPRT1* gene). There are three overlapping clinical syndromes associated with deficiencies in HGPRT activity. Individuals that have less than 1.5% residual enzyme activity exhibit debilitating neurologic disability, behavioral abnormalities that include impulsive and self-mutilating behaviors, and varying degrees of cognitive disability in addition to overproduction of uric acid. This most severe of the three clinical syndromes is Lesch-Nyhan syndrome. The second clinical syndrome represents patients who have 1.5–8% of residual enzyme activity. In this second grouping, patients exhibit neurologic disability that ranges from clumsiness to debilitating pyramidal (CNS neurons involved in voluntary motor movement) and extrapyramidal motor dysfunction in addition to overproduction of uric acid. In the third clinical grouping patients have at least 8% of normal HGPRT activity. This last grouping of patients exhibit overproduction of uric acid and associated hyperuricemia, renal lithiasis (kidney stones), and gout. The latter circumstance (partial deficiency with at least 8% enzyme activity) is associated with Kelley-Seegmiller syndrome. More than 270 different mutations in the *HPRT1* gene have been identified in LNS patients. Alterations to the gene include single-base insertions and deletions, large deletions, amino acid substitutions, and stop codon mutations. The characteristic clinical features of the Lesch-Nyhan syndrome are intellectual impairment, spastic cerebral palsy, choreoathetosis, uric acid urinary stones, and self-destructive biting of fingers and lips. The overall clinical features of LNS can be divided into three broad categories. These include uric acid overproduction and its associated consequences (eg, gouty arthritis and renal lithiasis), neurobehavioral dysfunction indicative of central nervous system involvement, and growth retardation. As indicated (and as expected from uric acid overproduction) LNS patients manifest with many of the symptoms of classic gout. All patients with Lesch-Nyhan syndrome manifest with profound motor dysfunction that is recognizable within the first 3–9 months of life. Infants fail to develop the ability to hold up their heads or to sit unaided. Further motor development will be delayed and the onset of pyramidal and extrapyramidal signs become evident by 1–2 years of age. In LNS patients there are three major signs of pyramidal dysfunction: spasticity,

CLINICAL BOX 20-3 (CONTINUED)

hyperreflexia, and the extensor plantar reflex (also known as the Babinski reflex: the great toe flexes toward the top of the foot and the other toes fan out after the sole of the foot has been firmly stroked). Extrapyramidal dysfunction in LNS patients is primarily evident as dystonia (sustained muscle contractions causing twisting and repetitive movements or abnormal postures) although many patients also exhibit choreoathetosis (involuntary movement disorder in association with slow continuous writhing particularly of the hands and feet). Most commonly associated with Lesch-Nyhan syndrome is the behavioral dysfunction manifest with impulsivity and self-mutilation particularly of the lips, fingers, and tongue. LNS patients will often strike out at people around them, spit on people, and use foul language. These symptoms are analogous to the uncontrollable compulsions associated with Tourette syndrome. The self-injury behavior is clearly an involuntary action as most LNS patients will learn to call out for help when they feel the compulsive behavior overtaking them, or they will sit on their hands or wear socks or gloves to limit the self-injurious behavior. Although the precise cause of the self-mutilating behavior in LNS patients is not clearly understood, it is most likely that it is a form of obsessive-compulsive disorder. In many circumstances the routine surgical removal of the adult teeth of LNS patients is considered most beneficial.

CLINICAL BOX 20-4 ADA DEFICIENT SCID

Severe combined immunodeficiency (SCID) refers to a group of potentially fatal disorders due to a combined loss of function of both T- and B-lymphocytes. There are at least 13 known and characterized genetic causes of SCID. The most common (45%) cause of SCID is the X-linked recessive disorder resulting from loss of function of the common gamma (γ) chain of the T-cell receptor and other interleukin (IL) receptors. The second most common (15%) form of SCID is caused by defects in the activity of the purine nucleotide catabolism enzyme, adenosine deaminase (ADA). This form of SCID is inherited as an autosomal recessive disorder with an incidence rate as high as 1:200,000, although some studies report an incidence of 1:1,000,000. More than 60 different mutations have been identified in the *ADA* gene resulting in immunodeficiency. Nearly 70% of all ADA mutations result in single amino acid substitutions with the rest being deletions and splicing mutations. In ADA deficiency there is an elevation in the level of adenosine and 2′-deoxyadenosine in the blood and 2′-deoxyadenosine levels in the urine are also elevated. The consequences of the elevations in these two ADA substrates are impaired lymphocyte differentiation, function, and viability which results in lymphopenia and severe immunodeficiency. Increases in 2′-deoxyadenosine, through the action of ubiquitous nucleoside phosphorylases, results in dramatic increases in cellular dATP pools. The consequences of increased dATP pools are an inhibition of ribonucleotide reductase (RR), the enzyme responsible for generating deoxyribonucleotides (necessary for DNA replication) from ribonucleotides. The inhibition of RR leads to a block to DNA replication which is critical for the expansion of lymphocytes in response to antigenic challenge. Deoxy-ATP also induces DNA strand breakage in nondividing lymphocytes via a direct activation of a major protease (caspase 9) involved in apoptosis (programmed cell death; see Chapter 31). In addition, *S* adenosylhomocysteine hydrolase activity is markedly inhibited by 2′-deoxyadenosine resulting in accumulation of *S*-adenosylhomocysteine which in turn results in reduced synthesis of *S*-adenosylmethionine (AdoMet), a critical substrate in transmethylation reactions. Infants with ADA-deficient SCID usually present within the first month of life with failure to thrive and life-threatening interstitial pneumonitis (inflammation of the walls of the airs sacs of the lungs). Pneumonia is often caused by *Pneumocystis carinii* or a viral infection. The gastrointestinal tract as well as the skin are also frequently involved in initial infections. Candidiasis is first observed as "diaper rash" but then progresses to an extensive infection involving the skin, oral, and esophageal mucosa, and the vagina in female patients. Persistent infections prompt most parents to have their baby examined and SCID is thus often diagnosed by 1–2 months of age from a determination of immune function. Most SCID patients lack both cell-mediated (T cell) and humoral (B cell) immunity and thus, the derivation of the disease name: severe combined immunodeficiency. Because this disease is so life-threatening most patients do not survive for more than a few months. If immunological function is not restored, SCID is always fatal by 1–2 years of age due to complications from infection with DNA or RNA viruses such as cytomegalovirus, varicella, and parainfluenza. The most effective treatment for SCID is bone marrow transplantation. However, many patients do not have a histocompatible sibling and thus other means of treatment were needed. Enzyme replacement therapy (ERT) has proved effective in treating some (but not all) ADA-deficient SCID patients. The most common treatment is to use intramuscular injection of highly purified bovine ADA coupled to the inert polymer, monomethoxypolyethylene glycol (PEG-ADA). The use of PEG-ADA therapy is sometimes warranted in SCID patients who are too ill to undergo bone marrow transplantation.

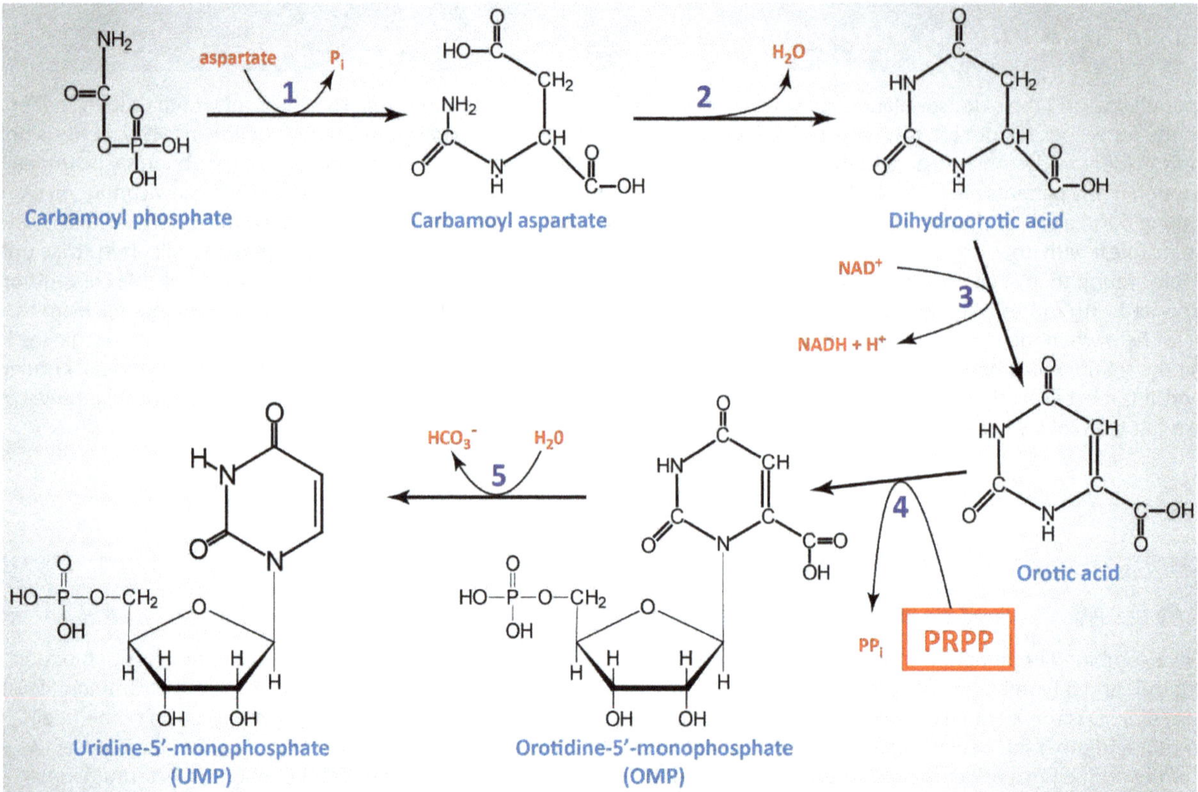

FIGURE 20–8 Synthesis of UMP from carbamoyl phosphate. Carbamoyl phosphate utilized in pyrimidine nucleotide synthesis is synthesized by the carbamoyl phosphate synthetase 2 (CPS2) activity of the CAD enzyme. The activities of CPS2 and reactions 1 and 2 of this figure are all catalyzed by the trifunctional enzyme encoded by the *CAD* gene. The activities of 4 and 5 are contained in a single bifunctional enzyme encoded by the uridine monophosphate synthetase (*UMPS*) gene. The numbers in the figure correspond to the following enzyme activity names:

1. aspartate transcarbamoylase (ATCase) activity of the *CAD* gene-encoded enzyme
2. dihydroorotase (previously called carbamoyl aspartate dehydratase) activity of the *CAD* gene encoded enzyme
3. dihydroorotate dehydrogenase (*DHODH* gene activity)
4. orotate phosphoribosyltransferase activity of the *UMPS* gene
5. orotidine-5′-phosphate decarboxylase (OMP decarboxylase) activity of the *UMPS* gene (Reproduced with permission from themedicalbiochemistrypage, LLC.)

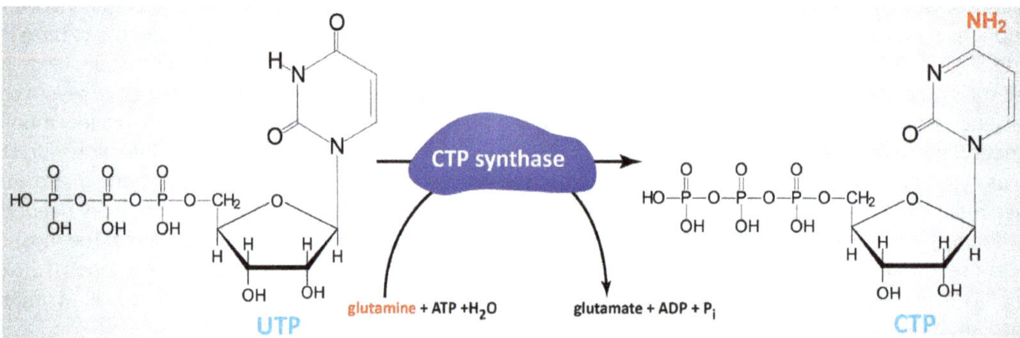

FIGURE 20–9 Synthesis of CTP from UTP. (Reproduced with permission from themedicalbiochemistrypage, LLC.)

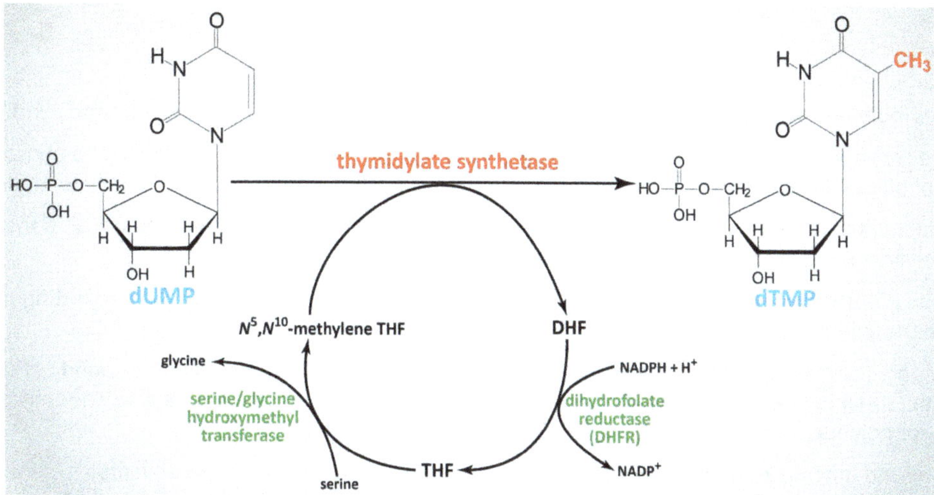

FIGURE 20–10 Pathway of thymidine synthesis. The synthesis of thymidine begins with dUMP. Thymidylate synthetase utilizes an active folate derivative, N^5,N^{10}-methylene tetrahydrofolate (methyleneTHF), as the methyl group donor in the synthesis of dTMP. In the process of thymidine synthesis, the THF derivative is converted to dihydrofolate (DHF). DHF is converted back to methyleneTHF in a two-step process requiring dihydrofolate reductase (DHFR) and serine/glycine hydroxymethyltransferase. (Reproduced with permission from themedicalbiochemistrypage, LLC.)

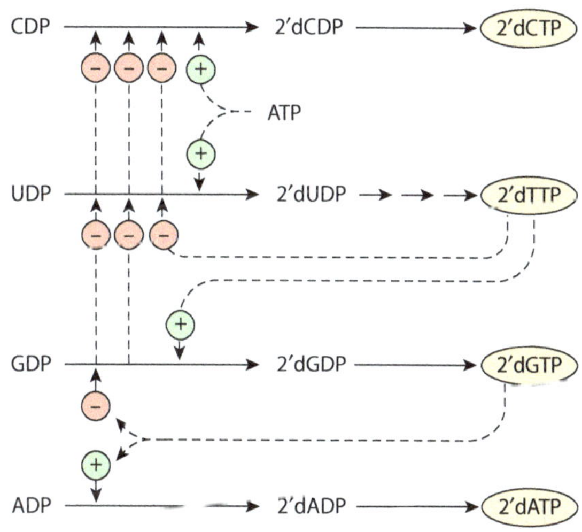

FIGURE 20–11 Regulation of ribonucleotide reductase. Solid lines represent direction of deoxynucleotide formation. Dashed lines represent either positive ⊕ or negative ⊖ feedback regulation. (Reproduced with permission from Rodwell VW, Bender DA, Botham KM, et al: *Harper's Illustrated Biochemistry*, 31st ed. New York, NY: McGraw Hill; 2018.)

CLINICAL BOX 20–5 CHEMOTHERAPEUTICS TARGETING THYMIDINE SYNTHESIS

Cells that are unable to regenerate THF, from the DHF generated during the thymidylate synthetase reaction, suffer defective DNA synthesis and eventual death. For this reason, as well as the fact that dTTP is utilized only in DNA, it is therapeutically possible to target rapidly proliferating cells over non-proliferating cells through the inhibition of thymidylate synthetase or through inhibition of DHFR. The class of molecules used to inhibit thymidylate synthetase are fluorinated pyrimidines. Molecules of this class include 5-fluorouracil (fluorouracil: 5-FU), 5-fluorodeoxyuridine (floxuridine; FUdR), and 5-fluoro-2′-deoxyuridine monophosphate (FUdR-MP). Fluorouracil within cells to numerous metabolic intermediates including FUdR-MP (also written FdUMP), 5-fluorodeoxyuridine triphosphate (FdUTP), and 5-fluorouridine triphosphate (FUTP). It is FUdR-MP (FdUMP) that inhibits thymidylate synthetase. The other major metabolites, FdUTP and FUTP, inhibit DNA synthesis and repair and RNA synthesis, respectively. The many different DHFR inhibitors are termed antifolates or antimetabolites and include methotrexate, aminopterin, trimethoprim, and pyrimethamine. Each of these is a structural analog of folic acid, hence the term antifolate.

CHECKLIST

- ☑ The nucleotides found in cells are derivatives of the heterocyclic, highly basic compounds purine and pyrimidine.
- ☑ Nucleosides are composed of a nucleobase (purine or pyrimidine) attached to ribose but containing no phosphate. Nucleotides are the result of phosphate addition to nucleosides and they can be either mono-, di-, or triphosphate modified.
- ☑ The triphosphate and diphosphate groups of nucleotides are phosphanhydride bonds imparting high transfer energy for participation in covalent bond synthesis, such as in the case of ATP.
- ☑ The nomenclature for the atoms in nucleosides and nucleotides includes a prime (′) designation to distinguish the atoms in the sugar from those in the base.
- ☑ Polynucleotides are composed of two or more nucleotides linked together via a phosphodiester bond between the 5′ phosphate of the sugar in one nucleotide and the 3′ hydroxyl of the sugar in another nucleotide. The common left-to-right nomenclature for polynucleotides is 5′ → 3′: eg, 5′-pApGpCpT-3′ or just 5′-AGCT-3′.
- ☑ Cyclic adenosine and guanine nucleotides act as second messengers in signal transduction events.
- ☑ Nucleotide analogs are used as antimicrobial and anticancer agents via their ability to interfere with nucleotide biosynthesis or DNA replication.
- ☑ Both purine and pyrimidine nucleotide biosynthesis involves the use of the activated form of ribose-5-phosphate, 5-phosphoribosyl-1-pyrophosphate (PRPP).
- ☑ Efficient dietary uptake, *de novo* synthesis, and intracellular salvage of nucleotides ensures that they are dietarily nonessential.
- ☑ Purine nucleotide synthesis proceeds with the initial construction of the nucleobase which is then added to PRPP. The first fully formed purine nucleotide is IMP which serves as a branch point for synthesis of AMP and GMP. ATP levels regulate GMP synthesis and GTP levels regulate AMP synthesis.
- ☑ The catabolism of purine nucleotides produces the insoluble product, uric acid. Excess purine degradation can lead to hyperuricemia and ultimately to gout.
- ☑ Purine nucleotides are efficiently savaged rendering *de novo* synthesis unnecessary except in conditions of rapid cell proliferation. Deficiencies in several salvage enzymes lead to a range of disorders from those with mild symptoms of hyperuricemia to potentially life-threatening immunodeficiency.
- ☑ Pyrimidine nucleotide synthesis proceeds via the construction of the nucleobase on PRPP. The first fully formed pyrimidine nucleotide is UMP. Following phosphorylation to UTP, some is converted to CTP via the action of CTP synthetase.
- ☑ Catabolism of pyrimidine nucleotides results in water-soluble products so there are no clinical manifestations of increased catabolism.
- ☑ Thymidine nucleotides are synthesized from dUMP. Since thymidine nucleotide is almost exclusively associated with DNA, the enzymes that are involved in its synthesis are targets of chemotherapeutic agents.
- ☑ Synthesis of the deoxynucleotides is catalyzed by ribonucleotide reductase (RR). RR activity is strongly inhibited by dATP.

REVIEW QUESTIONS

1. Following a relatively normal early developmental period, a 6-month-old boy becomes pale and lethargic and begins to show signs of deteriorating motor skill. The infant has severe megaloblastic anemia; however, serum measurements of iron, folate, vitamins B_{12} and B_6 demonstrate they are within normal range. Urine samples were clear when fresh, but when left to stand for several hours showed an abundant white precipitate that was composed of fine needle-shaped crystals. Analysis of the crystals identified them as orotic acid. Significant clinical improvement would be expected to be observed in this infant following oral administration of which of the following compounds?

(A) Adenosine
(B) Arginine
(C) Carbamoyl phosphate
(D) Guanosine
(E) Thymidine
(F) Uridine

2. The parents of a 1-year-old boy are alarmed at the increasing frequency of their child biting his lips and fingertips. In addition, on several occasions they have noticed what appears to be "orange sand" in their son's diapers. They report to their pediatrician that they believe their child is delayed in acquiring motor skills such as holding up his head and sitting unaided. Laboratory studies show a 10-fold elevation in the urinary ratio of uric acid to creatinine. These findings are most likely due to a defect in which of the following metabolic processes?

(A) Amino acid metabolism
(B) Galactose metabolism
(C) Glycosphingolipid metabolism
(D) Lysosomal glycogen metabolism
(E) Nucleotide metabolism

3. A 45-year-old man is being examined in the emergency department with a complaint of constant severe pain in his right ankle over the past 24 hours. His uncle also had episodes of pain in single joints. The ankle is swollen and warm. Serum analysis shows elevated urate. The attending physician prescribes an appropriate pharmaceutical intervention and asks that the patient report back in 1 week for a follow-up examination. Given the symptoms and treatment in this patient, which of the following is most likely?
(A) Lactic acidosis
(B) Hypertension
(C) Hypoglycemia
(D) Polydipsia
(E) Tachycardia

4. A 4-year-old child who has been afflicted with recurrent infections is being examined by his pediatrician. The child exhibits impaired development, weakness, and weight loss. Physical examination also shows absence of tonsils and no palpable lymph nodes. Analysis of blood finds that the levels of $CD3^+$, $CD4^+$, and $CD8^+$ T cells are markedly decreased. These signs and symptoms are most likely the result of which of the following disorders?
(A) Hyperuricemia
(B) Kelley-Seegmiller syndrome
(C) Lesch-Nyhan syndrome
(D) Orotic aciduria
(E) Severe-combined immunodeficiency (SCID)

5. A 7-year-old boy is being examined by his pediatrician. The child exhibits delayed motor development, overexaggerated reflexes, and spasticity. In addition, the boy has painful, swollen, inflamed joints. Given the most likely diagnosis in this case an analysis of blood from this patient would be expected to find elevated levels of which of the following compounds related to the observed findings?
(A) Citrulline
(B) Hypoxanthine
(C) Lactic acid
(D) Orotic acid
(E) Uric acid

6. The parents of a 5-year-old boy bring their son to his pediatrician because of their concern over his odd behavior that involves biting his lower lip to the point of bleeding as well as chewing on his fingertips. Physical examination demonstrates swollen tender joints and blood workup indicates elevated uric acid levels. These symptoms and lab results are indicative of a deficiency in which of the following enzymes?
(A) Adenosine deaminase
(B) Glucose-6-phosphate dehydrogenase
(C) Hypoxanthine-guanine phosphoribosyltransferase
(D) Ornithine transcarbamylase
(E) Thymidylate synthetase

7. A 37-year-old man is being examined in the emergency department with complaints of constant severe pain in his right ankle over the past 24 hours. His uncle also had episodes of pain in single joints. The attending physician prescribes allopurinol. Given this therapeutic intervention, which of the following is most likely to be observed in this patient?
(A) Decreased levels of PRPP
(B) Decreased thymidine synthesis
(C) Decreased xanthine in the blood
(D) Increased *de novo* synthesis of IMP
(E) Increased hypoxanthine in the urine
(F) Increased urate in the urine

8. Experiments are being carried out on the process of nucleotide metabolism using a cell line derived from a human hepatoma. Restriction of water-soluble vitamins from the culture medium appears to have little effect on the conversion of dUMP to dTMP. These results would suggest that the cancer cells have most likely lost the requirement for which of the following?
(A) Ascorbate
(B) Folate
(C) Niacin
(D) Pyridoxine
(E) Riboflavin
(F) Vitamin B_{12}

9. The parents of a 1-year-old boy are alarmed at the increasing frequency of their child biting his lips and fingertips. In addition, on several occasions they have noticed what appears to be "orange sand" in their son's diapers. They report to their pediatrician that they believe their child is delayed in acquiring motor skills such as holding up his head and sitting unaided. Which of the following laboratory findings would be most significant in this patient?
(A) Decreased serum alloisoleucine
(B) Decreased urinary lactate
(C) Decreased urinary urate
(D) Increased serum alloisoleucine
(E) Increased urinary lactate
(F) Increased urinary urate

10. A 48-year-old man presents with tophaceous deposits within the articular cartilage, synovium, tendons, tendon sheaths, pinnae, and the soft tissue on the extensor surface of the forearms. These clinical observations would most likely be found associated with which of the following?
(A) Adenosine deaminase deficiency
(B) Folate deficiency
(C) Hyperuricemia
(D) Orotic acidemia
(E) UMP synthase deficiency
(F) Vitamin B_{12} deficiency

11. A 6-month-old boy is brought to the physician because he is pale, lethargic, and showing deteriorating motor skills. He had a relatively normal early developmental period. Laboratory studies show a mean corpuscular volume (MCV) of 118 fL (N = 82–98 fL). Serum levels of iron, folate, cobalamin, and pyridoxine are within normal ranges. Urine samples are clear when fresh, but when left to stand for several hours, show an abundant white precipitate that is composed of fine needle-shaped crystals. Analysis of the crystals would most likely find them to be composed of which of the following?
(A) Bilirubin
(B) Cystine
(C) Lactate
(D) Orotic acid
(E) Urate

12. A 39-year-old man is being examined to determine the cause of his orotic aciduria. It is suspected that he suffers from a defect in pyrimidine nucleotide biosynthesis. However, aside

from the orotic aciduria there are no other classical symptoms apparent in this patient such as megaloblastic anemia. In addition, when assayed, it is found that the activity of UMP synthase is normal. Given these findings, which of the following is most likely deficient in this patient?
(A) Aspartate transcarbamoylase
(B) Carbamoyl phosphate synthetase 1 (CPS1)
(C) Hypoxanthine-guanine phosphoribosyltransferase (HGPRT)
(D) Ornithine transcarbamylase (OTC)
(E) 5'-Phosphoribosyl-1-pyrophosphate synthetase (PRPP synthetase)
(F) Thymidylate synthetase

13. Phase 1 clinical trials are being carried out on a potential new anticancer compound. Participants taking the compound are found to have elevated levels of serum urate compared to placebo control participants. This novel compound is most likely exerting which of the following effects?
(A) Inhibition of carbamoyl phosphate synthetase
(B) Inhibition of the conversion of dihydrofolate to tetrahydrofolate
(C) Inhibition of xanthine oxidase
(D) Interference with feedback control of 5-phosphoribosyl-1-pyrophosphate (PRPP) synthesis
(E) Interference with feedback control of thymidylate synthase

14. A 4-month-old infant is being examined by his pediatrician because his parents are concerned about his apparent failure to thrive since birth. Physical examination shows a doll-like face, thin extremities, and marked hepatomegaly. Serum studies show a below normal glucose concentration and increased concentrations of lactate, and triglycerides. Which of the following is most likely to also be found elevated in the serum of this patient?
(A) Adenosine
(B) Blood urea nitrogen
(C) Orotic acid
(D) Thymidine
(E) Uric acid

15. A 10-year-old boy who has begun chemotherapy for acute myelogenous leukemia awakens at night with a fever and severe pain in his ankles. Treatment with over-the-counter analgesics does not resolve the pain. The next morning, he has pain with urination and blood in the urine. Metabolism of which of the following is the most likely cause of this patient's symptoms?
(A) Lactic acid
(B) Leucine
(C) Fructose
(D) Guanine
(E) Phytanic acid
(F) Thymidine

16. A 6-year-old boy with moderate intellectual impairment is brought to the physician for a follow-up examination. He has had choreoathetoid movements since the age of 16 months. He has been biting his lips and fingers for the past 2 months. His older brother has a similar condition. Physical examination shows spasticity of the lower limbs. Laboratory studies show an increased serum uric acid concentration and an increased urinary excretion of uric acid. His increased serum uric acid concentration is most likely due to which of the following?
(A) Deficient amidophosphoribosyltransferase activity
(B) Deficient hypoxanthine guanine phosphoribosyltransferase activity
(C) Deficient xanthine oxidase activity
(D) Increased adenosine deaminase activity
(E) Increased adenosine phosphoribosyltransferase activity
(F) Increased purine nucleotide phosphorylase activity

17. A 4-month-old infant is being examined by his pediatrician because his parents are concerned about his apparent failure to thrive since birth. Physical examination shows a doll-like face, thin extremities, and marked hepatomegaly. Serum studies show a below normal glucose concentration and increased concentrations of lactate, triglycerides, and uric acid. Which of the following is the most likely mechanism for the increased serum uric acid concentration in this patient?
(A) Decreased adenosine deaminase activity
(B) Decreased glucose-6-phosphate dehydrogenase activity
(C) Decreased hypoxanthine-guanine phosphoribosyltransferase activity
(D) Increased malonyl-CoA decarboxylase activity
(E) Increased purine nucleotide catabolism
(F) Increased pyrimidine nucleotide catabolism

18. A 10-year-old boy who has begun chemotherapy for acute myelogenous leukemia awakens at night with fever and severe pain in the ankles. Treatment with over-the-counter analgesics does not resolve the pain. The next morning, he has pain with urination and blood in the urine. These signs and symptoms are most likely due to the fact that his treatment targeted which of the following pathways?
(A) Purine nucleotide synthesis
(B) Purine nucleotide catabolism
(C) Purine nucleotide salvage
(D) Pyrimidine nucleotide catabolism
(E) Thymidine nucleotide synthesis

19. A 4-year-old child who has been afflicted with recurrent infections is being examined by his pediatrician. The child exhibits impaired development, weakness, and weight loss. Physical examination also shows absence of tonsils and no palpable lymph nodes. Analysis of blood finds that the levels of $CD3^+$, $CD4^+$, and $CD8^+$ T cells are markedly decreased. These signs and symptoms are most likely the result of a defect in which of the following processes?
(A) Purine nucleotide catabolism
(B) Purine nucleotide synthesis
(C) Pyrimidine nucleotide catabolism
(D) Pyrimidine nucleotide synthesis

20. A 49-year-old man has a history of hyperuricemia which is exacerbated by his frequent consumption of alcohol. The evening following a birthday celebration, that included consumption of large amounts of alcohol and a dinner of lobster, shrimp, and steak, the man experienced excruciating pain and swelling in his knees, ankles, and great toes. Which of the following food components is most likely to have contributed to his symptoms?
(A) Cholesterol
(B) Glucose
(C) Glycolipid

(D) Nucleic acid
(E) Phospholipid
(F) Protein
(G) Triglyceride

21. A 58-year-old man is being examined by his physician with complaints of excruciating pain and swelling in his knees, ankles, and great toes. He reports he has been experiencing variable levels of pain in his joints and that the pain is most frequent following meals that include the consumption of red wine. The pain is stabbing in character and located on the right side of his back. Physical examination finds that his abdomen is mildly tender in the right lower quadrant with no rebound or guarding. His urine is positive (2+) for hematuria via a dipstick test. The physician makes a preliminary diagnosis and prescribes an appropriate medication. What is the most likely mechanism of action of the most likely drug prescribed for this patient?
(A) Activation of uric acid excretion from renal tubule cells
(B) Activation of xanthine oxidase
(C) Inhibition of renal tubule cell reabsorption of uric acid
(D) Inhibition of intestinal uptake of uric acid
(E) Specific activation of COX-2
(F) Specific inhibition of COX-2

22. A 58-year-old man is being examined by his physician with complaints of excruciating pain and swelling in his knees, ankles, and great toes. He reports he has been experiencing variable levels of pain in his joints and that the pain is most frequent following meals that include the consumption of alcohol. Physical examination finds that his abdomen is mildly tender in the right lower quadrant with no rebound or guarding. There is swelling and redness around the patient's first metatarsophalangeal joint of both feet. The swelling is tender to the touch and warm. The physician prescribes a medication that is the most appropriate for the long-term treatment of the primary cause of the patient's joint swelling and pain. The drug that is most likely prescribed is most likely targeting the activity of which of the following?
(A) Adenosine deaminase
(B) Glutamine phosphoribosylpyrophosphate amidotransferase
(C) Hypoxanthine-guanine phosphoribosyltransferase
(D) PRPP synthetase
(E) UMP synthase
(F) Xanthine oxidase

23. A 1-year-old boy is being examined by his pediatrician because his parents are concerned that he does not appear to be developing expected milestones such as those attained by their friend's son who is the same age. They report that their son is not able to sit by himself and does not appear to be attempting to talk. History reveals that the patient was born following an uncomplicated full-term pregnancy and that he has received all recommended vaccinations. Physical examination shows that the patient is at the 15th percentile for both weight and height, there is sparse hair on the infant's head, the liver is not palpable, and there are no signs of scleral icterus. The pediatrician orders a CBC and CMP, the results of which show hemoglobin 8.1 g/dL (N = 9.5–15 g/dL), MCV 112 fL (N = 70–84 fL), reticulocyte count 0.9% (N = 0.6–1.7%), glucose 80 mg/dL (N = 60–100 mg/dL), and ammonia 47 μmol/L (N = 15–55 μmol/L). Urinalysis finds an orotic acid level of 450 μmol/mmol creatinine (N = 0.76–4.1 μmol/mmol creatinine). The signs and symptoms in this patient are most likely the result of a deficiency in which of the following?
(A) Carbamoyl phosphate synthetase
(B) Folate
(C) Glucose-6-phosphate dehydrogenase
(D) Ornithine transcarbamylase
(E) Pyridoxine
(F) Pyruvate kinase deficiency
(G) UMP synthase
(H) Vitamin B_{12}

24. The parents of a 4-year-old boy bring their son to his pediatrician because of their concern over his odd behavior that makes them think he may be on the autism spectrum. Physical examination demonstrates hypotonia, swollen tender joints, and bite marks on his fingers and hands. Given the most likely diagnosis, which of the following processes is most likely impaired in this patient?
(A) Conversion of adenosine to inosine
(B) Conversion of hypoxanthine to xanthine
(C) Conversion of orotic acid to OMP
(D) Regulation of adenylosuccinate lyase activity
(E) Regulation of glutamine phosphoribosylpyrophosphate amidotransferase activity
(F) Regulation of PRPP synthetase activity

25. A 53-year-old man is being examined by his physician with complaints of intense pain in his back and pain and swelling in his knees and ankles. He reports he has been experiencing variable levels of pain in his joints and that the pain is most frequent following the consumption of alcohol. When asked, the patient states that he drinks at least two alcoholic drinks every day, and sometimes more. Physical examination finds that his abdomen is mildly tender in the right lower quadrant with no rebound or guarding. His urine is positive (2+) for hematuria via a dipstick test. The physician makes a preliminary diagnosis and prescribes an appropriate medication. What is the most likely negative consequence in this patient if he continues to drink heavily while on the medication most likely prescribed by his physician?
(A) High anion gap metabolic acidosis
(B) Hypokalemia
(C) Hypophosphatemia
(D) Metabolic alkalosis
(E) Renal lithiasis

ANSWERS

1. Correct answer is **F.** The infant is most likely exhibiting the typical findings of a megaloblastic anemia resulting from a mutation in the gene encoding UMP synthase. Two inherited disorders affecting pyrimidine biosynthesis are the result of deficiencies in the bifunctional enzyme, UMP synthase, catalyzing the last two steps of UMP synthesis, orotate phosphoribosyltransferase and OMP decarboxylase. These deficiencies result in two types of orotic aciduria (type 1 and type 2) that cause retarded growth, and severe anemia associated with hypochromic erythrocytes and megaloblastic bone marrow, both of which are the result of the block to DNA synthesis. Leukopenia is also common in with this particular orotic aciduria. These disorders can be treated with uridine and/or cytidine, which leads to increased UMP production via the action of nucleoside kinases and thymidine via dUMP. The UMP also inhibits the carbamoyl phosphate synthetase (CPS2) activity of the trifunctional pyrimidine biosynthesis enzyme encoded by the *CAD* gene. The reduced activity of the CAD enzyme results in the attenuation of orotic acid production. Adenosine (choice A) and guanosine (choice D) are purine nucleotides which would not be deficient in this patient and thus of no therapeutic benefit. Arginine supplementation (choice B) is useful in the treatment of urea cycle disorders but has no therapeutic benefit in a patient with a defect in pyrimidine nucleotide biosynthesis. Administration of carbamoyl phosphate (choice C) would not contribute to pyrimidine nucleotide biosynthesis due to the deficient UMP synthase but would exacerbate the orotic aciduria in this patient. Administration of thymidine (choice E) would only contribute to the production of deoxy thymidine but not to cytidine synthesis, therefore, DNA synthesis would still be impaired in this patient.

2. Correct answer is **E.** The patient is most likely experiencing the signs and symptoms of Lesch-Nyhan syndrome. Lesch-Nyhan syndrome (LNS) is an X-linked disorder resulting from the near complete lack of activity of the purine nucleotide salvage enzyme, hypoxanthine-guanine phosphoribosyltransferase, HGPRT (encoded by the *HPRT1* gene). The characteristic clinical features of the Lesch-Nyhan syndrome are intellectual impairment, spastic cerebral palsy, choreoathetosis, uric acid urinary stones, and self-destructive biting of fingers and lips. The overall clinical features of LNS can be divided into three broad categories. These include uric acid overproduction and its associated consequences (eg, gouty arthritis and renal lithiasis), neurobehavioral dysfunction indicative of central nervous system involvement, and growth retardation. Most commonly associated with Lesch-Nyhan syndrome is the behavioral dysfunction manifest with impulsivity and self-mutilation particularly of the lips, fingers, and tongue. Numerous disorders of amino acid metabolism (choice A) and glycosphingolipid metabolism (choice C) have been characterized by none are associated with the abnormal self-mutilation behavior evident in this patient. The most common disorder of galactose metabolism (choice B) is classic galactosemia. Classic galactosemia manifests by poor feeding behavior, a failure of neonates to thrive, and bleeding problems in untreated infants. In classic galactosemia, infants will exhibit vomiting and diarrhea rapidly following ingestion of lactose from breast milk or from lactose-containing formula. The glycogen storage disease, Pompe disease, is associated with abnormal lysosomal glycogen metabolism (choice D). Pompe disease patients usually die from severe cardiomyopathy between the second and third year of life.

3. Correct answer is **A.** The patient is most likely manifesting the symptoms resulting from chronic hyperuricemia. Treatments for chronic hyperuricemia and the resultant gout include the use of uricosuric drugs and drugs that inhibit the production of uric acid. The commonly prescribed uricosuric drug in the United States is probenecid. The use of two additional uricosurics, sulfinpyrazone and lesinurad, has been discontinued in the United States. These uricosuric drugs function, at high doses, by competing for urate reuptake from the glomerular filtrate via SLC22A12 (URAT1) and, therefore, reduce renal reabsorption of uric acid allowing for increased excretion in the urine. Transport of urate via SLC22A12 is selectively inhibited by lactate, succinate, β-hydroxybutyrate, and acetoacetate. Urate reabsorption is coupled to renal lactate reabsorption at the apical membrane of the proximal tubule cell via interactions between SLC22A12 and the lactate transporters encoded by the *SLC5A8* and *SCL5A12* genes. Due to this interaction, lactic acidemia impairs urate reabsorption and excretion while hyperuricemia results in impaired lactate excretion and reabsorption. The use of probenecid to treat hyperuricemia can lead to lactic acidosis as a contract indicating complication. None of the other symptoms (choices B, C, D, and E) would be apparent in a patient with hyperuricemia taking probenecid as a therapeutic.

4. Correct answer is **E.** The patient is most likely experiencing the signs and symptoms of adenosine deaminase (ADA) deficient severe combined immunodeficiency. Severe combined immunodeficiency (SCID) refers to a group of potentially fatal disorders due to a combined loss of function of both T- and B-lymphocytes. There are at least 13 known and characterized genetic causes of SCID. The most common (45%) cause of SCID is the X-linked disorder resulting from loss of function of the common gamma (γ) chain of the T-cell receptor and other interleukin (IL) receptors. The second most common (15%) form of SCID is caused by defects in the activity of the purine nucleotide catabolism enzyme, adenosine deaminase (ADA). Infants with ADA deficient SCID usually present within the first month of life with failure to thrive and life-threatening interstitial pneumonitis (inflammation of the walls of the airs sacs of the lungs). Pneumonia is often caused by *Pneumocystis carinii* or a viral infection. The gastrointestinal tract as well as the skin are also frequently involved in initial infections. Candidiasis is first observed as "diaper rash" but then progresses to an extensive infection involving the skin, oral, and esophageal mucosa, and the vagina in female patients. Persistent infections prompt most parents to have their baby examined and SCID is thus often diagnosed by 1–2 months of age from a determination of immune function. If not associated as a secondary complication, hyperuricemia (choice A) is usually not apparent until much later in life. Keeley-Seegmiller syndrome (choice B) and Lesch-Nyhan syndrome (choice C) are disorders that result from reduced, or no activity of the purine nucleotide salvage enzyme hypoxanthine guanine phosphoribosyltransferase (HGPRT), respectively. Both of these disorders have been associated with hyperuricemia. Orotic aciduria (choice D) is apparent in the urea cycle disorder resulting from deficiency in ornithine transcarbamylase as well as in the case of deficiency in the pyrimidine nucleotide biosynthetic enzyme UMP synthase.

5. Correct answer is **E.** The patient is most likely experiencing the signs and symptoms of Lesch-Nyhan syndrome. Lesch-Nyhan syndrome (LNS) is an X-linked disorder resulting from the near complete lack of activity of the purine nucleotide salvage enzyme, hypoxanthine-guanine phosphoribosyltransferase, HGPRT (encoded by the *HPRT1* gene). The characteristic clinical features of the Lesch-Nyhan syndrome are intellectual impairment, self-destructive biting of fingers and lips, spastic cerebral palsy, choreoathetosis, and hyperuricemia. The inability to salvage purine nucleotides results in the loss of the feedback regulation of the amidotransferase enzyme of purine nucleotide biosynthesis. The elevated synthesis of the purines leads to increased catabolism resulting in the hyperuricemia apparent in Lesch-Nyhan syndrome. Citrulline (choice A) is elevated in several urea cycle disorders.

Hypoxanthine (choice B) would not be elevated as its catabolism is not inhibited in Lesch-Nyhan syndrome. Lactic acid (choice C) can be elevated in individuals with hyperuricemia; however, this is not the most common finding in Lesch-Nyhan syndrome. Orotic acid (choice D) would be elevated in the pyrimidine nucleotide biosynthesis pathway as a result of mutations in the gene encoding UMP synthase. Orotic acid is also elevated in the urea cycle disorder resulting from mutations in the gene encoding ornithine transcarbamylase.

6. Correct answer is **C.** The patient is most likely experiencing the signs and symptoms of Lesch-Nyhan syndrome. Lesch-Nyhan syndrome (LNS) is an X-linked disorder resulting from the near complete lack of activity of the purine nucleotide salvage enzyme, hypoxanthine-guanine phosphoribosyltransferase, HGPRT (encoded by the *HPRT1* gene). The characteristic clinical features of the Lesch-Nyhan syndrome are intellectual impairment, self-destructive biting of fingers and lips, spastic cerebral palsy, choreoathetosis, and hyperuricemia. Adenosine deaminase (choice A) results in one form of severe combined immunodeficiency, SCID. Deficiency in glucose-6-phosphate dehydrogenase (choice B) is one of the most common inherited forms of hemolytic anemia. Deficiency in ornithine transcarbamylase (choice D) results in one of the urea cycle disorders. Deficiency in thymidylate synthetase (choice E) has not been observed in humans.

7. Correct answer is **E.** The patient is most likely experiencing the symptoms of gout resulting from hyperuricemia. Most forms of gout are the result of excess purine production and consequent catabolism or a partial deficiency in the salvage enzyme, hypoxanthine-guanine phosphoribosyltransferase, HGPRT. Most forms of gout can be treated by administering the antimetabolite allopurinol that strongly inhibits xanthine oxidase. The substrates for xanthine oxidase are hypoxanthine and xanthine, therefore, inhibition of the enzyme results in increased levels of hypoxanthine and xanthine in the blood and urine. None of the other observations (choices A, B, C, D, and F) would be apparent in a patient treated with allopurinol.

8. Correct answer is **B.** Thymidine nucleotides are synthesized from the terminal product of pyrimidine nucleotide biosynthesis, UMP. The *de novo* pathway to dTTP synthesis first requires the use of dUMP which is the result of the action of ribonucleotide reductase on UDP, generating dUDP, and then the transfer of phosphate via the action of ubiquitous nucleoside monophosphate or nucleoside diphosphate kinases generating dUMP. The synthesis of dTTP can also result from pyrimidine salvage reactions involving the conversion of cytidine to uridine or deoxycytidine to deoxyuridine, catalyzed by cytidine deaminase. The dUMP is converted to dTMP by the action of thymidylate synthase. The methyl group is donated by N^5,N^{10}-methylene tetrahydrofolate making folate a required vitamin in dTMP synthesis from dUMP. The thymidylate synthetase present in the hepatoma cells most likely lost the requirement for folate and is, therefore, utilizing some other methyl donor for the synthesis of dTMP. None of the other vitamins (choices A, C, D, E, and F) serve as the source of the cofactor required in the synthesis of dTMP from dUMP.

9. Correct answer is **F.** The patient is most likely experiencing the signs and symptoms of Lesch-Nyhan syndrome. Lesch-Nyhan syndrome (LNS) is an X-linked disorder resulting from the near complete lack of activity of the purine nucleotide salvage enzyme, hypoxanthine-guanine phosphoribosyltransferase, HGPRT (encoded by the *HPRT1* gene). The characteristic clinical features of the Lesch-Nyhan syndrome are intellectual impairment, self-destructive biting of fingers and lips, spastic cerebral palsy, choreoathetosis, and hyperuricemia, not decreased urate (choice C). Increases in serum alloisoleucine (choice D), but not decreases (choice A), are significant in patients suffering from defective metabolism of the branched-chain amino acid leucine as is typical in maple syrup urine disease. Changes in the levels of lactate (choices B and E) would not be significant in this patient.

10. Correct answer is **C.** The patient is most likely experiencing the symptoms of gout resulting from hyperuricemia. Most forms of gout are the result of excess purine production and consequent catabolism or to a partial deficiency in the purine nucleotide salvage enzyme, hypoxanthine-guanine phosphoribosyltransferase, HGPRT. Uric acid is very insoluble and when generated in large amounts will precipitate as uric acid crystals in the joints of the extremities and in renal interstitial tissue. These deposits are gritty or sandy in nature and thus are termed tophaceous deposits. Deficiency in adenosine deaminase (choice A) is the cause of the immunodeficiency identified as ADA deficient SCID. Folate deficiency (choice B) would manifest with megaloblastic anemia. Orotic acidemia (choice D) is found in the urea cycle and disorder resulting from deficiency in ornithine transcarbamylase. UMP synthase deficiency (choice E) will lead to megaloblastic anemia as well as orotic acidemia. Vitamin B_{12} deficiency (choice F) is characterized by megaloblastic anemia and methylmalonic acidemia.

11. Correct answer is **D.** The infant is most likely manifesting the signs and symptoms of the megaloblastic anemia that results from deficiency in pyrimidine nucleotide biosynthesis. Hereditary orotic aciduria results from mutations in the gene encoding UMP synthase which is required for *de novo* synthesis of pyrimidines. UMP synthase is a bifunctional enzyme that catalyzes the last two steps in pyrimidine synthesis, the conversion of orotic acid to OMP and OMP to UMP. Deficiencies in UMP synthase will, therefore, lead to increased urinary excretion of orotic acid. When present at high concentration in the urine, orotic acid will crystalize into long needle-shaped crystals. Bilirubin (choice A) and lactate (choice C) would not generate crystals in urine exposed to the air. Cystine (choice B) at high concentration in the glomerular filtrate can result in crystal formation but is not associated with the deteriorating motor skills evident in this patient. Uric acid (choice E) at high concentration, typical of hyperuricemia, will precipitate as crystals which usually form in synovial fluids not the urine.

12. Correct answer is **D.** The patient is most likely manifesting the signs and symptoms of a mild form of ornithine transcarbamylase deficiency. Orotic aciduria can be the result of a deficiency in the urea cycle enzyme ornithine transcarbamoylase, OTC. A deficiency in OTC results in the carbamoyl phosphate, produced by the urea cycle enzyme carbamoyl phosphate synthetase 1 (CPS1), being transported from the mitochondria to the cytosol. Within the cytosol the carbamoyl phosphate can serve as an intermediate in pyrimidine nucleotide synthesis bypassing the regulated rate-limiting steps catalyzed by the trifunctional enzyme encoded by the *CAD* gene. This will lead to synthesis of pyrimidine nucleotides in excess of the demands of the cells resulting in increased orotic acid production and excretion. Deficiency in none of the other enzymes (choices A, B, C, E, and F) would result in the orotic aciduria apparent in this patient.

13. Correct answer is **D.** Uric acid is the end product of purine nucleotide catabolism. Both the salvage and *de novo* synthesis pathways of purine metabolism utilize an activated sugar intermediate, 5-phosphoribosyl-1-pyrophosphate, PRPP. PRPP is generated by the action of PRPP synthetase. The activity of PRPP synthetase is feedback inhibited by purine-5′-nucleotides (predominantly AMP and GMP) and activated by ribose-5-phosphate. Inhibition of purine salvage pathways leads to a reduction in the production of purine-5′-nucleotides resulting in reduced inhibition of PRPP synthetase. Higher activity of PRPP synthetase results in excess purine nucleotide synthesis and as a consequence, increased catabolism to uric acid resulting in hyperuricemia. None of the other options (choices A, B, C, and E) would result in increased uric acid production as a result of the actions of the potential anticancer compound.

14. Correct answer is **E.** This patient most likely suffers from the glycogen storage disease known as von Gierke disease. von Gierke disease results from deficiency in glucose-6-phosphatase which is exclusively expressed in the liver, kidney, and small intestine. The inability of the liver, in particular, to release free glucose results in the diversion of excess glucose-6-phosphate into the pentose phosphate pathway resulting in increased production of ribose-5-phosphate. Ribose-5-phosphate activates PRPP synthetase leading to increased concentrations of the activated form of ribose, 5-phosphoribosyl-1-pyrophosphate (PRPP). PRPP, in turn, activates the rate-limiting enzyme of purine nucleotide synthesis, glutamine phosphoribosylpyrophosphate amidotransferase (commonly referred to simply as amidotransferase) resulting in elevated purine nucleotide synthesis. The purine nucleotides are not utilized for nucleic acid synthesis and are, therefore, catabolized leading to increased production of uric acid. The inability of the liver to release free glucose results in reduced gluconeogenesis and the consequent lactic acidemia of von Gierke disease. In addition hepatic glycolysis is increased ultimately resulting in increased concentrations of acetyl-CoA which are diverted into fatty acid biosynthesis which contributes to the elevated triglycerides seen in von Gierke disease. Adenosine (choice A) would not be elevated in this patient as there is no defect in purine catabolism. Blood urea nitrogen (choice B) would more likely be decreased, not increased, in a patient with von Gierke disease as a result of impaired hepatic function. Orotic acid (choice C) would accumulate as a result of a deficiency in pyrimidine nucleotide biosynthesis or a urea cycle defect, neither of which are apparent in this patient. Thymidine (choice D) is not likely to accumulate in von Gierke disease since its catabolism would be unaffected.

15. Correct answer is **D.** The patient is most likely experiencing one of the potentially serious complications of chemotherapy referred to as tumor lysis syndrome, TLS. TLS is a consequence of chemotherapy, radiotherapy, or immunotherapy. Tumor lysis syndrome is characterized by hyperuricemia, hyperkalemia, hyperphosphatemia, hypocalcemia, and higher than normal levels of blood urea nitrogen (BUN). These changes in blood electrolytes and metabolites are a result of the release of cellular contents into the bloodstream from breakdown of cells. Thymidine (choice F) is a pyrimidine nucleotide, and its catabolism does yield uric acid. Metabolism of none of the other compounds (choices A, B, C, and E) would result in the symptoms associated with tumor lysis syndrome.

16. Correct answer is **B.** The patient is most likely experiencing the signs and symptoms of Lesch-Nyhan syndrome. Lesch-Nyhan syndrome (LNS) is an X-linked disorder resulting from the near complete lack of activity of the purine nucleotide salvage enzyme, hypoxanthine-guanine phosphoribosyltransferase, HGPRT (encoded by the *HPRT1* gene). The characteristic clinical features of the Lesch-Nyhan syndrome are intellectual impairment, self-destructive biting of fingers and lips, spastic cerebral palsy, choreoathetosis, and hyperuricemia. The inability to salvage purine nucleotides results in the loss of the feedback regulation of the amidotransferase enzyme of purine nucleotide biosynthesis. The elevated synthesis of the purines leads to increased catabolism resulting in the hyperuricemia apparent in Lesch-Nyhan syndrome. None of the other options (choices A, C, D, E, and F) would result in the signs and symptoms observed in this patient that are typical of Lesch-Nyhan syndrome.

17. Correct answer is **E.** This patient most likely suffers from the glycogen storage disease known as von Gierke disease. von Gierke disease results from deficiency in glucose-6-phosphatase which is exclusively expressed in the liver, kidney, and small intestine. The inability of the liver, in particular, to release free glucose results in the diversion of excess glucose-6-phosphate into the pentose phosphate pathway resulting in increased production of ribose-5-phosphate. Ribose-5-phosphate activates PRPP synthetase leading to increased concentrations of the activated form of ribose, 5-phosphoribosyl-1-pyrophosphate (PRPP). PRPP, in turn, activates the rate-limiting enzyme of purine nucleotide synthesis, glutamine phosphoribosylpyrophosphate amidotransferase (commonly referred to simply as amidotransferase) resulting in elevated purine nucleotide synthesis. The purine nucleotides are not utilized for nucleic acid synthesis and are, therefore, catabolized leading to increased production of uric acid. The inability of the liver to release free glucose results in reduced gluconeogenesis and the consequent lactic acidemia of von Gierke disease. In addition of hepatic glycolysis is increased ultimately resulting in increased concentrations of acetyl-CoA which are diverted into fatty acid biosynthesis which contributes to the elevated triglycerides seen in von Gierke disease. None of the other options (choices A, B, C, D, and F) account for all of the signs and symptoms observed in this patient.

18. Correct answer is **E.** The patient is most likely experiencing one of the potentially serious complications of chemotherapy referred to as tumor lysis syndrome (TLS). TLS is a consequence of chemotherapy, radiotherapy, or immunotherapy. Tumor lysis syndrome is characterized by hyperuricemia, hyperkalemia, hyperphosphatemia, hypocalcemia, and higher than normal levels of blood urea nitrogen (BUN). These changes in blood electrolytes and metabolites are a result of the release of cellular contents into the bloodstream from breakdown of cells. Treatment of acute myelogenous leukemia involves an array of chemotherapeutic drugs including DNA synthesis inhibitors, mitotic inhibitors, and thymidine nucleotide synthesis inhibitors. None of the other processes (choices A, B, C, and D) represent common metabolic targets for the treatment of acute myeloid leukemias.

19. Correct answer is **A.** The patient is most likely experiencing the signs and symptoms of adenosine deaminase (ADA) deficient severe combined immunodeficiency. Severe combined immunodeficiency (SCID) refers to a group of potentially fatal disorders due to a combined loss of function of both T- and B-lymphocytes. There are at least 13 known and characterized genetic causes of SCID. The most common (45%) cause of SCID is the X-linked disorder resulting from loss of function of the common gamma (γ) chain of the T-cell receptor and other interleukin (IL) receptors. The second most common (15%) form of SCID is caused by defects in the activity of the purine nucleotide catabolism enzyme, adenosine deaminase (ADA). Infants with ADA deficient SCID usually present within the first month of life with failure to thrive and life-threatening interstitial pneumonitis (inflammation of the walls of the airs sacs of the lungs). Pneumonia is often caused by *Pneumocystis carinii* or a viral infection. The gastrointestinal tract as well as the skin are also frequently involved in initial infections. Candidiasis is first observed as "diaper rash" but then progresses to an extensive infection involving the skin, oral, and esophageal mucosa, and the vagina in female patients. Persistent infections prompt most parents to have their baby examined and SCID is thus often diagnosed by 1–2 months of age from a determination of immune function. Defects in none of the other processes (choices B, C, and D) are associated with the signs and symptoms of severe combined immunodeficiency.

20. Correct answer is **D.** The patient is most likely experiencing the symptoms of gout resulting from hyperuricemia. Most forms of gout are the result of excess purine production and consequent catabolism or to a partial deficiency in the salvage enzyme, hypoxanthine-guanine phosphoribosyltransferase, HGPRT. Red meats and shellfish are high in purine nucleotides and their consumption can exacerbate pre-existing hyperuricemia. The consumption of alcohol and its metabolism impairs gluconeogenesis resulting in elevated lactic acid in the blood. The excretion of lactate by the kidney interferes with the excretion of uric acid, therefore, alcohol consumption will result in exacerbation of pre-existing hyperuricemia. None of the other food components (choices A, B, C, E, F, and G) would contribute to the hyperuricemia present in this individual.

21. Correct answer is **C.** The patient is most likely experiencing the symptoms of gout as a result of hyperuricemia. Gout is a disorder that is related to excess production of uric acid and deposition of uric acid crystals. The root cause of gout is hyperuricemia, and it is characterized by recurrent attacks of acute inflammatory arthritis. The formation of urate crystals leads to the formation of tophaceous deposits (sandy, gritty, nodular masses of urate crystals), particularly in the joints, which precipitate the episodes of gouty arthritis. Gouty arthritis is the most painful manifestation of gout and is caused when urate crystals interact with neutrophils triggering an inflammatory response. Treatments for chronic hyperuricemia and the resultant gout include the use of uricosuric drugs and drugs that inhibit the production of uric acid. The commonly prescribed uricosuric drug in the United States is probenecid. The most commonly prescribed drug for reducing the production of uric acid is the xanthine oxidase inhibitor, allopurinol. Probenecid functions by inhibiting urate reuptake from the glomerular filtrate via the major renal urate-anion exchanger, URAT1, which is encoded by the *SLC22A12* gene and, therefore, reducing renal reabsorption of uric acid allowing for increased excretion in the urine. Treatments for hyperuricemia do not activate renal uric acid excretion (choice A) nor inhibit intestinal uptake (choice D). Activation of xanthine oxidase (choice B) would only result in increased levels of uric acid, exacerbating the hyperuricemia in this patient. Specific activation of COX-2 (choice E) would result in increased inflammation causing an increase in the inflammatory pain associated with gouty arthritis. Specific inhibition of COX-2 (choice F) would potentially treat the pain associated with gouty arthritis but would not treat the underlying cause of the hyperuricemia and therefore, would not likely be the type of medication prescribed for this patient.

22. Correct answer is **F.** The patient is most likely suffering from the consequences of chronic hyperuricemia which results in gout. Gout is a disorder that is related to the excess production of uric acid and deposition of uric acid crystals. Gout is characterized by recurrent attacks of acute inflammatory arthritis. The formation of urate crystals leads to the formation of tophaceous deposits (sandy, gritty, nodular masses of urate crystals), particularly in the joints, which precipitate the episodes of gouty arthritis. Gouty arthritis is the most painful manifestation of gout and is caused when urate crystals interact with neutrophils, triggering an inflammatory response. Long-term treatment of the consequences of hyperuricemia is primarily focused on reducing the production of uric acid from purine nucleotide catabolism. These drugs include the xanthine oxidase inhibitors, allopurinol and febuxostat. Of the two, allopurinol is the most commonly prescribed drug for the chronic treatment of the primary cause of the pathological consequences of hyperuricemia. Inhibition of enzymes of purine nucleotide biosynthesis (choices D and D) as well as enzymes of purine nucleotide catabolism (choice A) and salvage (choice C) would result in lower levels of uric acid production, however, none of these enzymes is currently a valid pharmacological target for the treatment of hyperuricemia. Inhibition of the pyrimidine nucleotide biosynthesis enzyme, UMP synthase (choice E) would have no direct effect on uric acid production.

23. Correct answer is **G.** The infant is most likely manifesting the signs and symptoms of a deficiency in the pyrimidine biosynthesis enzyme, UMP synthase. Two inherited disorders are the result of deficiencies in this bifunctional enzyme. One is the result of the loss of both activities of the enzyme, and is termed orotic aciduria type 1; the other is the result of the loss of the OMP decarboxylase activity of the enzyme, and this disorder is termed orotic aciduria type 2. Both disorders lead to impaired growth, and severe anemia associated with hypochromic erythrocytes and megaloblastic bone marrow, both of which are the result of the block to DNA synthesis. The megaloblastic anemia is apparent from the MCV value in this patient. Leukopenia is also common in these orotic acidurias. Deficiency in the urea cycle enzyme, carbamoyl phosphate synthetase 1 (choice A), would be associated with severely elevated levels of ammonia which is not the case in this patient. Orotic aciduria is also a feature of deficiency in the urea cycle enzyme, ornithine transcarbamylase (choice D), but in this situation there is an associated hyperammonemia, which is not found in this patient. Deficiency in either folate (choice B) or vitamin B_{12} (choice H) would be associated with megaloblastic anemia, such as in this patient, but would not be associated with elevated urinary orotic acid. Deficiency in glucose-6-phosphate dehydrogenase (choice C) or pyruvate kinase (choice F) would be associated with hemolytic anemia and not megaloblastic anemia as is the case for this patient. Pyridoxine (vitamin B_6) deficiency (choice) is not associated with impaired growth or megaloblastic anemia.

24. Correct answer is **E.** The patient is most likely suffering from Lesch-Nyhan syndrome (LNS) which is caused by mutations in the gene encoding hypoxanthine-guanine phosphoribosyltransferase (HGPRT). The characteristic clinical features of the Lesch-Nyhan syndrome are intellectual impairment, spastic cerebral palsy, choreoathetosis, uric acid urinary stones, and self-destructive biting of fingers and lips. The overall clinical features of LNS can be divided into three broad categories. These include uric acid overproduction and its associated consequences (eg, gouty arthritis and renal lithiasis), neurobehavioral dysfunction indicative of central nervous system involvement, and growth impairment. HGPRT represents one of the major enzymes involved in the salvage of purine nucleotides, allowing for the regeneration of IMP, GMP, and via IMP to AMP. All three of these nucleotides feed back and inhibit the rate-limiting enzyme of *de novo* purine nucleotide biosynthesis, glutamine phosphoribosylpyrophosphate amidotransferase, most often referred to simply as amidotransferase. Reduced levels of AMP, GMP, and IMP, therefore, lead to increased synthesis of the purine nucleotides and consequently, increased catabolism resulting in the hyperuricemia and the potential for gout that is typical in LNS. However, the bizarre self-mutilation behavior and the intellectual and developmental impairment are far more serious consequences of LNS. Impairment in none of the other processes (choices A, B, C, D, and F) would be associated with the symptoms of self-mutilation apparent in this patient. Impairment in the conversion of adenosine, as well as deoxyadenosine, to inosine and deoxyinosine (choice A) is one of the causes of severe combined immunodeficiency (SCID) that would manifest well before the age of this patient. Impairment in the conversion of orotic acid to OMP (choice C) results from mutations in the pyrimidine biosynthetic enzyme, UMP synthase, and is associated with megaloblastic anemia and impaired growth and development.

25. Correct answer is **A.** The patient is most likely experiencing the symptoms of gout as a result of hyperuricemia. Gout is a disorder that is related to excess production of uric acid and deposition of uric acid crystals. Gout is characterized by recurrent attacks of acute inflammatory arthritis. The formation of urate crystals leads to the formation of tophaceous deposits (sandy, gritty, nodular masses of urate crystals), particularly in the joints, which precipitate the episodes of gouty arthritis. Gouty arthritis is the most painful manifestation of gout and is caused when urate crystals interact with neutrophils triggering an inflammatory response. Treatments for chronic hyperuricemia and the resultant gout include the use of uricosuric drugs and drugs that inhibit the production of uric acid. The commonly prescribed uricosuric drug in the United States is probenecid. The most commonly prescribed drug for reducing the production of uric acid is the xanthine oxidase inhibitor, allopurinol. Probenecid functions by inhibiting urate reuptake from the glomerular filtrate via the major renal urate-anion exchanger, URAT1 which is encoded by the *SLC22A12* gene. This transporter exerts effects on the associated lactate efflux transporter, and thus, the inhibition of urate reabsorption results in inhibition of lactate efflux into the glomerular filtrate. Since alcohol metabolism (see Chapter 14) increases lactate production, the reduced lactate excretion from the kidneys as a result of probenecid can lead to lactic acidosis which is associated with high anion gap metabolic acidosis. High anion gap metabolic acidosis can cause hyperkalemia, not hypokalemia (choice B). The excess acid in the blood, due to the high anion gap, results in potassium movement from within cells to the bloodstream, causing hyperkalemia. Hypophosphatemia (choice C) and metabolic alkalosis (choice D) are not consequences of the pharmacologic treatment of hyperuricemia. Individuals with hyperuricemia are very susceptible to the formation of uric acid stones (lithiasis) in the kidneys (choice E), but the enhanced excretion of uric acid with probenecid treatment would reduce the likelihood of renal lithiasis, not increase it.

C H A P T E R

21

Heme Metabolism

High-Yield Terms

Porphyrin	A group of aromatic organic compounds composed of four modified pyrrole subunits interconnected at their α-carbon atoms via methine bridges
Porphyria	Any of a group of rare inherited or acquired disorders of enzymes involved in the production of the porphyrins and heme; the term porphyria is derived from the Greek term porphura which means "purple pigment" in reference to the coloration of body fluids in patients suffering from the originally described porphyria which is now known as porphyria cutanea tarda (PCT)
Hemin	Protoporphyrin IX containing a ferric (Fe^{3+}) iron, as opposed to heme which contains ferrous (Fe^{2+}) iron
Reticuloendothelial cells	A collective term for cells of the immune system that primarily comprises macrophages and monocytes but may include all phagocytic cells
Bilirubin	Open chain yellowish breakdown product of heme catabolism
Kernicterus	Bilirubin-induced brain dysfunction, also called bilirubin encephalopathy
Sideroblastic anemia	A disease in which the bone marrow produces ringed sideroblasts rather than healthy erythrocytes; sideroblasts are abnormal nucleated erythroblasts with granules of iron in perinuclear mitochondria

HEME

The heme molecules in biological systems consist of ferrous iron (Fe^{2+}) complexed with four nitrogens of the specific porphyrin molecule identified as protoporphyrin IX. The major function of heme in humans is its role in the coordination of O_2 molecules in hemoglobin.

There are three structurally distinct hemes in humans identified as heme *a*, heme *b*, and heme *c* (Figure 21–1). Heme *b* is the form of heme formed by the addition of Fe^{2+} to protoporphyrin IX. Heme *a* is synthesized from heme *b* by conversion of a methyl group to a formyl group and the addition of the isoprenoid molecule, farnesyl. Heme *c* is the same as heme *b* except that it is covalently attached to proteins through disulfide bonds to cysteines.

HIGH-YIELD CONCEPT

Clinical disorders associated with heme metabolism are of two types. Disorders that arise from defects in the enzymes of heme biosynthesis are termed the **porphyrias** (Table 21–1) and cause elevations in the levels of intermediates in heme synthesis in the serum and urine. Inherited disorders in bilirubin metabolism lead to **hyperbilirubinemia** which is the root cause of **jaundice**.

In addition to the role of heme in oxygen transport, heme is critical for the biological functions of several enzymes such as the cytochromes of oxidative phosphorylation and the xenobiotic metabolizing enzymes of the cytochrome P450 family (CYP).

HEME BIOSYNTHESIS

Heme biosynthesis occurs in both the mitochondria and the cytosol. The first reaction in heme biosynthesis takes place in the mitochondrion and involves the condensation of one glycine and one succinyl-CoA by the pyridoxal phosphate-containing enzyme, δ-aminolevulinic acid synthase, ALAS (Figure 21–2).

HIGH-YIELD CONCEPT

Deficiencies in ALAS2 result in a disorder called X-linked sideroblastic anemia, XLSA. Sideroblasts are erythroblasts with non-heme iron-containing organelles, called siderosomes. XLSA has also been called congenital sideroblastic anemia, hereditary sideroblastic anemia, hereditary iron-loading anemia, X-linked hypochromic anemia, hereditary hypochromic anemia, and hereditary anemia.

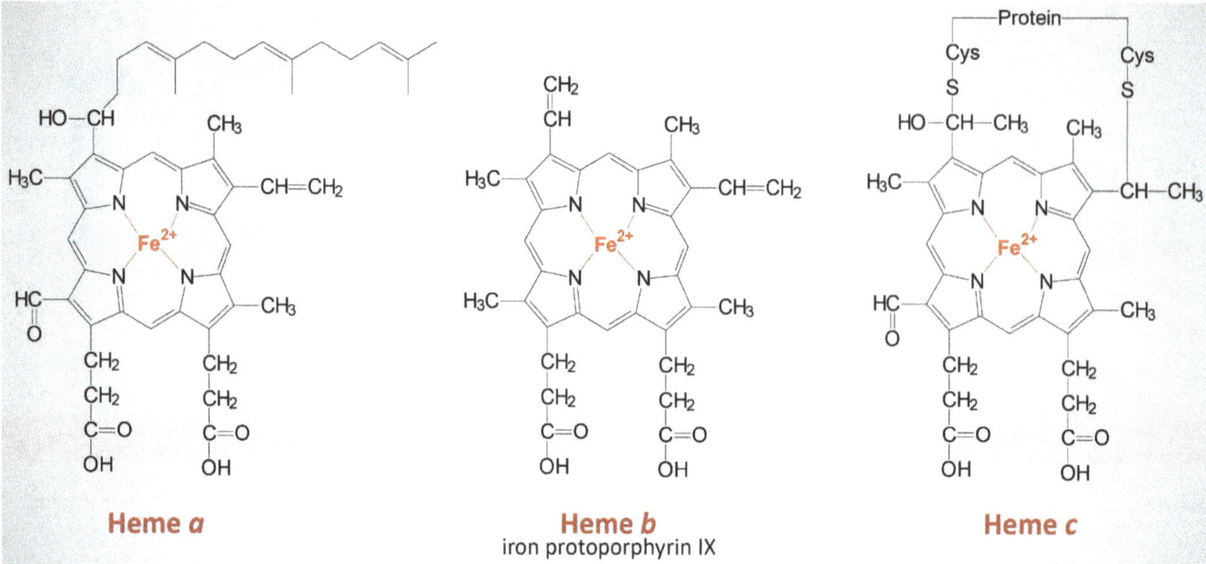

FIGURE 21–1 Structures of heme a, b, and c. (Reproduced with permission from themedicalbiochemistrypage, LLC.)

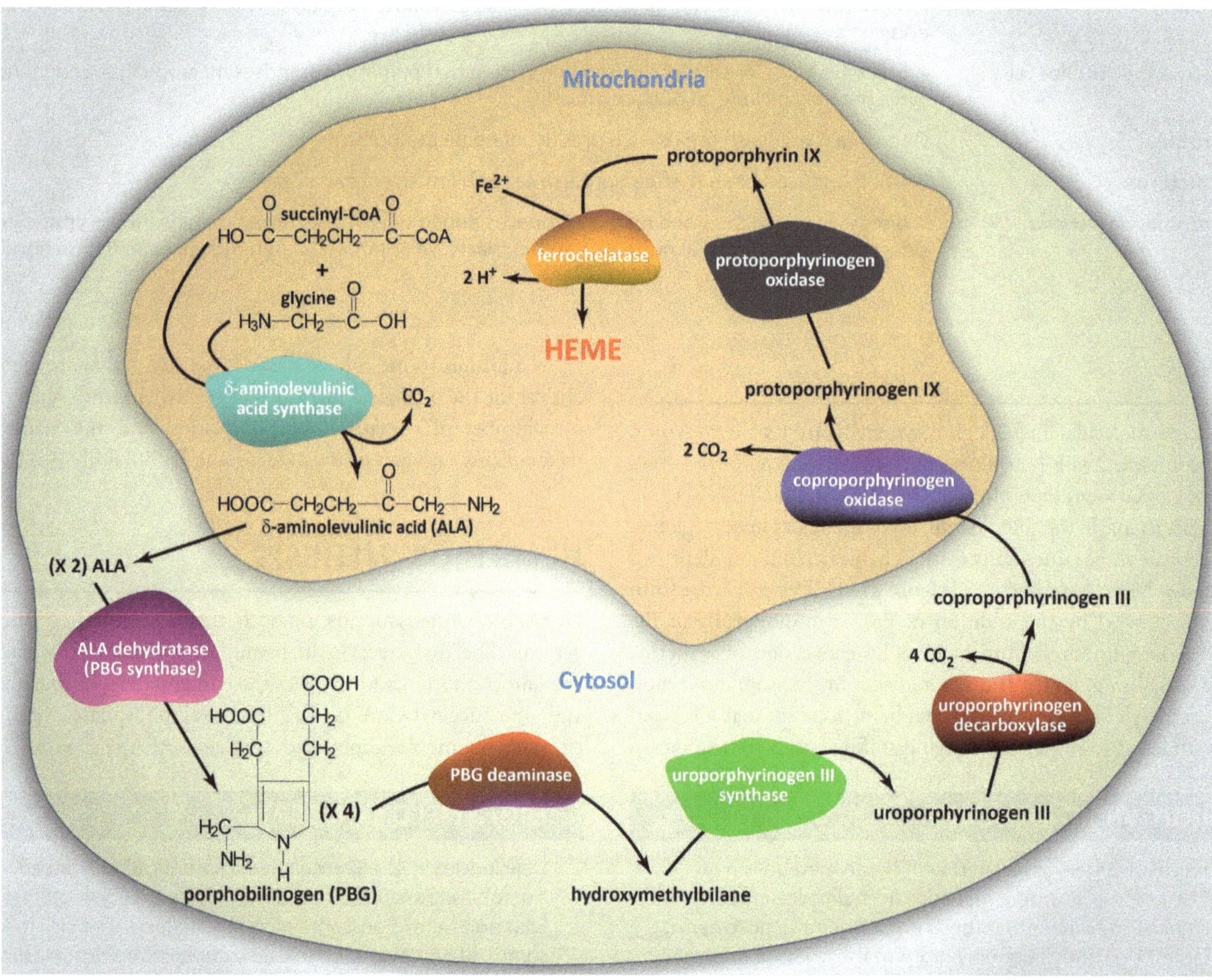

FIGURE 21–2 Pathway of heme biosynthesis. Heme biosynthesis begins in the mitochondria from glycine and succinyl-CoA, continues in the cytosol, and ultimately is completed within the mitochondria. The heme that is produced by this biosynthetic pathway is identified as heme *b*. PBG: porphobilinogen; ALA: δ-aminolevulinic acid. (Reproduced with permission from themedicalbiochemistrypage, LLC.)

TABLE 21–1 Erythroid and hepatic porphyrias.

Porphyria	Enzyme Defect – Gene	Primary Symptoms – Comments
Erythroid Class		
X-linked sideroblastic anemia, XLSA	δ-aminolevulinic acid synthase 2: ALAS2	Microcytic hypochromic anemia; sideroblasts are erythroblasts containing sidersomes (microscopic aggregates of hemosiderin); wide variability in age of presentation; progressive iron accumulation, fatal if not treated
Congenital erythropoietic porphyria, CEP (Gunther disease)	Uroporphyrinogen III synthase: UROS	Photosensitivity evidenced by blistering on the back of the hands and other sun-exposed areas of skin, skin friability after minor trauma, facial hypertrichosis (excessive hair growth), skin hyperpigmentation, reddish discoloration of the teeth (erythrodontia); mild to severe hemolytic anemia; wide variability in phenotypic presentation from fetal lethality to late onset
Erythropoietic protoporphyria, EPP	Ferrochelatase: FECH	Hypersensitivity to sunlight and fluorescent lighting resulting in burning and itching sensations in skin, severe blistering and scarring
Hepatic Class		
ALA dehydratase deficient porphyria, ADP	ALA dehydratase (also called porphobilinogen synthase): ALAD	Neurovisceral symptoms that are very similar to those experienced by acute intermittent porphyria patients
Acute intermittent porphyria, AIP (Clinical Box 21–1)	PBG deaminase (also called hydroxymethylbilane synthase or rarely uroporphyrinogen I synthase): HMBS	Neurovisceral symptoms including severe abdominal pain, nausea, vomiting, tachycardia, hypertension, anxiety, depression, convulsions, peripheral neuropathy; chronic complications include hepatocellular carcinoma (HCC) and renal failure
Hereditary coproporphyria, HCP	coproporphyrinogen III oxidase: CPOX	neurovisceral symptoms similar to those experienced by acute intermittent porphyria patients; seizures; peripheral neuropathy with ascending paralysis; some photosensitivity
Variegate porphyria, VP	Protoporphyrinogen IX oxidase: PPOX	Neurovisceral symptoms and photosensitivity; most commonly adult-onset; cutaneous blistering skin on photoexposed surfaces; crusty slowly healing skin lesions; occasional facial hypertrichosis (excessive hair growth) and hyperpigmentation; abdominal pain; constipation; back, chest, and extremity pain; anxiety; seizures; peripheral neuropathy associated with progressive muscle weakness that may progress to respiratory paralysis
Porphyria cutanea tarda type I, PCT type I, also called the sporadic type PCT (Clinical Box 21–2)	Hepatic uroporphyrinogen decarboxylase activity	Photosensitivity; referred to as the sporadic type of PCT; associated with reduced UROD activity in liver; not associated with direct mutations in the *UROD* gene; most likely due to multifactorial causes
Porphyria cutanea tarda type II, PCT type II, also called the familial type PCT, may also be referred to as hepatoerythropoietic porphyria, HEP	Uroporphyrinogen decarboxylase in nonhepatic tissues: UROD	Photosensitivity evidenced by blistering on the back of the hands and other sun-exposed areas of skin, skin friability after minor trauma, facial hypertrichosis (excessive hair growth), skin hyperpigmentation, severe thickening of affected skin areas (pseudoscleroderma)

This reaction is both the rate-limiting reaction of heme biosynthesis, and the most highly regulated reaction. There are two forms of ALAS. ALAS1 is considered a housekeeping gene and is expressed in all cells. ALAS2 is an erythroid-specific form of the enzyme and is expressed only in fetal liver and adult bone marrow.

Mitochondrial ALA is transported to the cytosol, where ALA dehydratase (also called porphobilinogen synthase) dimerizes two molecules of ALA to produce the pyrrole ring compound, porphobilinogen. The next step in the pathway involves the head-to-tail condensation of four molecules of porphobilinogen to produce hydroxymethylbilane catalyzed by porphobilinogen deaminase, PBG deaminase. PBG deaminase is also called hydroxymethylbilane synthase or uroporphyrinogen I synthase. Hydroxymethylbilane undergoes enzymatic conversion to uroporphyrinogen III, catalyzed by uroporphyrinogen III synthase. On exposure to light, hydroxymethylbilane can also undergo nonenzymatic cyclization forming uroporphyrinogen I.

Both uroporphyrinogen III and uroporphyrinogen I are decarboxylated by the enzyme uroporphyrinogen decarboxylase forming the coproporphyrinogens, with coproporphyrinogen III being the important normal intermediate in heme synthesis. Coproporphyrinogen III is transported back into the mitochondria, where the enzyme coproporphyrinogen III oxidase decarboxylates two propionate residues, yielding vinyl substituents. The product of this reaction is protoporphyrinogen IX.

CLINICAL BOX 21-1 ACUTE INTERMITTENT PORPHYRIA

Acute intermittent porphyria is inherited as an autosomal dominant disorder with late onset of symptoms. AIP is classified as an acute hepatic porphyria and results from defects in gene (*HMBS*) encoding the enzyme commonly called porphobilinogen deaminase (PBGD). PBGD is also known as hydroxymethylbilane synthase (HMBS). Mutations in the *HMBS* gene that result in 50% or less of normal enzyme activity cause the symptoms of AIP. The classic form of AIP results from mutations in the *HMBS* gene that alter the function of both the ubiquitous (housekeeping) nonerythroid cell form and the erythroid-specific form of the enzyme. A small percentage (5%) of AIP patients have functional erythroid-specific PBG deaminase but defective ubiquitous PBG deaminase. Mutations in the *HMBS* gene that result in AIP encompass splice site mutations, missense, frameshift, and nonsense mutations. Approximately 60% of all mutations are found in exons 10, 12, and 14. More than 150 mutations have been identified in the *HMBS* gene resulting in AIP. These mutations include missense, nonsense, and splicing mutations and insertions and deletions. Most of the identified mutations are unique to a given AIP patient. AIP is prevalent in Swedish populations, particularly northern Swedes where the frequency approaches 100 cases per 100,000 population. Because of this prevalence, AIP is also known as Swedish porphyria. Using immunological assays for the presence of PBGD activity, mutations in the *HMBS* gene have been classified into three distinct categories. Type I mutations result in about 50% detectable PBGD protein and enzyme activity. These mutations are referred to as CRIM-negative (or CRM-negative) mutations where CRIM means "cross-reactive immunologic material." Type I mutations represent the largest percentage of mutations in AIP patients, consisting of approximately 85% of mutations. Type II mutations are also CRIM-negative and result in absence of the housekeeping form of the enzyme but normal amounts of the erythroid-specific isozyme. These mutations are found in less than 5% of AIP patients. Type III mutations are CRIM-positive and result in decreased PBGD activity but do not alter the stability of the mutant enzyme. The clinical manifestations of AIP are related to the visceral, autonomic, peripheral, and central nervous system involvement of the disease. In fact almost all of the symptoms of AIP result from neurologic dysfunction, however, the exact mechanism leading to neural cell damage is not clearly understood. The pain associated with the neurologic dysfunction can be so severe as to require treatment with opiates. The symptoms of AIP result from a dramatic increase in the production and excretion of porphyrin precursors. A reduced ability to synthesize heme in a state of increased demand results in loss of heme-mediated control of the rate-limiting enzyme of heme synthesis, δ-aminolevulinc acid synthase, ALAS1. In this circumstance, unregulated ALAS1 results in large increases in synthesis of δ-aminolevulinic acid (ALA). The large increases in ALA drive the ALA dehydratase (also called porphobilinogen synthase) reaction to produce large amounts of porphobilinogen (PBG). With the block in heme synthesis at the PBG deaminase reaction the resulting increases in ALA and PBG synthesis lead to marked increases in urinary excretion of both compounds. Urinary ALA and PBG contribute to the deep red urine, a hallmark of AIP. Clinical manifestation in AIP becomes apparent in the event of an increased demand for hepatic heme production. This most often occurs due to drug exposure or some other precipitating factor such as an infection. In fact, an infection is the leading cause of attacks of acute porphyria. If a drug is the cause of an attack its use should be discontinued immediately. The neurovisceral signs and symptoms of AIP are nonspecific and highly variable resulting in patients being diagnosed with an unrelated illness. Because certain factors such as hormonal or nutritional influences or drug interactions can affect the clinical manifestation of AIP, as well as other hepatic porphyrias, these diseases are referred to as ecogenetic or pharmacogenetic disorders. Numerous drugs are known to lead to acute attacks of porphyria, in particular barbiturates. The use of barbiturates is strongly contraindicated for the treatment of pain in AIP patients, and for that matter, any individual with a porphyria. This is due to the inductive effect of barbiturates on the hepatic cytochrome P450 (CYP) drug metabolism pathway. Induction of CYP synthesis leads to increased utilization of heme which then results in reduced feedback inhibition of ALAS1. The de-repression of ALAS1 results in dramatic increases in the heme biosynthetic intermediates that were the cause of the porphyric symptoms. Other drugs that are known to exacerbate the symptoms of AIP include those used to treat hypertension such as ACE inhibitors (eg, enalapril: Vasotec) and calcium channel blockers (eg, nifedipine: Procardia), drugs used to treat hyperglycemia associated with type 2 diabetes such as the sulfonylureas (eg, glipizide: Glucotrol), and the sulfonamide class of antibiotics. The most common symptom (occurring in 85–95% of cases) during an acute attack is diffuse, poorly localized abdominal pain which can be quite severe. The abdominal pain is usually accompanied by constipation, nausea, and vomiting. The most common physical sign that is observed in up to 80% of AIP cases is tachycardia which may be due to sympathetic nervous system over activity. Additional symptoms of AIP are pain in the limbs, head, neck or chest, muscle weakness, and sensory loss. Often, without any precipitating influences, AIP remains latent and there may be no family history of the disease. The symptoms of AIP are almost never observed in pre-pubescent children and are seen more frequently in women than in men. Treating the symptoms of AIP involves a high carbohydrate diet and during a severe attack an infusion of 10% glucose is highly recommended. The metabolic and molecular logic behind the use of glucose infusion in acute porphyric attacks stems from the fact that hypoglycemia induces the expression of the transcriptional coactivator PGC-1α (peroxisome proliferator activated receptor-γ coactivator 1α). PCG-1α is a major transcriptional regulator of hepatic genes involved in gluconeogenesis and is also an activator of the *ALAS1* gene. Thus, hypoglycemia can precipitate acute attacks in AIP patients (as well as other porphyrias) due to increased synthesis of ALAS1. Hemin (Panhematin, a form of alkaline heme) is used to treat attacks of porphyria as it acts like heme to inhibit ALAS, thereby reducing the production of ALA and subsequently PBG. Many physicians with experience in treating porphyrias recommend early use of hemin without waiting to see if glucose administration alone eases symptoms.

CLINICAL BOX 21–2 PORPHYRIA CUTANEA TARDA

Porphyria cutanea tarda (PCT) is the result of deficiency in the activity of the heme biosynthetic enzyme, uroporphyrinogen decarboxylase. PCT is classified as an acquired porphyria given that even in individuals who inherit autosomal dominant mutations in the gene (*UROD*) encoding uroporphyrinogen decarboxylase, other susceptibility factors are needed to cause clinical symptoms. Deficiency in uroporphyrinogen decarboxylase activity can be acquired in the presence of iron overload, alcohol consumption, smoking, and many other susceptibility factors with as many as 80% of all PCT cases being sporadic. PCT is divided into two major subtypes: type 1 is the sporadic type with near normal levels of uroporphyrinogen decarboxylase protein, type 2 is the familial autosomal dominant type where individuals possess around 50% of normal uroporphyrinogen decarboxylase activity. Type 1 PCT accounts for approximately 80% of all PCT patients worldwide. Both types of PCT have similar clinical features. However, only type 2 PCT has been directly associated with mutations in the *UROD* gene and the disorder is an autosomal dominant inherited trait with the characteristic of incomplete penetrance. Type 1 PCT is the result of multifactorial effects on the level of activity of the UROD-encoded enzyme within hepatocytes. Hepatoerythropoietic porphyria (HEP) is the homozygous dominant form of type 2 PCT. HEP receives its name because the deficiency in UROD leads to the accumulation of porphyrins in both the liver and bone marrow. The symptoms of HEP are similar to those of congenital erythropoietic porphyria (CEP). At least 110 different mutations have been identified in the *UROD* gene resulting in type 2 autosomal dominant PCT. These mutations include missense, nonsense, and splicing mutations, as well as deletions and insertion. About 60% of the UROD mutations in type 2 PCT patients are missense mutations. Approximately 70% of all mutations in the *UROD* gene are found between exons 5 and 10. Most of the identified mutations are unique to a given PCT patient. PCT is a late-onset disease with most affected individuals manifesting symptoms in the 5th to 6th decade of life. The symptoms of PCT are characterized by blistering skin lesions on sun-exposed areas of the skin. Because of this characteristic feature, PCT is strongly indicated in persons who develop skin lesions, particularly on the back of the hands and back of the neck, on exposure to sunlight. In addition to blistering skin lesions, the typical sign of PCT is that which was originally described by Hippocrates, dark red or purple coloration of the urine. The reddish coloration of the urine in PCT patients is the result of the excretion of large amounts of uroporphyrin. Uroporphyrin is the product of hepatic CYP1A2 action on uroporphyrinogen which accumulates due to the reduced activity of uroporphyrinogen decarboxylase. Symptoms of PCT can be precipitated by excess hepatic iron, alcohol consumption, hepatitis C infection, estrogen administration, HIV infection, and by induction of cytochrome P450 (CYP) enzymes such as is typically seen in smokers. Alcohol consumption is a major susceptibility factor in PCT being associated with 60–90% of all cases of PCT. Persons harboring mutations in the *HFE1* gene which results in hemochromatosis are also highly predisposed to PCT. The blistering lesions of PCT rupture easily and heal slowly. The poor healing of the wounds can lead to secondary infections. Due to repeated blistering and rupture, the skin becomes thickened, scarred, and calcified resembling features of scleroderma (referred to as pseudoscleroderma). In addition to the cutaneous clinical features of PCT, there are also hepatic abnormalities that can be evidenced by abnormal liver function tests. Histologically the liver of PCT patients shows necrosis, inflammation, increased iron deposition, and increased fatty deposits. In spite of these hepatic findings cirrhosis is only reported in one-third of PCT patients. The specific treatment regimen for PCT patients depends on several factors. All patients need protection from sunlight while they are in the symptomatic phase. It is important to ensure that eliminate of known susceptibility factors is adhered to. These factors include alcohol consumption, smoking, oral estrogen use, and hepatotoxins. Reductions in total body iron stores and liver iron content may be necessary and is accomplished by phlebotomy and administration of low-dose antimalarial agents (chloroquine or hydroxychloroquine). Iron chelation therapy with the use of deferasirox, deferiprone, or desferrioxamine may be necessary if phlebotomy is contraindicated. Other porphyrias that cause blistering skin lesions, such as HEP, are not responsive to the same treatment regimen and, therefore, it is important to make a correct diagnosis of PCT before treatment is initiated.

Protoporphyrinogen IX is converted to protoporphyrin IX by protoporphyrinogen IX oxidase. The final reaction in heme synthesis involves the insertion of the Fe^{2+} into the ring system generating heme *b*. This last reaction is catalyzed by ferrochelatase.

HIGH-YIELD CONCEPT

The enzymes ferrochelatase, ALA synthase, and ALA dehydratase are highly sensitive to inhibition by heavy metals (eg, lead). Indeed, a characteristic of lead poisoning is an increase in ALA in the circulation in the absence of an increase in porphobilinogen.

REGULATION OF HEME BIOSYNTHESIS

The rate-limiting step in hepatic heme biosynthesis occurs at the ALAS catalyzed step, which represents the committed step in heme synthesis. The level of ALAS activity is negatively regulated by the end-product of the pathway, heme, in several ways. Heme represses expression of the *ALAS1* gene, induces degradation of ALAS mRNA, and inhibits translocation of the precursor enzyme into the mitochondria.

Control of heme biosynthesis in erythrocytes occurs at numerous sites other than at the level of ALAS. Control has been shown to be exerted at the level of both ferrochelatase and PBG deaminase.

HEME CATABOLISM: GENERATION OF BILIRUBIN

The largest repository of heme in the human body is in erythrocytes. The daily turnover of these cells results in the largest pool of heme that needs to be metabolized. Senescent erythrocytes, as well as heme from other sources, are engulfed by cells of the reticuloendothelial system. Once released from protein, heme degradation is initiated by heme oxygenase (Figure 21–3). The products of heme oxygenase are the linear tetrapyrrole biliverdin, ferric iron (Fe^{3+}), and carbon monoxide (CO). The next reaction is catalyzed by biliverdin reductase, producing bilirubin.

HIGH-YIELD CONCEPT

The heme oxygenase reaction is the only one that is known to produce CO. Most of the CO is excreted through the lungs, with the result that the CO content of expired air is a direct measure of the activity of heme oxygenase in an individual.

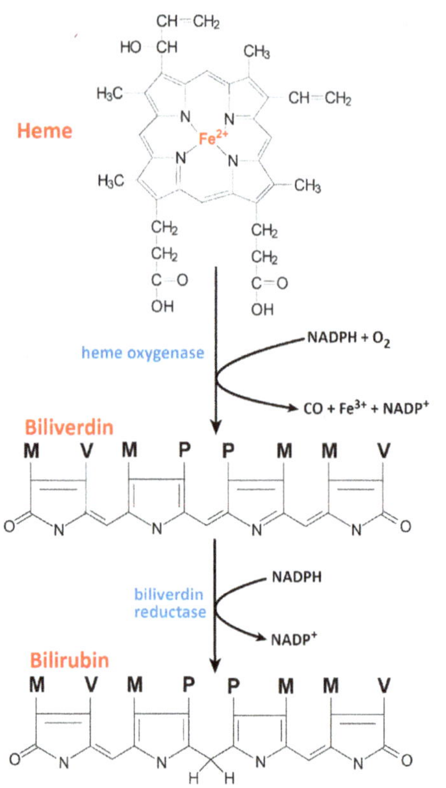

FIGURE 21–3 Heme catabolism initiated by the action of heme oxygenase. The heme ring is cleaved by heme oxygenase yielding biliverdin. Biliverdin is then converted to bilirubin via the action of biliverdin reductase. The side groups on biliverdin and bilirubin are abbreviated: M, methyl; V, vinyl; P, propyl. (Reproduced with permission from themedicalbiochemistrypage, LLC.)

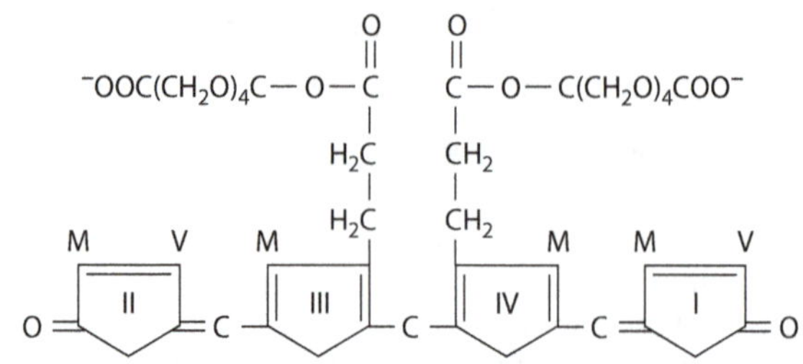

FIGURE 21–4 Structure of bilirubin diglucuronide (conjugated, "direct-reacting" bilirubin). Glucuronic acid is attached via ester linkage to the two propionic acid groups of bilirubin to form an acylglucuronide. (Reproduced with permission from Rodwell VW, Bender DA, Botham KM, et al: *Harper's Illustrated Biochemistry*, 31st ed. New York, NY: McGraw Hill; 2018.)

Bilirubin is significantly less conjugated than biliverdin causing a change in the color of the molecule from blue-green (biliverdin) to yellow-red (bilirubin). The latter catabolic processes are responsible for the progressive changes in the color of a hematoma, or bruise, in which the damaged tissue changes its color from an initial dark blue to a red-yellow and finally to a yellow color before all the pigment is transported out of the affected tissue. Peripherally arising bilirubin is transported to the liver in association with albumin, where the remaining catabolic reactions take place.

In hepatocytes, bilirubin-UDP-glucuronosyltransferase (bilirubin-UGT) adds two equivalents of glucuronic acid to bilirubin to produce the more water-soluble bilirubin diglucuronide derivative (Figure 21–4). The increased water solubility of bilirubin diglucuronide facilitates its excretion with bile. In the intestines, bilirubin and its catabolic products, generated by bacterial metabolism, are collectively known as the bile pigments.

CLINICAL SIGNIFICANCES OF BILIRUBIN

Increased production of bilirubin (eg, hemolytic pathologies) and/or decreased ability to dispose of bilirubin will result in increases in the circulation and accumulation in tissues. Any disorder resulting in plasma bilirubin more than 1 mg/dL is referred to as a hyperbilirubinemia. There are two major classes of hyperbilirubinemias: unconjugated and conjugated (Clinical Box 21–3). Because unconjugated bilirubin is not water soluble, and therefore much more toxic, the clinical symptoms of unconjugated hyperbilirubinemias can be severe and even fatal.

Several inherited disorders in bilirubin metabolism have been identified. Gilbert syndrome (Clinical Box 21–4) and the Crigler-Najjar syndromes (Clinical Box 21–5) result from predominantly unconjugated hyperbilirubinemia. Dubin-Johnson syndrome (Clinical Box 21–6) is a consequence of conjugated hyperbilirubinemia.

CLINICAL BOX 21–3 HYPERBILIRUBINEMIA CLASSIFICATION

There are two major classes of hyperbilirubinemias: unconjugated and conjugated. Bilirubin levels are measured in the serum by an assay utilizing Ehrlich diazo reagent and results in the formation of an azobilirubin product. Conjugated bilirubin does not require addition of alcohol to promote the azotization reaction and thus, this is referred to as measurement of **direct bilirubin**. The reaction with unconjugated bilirubin requires the addition of alcohol and thus, is referred to as the measurement of **indirect bilirubin**. Normal bilirubin measurements are 0.3–1.2 mg/dL for total (indirect + direct). Direct type bilirubin does not exist in the plasma; however, a small portion of indirect type bilirubin may present as direct reacting type and thus the serum measurement may show a direct bilirubin but this is never above 0.3 mg/dL in a normal individual. The mildest form of this condition is jaundice which is caused by a yellow-orange discoloration of the tissues and is most easily visible as icteric discoloration in the sclera of the eyes. Bilirubin toxicity (bilirubin encephalopathy) can be life-threatening in neonates. Bilirubin encephalopathy is characterized by yellow discoloration of the basal ganglia in babies with intense jaundice and is termed kernicterus. Any increase in plasma bilirubin above 20 mg/dL is considered dangerous in neonates. However, individual differences in bilirubin sensitivity can result in kernicterus at lower bilirubin levels. Kernicterus occurs in infants with severe unconjugated hyperbilirubinemia and in young adults with high serum levels of unconjugated bilirubin, with the latter the result of inherited deficiencies in bilirubin-UGT. Bilirubin has been shown to inhibit DNA synthesis, uncouple oxidative phosphorylation, and inhibit ATPase activity in brain mitochondria. Bilirubin also inhibits a variety of different classes of enzymes including dehydrogenases, electron transport proteins, hydrolases, and enzymes of RNA synthesis, protein synthesis, and carbohydrate metabolism. All of these toxic effects of bilirubin are reversed by binding to albumin. In fact, albumin plays a vital role in the disposition of bilirubin in the body by keeping the compound in solution and transporting it from its sites of production (primarily bone marrow and spleen) to its site of excretion which is the liver.

CLINICAL BOX 21–4 GILBERT SYNDROME

Gilbert (pronounced "zheel-BAIR") syndrome is an autosomal recessive disorder that results from mutation in a promoter element of the gene encoding bilirubin-UDP-glucuronosyltransferase (bilirubin-UGT). The human genome contains a complex locus on chromosome 2q37 that encodes several UDP-glucuronosyltransferase genes. This locus is referred to as the UDP-glucuronosyltransferase 1 family, polypeptide A complex locus (UGT1A). Several UGT1A enzymes, including bilirubin-UGT (identified as UGT1A1), are encoded by the *UGT1A* gene complex. The 5′ region of the UGT1A complex contains 13 tandemly arrayed first exons, including four pseudo exons. These tandemly arrayed exons are identified as 1A1, 1A2, 1A3, etc. Exons 2, 3, 4, and 5 are located in the UGT1A 3′ region. All UGT isoforms contain the same C-terminal domain encoded by exons 2 through 5. Each first exon has its own promoter element. The nine viable first exons are independently spliced to the common exons 2 through 5 to generate 9 UGT1A transcripts with unique 5′ ends and identical 3′ ends. The N-terminal region encoded by each unique first exon determines acceptor substrate specificity, while the 246-amino acid C-terminal region encoded by the four common exons specifies interactions with the common donor substrate, UDP-glucuronic acid. The wild-type UGT1A1 allele is identified as UGT1A1*1. Over 135 variants/polymorphisms have been identified in the UGT1A1 allele. The bilirubin-UGT isoform (UGT1A1) consists of 533 amino acids. The majority of patients with Gilbert syndrome inherit the disorder in an autosomal recessive manner. These individuals acquire the disorder as a result of mutations in the TATA-box of the promoter region upstream of exon 1 in the *UGT1A1* gene which results in reduced levels of expression of a normal bilirubin-UGT enzyme. The normal sequence of the UGT1A TATA-box is A(TA)6TAA. The most common mutations observed in patients with Gilbert syndrome is the addition of a T-A dinucleotide into the TATA-box resulting in the sequence: A(TA)7TAA. This mutation is referred to as the UGT1A1*28 allele. Additional TATA-box mutations, but much less common, result in A(TA)5TAA and A(TA)8TAA which are identified as the UGT1A1*36 and UGT1A1*37 alleles, respectively. The UGT1A1*36 allele is associated with increased promoter activity which is protective against hyperbilirubinemia. The UGT1A1*37 allele has promoter activity that is even less than the UGT1A1*28 allele. Both the UGT1A1*36 and UGT1A1*37 alleles are nearly exclusive to populations of African origin. Gilbert syndrome is also referred to as constitutional hepatic dysfunction and familial nonhemolytic jaundice. The syndrome is characterized by mild chronic, unconjugated hyperbilirubinemia. Almost all afflicted individuals have a degree of icteric discoloration in the eyes typical of jaundice. Serum bilirubin levels in Gilbert syndrome patients is usually less than 3 mg/dL. Many patients manifest with fatigue and abdominal discomfort, symptoms that are ascribed to anxiety, but are not due to bilirubin metabolism. Expression of the Gilbert phenotype requires a relatively high level of bilirubin production. This is evident from the fact that persons homozygous for the UGT1A TATA-box mutation do not exhibit hyperbilirubinemia. Presentation of Gilbert syndrome symptoms also occurs more frequently in men than in women because the production of bilirubin is higher in males.

CLINICAL BOX 21-5 CRIGLER-NAJJAR SYNDROMES

The Crigler-Najjar syndromes (CNS) belong to a family of autosomal recessive disorders that result as a consequence of mutations in the coding region of the gene encoding bilirubin-UDP-glucuronosyltransferase (bilirubin-UGT). There are two forms of Crigler-Najjar syndrome: type 1 (CN1) results from mutations in the bilirubin-UGT gene that result in complete loss of enzyme activity, whereas, type 2 (CN2) is the result of mutations that cause reduced levels of enzyme activity. At least 37 mutations identified in UGT1A1 have been shown to be associated with type 1 Crigler-Najjar syndrome and at least 16 mutations shown to be associated with type 2 Crigler-Najjar syndrome. UGT1A1 mutations found in the Crigler-Najjar syndromes include deletions, insertions, missense mutations, and premature stop codons in any of the five exons encoding the UGT1A1 mRNA. All UGT1A1 mutations that are associated with type 1 Crigler-Najjar result in inactive enzyme or no enzyme production. In type 2 Crigler-Najjar syndrome, the UGT1A1 mutations result in reduced level of enzyme activity that has been shown to vary from as little as 4% to as much as 80% of the normal level.

CNS Type I: In patients with very high levels of unconjugated bilirubin, but with normal liver function tests, Crigler-Najjar syndrome type 1 is indicated. Almost all afflicted infants manifest with severe nonhemolytic icterus within the first few days of life. The jaundice in these patients is characterized by increased concentrations of indirect-reacting bilirubin in the plasma. The advent of phototherapy has allowed for greater survival in type 1 patients, in fact without this therapy infants will succumb to kernicterus by the age of 15 months. Use of phototherapy and intermittent plasmapheresis has allowed many type I infants to survive until puberty without significant brain damage. The risk for kernicterus persists following puberty, however, because phototherapy is less effective at this age. Liver transplantation is considered the only definitive treatment for type 1 Crigler-Najjar syndrome.

CNS Type II: The clinical manifestations of type 2 disease are similar to those of type I except that serum bilirubin levels are much lower, generally below 20 mg/dL. The prognosis for type II patients is also much better than for type 1 patients. Induction of bilirubin-UGT by drugs such as phenobarbitol can lead to reductions in serum bilirubin levels in type 2 patients. Given that type 1 Crigler-Najjar results from complete loss of functional bilirubin-UGT, it is not surprising that phenobarbitol has no effect in those patients. Type 2 Crigler-Najjar syndrome was first described by I. M. Arias and, thus, this form of the disease is also sometimes referred to as Arias syndrome.

CLINICAL BOX 21-6 DUBIN JOHNSON SYNDROME

Dubin-Johnson syndrome is an autosomal recessive disorder that results from defects in the canalicular multispecific organic anion transporter (CMOAT) that is encoded by the *ABCC2* (ATP-binding cassette subfamily C member 2) gene. The CMOAT protein has also been called multidrug resistance-associated protein 2 (MRP2). Most of the mutations in the *ABCC2* gene resulting in Dubin-Johnson syndrome are found in the exons encoding the cytoplasmic portion of the protein. This is the region that contains the ATP-binding cassettes. The defect causing Dubin-Johnson syndrome leads to an abnormality in porphyrin metabolism such that more than 80% of the urinary compound from this pathway is coproporphyrin I, whereas in a normal individual it is usually less than 35%. Due to impaired transport of epinephrine metabolites to the bile canaliculi, melanin-like pigments accumulate in the liver such that there is a characteristic black appearance to the organ but with normal histology. Jaundice is usually the only physical symptom detected in this disease. Most patients remain asymptomatic although some complain of weakness and abdominal pains. Only occasionally do patients develop hepatosplenomegaly. In many cases, individuals with the disorder remain undiagnosed due to lack of obvious signs and symptoms. Women may exhibit overt symptoms for the first time when taking oral contraceptives or when pregnant.

CHECKLIST

- ☑ Heme-containing proteins include hemoglobin, cytochromes of the electron transport chain, and the cytochrome P450 enzymes. Heme is composed of iron and the tetrapyrrole compound protoporphyrin IX.
- ☑ Protoporphyrin IX is synthesized via the porphyrin biosynthetic pathway that takes place in the mitochondria and the cytosol utilizing glycine and succinyl-CoA. The initial reaction is catalyzed by the rate-limiting and highly regulated enzyme δ-aminolevulinic acid synthase (ALAS).
- ☑ Iron is inserted into protoporphyrin IX by ferrochelatase.

- ☑ Defects in enzymes of porphyrin synthesis result in a family of disorders called the porphyrias. The porphyrias can be divided into erythroid and hepatic forms dependent on the tissue most affected by the deficiency. Common symptoms of the porphyrias are photosensitivity and variable levels of neurologic deficit.
- ☑ The major site of heme utilization is in erythrocytes. Erythrocytes are in continual flux, dying after approximately 120 days in the circulation. The turnover of erythrocytes creates a significant demand for the degradation of the heme in hemoglobin. Heme degradation occurs primarily in the liver and is initiated via the action of heme oxygenase, the only enzyme in the body to produce carbon monoxide.
- ☑ The byproduct of heme catabolism is bilirubin. Bilirubin is insoluble in the aqueous environment so the liver conjugates it to glucuronic acid to increase its solubility. This reaction is catalyzed by bilirubin DP-glucuronosyltransferase.
- ☑ Elevated levels of bilirubin in the blood (hyperbilirubinemia) and tissues is the cause of jaundice, characterized by yellowing skin and sclera of the eyes. Conjugated hyperbilirubinemias are not as toxic as the unconjugated hyperbilirubinemias due to its increased solubility. Excessive hyperbilirubinemia, especially in the neonate, can lead to the potential for severe neurologic impairment; this is referred to as kernicterus (bilirubin encephalopathy).
- ☑ There are numerous causes of hyperbilirubinemia including anemias and hepatic dysfunction. Several hyperbilirubinemias are due to inherited defects in bilirubin metabolism and include Crigler-Najjar syndrome, Gilbert syndrome, Dubin-Johnson syndrome, and Rotor syndrome.

REVIEW QUESTIONS

1. A 37-year-old male patient is being examined by his physician with complaints of persistent abdominal discomfort. Physical examination shows mildly icteric sclera. Blood work shows elevated serum total bilirubin of 2.4 mg/dL (N = 0.3–1.0 mg/dL) of which 95% was unconjugated. Liver enzyme tests were normal. With respect to the mRNA encoding the primary bilirubin metabolic enzyme, which of the following most likely represents the situation in this patient?

	Size	Synthesis Rate
A.	Larger	Increased
B.	Larger	Unaffected
C.	Smaller	Decreased
D.	Smaller	Increased
E.	Unaffected	Decreased
F.	Unaffected	Unaffected

2. A 38-year-old woman is being examined by her physician with complaints of 1 week history of fever and malaise. Physical examination shows that the patient has a temperature of 38.3°C and icteric sclera. Blood work finds her hemoglobin concentration is 13.8 g/dL (N = 12.0–15.0 mg/dL), WBC of 13×10^9/L (N = 4.5–10×10^9/L), and bilirubin concentration of 2.7 mg/L (N = 0.3–1.0 mg/L), of which 95% was unconjugated. Liver enzyme tests were normal. Which of the following is the most likely cause of these signs and symptoms?

(A) Decreased UDP-glucuronosyltransferase
(B) Excessive hemolysis
(C) Hepatobiliary obstruction
(D) Thiamine deficiency
(E) Vitamin B_6 deficiency

3. A 2-day-old male neonate is undergoing a routine postnatal examination. The infant was born with no identified complications following a complete term. Physical examination finds icteric sclera and yellowish looking skin. The physician recommends at-home treatment with a biliblanket which resolved the observed scleral and skin issues. A reduced level of which of the following enzymes most likely accounted for the symptoms observed in this infant?

(A) δ-Aminolevulinate synthase
(B) Ceruloplasmin
(C) Ferrochelatase
(D) Ferroportin
(E) Porphobilinogen deaminase
(F) UDP-glucuronosyltransferase

4. A 47-year-old man has experienced chronic blistering and scarring of his skin when exposed to sunlight. This man is a smoker and drinks heavily, both of which exacerbate his responses to sun light. Analysis of his urine and plasma indicates a high accumulation of complex porphyrins, predominantly uroporphyrinogens. The symptoms and clinical signs displayed by this patient indicate that he is most likely suffering from which of the following disorders?

(A) Acute intermittent porphyria
(B) Hereditary coproporphyria
(C) Porphyria cutanea tarda
(D) Variegate porphyria
(E) X-linked sideroblastic anemia

5. A 12-year-old boy was referred to the pediatrics clinic because of persistent anemia, irritability, sudden loss of weight accompanied by loss of appetite, and complaints of stomach pain. Laboratory analysis indicates an MCV of 67 fL (N = 82–98 fL). The child's pediatrician suspects the signs and symptoms are due to external factors. To confirm her suspicions, the physician orders a specific laboratory study to be undertaken. Which of the following is most likely the assay the physician orders in this case?

(A) Blood zinc protoporphyrin analysis
(B) Plasma antinuclear antigen level

(C) Red blood cell transketolase activity
(D) Serum diphtheria antitoxoid antibody titer
(E) Stool culture on thiosulfate-citrate-bile salts agar

6. A 32-year-old man has suffered from chronic blistering and scarring of his skin following periods of unprotected exposure to sunlight. History reveals that the symptoms that occur following sun exposure are worse when he has been drinking heavily and smoking. The doctor orders blood and urine tests. Analysis of urine samples upon exposure to a UV-A lamp (Wood's lamp) shows a distinctive pink fluorescence. Which of the following metabolic processes would be expected to be most abnormal in the liver of this patient?
(A) Bile acid synthesis
(B) Branched-chain amino acid catabolism
(C) Glycogen homeostasis
(D) Heme biosynthesis
(E) Purine nucleotide catabolism
(F) Pyrimidine nucleotide biosynthesis

7. A 3-month-old infant who suffered bouts of jaundice and was diagnosed with severe nonhemolytic icterus shortly after birth has succumbed to the complications associated with kernicterus. Prior to the infant's death serum studies showed an increased concentration of indirect-reacting bilirubin with no detection of conjugated bilirubin. The premature death and early clinical findings in this infant were most likely due to which of the following?
(A) Bile duct obstruction
(B) Glucose-6-phosphate dehydrogenase deficiency
(C) Hepatic glucuronidation deficiency
(D) Hereditary spherocytosis
(E) Paroxysmal nocturnal hemoglobinuria
(F) Splenic red blood cell turnover

8. A 21-year-old woman is being examined by her physician with a complaint of a week-long fever, weakness, and tiredness. Physical examination finds a temperature of 38.3°C and icteric sclera. Blood work finds her hemoglobin concentration is 13.8 g/dL (N = 12.0–15.0 mg/dL), WBC of 13 × 10^9/L (N = 4.5–10 × 10^9/L), and bilirubin concentration of 2.3 mg/L (N = 0.3–1.0 mg/L), of which 95% was unconjugated. Liver enzyme tests were normal. Which of the following is the most likely cause of these signs and symptoms?
(A) Decreased glucose-6-phosphate dehydrogenase activity
(B) Decreased glucuronosyltransferase activity
(C) Decreased heme oxygenase activity
(D) Excessive hemolysis
(E) Excessive glucose-6-phosphate dehydrogenase activity
(F) Excessive glucuronosyltransferase activity

9. An 18-month-old boy was referred to the pediatrics clinic because of persistent anemia and associated failure to thrive. Analysis of blood confirmed a microcytic anemia and revealed a blood lead level twice the normal levels. Urine analysis found high levels of coproporphyrinogen III. The child was put on chelation therapy and recovered uneventfully. The cause of the child's difficulty was most likely due to the effect of lead on which of the following?
(A) Alcohol dehydrogenase
(B) δ-Aminolevulinic acid (ALA) synthase
(C) Ferrochelatase
(D) Heme oxygenase
(E) Porphobilinogen (PBG) deaminase
(F) Glucose-6-phosphate dehydrogenase

10. Experiments are being carried out using cultured hepatocytes isolated from a human hepatoma. Results from these experiments find that the addition of hematin (ferric iron heme with an additional chloride ligand) does not result in reduction in protoporphyrin IX synthesis as is the case in normal hepatocytes. Given this observation it is most likely that the hepatoma-derived hepatocytes harbor a mutation in which of the following?
(A) δ-Aminolevulinic acid (ALA) dehydratase
(B) δ-Aminolevulinic acid (ALA) synthase
(C) Ferrochelatase
(D) Heme oxygenase
(E) PBG deaminase

11. A 47-year-old man has experienced chronic blistering and scarring of his skin when exposed to sunlight. This man is a smoker and drinks heavily, both of which exacerbate his responses to sunlight. Analysis of his urine and plasma indicates a high accumulation of complex porphyrins, predominantly uroporphyrinogens. The symptoms and clinical signs displayed by this patient indicate he is most likely suffering from which of the following?
(A) Acute intermittent porphyria
(B) Erythrocyte pyruvate kinase deficiency
(C) Glucose-6-phosphate dehydrogenase deficiency
(D) Porphyria cutanea tarda
(E) Variegate porphyria
(F) X-linked sideroblastic anemia

12. A 32-year-old man has suffered from chronic blistering and scarring of his skin following periods of unprotected exposure to sunlight. History reveals that the symptoms that occur following sun exposure are worse when he has been drinking heavily and smoking. The doctor orders blood and urine tests to aid in her diagnosis. Analysis of a urine sample, upon exposure to a UV-A lamp (Wood lamp), shows a distinctive pink fluorescence. Which of the following metabolic processes would be expected to be most abnormal in the liver of this patient?
(A) Bile acid synthesis
(B) Branched-chain amino acid catabolism
(C) Glycogen homeostasis
(D) Heme biosynthesis
(E) Purine nucleotide catabolism
(F) Pyrimidine nucleotide biosynthesis

13. A 3-month-old infant who suffered bouts of jaundice and was diagnosed with severe non-hemolytic icterus shortly after birth has succumbed to the complications associated with kernicterus. Prior to the infant's death, serum studies showed an increased concentration of indirect, reacting bilirubin with no detection of conjugated bilirubin. This infant's symptoms were most likely due to a defect in which the following enzymes?
(A) Ferrochelatase
(B) Glucose 6-phosphate dehydrogenase
(C) Porphobilinogen deaminase
(D) Pyruvate kinase
(E) UDP-glucuronosyltransferase

14. A 59-year-old man is being examined in the emergency department with a complaint of the recent onset of excruciating abdominal pain, nausea, and vomiting. History reveals the patient has been experiencing mood changes over the past several months which has led him to begin drinking heavily.

The patient has been hypertensive for several years and has been taking enalapril for management of his blood pressure for the past 3 months. Physical examination shows the patient is tachycardic and is experiencing numbness and tingling in his hands and feet. A deficiency in which of the following is the most likely cause of this patient's signs and symptoms?
(A) Alcohol dehydrogenase
(B) δ-Aminolevulinic acid (ALA) synthase
(C) Ferrochelatase
(D) Glucose-6-phosphate dehydrogenase
(E) Porphobilinogen deaminase
(F) UDP-glucuronosyltransferase

15. Experiments are being carried out using cultured hepatocytes isolated from a human hepatoma. Results from these experiments find that the level of measurable carbon monoxide produced by these cells is three times higher than those of normal hepatocytes. These results suggest that the hepatoma-derived cell line most likely harbors an activated form of which of the following?
(A) Biliverdin reductase
(B) Glucose-6-phosphate dehydrogenase
(C) Heme oxygenase
(D) Ferrochelatase
(E) UDP-glucuronosyltransferase

16. A 47-year-old man is being examined in the emergency department with a complaint of the recent onset of excruciating abdominal pain, nausea, and vomiting. History reveals the patient is a smoker and has recently begun taking an ACE inhibitor to treat his hypertension. Physical examination shows the patient is tachycardic and is experiencing numbness and tingling in his hands and feet. The attending physician makes a diagnosis and orders an IV. Which of the following represents the most likely substance added to the patient's IV solution?
(A) Ferrous glycinate
(B) Hematin
(C) Ibuprofen
(D) Phenobarbital
(E) Thiamine

17. A 12-year-old boy was referred to the pediatrics clinic because of persistent anemia, irritability, sudden loss of weight accompanied by loss of appetite, and complaints of stomach pain. Laboratory analysis indicates an MCV of 67 fL (N = 82–98 fL). The child's pediatrician suspects the signs and symptoms are due to external factors. Assay for a decreased serum level of which of the following would most likely confirm the pediatrician's suspicions?
(A) δ-Aminolevulinic acid (ALA)
(B) Ferritin
(C) Free Iron
(D) Protoporphyrin IX
(E) Pyridoxal phosphate

18. A 59-year-old man is being examined in the emergency department with a complaint of the recent onset of excruciating abdominal pain, nausea, and vomiting. History reveals the patient has been experiencing mood changes over the past several months which has led him to begin drinking heavily. The patient has been hypertensive for several years and has been taking enalapril for management of his blood pressure for the past 3 months. Physical examination shows the patient is tachycardic and is experiencing numbness and tingling in his hands and feet. Assay for which of the following is most likely to show elevated levels in the blood of this patient?
(A) δ-Aminolevulinic acid (ALA)
(B) Coproporphyrinogen
(C) Hydroxymethylbilane
(D) Protoporphyrin IX
(E) Uroporphyrinogen

19. An elderly homeless woman is being examined in the emergency department. Physical examination shows a yellowish color of her skin. From her somewhat incoherent story, it can be determined that she has consumed substantial amounts of alcohol over the past three decades. The physician made the diagnosis of alcoholic liver cirrhosis, associated with extensive liver fibrosis. Which of the following changes in plasma and urinary levels of bilirubin are most likely?

	Unconjugated Bilirubin in Plasma	Conjugated Bilirubin in Plasma	Conjugated Bilirubin in Urine
A.	↓	↓	↓
B.	↓	↔ or ↑	↑
C.	↑	↓	↑
D.	↑	↔	↑
E.	↔ or ↑	↑	↑

20. A 37-year-old woman visits her primary care physician after developing jaundice and scleral icterus. She is diagnosed with paroxysmal nocturnal hemoglobinuria. Which of the following metabolites would most likely be increased in her urine?
(A) Chenodeoxycholate
(B) Protoporphyrin IX
(C) Stercobilin
(D) Unconjugated bilirubin
(E) Urobilin

21. A 20-year old woman is being examined by her physician due to her concerns about her increased level of fatigue and the discoloration she has noted in her eyes. Physical examination shows clear icteric sclera. History reveals that she does not drink alcohol and that she has not experienced any changes in her stool. Blood work found normal liver enzyme profile and increased total bilirubin level with the majority being direct bilirubin. Which of the following would most closely explain the observations in this patient?
(A) Defect in hepatocyte bile acid synthesis
(B) Gallstones
(C) Increased rate of hemolysis
(D) Tumor obstructing bile duct
(E) Vitamin B_{12} deficiency

22. A 37-year-old man comes to his physician because of chronic fatigue and persistent abdominal discomfort. He reports that these symptoms began following a particularly severe episode of the flu. Physical examination shows mildly icteric sclera. Laboratory studies show unconjugated bilirubin levels are 3 mg/dL (N = 0.2–0.7 mg/dL). Which of the following is the most likely diagnosis in this patient?
(A) Acute intermittent porphyria
(B) Crigler-Najjar syndrome, type 1
(C) Dubin-Johnson syndrome
(D) Gilbert syndrome
(E) X-linked sideroblastic anemia

23. A 2-day-old infant is being treated for severe jaundice. Blood work shows an indirect bilirubin level of 17 mg/dL (neonatal normal = 5–10 mg/dL). Given the age of onset and the severity of the hyperbilirubinemia in this infant, which of the following would represent the most likely diagnosis?
(A) Acute intermittent porphyria
(B) Crigler-Najjar syndrome, type 1
(C) Dubin-Johnson syndrome
(D) Gilbert syndrome
(E) Rotor syndrome

24. A 47-year-old man is being examined in the emergency department with a complaint of the recent onset of excruciating abdominal pain, nausea, and vomiting. History reveals the patient is a smoker and has recently begun taking an ACE inhibitor to treat his hypertension. Physical examination shows the patient is tachycardic and is experiencing numbness and tingling in his hands and feet. The attending physician makes a diagnosis and administers an IV of 5% dextrose and the patient's nausea and abdominal pain lessen within 2 hours. Which of the following represents the most likely benefit associated with the administration of the dextrose?
(A) Activated expression of the δ-aminolevulinic acid synthase gene
(B) Activated expression of the heme oxygenase gene
(C) Activated expression of the UDP-glucuronosyltransferase gene
(D) Reduced expression of the δ-aminolevulinic acid synthase gene
(E) Reduced expression of the heme oxygenase gene
(F) Reduced expression of the UDP-glucuronosyltransferase gene

25. A 59-year-old man is being examined in the emergency department with a complaint of the recent onset of excruciating abdominal pain, nausea, and vomiting. History reveals the patient has been experiencing mood changes over the past several months which has led him to begin drinking heavily. The patient has been hypertensive for several years and has been taking enalapril for management of his blood pressure for the past 3 months. Physical examination shows the patient is tachycardic and is experiencing numbness and tingling in his hands and feet. Infusion of which of the following would be most useful in the treatment of this patient?
(A) Glucagon
(B) Glucose
(C) Ibuprofen
(D) Insulin
(E) Oxycodone
(F) Phenobarbital

26. A 26-year-old man is seen by his physician complaining of weakness, abdominal pain, nausea, and hair loss. Analysis of blood finds the patient has a hypochromic and microcytic anemia and a transferrin saturation value of 67% (N = 15–50%). Histological examination of the patient's blood shows iron deposits around perinuclear mitochondria. These signs and symptoms are most likely the result of which of the following?
(A) Acute intermittent porphyria
(B) Erythropoietic porphyria
(C) Porphyria cutanea tarda
(D) Variegate porphyria
(E) X-linked sideroblastic anemia

27. A 9-month-old infant who suffered bouts of jaundice and was diagnosed with severe non-hemolytic icterus shortly after birth has succumbed to the complications associated with kernicterus. Prior to the infant's death serum studies showed an increased concentration of indirect-reacting bilirubin with no detection of conjugated bilirubin. The premature death and early clinical findings in this infant were most likely due to which of the following?
(A) Bile duct obstruction
(B) Glucose-6-phosphate dehydrogenase deficiency
(C) Hepatic glucuronidation deficiency
(D) Hereditary spherocytosis
(E) Paroxysmal nocturnal hemoglobinuria

28. A 38-year-old woman is undergoing exploratory laparotomy in order to determine the cause of her chronic abdominal pain. Physical examination of the patient found no overt potential cause for her symptoms. Her physician does note that she is mildly icteric. Routine blood work done prior to scheduling the surgery found no abnormalities. Upon commencement of the surgery it is discovered that there is a blackish sheen over the surface of her liver. Which of the following disorders most likely explains the signs and symptoms in this patient?
(A) Acute intermittent porphyria
(B) Crigler-Najjar syndrome, type 1
(C) Dubin-Johnson syndrome
(D) Gilbert syndrome
(E) Rotor syndrome

29. A 40-year-old man is being examined by his physician to determine the cause of his blistering sunburn after a brief 15-minute exposure. History reveals that the patient is a smoker and that he has always been highly sensitive to the sun. Physical examination shows several areas of scaly thickened skin on his forearms and his teeth appear reddish brown. Which of the following metabolic pathways is most likely defective in this patient?
(A) Cholesterol biosynthesis
(B) Glycogen metabolism
(C) Lysosomal ganglioside catabolism
(D) Porphyrin synthesis
(E) Ubiquinone synthesis

30. A 3-day-old boy born at full-term is brought to his physician because of a 24-hour history of a yellowish coloration of his skin. Physical examination shows a generally healthy baby exhibiting mild jaundice. Laboratory studies show a hemoglobin concentration of 17 g/dL (N = 14–24 g/dL) and a total serum bilirubin concentration of 11 mg/dL (neonatal normal = 5–10 mg/dL). The jaundice resolves on its own within 48 hours. A reduced level of which of the following enzymes is the most likely cause of the jaundice in this patient?
(A) Erythrocyte δ-aminolevulinic acid synthase
(B) Erythrocyte glutathione peroxidase
(C) Erythrocyte pyruvate kinase
(D) Hepatic aldolase B
(E) Hepatic δ-aminolevulinic acid synthase
(F) Hepatic UDP-glucuronosyltransferase

31. A 38-year-old woman was being examined by her physician with complaints of chronic fatigue and abdominal discomfort. Serum studies find an indirect bilirubin level of 2.7 mg/dL (N = 0.2–0.7 mg/dL). Liver function enzymes (AST and ALT) were not elevated. Blood work-up indicated that these symptoms were not due to hemolytic anemia. Molecular analysis of her bilirubin UDP-glucuronosyltransferase gene was carried out and the protein coding sequences were determined to be normal. However, in an upstream region of the gene (between −25 and −40), two additional nucleotides (TA) were found. Which of the following represents the most likely result of the addition of these two nucleotides?

(A) An enhancer-binding factor fails to recognize and bind to the gene
(B) In-frame mutation of the reading frame of the gene
(C) Missense mutation resulting in a less than normally functional enzyme
(D) Nonsense mutation resulting in a truncated enzyme
(E) Suboptimal binding of RNA polymerase to the gene

32. An 8-year-old boy is being examined by his pediatrician because his parents are concerned about his irritability, sudden loss of weight accompanied by loss of appetite, and complaints of stomach pain. Physical examination shows that he is afebrile, and all vital signs are within normal limits. Although the patient's history reveals that he has consistently been at the 60th percentile for both weight and height, at today's examination he is at the 35th percentile for height. Laboratory analysis indicates an MCV of 67 fL (N = 82–98 fL). X-rays showed transverse bands at the distal ulnar and proximal fibular metaphyses. Given the signs and symptoms in this patient, which of the following represents the most likely histopathological finding from a peripheral blood smear?

(A) Basophilic stippling
(B) Bite cells
(C) Heinz bodies
(D) Howell-Jolly bodies
(E) Target cells

33. An 18-year-old man is rushed to the Emergency Department by his father because he is experiencing a constant, sharp, stabbing pain in his lower right abdominal region. Examination by the attending physician finds that the patient is experiencing worsening pain with palpation and demonstrable rebound tenderness. The physician also notes that the patient is exhibiting mild scleral icterus. Suspecting appendicitis, an ultrasound is ordered which confirms the diagnosis. During the laparoscopic removal of the appendix, the surgeon notes that the patient's liver appears to have an almost blackish appearance. Blood drawn prior to surgery is tested and shows that the level of total bilirubin is 3.1 mg/dL (N = 0.2–1.3 mg/dL) and direct bilirubin is 1.5 mg/dL (N = <0.3 mg/dL). There is no evidence of any hemolysis from the blood work performed prior to surgery. Which of the following would most likely account for the observations in this patient?

(A) Defective efflux of bilirubin into bile canaliculi
(B) Defective hepatic uptake of plasma bilirubin diglucuronide
(C) Deficiency in bilirubin-UDP-glucuronosyltransferase
(D) Deficiency in heme oxygenase
(E) Excessive hepatic copper accumulation
(F) Excessive hepatic iron accumulation

34. A 34-year-old man admits himself to the Emergency Department because of the acute onset of excruciating abdominal pain combined with confusion. The patient reports that he used to experience nausea and abdominal pain when he drank alcohol, and as a result, he no longer consumes alcohol. He notes that for the past several days his urine has had a reddish color. Physical examination finds that his vital signs are stable, but that he experiences mild tenderness to abdominal palpation, although his abdomen is soft and nondistended. Given the most likely diagnosis in this patient, which of the following substances is most likely to be found elevated in his urine?

(A) δ-Aminolevulinic acid
(B) Bilirubin
(C) Lactate
(D) Porphobilinogen
(E) Uric acid

35. A 34-year-old man is being examined by his physician for evaluation of the cause of his intermittent severe abdominal pain that he has been experiencing over the past 72 hours. He reports that he has been experiencing constipation for the past 3 days but has not had any nausea or vomiting. When asked, he reports that he has not observed any blood in his stools. He also states that he has been experiencing worsening fatigue and decreased concentration. History reveals that the patient works as a home restorer and has recently been involved in the complete renovation of a mansion built in 1936. The patient has no prior history of serious illness, and he drinks only occasionally and does not smoke cigarettes or use illegal drugs. Physical examination shows mild tenderness to abdominal palpation without rebound or guarding. Laboratory analysis indicates an MCV of 67 fL (N = 82–98 fL), and a peripheral blood smear analyzed by Wright-Giemsa staining shows small blue granules. The signs and symptoms in this patient are most likely due to inhibition of which of the following?

(A) δ-Aminolevulinic acid synthase
(B) Bilirubin UDP-glucuronosyltransferase
(C) Ferrochelatase
(D) Glucose-6-phosphate dehydrogenase
(E) Heme oxygenase
(F) Porphobilinogen deaminase

ANSWERS

1. Correct answer is **E.** The patient is most likely exhibiting the classic signs associated with the unconjugated hyperbilirubinemia called Gilbert syndrome. Gilbert syndrome is the result of a mutation in the TATA-box of the UDP-glucuronosyltransferase 1A (*UGT1A*) gene. The specific mutation converts the normal $A(TA)_6TAA$ of the TATA-box of the *UGT1A* gene to $A(TA)_7TAA$. This change causes a reduced ability of the gene to be transcriptionally active, thus less mRNA is made but the resulting translated protein has normal enzymatic activity, albeit there is a reduced amount of this active enzyme. None of the other options (choices A, B, C, D, and F) relate to the relationship between the mRNA transcribed from the *UGT1A* gene in Gilbert syndrome.

2. Correct answer is **A.** The patient is most likely exhibiting the classic signs associated with the unconjugated hyperbilirubinemia called Gilbert syndrome. Gilbert syndrome is the result of a mutation in the TATA-box of the UDP-glucuronosyltransferase 1A (*UGT1A*) gene. The specific mutation converts the normal $A(TA)_6TAA$ of the TATA-box of the *UGT1A* gene to $A(TA)_7TAA$. This change causes a reduced ability of the gene to be transcriptionally active, thus less mRNA is made but the resulting translated protein has normal enzymatic activity, albeit there is a reduced amount of this active enzyme. Numerous disorders can result in excessive hemolysis (choice B) but are primarily associated with increased conjugated bilirubin. Hepatobiliary obstruction (choice C) can result from numerous pathologies such as pancreatitis, cholelithiasis, choledochal cysts, or cancer. Common symptoms of hepatobiliary obstruction include increased direct and indirect bilirubin in the blood, steatorrhea, and increased liver enzymes in the blood. Thiamine deficiency (choice D) affects energy production and can manifest with neurologic deficit primarily due to reduced pyruvate dehydrogenase activity. Vitamin B_6 deficiency (choice E) is associated with microcytic anemia due to reduced capacity to synthesize heme.

3. Correct answer is **F.** Following birth the red blood cells that contain fetal hemoglobin (HbF) are rapidly replaced by red blood cells containing adult hemoglobin, HbA_1. The increased hemolysis associated with this change of hemoglobin type results in a temporary but a significant increase in serum bilirubin in neonates resulting in hyperbilirubinemia. The expression of the UDP-glucuronosyltransferase gene is activated at birth so there is always a lag in the rate of bilirubin conjugation and removal in neonates. In some infants the level of UDP-glucuronosyltransferase is insufficient to handle all the bilirubin and can result in potentially pathologic levels in the blood. To aid in the removal of the serum bilirubin a common therapeutic intervention is the use of bililights or biliblankets. The blue wavelength light that is emitted from these devices aids in the degradation of bilirubin and its excretion. A reduced level of none of the other enzymes (choices A, B, C, D, and E) account for the hyperbilirubinemia in the neonate.

4. Correct answer is **C.** The patient is most likely suffering from the symptoms of porphyria cutanea tarda, PCT. PCT is the most common of all the porphyrias. PCT is the result of deficiency in the activity of the heme biosynthetic enzyme, uroporphyrinogen decarboxylase. PCT is classified as an acquired porphyria given that even in individuals who inherit autosomal dominant mutations in the gene (*UROD*) encoding uroporphyrinogen decarboxylase, other susceptibility factors are needed to cause clinical symptoms. Symptoms of PCT include cutaneous involvement and liver abnormalities. Cutaneous features include chronic blistering lesions on sun-exposed skin. These lesions lead to skin thickening, scarring, and calcification. Symptoms usually develop in adults and are exacerbated by excess hepatic iron, alcohol consumption, induction of cytochrome P450 (CYP) enzymes as occurs in smokers. Symptoms of acute intermittent porphyria, AIP (choice A) usually appear after puberty and are more frequent in females than in males. The majority of AIP carriers (>80%) do not exhibit symptoms, those that do manifest intermittent neurologic complications with no cutaneous photosensitivity. Hereditary coproporphyria, HCP (choice B) has clinical features and precipitating factors that are essentially identical to those of AIP with the addition of occasional skin photosensitivity. Variegate porphyria, VP (choice D), symptoms are also very similar to those of AIP and HCP, but photosensitivity is more common than in HCP. X-linked sideroblastic anemia (choice E) is due to a defect in the erythroid-specific form of δ-aminolevulinic acid synthase (ALAS2). With defects in ALAS2 there is a reduction in erythroblast heme synthesis in affected individuals leading to erythropoiesis which is ineffective. The consequences of ALAS2 deficiency are non-ferritin iron accumulation in and on the mitochondria of erythroblasts giving rise to the characteristic ring siderosomes and the resulting cells are referred to as sideroblasts.

5. Correct answer is **A.** The child is most likely suffering from the effects of lead poisoning. Lead poisoning interferes with the function of several enzymes of heme metabolism including ALA synthase, ALA dehydratase, and ferrochelatase. The effect on ferrochelatase is much more pronounced than its effects on ALA synthase and ALA dehydratase. The inhibition of ferrochelatase results in the inability to insert Fe^{2+} into protoporphyrin IX, therefore heme is not produced. In erythroid progenitor cells the lack of heme activates the heme-regulated inhibitor (HRI) which phosphorylates the translation initiation factor, eIF-2 resulting in inhibition of protein synthesis. The consequences of inhibited protein synthesis are erythroid progenitor cells smaller than normal resulting in the microcytic anemia evident by the patient's MCV value. The lack of Fe^{2+} incorporation into protoporphyrin IX allows for nonenzymatic insertion of zinc (Zn^{2+}). The analysis of zinc protoporphyrin, referred to as the ZPP assay, is diagnostic for heavy metal poisoning such as lead. The analysis of plasma antinuclear antigen (choice B) is done in patients suspected of having systemic lupus erythematosus, SLE. Assay for red blood cell transketolase (choice C) is the recommended screening test in patients suspected of having a thiamine deficiency. The serum diphtheria antitoxoid antibody test (choice D) is carried out to assay for the presence of the bacterium, *Corynebacterium diphtheriae*. A stool culture on thiosulfate citrate bile salt agar (choice E) is the assay to test for the presence of the bacterium, *Vibrio cholerae*.

6. Correct answer is **D.** The patient is most likely suffering from the symptoms of porphyria cutanea tarda, PCT. PCT is associated with deficiency in the function of the heme biosynthesis enzyme, uroporphyrinogen decarboxylase, UROD. PCT is the most common of all the porphyrias. Symptoms of PCT include cutaneous involvement and liver abnormalities. Cutaneous features include chronic blistering lesions on sun-exposed skin. These lesions lead to skin thickening, scarring, and calcification. Symptoms usually develop in adults and are exacerbated by excess hepatic iron, alcohol consumption, induction of cytochrome P450 (CYP) enzymes as occurs in smokers. None of the other metabolic processes (choices A, B, C, E, and F) would be found to be abnormal in this patient.

7. Correct answer is **C.** The infant most likely suffered from the pathology associated with Crigler-Najjar syndrome type 1. Crigler-Najjar syndrome results from mutations in the UDP glucuronosyltransferase gene. The function of UDP-glucuronosyltransferase is the glucuronidation of bilirubin in the liver. In Crigler-Najjar syndrome type 1 there is essentially no functional enzyme. The consequences of this disorder are extremely high levels of unconjugated bilirubin resulting in the lethal consequences in the brain referred to as kernicterus. None of the other options (choice A, B, D, E, and F) would be relevant clinical findings in this infant.

8. Correct answer is **B.** The patient is most likely exhibiting classic signs associated with the unconjugated hyperbilirubinemia called Gilbert syndrome. Gilbert syndrome is the result of a mutation in the TATA-box of the UDP-glucuronosyltransferase 1A (*UGT1A*) gene. The specific mutation converts the normal $A(TA)_6TAA$ of the TATA-box of the *UGT1A* gene to $A(TA)_7TAA$. This change causes a reduced ability of the gene to be transcriptionally active, thus less mRNA is made but the resulting translated protein has normal enzymatic activity, albeit there is a reduced amount of this active enzyme, not an

excessive amount (choice F). Decreased glucose-6-phosphate dehydrogenase activity (choice A) causes a hemolytic anemia where the red blood cells contain Heinz bodies that are visible in a blood smear. Excessive hemolysis (choice D) will always be associated with elevated levels of serum bilirubin but is more likely to be conjugated bilirubin not unconjugated bilirubin. None of the other options (choices C and E) would result in the signs and symptoms presenting in this patient.

9. Correct answer is **C.** The child is most likely suffering from the effects of lead poisoning. Lead poisoning interferes with the function of several enzymes of heme of metabolism including ALA synthase, ALA dehydratase, and ferrochelatase. The effect on ferrochelatase is much more pronounced than its effects on ALA synthase and ALA dehydratase. The inhibition of ferrochelatase results in the inability to insert Fe^{2+} into protoporphyrin IX, therefore heme is not produced. The appearance of coproporphyrinogen III in the urine of this patient indicates that the inhibition of ferrochelatase is profound whereas ALA synthase (choice B) and ALA dehydratase are minimally inhibited. Heavy metal inhibition of heme oxygenase (choice D) is not associated with microcytic anemia. Heavy metals, such as lead, do not significantly impair the activity of the other enzymes (choices A, E, and F).

10. Correct answer is **B.** In the liver, heme acts as a feedback inhibitor of the first enzyme of heme biosynthesis which is also the rate-limiting enzyme of the pathway, ALA synthase. In addition, heme acts to repress transport of ALA synthase into the mitochondria as well as repressing synthesis of the enzyme. Therefore, a continued synthesis of protoporphyrin IX in the presence of heme indicates that ALA synthase is active but nonresponsive to the normally inhibitory action of heme. None of the other enzymes (choices A, C, D, and E) are subject to inhibition by heme.

11. Correct answer is **D.** The patient is most likely suffering the consequences of the porphyria called porphyria cutanea tarda, PCT. PCT is the most common porphyria. Symptoms of PCT include cutaneous involvement and liver abnormalities. Cutaneous features include chronic blistering lesions on sun-exposed skin. These lesions lead to skin thickening, scarring, and calcification. Symptoms usually develop in adults and are exacerbated by excess hepatic iron, alcohol consumption, induction of cytochrome P450 (CYP) enzymes as occurs in smokers. Acute intermittent porphyria, AIP (choice A) results from mutations in the PBG deaminase gene. Clinical manifestation in AIP becomes apparent in the event of an increased demand for hepatic heme production. The clinical manifestations of AIP are related to the visceral, autonomic, peripheral, and central nervous system involvement of the disease. Both erythrocyte pyruvate kinase deficiency (choice B) and glucose-6-phosphate dehydrogenase deficiency (choice C) are associated with hemolytic anemia. Variegate porphyria (choice E) results from mutations in the protoporphyrinogen IX oxidase gene. Common symptoms of variegate porphyria include cutaneous photosensitivity, abdominal pain, constipation, nausea, vomiting, hypertension, tachycardia, neuropathy, and back pain. X-linked sideroblastic anemia, XLSA (choice F) is a heme biosynthesis disorder resulting from mutations in the erythroid specific ALA synthase, encoded by the *ALAS2* gene. Symptoms of XLSA usually appear in the second or third decade of life and include hepatomegaly and/or splenomegaly, hepatocellular carcinoma, diabetes, body hair loss, nausea and abdominal pain, cirrhosis, growth delay, and arthropathy.

12. Correct answer is **D.** The patient is most likely suffering from the symptoms of porphyria cutanea tarda, PCT. PCT is associated with deficiency in the function of the heme biosynthesis enzyme, uroporphyrinogen decarboxylase, UROD. PCT is the most common of all the porphyrias. Symptoms of PCT include cutaneous involvement and liver abnormalities. Cutaneous features include chronic blistering lesions on sun-exposed skin. These lesions lead to skin thickening, scarring, and calcification. Symptoms usually develop in adults and are exacerbated by excess hepatic iron, alcohol consumption, induction of cytochrome P450 (CYP) enzymes as occurs in smokers. Porphyrias can be detected with the use of the Wood lamp due to the pink fluorescence of the accumulating compounds. The test can be performed on the skin or the urine. Abnormalities in none of the other metabolic processes (choices A, B, C, E, and F) would manifest with the symptoms observed in this patient.

13. Correct answer is **E.** The infant most likely suffered from the pathology associated with Crigler-Najjar syndrome type 1. Crigler-Najjar syndrome results from mutations in the UDP-glucuronosyltransferase gene. The function of UDP-glucuronosyltransferase is the glucuronidation of bilirubin in the liver. In Crigler-Najjar syndrome type 1 there is essentially no functional enzyme. The consequences of this disorder are extremely high levels of unconjugated bilirubin resulting in the lethal consequences in the brain referred to as kernicterus. Deficiencies in ferrochelatase (choice A) and porphobilinogen deaminase (choice C) result in disorders of heme biosynthesis referred to as the porphyrias. Deficiencies in glucose-6-phosphate dehydrogenase (choice B) and pyruvate kinase (choice D) result in hemolytic anemias.

14. Correct answer is **E.** The patient is most likely experiencing the symptoms of acute intermittent porphyria, AIP. AIP results from mutations in the porphobilinogen deaminase (PBG deaminase) gene. PBG deaminase (also called hydroxymethylbilane synthase) catalyzes the heme biosynthesis reaction involving the head-to-tail condensation of four molecules of porphobilinogen to produce the linear tetrapyrrole intermediate, hydroxymethylbilane. The clinical manifestations of AIP are related to the visceral, autonomic, peripheral, and central nervous system involvement of the disease. In fact, almost all of the symptoms of AIP result from neurologic dysfunction. Certain factors such as hormonal or nutritional influences or drug interactions can affect the clinical manifestation of AIP. Drugs known to trigger acute attacks in AIP patients include those used to treat hypertension such as ACE inhibitors (eg, enalapril) and calcium channel blockers (eg, nifedipine), drugs used to treat hyperglycemia associated with type 2 diabetes such as the sulfonylureas, and the sulfonamide class of antibiotics. Deficiencies in none of the other enzymes (choices A, B, C, D, and F) would result in the symptoms manifesting in this patient.

15. Correct answer is **C.** During the catabolism of heme the molecule is first oxidized, with the heme ring being opened by the endoplasmic reticulum enzyme, heme oxygenase. The oxidation step requires heme as a substrate, and any hemin (Fe^{3+}) is reduced to heme (Fe^{2+}) prior to oxidation by heme oxygenase. The oxidation occurs on a specific carbon producing the linear tetrapyrrole biliverdin, ferric iron (Fe^{3+}), and carbon monoxide (CO). This is the only enzyme in the body that is known to produce CO. Most of the CO is excreted through the lungs, with the result that the CO content of expired air is

a direct measure of the activity of heme oxygenase in an individual. The activity of none of the other enzymes (choices A, B, D, and E) produce carbon monoxide as a byproduct of their reactions.

16. Correct answer is **B.** The patient is most likely experiencing the symptoms of acute intermittent porphyria, AIP. AIP results from mutations in the porphobilinogen deaminase (PBG deaminase) gene. The clinical manifestations of AIP are related to the visceral, autonomic, peripheral, and central nervous system involvement of the disease. In fact, almost all the symptoms of AIP result from neurologic dysfunction. Certain factors such as hormonal or nutritional influences or drug interactions can affect the clinical manifestation of AIP. Drugs known to trigger acute attacks in AIP patients include those used to treat hypertension such as ACE inhibitors. Hematin is a hydroxylated form of ferrous iron heme. The benefit of hematin infusion during the acute attacks in AIP patients relates to the fact that the rate-limiting enzyme of heme biosynthesis, δ-aminolevulinic acid synthase (ALAS), is inhibited by heme. The hematin-mediated inhibition of ALAS reduces the accumulation of the intermediates of heme biosynthesis that induce the acute pathology in AIP. Administration of none of the other substances (choices A, C, D, and E) would be beneficial in treating the acute symptoms in AIP patients. Indeed, administration of phenobarbital (choice D) is strongly contraindicated for porphyria patients because the drug is metabolized by the hepatic CYP system. Enhanced CYP utilization leads to reduced levels of heme in hepatocytes and heme serves as a feedback inhibitor of δ-aminolevulinic acid synthase, the rate-limiting enzyme of heme synthesis. Therefore, administration of phenobarbital to AIP patients would precipitate a worsening of pathology.

17. Correct answer is **A.** The child is most likely suffering from the effects of lead poisoning. Lead poisoning interferes with the function of several enzymes of heme of metabolism including ALA synthase, ALA dehydratase, and ferrochelatase. The inhibition of ALA synthase would, therefore, result in reduced levels of δ-aminolevulinic acid. Protoporphyrin IX (choice D) levels would also be reduced in this patient, but the more accurate assay would be determination of δ-aminolevulinic acid levels. The inability to generate sufficient protoporphyrin IX would result in increased, not decreased (choice C) free iron. The increase in free iron would result in increased iron storage in ferritin. As iron storage in ferritin rises more ferritin, not less (choice B), would be detectable in the blood. Vitamin B_6, the precursor to pyridoxal phosphate, is a water-soluble vitamin, therefore even in the presence of less functional δ-aminolevulinic acid synthase, which requires pyridoxal phosphate, there would be no significant increase (choice E) in pyridoxal phosphate in the blood.

18. Correct answer is **A.** The patient is most likely experiencing the symptoms of acute intermittent porphyria, AIP. AIP results from mutations in the porphobilinogen deaminase (PBG deaminase) gene. PBG deaminase (also called hydroxymethylbilane synthase) catalyzes the heme biosynthesis reaction involving the head-to-tail condensation of four molecules of porphobilinogen to produce the linear tetrapyrrole intermediate, hydroxymethylbilane. δ-Aminolevulinic acid (ALA) is the precursor for porphobilinogen, thus a defect in PBG deaminase would lead to excess ALA excretion. The deficiency of PBG deaminase function in AIP patients would lead to reduced, not elevated, levels of all of the subsequent intermediates in heme biosynthesis (choices B, C, D, and E).

19. Correct answer is **E.** Excessive and long-term alcohol consumption damages hepatocytes and leads to increased total bilirubin, both unconjugated and conjugated, in plasma, with the majority being conjugated. Although the mechanism is not fully defined, the increase in conjugated plasma bilirubin is most likely to be due to release from damaged hepatocytes, reduced disposition within hepatocytes, and reduced secretion from hepatocytes. It is also possible that the liver damage resulted in obstruction of bile flow, which leads to a backup of largely conjugated bilirubin in the blood stream. The increase in the serum of unconjugated bilirubin is the result of reduced hepatic conjugation capacity as a consequence of the ethanol-mediated damage to hepatocytes. Conjugated bilirubin is eventually removed by the kidneys and results in increased conjugated bilirubin in urine. Alcoholism might also lead to an increase in unconjugated plasma bilirubin, in the case that the ability of hepatocytes to remove unconjugated bilirubin from plasma is grossly impaired. As with all chronic diseases, alcoholism may present with a wide spectrum of symptoms. None of the other options (choices A, B, C, and D) correctly reflect the changes in the serum and urine bilirubin levels with respect to the effects of chronic alcohol consumption on liver function.

20. Correct answer is **E.** Paroxysmal nocturnal hemoglobinuria (PNH) is a hemolytic anemia in which an acquired cell membrane defect increases red blood cell susceptibility to lysis by endogenous complement. PNH is principally due to the lack of the complement inhibitor proteins CD55 and CD59, which are GPI-anchored, on the surface of erythrocytes. Intravascular hemolysis overwhelms the capacity of hepatic UDP-glucuronosyltransferase conjugation capability and leads to an increase in unconjugated bilirubin (water-insoluble) in serum. The liver enzyme, UDP-glucuronosyltransferase converts unconjugated bilirubin into conjugated bilirubin (now water-soluble), which is then excreted by hepatocytes into the bile. After secretion of bile into the intestine, ileal and colonic bacteria convert conjugated bilirubin into urobilinogen. A fraction of urobilinogen is oxidized to stercobilin and directly excreted in feces, thus, would not be a urinary metabolite. The remaining urobilinogen is reabsorbed from the intestine and re-enters the portal circulation where a portion is taken up by the liver and re-excreted into bile, while the rest bypasses the liver and is excreted by the kidney as urobilin. Therefore, in hemolytic anemias, increased liver excretion of conjugated bilirubin will lead to an increase in urinary urobilin levels. Note that this is in contrast to biliary tract obstruction in which failure of conjugated bilirubin to enter the intestine would lead to decreased levels of both fecal stercobilin and urinary urobilin. Unconjugated bilirubin (choice D) is lipid soluble and cannot be excreted by the kidneys. None of the other compounds (choices A, B, and C) would be elevated in the urine in this patient.

21. Correct answer is **D.** The icteric sclera present in this patient is evidence of elevated serum levels of bilirubin. In a patient with jaundice resulting primarily from conjugated bilirubin, where liver function assays are normal, this is an indication of pathology associated with hepatobiliary circulation. Hemolysis of large numbers of erythrocytes (choice C) can result in jaundice in the absence of any liver disease due to the amount of bilirubin exceeding overall capacity of hepatocytes to conjugate all of it. However, there are no signs or symptoms in this patient indicative of hemolytic anemia. None of the other options (choices A, B, and E) would be associated with the jaundice in this seemingly otherwise healthy patient.

22. Correct answer is **D.** The patient is most likely exhibiting classic signs associated with the unconjugated hyperbilirubinemia called Gilbert syndrome. Gilbert syndrome is the result of a mutation in the TATA-box of the UDP-glucuronosyltransferase 1A (*UGT1A*) gene. The specific mutation converts the normal $A(TA)_6TAA$ of the TATA-box of the *UGT1A* gene to $A(TA)_7TAA$. This change causes a reduced ability of the gene to be transcriptionally active, thus less mRNA is made but the resulting translated protein has normal enzymatic activity. Gilbert syndrome is characterized by mild chronic, unconjugated hyperbilirubinemia. Almost all afflicted individuals have a degree of icteric discoloration in the eyes typical of jaundice. Serum bilirubin levels in Gilbert syndrome patients are usually less than 3 mg/dL. Many patients manifest with fatigue and abdominal discomfort, symptoms that are ascribed to anxiety, but are not due to bilirubin metabolism. Acute intermittent porphyria, AIP (choice A) results from mutations in the heme biosynthetic enzyme, PBG deaminase. The clinical manifestations of AIP are related to the visceral, autonomic, peripheral, and central nervous system involvement of the disease. In fact, almost all the symptoms of AIP result from neurologic dysfunction. Crigler-Najjar syndrome, type 1 (choice B) is usually a neonatal lethal disorder of severe unconjugated hyperbilirubinemia resulting in kernicterus. Dubin-Johnson syndrome (choice C), like Gilbert syndrome, is a relatively benign disorder of bilirubin metabolism. Dubin-Johnson syndrome results from mutations in the gene encoding the bile canalicular multispecific organic anion transporter. This transporter is involved in the excretion of many non-bile organic anions by an ATP-requiring process. Jaundice is usually the only physical symptom detected in Dubin-Johnson syndrome. Most patients remain asymptomatic although some complain of weakness and abdominal pains. X-linked sideroblastic anemia, XLSA (choice E) is a form of anemia resulting from mutations in the erythroid specific δ-aminolevulinic acid synthase encoded by the *ALAS2* gene. Clinical manifestations of XLSA include hepatomegaly and/or splenomegaly, hepatocellular carcinoma, diabetes, body hair loss, nausea, and abdominal pain, cirrhosis, growth delay, and arthropathy (disease of the joints). Weakness, fatigue, and palpitations are due to cardiac involvement.

23. Correct answer is **B.** The infant most likely suffered from the pathology associated with Crigler-Najjar syndrome type 1. Crigler-Najjar syndrome results from mutations in the UDP-glucuronosyltransferase gene. The function of UDP-glucuronosyltransferase is the glucuronidation of bilirubin in the liver. In Crigler-Najjar syndrome type 1 there is essentially no functional enzyme. The consequences of this disorder are extremely high levels of unconjugated bilirubin resulting in the lethal consequences in the brain referred to as kernicterus. Acute intermittent porphyria, AIP (choice A) results from mutations in the heme biosynthetic enzyme, PBG deaminase. The clinical manifestations of AIP are related to the visceral, autonomic, peripheral, and central nervous system involvement of the disease. In fact, almost all the symptoms of AIP result from neurologic dysfunction. Dubin-Johnson syndrome (choice C) is a relatively benign disorder of bilirubin metabolism. Dubin-Johnson syndrome results from mutations in the gene encoding the bile canalicular multispecific organic anion transporter. This transporter is involved in the excretion of many non-bile organic anions by an ATP-requiring process. Jaundice is usually the only physical symptom detected in Dubin-Johnson syndrome. Most patients remain asymptomatic although some complain of weakness and abdominal pains. Gilbert syndrome (choice D), like Dubin-Johnson syndrome, is a relatively benign disorder of bilirubin metabolism. The disorder results from a mutation in the TATA-box of the UDP-glucuronosyltransferase 1A (*UGT1A*) gene. Gilbert syndrome is characterized by mild chronic, unconjugated hyperbilirubinemia. Almost all afflicted individuals have a degree of icteric discoloration in the eyes typical of jaundice. Rotor syndrome (choice E) is conjugated hyperbilirubinemia resulting from mutations in two genes encoding transport proteins. These two transport proteins are responsible for the uptake of bilirubin by the liver. The symptoms of Rotor syndrome are similar to those of Dubin-Johnson syndrome except that there is no liver discoloration in the Rotor syndrome.

24. Correct answer is **D.** The patient is most likely experiencing the symptoms of acute intermittent porphyria, AIP. AIP results from mutations in the porphobilinogen deaminase (PBG deaminase) gene. The clinical manifestations of AIP are related to the visceral, autonomic, peripheral, and central nervous system involvement of the disease. In fact, almost all the symptoms of AIP result from neurologic dysfunction. Certain factors such as hormonal or nutritional influences or drug interactions can affect the clinical manifestation of AIP. Drugs known to trigger acute attacks in AIP patients include those used to treat hypertension such as ACE inhibitors. The benefit of glucose (dextrose) infusion during the acute attacks in AIP patients relates to the expression of the transcription factor PGC-1α. In the fasted state the expression of PGC-1α increases as a means to increase the expression of genes encoding enzymes required for gluconeogenesis. In the case of AIP patients, as well as in other porphyrias, the activity of PGC-1α enhances the expression of the *ALAS1* gene encoding the rate-limiting enzyme of heme biosynthesis. This results in enhanced accumulation of heme biosynthetic intermediates which exacerbate the acute pathology of AIP. Therefore, glucose infusion lowers the expression of PGC-1α and, consequently, the reduced expression of the *ALAS1* gene. None of the other options (choices A, B, C, E, and F) correctly correlate to the beneficial effects of dextrose infusion in AIP patients.

25. Correct answer is **B.** The patient is most likely experiencing the symptoms of acute intermittent porphyria, AIP. AIP results from mutations in the porphobilinogen deaminase (PBG deaminase) gene. The clinical manifestations of AIP are related to the visceral, autonomic, peripheral, and central nervous system involvement of the disease. In fact, almost all the symptoms of AIP result from neurologic dysfunction. Certain factors such as hormonal or nutritional influences or drug interactions can affect the clinical manifestation of AIP. Drugs known to trigger acute attacks in AIP patients include those used to treat hypertension such as ACE inhibitors (eg, enalapril) and calcium channel blockers (eg, nifedipine), drugs used to treat hyperglycemia associated with type 2 diabetes such as the sulfonylureas, and the sulfonamide class of antibiotics. The benefit of glucose infusion during the acute attacks in AIP patients relates to the expression of the transcription factor PGC-1α. In the fasted state the expression of PGC-1α increases as a means to increase the expression of genes encoding enzymes required for gluconeogenesis. In the case of AIP patients, as well as in other porphyrias, the activity of PGC-1α enhances the expression of the *ALAS1* gene encoding the rate-limiting enzyme of heme biosynthesis.

This results in enhanced accumulation of heme biosynthetic intermediates which exacerbates the acute pathology of AIP. Therefore, glucose infusion lowers expression of PGC-1α and, consequently, the expression of ALAS1. Administration of none of the other substances (choices A, C, D, E, and F) would be beneficial in treating the acute symptoms in AIP patients. Indeed, administration of phenobarbital (choice F) is strongly contraindicated for porphyria patients because the drug is metabolized by the hepatic CYP system. Enhanced CYP utilization leads to reduced levels of heme in hepatocytes and heme serves as a feedback inhibitor of δ-aminolevulinic acid synthase, the rate-limiting enzyme of heme synthesis. Therefore, administration of phenobarbital to AIP patients would precipitate a worsening of pathology.

26. Correct answer is **E.** The patient is most likely experiencing the signs and symptoms of X-linked sideroblastic anemia, XLSA. XLSA is a form of porphyria that results from mutations in the gene, *ALAS2*, encoding the erythroid-specific form of δ-aminolevulinic acid synthase. The *ALAS2* gene is located on the X chromosome. As a result of defective ALAS2 activity there is reduced protoporphyrin IX synthesis in erythroid progenitor cells. The lack of ability to synthesize heme in these cells results in a block to protein synthesis resulting in a microcytic hypochromic anemia. In the absence of sufficient protoporphyrin IX, iron accumulates in the erythroid progenitor cells. This excess iron deposits as non-ferritin iron in the mitochondria that surround the nuclei. These deposits give the cells a distinctive pathologic appearance referred to as ring sideroblasts hence the name of the disorder as X-linked sideroblastic anemia. Acute intermittent porphyria, AIP (choice A) results from mutations in the porphobilinogen deaminase (PBG deaminase) gene. The clinical manifestations of AIP are related to the visceral, autonomic, peripheral, and central nervous system involvement of the disease. In fact, almost all the symptoms of AIP result from neurologic dysfunction. Erythropoietic porphyria (choice B) results from defects in ferrochelatase. Light-sensitive dermatitis commencing in childhood, usually before 10 years of age, is the presenting finding in erythropoietic protoporphyria. Porphyria cutanea tarda, PCT (choice C) is the result of deficiency in the activity of the heme biosynthetic enzyme, uroporphyrinogen decarboxylase, UROD. Symptoms of PCT include cutaneous involvement and liver abnormalities. Cutaneous features include chronic blistering lesions on sun-exposed skin. Variegate porphyria (choice D) results from mutations in the protoporphyrinogen IX oxidase gene. Common symptoms of variegate porphyria include cutaneous photosensitivity, abdominal pain, constipation, nausea, vomiting, hypertension, tachycardia, neuropathy, and back pain.

27. Correct answer is **C.** The infant most likely suffered from the pathology associated with Crigler-Najjar syndrome type 1. Crigler-Najjar syndrome results from mutations in the UDP-glucuronosyltransferase gene. The function of UDP-glucuronosyltransferase is the glucuronidation of bilirubin in the liver. In Crigler-Najjar syndrome type 1 there is essentially no functional enzyme. The consequences of this disorder are extremely high levels of unconjugated bilirubin resulting in the lethal consequences in the brain referred to as kernicterus. Bile duct obstruction (choice A) would result in hyperbilirubinemia but is not a lethal condition in the neonatal period. Glucose-6-phosphate dehydrogenase (G6PDH) deficiency (choice B) is one of the most common inherited hemolytic anemias. As a result of hemolysis in G6PDH deficiency there would be hyperbilirubinemia, however, this disorder is not lethal in the neonatal period. Hereditary spherocytosis (choice D) is a term relating to hemolytic anemias resulting from loss of the normal biconcave structure of erythrocytes. The most common cause of hereditary spherocytosis is mutations in the gene encoding the cytoskeletal protein, spectrin. Typical symptoms of hereditary spherocytosis are hyperbilirubinemia and splenomegaly, but the disease is not lethal. Paroxysmal nocturnal hemoglobinuria, PNH (choice E) is a disorder where the cells lack GPI-anchored proteins. This disorder is characterized by intravascular hemolysis of erythrocytes by complement system proteins. This phenotype is principally due to the lack of the complement inhibitor proteins CD55 and CD59, which are GPI-anchored, on the surface of erythrocytes. PNH is a potentially lethal disorder but not in the neonatal period.

28. Correct answer is **C.** The patient is most likely exhibiting one of the signs of Dubin-Johnson syndrome. Dubin-Johnson syndrome results from mutations in the gene encoding the bile canalicular multispecific organic anion transporter. This transporter is involved in the excretion of many non-bile organic anions by an ATP-requiring process. Jaundice is usually the only physical symptom detected in Dubin-Johnson syndrome. Most patients remain asymptomatic although some complain of weakness and abdominal pains. Due to impaired transport of epinephrine metabolites to the bile canaliculi, melanin-like pigments accumulate in the liver such that there is a characteristic black appearance to the organ but with normal histology. Acute intermittent porphyria, AIP (choice A) results from mutations in the porphobilinogen deaminase (PBG deaminase) gene. The clinical manifestations of AIP are related to the visceral, autonomic, peripheral, and central nervous system involvement of the disease. In fact, almost all the symptoms of AIP result from neurologic dysfunction. Crigler-Najjar syndrome, type 1 (choice B) results from mutations in the UDP-glucuronosyltransferase gene. The function of UDP-glucuronosyltransferase is the glucuronidation of bilirubin in the liver. In Crigler-Najjar syndrome type 1 there is essentially no functional enzyme. The consequences of this disorder are extremely high levels of unconjugated bilirubin resulting in the lethal consequences in the brain referred to as kernicterus. Gilbert syndrome (choice D) is a relatively benign disorder of bilirubin metabolism. The disorder results from a mutation in the TATA-box of the UDP-glucuronosyltransferase 1A (*UGT1A*) gene. Gilbert syndrome is characterized by mild chronic, unconjugated hyperbilirubinemia. Almost all afflicted individuals have a degree of icteric discoloration in the eyes typical of jaundice. Rotor syndrome (choice E) is conjugated hyperbilirubinemia resulting from mutations in two genes encoding transport proteins. These two transport proteins are responsible for the uptake of bilirubin by the liver. The symptoms of Rotor syndrome are similar to those of Dubin-Johnson syndrome except that there is no liver discoloration in the Rotor syndrome.

29. Correct answer is **D.** The patient is most likely suffering from the symptoms of porphyria cutanea tarda, PCT. PCT is associated with deficiency in the function of the heme biosynthesis enzyme, uroporphyrinogen decarboxylase, UROD. PCT is the most common of all the porphyrias. Symptoms of PCT include cutaneous involvement and liver abnormalities. Cutaneous features include chronic blistering lesions on sun-exposed skin. These lesions lead to skin thickening, scarring, and calcification. Symptoms usually develop in adults and are exacerbated by induction of cytochrome P450 (CYP) enzymes as occurs in smokers. The heme biosynthetic intermediates that accumulate in PCT patients turn the urine red and when deposited in the teeth turn them reddish brown. Accumulation of these byproducts in the skin renders it extremely sensitive to sunlight causing ulceration and disfiguring scars. Defects in none of the other pathways (choices A, B, C, and E) would account for the signs and symptoms in this patient.

30. Correct answer is **F.** Following birth, the red blood cells that contain fetal hemoglobin (HbF) are rapidly replaced by red blood cells containing adult hemoglobin, HbA_1. The increased hemolysis associated with this change of hemoglobin type results in a temporary but a significant increase in serum bilirubin in neonates resulting in hyperbilirubinemia. The expression of the UDP-glucuronosyltransferase gene is activated at birth so there is always a lag in the rate of bilirubin conjugation and removal in neonates. In some infants the level of UDP-glucuronosyltransferase is insufficient to handle all the bilirubin and can result in potentially pathologic levels in the blood. A reduced level of none of the other enzymes (choices A, B, C, D, and E) would be associated with the temporary hyperbilirubinemia seen in this neonate.

31. Correct answer is **E.** The patient is most likely exhibiting classic signs associated with the unconjugated hyperbilirubinemia called Gilbert syndrome. Gilbert syndrome is the result of a mutation in the TATA-box of the UDP-glucuronosyltransferase 1A (*UGT1A*) gene. The specific mutation converts the normal $A(TA)_6TAA$ of the TATA-box of the *UGT1A* gene to $A(TA)_7TAA$. This change causes a reduced ability of the gene to be transcriptionally active, thus less mRNA is made but the resulting translated protein has normal enzymatic activity, albeit there is a reduced amount of this active enzyme. The loss of an enhancer binding factor (choice A) does not correspond to the position of the additional nucleotides identified in the UDP-glucuronosyltransferase gene. Each of the other options (choices B, C, and D) are related to coding region mutations which are not possible in this patient given that the additional nucleotides were identified upstream of the transcriptional start site of the UDP glucuronosyltransferase gene.

32. Correct answer is **A.** The child is most likely suffering from the effects of lead poisoning. Lead poisoning interferes with the function of several enzymes of heme metabolism including ALA synthase, ALA dehydratase, and ferrochelatase. The effect on ferrochelatase is much more pronounced than its effects on ALA synthase and ALA dehydratase. The inhibition of ferrochelatase results in the inability to insert Fe^{2+} into protoporphyrin IX, therefore, heme is not produced. In erythroid progenitor cells, the lack of heme activates the heme-regulated inhibitor (HRI) which phosphorylates the translation initiation factor, eIF-2 resulting in inhibition of protein synthesis. The consequences of inhibited protein synthesis are erythroid progenitor cells that are smaller than normal resulting in the microcytic anemia evident by the patient's MCV value. The lack of protein synthesis causes RNA and ribosomes to aggregate into small granules scattered throughout the cell giving the cell a stippled appearance, referred to as basophilic stippling. Bite cells (choice B) and Heinz bodies (choice C) are characteristic features of red blood cells in patients with glucose-6-phosphate dehydrogenase (G6PDH) deficiency. Red blood cells containing Heinz bodies interact with splenic macrophages which remove the membrane-localized Heinz bodies generating cells that histopathologically look like there has been a "bite" taken out of them. Bite cells are also known as degmacytes. Howell-Jolly bodies (choice D) are nuclear remnants found in peripheral blood smears from individuals with megaloblastic anemias due to vitamin B_{12} or folate deficiency or due to splenic dysfunction. Target cells (choice E), also termed codocytes, are abnormal red blood cells that look like the bullseye on a target, hence the nomenclature. Target cells are characteristic of thalassemia but are also observed in patients with hemoglobin C or following splenectomy.

33. Correct answer is **A.** The observations made of the patient's liver during the appendectomy, together with the serum bilirubin levels, indicate that the patient is most likely to have Dubin-Jonson syndrome (DJS). DJS is an autosomal recessive disorder that is a member of the conjugated hyperbilirubinemia family. DJS results from mutations in the gene (*ABCC2*) encoding the bile canalicular multispecific organic anion transporter. This transporter is involved in the excretion of not only conjugated bilirubin, but also many non-bile organic anions by an ATP-requiring process. characterized by mild, predominantly conjugated hyperbilirubinemia. Due to impaired transport of epinephrine metabolites to the bile canaliculi, melanin-like pigments accumulate in the liver such that there is a characteristic black appearance to the organ but with normal histology. Jaundice is usually the only physical symptom detected in this disease. Most patients remain asymptomatic, although some complain of weakness and abdominal pains. None of the other processes (choices B, C, D, E, and F) would account for the characteristic blackish surface of the liver seen in DJS patients. Deficiency in bilirubin-UDP-glucuronosyltransferase activity (choice C), associated with Crigler-Najjar syndromes, would be associated with symptoms in the early post-natal period and with greatly elevated levels of indirect (unconjugated) bilirubin. In the case of Gilbert syndrome, the level of bilirubin-UDP-glucuronosyltransferase activity is only partially reduced, and patients live with chronic mild elevation (usually less than 3 mg/dL) in indirect bilirubin levels.

34. Correct answer is **D.** The patient is most likely experiencing the symptoms of acute intermittent porphyria (AIP). AIP results from mutations in the porphobilinogen deaminase (PBG deaminase) gene. The clinical manifestations of AIP are related to the visceral, autonomic, peripheral, and central nervous system involvement of the disease. In fact, almost all the symptoms of AIP result from neurologic dysfunction. Certain factors such as hormonal or nutritional influences or drug interactions, such as occurs with alcohol consumption, can affect the clinical manifestation of AIP. The deficiency in PBG deaminase results in the progressive accumulation of heme biosynthesis intermediates, such as porphobilinogen, accumulates in the blood and urine. Although there is the possibility for a slight increase in the urinary level of δ-aminolevulinic acid (choice A) due to PBG deaminase deficiency, the normal activity of the enzymes prior to PBG deaminase means that the majority is converted to porphobilinogen. Bilirubin (choice B) will accumulate in numerous conditions but is not associated with the typical late-onset and drug-induced (ie, ethanol) symptoms of AIP. Lactate accumulation (choice C) is associated with symptoms of high anion gap metabolic acidosis and not the symptoms observed in this patient. Accumulation of uric acid (choice E) typically manifests with acute-onset gouty arthritis, not the symptoms observed in this patient.

35. Correct answer is **C.** The child is most likely suffering from the effects of lead poisoning. Lead poisoning interferes with the function of several enzymes of heme metabolism including ALA synthase, ALA dehydratase, and ferrochelatase. The effect on ferrochelatase is much more pronounced than its effects on ALA synthase and ALA dehydratase. The inhibition of ferrochelatase results in the inability to insert Fe^{2+} into protoporphyrin IX; therefore, heme is not produced. In erythroid progenitor cells the lack of heme activates the heme-regulated inhibitor (HRI) which phosphorylates the translation initiation factor, eIF-2 resulting in inhibition of protein synthesis. The consequences of inhibited protein synthesis are erythroid progenitor cells that are smaller than normal resulting in the microcytic anemia evident by the patient's MCV value. The lack of protein synthesis causes RNA and ribosomes to aggregate into small granules scattered throughout the cell giving the cell a stippled appearance, referred to as basophilic stippling, which is evidenced as dark blue granules with Wright-Giemsa staining. Although the activity of δ-aminolevulinic acid synthase (ALA synthase; choice A) is affected by lead, it is not as sensitive to this inhibition as is ferrochelatase, and the microcytic anemia typical of lead poisoning results from the inhibition of ferrochelatase. Inhibition of enzymes of heme metabolism (choices B and E) is not associated with microcytic anemia. Inhibition of glucose-6-phosphate dehydrogenase (choice D) causes hemolytic anemia with histopathology of blood smears showing Heinz bodies and bite cells (degmacytes). Deficiency in porphobilinogen deaminase (choice F) is the cause of acute intermittent porphyria (AIP), a disorder with characteristic neurovisceral symptoms but with normal red blood cells.

PART III CELLULAR AND MOLECULAR BIOLOGY

CHAPTER 22

DNA

High-Yield Terms

Phosphodiester bond Chemical bond between the 5′-phosphate of one base and the 3′-hydroxyl of an adjacent base in nucleic acids

Watson-Crick base-pair Refers to the normal hydrogen bonding that occurs where A bonds to T and G bonds to C; occurs in a DNA duplex, or an RNA-DNA duplex, or an RNA-RNA duplex

Nucleosome A structure formed by DNA and protein interaction that consists of an octamer protein structure composed of two subunits each of histones H2A, H2B, H3, and H4

Chromatin The combination of DNA and proteins that make up the contents of the nucleus of a cell

Heterochromatin Densely packed region of a chromosome often found near the centromeres, is generally transcriptionally silent

Euchromatin Loosely packed regions of a chromosome where active gene transcription can occur

Centromere Chromosomal structure separating the p and q arms of chromosomes; proteins of kinetochore nucleate at the centromere

Telomere A region of repetitive nucleotide sequences at each end of a chromatid

Cyclin Any of a number of proteins whose levels fluctuate during the eukaryotic cell cycle; these proteins regulate the activity of a family of kinases involved in controlling passage through the cell cycle

Proof-reading In the process of DNA replication this refers to the 3′ → 5′ exonuclease activity of DNA polymerase which allows it to remove an incorrectly incorporated nucleotide, recognized by non-Watson-Crick base-pairing

Epigenetics Defines the mechanism by which changes in the pattern of inherited gene expression occur in the absence of alterations or changes in the nucleotide composition of a given gene

Imprinting Parental-specific patterns of expression; control exerted by state of DNA methylation of the parental alleles

Trinucleotide repeats Are sequences of three nucleotides repeated in tandem on the same chromosome a number of times; abnormal expansion of the repeat is associated with the genesis of disease

DNA STRUCTURE

DNA exists as a helix of two complementary antiparallel polynucleotide strands, wound around each other in a rightward antiparallel direction and stabilized by hydrogen bonding (H-bonds) between the nucleotides in adjacent strands (Figure 22–1). The H-bonding between two complimentary nucleotide (A with T and G with C) constitutes what is referred to as **Watson-Crick base-pairing**. The nucleobases are in the interior of the helix aligned at a nearly 90-degree angle relative to the axis of the helix, while the phosphates of the phosphodiester bonds face the outer surface of the DNA helix. Given that purine bases form H-bonds with pyrimidines, in any given molecule of DNA the concentration of adenine (A) is equal to thymine (T) and the concentration of cytidine (C) is equal to guanine (G).

The antiparallel nature of the helix stems from the orientation of the individual strands. From any fixed position in the helix,

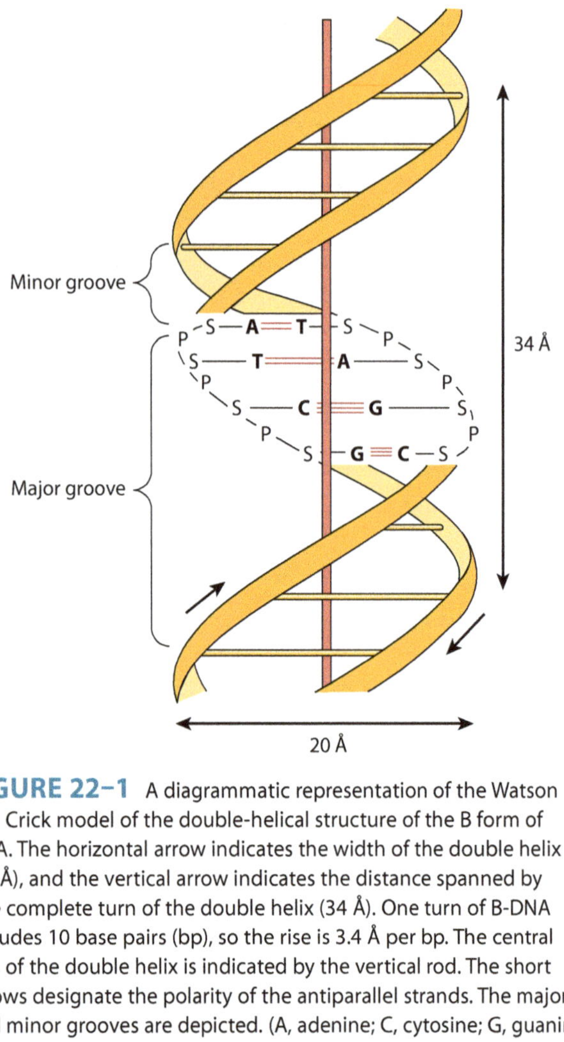

FIGURE 22–1 A diagrammatic representation of the Watson and Crick model of the double-helical structure of the B form of DNA. The horizontal arrow indicates the width of the double helix (20 Å), and the vertical arrow indicates the distance spanned by one complete turn of the double helix (34 Å). One turn of B-DNA includes 10 base pairs (bp), so the rise is 3.4 Å per bp. The central axis of the double helix is indicated by the vertical rod. The short arrows designate the polarity of the antiparallel strands. The major and minor grooves are depicted. (A, adenine; C, cytosine; G, guanine; P, phosphate; S, sugar [deoxyribose]; T, thymine.) Hydrogen bonds between A/T and G/C bases indicated by short, red, horizontal lines. (Reproduced with permission from Rodwell VW, Bender DA, Botham KM, et al: *Harper's Illustrated Biochemistry*, 31st ed. New York, NY: McGraw Hill; 2018.)

one strand is oriented in the 5′→3′ direction and the other in the 3′→5′ direction. On its exterior surface, the double helix of DNA contains two deep grooves termed the major and minor grooves (see Figure 22–1).

The double helix of DNA has been shown to exist in several different forms, depending on sequence content and ionic conditions of crystal preparation. The B-form of DNA prevails under physiologic conditions of low ionic strength and a high degree of hydration. Regions of the helix that are rich in CG dinucleotides can exist in a novel left-handed helical conformation termed Z-DNA. This conformation results from a 180-degree change in the orientation of the bases relative to that of the more common A- and B-DNA.

In order for the process of DNA replication to proceed, the two strands of the helix must first be separated, in a process termed denaturation. Because A-T base-pairs are formed from only two H-bonds and G-C base-pairs are formed from three H-bonds, regions of DNA that have predominantly A-T base-pairs will be less thermally stable than those rich in G-C base-pairs. When denatured DNA strands reform a stable duplex, the process is termed annealing or hybridization.

CHROMATIN STRUCTURE

Chromatin is a term designating the structure in which DNA exists within cells. The structure of chromatin is determined and stabilized through the interaction of the DNA with DNA-binding proteins. There are two classes of DNA-binding proteins, the histones and non-histone proteins. The histones are the major class of DNA-binding proteins involved in maintaining the compacted structure of chromatin. There are five different histone proteins identified as H1, H2A, H2B, H3, and H4.

The binding of DNA by the histones generates a structure called the nucleosome (Figure 22–2). The nucleosome core is composed of an octameric protein structure consisting of two subunits each of H2A, H2B, H3, and H4. Histone H1 occupies the inter-nucleosomal DNA and is identified as the linker histone.

The nucleosome cores themselves promote further compaction of chromatin such that in most compact state, as occurs during metaphase of the cell cycle there is the characteristic chromatin structure seen in a typical karyotype analysis (Figure 22–3).

In a broad consideration of chromatin structure there are two forms: **heterochromatin** and **euchromatin**. Heterochromatin is more densely packed than euchromatin and is often found near the centromeres of the chromosomes. Heterochromatin is generally transcriptionally silent. Euchromatin on the other hand is more loosely packed and is where active gene transcription can occur.

MODIFYING CHROMATIN STRUCTURE

Posttranslational modifications to histone proteins and postreplicative modifications to DNA represent the mechanisms by which the overall structure of chromatin is altered. Alterations in chromatin

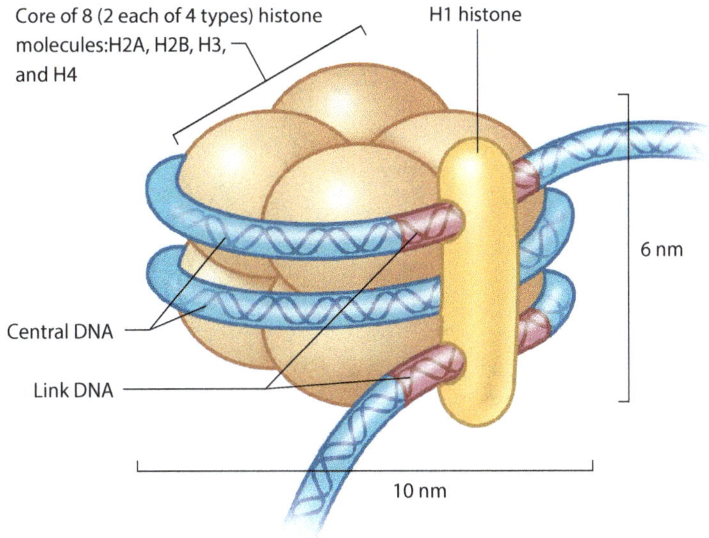

FIGURE 22–2 Components of a nucleosome. Nucleosome is a structure that produces the initial organization of free double-stranded DNA into chromatin. Each nucleosome has an octameric core complex made up of four types of histones, two copies each of H2A, H2B, H3, and H4. Around this core is wound DNA approximately 150 bp in length. One H1 histone is located outside the DNA on the surface of each nucleosome. DNA associated with nucleosomes in vivo thus resembles a long string of beads. Nucleosomes are very dynamic structures, with H1 loosening and DNA unwrapping at least once every second to allow other proteins, including transcription factors and enzymes, access to the DNA. (Reproduced with permission from Mescher AL. *Junqueira's Basic Histology Text and Atlas*, 16th ed. New York, NY: McGraw Hill; 2021.)

HIGH-YIELD CONCEPT

There are two primary mechanisms operating in a dynamic manner to alter the structure of chromatin. These mechanisms are methylation of cytidine residues in specific locations in the DNA and histone modification. Histone modifications are quite diverse and include, but are not limited to, acetylation, methylation, phosphorylation, ubiquitylation, O-GlcNAcylation, β-hydroxybutyrylation, lactylation, and dopaminylation.

structure allow for changes in the accessibility of DNA to the transcriptional machinery and thus, structural changes to chromatin represent major mechanism for regulation of gene expression.

Changes to chromatin structure can alter the phenotype of cells in the absence of changes to the coding capacity of the DNA. These types of gene expression changes are referred to as **epigenetic**. The classic definition of epigenetics states changes in phenotype are brought about by changes ON the DNA as opposed to changes BY the DNA.

One of the highest yield histone modifications is acetylation. This is because evidence has demonstrated a consistent correlation between activation of gene expression and histone acetylation. Histone acetylation results in a more open chromatin structure and these modified histones are found in regions of the chromatin that are transcriptionally active. Conversely, deacetylation of histones leads to a more compact less transcriptionally active chromatin structure. Transcriptional repressor complexes contain histone deacetylases (HDAC), while transcriptional activator complexes contain histone acetyltransferases (HAT).

EUKARYOTIC CELL CYCLES

The eukaryotic cell cycle refers to the ordered series of events that lead to duplication of DNA content and eventual separation into two identical progeny cells. In order to maintain the fidelity of the developing organism this process of cell division in multicellular organisms must be highly ordered and tightly regulated. The eukaryotic cell cycle is composed of four steps, or phases identified as G_1, S, G_2, and M (Table 22–1).

Not all cells continue to divide during the life span of an organism. The vast majority of the cells in the adult have undergone what is referred to as **terminal differentiation** and become quiescent and no longer divide. The cells reside in a cell cycle phase termed G_0.

CHECKPOINTS AND CELL CYCLE REGULATION

The processes that drive a cell through the cell cycle must be highly regulated so as to ensure that the resultant daughter cells are viable and each contains the complement of DNA found in the original parental cell. Many important genes involved in the regulation of cell cycle transit have been identified with some of the most important termed the cyclins and the cyclin-dependent kinases, CDK (Table 22–2). Different CDKs operate at different points in the cell cycle. The cyclical activity of each CDK is controlled by interactions with a specific cyclin partner. The cyclins are so-called because their levels cycle up and down as the cell progresses through the phases of the cell cycle.

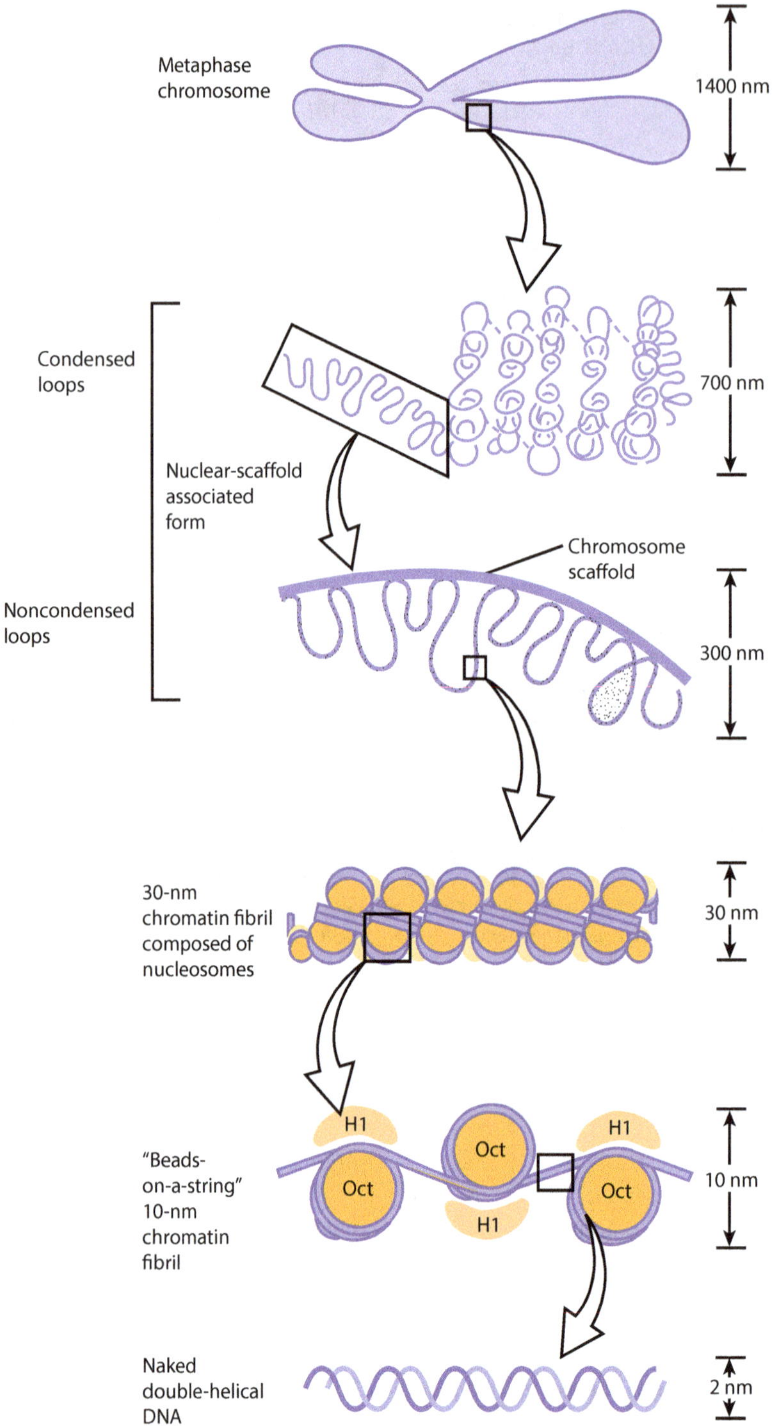

FIGURE 22–3 Levels of DNA packing in a typical metaphase chromosome (top) down to a naked duplex of DNA (bottom). The "beads-on-a-string" structure, formed as histones form nucleosomes and become wrapped by the DNA, is visible as such under electron microscopy. The DNA-protein complex within the cell is attached to a scaffold composed of highly specialized DNA-binding proteins that aid in the condensation of the chromosome to the metaphase stage. (Reproduced with permission from Rodwell VW, Bender DA, Botham KM, et al: *Harper's Illustrated Biochemistry*, 31st ed. New York, NY: McGraw Hill; 2018.)

TABLE 22–1 Overview of the cell cycle.

	Phase	Description
Interphase	G_0	Period of no cell replication/division, usually entered from G_1 restriction checkpoint. Cell cycle progression is halted by an inhibitory protein cyclin-dependent kinase inhibitor 2A that blocks the interaction of CDK4 with cyclin D. G_0 cells lose cell cycle proteins, including cyclins and CDKs.
	G_1	Period of high rate of cell growth/protein production in preparation for DNA synthesis. Entry into G_1 relies on the G_1 restriction checkpoint in which the binding of CDK4 to cyclin D leads to phosphorylation of the tumor suppressor retinoblastoma (Rb) protein. Phosphorylated Rb dissociates from the E2F transcription promoter, leading to the expression of cyclin E. Cyclin E activates CDK2, allowing progression into S-phase. These checks prepare the cell for DNA synthesis and cell cycle continuation.
	S	Synthesis phase during which DNA replication occurs. RNA transcription is very low except for that involved in histone production.
	G_2	Second period of cell growth between DNA synthesis and cell division (mitosis), mainly involving synthesis of microtubules for the mitotic spindle and chromosome condensation. The G_2 checkpoint prepares the cell for cell division and cell cycle continuation. This process is controlled by dephosphorylation of tyrosine residues in the maturation/mitosis-promoting factor complex, made of cyclin B (or A) and CDK1. CDK1 is activated, causing irreversible progression to mitosis. When the cell is unprepared for mitosis, Cdc25 can be inactivated by phosphorylation by a protein kinase.
Cell Division	M	No cell growth. Alignment of the replicated chromosomes and the tension created by the protein attachment of the mitotic spindle to the centromeres and the mitotic plate initiate mitosis. When the tension is sufficient, cyclin B is degraded, allowing activity of the anaphase-promoting complex (APC). Activated APC leads to degradation of the kinetichore structural protein securin, releasing its inhibition on separase, the protein that leads to the separation of the sister chromatids.

CDK, cyclin-dependent kinase; DNA, deoxyribonucleic acid.

Reproduced with permission from Janson LW, Tischler ME. *The Big Picture: Medical Biochemistry*. New York, NY: McGraw Hill; 2012.

In addition to control of CDK activity by cyclin binding, control is exerted to inhibit CDK activity through interaction with inhibitory proteins (Figure 22–4). Proteins that bind to and inhibit cyclin-CDK complexes are members of the cyclin-dependent kinase inhibitor (CDKN) family. Mammalian cells express two subclasses of CDKN proteins. These are commonly referred to as CIP for CDK inhibitory proteins and INK4 for inhibitors of kinase 4. The CIP bind and inhibit CDK1, CDK2, CDK4, and CDK6 complexes, whereas the INK4 bind and inhibit only the CDK4 and CDK6 complexes. There are at least three CIP proteins (p21, p27, and p57) and four INK proteins (p15, p16, p18, and p19) in mammalian cells.

TABLE 22–2 Cyclins and cyclin-dependent kinases involved in cell-cycle progression.

Cyclin	Kinase	Function
D	CDK4, CDK6	Progression past restriction point at G_1/S boundary
E, A	CDK2	Initiation of DNA synthesis in early S phase
B	CDK1	Transition from G_2 to M

Reproduced with permission from Rodwell VW, Bender DA, Botham KM, et al: *Harper's Illustrated Biochemistry*, 31st ed. New York, NY: McGraw Hill; 2018.

DNA REPLICATION

Replication of DNA occurs during S-phase of normal cell division cycles. The entire process of DNA replication is complex and involves multiple enzymatic activities (Table 22–3) with the actual replication being catalyzed by DNA polymerases.

Eukaryotic cells express several DNA polymerases that function in distinct types of DNA replication. For example, DNA polymerase α functions in with a complex of activities that are required for the synthesis of the mixed DNA-RNA primer required for DNA replication, and DNA polymerase δ also functions in a complex and is the major DNA replication enzyme.

The process of DNA replication begins at specific sites in the chromosomes termed origins of replication, requires a primer bearing a free 3′–OH, proceeds specifically in the 5′→3′ direction on both strands of DNA concurrently, and results in the copying of the template strands in a semiconservative manner. The semiconservative nature of DNA replication means that the newly synthesized daughter strands remain associated with their respective parental template strands. At each origin of replication the strands of DNA are dissociated and unwound in order to allow access to DNA polymerase. The site of the unwound template strands is termed the replication fork (Figure 22–5).

Synthesis of DNA proceeds in the 5′→3′ direction through the attachment of the 5′–phosphate of an incoming dNTP to the existing 3′–OH in the elongating DNA strands with the

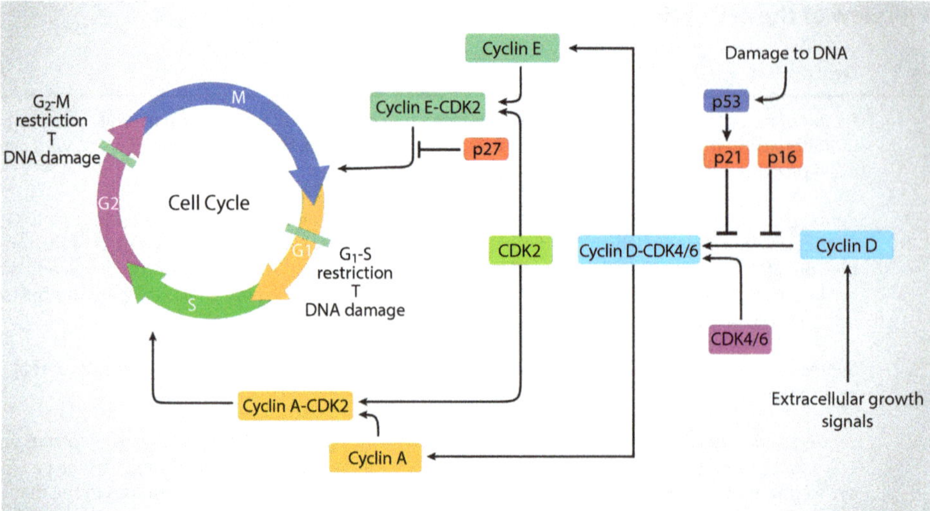

FIGURE 22–4 Overview of cell cycle control. Cells enter the cell cycle in response to various growth and mitogenic signals. These signals activate the modification of preexisting regulatory proteins and also induce the expression of genes encoding regulatory proteins. If a cell sustains DNA damage, cell cycle inhibitors can be activated to ensure that the cell does not enter S-phase until the damage has been repaired. (Reproduced with permission from themedicalbiochemistrypage, LLC.)

concomitant release of pyrophosphate. While incorporating dNTP into DNA in the 5′→3′ direction, DNA polymerases move in the 3′→5′ direction with respect to the template strand.

Synthesis proceeds bidirectionally, with one strand in each direction being copied continuously and one strand in each direction being copied discontinuously. The strand of DNA synthesized continuously is termed the **leading strand**, and the discontinuous strand is termed the **lagging strand**, commonly referred to **Okazaki fragments**. The gaps that exist between the 3′–OH of one leading strand and the 5′–phosphate of another as well as between one Okazaki fragment and another are repaired by DNA ligases, thereby completing the process of replication.

TABLE 22–3 Classes of proteins involved in replication.

Protein	Function
DNA polymerases	Deoxynucleotide polymerization
Helicases	Processive unwinding of DNA
Topoisomerases	Relieve torsional strain that results from helicase-induced unwinding
DNA primase	Initiates synthesis of RNA primers
Single-strand binding proteins	Prevent premature reannealing of dsDNA
DNA ligase	Seals the single-strand nick between the nascent chain and Okazaki fragments on lagging strand

Reproduced with permission from Rodwell VW, Bender DA, Botham KM, et al: *Harper's Illustrated Biochemistry*, 31st ed. New York, NY: McGraw Hill; 2018.

TOPOISOMERASES

The progression of the replication fork requires that the DNA ahead of the fork be continuously unwound. Due to the fact that eukaryotic chromosomal DNA is attached to a protein scaffold, the progressive movement of the replication fork introduces severe torsional stress into the duplex ahead of the fork. This torsional stress is relieved by DNA topoisomerases. Topoisomerases relieve torsional stresses in duplexes of DNA by introducing either double- (topoisomerases II) or single-stranded (topoisomerases I) breaks into the backbone of the DNA.

The clinical significance of topoisomerase activity is that it can be targeted pharmacologically in the treatment of cancers. The camptothecin class of drugs (eg, irinotecan) inhibit the activities of topoisomerase I, while the anthracycline class of drugs (eg, doxorubicin) inhibit the activities of topoisomerase II.

ADDITIONAL DNA POLYMERASE ACTIVITIES

The main enzymatic activity of DNA polymerases is the 5′→3′ synthetic activity. However, DNA polymerases possess two additional activities of importance for both replication and repair. These additional activities include a 5′→3′ exonuclease function and a 3′→5′ exonuclease function. The 3′→5′ exonuclease function is utilized during replication to allow DNA polymerase to remove mismatched bases, a process referred to as "**proof-reading**."

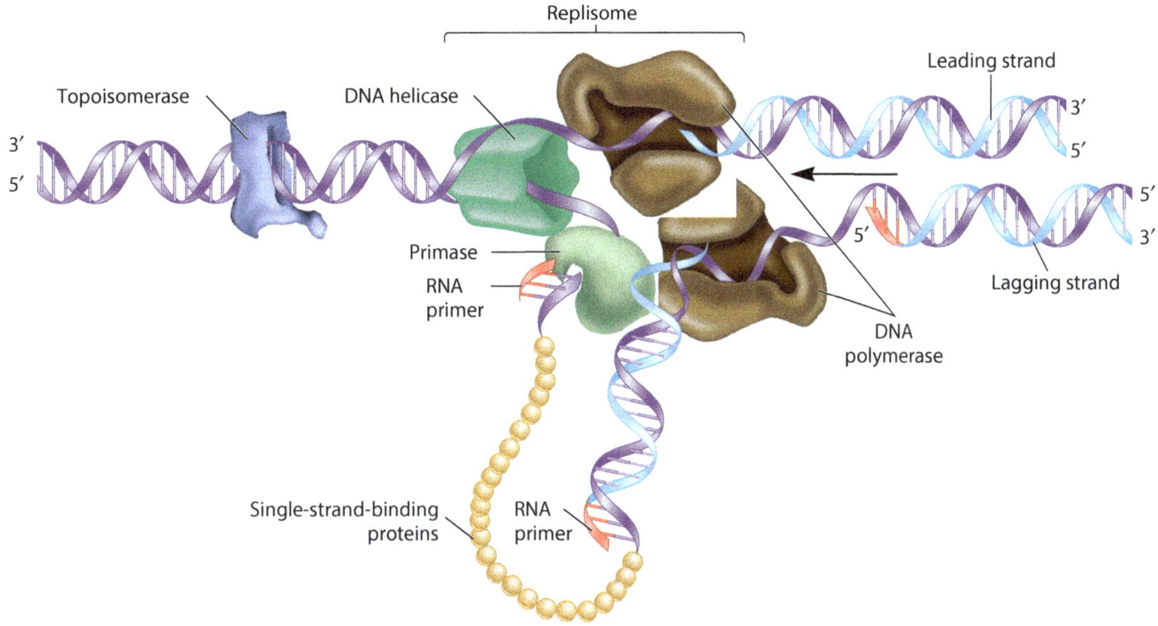

FIGURE 22–5 During DNA replication, the helicase and primase form a primasome, which associates with two molecules DNA polymerase. One of these synthesizes a new strand continuously on the leading strand, but the other synthesizes new fragments in discontinuous bursts on the lagging strand. The primasome plus the two polymerases make up the replisome. (Adapted with permission from Brooker RJ: *Genetics: Analysis & Principles*, 7th ed. New York, NY: McGraw Hill, 2021.)

TELOMERE REPLICATION

Telomeres are the specialized DNA structures at the ends of all chromosomes. Telomeres consist of repetitive DNA sequences and nucleoproteins. The DNA repeat of human telomeres is 5′–TTAGGG–3′. The telomeric repeat sequence spans up to several kilobases and is involved in protecting the ends of the chromosomes from exonuclease activity.

The telomeric ends of the lagging strand of each chromosome require a unique method of replication which involves the activity of the enzyme complex called **telomerase**. Telomerase is a complex composed of several proteins, an RNA with sequence complimentary to the telomeric repeats, and a reverse transcriptase activity that extends the 3′-end of the lagging strands using the telomerase RNA as the template (Figure 22–6). The reverse transcriptase activity of telomerase is encoded by the TERT gene (**te**lomerase **r**everse **t**ranscriptase), and the RNA component is encoded by the TERC gene (**te**lomerase **R**NA **c**omponent).

TRINUCLEOTIDE REPEAT DISORDERS

The trinucleotide repeat disorders (also known as trinucleotide repeat expansion disorders or triplet repeat expansion disorders) are a family of unrelated genetic disorders caused by an increase in

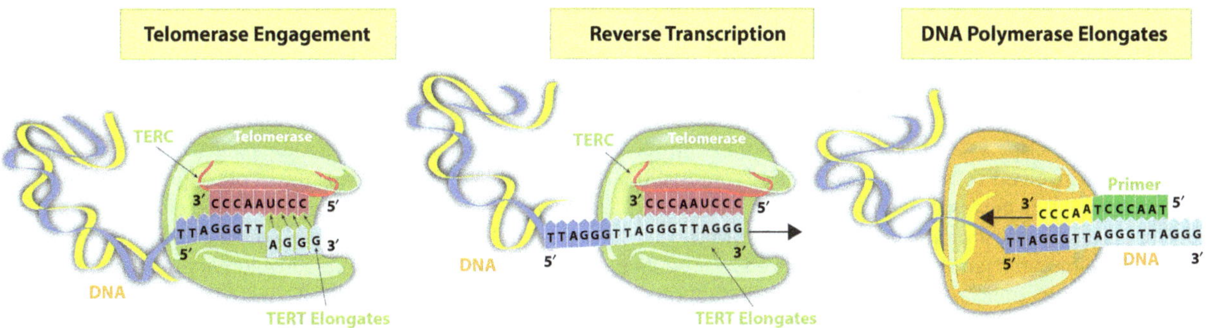

FIGURE 22–6 Steps in telomere replication by telomerase. The repeat element of the telomere is recognized by the RNA encoded by the *TERC* gene providing a free 3′-OH for use by the reverse transcriptase encoded by the *TERT* gene. Following reverse transcription and telomere extension, a primer for DNA replication can be introduced by the primase complex allowing for partial to complete replication of the 3′-end of each telomere. (Reproduced with permission from themedicalbiochemistrypage, LLC.)

the number of trinucleotide repeats, in certain genes, that exceeds the normal, stable, threshold. Each gene affected by trinucleotide repeat expansion has a different number of repeats that constitutes the normal threshold and the number that results in manifestation of disease.

The trinucleotide repeat disorders are divided into three categories determined by the type of repeat. When the repeat is the triplet CAG and is in the coding region of the gene the disorders are referred to as the polyglutamine (polyQ) disorders. The best-known disorder of this type is Huntington disease (Clinical Box 22–1). The second category of disorders either do not involve the CAG triplet, or the CAG triplet is not in the coding region of the gene and therefore, these disorders are referred to as the non-polyglutamine disorders. Myotonic dystrophy type 1 (Clinical Box 22–2) and Fragile X syndrome (Clinical Box 22–3) are well known forms of the non-polyglutamine expansion disorders. The third category of trinucleotide repeat expansion disorder consists of the diseases associated with expansion of a polyalanine tract (PA) or alterations in genes harboring a polyalanine tract.

Although trinucleotide repeat expansion encompasses the vast majority of repeat expansion diseases, there are other diseases caused by repeat expansion where the repeat size is four (tetranucleotide), five (pentanucleotide), or 10 (dodecanucleotide) nucleotides in length. A second genetic cause of myotonic dystrophy, identified as myotonic dystrophy type 2 (also identified as dystrophia myotonica 2, Ricker syndrome, or proximal myotonic myopathy) results from the expansion of the tetranucleotide, CCTG. The CCTG repeat resides in the first intron of the zinc finger protein 9 (*ZNF9*) gene.

CLINICAL BOX 22–1 HUNTINGTON DISEASE

Huntington disease (HD) is inherited as an autosomal dominant, late-onset disorder characterized by slowly progressive neurodegeneration associated with choreic movements (abnormal involuntary movements) and dementia. The disease is named after George Huntington who provided the classical account of the disease in 1872. The pathology of HD reveals neurodegeneration in the corpus striatum and shrinkage of the brain. HD is caused by expansion of a CAG trinucleotide repeat in the first exon of the huntingtin gene (*HTT*). In the normal non-triplet expanded state, the *HTT* gene encodes a protein of approximately 3145 amino acids. Due to individual differences in the number of Gln (Q) residues in the N-terminus of the huntingtin protein, the total number of amino acids in unaffected individuals ranges between 3144 and 3172. The CAG repeat resides 17 codons downstream of the initiator AUG codon. The range of CAG repeat size in normal individuals is 6–34 and in affected individuals it is 36–121. The longer the length of the CAG repeat the earlier is the onset of symptoms. However, there is a wide degree of variation in age of onset for any given length of CAG repeat. Thus, the CAG repeat number itself is not predictive for age of onset. The variation in age of onset is related to the effects of other modifying genes, the environment, and the length of the CAG repeat. In addition, HD exhibits a genetic phenomenon termed "anticipation" which means that the symptoms of the disease appear earlier and are more severe in subsequent generations. Anticipation was first identified in families with myotonic dystrophy, type 1 (see Clinical Box 22–2). With HD the phenomenon of anticipation is explained by meiotic instability which increases the CAG repeat number and is greater in spermatogenesis than in oogenesis. Therefore, anticipation is mainly observed when the mutation is inherited through the paternal line. The huntingtin protein is unrelated to any other protein. The polyglutamine tract begins at codon 18 and is followed by a stretch of 29 consecutive proline residues. Wild-type huntingtin protein is found primarily in the cytoplasm with a small percentage being intranuclear. The protein is also found associated with the plasma membrane, the endoplasmic reticulum (ER), the Golgi apparatus, endocytic vesicles, the mitochondria, and microtubules. In addition to the polyglutamine and polyproline motifs, huntingtin contains 28–36 repeats, termed HEAT motifs, dispersed throughout the length of the protein. The HEAT motif is approximately 50 amino acids in length and is composed of two anti-parallel α-helices that form a hairpin structure. HEAT motifs are involved in protein-protein interactions and serve roles in intracellular transport, chromosome segregation, and microtubule dynamics. Huntingtin is also fatty acid modified at cysteine 214 (C214) with palmitic acid. The acylation is catalyzed by Hip14 (huntingtin interacting protein 14). This modification regulates huntingtin function and trafficking. The significance of the palmitoylation is demonstrated by the fact that huntingtin protein with an expanded polyglutamine tract is a much poorer substrate for Hip14 than is wild-type protein. Huntingtin is essential for early embryonic development as evidenced by lethality in embryonic mice lacking functional protein. The protein is known to be important in adult neurons and testes for cellular viability. If the level of the protein is reduced, it leads to developmental defects and disruptions in iron homeostasis. Huntingtin also has a role in regulation of transcription through its interaction with numerous transcription factors and other proteins involved in the regulation of mRNA production. The classical symptoms of HD consist of progressive dementia, evolving involuntary movements and psychiatric disturbances that include personality changes and mood disorder. Choreiform movements are the most prominent physical abnormality in HD and as such the disease was early on referred to as Huntington chorea. Choreiform movements are characterized by repetitive, brief, irregular, somewhat rapid involuntary movements typically in the face, mouth, trunk, and limbs. The earliest indication of HD is the appearance of spasmodic twitching of the extremities, generally beginning with the fingers. Additional early physical manifestations of HD are clumsiness, hyperreflexia, and eye movement disturbances. Positron-emission tomography (PET scanning) is used to demonstrate a loss of uptake of glucose in the caudate nuclei and is a valuable indication of affectation in the presymptomatic period in HD patients. There is no cure for HD and all afflicted individuals will succumb to the disease. The age of death in HD is related to the age of onset, that is, the earlier the onset, the earlier an individual will die.

CLINICAL BOX 22–2 MYOTONIC DYSTROPHY TYPE 1

Type 1 myotonic dystrophy (originally abbreviated DM1 for the Latin *dystrophia myotonica*) is the most commonly occurring form of muscular dystrophy in adults. The disease manifests in nearly 1 in 8000 individuals. DM1 is an autosomal dominant disorder resulting from the expansion of a CTG trinucleotide repeat in the dystrophia myotonica protein kinase gene (also called myotonin-protein kinase). The CTG repeat (CUG in the mRNA) resides in the 3′-untranslated region of the mRNA. Normal individuals have 5–37 repeats and affected individuals have repeats ranging from 50 to several thousand. Like many trinucleotide repeat disorders DM1 exhibits the genetic phenomena of anticipation which refers to the appearance of symptoms earlier and with more severity in subsequent generations. Of note is that myotonic dystrophy is the first disorder in which anticipation was demonstrated as the clinical basis of the course of the disease. The dystrophia myotonica protein kinase gene (*DMPK*, also identified as Mt-PK) encodes a protein (isoform 1) of 639 amino acids in length and contains an N-terminal domain that shares strong homology to the cAMP-dependent serine-threonine protein kinase family. The DMPK protein is predominantly localized at sites of neuromuscular and myotendinous junctions of skeletal muscles. In patients with DM1 the levels of detectable DMPK in skeletal and cardiac muscle are much lower than in unaffected individuals. The mechanism of disease development in DM1, as a consequence of expansion of the CTG triplet in the *DMPK* gene, is related to disruption in mRNA metabolism. The expansion of the CUG repeat in DMPK RNA leads to abnormal regulation of alternative splicing events. The negative effect on RNA splicing occurs in *trans*. The mutant DMPK RNA is normally spliced but the presence of the expansion alters the splicing of other mRNAs. These aberrant splicing effects have been identified in at least 13 different mRNAs from three different tissues. Several of the mRNAs found to be affected by the altered RNA processing events correlate well with the symptoms seen in DM1. These include the insulin receptor (resulting in insulin resistance and diabetes), cardiac troponin T (leading to cardiac abnormalities), voltage-gated chloride channel 1 (CLCN1, resulting in myotonia), as well as RYR1 (ryanodine receptor 1), MTMR1 (myotubularin-related protein 1; is a member of the Tyr/dual-specificity phosphatase superfamily) and ATP2A1 (ATPase, Ca^{2+} transporting, cardiac muscle, fast twitch; also called SERCA1) leading to muscle wasting. As the name of the disorder implies the characteristic clinical manifestation in DM1 is myotonia (muscle hyperexcitability) and muscle degeneration. Affected individuals will also develop insulin resistance, cataracts, heart conduction defects, testicular atrophy, hypogammaglobulinemia, and sleep disorders. Symptoms of myotonic dystrophy can manifest in the adult or in childhood. The childhood onset form of the disease is often associated with intellectual impairment. In addition, there is a form of the disease referred to as congenital myotonic dystrophy. This latter form of the disease is frequently fatal and is seen almost exclusively in children born of mothers who themselves are mildly affected by the disease. In congenital DM1 the facial manifestations are distinctive due to bilateral facial palsy and marked jaw weakness. Many infants with congenital myotonic dystrophy die due to respiratory insufficiency before a proper diagnosis of the disease is made. Manifestation of DM1 initially involves the distal muscles of the extremities and only as the disease progresses do proximal muscles become affected. In addition, muscles of the head and neck are affected early in the course of the disease. Weakness in eyelid closure, limited extraocular movement, and ptosis result from involvement of the extraocular muscles. Many individuals with DM1 exhibit a characteristic "haggard" appearance that is the result of atrophy of the masseters (large muscles that raise and lower the jaw), sternocleidomastoids (large, thick muscles that pass obliquely across each side of the neck and contribute to arm movement), and the temporalis muscle (muscle involved in chewing).

CLINICAL BOX 22–3 FRAGILE X SYNDROME

Fragile X syndrome is an X-linked dominant disorder representing the most common form of inherited intellectual impairment. Fragile X syndrome occurs with a frequency of approximately 1 in 4000 males and 1 in 8000 females. Affected males will exhibit moderate to severe intellectual impairment as well as a speech delay, hyperactivity, and behavioral and social difficulties. The fragile X syndrome gene (*FRAXA*; also referred to as *FMR1*) belongs to the class of folate-sensitive rare fragile sites. Fragile X syndrome results from the expansion of a CGG trinucleotide repeat in the *FRAXA* gene which encodes the FMRP protein. The CGG repeat resides in the 5′-untranslated region (UTR) of the *FRAXA* gene. Normal individuals have 6–53 CGG repeats and the premutation size is between 55 and 230 repeats. A full mutation in affected individuals is more than 200 repeats. Males with the premutation sized expansion develop a late-onset neurodegenerative condition termed fragile X-associated tremor/ataxia syndrome (FXTAS). In females with the premutation expansion there is a 25% chance of their developing ovarian failure. The molecular consequences of the amplification of the CGG repeat are the presentation of CpG dinucleotide sites that can be methylated on the cytidine. Indeed, the repeat expansion in the *FRAXA* gene leads to epigenetic transcriptional silencing due to hypermethylation of the promoter region of the gene. The *FRAXA* gene is located on the X chromosome at Xq27.3. The FMRP protein is an RNA-binding protein found in ribonucleoprotein complexes. Early during human fetal development the *FRAXA* gene is expressed at highest levels in cholinergic neurons of the nucleus basalis magnocellularis and in pyramidal neurons of the hippocampus which may contribute to the pathogenesis of fragile X syndrome. The *FRAXA* gene is also expressed in the mature testes at high levels in spermatogonia. FMRP has been shown to bind to approximately 4% of fetal human brain mRNAs. In addition, FMRP can bind

CLINICAL BOX 23–3 (CONTINUED)

to its own mRNA. Mutations in the RNA-binding domains of FMRP have been associated with fragile X syndrome. One important pathway involving the activity of FMRP is the metabotropic glutamate receptor-(mGluR) dependent long-term depression (LTD) pathway. Stimulation of the mGluR pathway leads to increased translation of FMRP, which subsequently suppresses the translation of other proteins at the synapse. The characteristic symptoms of fragile X syndrome in males is moderate to severe intellectual impairment. In males with the full mutation (ie, >200 CGG repeats) the physical hallmarks of the disorder include a long narrow face, prominent ears, and macroorchidism (large testicles). These physical signs are most apparent in postpubertal males. Additional physical findings can include hyperextensible finger joints, flat feet, double jointed thumbs, and a high arched plate. Fragile X syndrome also manifests with distinct behavioral abnormalities that include hyperactivity, anxiety, extreme sensitivity to stimulation and sensations, hyperarousal, and occasionally aggressive tendencies. The behavioral anomalies overlap with those of autism such as impaired verbal and nonverbal communication, difficulty with social interactions, poor eye contact, tactile defensiveness, hand flapping, and hand biting. Females with a full mutation are less affected with respect to all aspects of the mental and physical characteristics of fragile X syndrome. This is, of course, due to the process of X chromosome inactivation.

DNA METHYLATION

One of the major postreplicative reactions that modifies the DNA is methylation. However, not all DNA methylation is dependent on, nor occurs in relationship to replication. Regardless, the sites of natural methylation (ie, not chemically induced) of eukaryotic DNA are almost always on cytidine residues and these cytidines are almost always present in CpG (also written CG) dinucleotides. The cytidine is methylated at the 5 position of the pyrimidine ring generating 5-methylcytidine (5mC). Not all cytidines present in CpG dinucleotides are methylated at the C residue. However, in the human genome it has been shown that 60–80% of all the CpG dinucleotides present in the genome contain 5mC. Methylation of cytidines in CA dinucleotides has also been demonstrated with these methylation sites being most abundant in postmitotic neurons.

Methylation of cytidine residues alters the structure of chromatin such that when regions of a gene that can be methylated are, the associated gene is transcriptionally silent, and when the region is under-methylated the gene is transcriptionally active or can be activated. Methylated cytidine residues are recognized by specific proteins. Clinical significance of proteins that interact with 5mC residues in DNA can be seen in the disorder called Rett syndrome (Clinical Box 22–4)

The methylation of DNA is catalyzed by several different DNA methyltransferases (abbreviated Dnmt). When cells divide, the DNA contains one strand of parental DNA and one strand of the newly replicated DNA. If the parental DNA contains 5mC the daughter strand must undergo methylation in order to maintain the parental pattern of methylation. This "maintenance" methylation is catalyzed by Dnmt1 and thus, this enzyme is called the maintenance methylase (Figure 22–7).

CLINICAL BOX 22–4 RETT SYNDROME

Rett syndrome is a monogenic X-linked dominant disorder that occurs with a frequency of 1 in 10,000 live births. This disorder was first described by Andreas Rett, an Austrian pediatric neurologist. Rett syndrome is one of the most common causes of complex disability in females. Rett syndrome is characterized by early neurologic regression that severely affects motor, cognitive, and communication skills, by autonomic dysfunction and often a seizure disorder, microcephaly, and arrested development. Characteristic of Rett syndrome is a delay in acquiring new skills, absence of speech, emergence of autistic features, loss of purposeful manipulation skills along with other motor abnormalities that include abnormal muscle tone, ataxia, and apraxia. Rett syndrome results from mutations in the *MECP2* gene encoding methyl-CpG-binding protein MeCP2. The MeCP2 protein binds to 5mC found in the trinucleotide sequence, 5mCAC. Mutations in the *MECP2* gene arise predominantly in the sperm. The vast majority of mutations in the *MECP2* gene that lead to Rett syndrome are new somatic mutations and not inherited. Although hundreds of different mutations have been identified in the *MECP2* gene in Rett syndrome patients, eight hotspots for mutation have been identified in 60% of patients. Rett syndrome patients that harbor mutations in the *MECP2* gene are heterozygous, containing only one mutant gene. The reason that mutations in the X-linked *MECP2* gene manifest with disease almost exclusively in females is that these mutations are lethal to male fetuses. In live born males with MECP2 mutations there will be severe congenital encephalopathy and death within 2 years. The MeCP2 protein is ubiquitously present but is most abundantly expressed in the brain. The primary function of MeCP2 is as a transcriptional repressor through its interactions with members of the histone deacetylase family. Loss of function of MeCP2 in differentiated postmitotic neurons is likely to result in the inappropriate overexpression of MeCP2 target genes, with potentially damaging effects during central nervous system maturation.

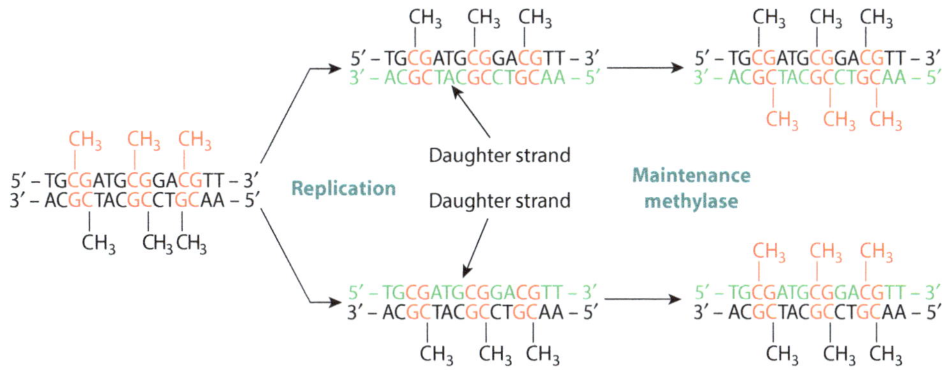

FIGURE 22–7 Process of DNA methylation following DNA replication. Sites of DNA methylation have two fates following the process of DNA replication: they can be maintained or they can be progressively removed. Following replication the parental (template) strands of DNA contain 5mCpG, whereas the reciprocal C residue in the daughter strand is not methylated. If the methylation state of the gene is to be maintained then the maintenance methylase, Dnmt1, incorporates a methyl group into the C residue of the daughter strand CpG dinucleotide. (Reproduced with permission from themedicalbiochemistrypage, LLC.)

DNA METHYLATION AND IMPRINTING

The phenomenon of genomic imprinting refers to the fact that the expression of some genes depends on whether or not they are inherited maternally or paternally. The allele-specific expression of imprinted genes is regulated by epigenetic modifications of which DNA methylation is the controlling modification. Thus, these imprinted alleles are "marked" by their state of methylation. The methylated CpG-rich regions of imprinted loci contain the methylation state on only one of the two parental chromosomes. For this reason, these imprinted domains are referred to as differentially methylated regions, DMR. Several hundred different imprinted loci have been identified in the human genome. Incorrect inheritance of, or mutations/deletions in, imprinted loci is associated with pathology. The highest yield imprinted disorders are Prader-Willi syndrome(Clinical Box 22–5) and Angelman syndrome (Clinical Box 22–6).

CLINICAL BOX 22–5 PRADER-WILLI SYNDROME

Prader-Willi syndrome (PWS) was first described in 1887 by John Langdon Down who also identified Down syndrome. The full spectrum of PWS was reported in 1956 by Andrea Prader, Alexis Labhart, and Heinrich Willi, hence the current name of the disorder. Prader-Willi syndrome and Angelman syndrome (AS; Clinical Box 22–6) were the first diseases associated with the process of genomic imprinting. Although the symptoms of these two disorders are quite different it was shown in 1989 that both are caused by alterations in the pattern of genomic imprinting in the same region of chromosome 15. However, the distinct clinical spectrum of PWS and AS results as a consequence of the parental origin of the chromosome 15 alteration. Chromosomal region 15q11.2-q13 contains a cluster of imprinted genes with relevance to these two distinct neurogenetic disorders. PWS results from the loss of a group of paternal-specific expressed genes in the chromosome 15q11.2-q13 region. Analysis of the region of chromosome 15q11.2-q13 has identified several imprinted and nonimprinted genes as well as the AS imprinting control (AS-IC) region and the Prader-Willi imprinting control (PW-IC) region. There are 16 characterized genes in this region of chromosome 15 and a complex locus identified as small nucleolar RNA host gene 14 (*SNHG14*). Of these 16 genes, 10 are expressed from both the paternal and maternal chromosomes. Causes of PWS have been shown to be the result of three primary mechanisms. The most common cause (65–75% of cases) of PWS is deletion of a 5–7 Mb region from the paternal chromosome 15q11.2-q13 domain. The deletions are the result of nonhomologous recombination events that are mediated by repetitive sequence elements that define a series of breakpoint cluster regions on either side of the imprinted chromosome 15q11.2-q13 domain. In 20–30% of PWS patients the disorder is the result of maternal uniparental disomy (UPD; see Chapter 35). A small percentage (1–3%) of PWS patients are the result of defects in the Prader-Willi imprinting control region (PW-IC) that controls the imprinting process. PWS is characterized by a failure to thrive in the neonatal period accompanied by muscular hypotonia. During early childhood PWS patients exhibit hyperphagia (excessive hunger and abnormally large intake of solid foods), obesity, hypogonadism, sleep apnea, behavior problems, and mild to moderate intellectual impairment. Hypogonadism is present in both males and females. The characteristics of the hypogonadism are genital hypoplasia, incomplete pubertal development, and, in most patients there is infertility. A distinctive behavioral phenotype of PWS is temper tantrums, stubbornness, and manipulative and compulsive behaviors. Additionally, PWS children have small hands and feet. In prepubertal males the hypogonadism results in sparse body hair, poor development of skeletal muscles, and delay in epiphyseal closure resulting in long arms and legs. Short stature is common in PWS patients as a result of insufficiency in growth hormone (GH) production and secretion. PWS patients often present with characteristic facial features, strabismus, and scoliosis. The tendency to obesity is highly correlated to the development of type 2 diabetes in PWS patients.

CLINICAL BOX 22–6 ANGELMAN SYNDROME

Angelman syndrome (AS) is named after the English physician Harry Angelman who first described the disorder in 1965. He observed three children with a similar constellation of symptoms and he referred to these symptoms as the "happy puppet syndrome" because of their smiling and laughing demeanor and jerky gait. The disease is now known to occur with a frequency of 1 in 15,000–20,000 persons worldwide. Angelman syndrome results from loss of neuron-specific maternal expression of a ubiquitin ligase gene (*UBE3A*) in the imprinted locus of chromosome 15q11.2-q13. As indicated in Clinical Box 22–5, there are 16 genes in the imprinted locus of which 10 are expressed from both the paternal and maternal chromosomes. All but the *UBE3A* gene are hypermethylated on the maternal chromosome and as a result are only expressed from the paternal chromosome. The parent-of-origin specific expression in the *UBE3A* gene is not the result of differential DNA methylation of the gene but through the imprinted expression of a complex locus in the imprinted region of chromosome 15 identified as small nucleolar RNA host gene 14 (SNHG14). The SNHG14 locus contains 148 exons and undergoes complex alternative splicing. In addition to the transcriptional complexity of the *SNHG14* gene, the introns of the SNHG14 locus encode several small nucleolar RNAs (snoRNAs). The promoter region controlling expression of both the SNRPN and the SNHG14 locus is methylated on the maternal chromosome and therefore not expressed. Of particular significance to the clinical manifestation of AS is the fact that imprinted UBE3A expression is restricted to neurons in the brain. At least four known genetic mechanisms can result in AS. The vast majority of cases (~75%) result from *de novo* maternal deletion of 5–7 Mb of the chromosome 15q11.2–q13 region. The deletions are the result of nonhomologous recombination events that are mediated by repetitive sequence elements that define a series of breakpoint cluster regions on either side of the imprinted domain. Approximately 2% of AS cases involve paternal uniparental disomy (UPD; see Chapter 35). Genomic imprinting defects lead to an additional 2–3% of AS cases. The imprinting defect can be caused by genetic or epigenetic factors that lead to gene expression throughout the imprinted domain. AS patients in this classification exhibit inheritance of chromosome 15 from both parents but in the maternal copy the normal methylation state of the SNRPN promoter region is absent resulting in expression of the complex SNHG14 locus which in turn suppresses the expression of the *UBE3A* gene. The remaining, approximately 25% of AS patients, will harbor mutations in the *UBE3A* gene. The majority of UBE3A mutations found in AS patients are nonsense mutations. To date 73 different pathogenic variants affecting the maternal allele of UBE3A have been characterized. The characteristic clinical spectrum of Angelman syndrome include microcephaly, seizure disorder, ataxia, muscular hypotonia with hyperreflexia, and motor delay. The psychomotor delay in AS patients is evident by 6 months of age and is associated with hypotonia and feeding difficulties. The microcephaly is not apparent at birth but develops within the first 3 years. The seizure disorder associated with AS typically develops between the first and third years of life. When AS patients are examined with an MRI of the brain it will show delayed myelination but with no structural abnormalities or gross pathology. Limb movement tremors, typical of AS patients, usually begin in infancy and will progress to ataxia in the trunk. The tremors result in AS infants exhibiting difficulty with crawling. Most children with AS will not begin walking until they are 3–4 years of age and they will have a distinctive marionette-like jerky aspect to their walking. Individuals with AS can develop sufficiently enough to be able to establish intentional relationships such as with their parents and siblings although they generally do not develop expressive speech. Angelman syndrome children are active explorers such that a common description is that they are in constant motion and into everything. The constant motion, laughter, and tremulous movements characterize the distinctive behavioral phenotype of AS children. The clinical problems associated with AS persist into adulthood. The seizure disorder will diminish in frequency and intensity over time but will not disappear altogether. Physical activity will diminish as AS patients age accompanied by increases in muscle rigidity and/or quivering movements. The life span of AS patients can be quite long as there are individuals with this disorder who are in their 60s and 70s. Early mortality associated with AS can be related to the severity of the seizure disorder as well as to accidental injury due to their hyperactivity coupled with diminished cognitive skills.

X CHROMOSOME INACTIVATION

The fact that mammalian females harbor two copies of the X chromosome has led to the potential for differences in X-linked gene dosage between females and males. These potential gene dosage differences are compensated for through the process of X chromosome inactivation (XCI), a process first characterized in 1961 by Mary Lyon. As a result of her discovery, the process of XCI is often referred to as lyonization.

The process of XCI takes place very early in development and ensures equivalent X chromosome gene expression levels throughout development in both males and females. In eutherian mammals, such as humans, the process of XCI is random such that in human females roughly half of the cells in her body have inactivated the paternal X chromosome (Xp) and the other half have inactivated the maternal X chromosome (Xm). This results in all human females being mosaic for all cell populations within the same tissues where either the Xp or the Xm chromosome is inactive. Once a human X chromosome is inactivated, it remains inactive in all the progeny cells throughout life.

Although one of the two X chromosomes in females is randomly inactivated, not all of the genes on the inactive X chromosome (Xi) are in fact transcriptionally silent. Several of the genes that remain active are found in the pseudo-autosomal region, PAR. The X chromosome PAR is a region of the X chromosome that is homologous to a region in the Y chromosome and is responsible for the X and Y chromosomes pairing up during meiosis. In addition to the genes in the PAR, several other genes on the Xi remain transcriptionally active. These latter genes are referred to as escape genes and approximately 15–20% of human X-linked genes completely escape inactivation while another 10% partially escape inactivation.

XCI requires a family of long noncoding RNAs (lncRNA) with the central regulatory lncRNA being encoded by the *XIST* gene (X-inactive specific transcript). The *XIST* gene resides in a region on the X chromosome called the X inactivation center (XIC). Expression of the *XIST* gene is exclusive to the future inactive X chromosome (Xi) and the encoded XIST lncRNA coats the X chromosome.

Within the context of the process of XCI, the state of CpG methylation can be highly correlated to gene expression levels. The level of CpG methylation in the promoter regions of most of the genes on the X chromosome is higher on the Xi when compared to the same genes on the Xa. However, in the promoter regions of genes in the PAR and of escape genes, the CpG methylation state is lower overall than the level of methylation of XCI-associated silenced genes. Although CpG methylation can be highly correlated to transcriptional silencing associated with XCI, overall chromatin structure also plays an important role in the transcriptional silencing as well as in the escape of certain genes from XCI.

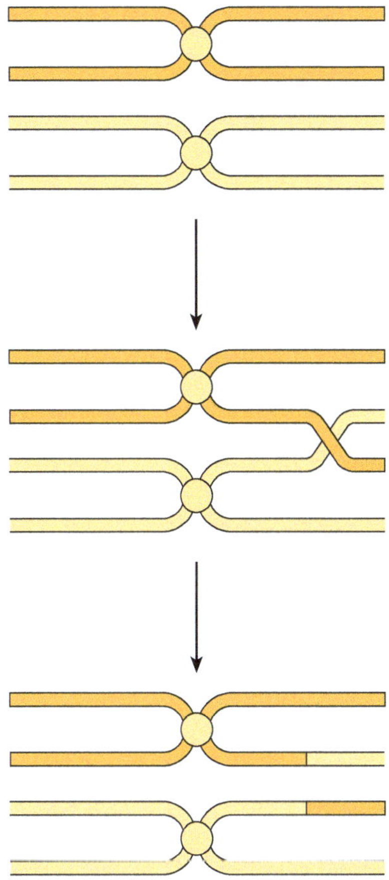

FIGURE 22–8 The process of crossing over between homologous metaphase chromosomes to generate recombinant chromosomes. (Reproduced with permission from Rodwell VW, Bender DA, Botham KM, et al: *Harper's Illustrated Biochemistry*, 31st ed. New York, NY: McGraw Hill; 2018.)

DNA RECOMBINATION

DNA recombination refers to the phenomenon whereby two parental strands of DNA are spliced together resulting in an exchange of portions of their respective strands. This process leads to new molecules of DNA that contain a mix of genetic information from each parental strand.

Homologous recombination is the most common type of DNA recombination occurring in eukaryotic cells (Figure 22–8). Homologous recombination is a critical component of mechanisms that repair damaged DNA. Another critical role for homologous recombination occurs during gametogenesis. During prophase of meiosis I (specifically during the substage referred to as leptotene) homologous recombination contributes to the genetic diversity of the offspring but also ensures the proper segregation of chromosomes at the end of meiosis I.

REPAIR OF DAMAGED DNA

DNA damage (Table 22–4) can occur as the result of exposure to environmental stimuli such as alkylating chemicals, ultraviolet or radioactive irradiation, and reactive oxygen species (ROS). These phenomena can, and do, lead to the introduction of mutations in the coding capacity of the DNA. Single nucleotide mutations in DNA are of two types. Transition mutations result from the exchange of one purine for another purine or one pyrimidine for another pyrimidine. Transversion mutations result from the exchange of a purine for a pyrimidine or *vice versa*.

TABLE 22–4 Types of damage to DNA.

Single-base alteration
A. Depurination
B. Deamination of cytosine to uracil
C. Deamination of adenine to hypoxanthine
D. Alkylation of base
E. Insertion or deletion of nucleotide
F. Base-analog incorporation
Two-base alteration
A. UV light-induced thymine—thymine (pyrimidine) dimer
B. Bifunctional alkylating agent cross-linkage
Chain breaks
A. Ionizing radiation
B. Radioactive disintegration of backbone element
C. Oxidative free radical formation
Cross-linkage
A. Between bases in same or opposite strands
B. Between DNA and protein molecules (eg, histones)

Reproduced with permission from Rodwell VW, Bender DA, Botham KM, et al: *Harper's Illustrated Biochemistry*, 31st ed. New York, NY: McGraw Hill; 2018.

TABLE 22–5 Human diseases of DNA damage repair.

Defective Non-homologous End Joining Repair (NHEJ)
Severe combined immunodeficiency disease (SCID)
Radiation-sensitive severe combined immunodeficiency disease (RS-SCID)
Defective Homologous Repair (HR)
AT-like disorder (ATLD)
Nijmegen breakage syndrome (NBS)
Bloom syndrome (BS)
Werner syndrome (WS)
Rothmund-Thomson syndrome (RTS)
Breast cancer susceptibility 1 and 2 (BRCA1, BRCA2)
Defective DNA Nucleotide Excision Repair (NER)
Xeroderma pigmentosum (XP)
Cockayne syndrome (CS)
Trichothiodystrophy (TTD)
Defective DNA Base Excision Repair (BER)
MUTYH-associated polyposis (MAP)
Defective DNA Mismatch Repair (MMR)
Lynch syndrome (also known as hereditary non-polyposis colorectal cancer, HNPCC)

Reproduced with permission from Rodwell VW, Bender DA, Botham KM, et al: *Harper's Illustrated Biochemistry*, 31st ed. New York, NY: McGraw Hill; 2018.

One by-product from UV irradiation of DNA is the formation of pyrimidine dimers (most often thymidine dimers) between two adjacent pyrimidines in the same strand of DNA. Thymidine dimers, as well as other damaged nucleotides are removed via a process termed base excision repair (BER). This repair mechanism is initiated by one of eleven glycohydrolases followed by repair polymerases and DNA ligases. Thymidine dimers are removed by the glycohydrolase identified as uracil DNA glycosylase, encoded by the *UNG* gene.

In addition to BER, the process referred to as nucleotide excision repair (NER) functions to repair DNA damage. NER involves the removal of a wide array of structurally unrelated DNA lesions and is catalyzed by a large family of nucleotide excision repair enzymes. Another DNA damage repair system involves the repair of double-strand breaks (DSB) in the DNA. DSB repair involves the process of nonhomologous end joining (NHEJ).

When DNA damage exceeds the capacity of the cell to repair it, a series of reactions is activated leading to apoptosis, a process of programmed cell death (see Chapter 34). DNA damage results in the activation of the tumor suppressor, p53 (see Figure 34–7) which in turn transcriptionally activates numerous genes whose encoded proteins participate in the activation of apoptosis. Expression of the PMAIP1 (phorbol-12-myristate-13-acetate-induced protein 1; commonly called NOXA), the BBC3 (BCL-2 binding component 2; commonly referred to as PUMA), and the *BAX* genes are all induced by activated p53. The PUMA and NOXA encoded proteins are BH3-only BCL-2 homology family proteins termed apoptosis initiators.

Defective DNA repair processes can result in potentially devastating disorders (Table 22–5) such as cancers (see Chapter 34), ataxia telangiectasia, AT (Clinical Box 22–7), and xeroderma pigmentosum, XP (Clinical Box 22–8).

CLINICAL BOX 22–7 ATAXIA TELANGIECTASIA

Ataxia telangiectasia (AT) is an autosomal recessive disorder that is characterized by hypersensitivity to ionizing radiation, progressive truncal ataxia affecting the gait with onset by 1–3 years of age, slurring of speech, oculocutaneous telangiectasias that begin to develop by age 6, frequent infections and cellular immunodeficiencies, and susceptibility to leukemias and lymphomas. Telangiectasias are areas of the skin under which there are dilated superficial vessels resulting in an appearance similar to that in patients with rosacea or scleroderma. In addition, as is common in AT, the telangiectasias can develop in the eye.
The AT syndrome results from mutations in the ataxia telangiectasia mutated (*ATM*) gene. The ATM protein is a member of the large molecular weight protein kinase family. Specifically, ATM is a member of the phosphatidylinositol-3-kinase (PI3K) family of kinases. The ATM kinase responds to DNA damage (specifically double-strand DNA breaks) by initiating the phosphorylation of several hundred proteins involved in DNA repair and/or cell cycle control. In the presence of mutant ATM, cell cycle arrest does not occur and damaged DNA does not get repaired prior to replication leading to the propagation of potentially cancer-causing mutations. ATM is known to phosphorylate the tumor suppressors p53 (a pivotal protein in cell cycle control) and BRCA1. In addition, ATM phosphorylates many other proteins involved in the control of cell cycle progression. AT is a highly pleiotropic disease reflecting the numerous pathways requiring the ATM kinase. The most striking and obvious clinical manifestations seen in AT is progressive cerebellar ataxia. On postmortem examination, it is observed that there is significant loss of Purkinje cells in the cerebellum. During development the Purkinje cells degenerate and migrate abnormally in the cerebellum. Changes are also seen in the dentate and olivary nuclei along with degeneration in the substantia nigra and neuroaxonal dystrophy in the medulla. Additional organ involvement is seen in the thymus which remains embryonic. The growth deficit in the thymus is responsible, in part, for the immunodeficiency seen in AT patients. Many other organs show nuclear changes resulting in nucleomegaly. An additional characteristic observation in 95% of AT patients is an elevation in serum α-fetoprotein (AFP). Children suffering from AT may begin to learn to walk but will shortly begin to stagger and eventually will be confined to a wheelchair by the age of 10. Two additional classic symptoms in AT patients is slurred speech and oculomotor apraxia (difficulty in moving the eyes from side to side). All teenage AT patients will need help with eating, getting dressed, and using the bathroom. Uncontrolled drooling is a frequent complaint with AT patients. Although neurologic status may appear to improve between the ages of 3 and 7 years, it begins to progressively deteriorate again. As implied by the name of this disorder, individuals exhibit a typical distribution

CLINICAL BOX 22–7 (CONTINUED)

of telangiectasias. These generally appear between the ages of 4 and 6 years and are found on the conjunctiva of the eye, the bridge of the nose, on the ears, and in the antecubital fossae (the triangular area on the anterior side of the elbow joint). Approximately 35–40% of AT patients will develop cancers within their shortened life spans and approximately 85% of these cancers are leukemias or lymphomas. The propensity for cancer in these patients is partly related to the increased frequency of chromosomal translocations seen in AT patients. These translocations involve chromosomes 14q11–q12, 14q32, 7q35, and 7p14. Treatment for AT is restricted to supportive care. The use of free-radical scavengers is highly recommended and includes vitamin E, coenzyme Q10 (CoQ10), and α-lipoic acid. Daily administration of folic acid has been associated with a reduction in chromosomal breakage in these patients.

CLINICAL BOX 22–8 XERODERMA PIGMENTOSUM

Xeroderma pigmentosum defines a class of autosomal recessive inherited diseases that are characterized clinically by sun sensitivity that results in progressive degeneration of sun-exposed areas of the skin and eyes. Often these changes will result in neoplasia. Some XP patients also manifest with progressive neurologic degeneration. There are currently eight alleles whose mutations result in manifestation of XP. Seven of the genes are involved in processes of nucleotide excision repair, NER. These seven genes represent XP complementation groups that are identified as XPA (*XPA* gene), XPB (*ERCC3* gene; excision-repair cross complementing 3), XPC (*XPC* gene), XPD (*ERCC2* gene), XPE (*DDB2* gene; damage-specific DNA-binding protein 2), XPF (*ERCC4* gene), and XPG (*ERCC5* gene). An additional class of XP patients, referred to as XP variants (XPV), results from mutations in the gene encoding DNA polymerase H (POLH). In most XP patients the initial symptoms are an abnormal reaction to sun exposure which includes severe sunburn with blistering and persistent erythema with minimal exposure to the sun. These symptoms most often manifest between 1 to 2 years of age although some patients do not exhibit symptoms until the teens. Most XP patients will develop xerosis (dry skin) and poikiloderma. Poikiloderma is defined as areas of the skin exhibiting increased pigment alternating with areas of reduced pigment, atrophy, and telangiectasias. Telangiectasias are areas of the skin under which there are dilated superficial vessels resulting in an appearance similar to that in patients with rosacea or scleroderma. This constellation of skin manifestations gave rise to the name of this disease. The skin of affected patients will appear similar to that of a person exposed to the sun for many years even though they are very young. Additional benign lesions in the skin include actinic keratoses (scaly crusty bumps), keratoacanthomas (well-differentiated squamous cell carcinoma), angiomas (benign tumors composed of blood vessels at or near the surface of the skin) and fibromas (benign tumors of connective tissue). Patients with XP who are younger than 20 years have a greater than 1000-fold increase in developing cancer at UV-exposed areas of the skin relative to unaffected individuals. Nonmelanoma skin cancer in XP patients appears with a median age of 10 years. In addition to photophobia, XP-related ocular symptoms are restricted to the sun-exposed anterior portion of the eye. The anterior portion of the eye includes the lid, cornea, and conjunctiva and these protect the posterior eye (uveal tract and retina) from UV radiation. Only visible light reaches the photosensitive areas of the retina. The ocular symptoms include conjunctivitis, ectropion (eyelids that turn outward) due to atrophy of the skin of the eyelids, exposure keratitis, and benign and malignant neoplasms of the eyelids. In XP patients with neurologic symptoms there is variation in age of onset and severity. However, all are characterized by progressive deterioration. Frequently observed symptoms are sensorineural deafness and diminished deep tendon reflexes. In some patients progressive intellectual impairment is evident but usually is not evident until the second decade of life.

CHEMOTHERAPIES TARGETING REPLICATION AND THE CELL CYCLE

Inhibition of Thymidine Synthesis

Drugs that interfere with aspects of nucleotide metabolism are known as the antimetabolites. There are two major types of antimetabolites: compounds that inhibit thymidylate synthetase and compounds that inhibit dihydrofolate reductase (DHFR). Drugs that inhibit thymidylate synthetase include 5-fluorouracil and 5-fluorodeoxyuridine. Those that inhibit DHFR are analogs of folic acid and include methotrexate, pyrimethamine, and trimethoprim.

Alkylating Drugs

Alkylating agents function by reacting with and disrupting the structure of DNA. Commonly used alkylating agents include cyclophosphamide, ifosfamide, dacarbazine, chlorambucil, and procarbazine.

Topoisomerase Inhibitors

Topoisomerase inhibitors inhibit either topoisomerase I or II. Two of these classes are the anthracyclines and the camptothecins. The camptothecins inhibit topoisomerase I and include irinotecan and topotecan. The anthracyclines inhibit topoisomerase II and include doxorubicin, daunorubicin, and mitoxanthrone. In addition to the anthracyclines the anticancer compound, etoposide, is also a topoisomerase II inhibitor.

Vinca Alkaloids

Anticancer compounds that are extracted from the periwinkle plant, *Vinca rosea*, are called the vinca alkaloids. These compounds bind to tubulin monomers leading to the disruption of the microtubules of the mitotic spindle fibers that are necessary for cell division during mitosis. The vinca alkaloids include vincristine, vinblastine, vinorelbin, and vindesine.

Taxanes

The taxanes are another class of plant-derived compounds that act via interference with microtubule function. These compounds function by hyperstabilizing microtubules which prevents cell division. The taxanes include paclitaxel and docetaxel.

CHECKLIST

- ☑ DNA present in eukaryotic cells is complexed with a variety of proteins forming a structure referred to as chromatin.
- ☑ The major proteins associated with DNA in chromatin are the histones. An octamer core composed of two copies of each of four different histone proteins is wrapped by approximately 150 bp of DNA.
- ☑ The histone proteins are subject to a wide variety of posttranslational modifications, the consequences of which dynamically alter the structure of chromatin. These dynamic changes result in variable access of the DNA to the transcriptional machinery.
- ☑ Transcriptional activity is controlled, in part, by the overall structure of chromatin, which itself is regulated by the state of histone modifications and DNA methylation. Histone acetylation is associated with activation of transcription, whereas, deacetylation is associated with transcriptional silencing.
- ☑ Actively dividing eukaryotic cells progress through a higher-order series of events referred to as the cell cycle. The cell cycle consists of an initial stage called G1, then DNA is synthesized in S-phase, the cell pauses again in G2, and then cytokinesis occurs in M-phase.
- ☑ The ability of cells to progress through the different phases of the cell cycle requires a specialized set of proteins known as cyclins, and the kinase the cyclins regulate are called cyclin-dependent kinases, CDKs. The cyclins are so-called because their levels fluctuate during the cell cycle phases due to repeated ubiquitin-mediated degradation and transcription of the corresponding gene.
- ☑ DNA replication occurs during the S-phase of the cell cycle and involves a wide array of different protein activities including polymerases, various types of DNA-unwinding proteins, primer synthesizing enzymes, single-strand stabilizing proteins, and DNA ligases.
- ☑ Replication is initiated at multiple locations in each chromosome termed origins of replication and proceeds along both strands simultaneously in both directions from the origin. The leading edge of the replication process is referred to as the replication fork.
- ☑ Given the restrictions on the process of DNA synthesis catalyzed by DNA polymerases, one of the two strands can be synthesized continuously (called the leading strand), the other discontinuously (called the lagging strand). The fragments of new DNA from the lagging strand of synthesis are called Okazaki fragments.
- ☑ Due to the process of replication the ends of the lagging strand of each chromosome cannot be replicated by DNA polymerase. The ends of the chromosomes are called telomeres and they contain highly repeated sequences that are recognized by the enzyme complex called telomerase. Telomerase aids in the extension of the lagging strand so that DNA polymerase can carry out replication. The process is never complete such that the telomeric ends of the chromosomes shorten with each cell cycle.
- ☑ DNA can be posttranscriptionally modified by DNA methyltransferases that methylate the 5-position of cytosine residues present in a CpG dinucleotide.
- ☑ The state of DNA methylation can affect chromatin structure and consequently the level of transcriptional activity. DNA methylation is also associated with the phenomenon of genomic imprinting.
- ☑ Remodeling of DNA can occur via the actions of recombination or transposition. The primary form of recombination in eukaryotic DNA is between regions of homology in sister chromatids.
- ☑ Several genes contain regions of trinucleotide repeats that can become abnormally expanded (amplified) resulting in the development of disease, such as is the case in Huntington disease. These diseases are all referred to as trinucleotide repeat diseases.
- ☑ Numerous events of the cell cycle, such as DNA synthesis and cytokinesis, are the targets of various chemotherapeutic drugs used to treat various forms of cancer.

REVIEW QUESTIONS

1. Experiments are being conducted on the effects of various compounds on cultures of cells derived from a melanoma. One of the compounds being tested has been shown to enhance the activity of a member of the sirtuin family of proteins. Based on these results, which of the following is most likely to be observed in these cells with respect to the process of DNA replication?
   (A) Decrease in the rate
   (B) Destabilization of the double helix allowing access to the primase activity
   (C) Enhancement in the formation of new chromatin following completion of replication
   (D) Increase in the rate
   (E) No effect on activity or rate

2. Experiments are being carried out on the process of DNA replication using cultures of cells isolated from the biopsy of a breast cancer tumor. Results of the experiments find that the process of replication proceeds normally except in regions where the DNA is attached to the chromatin scaffold. Given these observations, which of the following activities of DNA replication is most likely to be defective in these cells?
   (A) DNA ligase
   (B) Helicase
   (C) Polymerase-α
   (D) Single-strand binding proteins
   (E) Topoisomerase

3. A 6-year-old girl is brought to the physician because her parents are concerned about the severe skin blistering on her arms and back of her neck a few days after she played in the sun for 15 minutes without sunscreen. Physical examination shows the girl has numerous freckles on her face, neck, arms, and hands. In addition, she has numerous telangiectasias on her arms as well as crusty and scaly patches of skin. Which of the following processes is most likely defective in this patient?
   (A) Base excision repair
   (B) DNA double-strand break repair
   (C) DNA mismatch repair
   (D) Nucleotide excision repair
   (E) Pyrimidine nucleotide biosynthesis
   (F) Telomere replication

4. A 35-year-old man comes to the physician because of concern regarding his potential risk of developing cancer. Both his father and his father's sister developed gastrointestinal cancer in their late twenties. Histopathology of biopsy samples taken during the patient's disease is shown. Which of the following processes would most likely have become defective leading to the initiation of the events that ultimately resulted in the findings in this histopathologic section?

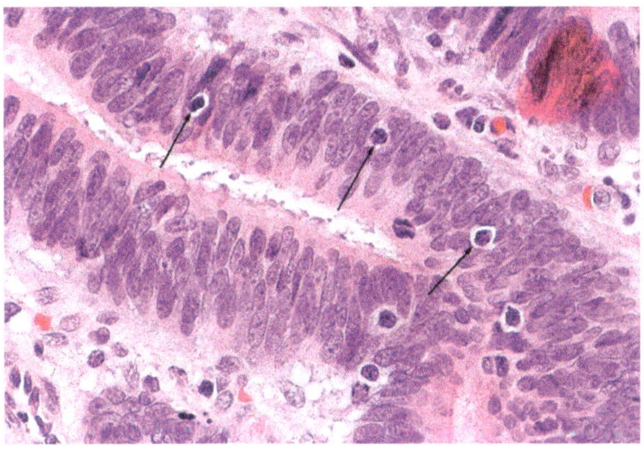

   (A) Cell cycle checkpoint monitoring
   (B) DNA mismatch repair
   (C) DNA proof-reading during replication
   (D) Growth factor synthesis
   (E) Nuclear receptor phosphorylation
   (F) Tumor-suppressor synthesis
   (G) Tyr kinase receptor downregulation

5. Experiments are being conducted that are aimed at defining the defect(s) in the processes of DNA replication in a cell line derived from biopsy of a colon carcinoma. Results of these experiments demonstrate that the replication process is incapable of duplicating an entire chromosome. Microscopic examination of the cells finds that the DNA that is not replicated resides near to the scaffold. Given these observations, which of the following chemicals would be most likely to exert the same effects observed in these cells?
   (A) Bleomycin
   (B) Cisplatin
   (C) Cyclophosphamide
   (D) Irinotecan
   (E) Vinblastine

6. A 66-year-old man presented to an urgent care clinic with a 4-day history of dry cough, progressing to rusty colored sputum and the sudden onset of chills the previous evening. The patient thought he had a cold, but the symptoms have worsened, and he reports that he barely slept last night due to persistent coughing. He indicates that he has experienced some sharp right-sided pain but no shortness of breath, no leg swelling, no left-sided chest pain, and no gastrointestinal issues. Medical history reveals the patient is diabetic and hypertensive and he is taking metformin and lisinopril. He reported no antibiotic use in the previous 3 months. Vital signs include a temperature of 100.2°F, blood pressure 128/76, heart rate of 102 bpm with regular rhythm, and O_2 saturation of 90%. Physical examination reveals mild tachypnea with dullness to percussion over the lower-right lung. The attending physician orders a chest X-ray and a prescription for antibiotics. Given the signs and symptoms in this patient which of the following is the most likely target of the drug prescribed for this patient?
   (A) Cell wall synthesis
   (B) DNA replication
   (C) Nucleotide synthesis
   (D) Peptidoglycan synthesis
   (E) RNA synthesis

7. A 51-year-old man has been diagnosed with colorectal carcinoma. Biopsy tissue has been analyzed via whole exome sequencing, and it has been found that there is a 10-fold higher level of expression of the thymidylate synthase gene when compared to normal tissue. Given these findings, which of the following would be the most useful in the treatment regimen for this patient?
   (A) Doxorubicin
   (B) Fluorouracil
   (C) Irinotecan
   (D) Methotrexate
   (E) Vincristine

8. A 7-year-old boy is being examined by his pediatrician due to concerns of his parents about the many patches of dry scaly skin on the back of his hands, his neck, and ears. The pediatrician excises a skin sample for biopsy. Results of the biopsy show the presence of basal and squamous cell carcinoma. Given these findings, and the age of the patient, which of the following processes is most likely to be deficient?

(A) DNA repair
(B) DNA replication
(C) RNA splicing
(D) Transcription
(E) Translation

9. Experiments are being conducted on the effects of ultraviolet radiation on the processes of DNA replication. These experiments are being conducted on normal skin fibroblasts in culture. Following exposure of these cells to an ultraviolet light source, the activity of which of the following proteins is most likely to enhanced?
(A) CDK2
(B) Cyclin A
(C) Cyclin D
(D) E2F
(E) p53

10. A clinical study is being carried out to examine the relationship between telomere length and pathology. Participants in this study group include developmentally normal children and adults, individuals with various cancers, and individuals with various developmental abnormalities. Which of the following observations would most closely reflect the findings of this clinical study?
(A) Longer telomeres in all the abnormal individuals
(B) Longer telomeres in individuals who have cancer and in those who are developmentally abnormal
(C) Longer telomeres only the young individuals
(D) Shorter telomeres in the older individuals and the developmentally abnormal individuals
(E) Shorter telomeres in the older individuals only
(F) Shorter telomeres in only the young and developmentally normal individuals

11. A 5-year-old man is being examined to ascertain the possible cause of his apparent intellectual impairment. Physical examination finds the child is of short stature, has small hands and feet, is slightly hypotonic, and is well above expected weight for age. Genetic studies identify the child harbors a chromosome 15 with a large deletion in the q arm. The symptoms and genetic data indicate the child is most likely suffering from which of the following disorders?
(A) Angelman syndrome
(B) Ataxia telangiectasia
(C) Beckwith-Wiedemann syndrome
(D) Prader-Willi syndrome
(E) Rett syndrome

12. Experiments are being conducted on the effects of various compounds on the process of DNA replication in cells in culture. One of the compounds being tested is structurally related to irinotecan. Which of the following is the most likely activity that would be inhibited when this compound is added to the cell culture?
(A) ATP-dependent DNA helicase
(B) DNA ligase
(C) DNA polymerase
(D) Single-strand DNA-binding
(E) Topoisomerase

13. Experiments are being conducted on the effects of various compounds on the process of DNA replication in cells in culture. One of the compounds being tested is related to 5-azacytidine. Which of the following is the most likely effect of the addition of this compound to the cultured cells?
(A) Decreased mutagenesis
(B) Hypermethylation
(C) Hypomethylation
(D) Increased mutagenesis
(E) Increased replication
(F) Inhibition of replication

14. Experiments are being conducted on the effects of various compounds on the process of DNA replication in cells in culture. One of the compounds being tested is structurally related to docetaxel. If this compound is added to the cells in culture, which of the following would be its most likely mode of action?
(A) Binds to, and stabilizes microtubules, preventing their shortening and interfering with cell division
(B) Binding to the activated form of the RAS protein which in turn interferes with the signaling cascades involving this protein
(C) Interaction with the tumor suppressor protein (pRB) inducing its suppressive activity
(D) Interaction with topoisomerase II preventing its role in DNA synthesis
(E) Interference with retinoic acid receptor interaction with DNA, thus preventing the growth induction by this hormone

15. Experiments are being conducted on the effects of various compounds on the process of DNA replication in cells in culture. One of the compounds being tested is structurally related to doxorubicin. Which of the following is the most likely effect of the addition of this compound to the cultured cells?
(A) DNA ligase
(B) DNA polymerase α
(C) Primase
(D) Topoisomerase
(E) Uracil *N*-glycosylase

16. Experiments are being conducted with cells in culture that were derived from a human hepatoma. When analyzing DNA synthesis in these cells, it is discovered that errors are found in the daughter strand of DNA with a much higher frequency than in normal hepatocytes in culture. Based on these findings, which of the following is most likely defective in the hepatoma-derived cells?
(A) Exonuclease activity in the 3′ to 5′ direction
(B) Exonuclease activity in the 5′ to 3′ direction
(C) Insertion of nucleotides in 5′ to 3′ orientation
(D) Synthesis of the mixed RNA-DNA primers
(E) Topoisomerase-mediated cleavage of the DNA backbone

17. A 4-year-old girl is undergoing examination following a seizure. History reveals that the child started to crawl, grasp items with her hands, and made babbling attempts at speech. However, these skills never progressed and now the child does not attempt speech at all, exhibits unusual hand and eye movements, and has trouble breathing. Physical examination finds that the girls head circumference is smaller than expected for her age. Which of the following is the most likely mechanism by which this child acquired the disorder?
(A) A new mutation
(B) Autosomal dominant inheritance
(C) Autosomal recessive inheritance
(D) Mitochondrial inheritance
(E) X-linked recessive inheritance

18. Experiments are being conducted on the effects of various compounds on the process of DNA replication in lung tumor-derived cells in culture. One of the compounds being tested has been shown to alter the activity of topoisomerase II. The results find that this altered topoisomerase activity is not inhibited by typical topoisomerase targeting anticancer drugs. Given these findings, which of the following would most likely be ineffective in targeting this enzyme to inhibit the growth of these tumor cells?
(A) A taxane
(B) A vinca alkaloid
(C) An alkylating compound
(D) An anthracycline
(E) An antimetabolite

19. A 57-year-old man is being examined by his physician with concerns about his unstable posture and difficulty walking. The patient reports that he has been very moody lately and has been overcome with a sensation of great depression on numerous occasions. Physical examination finds the patient has difficulty swallowing and slightly slurred speech. History reveals that the patient's father had similar physical difficulties and died when he was 63. Which of the following is the most likely cause of the symptoms in this patient?
(A) Chromosomal deletion
(B) Chromosomal duplication
(C) DNA methylation error
(D) DNA repair error
(E) Trinucleotide repeat expansion

20. Experiments are being carried out to characterize nucleic acids in various cells isolated from several different normal tissues. The results of these studies find that the molar amount of adenosine in the double-stranded DNA extracted from these various cells is 20%. Given these findings, which of the following is the most likely molar amount of cytidine in these DNA molecules?
(A) 10%
(B) 20%
(C) 30%
(D) 40%
(E) 60%

21. A 5-year-old man is being examined to ascertain the possible cause of his apparent intellectual impairment. Physical examination finds the child is of short stature, has small hands and feet, is slightly hypotonic, and is well above expected weight for age. Genetic studies identify the child harbors a chromosome 15 with a large deletion in the q arm. Which of the following most correctly defines the molecular mechanism that underlies the manifestation of the phenotypes in this child?
(A) Activation of expression by hypermethylation of genomic DNA sites
(B) Activation of expression by hypomethylation of genomic DNA sites
(C) Expansion of trinucleotide repeats in regulated genes resulting in dysregulated expression
(D) Inhibition of expression by hypomethylation of genomic DNA sites
(E) Regulated expression dependent on parental origin of regulated genes

22. Experiments are being conducted on the effects of a novel compounds on various cellular processes with the use of cells in culture. The compound has been shown to interfere with the normal function of cyclin D. Given these findings, which of the following is most likely to exhibit reduced activity in the presence of this compound?
(A) Cyclin-dependent kinase 2 (CDK2)
(B) E2F
(C) MDM2
(D) $p21^{CIP}$
(E) p53

23. A 10-month-old infant has been rushed to the emergency department following a seizure. History reveals that the child has had difficulty feeding for the past several weeks and has difficulty learning to crawl with tremors apparent in her legs when she attempts to crawl. Physical examination finds hypotonia, a head circumference smaller than expected for age, and hyperreflexia. Which of the following most closely explains the observed symptoms in this patient?
(A) Angelman syndrome
(B) Huntington disease
(C) Mitochondrial DNA depletion syndrome
(D) Myotonic dystrophy type 1
(E) Prader-Willi syndrome

24. Experiments are being conducted on the effects of various compounds on the growth properties of lung tumor-derived cells in culture. One of the compounds being tested has been shown to result in mitotic arrest. This mitotic arrest is not associated with any defects in microtubule function. Given these results, which of the following is the most likely target of the compound?
(A) Anaphase promoting complex (APC)
(B) Cyclin D
(C) Cyclin E
(D) E2F
(E) Securin

25. Experiments are being carried out to identify the defect resulting in the development of a squamous cell carcinoma. When these cells are exposed to a brief dose of gamma irradiation it is found that there is a high rate of incorporation of structurally altered nucleotides into the daughter strand of DNA following replication. Given these findings, which of the following is most likely defective in these cancer-derived cells?
(A) Anaphase promoting complex (APC)
(B) CDK4/6
(C) Cyclin D
(D) DNA polymerase-α
(E) p53

26. A 3-year-old boy is being examined by his pediatrician due to the onset of ataxia that has made it nearly impossible for the child to walk. History reveals that the child has had numerous infections over the past 2 years. Physical examination finds numerous areas of dilated superficial vessels leading to the appearance of rosacea. Blood work finds high levels of serum α-fetoprotein. A defect in which of the following processes best explains the signs and symptoms in this patient?
(A) DNA methylation
(B) DNA repair
(C) DNA replication
(D) Protein glycosylation
(E) Protein targeting
(F) RNA splicing

27. Experiments are being conducted on the effects of a novel compound using cultures of human skin fibroblasts. The compound is found to inhibit the function of pRB. Given these results, which of the following is most likely to exhibit increased activity in the presence of this compound?
(A) Cyclin D
(B) E2F
(C) $p21^{CIP}$
(D) p53
(E) Topoisomerase

28. Regions of genes in the human genome that contribute to transcriptional regulation have been shown to be enriched in 5′-CpG-3′ dinucleotides. Very often the C residue is methylated at the 5′ position of the nucleobase (m^5CpG). Evidence has found that these methylated regions of the genome are highly prone to mutation. Which of the following is the best explanation of this observation?
(A) Deamination of m^5C results in replacement with thymine
(B) Histones bind less tightly to m^5C sequences than to other sequences
(C) Homologous recombination occurs preferentially at m^5C sequences
(D) Methylation of C interferes with base pairing to G during DNA replication
(E) Nonhomologous end joining (NHEJ) is stimulated by the presence of m^5C residues

29. Which of the following best describes the term, epigenetics?
(A) Gene expression results from regulated levels of DNA methylation
(B) Gene expression that is restricted to a specific cell lineage
(C) Gene regulation is exerted by sex-type specific factors
(D) Genotype differences are not reflected by phenotype differences
(E) Phenotype differences are independent of genotype variation

30. A 4-year-old girl is undergoing examination following a seizure. History reveals that the child started to crawl, grasp items with her hands, and made babbling attempts at speech. However, these skills never progressed and now the child does not attempt speech at all, exhibits unusual hand and eye movements, and has trouble breathing. Physical examination finds that the girl's head circumference is smaller than expected for her age. Which of the following processes is most likely defective in this child resulting in the observed symptoms?
(A) DNA repair
(B) DNA replication
(C) Protein glycosylation
(D) Protein targeting
(E) Regulation of transcription
(F) RNA splicing

31. A 57-year-old man is being examined by his physician with concerns about his unstable posture and difficulty walking. The patient reports that he has been very moody lately and has been overcome with a sensation of great depression on numerous occasions. Physical examination finds the patient has difficulty swallowing and slightly slurred speech. History reveals that the patient's father had similar physical difficulties and died when he was 63. Which of the following represents the most likely cause of the patient's symptoms?
(A) Fragile X syndrome
(B) Huntington disease
(C) Mitochondrial DNA depletion syndrome
(D) Myotonic dystrophy type 1
(E) Prader-Willi syndrome

32. An 8-year-old girl, who recently moved to a new city, is being examined by a pediatrician as a new patient. History reveals that the patient is in special education due to her intellectual impairment. Her parents state that they have always had difficulty keeping their daughter's weight down due to her habit of over-eating and sneaking food when they are not watching. In addition, they state their daughter has frequent tantrums and exhibits stubbornness and compulsive behaviors. Physical examination finds that the patient exhibits a diffuse level of hypotonia and is at the 95th percentile for body weight. The signs and symptoms exhibited in this patient are most likely due to which of the following molecular properties?
(A) Deletion from the p arm of chromosome 5
(B) Deletion from the p arm of chromosome 11 of the maternal allele
(C) Deletion from the p arm of chromosome 11 of the paternal allele
(D) Deletion from the q arm of chromosome 15 of the maternal allele
(E) Deletion from the q arm of chromosome 15 of the paternal allele
(F) CCG trinucleotide repeat in *FMR1* gene
(G) Trisomy 21

33. A 7-year-old boy is being examined by his pediatrician because his parents are concerned about his behavioral issues that include frequent tantrums, stubbornness, and compulsive activities. Physical examination finds that the patient exhibits a diffuse level of hypotonia, has small hands and feet, arms and legs that are longer than normal, and sparse body hair. Given the most likely diagnosis, which of the following is one of the most likely additional clinical features that will present in this patient?
(A) Choreiform movements
(B) Hemolytic anemia
(C) Intention tremors
(D) Macroorchidism
(E) Obesity

34. A 4-year-old girl has been taken to the Emergency Department by her parents following a particularly lengthy seizure. The parents report that their daughter has had several smaller, less pronounced seizures over the prior 6 months for which she was prescribed valproic acid. During this most recent event, the parents stated that their daughter had severe contractions of her limbs and she lost consciousness. Physical examination shows the child has a prominent nose, broad forehead, and microcephaly. While observing the patient, the attending physician notes that the patient continuously claps her hands, smiles, and laughs. Which of the following is the most likely underlying genetic mechanism accounting for the signs and symptoms in this patient?
(A) Deletion from the p arm of chromosome 11 of the maternal allele
(B) Deletion from the p arm of chromosome 11 of the paternal allele
(C) Mutated *UBE3A* gene on maternal chromosome 15
(D) Mutated *UBE3A* gene on paternal chromosome 15
(E) Trinucleotide repeat within the *DMPK* gene
(F) Trinucleotide repeat within the *FMR1* gene

35. A 9-year-old boy is being examined by his pediatrician because his parents are concerned about the amount of dry skin and abnormal pigmentation, as well as his extreme sensitivity to the sun. Physical examination finds xerosis and poikiloderma with several actinic keratoses. One well-defined lesion on the patient's left forearm is removed for biopsy, which confirms that it is keratoacanthoma. Given the signs and symptoms in this patient, which of the following is most likely to be deficient?

(A) Base excision repair
(B) Double-strand break repair
(C) Mismatch repair
(D) *NF1* gene
(E) Nucleotide excision repair
(F) *RB1* gene
(G) *TP53* gene

ANSWERS

1. Correct answer is **E.** Histone deacetylation is necessary to regulate the positive or negative effects on gene expression exerted by histone acetylation. The deacetylation of histones is catalyzed by a large superfamily of enzymes that is composed of the sirtuin (*SIRT*) genes and the histone deacetylase (*HDAC*) genes. The consequences of reduced histone acetylation are altered chromatin structure making it difficult for the transcriptional machinery to engage the DNA. Thus, the activation of a member of sirtuin family of histone deacetylases would be associated with reduced transcription but would not appreciably, or at all, affect DNA replication. None of the other options (choices A, B, C, and D) related to the role of histone deacetylases in the process of DNA replication.

2. Correct answer is **E.** The progression of the replication fork requires that the DNA ahead of the fork be continuously unwound. Due to the fact that eukaryotic chromosomal DNA is attached to a protein scaffold, the progressive movement of the replication fork introduces severe torsional stress into the duplex ahead of the replication fork. This torsional stress is relieved by enzymes of the DNA topoisomerase family. Topoisomerases relieve torsional stresses in duplexes of DNA by introducing either double-stranded (topoisomerases II) or single-stranded (topoisomerases I) breaks into the backbone of the DNA. These breaks allow unwinding of the duplex and removal of the replication-induced torsional strain. The nicks are then resealed by the topoisomerases. Therefore, the inability to fully replicate DNA where it is attached to the scaffold would most likely be due to lack of adequate topoisomerase activity. Defects in DNA ligase (choice A) would result in a lack of ability to generate a phosphodiester bond between any given 3′-hydroxyl and 5′-phosphate, therefore global DNA replication would be severely impaired. Defects in helicase activity (choice B) would prevent unwinding of the duplex of DNA and would, therefore reduce global DNA replication. Defects in polymerize-α (choice C), which is the enzyme that synthesizes the mixed RNA-DNA primers required for DNA replication would be prevent replication from occurring at all. Defects in single-strand binding proteins (choice D) would prevent the maintenance of the separated strands of DNA, which is required for the function of DNA polymerases, and as a consequence would interfere with global replication.

3. Correct answer is **D.** The patient is most likely experiencing the symptoms of xeroderma pigmentosum. Xeroderma pigmentosum (XP) defines a class of autosomal recessive inherited diseases that are characterized clinically by sun sensitivity that results in progressive degeneration of sun-exposed areas of the skin and eyes. Often these changes will result in neoplasia. Some XP patients also manifest with progressive neurologic degeneration. There are currently eight alleles whose mutations result in manifestation of XP. Seven of the genes are involved in processes of nucleotide excision repair, NER. Defects in none of the other processes (choices A, B, C, E, and F) are associated with the causation of xeroderma pigmentosum.

4. Correct answer is **B.** Given the presence of tumor infiltrating lymphocytes (arrows in image), observed in the histopathology of a biopsy specimen taken from the patient's father, there is a strong indication that the father most likely had Lynch syndrome, also known as hereditary nonpolyposis colorectal carcinoma, HNPCC. Lynch syndrome is an autosomal dominant condition that represents the most common cause of hereditary colorectal carcinoma. Family members are also at increased risk for cancers of the small intestine, stomach, brain, skin, ovary, and endometrium. The hallmark of Lynch syndrome is a deficiency in DNA mismatch repair. Mutations in any one of four mismatch repair genes, identified as MLH1, MSH2, PMS2, and MSH6, are highly correlated to Lynch syndrome. Functionally, MLH1 dimerizes with PMS2 and MSH2 dimerizes with MSH6. Defects in none of the other processes (choices A, C, D, E, F, and G) correlate to the inherited colorectal carcinoma in this family.

5. Correct answer is **D.** The progression of the replication fork requires that the DNA ahead of the fork be continuously unwound. Due to the fact that eukaryotic chromosomal DNA is attached to a protein scaffold, the progressive movement of the replication fork introduces severe torsional stress into the duplex ahead of the replication fork. This torsional stress is relieved by enzymes of the DNA topoisomerase family. Topoisomerases relieve torsional stresses in duplexes of DNA by introducing either double-stranded (topoisomerases II) or single-stranded (topoisomerases I) breaks into the backbone of the DNA. These breaks allow unwinding of the duplex and removal of the replication-induced torsional strain. The nicks are then resealed by the topoisomerases. Therefore, the inability to fully replicate DNA where it is attached to the scaffold strongly suggests that the experimental compound is inhibiting topoisomerase activity. Several classes of anticancer drugs function through interference with the actions of the topoisomerases. Two of these classes are the anthracyclines and the camptothecins. The anthracyclines inhibit the actions of topoisomerase II whereas the camptothecins inhibit the action of topoisomerase I. Irinotecan and topotecan are two commonly used members of the camptothecin family. Bleomycin (choice A) is a nonheme iron protein that induces DNA strand breakage by intercalating into double-stranded DNA. Cisplatin (choice B) is a member of the platinum-based anticancer drugs that function by inducing intrastrand DNA crosslinking at purine residues. Cyclophosphamide (choice C) is a member of the alkylating family of anticancer drugs that induce DNA crosslinking within and between DNA strands at guanine residues. Vinblastine (choice E) is a member of the vinca alkaloids family of anticancer drugs. The vinca alkaloids inhibit cell growth by inhibiting the polymerization of microtubule machinery of the cell preventing mitosis.

6. Correct answer is **B.** The patient most likely has community acquired pneumonia (CAP) but is not compromised enough to warrant hospitalization. However, the patient does have the comorbidity of hypertension. The most common bacterium involved in CAP is *Streptococcus pneumoniae.* In patients with CAP, who do not require hospitalization but also have additional comorbidities, the most common recommendation is the use of an antibiotic of the fluoroquinolone family such as levofloxacin. Other options, but not as common, are the use of a beta-lactam plus a macrolide or a beta-lactam plus doxycycline. The mode of action of the fluoroquinolone drugs is the inhibition of bacterial DNA gyrase, the equivalent of eukaryotic topoisomerase. Therefore, the mode of action is the inhibition of DNA replication. Inhibition of cell wall synthesis (choice A) as well as peptidoglycan synthesis (choice D) is the mode of action of beta-lactam family drugs as well as many other drugs such as bacitracin and tunicamycin. Several antibiotics, such as trimethoprim and pyrimethamine, inhibit nucleotide synthesis (choice C). Inhibitors of prokaryotic RNA synthesis (choice E) include rifampicin and rifamycin.

7. Correct answer is **B.** Given the elevated level of expression of the thymidylate synthetase (also called thymidylate synthase) in this patient's cancer the use of anticancer drugs that target the function of this enzyme would be recommended. Drugs that inhibit thymidylate synthetase include 5-fluorouracil and 5-fluorodeoxyuridine. Doxorubicin (choice A) is an anthracycline class drug that inhibits topoisomerase II. Irinotecan (choice C) is a camptothecin class drug that inhibits topoisomerase I. Methotrexate (choice D) inhibits dihydrofolate reductase. Vincristine (choice E) is a member of the vinca alkaloid class of drug that inhibit microtubule polymerization.

8. Correct answer is **A.** The patient is most likely experiencing the symptoms of xeroderma pigmentosum. Xeroderma pigmentosum (XP) defines a class of autosomal recessive inherited diseases that are characterized clinically by sun sensitivity that results in progressive degeneration of sun exposed areas of the skin and eyes. Often these changes will result in neoplasia. Some XP patients also manifest with progressive neurologic degeneration. There are currently eight alleles whose mutations result in manifestation of XP. Seven of the genes are involved in processes of nucleotide excision repair (NER) of DNA damage. None of the other processes (choices B, C, D, and E) would be defective in a patient with XP.

9. Correct answer is **E.** One major function of the p53 protein is to serve as a component of the checkpoint that controls whether cells enter, as well as progress through, S-phase of the cell cycle. The action of p53 is induced in response to DNA damage. Under normal circumstances p53 is in the cytosol and its levels remain very low due to its interaction with a member of the ubiquitin ligase family called MDM2. In response to DNA damage, such as resulting from UV irradiation or γ-irradiation, cells activate several kinases including checkpoint kinase 2 (CHK2) and ataxia telangiectasia mutated (ATM). One target of these kinases is p53. ATM also phosphorylates MDM2. When p53 is phosphorylated, it is released from MDM2 and migrates into the nucleus where it can carry out its transcriptional activation functions. One target of p53 is the gene encoding the cyclin inhibitor, $p21^{Cip1}$. Activation of $p21^{Cip1}$ leads to increased inhibition of the cyclin D1-CDK4 and cyclin E-CDK2 complexes thereby halting progression through the cell cycle either prior to S-phase entry or during S-phase. Enhanced activity of none of the other cell cycle regulating proteins (choices A, B, C, and D) is directly affected by UV irradiation and the consequent DNA damage.

10. Correct answer is **D.** Numerous studies have demonstrated a correlation between telomere shortening and human aging, disease progression, and developmental delay. Decreased telomere length in peripheral blood leukocytes has been shown to correlate with higher mortality rates in older (more than 60 years of age) individuals. This is contrasted by studies in centenarians and their offspring that have shown a positive link between telomere length and longevity. There is also an intriguing correlation between telomere length and psychological stress and the risk for development of psychiatric disease. The level of telomerase activity in peripheral blood leukocytes has been shown to be lowest in individuals with the highest levels of stress which also coincided with the highest levels of oxidative stress. This correlation between stress and telomerase activity and telomere length is quite intriguing given that it is known that individuals subject to chronic psychological stress show a shortened lifespan and more rapid onset of diseases that are more typical of an aged population such as cardiovascular disease. None of the other options (choices A, B, C, E, and F) correctly correlate with telomere length as it relates to aging, potential for cancer, or association with development.

11. Correct answer is **D.** The patient is most likely manifesting the signs and symptoms of Prader-Willi syndrome. Prader-Willi syndrome (PWS) is characterized by a failure to thrive in the neonatal period accompanied by muscular hypotonia. During early childhood PWS patients exhibit hyperphagia (excessive hunger and abnormally large intake of solid foods), obesity, hypogonadism, sleep apnea, behavior problems, and mild to moderate intellectual impairment. Additionally, PWS children have small hands and feet. In prepubertal males the hypogonadism results in sparse body hair, poor development of skeletal muscles, and delay in epiphyseal closure resulting in long arms and legs. PWS results from the loss of a group of genes exclusively expressed from the paternal genome due to a deletion of a region of the q arm of the paternal chromosome 15. These genes are hypermethylated on the q arm of the maternal chromosome 15 and are, therefore, not expressed from this chromosome. Angelman syndrome (choice A) is the result of mutations or deletions in the gene, *UBE3A*, encoding a ubiquitin ligase. This gene resides in the same region of the q arm of chromosome 15 that is associated with Prader-Willi syndrome. The gene is hypermethylated on the paternal chromosome and, therefore, is not expressed. Ataxia telangiectasia (choice B) is a disorder associated with defective DNA damage repair. Beckwith-Wiedemann syndrome (choice C) is another imprinting-related disorder associated abnormal regulation of imprinted genes on chromosome 11. Rett syndrome (choice E) manifests almost exclusively in females due to in utero or early and postnatal lethality. Rett syndrome results from loss of function of a protein, MECP2, responsible for the recognition of methylated DNA.

12. Correct answer is **E.** Irinotecan is a drug that is a member of the camptothecin family of topoisomerase inhibitors. None of the other enzymes (choices A, B, C, and D) are the target of the camptothecin family of drugs such as irinotecan.

13. Correct answer is **C.** The nucleotide analog, 5-azacytidine (5-azaC), is incorporated into replicating DNA when DNA polymerase would normally use deoxycytidine as the substrate.

The incorporation of a nitrogen instead of carbon at position 5 of the nucleobase prevents subsequent methylation of 5-azaC in the DNA when it is inserted into positions where the template strand of DNA contains a 5-methyl cytidine (m^5C) in the context of the dinucleotide, CpG. Thus, the incorporation of 5-azaC prevents conservation of methylation status in newly synthesized DNA which results in hypomethylation of the newly synthesized DNA. None of the other options (choices A, B, D, E, and F) correctly correlates to DNA hypomethylation as would be induced in the presence of 5-aza C.

14. Correct answer is **A.** The taxanes are a class of plant-derived compounds that act via interference with microtubule function. These compounds include paclitaxel (Taxol) and docetaxel (Taxotere). The taxanes function by hyperstabilizing microtubules which prevents cell division. Specifically, the taxanes bind to the tubulin protein of microtubules and locks them in place. The resulting microtubule/taxane complex does not have the ability to disassemble. This adversely affects cell function because the shortening and lengthening of microtubules (termed dynamic instability) is necessary for their function as a transportation highway for the cell. Chromosomes, for example, rely on this property of microtubules during mitosis. Therefore, the inability of cells to organize and undertake the necessary movements of mitosis prevents cell division. These compounds are used to treat a wide range of cancers including head and neck, lung, ovarian, breast, bladder, and prostate cancers. None of the other options (choices B, C, D, and E) represent the processes that are disrupted in the presence of drugs of the taxane family.

15. Correct answer is **D.** Doxorubicin is a drug that is a member of the anthracycline family of topoisomerase II inhibitors. None of the other enzymes (choices A, B, C, and E) are the target of the anthracycline family of drugs such as doxorubicin.

16. Correct answer is **A.** The main enzymatic activity of DNA polymerases is the 5′→3′ synthetic activity. However, DNA polymerases possess two additional activities of importance for both replication and repair. These additional activities include a 5′→3′ exonuclease function and a 3′→5′ exonuclease function. The 3′→5′ exonuclease function is utilized during replication to allow DNA polymerase to remove non-Watson-Crick base paired nucleotides and is referred to as the proof-reading activity of DNA polymerase. It is possible (but rare) for DNA polymerases to incorporate an incorrect base during replication. These mismatched bases are recognized by the polymerase immediately due to the lack of correct Watson-Crick base-pairing. The mismatched base is then removed by the 3′→5′ exonuclease activity and the correct base inserted prior to progression of replication. Therefore, the high rate of nucleotide error incorporation during DNA replication would most likely be associated with a defect in the proofreading activity of DNA polymerase. Defects in none of the other processes (choices B, C, D, and E) would correlate with a higher rate of nucleotide errors in the daughter strand during DNA replication.

17. Correct answer is **A.** The patient is most likely exhibiting the signs and symptoms of Rett syndrome. Rett syndrome is an X-linked disorder resulting from mutations in gene (*MECP2*) encoding the protein identified as methyl-CpG binding protein 2. Rett syndrome is a neurodevelopmental disorder that occurs almost exclusively in females manifesting as intellectual impairment, seizures, microcephaly, arrested development, and loss of speech. The vast majority of mutations in the *MECP2* gene that lead to Rett syndrome are new somatic mutations and not inherited. Rett syndrome patients, that harbor mutations in the *MECP2* gene, are heterozygous containing only one mutant gene. The reason that mutations in the X-linked *MECP2* gene manifest with disease almost exclusively in females is that these mutations are almost always lethal to male fetuses. None of the other options (choices B, C, D, and E) correlate the primary mode of acquisition of Rett syndrome.

18. Correct answer is **D.** Several classes of anticancer drugs function through interference with the actions of the topoisomerases. Two of these classes are the anthracyclines and the camptothecins. The anthracyclines inhibit the actions of topoisomerase II whose function is to introduce double-strand breaks in DNA during the process of replication as a means to relive torsional stresses. Anthracyclines also function by inducing the formation of oxygen free radicals that cause DNA strand breaks resulting in inhibition of replication. The taxanes (choice A) interfere with microtubule function causing inhibition of cytokinesis. The vinca alkaloids (choice B) also interfere with microtubule function. Alkylating drugs, such as cyclophosphamide, (choice C) induce intra-and inter-strand cross-linking of DNA resulting global loss of DNA replication. An antimetabolite (choice E) is a drug that interferes with nucleotide biosynthesis.

19. Correct answer is **E.** The patient is most likely experiencing the symptoms of Huntington disease. Huntington disease is caused by expansion of a CAG trinucleotide repeat in the first exon of the huntingtin gene (*HTT*). The range of CAG repeat size in normal individuals is 6–34 and in affected individuals it is 36–121. The longer the length of the CAG repeat the earlier is the onset of symptoms. None of the other options (choices A, B, C, and D) correlate to the cause of Huntington disease.

20. Correct answer is **C.** The molar ratio of adenosine (A) in any molecule of double-stranded DNA will be equivalent to that of thymidine (T), since these two nucleotides hydrogen bond to form base-pairs. Therefore, the total amount of the DNA accounted for in A-T base-pairs would be 40%. Since guanosine (G) and cytidine (C) hydrogen bond to form base-pairs, they too contribute an equivalent molar ratio in double-stranded DNA. In double-stranded DNA with 40% A-T composition, the molar ratio of cytidine would be half of the remaining 60% of the DNA, or 30%. None of the other options (choices A, B, D, and E) correctly corresponds to the amount of cytidine that would be present in a DNA molecule containing 20% adenine.

21. Correct answer is **E.** The patient is most likely manifesting the signs and symptoms of the Prader-Willi syndrome. Prader-Willi syndrome (PWS) is characterized by a failure to thrive in the neonatal period accompanied by muscular hypotonia. During early childhood PWS patients exhibit hyperphagia (excessive hunger and abnormally large intake of solid foods), obesity, hypogonadism, sleep apnea, behavior problems, and mild to moderate intellectual impairment. Additionally, PWS children have small hands and feet. In prepubertal males the hypogonadism results in sparse body hair, poor development of skeletal muscles, and delay in epiphyseal closure which resulting in long arms and legs. PWS results from the loss of a group of genes exclusively expressed from the paternal genome due to a deletion of a region of the q arm of the paternal chromosome 15. These genes are hypermethylated on the q arm of the maternal chromosome 15 and are, therefore, not expressed from this chromosome. This phenomenon of DNA methylation regulated, and parental origin-specific gene expression is referred to as genomic imprinting. None of the other options (choices A, B, C, and D) correctly underlies the phenomenon of genomic imprinting and is associated parental-specific origin of gene expression.

22. Correct answer is **B.** Cyclin D activates the cyclin dependent kinases, CDK4 and CDK6 (most often designated as CDK4/6). One of the functions of the cyclin D-CDK4 complex is to phosphorylate the tumor suppressor protein pRB. The normal function of pRB is to prevent the transcriptional activity of members of the E2F family through the formation of a complex with E2F. Phosphorylation of pRB results in release of E2F, thereby, allowing E2F to transcriptionally activate target genes. In the context of cell cycle regulation, the transcription factor E2F activates the expression of cyclin A, cyclin E, and CDK2. Therefore, loss of cyclin D activity by addition of the novel compound would lead to reduced levels of active E2F. None of the other proteins (choices A, C, D, and E) would be directly affected by inhibition of cyclin D.

23. Correct answer is **A.** The patient is most likely exhibiting the signs and symptoms of Angelman syndrome. The characteristic clinical spectrum of Angelman syndrome include microcephaly, seizure disorder, ataxia, muscular hypotonia with hyperreflexia, and motor delay. The psychomotor delay in AS patients is evident by 6 months of age and is associated with hypotonia and feeding difficulties. Angelman syndrome is the result of mutations or deletions in the gene, *UBE3A*, encoding a ubiquitin ligase. This gene resides in the same region of the q arm of chromosome 15 that is associated with Prader-Willi syndrome (choice E). The gene is hypermethylated on the paternal chromosome and, therefore, is not expressed. Huntington disease (choice B) is a late-onset disorder associated with trinucleotide repeat expansion in the *HTT* gene. Mitochondrial depletion syndrome (choice C) represents a constellation of mitochondrial encephalomyopathies resulting from deletions of DNA from the mitochondrial genome, mtDNA. Myotonic dystrophy type 1 (choice D) is a disorder caused by trinucleotide repeat expansion in the *DM1* gene. The characteristic clinical manifestation in myotonic dystrophy is myotonia (muscle hyperexcitability) and muscle degeneration. Affected individuals will also develop insulin resistance, cataracts, heart conduction defects, testicular atrophy, hypogammaglobulinemia, and sleep disorders. Symptoms of myotonic dystrophy can manifest in the adult or in childhood.

24. Correct answer is **A.** The anaphase promoting complex (APC) is a ubiquitin ligase that controls the levels of the M-phase cyclins as well as other regulators of mitosis. One important function of APC is to control the initiation of sister chromatid separation which begins at the metaphase-anaphase transition. The attachment of the sister chromatids to the opposite poles of the mitotic spindles occurs early during mitosis. The ability of the sister chromatids to be pulled apart is initially inhibited because they are bound together by a protein complex termed the cohesin complex. The cohesin complex is deposited along the chromosomes as they are duplicated during S-phase. Anaphase can only begin with the disruption of the cohesin complex. The breakdown of the cohesin complex is brought about as a consequence of the activation of the ubiquitin ligase activity of the APC. APC targets a protein called securin. Securin functions to inhibit the protease called separase and the action of separase is to degrade the proteins of the cohesin complex, thus allowing sister chromatid separation. Therefore, the induced mitotic arrest in these cells is most likely the result of interference with the function of functional APC. Given the associated mitotic arrest, none of the other proteins (choices B, C, D, and E) are likely to be the targets of the compound used in these studies.

25. Correct answer is **E.** One major function of the p53 protein is to serve as a component of the checkpoint that controls whether cells enter, as well as progress through, S-phase of the cell cycle. The action of p53 is induced in response to DNA damage. Under normal circumstances p53 is in the cytosol and its levels remain very low due to its interaction with a member of the ubiquitin ligase family called MDM2. In response to DNA damage, such as resulting from UV irradiation or γ-irradiation, cells activate several kinases including checkpoint kinase 2 (CHK2) and ataxia telangiectasia mutated (ATM). One target of these kinases is p53. ATM also phosphorylates MDM2. When p53 is phosphorylated, it is released from MDM2 and migrates into the nucleus where it can carry out its transcriptional activation functions. One target of p53 is the gene encoding the cyclin inhibitor, $p21^{Cip1}$. Activation of $p21^{Cip1}$ leads to increased inhibition of the cyclin D1-CDK4 and cyclin E-CDK2 complexes thereby halting progression through the cell cycle either prior to S-phase entry or during S-phase. Defects in none of the other activities (choices A, B, C, and D) would result in unregulated replication of damaged DNA.

26. Correct answer is **B.** The patient is most likely exhibiting the symptoms associated with the disorder known as ataxia telangiectasia, AT. AT is an autosomal recessive disorder that is characterized by hypersensitivity to ionizing radiation, progressive truncal ataxia affecting the gait with onset by 1–3 years of age, slurring of speech, oculocutaneous telangiectasias that begin to develop by age 6, frequent infections and cellular immunodeficiencies, and susceptibility to leukemias and lymphomas. Telangiectasias are areas of the skin under which there are dilated superficial vessels resulting in an appearance similar to that in patients with rosacea or scleroderma. AT results from mutations in the ataxia telangiectasia mutated (*ATM*) gene. The ATM protein is a member of the large molecular weight protein kinase family. Specifically, ATM is a member of the phosphatidylinositol-3-kinase (PI3K) family of kinases. The ATM kinase responds to DNA damage (specifically double-strand DNA breaks) by initiating the phosphorylation of several hundred proteins involved in DNA repair and/or cell cycle control. Defects in none of the other processes (choices A, C, D, E, and F) are associated with the signs and symptoms of ataxia telangiectasia.

27. Correct answer is **B.** The normal function of pRB is to prevent the transcriptional activity of members of the E2F family through the formation of a complex with E2F. Phosphorylation of pRB results in release of E2F, thereby, allowing E2F to transcriptionally activate target genes. In the context of cell cycle regulation, the transcription factor E2F activates the expression of cyclin A, cyclin E, and CDK2. Therefore, loss of pRB function would result in increased activity of E2F. Interference with the function of pRB would not lead to increased activity of any of the other proteins (choices A, C, D, and E).

28. Correct answer is **A.** The majority of C to T transition mutations found in cancers are located to CpG dinucleotides.

Many of the C residues, in these CpG dinucleotides, are methylated (m^5CpG). Cytosine in DNA can undergo spontaneous hydrolytic deamination resulting in conversion of the nucleotide to uracil. This deamination gives rise to G-U mispairs. Spontaneous hydrolytic deamination of 5-methylcytosine gives rise to G-T mispairs. These mispairs need to be repaired to G-C in order to avoid the C to T transition mutation. Restoration of both G-T and G-U mismatches is mediated by a short-patch excision repair pathway. There are two enzymes in this pathway, one is uracil DNA glycosylase, and the other is thymine DNA glycosylase. The thymine DNA glycosylase has been shown to have the potential to specifically remove thymine and uracil bases mispaired with guanine. None of the other options (choices B, C, D, and E) correctly defines high rate of mutation at m^5CpG dinucleotides.

29. Correct answer is **E.** The term epigenetics was first coined by Conrad Waddington in 1939 to define the unfolding of the genetic program during development. In addition, he coined the term epigenotype to define "the total developmental system consisting of interrelated developmental pathways through which the adult form of an organism is realized." Clearly this definition encompasses a broad range of concepts dealing with genetics, inheritance, and development. Today the term epigenetics is used to define the mechanism by which changes in the pattern of inherited gene expression occur in the absence of alterations or changes in the nucleotide composition of a given gene. A literal interpretation is that epigenetics means "in addition to changes in genome sequence." None of the other options (choices A, B, C, and D) correctly define the meaning of epigenetics.

30. Correct answer is **E.** The patient is most likely exhibiting the signs and symptoms of Rett syndrome. Rett syndrome is an X-linked disorder resulting from mutations in gene (*MECP2*) encoding the protein identified as methyl-CpG binding protein 2 (MeCP2). Rett syndrome is a neurodevelopmental disorder that occurs almost exclusively in females manifesting as intellectual impairment, seizures, microcephaly, arrested development, and loss of speech. The function of the MeCP2 protein is exerted through its ability to recognize and bind to regions of methylated DNA. When MeCP2 binds to methylated CpG dinucleotides the DNA takes on a closed chromatin structure and leads to transcriptional repression. Defects in the role of MECP2 in the control of transcriptional regulation is the molecular basis of the phenotype of Rett syndrome patients. Defects in none of the other processes (choices A, B, C, D, and F) are associated with the pathology of Rett syndrome.

31. Correct answer is **B.** The patient is most likely experiencing the symptoms of Huntington disease. Huntington disease is caused by expansion of a CAG trinucleotide repeat in the first exon of the huntingtin gene (*HTT*). The range of CAG repeat size in normal individuals is 6–34 and in affected individuals it is 36–121. The longer the length of the CAG repeat the earlier is the onset of symptoms. The classical symptoms of Huntington disease consist of progressive dementia, evolving involuntary movements and psychiatric disturbances that include personality changes and mood disorder. Choreiform movements are the most prominent physical abnormality in HD and as such the disease was early on referred to as Huntington chorea. Fragile X syndrome (choice A) results from expansion of a trinucleotide repeat in the promoter region of the *FMR1* gene. The characteristic symptoms of fragile X syndrome in males are moderate to severe intellectual impairment, a long narrow face, prominent ears, and macroorchidism (large testicles). Mitochondrial depletion syndrome (choice C) represents a constellation of mitochondrial encephalomyopathies resulting from deletions of DNA from the mitochondrial genome, mtDNA. Myotonic dystrophy type 1 (choice D) is a disorder caused by trinucleotide repeat expansion in the *DM1* gene. The characteristic clinical manifestation in myotonic dystrophy is myotonia (muscle hyperexcitability) and muscle degeneration. Affected individuals will also develop insulin resistance, cataracts, heart conduction defects, testicular atrophy, hypogammaglobulinemia, and sleep disorders. Symptoms of myotonic dystrophy can manifest in the adult or in childhood. Prader-Willi syndrome, PWS, (choice E) is characterized by childhood obesity, hypogonadism, sleep apnea, behavior problems, and mild to moderate intellectual impairment. PWS results from the loss of a group of genes exclusively expressed from the paternal genome due to a deletion of a region of the q arm of the paternal chromosome 15. These genes are hypermethylated on the q arm of the maternal chromosome 15 and are, therefore, not expressed from this chromosome.

32. Correct answer is **E.** The patient is most likely exhibiting the signs and symptoms of Prader-Willi syndrome (PWS). PWS and Angelman syndrome (AS) were the first diseases associated with the process of genomic imprinting. PWS results from the loss of a group of paternal-specific expressed genes in the chromosome 15q11.2-q13 region, whereas, AS results from loss of a maternal-specific expression, within neurons, of a ubiquitin ligase gene (*UBE3A*) in the same chromosomal region. PWS is characterized by failure to thrive in the neonatal period accompanied by muscular hypotonia. During early childhood, PWS patients exhibit hyperphagia (excessive hunger and abnormally large intake of solid foods), obesity, hypogonadism, sleep apnea, behavior problems, and mild to moderate intellectual impairment. Hypogonadism is present in both males and females. A distinctive behavioral phenotype of PWS is temper tantrums, stubbornness, and manipulative and compulsive behaviors. Additionally, PWS children have small hands and feet. In prepubertal males the hypogonadism results in sparse body hair, poor development of skeletal muscles, and delay in epiphyseal closure resulting in long arms and legs. Deletions from the p arm of chromosome 5 (choice A) are the cause of cri-du-chat syndrome. Patients with cri-du-chat syndrome typically present with a high-pitched, cat-like cry, intellectual disability, delayed development, and distinctive facial features that include widely spaced eyes, a broad, flattened bridge of the nose, and a round face. Deletion of a portion of the p arm of chromosome 11 (choices B and C) is the cause of Beckwith-Weideman syndrome, BWS. The cardinal features of BWS are exomphalos (an umbilical hernia at birth in which some abdominal organs push into the umbilical cord), macroglossia (an enlarged tongue), and gigantism (specifically embryonic and placental overgrowth). These three cardinal symptoms led to an original designation of this disorder as EMG syndrome. Expansion of the CCG trinucleotide repeat in the *FMR1* gene (choice F) is the cause of fragile X syndrome. The characteristic symptom observed in males with fragile X syndrome is moderate to severe intellectual impairment. The physical hallmarks of the disorder include a long narrow face, prominent ears, and macroorchidism (large testicles). Fragile X syndrome also manifests with distinct behavioral abnormalities that include hyperactivity, anxiety, extreme sensitivity to stimulation and

sensations, hyperarousal and occasionally aggressive tendencies. Trisomy 21 (choice G) is the cause of Down syndrome. Down syndrome patients present with short stature, delayed speech, developmental delay, learning disability, and characteristic facial features that include down-slanting eyes, a flat nasal bridge, and small ears.

33. Correct answer is **E.** The patient is most likely exhibiting the signs and symptoms of Prader-Willi syndrome (PWS). PWS results from the loss of a group of paternal-specific expressed genes in the chromosome 15q11.2-q13 region. During early childhood PWS patients exhibit hyperphagia (excessive hunger and abnormally large intake of solid foods), obesity, hypogonadism, sleep apnea, behavior problems, and mild to moderate intellectual impairment. PWS is also characterized by failure to thrive in the neonatal period accompanied by muscular hypotonia. Hypogonadism is present in both males and females. A distinctive behavioral phenotype of PWS is temper tantrums, stubbornness, and manipulative and compulsive behaviors. Additionally, PWS children have small hands and feet. In prepubertal males the hypogonadism results in sparse body hair, poor development of skeletal muscles, and delay in epiphyseal closure resulting in long arms and legs. Choreiform movements (choice A) are associated with Huntington disease, tardive dyskinesia, and Sydenham's chorea. Choreiform movements are characterized by brief, rapid, irregular, and jerky involuntary movements. Hemolytic anemia (choice B) is not found associated with PWS. Intention tremors (choice C) are associated with disorders that affect the cerebellum, but they are not associated with PWS. Intention tremors are a type of tremors that worsens with movement toward a target. PWS is associated with microorchidism (hypogonadism) not macroorchidism (choice D). Macroorchidism is a common feature of the trinucleotide repeat disorder, fragile X syndrome.

34. Correct answer is **C.** The patient is most likely exhibiting the signs and symptoms of Angelman syndrome (AS). Angelman syndrome, as well as Prader-Willi syndrome, was one of the first diseases associated with the process of genomic imprinting. AS results from loss of neuron-specific maternal, not paternal (choice D) expression of a ubiquitin ligase gene (*UBE3A*) in the chromosome 15q11.2-q13 region. The characteristic clinical spectrum of Angelman syndrome includes microcephaly, seizure disorder, ataxia, muscular hypotonia with hyperreflexia, and motor delay. The psychomotor delay in AS patients is evident by 6 months of age and is associated with hypotonia and feeding difficulties. The microcephaly is not apparent at birth but develops within the first 3 years. The seizure disorder associated with AS typically develops between the first and third years of life. Deletion of a portion of the p arm of chromosome 11 (choices A and B) is the cause of Beckwith-Weideman syndrome (BWS). The cardinal features of BWS are exomphalos (an umbilical hernia at birth in which some abdominal organs push into the umbilical cord), macroglossia (an enlarged tongue), and gigantism (specifically embryonic and placental overgrowth). These three cardinal symptoms led to an original designation of this disorder as EMG syndrome. Trinucleotide repeat within the *DMPK* gene (choice E) is the cause of myotonic dystrophy, type 1. The characteristic clinical manifestation in myotonic dystrophy is myotonia (muscle hyperexcitability) and muscle degeneration. Symptoms of myotonic dystrophy can manifest in the adult or in childhood. Trinucleotide repeat within the *FMR1* gene (choice F) is the cause of fragile X syndrome. The characteristic symptom observed in males with fragile X syndrome is moderate to severe intellectual impairment. The physical hallmarks of the disorder include a long narrow face, prominent ears, and macroorchidism (large testicles). Fragile X syndrome also manifests with distinct behavioral abnormalities that include hyperactivity, anxiety, extreme sensitivity to stimulation and sensations, hyperarousal and occasionally aggressive tendencies.

35. Correct answer is **E.** The patient is most likely experiencing the signs and symptoms of xeroderma pigmentosa (XP). Xeroderma pigmentosum defines a class of autosomal recessive inherited diseases that are clinically characterized by sun sensitivity that results in progressive degeneration of sun-exposed areas of the skin and eyes. There are currently eight alleles whose mutations result in manifestation of XP. Seven of the genes are involved in processes of nucleotide excision repair (NER). NER involves the removal of a wide array of structurally unrelated DNA lesions including thymine (pyrimidine) dimers that are produced in human skin by shortwave UV light. Most often the skin changes in XP patients will result in neoplasia. In most XP patients the initial symptoms are an abnormal reaction to sun exposure which includes severe sunburn with blistering and persistent erythema with minimal exposure to the sun. Most XP patients will develop xerosis (dry skin) and poikiloderma. Poikiloderma is defined as areas of the skin exhibiting increased pigment alternating with areas of reduced pigment, atrophy, and telangiectasias. Telangiectasias are areas of the skin under which there are dilated superficial vessels resulting in an appearance similar to that in patients with rosacea or scleroderma. Additional benign lesions in the skin include actinic keratoses (scaly crusty bumps), keratoacanthomas (well-differentiated squamous cell carcinoma), angiomas (benign tumors composed of blood vessels at or near the surface of the skin), and fibromas (benign tumors of connective tissue). Base excision repair, BER (choice A) is a process of removing many types of DNA lesions including alkylations, oxidations, deaminations and depurinations, as well as single-strand breaks (SSB). Defects in BER are associated with premature aging and cancers, but generally not skin cancers. Double-strand break (DSB) repair (choice B) is the process that repairs DNA lesions where the phosphate-sugar backbones of both DNA strands are broken at the same position (or in close proximity to each other) which allows for physical dissociation of the double helix into two separate molecules. Mutations in any of the genes responsible for DSB are associated with increased cancer susceptibility, neurological defects, and/or immunodeficiencies. Several disease syndromes such as ataxia telangiectasia (AT), Nijmegen breakage syndrome, and some forms of severe combined immunodeficiency (SCID) are associated with defects in DSB repair. Defects in the mismatch repair process (choice C) is a common feature of Lynch syndrome, a disorder typified by colorectal carcinoma. Defects in the *NF1* gene (choice D) are the causes of neurofibromatosis type 1 (NF1) which is also known as von Recklinghausen disease. NF1 is classified as a tumor predisposition syndrome characterized by the development of multiple neurofibromas, café-au-lait spots, and Lisch nodules. Defects in the *RB1* gene (choice F) result in the childhood cancer, retinoblastoma. Inherited defects in the *TP53* gene (choice G) are the cause of Li Fraumeni syndrome (LFS), a disorder associated with brain tumors, sarcomas, leukemia, and breast cancer.

C H A P T E R

23

Eukaryotic RNA

High-Yield Terms

Promoter	Sequences in the gene that promote the ability of RNA polymerases to recognize the nucleotide at which initiation begins, must reside close to the gene and in a specific orientation for activity
Enhancer	Sequences that act in *cis* by binding proteins that result in enhancement of transcription, can be located long distance from the gene or even on different chromosomes, also do not require orientation for activity
RNA editing	A novel enzymatic mechanism for the modification of nucleotide sequences of RNA resulting in altered coding capacity
Small non-coding RNAs	Includes the small nuclear RNAs (snRNAs) of the splicing machinery, the microRNAs (miRNAs) derived from noncoding genes that are involved in processes of expression control, and the small interfering RNAs (siRNAs) responsible for the process of RNA-mediated interference (RNAi) in gene expression
Ribozyme	An enzyme activity solely associated with an RNA molecule, such as the peptidyltransferase activity of the large ribosomal subunit

CLASSES OF EUKARYOTIC RNA

Eukaryotic RNAs exist in a wide array of functional sizes from tens of ribonucleotides to several thousand (Table 23–1). The vast array of RNAs serve numerous functions including the regulation of X chromosome inactivation, the control of transcription and RNA processing, control of translation, and the actual synthesis of proteins.

The broad classifications of RNAs include ribosomal RNAs (rRNA), transfer RNAs (tRNA), messenger RNAs (mRNA), small noncoding RNAs (sncRNA), and long noncoding RNAs (lncRNA). Whereas each of these broad classifications includes many different RNAs, the rRNA family in humans is composed of four members. The 28*S*, 5*S*, and 5.8*S* rRNAs are associated with the large ribosomal subunit and the 18*S* rRNA is associated with the small ribosomal subunit.

EUKARYOTIC RNA POLYMERASES

In eukaryotic cells there are three distinct classes of RNA polymerase, RNA polymerase I (po I), RNA pol II, and RNA pol III. Each polymerase is responsible for the synthesis of specific subsets RNAs. In a general sense RNA pol I is responsible for rRNA synthesis, RNA pol II is responsible for mRNA synthesis, and RNA pol III is responsible for tRNA synthesis. The vast majority of sncRNAs and lncRNAs are transcribed by RNA pol II.

TRANSCRIPTION OF EUKARYOTIC RNA

RNA synthesis requires accurate and efficient initiation, elongation proceeds in the 5′→3′ direction (ie, the polymerase moves along the template strand of DNA in the 3′→5′ direction), and requires distinct and accurate termination.

Initiation of transcription, particularly the transcription of mRNA genes, is tightly regulated by transcription factors, some of which bind directly to DNA sequences (Figure 23–1). Sequences in the template DNA act in *cis* to stimulate the initiation of transcription. These sequence elements are termed **promoters** and **enhancers**.

Promoter sequences are generally found in all mRNA genes, are most often closely associated with the transcriptional start site, and they are binding sites for transcription factors that are not cell type or tissue specific. Two promoter elements found in almost all mRNA genes upstream of the transcription start site are the TATA-box and the CAAT-box (see Figure 23–1). Because the start site for transcription is identified as the +1 nucleotide, the position of promoter elements is denoted by a minus sign such as −25 typical of the location of the TATA-box.

TABLE 23–1 Classes of eukaryotic RNA.

RNA	Types	Abundance	Stability
Ribosomal (rRNA)	28S, 18S, 5.8S, 5S	80% of total	Very stable
Messenger (mRNA)	~10^5 Different species	2–5% of total	Unstable to very stable
Transfer (tRNA)	~60 Different species	~15% of total	Very stable
Small RNAs			
Small nuclear (snRNA)	~30 Different species	≤1% of total	Very stable
Micro (miRNA)	100s-1000	<1% of total	Stable

Adapted with permission from Rodwell VW, Bender DA, Botham KM, et al: *Harper's Illustrated Biochemistry*, 31st ed. New York, NY: McGraw Hill; 2018.

TABLE 23–2 Summary of the properties of enhancers to work when located long distances from the promote.

- Work when located long distances from the promoter
- Work when upstream or downstream from the promoter
- Work when oriented in either direction
- Can work with homologous or heterologous promoters
- Work by binding one or more proteins
- Work by facilitating binding of the basal transcription complex to the cis-linked promoter
- Work by recruiting chromatin-modifying coregulatory complexes

Reproduced with permission from Rodwell VW, Bender DA, Botham KM, et al: *Harper's Illustrated Biochemistry*, 31st ed. New York, NY: McGraw Hill; 2018.

Enhancer sequences (Table 23–2), on the other hand, are generally specific to a particular gene, do not reside near the start site for transcription (indeed can even reside within a gene), and are binding sites for cell type and/or tissue-specific transcriptional factors.

Eukaryotic mRNA transcriptional initiation is an extremely complex process that includes proteins common to all mRNA genes as well as cell-type specific proteins. The common (basal) transcription factors for RNA pol II were originally identified with the TFII designation (Figure 23–2). Although the TFII designation is still in wide use, the accepted nomenclature now uses the GTF acronym for general transcription factor.

Some of the TFII proteins bind directly to DNA, such as TFIID (also called TATA-box binding protein, TBP), while other TFII proteins interact with other transcription factors or RNA pol II itself.

One of the TFII factors, TFIIH, is actually a complex of many proteins. The TFIIH complex contains the kinase,

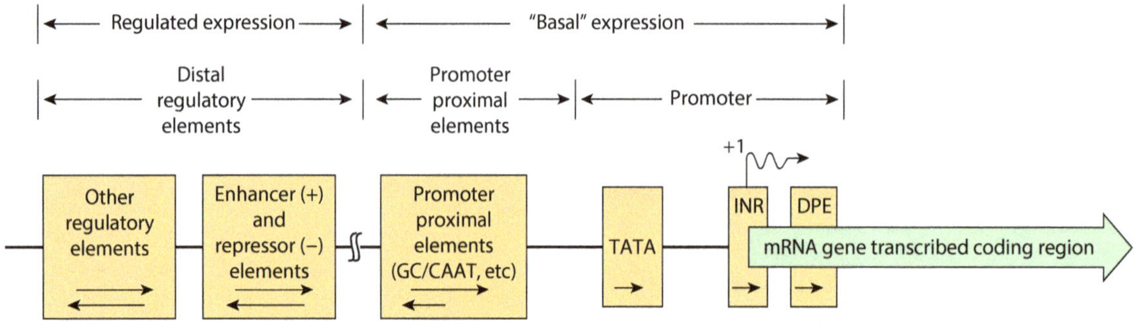

FIGURE 23–1 Schematic diagram showing the transcription control regions in a hypothetical mRNA-producing, eukaryotic gene transcribed by RNA polymerase II. Such a gene can be divided into its coding and regulatory regions, as defined by the transcription start site (arrow; +1). The coding region contains the DNA sequence that is transcribed into mRNA, which is ultimately translated into protein. The regulatory region consists of two classes of elements. One class is responsible for ensuring basal expression. The "promoter," is often composed of the TATA box and/or INR and/or DPE elements direct RNA polymerase II to the correct site (fidelity). However, in certain genes that lack TATA, the so-called TATA-less promoters, an initiator (INR) and/or DPE elements may direct the polymerase to this site. Another component, the upstream elements, specifies the frequency of initiation; such elements can either be proximal (50–200 bp) or distal (1000–105 bp) to the promoter as shown. Among the best studied of the proximal elements is the CAAT box, but several other elements (bound by the transactivator proteins Sp1, NF1, AP1, etc.) may be used in various genes. The distal elements enhance or repress expression, several of which mediate the response to various signals, including hormones, heat shock, heavy metals, and chemicals. Tissue-specific expression also involves specific sequences of this sort. The orientation dependence of all the elements is indicated by the arrows within the boxes. For example, the proximal promoter elements (TATA box, INR, DPE) must be in the 5′–3′ orientation, while the proximal upstream elements often work best in the 5′–3′ orientation, but some can be reversed. The locations of some elements are not fixed with respect to the transcription start site. Indeed, some elements responsible for regulated expression can be located interspersed with the upstream elements or can be located downstream from the start site. (Reproduced with permission from Rodwell VW, Bender DA, Botham KM, et al: *Harper's Illustrated Biochemistry*, 31st ed. New York, NY: McGraw Hill; 2018.)

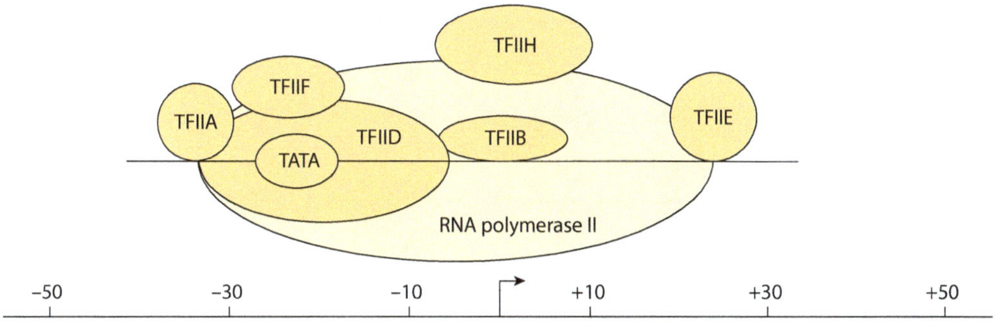

FIGURE 23–2 The eukaryotic basal transcription complex. Formation of the basal transcription complex begins when TFIID binds to the TATA box. It directs the assembly of several other components by protein-DNA and protein-protein interactions; TFIIA, B, E, F, H, and polymerase II (pol II). The entire complex spans DNA from position −30 to +30 relative to the transcription start site (TSS; +1, marked by bent arrow). The atomic level, x-ray-derived structures of RNA polymerase II alone and of the TBP subunit of TFIID bound to TATA promoter DNA in the presence of either TFIIB or TFIIA have all been solved at 3 Å resolution. The structures of TFIID and TFIIH complexes have been determined by electron microscopy at 30 Å resolution. Thus, the molecular structures of the transcription machinery are beginning to be elucidated. Much of this structural information is consistent with the models presented here. (Reproduced with permission from Murray RK, Bender DA, Botham KM, et al: *Harper's Illustrated Biochemistry*, 29th ed. New York, NY: McGraw Hill; 2012.)

cyclin-dependent kinase 7 (CDK7), that phosphorylates a specific serine residue in the C-terminal domain (CTD) of the large subunit of RNA pol II. The phosphorylation of the CTD of RNA pol II is required for mRNA transcription to initiate.

Elongation involves the addition of the 5′–phosphate of ribonucleotides to the 3′–OH of the elongating RNA with the concomitant release of pyrophosphate. Nucleotide addition pauses when the nascent mRNA is 20–30 nucleotides long. This pausing, a form of transcriptional attenuation, is required for the cap structure (see next section) to be added to the 5′-end of the new mRNA. Once the cap structure is added, transcription continues until specific termination signals are encountered. Following termination the core polymerase dissociates from the template.

CAPPING OF mRNA

The 5′ end of the vast majority of eukaryotic mRNAs is capped with a unique 5′→5′ linkage to a 7-methylguanosine residue (Figure 23–3). The capping process occurs when the nascent mRNA is around 20–30 bases long and RNA pol II pauses. Following cap addition, cyclin-dependent kinase 9 (CDK9) phosphorylates RNA pol II on a serine residue (different from that phosphorylated by CDK7) in the CTD of the large subunit of the enzyme. CDK9 is part of a complex called positive transcription elongation factor b (P-TEFB).

There are two critical functions of the 5′-cap on mRNAs. One is protection of the mRNA from ribonucleases and the

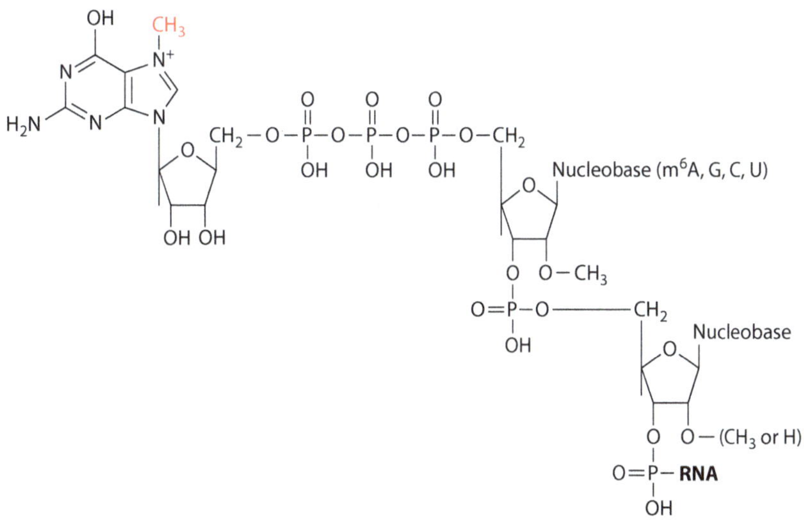

FIGURE 23–3 Structure of the 5′ cap found on eukaryotic mRNAs. (Reproduced with permission from King MW: *Integrative Medical Biochemistry Examination and Board Review*. New York, NY: McGraw Hill; 2014.)

other, more important function, is recognition of the mRNA by a specific protein complex of the translation machinery (see Chapter 24).

TERMINATION OF TRANSCRIPTION

Transcriptional termination of eukaryotic mRNA genes occurs when RNA pol II encounters the sequence, 3′-TTATTT-5′, in the template DNA which directs the incorporation of the termination and polyadenylation [poly(A)] signal, 5′-AAUAAA-3′ in the mRNA.

Following incorporation of the AAUAAA element into the mRNA, the cleavage and polyadenylation specificity complex, which is associated with the RNA pol II complex, recruits other proteins to the site. The proteins that are recruited then cleave the mRNA freeing it from the transcription complex and transcription terminates.

Termination of RNA pol I transcription requires an RNA pol I specific termination factor that is a DNA-binding protein. Termination of RNA pol III transcription occurs following the incorporation of a series of U residues in the transcript.

mRNA 3′-END POLYADENYLATION

Almost all mammalian mRNAs are polyadenylated at the 3′-end. A specific sequence, AAUAAA, is the primary sequence recognized by one of several proteins and multiprotein complexes. These protein complexes are responsible for catalyzing the mRNA cleavage and subsequent polyadenylation reactions. In mammals, the 3′-end cleavage and polyadenylation reactions are regulated by the interactions of several multiprotein complexes and the poly(A) polymerases (PAP).

SPLICING OF EUKARYOTIC RNA

Almost all mRNA, tRNA, and rRNA genes contain introns. The sequences encoded by introns become part of the newly synthesized RNAs and they must be removed to generate a functional RNA. The process of intron removal is referred to as RNA splicing.

Mammalian mRNA genes contain highly conserved consensus sequences that ultimately reside at the 5′ and 3′ ends of the introns in the mRNA (Figure 23–4). The process of intron removal is catalyzed by a specialized RNA–protein complex called the spliceosome. The spliceosome is composed of small nuclear ribonucleoprotein particles (snRNP, pronounced "snurp") that contain proteins and several sncRNAs identified as U1, U2, U4, U5, and U6.

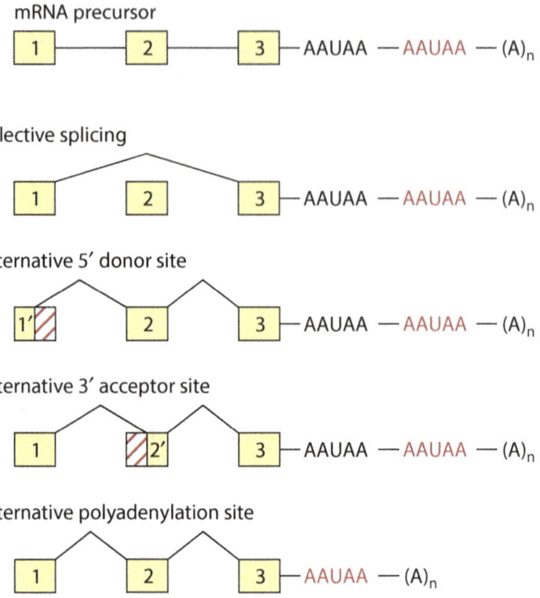

FIGURE 23–5 Mechanisms of alternative processing of mRNA precursors. This form of mRNA processing involves the selective inclusion or exclusion of exons, the use of alternative 5′ donor or 3′ acceptor sites, and the use of different polyadenylation sites. (Reproduced with permission from Rodwell VW, Bender DA, Botham KM, et al: *Harper's Illustrated Biochemistry*, 31st ed. New York, NY: McGraw Hill; 2018.)

ALTERNATIVE SPLICING

The presence of introns in RNAs allow for alternative splicing to occur, the result of which is the potential for an increase in phenotypic diversity without increasing the overall number of genes. By altering the pattern of exons that are spliced together, different proteins can arise from the processed mRNA from a single gene (Figure 23–5).

Alternative splicing allows for the generation of protein isoforms that exhibit different biological properties, that differ in protein-protein interaction, that are localized to different

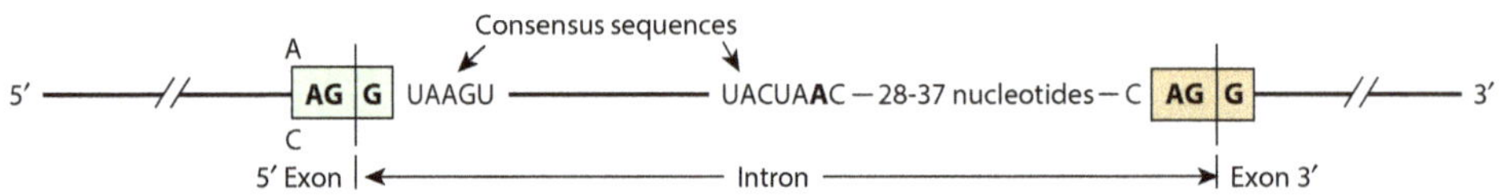

FIGURE 23–4 Consensus sequences at splice junctions. The 5′ (donor; left) and 3′ (acceptor; right) sequences are shown. Also shown is the yeast consensus sequence (UACUA A C) for the branch site. In mammalian cells, this consensus sequence is PyNPyPyPuAPy, where Py is a pyrimidine, Pu is a purine, and N is any nucleotide. The branch site is located at 20-40 nucleotides upstream from the 3′ splice site. (Reproduced with permission from Rodwell VW, Bender DA, Botham KM, et al: *Harper's Illustrated Biochemistry*, 31st ed. New York, NY: McGraw Hill; 2018.)

subcellular locations, or that exhibit different catalytic activities and/or abilities. The process of alternative splicing has been identified to occur in the primary transcripts from at least 80% of all human protein coding (mRNA) genes.

RNA EDITING

RNA editing refers to a process by which posttranscriptional change of nucleotide sequences of a given mRNA occurs via an enzymatic reaction involving deamination. There are two primary mRNA editing reactions that occur in mammalian cells. One involves deamination of cytidine (C) generating uridine (U) and the other involves the deamination of adenine (A) generating inosine (I). The deamination of C residues is catalyzed by cytidine deaminases, while deamination of A residues involves adenosine deaminases acting on RNA (ADAR).

An example of a physiologically and clinically significant C-to-U editing involves the apolipoprotein B (apoB) mRNA in humans (Figure 23–6). ApoB-100 is produced in the liver and apoB-48 is produced in the intestines. Following processing and splicing of the apoB mRNA in the liver, no further changes occur and the full-length apoB-100 protein is encoded. In the intestines, following processing and splicing of the apoB mRNA, the specific C residue is deaminated creating the stop codon. This results in the apoB-48 protein being encoded with the terminology reflecting that the protein is 48% of the full-length (apoB-100) protein.

SMALL NONCODING RNA (sncRNA)

The term noncoding RNA refers to any functional RNA that is not a protein coding RNA (mRNA). Both rRNA and tRNA are members of the large family of noncoding RNAs. Small noncoding RNA (sncRNA) refers to any functional endogenous RNA that is, generally, less than 200 nucleotides.

One class of sncRNA is the microRNA (miRNA or simply miR) family (Figure 23–7). This RNA family is a large subclass of sncRNA that are composed of approximately 22–25 nucleotides. The human genome contains more than 1900 miRNA genes. The processing and functioning of miRNAs is similar to that of the RNA silencing pathway identified in plants known as the posttranscriptional gene silencing (PTGS) pathway and the RNA inhibitory (RNAi) pathway activated on viral infection.

miRNAs interfere with the expression of target genes by forming RNA-RNA duplexes with specific regions of a target mRNA. The result of the interaction of a miRNA with a target mRNA can include inhibition of translation and/or directing the degradation of the target mRNA via recruitment of the RNA-induced silencing complex (RISC). In addition, miRNAs have been shown to interfere with gene expression through alterations in the processes of histone modification and DNA methylation at promoter sites in target genes. These effects represent a form of epigenetic regulation of gene expression.

The role of miRNA in the inhibition of gene expression has allowed for the development of a whole new class of pharmaceutical. The ability to introduce an miRNA-expressing construct

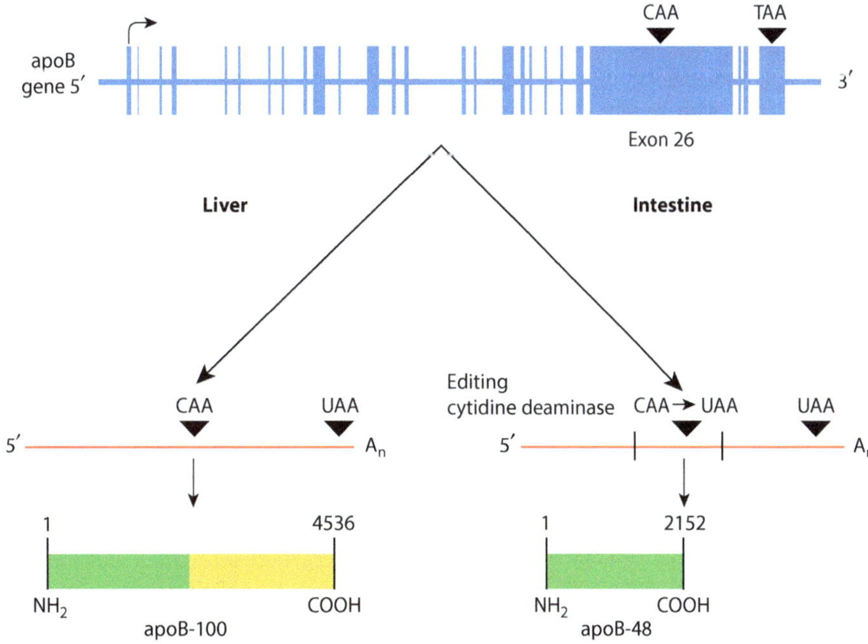

FIGURE 23–6 C-to-U editing of the apoB mRNA. In humans (and other mammals) the *apoB* gene is expressed in both hepatocytes and intestinal epithelial cells. In liver cells, the protein product is a 500-kD protein identified as apoB-100, whereas in intestinal cells the protein product is a smaller protein identified as apoB-48. The apoB-100 protein is translated from a nonedited mRNA, but the apoB-48 is translated from an edited mRNA. The C-to-U editing occurs in a CAA codon in exon 26 that results in the generation of a stop codon at that location in the edited mRNA, resulting in the truncation apoB-48 protein. The editing of the apoB mRNA is catalyzed by a cytidine deaminase. (Reproduced with permission from themedicalbiochemistrypage, LLC.)

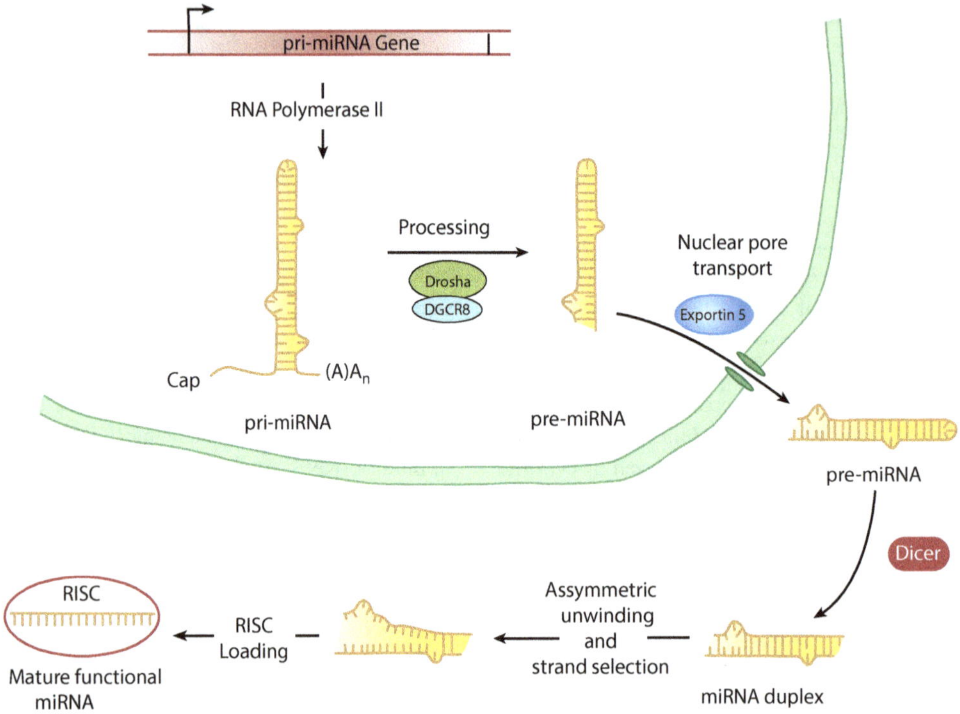

FIGURE 23–7 Biogenesis of miRNAs. miRNA-encoding genes are transcribed by RNA pol II into a primary miRNA transcript (pri-miRNA), which is 5′-capped and polyadenylated as is typical of mRNA coding primary transcripts. This pri-miRNA is subjected to processing within the nucleus by the action of the Drosha-DGCR8 nuclease, which trims sequences from both 5′ and 3′ ends, generating the pre-miRNA. This partially processed double-stranded RNA is transported through the nuclear pore by exportin-5. The cytoplasmic pre-miRNA is then trimmed further by the action of the multi-subunit nuclease termed Dicer, to form the miRNA duplex. One of the two resulting 21-22 nucleotide-long RNA strands is selected, the duplex unwound, and the selected strand loaded into the RISC complex, thereby generating the mature, functional miRNA. (Reproduced with permission from Murray RK, Bender DA, Botham KM, et al: *Harper's Illustrated Biochemistry*, 29th ed. New York, NY: McGraw Hill; 2012.)

into the body can result in a significant reduction in the expression of abnormal proteins associated with certain disease states (Table 23–3).

Equally important is the role of miRNAs in the development and progression of cancer. miRNAs, whose expression promotes cancer, are commonly referred to as onco-miRNA (or oncomiR), conversely there are miRNAs that function as tumor suppressors. The identification of circulating onco-miRNA may prove invaluable as biomarkers for classification of certain types of cancer.

TABLE 23–3 Diseases targeted for miRNA therapy.

Target RNA	Disease Indication
p53	Delayed graft function, acute kidney injury
SYK kinase	Asthma
VEGF	Primary and secondary liver cancer
VEGFR1	AMD
Bcr-abl oncogene	CML
β_2-adrenergic receptor	Glaucoma
ApoB	Hypercholesterolemia

Reproduced with permission from King MW: *Integrative Medical Biochemistry Examination and Board Review*. New York, NY: McGraw Hill; 2014.

LONG NONCODING RNAs (lncRNA)

The distinction for the term long noncoding RNA is that these RNA molecules are greater than 200 nucleotides. Most of the lncRNAs are posttranscriptionally processed like mRNAs, that is, they are capped, polyadenylated, and spliced. The subcellular localization of lncRNAs are diverse including nuclear, cytoplasmic, and extracellular. In addition to diverse localization, the functions of this class of RNA are also highly diverse.

Most of the lncRNAs (representing the two major classes of lncRNA) are transcribed from either intergenic regions (ie, between mRNA genes) or from the opposite strand of protein coding mRNA genes. The intergenic lncRNAs are referred to as large intergenic noncoding RNAs and given the designation, lincRNA. The lncRNAs that are transcribed across protein coding mRNA genes but in the opposite direction utilizing the opposite strand of DNA are referred to as natural antisense transcripts and given the designation, NAT. Of the two major lncRNA classes, the lincRNA class is by far the largest with over 10,000 identified genes.

lncRNAs, like the miRNAs, have important roles in the regulation of gene expression at both the transcriptional and post-transcriptional levels in diverse cellular contexts and in a variety of biological processes. The lncRNAs that remain in the nucleus have been shown to play roles in the integrity of the structure of the nucleus and in the regulation of expression of nearby genes. The lncRNAs localized to the cytosol exert *trans*-acting effects on gene expression by interacting with proteins and mRNAs. In the context of X chromosome inactivation the *XIST* gene encodes a lnRNA, the expression of which is absolutely required for X chromosome inactivation in females.

Mutations in *lncRNA* genes, as well as dysregulation in lncRNA functions, have been correlated to numerous disease states in humans. Indeed, the progression of diabetes, breast cancer, ovarian cancer, prostate cancer, hepatocellular cancer, colon cancer, lung cancer, and bladder cancer has been associated with abnormal lncRNA activity. Indeed, more than 200 human diseases have been shown to be associated with lncRNA activity.

CATALYTICALLY ACTIVE RNAs: RIBOZYMES

Ribozymes are RNAs with catalytic activity. Ribozymes function during protein synthesis in RNA-processing reactions and in the regulation of gene expression. Almost all ribozymes carry out a phosphoryl transfer reaction, catalyzing the cleavage or ligation of the RNA phosphodiester backbone. A notable exception is the peptidyl transferase activity of the ribozyme activity associated with the 28*S* subunit of the ribosome.

REGULATION OF EUKARYOTIC TRANSCRIPTION

The controls that act on eukaryotic gene expression are highly complex and occur at multiple points from the DNA and its structure to the biologically active protein (Table 23–4).

In order for RNA polymerases to access the transcriptional start site of a given gene they must obtain access to the DNA template. Due to the organization of chromatin which is regulated by the state of DNA methylation and the state of histone modification, as well as the presence or absence of transcriptional accessory proteins (transcription factors), RNA polymerase may or may not be able to activate transcription.

As outlined in Chapter 22, chromatin structure can be modified from a state which prevents transcription to one which promotes transcription by either of two major mechanisms: DNA methylation and/or histone modification. The CpG dinucleotides that can become methylated are found with much higher frequency in the regulatory regions of genes when compared to the rest of the genome. Histone acetylation is another major regulator

TABLE 23–4 Overview of gene expression control in eukaryotes.

Control Point	Properties
Chromatin structure	The physical structure of chromatin can affect the ability of transcriptional regulatory proteins and RNA polymerases to find access to specific genes and to activate transcription
Epigenetic	Refers to changes in the pattern of gene expression that are not due to changes in the nucleotide composition of the genome; involves DNA methylation and histone modifications
Transcriptional initiation	Specific factors that exert control include the strength of promoter elements, the presence or absence of enhancer sequences, and the interaction between multiple activator and inhibitor proteins
RNA processing and modification	mRNAs are capped, polyadenylated, and the introns must be accurately removed from all RNA classes
RNA transport	A fully processed mRNA must leave the nucleus in order to be translated into protein
RNA stability	Certain mRNAs have sequences that are signals for rapid degradation
Small noncoding RNAs (sncRNA)	sncRNA-mediated control can be exerted at numerous levels such as the translatability of the mRNA, the stability of the mRNA, the processing of mRNA, or via changes in chromatin structure
Long noncoding RNAs (lncRNA)	Function to regulate gene expression in both the nucleus and the cytosol; also involved in process of X chromosome inactivation (XCI)
Translational initiation	Many mRNAs have multiple methionine codons, the ability of ribosomes to recognize and initiate synthesis from the correct AUG codon can affect the expression of a gene product
Posttranslational modification	Multiple types of modifications including glycosylation, acetylation, fatty acylation, disulfide bond formations, etc.
Protein transport	To be biologically active, proteins must be transported to their site of action
Protein stability	Many proteins are rapidly degraded, whereas others are highly stable

of transcriptional initiation where the presence of acetylation is associated with higher transcriptional activity. Many transcriptional activator complexes contain histone acetyltransferase (HAT) activity, whereas transcriptional repressor complexes contain histone deacetylase (HDAC) activity.

The most complex controls observed in eukaryotic genes are those that regulate the expression of RNA pol II-transcribed genes, the mRNA genes. Eukaryotic mRNA genes contain a basic structure (see Figure 23–1) consisting of coding exons and noncoding introns and any number of different transcriptional regulatory domains that are sites for the interaction of various classes of transcription factor (Table 23–5). Several conserved structural motifs are found in most transcription factors including the helix-loop-helix, the zinc finger, and the leucine zipper.

The helix-loop-helix (HLH) domain is involved in protein homo- and heterodimerization. The HLH motif is composed of two regions of α-helix separated by a region of variable length which forms a loop between the two α-helices. The HLH class of transcription factor most often contains a region of basic amino acids located on the N-terminal side of the HLH domain (termed bHLH proteins) that is necessary in order for the protein to bind DNA at specific sequences.

The zinc finger domain is a DNA-binding motif consisting of specific spacing of cysteine and histidine residues that allow the protein to bind zinc atoms. The metal atom coordinates the sequences around the cysteine and histidine residues into a finger-like domain. The finger domains can lie within the major groove of the DNA helix.

The leucine zipper domain is necessary for protein homo- and heterodimerization. It is a motif generated by a repeating distribution of leucine residues spaced seven amino acids apart within α-helical regions of the protein. These leucine residues end up with their R-groups protruding from the α-helical domain and are thought to interdigitate with leucine R groups of another leucine zipper domain, thus stabilizing homo- or heterodimerization.

TABLE 23–5 Three classes of transcription factors involved in mRNA gene transcription.

General Mechanisms	Specific Components
Basal components	RNA Polymerase II, TBP, TFIIA, B, D, E, F, and H
Coregulators	TAFs (TBP + TAFs) = TFIID; certain genes Mediator, Meds Chromatin modifiers Chromatin remodelers
Activators	SP1, ATF, CTF, AP1, etc

Reproduced with permission from Rodwell VW, Bender DA, Botham KM, et al: *Harper's Illustrated Biochemistry*, 31st ed. New York, NY: McGraw Hill; 2018.

CHECKLIST

- ☑ RNAs are synthesized from a template of DNA by the action of RNA polymerases in a process termed transcription.
- ☑ Mammalian cells contain three distinct RNA polymerases involved in the transcription of nuclear DNA, identified as pol I, pol II, and pol III. Each polymerase transcribes a unique set of genes.
- ☑ The rate of transcription is controlled by a series of basal transcription factors and the concerted actions of gene specific transcriptional regulators (both activators and repressors).
- ☑ The basal transcription factors of RNA polymerase II are called TFII proteins. Two promoter elements that are present upstream of almost all mRNA genes (called the TATA-box and the CAAT-box) interact with members of the TFII family of basal factors.
- ☑ Transcription involves efficient, accurate, and regulated initiation, followed by elongation, and termination.
- ☑ Almost all eukaryotic RNAs (mRNA, tRNA, and rRNA) are synthesized as precursor molecules that undergo various post-transcriptional processing that includes intron removal (all classes), nucleotide modification (all tRNAs), capping, and polyadenylation (almost all mRNAs)
- ☑ Some mRNAs are edited following transcription which is an enzymatic modification of some of the nucleotides, resulting in altered coding capacity of the edited RNA.
- ☑ Ribozymes are a highly specialized class of RNA that possess enzymatic activity.
- ☑ Regulation of gene expression is a term that relates to the multiple processes that control the ability of a gene to be converted into a biologically active protein. Regulation of eukaryotic transcription is the most important mechanism for the regulation of gene expression.
- ☑ Numerous small noncoding RNAs and large noncoding RNAs are involved in the regulating gene expression. These include the small nuclear RNAs (snRNAs) that are involved in mRNA splicing, the micro RNAs (miRNAs)-directed mRNA degradation and translation repression processes, and the long noncoding RNA, encoded by the *XIST* gene, required for X chromosome inactivation.

REVIEW QUESTIONS

1. A mutant gene, suspected of causing a form of ovarian cancer, is being characterized. Analysis indicates that the gene is approximately 35 kilobases (kb) in length. Transcriptional studies show that there are several discrete mRNAs produced by this gene ranging in length from 4.0 to 5.5 kb in these cancerous cells. Which of the following processes is the most likely cause of the difference in size of the mRNAs produced by this gene?
   (A) Alternative splicing
   (B) Poly(A) addition
   (C) Posttranscriptional RNA processing
   (D) Recombination
   (E) RNA editing

2. A 34-year-old woman had chronic, mild hyperbilirubinemia (1.5–4.0 mg/dL) consisting of 90% unconjugated bilirubin (N = 0.2–0.7 mg/dL). Serum alanine aminotransferase (ALT) and aspartate aminotransferase (AST) levels were normal. Hemolysis was excluded as a cause of her condition. All five exons including the exon–intron junctions of the gene (*UGT1A*) encoding bilirubin UDP-glucuronosyltransferase were sequenced and found to be normal. A 247-nucleotide segment of the gene was sequenced and found to contain two additional nucleotides (TA) between nucleotides −23 and −38. Which of the following represents the most likely result of the observed mutation in this patient's *UGT1A* gene?
   (A) Frameshift mutation of the reading frame of the gene
   (B) In-frame mutation of the reading frame of the gene
   (C) Less than optimal binding RNA polymerase to the promoter
   (D) Missense mutation resulting in a one–amino acid change in the enzyme
   (E) Nonsense mutation resulting in a truncated enzyme

3. Experiments are being performed in order to characterize the products of *in vitro* transcription reactions. In one series of experiments, the following synthetic template of DNA is utilized. Which of the following is most likely the sequence of the resultant RNA after the *in vitro* transcription reaction in this system?

   Synthetic template: GCAATTGCAATTGCAATT
   (A) 3′-AAUUGCAAUUGCAAUUGC-5′
   (B) 5′-AAUUGCAAUUGCAAUUGC-3′
   (C) 3′-GCTTAAGCTTAAGCUUAA-5′
   (D) 5′-CGUUAACGUUAACGUUAA-3′
   (E) 3′-GCAAUUGCAAUUGCAAUU-5′
   (F) 5′-CGAAUUCGAAUUCGAAUU-3′

4. A 27-year-old man, who was diagnosed as HIV positive 2 years ago, is being examined by his physician with complaints of severe fatigue and a persistent cough for the past 3 weeks. During periods of coughing the patient reports that he often spits up bloody phlegm. The patient also reports that he has no appetite, has lost 6 lb in the past 3 weeks, and experiences night chills and night sweats. The physician makes a diagnosis and prescribes an appropriate pharmacologic intervention. Given the symptoms and treatment in this patient, which of the following is most likely to be observed?
   (A) Persistent diarrhea
   (B) Reddish colored urine
   (C) Renal failure
   (D) Severe skin rashes on sunlight exposed surfaces
   (E) Vestibular disturbances

5. Experiments are being performed to study lipoprotein metabolism utilizing cells in culture that are derived from an intestinal biopsy of a patient with a duodenal carcinoma. Results of these experiments find that the cancer-derived cells synthesize the same apolipoprotein composition contained in lipoproteins made in hepatocytes from the same patient. This contrasts with the different sizes generated from normal duodenal cells and normal hepatocytes. Which of the following processes is most defective accounting for the observations in the cancer-derived cells?
   (A) Alternative mRNA polyadenylation
   (B) Alternative mRNA splicing
   (C) Differential promoter utilization
   (D) mRNA 5′-capping
   (E) RNA editing

6. Experiments are being carried out to study the processes of RNA transcription utilizing cultures of cells derived from a patient with breast cancer. One result from these studies shows that whereas RNA polymerase II normally pauses shortly after the initiation of transcription to allow the mRNA to be modified at the 5′ end, the expected pausing does not occur in these cancer cells. The transcriptional pausing is triggered by the modification of RNA polymerase which the experiments find does not occur in the cancer cells. Which of the following most likely represents the modification that is lacking in these cancer cells?
   (A) Acetylation
   (B) Deacetylation
   (C) Demethylation
   (D) Dephosphorylation
   (E) Methylation
   (F) Phosphorylation

7. Experiments are being carried out to study the processes of RNA metabolism utilizing cultures of cells derived from a patient with pancreatic cancer. One result from these studies shows that these cells have a greatly reduced concentration of the U1 small nuclear RNA (snRNA). Which of the following is most likely to be impaired in these cells?
   (A) 5′-Capping of mRNAs
   (B) mRNA splicing
   (C) mRNA synthesis
   (D) Poly-A tail addition
   (E) rRNA synthesis

8. Experiments are being carried out to study the processes of RNA metabolism utilizing cultures of cells derived from a patient with duodenal cancer. Results from these experiments find that the gene encoding a cytidine deaminase (APOBEC1) is not expressed in these cells. Given these findings, which of the following is most likely to be absent from these cells?
   (A) ApoB-48
   (B) Ferritin
   (C) Ferroportin
   (D) Glutamate dehydrogenase
   (E) Hephaestin

9. Experiments are being carried out using a novel compound on cells in culture. The compound being tested is structurally related to suberoylanilide hydroxamic acid, a known histone

deacetylase inhibitor. Addition of this novel compound to the culture cells would most likely result in which of the following effects?
(A) Conversion of transcriptional coactivators into corepressors
(B) Conversion of transcriptional corepressors into coactivators
(C) General enhanced rate of transcription of numerous genes
(D) General reduced rate of transcription of numerous genes
(E) Would be expected to have no effect on transcription

10. *Experiments are being performed in order* to characterize the products of *in vitro* transcription reactions. In one series of experiments, the following RNA is generated in this system. Which of the following is most likely the sequence of the template strand of DNA from which this RNA was generated?

RNA: 5′-GCAAUUGCAATTGCAAUU-3′
(A) 3′-AATTGCAATTGCAATTGC-5′
(B) 5′-AATTGCAATTGCAATTGC-3′
(C) 3′-GCTTAAGCTTAAGCTTAA-5′
(D) 5′-CGTTAACGTTAACGTTAA-3′
(E) 3′-GCAATTGCAATTGCAATT-5′
(F) 5′-CGAATTCGAATTCGAATT-3′

11. Experiments have been carried out to develop a strain of transgenic mice that express a human β-globin gene. The transgenic construct includes all three exons of the human β-globin gene plus 500 nucleotides of both 5′- and 3′-flanking sequences. Examination of these transgenic mice shows that the human β-globin construct generates about 10-fold lower amounts of mRNA than the endogenous mouse β-globin gene. These results are most likely indicative of the lack of which of the following in the human DNA construct used to generate the transgenic mice?
(A) Gene-specific enhancer elements
(B) Polyadenylation signals
(C) Splice donor sequences
(D) Transcriptional silencing sequences
(E) Ubiquitous promoter elements

12. Experiments are being carried out on the effects of a novel compound on the activity of the glucocorticoid receptor (GR). Results from these experiments find that the compound prevents the chaperone, hsp90, from interacting with the GR. Given the results of this experiment, which of the following represents the most likely cellular location of the GR in the presence of this novel compound?
(A) Cytoplasmic surface of the plasma membrane
(B) Endoplasmic reticulum
(C) Golgi apparatus
(D) Nucleus bound to DNA
(E) Nucleus bound to pre-mRNAs

13. Experiments are being carried out in a cell-free system on the processes of tRNA synthesis and processing. The results of these experiments find that when a polymerase with tRNA nucleotidyltransferase activity is added to the system, the sequence, CCA, is added to the 3′ end of a synthetic tRNA. Which of the following characteristics best distinguishes this polymerase from eukaryotic RNA polymerase II?
(A) Can function in both the 5′ to 3′ and 3′ to 5′ directions
(B) Can use both mRNA and tRNA as substrates
(C) Performs its function without a template
(D) Requires only a GGU template
(E) Uses nucleoside monophosphate as substrates

14. Experiments are being carried out to determine the role of RNA processing using a compound designed to interfere with ribosomal RNA (rRNA) maturation. Results from these studies find that addition of the compound causes a significantly reduced amount of correctly processed 45S rRNA precursor. Failure of the precursor rRNA to be localized to which of the following subcellular locations is the most likely explanation of the inefficient processing?
(A) Cytosol
(B) Endoplasmic reticulum
(C) Golgi apparatus
(D) Nuclear matrix
(E) Nucleolus

15. Experiments are being conducted with a novel compound utilizing cultures of human fibroblasts. Results of the experiments show that when the compound is added to the cultures the level of expression of the *COL1A1* gene encoding a type 1 collagen increases by twofold but that the level of the encoded collagen protein increases 5-fold when compared to control untreated cells. Which of the following best explains these results?
(A) Enhanced polyadenylation of pre-mRNA
(B) Increased export of pre-mRNA to the cytosol
(C) Inhibition of mRNA degradation
(D) Inhibition of pre-mRNA splicing
(E) Retention of mRNA in the nucleus

16. A 47-year-old woman who is 16-weeks pregnant is undergoing amniocentesis to determine the likelihood her fetus will harbor trisomy 21. Analysis of the fetal chromosomes shows a normal complement of two copies of chromosome 21 but that there is an apparent amplification of the p arm of one of the two chromosomes. Which of the following is most likely to be increased in the cells of the fetus as a result of this amplification?
(A) Histone H1 mRNAs
(B) micro RNAs (miRNAs)
(C) Polyadenylated mRNAs
(D) Pre-ribosomal RNAs
(E) tRNAs

17. A 10-month-old infant has been rushed to the emergency department following a seizure. History reveals that the child has had difficulty feeding for the past several weeks and has had difficulty learning to crawl with tremors apparent in her legs when she attempts to crawl. Physical examination finds hypotonia, a head circumference smaller than expected for age, and hyperreflexia. Which of the following molecular mechanisms most likely accounts for the symptoms in this infant?
(A) Aberrant dissociation of RNA pol II from a critical gene
(B) Altered methylation of cytosine residues within a critical gene
(C) Alternative splicing of a critical gene
(D) Deletion of the promoter region of a critical gene
(E) Inhibition of mRNA splicing

18. Experiments are being caried out to examine the changes that have occurred in the genomes of members of a family susceptible to an inherited form of liver cancer. A candidate gene has been identified, and it harbors a deletion of a domain of the encoded protein that is predicted to interact with zinc ions. Which of the following is the most likely result of this mutation?

(A) Decreased binding of the protein to DNA
(B) Decreased binding of the protein to RNA
(C) Enhanced binding of a hormone to its receptor
(D) Interference with localization of the protein to the nucleus
(E) Retention of the protein in the endoplasmic reticulum

19. Experiments are being conducted to identify compounds that can interfere with the process of X chromosome inactivation. A candidate molecule has been identified based upon observations of its binding to an RNA molecule that is known to participate in X inactivation. Which of the following is the most likely type of RNA molecule to which the compound binds?
(A) Long noncoding RNA (lncRNA)
(B) Micro RNA (miRNA)
(C) mRNA
(D) rRNA
(E) tRNA

20. A 57-year-old man is being examined by his physician with concerns about his unstable posture and difficulty walking. The patient reports that he has been very moody lately and has been overcome with a sensation of great depression on numerous occasions. Physical examination finds the patient has difficulty swallowing and slightly slurred speech. History reveals that the patient's father had similar physical difficulties and died when he was 63. Therapeutic intervention based on the overexpression of which type of RNA molecule would prove most useful in this patient?
(A) Long noncoding RNA (lncRNA)
(B) Micro RNA (miRNA)
(C) mRNA
(D) rRNA
(E) tRNA

21. A 2-year-old boy is brought to the physician's office for evaluation of severe developmental delay. The parents say that his urine has always had a strange musty odor. Physical examination shows the boy has fair colored hair, pale skin, and pale blue irises. Molecular studies have determined that both alleles of the boy's phenylalanine hydroxylase (*PAH*) genes harbor a deletion of five nucleotides at the 5′-end of the second intron. Which of the following is the most likely result of this deletion?
(A) Inability of RNA polymerase II to complete transcription of the *PAH* gene
(B) Inability of RNA polymerase II to initiate transcription of the *PAH* gene
(C) Increased size of the PAH mRNA
(D) Loss of polyadenylation resulting in rapid degradation of the PAH mRNA
(E) Truncated size of the PAH mRNA

ANSWERS

1. Correct answer is **A.** The major mechanisms that result in multiple different sized mRNAs being produced from a single gene are alternative splicing, alternative promoter usage, and alternative polyadenylation signal sequence recognition. Of these three mechanisms, alternative splicing represents the major process by which different sized mRNAs result from the transcription of a single gene. Indeed, greater than 80% of all mRNAs undergo alternative splicing. Poly(A) addition (choice B) only adds up to several hundred adenine residues to the 3′ end of most mRNAs and, therefore, would not account for 1.5 kb differences in the mRNAs characterized in these cancer cells. Posttranscriptional RNA processing (choice C) includes both mRNA splicing and 3′ polyadenylation but since neither is specified this option is not the most correct answer. Recombination (choice D) can occur during meiosis as well as in somatic cells. In the context of somatic cells recombination predominantly occurs only in developing lymphocytes during B-cell maturation. RNA editing (choice E) only results in the modification of a single nucleotide within the edited mRNA and could not account for size differences of 1.5 kb.

2. Correct answer is **C.** The patient is most likely exhibiting the classic signs associated with the unconjugated hyperbilirubinemia called Gilbert syndrome. Gilbert syndrome is the result of a mutation in the TATA-box of the UDP-glucuronosyltransferase 1A (*UGT1A*) gene. The specific mutation converts the normal $A(TA)_6TAA$ of the TATA-box of the *UGT1A* gene to $A(TA)_7TAA$. This change causes a reduced ability of the gene to be transcriptionally active, thus less mRNA is made but the resulting translated protein is of normal size and function. All of the other options (choices A, B, D, and E) relate to protein synthesis which do not correlate to mutations upstream of the transcriptional start site as identified in the *UGT1A* gene in this patient.

3. Correct answer is **B.** Nucleic acid sequences are always presented in the 5′ to 3′ orientation unless specifically designated by inclusion of the 5′ and 3′ symbols. Therefore, the synthetic template is written 5′ to 3′. RNA is synthesized in the 3′ to 5′ direction with respect to the template DNA sequence which means that the 5′ nucleotide of the RNA is complementary to the last T residue (the 3′ nucleotide) in the template DNA and is, therefore an A residue. Since it is a given that the 5′ nucleotide of the RNA has to be an A there are only two RNAs that satisfy this requirement but the order of the G and C residues in choice C are incorrect. None of the other options (choices A, D, E, and F) correctly represent the RNA that would be transcribed from the synthetic template.

4. Correct answer is **B.** A very common complication in AIDS patients, due to their immunocompromised state, is infection with *Mycobacterium tuberculosis*. Symptoms of tuberculosis are cough (sometimes blood-tinged), weight loss, night sweats, and fever typical of the symptoms in this patient. The most common treatment for tuberculosis in AIDS patients is the use of the combination of isoniazid, rifampin, and ethambutol. The bactericidal function of rifampin is through its ability to inhibit prokaryotic RNA synthesis. One side effect of rifampin therapy is that urine appears reddish in coloration. Persistent diarrhea (choice A) is a side effect of many antibiotics but is not commonly observed with the drugs used to treat tuberculosis. Renal failure (choice C) is a complication associated with long-term use of aminoglycoside antibiotics. Severe skin rashes on sun exposed skin (choice D) can occur in patients using tetracyclines as an antibiotic. Vestibular disturbances (choice E) are the most common early onset complication of aminoglycoside use.

5. Correct answer is **E.** RNA editing is a molecular process through which some cells can make discrete changes to specific nucleotide sequences within a mRNA molecule after it has been generated by RNA polymerase and processed.

There are two major types of RNA editing with one being a C to U change catalyzed by cytidine deaminase that deaminates a cytidine base into a uridine base. An example of C-to-U editing is with the mRNA derived from the *APOB* gene. When the *ABOB* gene is transcribed in the liver the fully processed mRNA is translated into a protein identified as apoB-100 indicating that it contains 100% of the coding capacity of the mRNA. When the *APOB* gene is transcribed in intestinal enterocytes the resulting mRNA undergoes a C to U edit that introduces a stop codon into the mRNA. The result of this editing process is that the intestinal protein is shorter and is identified as apoB-48 indicating that it contains 48% of the original coding capacity of the mRNA. Given that the lipoprotein composition in cancer cells is identical to that of normal hepatocytes, it indicates that the process of RNA editing is defective. None of the other processes (choices A, B, C, and D) would effectively account for the observations in the cancer cells if they were abnormal.

6. Correct answer is **F.** The cancer cell derived RNA polymerase (pol) is most likely unable to be phosphorylated as normally occurs shortly after transcription begins. The 5′ ends of nearly all eukaryotic mRNAs are capped with a unique 5′→5′ linkage to a 7-methylguanosine residue. The capping process occurs after the newly synthesizing mRNA is around 20–30 bases long, at which point RNA pol II pauses. While RNA pol II is paused on the template, the kinase complex, known as positive transcription elongation factor b (P-TEFb), phosphorylates the catalytic enzyme of the RNA pol II complex (the *POLR2A* encoded enzyme) on the serine-2 residue (Ser2) in the repeat unit of the C-terminal domain (CTD). The P-TEFb complex is composed of cyclin-dependent kinase 9 (CDK9) and either cyclin T1, T2, or K. The complex is also called C-terminal domain kinase 1 (CTDK1). There are two isoforms of the T2 cyclin identified as T2a and T2b. All four of these cyclins can associate with CDK9 resulting in the formation of multiple different forms of P-TEFb. This pausing and regulatory phosphorylation event allows for the potential of attenuation in the rate of transcription. These cancer cells have most likely sustained a mutation in the *POLR2A* gene resulting in a catalytic subunit that does not become phosphorylated on the Ser2 residue typical of wild type catalytic subunit. None of the other modifications (choices A, B, C, D, and E) represent the modification that results in attenuated activity of RNA pol II.

7. Correct answer is **B.** The vast majority of mRNA encoding genes contain introns, the sequences of which are removed during the processing of the mRNAs. The removal of intronic RNA from precursor mRNA molecules requires a complex machinery termed the spliceosome. The spliceosome is composed of numerous small nuclear RNAs (snRNAs) and numerous proteins. The spliceosome catalyzes the reactions that result in intron removal and the joining together of the protein-coding exons. The spliceosome has been shown to be composed of as many as 300 distinct proteins and five RNAs. The five small nuclear RNAs (snRNAs) that constitute the spliceosome RNAs are identified as U1, U2, U4, U5, and U6. Lack of sufficient amounts of the U1 snRNA would ultimately result in a failure to properly splice mRNAs. None of the other processes (choices A, C, D, and E) would be significantly impaired in the absence of sufficient U1 snRNA.

8. Correct answer is **A.** The cytidine deaminase that is encoded by *APOBEC1* gene is involved in the process of RNA editing. RNA editing systems have been identified that result in changes in A residues to I residues, referred to as A-to-I editing systems, or changes in C residues to U residues, referred to as C-to-U editing systems. The enzymes that catalyze the A-to-I edits are members of a family of adenosine deaminases that act on RNA (ADAR). This distinguishes these enzymes from the adenosine deaminase involved in the catabolism and salvage of purine nucleotides. The enzymes that catalyze C-to-U edits are called cytosine deaminases that act on RNA (CDAR). The first identified C-to-U editing was within the mRNA encoding apolipoprotein B (apoB). Editing of the apoB mRNA changes a CAA codon (at amino acid 2180) to a UAA translational stop codon leading to premature termination of protein synthesis. When the apoB gene is transcribed within hepatocytes the mRNA is not edited and a full-length (100%) apoB protein is generated called apoB-100. Within intestinal enterocytes, the apoB mRNA is edited resulting in the generation of a smaller protein (48% of full-length) called apoB-48. The C-to-U editing of the apoB mRNA requires a functional complex that includes the editing enzyme, catalytic polypeptide 1 (APOBEC-1; the catalytic deaminase). Lack of expression of the *APOBEC1* gene would result in an inability of apoB mRNA editing. None of the other proteins (choices B, C, D, and E) are derived from edited mRNAs.

9. Correct answer is **C.** Modification of histone proteins is one of several mechanisms that confer control over the transcriptional activity of genes. One type of histone modification is acetylation and deacetylation. Histone acetylation is known to result in a more open chromatin structure and these modified histones are found in regions of the chromatin that are transcriptionally active. Conversely, under acetylation (deacetylation) of histones is associated with closed chromatin and transcriptional inactivity. A direct correlation between histone acetylation and transcriptional activity was demonstrated when it was discovered that protein complexes, previously known to be transcriptional activators, were found to have histone acetyltransferase (HAT) activity. And as expected, transcriptional repressor complexes were found to contain histone deacetylase (HDAC) activity. The inhibition of histone deacetylation would, therefore, be expected to be associated with an overall enhancement of transcription. None of the other options (choices A, B, D, and E) would be associated with the inhibition of histone deacetylation.

10. Correct answer is **B.** RNA is synthesized in the 3′ to 5′ direction with respect to the template DNA sequence which means that the 3′ nucleotide of the RNA (U) would be complementary to the 5′ nucleotide in the template DNA. Any U residue in an RNA is complementary to an A residue in the template strand of DNA. Therefore, the 5′ end of the template strand of DNA from which the RNA was derived must start with an A which is found in only choice B and choice C. However, the order of the G and C residues in choice C are incorrect. None of the other options (choices A, D, E, and F) correctly represent the template strand of DNA from which the RNA was transcribed.

11. Correct answer is **A.** Control of transcription can be exerted by the presence of specific DNA sequences identified as promoters and enhancers. Enhancer elements are *cis*-acting DNA sequences that can increase transcription of genes. Enhancers can usually function in either orientation as well as at various distances from the start site of transcription, or even from within the regulated gene itself. The β-globin construct

used to create the transgenic mice most likely did not include the appropriate enhancer element(s) that are present in the endogenous mouse β-globin gene, thereby accounting for the reduced expression of the transgene. Lack of none of the other mechanisms (choices B, C, D, and E) would correctly explain the transcriptional differences between the human β-globin construct and the endogenous mouse β-globin gene.

12. Correct answer is **D.** In the absence of ligand, the glucocorticoid receptor (GR) remains in the cytosol contained within multiprotein chaperone complexes. The cytosolic GR-containing complex includes heat-shock protein 90 (hsp90), hsp70, the co-chaperone identified as p23 (encoded by the prostaglandin E synthase 3, *PTGES3* gene), and various immunophilins (eg, FKBP51 and FKBP52), all of which prevent its degradation and assist in its maturation. In addition to maintaining the GR in the cytosol, the multiprotein complex facilitates high-affinity ligand binding. Upon ligand binding, the GR complex changes its conformation leading to release of the ligand-bound receptor and exposure of the two nuclear localization signals in the GR allowing for rapid transport into the nucleus. A compound that prevented the interaction of GR with hsp90 would most likely result in localization of the receptor to the nucleus. The GR would not likely be localized to any of the other locations (choices A, B, C, and E) in the absence of interaction with hsp90.

13. Correct answer is **C.** The posttranscriptional addition of the CCA trinucleotide to the 3′-end of all tRNAs is carried out by an RNA polymerase identified as tRNA nucleotidyltransferase 1 that is also referred to as ATP(CTP):tRNA nucleotidyltransferase or simply as CCase. The enzyme catalyzes the sequential addition of the CCA nucleotides in a template-independent but sequence-specific nucleotide polymerization reaction. This polymerase sequentially adds these three nucleotides to every tRNA transcript. The CCA terminus of all tRNAs is subjected to frequent turnover such that tRNA nucleotidyltransferase 1 has the additional responsibility to regenerate the CCA terminus and thus, the maintenance of the proper tRNA terminus. None of the other options (choices A, B, D, and E) correctly define the unique property of this RNA polymerase that distinguishes it from RNA pol II.

14. Correct answer is **E.** Ribosomal RNAs (rRNAs) are the most abundant noncoding RNAs. Transcription of ribosomal RNA genes, processing of pre-rRNA, and assembly of precursor 60S and 40S subunits occur in the nucleolus. In eukaryotes, three of the four ribosomal RNAs forming the 40S and 60S subunits are derived from a long polycistronic pre-ribosomal RNA. A complex sequence of processing steps is required to gradually release the mature RNAs from this precursor. Within the eukaryotic primary rRNA transcript, the mature 18S, 5.8S, and 28S rRNAs are separated by the internal transcribed spacers 1 (ITS1) and 2 (ITS2) and flanked by the 5′ and 3′ external transcribed spacers (5′-ETS and 3′-ETS). The nascent primary transcripts associate co-transcriptionally with numerous pre-ribosomal factors (PRFs), and small nucleolar ribonucleoprotein particles (snoRNPs). This complex carries out the sequential removal of the transcribed spacers through a complex series of endonucleolytic and exonucleolytic cleavages. None of the other subcellular locations (choices A, B, C, and D) represent the correct location of rRNA synthesis and processing.

15. Correct answer is **C.** Regulation of gene expression refers to the collective processes that control the amount of functional protein generated from a given gene. These regulatory processes include, but is not limited to, activation of transcription, processing of mRNA, stability of the mRNA, regulation of translational initiation, processing of protein, localization of protein, and stability of the protein. The disconnect between the level of gene expression which results in mRNA increases and the level of protein increases from the resultant mRNAs can be accounted for by numerous consequences. The observed consequence of the added compound is most likely the result of enhanced stabilization of the mRNA or conversely inhibition of degradation of the mRNA. The more long-lasting the mRNA the more often it can be engaged by the translational machinery resulting in more protein being made. Therefore, the test compound is most likely inhibiting the degradation of mRNAs by ribonucleases. None of the other options (choices A, B, D, and E) can more correctly account for the observations in this experiment.

16. Correct answer is **D.** Chromosome 21 is one of the five acrocentric chromosomes. The acrocentric chromosomes are unique among the autosomes in that they have nearly nonexistent p arms. Human ribosomal RNA gene repeats are distributed among nucleolar organizer regions (NOR) on the p arms of the five acrocentric chromosomes. Each acrocentric p arm contains 30–40 tandem repeats that each contain genes encoding the 45*S* rRNA precursor for the 5.8*S*, 18*S*, and 28*S* rRNAs. The repeats that contain the genes for the 5*S* rRNA are contained on the q arm of chromosome 1. None of the other RNA species (choices A, B, C, and E) would be affected by an amplification of the p arm of chromosome 21.

17. Correct answer is **B.** The patient is most likely suffering from Angelman syndrome. The characteristic clinical spectrum of Angelman syndrome include microcephaly, seizure disorder, ataxia, muscular hypotonia with hyperreflexia, and motor delay. The psychomotor delay in these patients is evident by 6 months of age and is associated with hypotonia and feeding difficulties. The microcephaly is not apparent at birth but develops within the first 3 years. Angelman syndrome was one of the first diseases demonstrated to be the result of the process of genomic imprinting. Angelman syndrome results from loss of the maternal expression of a neuron-specific ubiquitin ligase gene (*UBE3A*). Genomic imprinting refers to a genetic phenomenon whereby there is preferential expression of a gene (or cluster of genes) from only one of the two parental alleles. This phenomenon of allele-specific expression results from allele-specific epigenetic modifications such as CpG dinucleotide methylation. These modifications are referred to as epigenetic modifications (also referred to as epigenetic "marks"). None of the other molecular processes (choices A, C, D, and E) correctly correlates to the manifestations of the pathology of Angelman syndrome.

18. Correct answer is **A.** Protein domains that interact with zinc ions are referred to as zinc finger domains. The zinc finger domain is a DNA-binding motif consisting of specific spacings of cysteine and histidine residues that allow the protein to bind zinc atoms. The metal atom coordinates the sequences around the cysteine and histidine residues into a finger-like domain. The finger domains can interdigitate into the major groove of the DNA helix. The spacing of the zinc finger domain in this class of transcription factor coincides with a half-turn of the double helix. Proteins of the steroid and thyroid hormone superfamily of transcription factors contain zinc finger domains. None of the other options (choices B, C, D, and E) correctly explain the consequence of the deletion of a domain related to interact with zinc ions.

19. Correct answer is **A.** The process of X chromosome inactivation (XCI) takes place very early in development and ensures equivalent X chromosome gene expression levels throughout development in both males and females. The process of XCI in humans is random such that in roughly half of the cells in a female have inactivated the paternal X chromosome (Xp) and the other half have inactivated the maternal X chromosome (Xm). Once a human X chromosome is inactivated it remains inactive in all the progeny cells throughout life. X chromosome inactivation requires a family of long noncoding RNAs (lncRNA) with the central regulatory lncRNA being encoded by the *XIST* gene (X-inactive specific transcript). Like most lncRNA, the primary XIST transcript is spliced and polyadenylated. The *XIST* gene resides in a region on the X chromosome called the X inactivation center (XIC). None of the other types of RNA (choices B, C, D, and E) significantly contribute to the processes of X chromosome inactivation.

20. Correct answer is **B.** The patient is most likely experiencing the signs and symptoms of Huntington disease. Huntington disease is an autosomal dominant disorder meaning only one of two mutant alleles is necessary in order to manifest disease. Huntington disease is caused by expansion of a CAG trinucleotide repeat in the first exon of the huntingtin gene. The CAG repeat resides 17 codons downstream of the initiator AUG codon such that the result is a polyglutamine stretch in the N-terminus of the huntingtin protein. The expansion of the polyglutamine stretch results in loss of proper huntingtin protein function. Given that Huntington disease is an autosomal dominant disorder, the ability to remove or reduce the abnormal protein would afford therapeutic benefit since there is wild-type protein expressed from the allele in which the CAG repeat has not expanded. RNA interference (RNAi) refers to a process involving small (~21–22 bp) double-stranded RNA (dsRNA) molecules that trigger homology-dependent control of gene activity through interference with protein synthesis as well as activating RNA degradation. These RNAs are also known as small interfering RNAs, siRNA. An important form of RNAi involves the microRNA (miRNA) encoding genes in the human genome that regulate gene expression. This miRNA mechanism for sequence-specific gene silencing is the basis of current approaches to therapeutic intervention in numerous disorders such as Huntington disease. The important consideration for the use of RNAi technology is that it is utilized to remove, as opposed to replace, an abnormal gene product. None of the other RNA molecules (choices A, C, D, and E) reflect the basis of an RNA-mediated therapeutic approach to disease.

21. Correct answer is **C.** Highly conserved sequences at both the 5′ and 3′ ends of introns are required for proper control of RNA splicing. Loss of the five nucleotides at the 5′ end of the second intron of the PAH gene would most likely result in the loss of correct splicing together of the first and second exons. The result of this altered splicing is most likely to be an mRNA that is larger than the mRNA from the wild -type *PAH* gene. None of the other options (choices A, B, D, and E) correctly define the most likely result of the five-nucleotide deletion identified in this patient's *PAH* gene.

CHAPTER

24

Protein Synthesis, Modification, and Targeting

High-Yield Terms

Genetic code	The genetic code defines the set of rules (the nucleotide triplets) by which information encoded within the genes is translated into proteins
Wobble hypothesis	Explains the non-Watson-Crick base pairing that can occur between the 3′-nucleotide of a codon and the 5′-nucleotide of an anticodon
Peptidyltransferase	Is an RNA-mediated (ribozyme) enzymatic activity of the 60*S* ribosome that catalyzes transpeptidation during protein elongation
Selenoprotein	Any of a family of proteins that contain a selenocysteine (Sec) amino acid
Signal sequence	The N-terminal 15-25 hydrophobic amino acids in proteins that are destined for secretion of membrane insertion; the sequences are recognized by the signal recognition particle which assists in binding of the ribosome to the ER membrane
Ubiquitin	A 76-amino-acid peptide enzymatically attached to proteins which, in most cases, targets the modified protein for degradation in the proteasome
Proteasome	A large protein complex whose function is to proteolytically degrade damaged or unneeded proteins
Hexosamine biosynthesis pathway, HBP	Pathway for conversion of glucose to *O*-GlcNAc which is important for the carbohydrate modification of numerous cytoplasmic and nuclear proteins
Lectin	Any of a family of proteins that contain a carbohydrate-binding domain; lectin is derived from the Latin word meaning "to select"
Mucin	Any of a family of high molecular weight, heavily glycosylated proteins with the ability to form gels that lubricate and form chemical barriers
Congenital disorders of glycosylation, CDG	A family of diseases resulting from inherited defects in the synthesis, processing, and modification of both *N*-linked and *O*-linked glycoproteins and related glycan modified molecules

Translation is the RNA-directed synthesis of proteins. The process requires not only the template mRNA but also the participation of the tRNAs and rRNAs. The tRNAs are necessary to carry activated amino acids into the ribosome which itself is composed of rRNAs and ribosomal proteins. The process of translation starts somewhere near the 5′ end of the mRNA which is determined by the recognition of a translation start codon. Translation proceeds along the mRNA in the 5′ → 3′ direction until a translation stop codon in encountered. The directionality of the mRNA corresponds to the N-terminal to C-terminal direction of the amino acid sequences within proteins.

Translation proceeds in an ordered process. First, accurate and efficient **initiation** must take place, then peptide **elongation**, and finally accurate and efficient **termination** must occur. All three of these processes require specific proteins, some of which are ribosome associated and some of which are separate from the ribosome but may be temporarily associated with it.

THE GENETIC CODE

The genetic code consists of triplets of nucleotides in the mRNA (Table 24–1). The fact that there are more triplets (64 in all) possible than there are amino acids in proteins (20 in all) defines the basis for the degeneracy of the genetic code. The degeneracy refers to the fact that there are multiple possible triplet nucleotides for a given amino acid.

TABLE 24–1 The genetic code[1] (Codon Assignments in Mammalian Messenger RNAs).

First Nucleotide			Second Nucleotide		Third Nucleotide
	U		C	A	G
U	Phe	Ser	Tyr	Cys	U
	Phe	Ser	Tyr	Cys	C
	Leu	Ser	Term	Term[2]	A
	Leu	Ser	Term	Trp	G
C	Leu	Pro	His	Arg	U
	Leu	Pro	His	Arg	C
	Leu	Pro	Gln	Arg	A
	Leu	Pro	Gln	Arg	G
A	Ile	Thr	Asn	Ser	U
	Ile	Thr	Asn	Ser	C
	Ile[2]	Thr	Lys	Arg[2]	A
	Met	Thr	Lys	Arg[2]	G
G	Val	Ala	Asp	Gly	U
	Val	Ala	Asp	Gly	C
	Val	Ala	Glu	Gly	A
	Val	Ala	Glu	Gly	G

[1] The terms first, second, and third nucleotide refer to the individual nucleotides of a triplet codon read $5' \rightarrow 3'$, left to right. A, adenine nucleotide; C, cytosine nucleotide; G, guanine nucleotide; Term, chain terminator codon; U, uridine nucleotide. AUG, which codes for Met, serves as the initiator codon in mammalian cells and also encodes for internal methionines in a protein. (Abbreviations of amino acids are explained in Chapter 3.)

[2] In mammalian mitochondria, AUA codes for Met and UGA for Trp, and AGA and AGG serve as chain terminators.

CHARACTERISTICS OF tRNAs

More than 300 different tRNAs have been characterized and shown to have extensive similarities. They vary in length from 60–95 nucleotides and exhibit a cloverleaf-like secondary structure that is composed of an anticodon loop, a D loop, and a TψC loop (Figure 24–1). These terms derive from the fact that the D loop contains the modified nucleotide, dihydrouridine, and the TψC loop contains pseudouridine (designated by the Greek ψ). All tRNAs also have the trinucleotide sequence, CCA, added to their 3′-ends posttranscriptionally. The A residue serves as the acceptor site for attachment of the appropriate amino acid.

AMINO ACID ACTIVATION

Activation of amino acids is carried out by a family of enzymes termed aminoacyl-tRNA synthetases (Figure 24–2). Humans express 38 genes encoding these enzymes, several of which are responsible for mitochondrial protein synthesis. Accurate recognition of the correct amino acid as well as the correct tRNA by a given aminoacyl-tRNA synthetase to ensure correct amino acid incorporation into proteins.

Given the high degree of nucleotide modifications that occur in tRNAs, it is possible for non-Watson-Crick base pairing to occur at the third codon position, that is, the 3′ nucleotide of the mRNA codon and the 5′ nucleotide of the tRNA anticodon. This phenomenon is referred to as the **wobble hypothesis.**

TRANSLATION INITIATION

Initiation of translation requires numerous components including an mRNA, a pool of amino acid charged tRNAs including a specific initiator tRNA, $tRNA_i^{met}$, the ribosome, and numerous nonribosomal proteins termed initiation factors (Table 24–2). Eukaryotic translational initiation factors are identified by the abbreviation: eIF.

Initiation of translation requires four specific steps: (1) a ribosome must dissociate into its' 40*S* and 60*S* subunits; (2) a ternary complex (termed the preinitiation complex) consisting of the initiator met-tRNA, eIF-2 and GTP must engage the dissociated

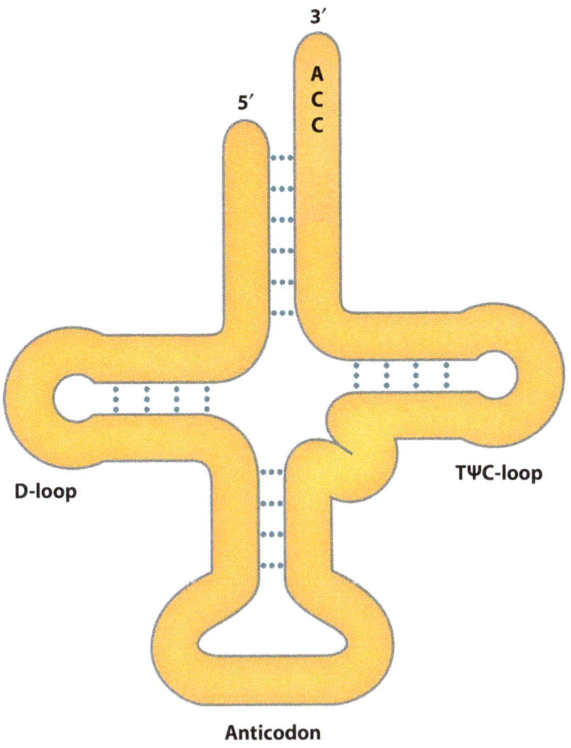

FIGURE 24–1 Structure of a typical tRNA molecule. The common stem-loop domains that form the anticodon loop, the D loop, and the TψC loop are highlighted. The –CCA– nucleotides shown at the 3′ end of the tRNA are added posttranscriptionally to all eukaryotic tRNAs. (Reproduced with permission from themedicalbiochemistrypage, LLC.)

40*S* subunit; (3) the mRNA is then bound to the preinitiation complex; and (4) the 60*S* subunit must associate with the preinitiation complex to form the 80*S* initiation complex (Figure 24–3).

The large ribosomal subunit contains domains termed the A-site, P-site, and E-site. The A-site resides over the next codon to be recognized in the mRNA and each incoming aminoacyl-tRNA enters the ribosome at this site. The P-site is where the elongating protein, attached to a tRNA, will reside following each round of elongation. The E-site is where the protein is ejected from the ribosome upon completion of translation.

The hydrolysis of the GTP associated with eIF-2 stimulates the formation of the 80*S* initiation complex. The GDP bound form of eIF-2 then binds to eIF-2B which stimulates the exchange of GTP for GDP. The overall process of eIF-2B-mediated GTP for GDP exchange in eIF-2 is termed the eIF-2 cycle (Figure 24–3). The activity called eIF-2B is actually a complex of five subunits identified as α, β, γ, δ, and ε, each encoded by a separate gene. Inherited mutations in any one of these five genes results in a severe neurodegenerative disorder termed leukoencephalopathy with vanishing white matter (Clinical Box 24–1).

REGULATION OF TRANSLATION INITIATION: THE eIF-2α KINASES

Regulation of initiation in eukaryotes is primarily controlled by phosphorylation of Ser (S) residues in the α-subunit of eIF-2 (Figure 24–4). Phosphorylated eIF-2α, in the absence of eIF-2B, is just as active an initiator as nonphosphorylated eIF-2. However, when eIF-2α is phosphorylated the GDP-bound complex is stabilized and exchange for GTP is inhibited. A number of different conditions, including endoplasmic reticulum (ER) stress, nutrient stress (deprivation or restriction), viral infection, and heme levels in erythrocytes lead to activation of kinases that phosphorylate eIF-2α.

Proteins that are destined for secretory vesicles are translated while associated with ER membranes. During translation secreted proteins are transported into the lumen of the ER in an unfolded state. Proper folding occurs prior to the transfer of the protein to the Golgi apparatus. Under certain conditions the secretory responses of a cell can exceed the capacity of the folding processes of the ER. Accumulation of unfolded proteins triggers the unfolded protein response (UPR) which is a form of ER stress. The UPR activates an eIF-2α kinase termed PERK [RNA-dependent protein kinase (**PK**R)-like **ER** **k**inase].

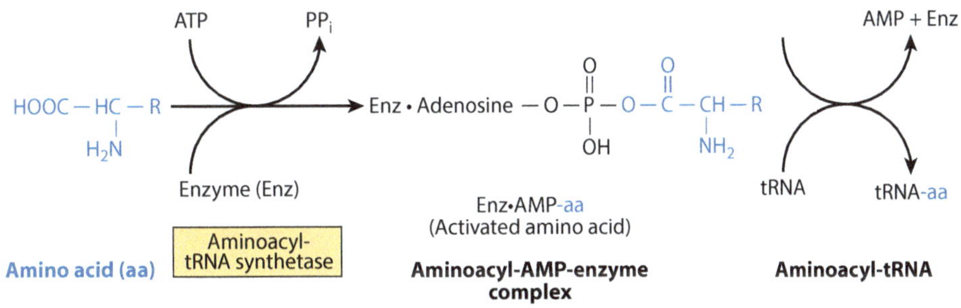

FIGURE 24–2 Formation of aminoacyl-tRNA. A two-step reaction involving the enzyme amino-acyl-tRNA synthetase results in the formation of aminoacyl-tRNA. The first reaction involves the formation of an AMP-amino acid–enzyme complex. This activated amino acid is next transferred to the corresponding tRNA molecule. The AMP and enzyme are released, and the latter can be reutilized. The charging reactions have an error rate (ie, esterifying the incorrect amino acid on tRNAx) of less than 10–4. (Reproduced with permission from Rodwell VW, Bender DA, Botham KM, et al: *Harper's Illustrated Biochemistry*, 31st ed. New York, NY: McGraw Hill; 2018.)

TABLE 24–2 Important eukaryotic translation initiation factors.

Initiation Factor	Activity
eIF-1	Repositioning of met-tRNA to facilitate mRNA binding; encoded by the *EIF1* gene
eIF-2	Heterotrimeric G-protein composed of α, β, and γ subunits; formation of ternary complex consisting of eIF2-GTP + initiator methionine tRNA (met-tRNA^{imet}); AUG-dependent met-tRNA^{imet} binding to 40S ribosome; α-subunit encoded by the *EIF2S1* gene, β-subunit encoded by the *EIF2S2* gene, γ-subunit encoded by the *EIF2S3* gene
eIF-2B	Composed of five subunits: α, β, γ, δ, ε; functions in GTP/GDP exchange during eIF-2 recycling; genes encoding the subunits identified as EIF2B1–EIF2B5, mutations in any one of which causes the severe autosomal recessive neurodegenerative disorder called leukoencephalopathy with vanishing white matter (VWM: see Clinical Box 24–1)
eIF-3	Is a complex composed of 13 subunits; ribosome subunit anti-association by binding to 40S subunit; eIF-3E and eIF-3I subunits transform normal cells when overexpressed, eIF-3A (also called eIF3 p170) overexpression has been shown to be associated with several human cancers
eIF-4F	Is a complex composed of three primary subunits: eIF-4E, eIF-4A, eIF-4G, and at least two additional factors: polyA-binding protein, Mnk1 (or Mnk2); mRNA binding to 40S subunit, ATPase-dependent RNA helicase activity, interaction between polyA tail and cap structure; eIF-4A encoded by one of three genes (EIF4A1, EIF4A2, or EIF4A3); eIF-4E encoded by EIF4E gene; eIF-4G encoded by one of three genes (EIF4G1, EIF4G2, or EIF4G3)
PABPC1	polyA-binding protein C1; principal cytoplasmic polyA-binding protein of mRNA translation; binds to the polyA tail of mRNAs and provides a link to eIF-4G; encoded by the *PABPC1* gene; humans express several cytoplasmic (PABPC) and at least one nuclear (PABPN) polyA-binding protein; the PABPN1-encoded protein is involved in polymerization of the polyA tail
Mnk1 and Mnk2	Are eIF-4E kinases; phosphorylate eIF-4E increasing association with cap structure; Mnk1 is encoded by the MKNK1 (MAPK interacting serine/threonine kinase 1) gene; Mnk2 is encoded by the *MKNK2* gene
eIF-4A	ATPase-dependent RNA helicase; encoded by one of three genes (*EIF4A1*, *EIF4A2*, or *EIF4A3*)
eIF-4E	5′ cap recognition; encoded by the *EIF4E* gene; frequently found over-expressed in human cancers, inhibition of eIF4E is currently a target for anticancer therapies
4E-BP	Humans express 9 eIF-4 binding protein genes (EIF4BP1–EIF4BP9); original eIF-4BP (EIF4BP1) was called phosphorylated heat- and acid-stable protein 1 (PHAS1); when dephosphorylated 4E-BP binds eIF-4E and represses its' activity, phosphorylation of 4E-BP occurs in response to many growth stimuli leading to release of eIF-4E and increased translational initiation
eIF-4G	Encoded by one of three genes (*EIF4G1*, *EIF4G2*, or *EIF4G3*); acts as a scaffold for the assembly of eIF-4E and -4A in the eIF-4F complex; interaction with PABP family member proteins allows 5′-end and 3′-ends of mRNAs to interact
eIF-5A	Binds to the ribosome between the P-site and the tRNA exit site (E-site); promotes peptide bond formation by preventing ribosome stalling in mRNAs containing proline repeats as well as many other ribosome stalling sites; also enhances translation termination; only human protein that contains a modified lysine residue called hypusine (derived from **h**ydroxy**pu**trescine and ly**sine**); synthesis of the hypusine involves the polyamine, spermidine

Deficiencies in PERK result in the extremely rare autosomal recessive disorder known as Wolcott-Rallison syndrome, WRS (Clinical Box 24–2).

REGULATION OF eIF-4E ACTIVITY

The level and activity of eIF-4E is controlled at the level of transcription of the eIF-4E gene, posttranslational modification via phosphorylation, and inhibition by interaction with binding proteins (Figure 24–5). The principal regulatory mechanism involves a family of binding/repressor proteins termed 4E-binding proteins (4EBP). Humans express nine 4EBP genes. Binding of 4EBP to eIF-4E prevents the interaction of eIF-4E with eIF-4G which in turn suppresses the formation of the eIF-4F complex.

The ability of the various 4EBP to interact with eIF-4E is controlled via their state of phosphorylation. Numerous growth and signal transduction stimulating effectors lead to phosphorylation of 4EBP as one mechanism to increase the rate of protein synthesis. Phosphorylated 4EBP dissociates from eIF-4E allowing eIF-4E to interact with eIF-4G and the formation of a functional eIF-4F complex.

TRANSLATION ELONGATION

Elongation of proteins requires specific nonribosomal proteins termed eEFs. Protein elongation occurs in a cyclic manner such that at the end of one complete round of amino acid addition the A-site will be empty and ready to accept the

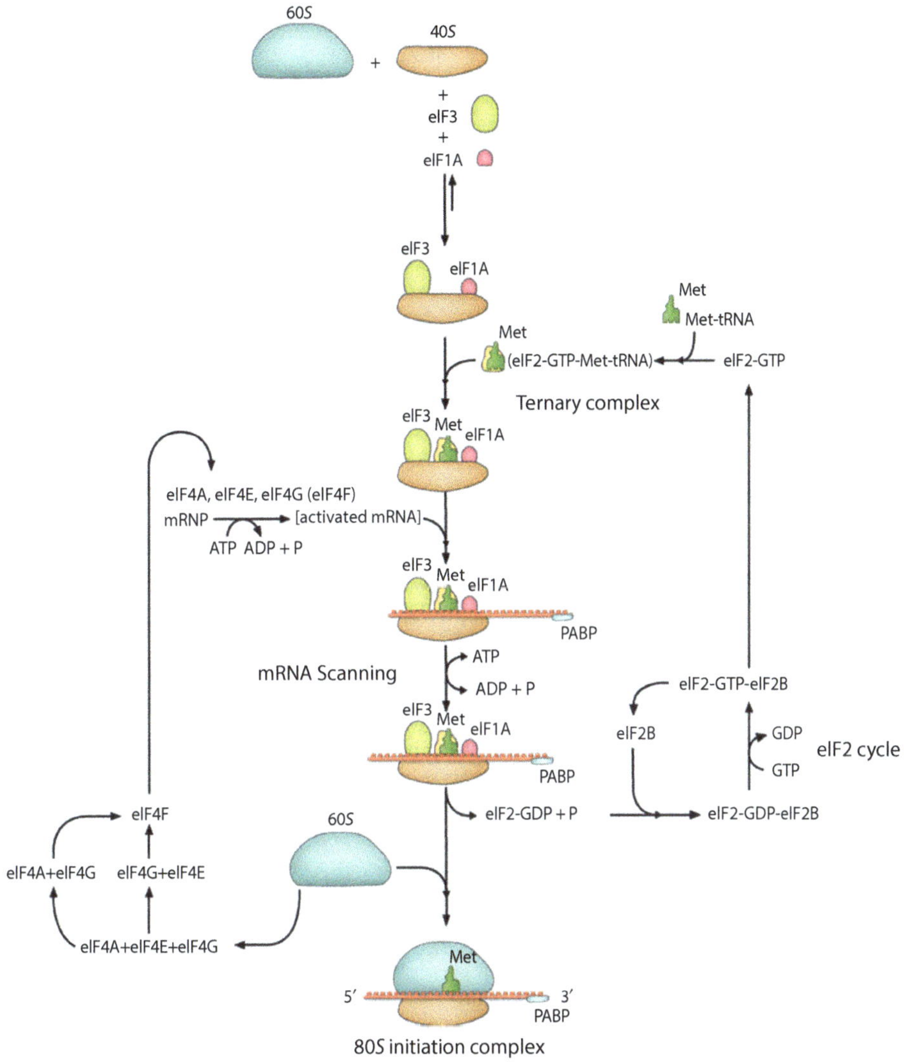

FIGURE 24–3 Details of the complex processes required for accurate and efficient initiation of translation. Several initiation factors (eg, eIF-1 and eIF-3) are required to ensure that the 60*S* and 40*S* ribosomal subunits remain separated (antiassociation) so that new rounds of translation can begin. The ternary complex, composed of GTP bound to the α-subunit of eIF2 and the initiator methionyl-tRNA^{met}, can engage the 40*S* subunit. The eIF-4F complex, which comprises the cap-binding factor, eIF-4E, the RNA helicase eIF-4A, and the scaffold subunit, eIF-4G, captures an mRNA and brings it to the 40*S* subunit and the ternary complex. Once the mRNA, 40*S* and 60*S* subunits, and the ternary complex are integrated, the resulting 80*S* initiation complex constitutes the completion of the process of translation initiation. PABP, polyA binding protein. (Reproduced with permission from themedicalbiochemistrypage, LLC.)

CLINICAL BOX 24–1 EIF-2B AND LEUKOENCEPHALOPATHY

Leukoencephalopathy with vanishing white matter (VWM), also referred to as childhood ataxia with central hypomyelination and myelinopathia centralis diffusa, is one of the most prevalent inherited white matter disorders of childhood but it can affect people of all ages, including neonates and adults. Although other tissues are affected, VWM is primarily a brain disorder in which oligodendrocytes and astrocytes are selectively affected. VWM is a progressive disorder clinically dominated by cerebellar ataxia and in which minor stress conditions, such as fever or mild trauma, can induce major episodes of neurologic deterioration. Typical pathologic findings are diminishing white matter, the gross pathology that lends its name to this disorder. Additional pathology includes cystic degeneration, oligodendrocytosis with highly characteristic foamy oligodendrocytes, limited astrogliosis with dysmorphic astrocytes, and apoptotic loss of oligodendrocytes. VWM is caused by mutations in any of the five genes (EIF2B1–EIF2B5) encoding the subunits (α, β, γ, δ, and ε) of initiation factor 2B (eIF-2B). All identified mutations in these genes result in eIF-2B complexes with diminished activity and impair its function to couple protein synthesis to the cellular demands in basal conditions and during stress. The reduction in eIF-2B function results in a sustained inappropriate activation of the unfolded protein response (UPR). Sustained activation of the UPR triggers an apoptotic process leading to the observed apoptotic loss of oligodendrocytes.

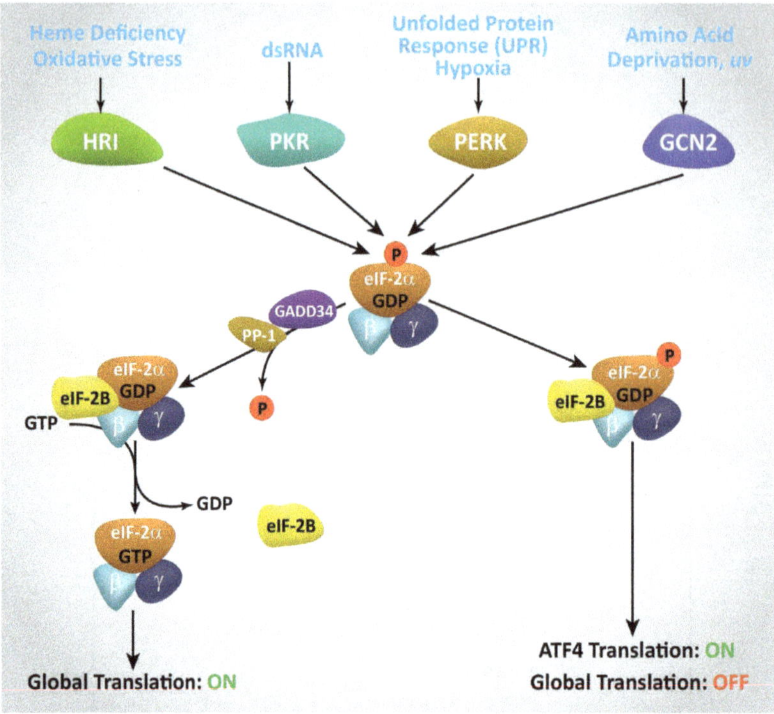

FIGURE 24–4 Each of the various eIF-2α kinases responds to different physiologic and/or environmental stressors and induces the phosphorylation of the α-subunit of eIF-2. In the case of nutritional stress or the unfolded protein response (UPR), the phosphorylation of eIF-2α results in the preferential translation of transcription factors (eg, ATF4) that initiate a pattern of gene expression that allows the cell to respond to the stress or in the case of severe and damaging stress the apoptotic program is triggered. GADD34 is a regulatory subunit of protein phosphatase-1 (PP-1). Transcription of the *GADD34* gene by ATF4 allows for a feedback control loop on the level of eIF-2α phosphorylation. (Reproduced with permission from themedicalbiochemistrypage, LLC.)

next incoming aminoacyl-tRNA dictated by the next codon of the mRNA (Figure 24–6). Each incoming aminoacyl-tRNA is brought to the ribosome by an eEF-1α-GTP complex. When the correct tRNA is deposited into the A-site the GTP is hydrolyzed and the eEF-1α-GDP complex dissociates. In order for additional translocation events, the GDP must be exchanged for GTP. This is carried out by eEF-1βγ similarly to the GTP exchange that occurs with eIF-2α catalyzed by eIF-2B.

The peptide attached to the tRNA in the P-site is transferred to the amino acid on the aminoacyl-tRNA in the A-site forming a new peptide bond. This reaction is catalyzed by the peptidyltransferase activity which resides in what is termed

CLINICAL BOX 24–2 WOLCOTT-RALLISON SYNDROME

Wolcott-Rallison syndrome (WRS) is a rare autosomal recessive disease, characterized by neonatal/early-onset non-autoimmune insulin-requiring diabetes associated with skeletal dysplasia and growth retardation. WRS is the most frequent cause of neonatal/early-onset diabetes in patients with consanguineous parents. WRS should be suspected as the cause of diabetes mellitus occurring neonatally or before 6 months of age and originating from a population where there is a high prevalence of consanguinity. Additional signs in these children are skeletal dysplasia and/or episodes of acute liver failure. Other symptoms show variability in their nature and severity between patients with WRS. These additional symptoms include frequent episodes of acute liver failure, renal dysfunction, exocrine pancreas insufficiency, intellectual deficit, hypothyroidism, neutropenia, and recurrent infections. WRS is caused by mutations in the gene encoding the eIF-2α kinase, PERK (PKR-like endoplasmic reticulum kinase). PERK plays a key role in translation control during the unfolded protein response (UPR). Indeed, ER dysfunction is central to the disease processes in WRS. Molecular genetic testing confirms the diagnosis in patients suspected of having WRS. Aggressive therapeutic monitoring and interventional treatment of the diabetes with an insulin pump is highly recommended because of the risk of acute episodes of hypoglycemia and ketoacidosis. The prognosis for WRS patients is poor and most patients die at a young age.

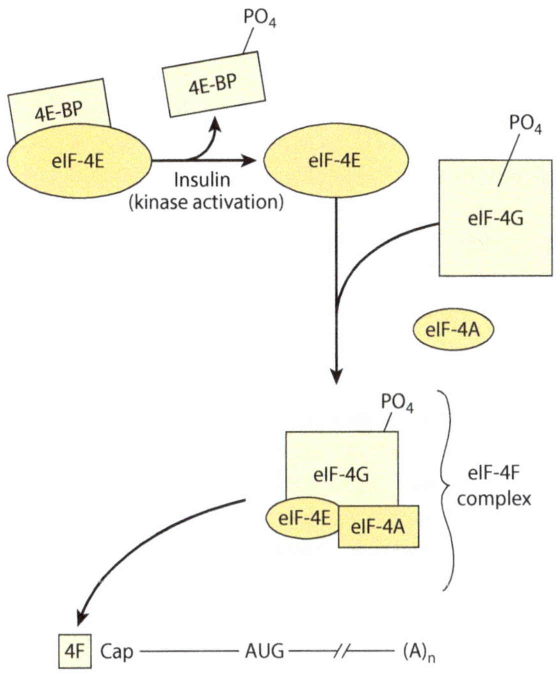

FIGURE 24–5 Activation of eIF-4E by insulin and its subsequent incorporation into the functional eIF-4F cap-binding complex. When 4E-BP is phosphorylated by insulin (as well as numerous other growth factors and mitogens), it dissociates from eIF-4E which allows the latter factor to interact with eIF-4G and then form the eIF-4F complex. Growth factors also induce phosphorylation of eIF-4G, generating a phosphorylated eIF-4F complex that interacts with the cap with higher affinity than nonphosphorylated eIF-4F. (Reproduced with permission from Murray RK, Bender DA, Botham KM, et al: *Harper's Illustrated Biochemistry*, 29th ed. New York, NY: McGraw Hill; 2012.)

the peptidyltransferase center (PTC) of the large ribosomal subunit (60*S* subunit). Peptide bond formation is catalyzed by the ribozyme activity of the large ribosomal RNA (28*S*) contained in the 60*S* subunit.

The process of moving the peptidyl-tRNA from the A-site to the P-site is termed translocation and is catalyzed by eEF-2 coupled to GTP hydrolysis. Following translocation eEF-2 is released from the ribosome. The ability of eEF-2 to carry out translocation is regulated by its state of phosphorylation; when phosphorylated the eEF-2 activity is inhibited. Phosphorylation of eEF-2 is catalyzed by the enzyme eEF-2 kinase (eEF2K). Regulation of eEF2K activity is normally under the control of insulin and Ca^{2+} fluxes. The Ca^{2+}-mediated effects are the result of calmodulin interaction with eEF2K. Activation of eEF2K in skeletal muscle by Ca^{2+} is important to reduce consumption of ATP in the process of protein synthesis during periods of exertion.

TERMINATION

Translational termination in eukaryotic cells requires only one factor, termed eRF (eukaryotic releasing factor). The signals for translation termination are the three termination codons, UAG, UAA, and UGA. The binding of eRF to the ribosome stimulates the peptidytransferase activity to transfer the protein to water instead of an aminoacyl-tRNA (Figure 24–7). The resulting uncharged tRNA left in the P site is expelled with concomitant hydrolysis of GTP. The inactive ribosome then releases its mRNA and the 80*S* complex dissociates into the 40*S* and 60*S* subunits ready for another round of translation.

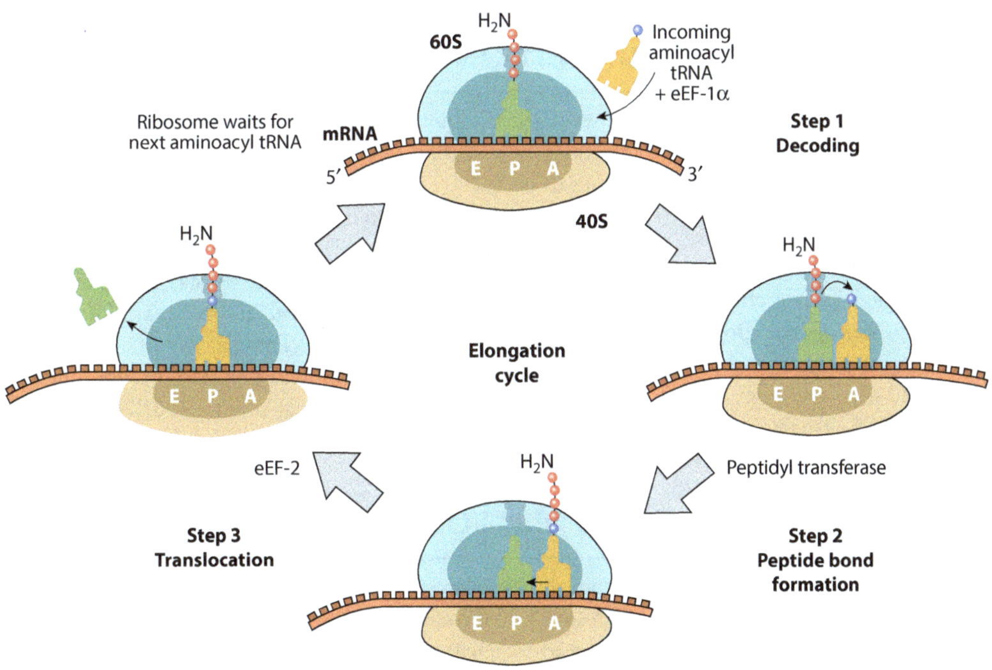

FIGURE 24–6 The cyclical steps of elongation. The elongation factor eEF-1α carries each incoming aminoacyl-tRNA to the A-site. The peptide in the P-site is transferred to the amino acid in the A-site through the action of peptidyltransferase. Following peptide transfer the elongation factor eEF-2 induces translocation of the ribosome along the mRNA such that the naked tRNA is temporarily within the E-site and the peptidyl-tRNA is moved to the P-site leaving the A-site empty and residing over the next codon of the mRNA. (Reproduced with permission from themedicalbiochemistrypage, LLC.)

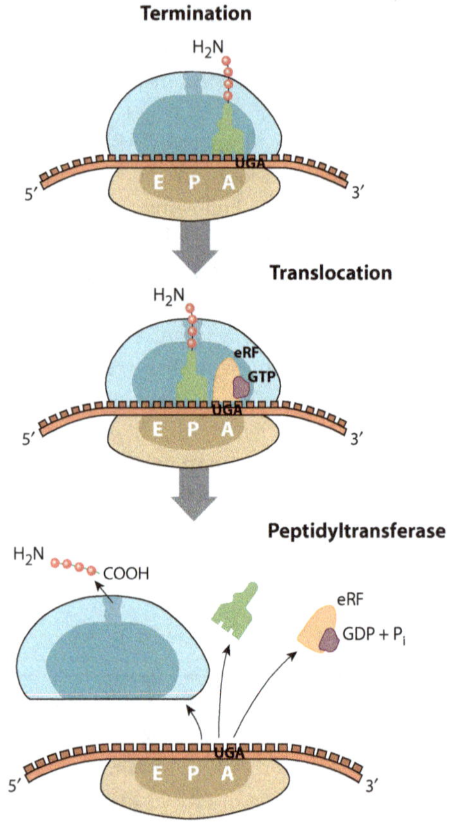

FIGURE 24–7 Translation termination occurs when a stop codon is encountered. The termination factor eRF, which binds GTP, then stimulates the peptidyltransferase to transfer the peptide, from the tRNA in the P-site to H_2O coupled with the hydrolysis of GTP. The peptide is released from the ribosome along with the naked tRNA and eRFGDP complex. (Reproduced with permission from themedicalbiochemistrypage, LLC.)

CAP-INDEPENDENT TRANSLATIONAL INITIATION

Cap-dependent translational initiation involves the recognition of an internal ribosome entry site (IRES). An IRES is an RNA structure that directly recruits the 40*S* ribosomal subunits via a mechanism that is independent of the cap structure. IRES elements function via interactions with several of the initiation factors (eIFs) required for cap-dependent initiation, such as eIF4G.

Several eukaryotic genes encoding proto-oncogenes, growth factors, proteins involved in the regulation of programmed cell death (apoptosis), cell-cycle progression, and stress responses have been shown to express mRNA that contain IRES elements in their 5′ untranslated regions (UTRs). The presence of IRES elements in these mRNAs allows translation to proceed under conditions where cap-dependent translational initiation is repressed. Thus, the hallmark of IRES-mediated translation is that it allows for enhanced or continued gene expression (at the level of protein synthesis) under conditions where normal, cap-dependent translation is shut-off or compromised.

SELENOCYSTEINE INCORPORATION

Humans express several genes whose encoded enzymes contain a selenocysteine (Sec) residue. A particularly important group of Sec containing enzymes are the glutathione peroxidases (GPx) which are critical antioxidant enzymes. The Sec is incorporated into the protein during translation through recognition of specific UGA codons (normally stop codons) and mRNA secondary structures by a number of specialized proteins and protein complexes (Figure 24–8).

IRON CONTROL OF TRANSLATION

Regulation of the translation of certain mRNAs occurs via the interaction of specific RNA-binding proteins to sequences in either the 5′ nontranslated region (5′-UTR) or 3′-UTR (Figure 24–9). These mRNA structures are referred to as iron-response elements, and the proteins that bind them are called iron-response element-binding proteins (IRBP).

Two particularly interesting and important regulatory schemes related to iron homeostasis encompass an RNA-binding protein that binds to IRE in the 5′-UTR of the ferritin mRNAs or to the IRE in the 3′-UTR of the transferrin receptor mRNA. In addition to the ferritin and transferrin receptor mRNAs, additional mRNAs encoding proteins involved in overall iron homeostasis also contain an IRE.

When iron levels are low the rate of synthesis of the transferrin receptor increases so that cells can take up more iron, whereas translation of the ferritin mRNA is inhibited in order to restrict intracellular storage of iron. The IRBP that recognizes the IRE in these various mRNAs is an iron-binding protein and interaction with an IRE is controlled by the state of iron binding. When iron levels are low, IRBP is free of iron and can therefore, interact with the IREs. Conversely, when iron levels are high, IRBP binds iron and then cannot interact with the IRE.

INHIBITION OF PROTEIN SYNTHESIS

Many of the antibiotics utilized for the treatment of bacterial infections, as well as certain toxins produced by bacteria that contribute to pathology, function through the inhibition of translation (Clinical Boxes 24–3 and 24–4).

Antibiotics are broadly divided into two categories, the bactericidal and bacteriostatic compounds. Bacteriostatic compounds do not kill bacteria but instead prevent them from reproducing. The bactericidal agents do kill bacteria. The majority of antibiotics in use interfere with prokaryotic protein synthesis by either inhibiting functions of the large ribosomal subunit (50*S*) or the small ribosomal subunit (30*S*).

PROTEIN FOLDING

Within the environment of the cell, newly synthesized proteins are at great risk of aberrant folding and aggregation. Improper folding and protein aggregation can lead to the formation of potentially

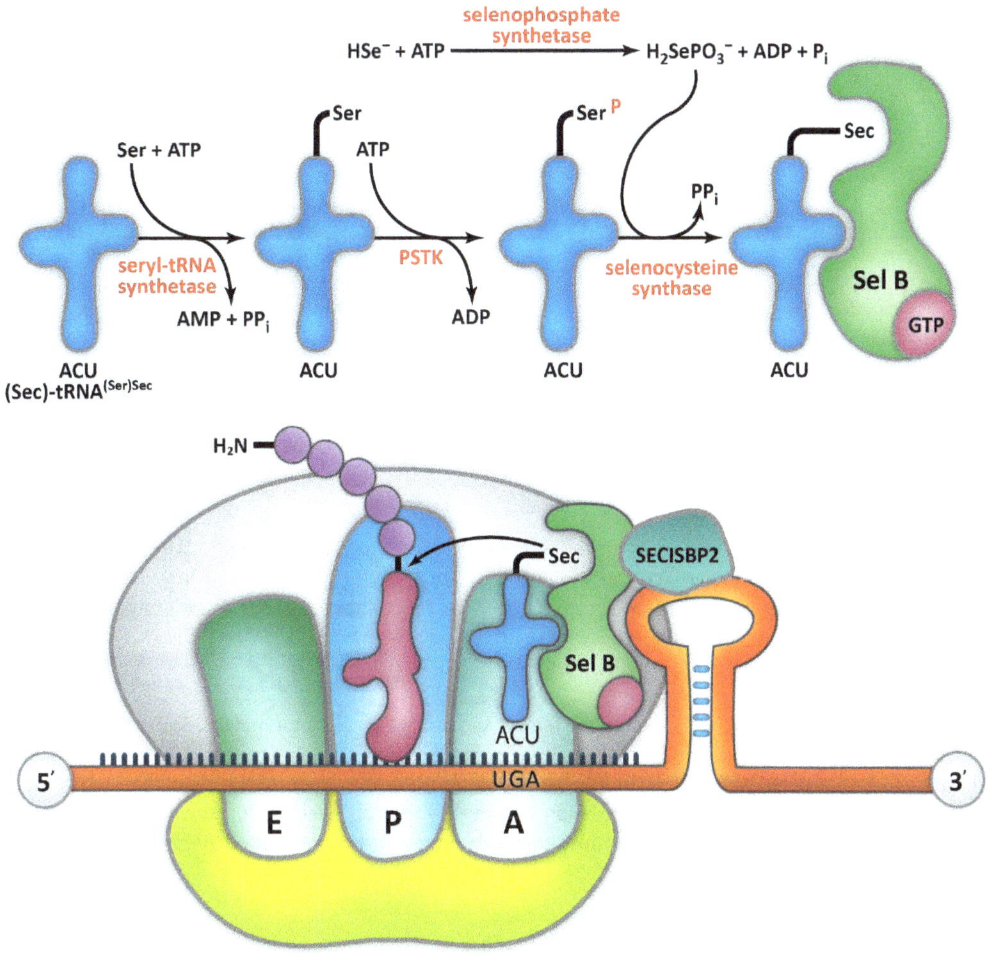

FIGURE 24–8 Selenocysteine biosynthesis and incorporation. The first step in the incorporation of a selenocysteine residue involves the activation of the specialized tRNA, (Sec)-tRNA$^{(Ser)Sec}$. This tRNA is recognized by seryl-tRNA synthetase (encoded by the *SARS* gene) which incorporates a Ser residue to the 3′-end of the tRNA in a standard activation reaction. The Ser residue is then phosphorylated by the enzyme phosphoseryl-tRNA kinase encoded by the *PSTK* gene. The phosphoserine is then converted to selenocysteine in a two-step process that first involves the synthesis of selenophosphate by the enzyme selenophosphate synthetase. Humans express two selenophosphate synthetase genes identified as *SEPHS1* and *SEPHS2*. The *SEPH2* encoded selenophosphate synthetase is itself a selenocysteine-containing protein. The *SEPHS1* encoded enzyme functions in a pathway that is unrelated to selenoprotein synthesis but is likely to be involved in Sec recycling in a selenium salvage pathway. The selenophosphate generated by selenophosphate synthetase 2 is utilized by selenocysteine synthase to convert the phosphoserine on the Sec-tRNA to selenocysteine. Selenocysteine synthase is encoded by the *SEPSECS* [Sep (O-phosphoserine) tRNA:Sec (selenocysteine) tRNA synthase] gene. Following the formation of (Sec)-tRNASec this specialized tRNA is bound by SelB and the complex is incorporated into the translational machinery aided by SECISBP2, eIF-4A3, and nucleolin. The elongating protein is transferred to the selenocysteinyl-tRNA via the action of peptidyltransferase as for any other incoming amino acid and normal elongation continues. (Reproduced with permission from themedicalbiochemistrypage, LLC.)

toxic species. To reduce and prevent these negative outcomes, cells harbor a complex network of molecular chaperones whose functions are to promote efficient folding and to prevent protein aggregation.

Human cells express several families of molecular chaperones that includes members of the heat shock protein (Hsp) family. The Hsp superfamily is composed of multiple protein subfamilies that are loosely designated by molecular weights. These Hsp families include the Hsp40, Hsp60, Hsp70, Hsp90, and Hsp100 families. Two additional folding chaperones are calnexin and calreticulin that function in the ER in the processes of glycoprotein maturation. Additional ER folding chaperones that possess intrinsic enzymatic activity are the protein disulfide isomerases (PDI) and the peptidylprolyl cis-trans isomerases (PPI). The PDI catalyze the formation of disulfide bonds between cysteine residues in a substrate protein, while the peptidylprolyl cis-trans isomerases (PPI) catalyze isomerization of peptide bonds involving proline residues.

Disturbances in the function of molecular chaperones contribute to a plethora of disease states as well as disturbance in the normal processes of cellular aging. Mutations in genes encoding members of the PDI family and the PPI family are associated with age-related diseases including cardiovascular diseases (CVD), atherosclerosis, type 2 diabetes (T2D), chronic kidney disease (CDK), neurodegeneration, cancer, and age-related macular degeneration (AMD).

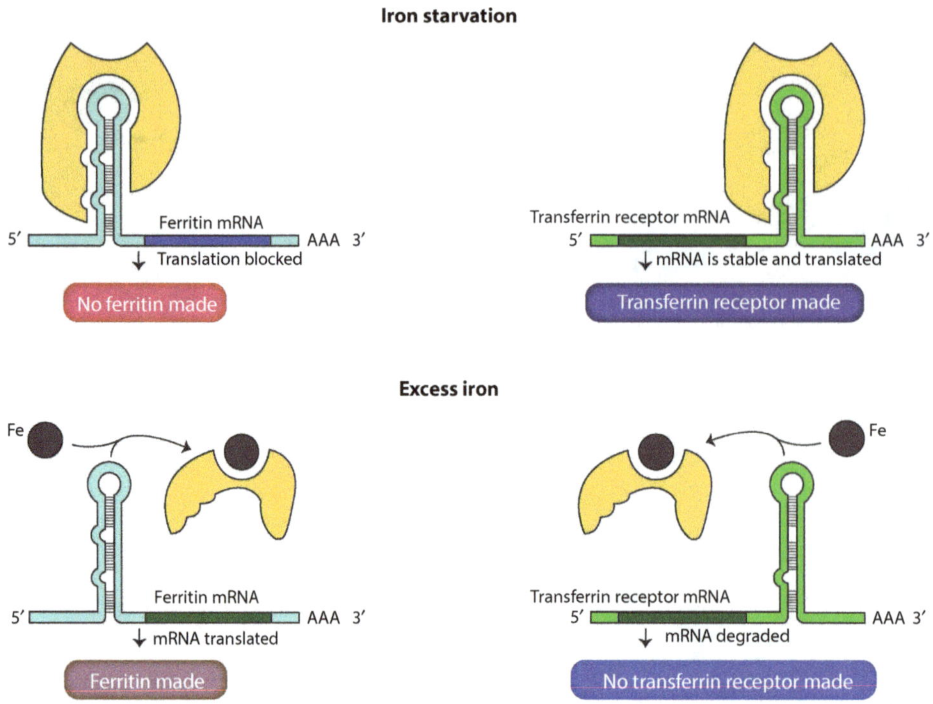

FIGURE 24–9 Iron-mediated regulation of translation of the ferritin and transferrin receptor mRNAs. Both mRNAs contain stem-loop structures that form an iron response element (IRE) that binds the iron response-element binding protein (IRBP). In the case of ferritin mRNA this IRBP stem-loop is in the 5′–untranslated region (5′-UTR), whereas in the transferrin receptor mRNA it is in the 3′-UTR. When iron levels are low, IRBP interacts with the IRE and exerts control on translation. However, when iron levels are low the excess iron is bound by the IRBP which causes it to be released from the mRNA and the opposite effects on translation are exerted. (Reproduced with permission from themedicalbiochemistrypage, LLC.)

CLINICAL BOX 24–3 ANTIBIOTICS

Macrolides: The macrolides belong to the polyketide class of naturally occurring compounds. The specific classifications of the macrolides are determined on the basis of the number of atoms in the ring of the macrocyclic lactone which can range from 12 to 17. However, the macrolides used as antibiotics in humans are all derived from the 14-, 15-, or 16-membered macrocyclic lactones. The deoxy sugars attached to the macrocyclic ring include either cladinose or desosamine. All of the macrolides, and semi-synthetic macrolide derivatives, that are formed from the 14- and 15-membered rings contain the suffix -thromycin in the drug name. The macrolides that contain a 14-membered ring include clarithromycin, erythromycin, roxithromycin, and the ketolide semi-synthetic derivatives such as telithromycin. The ketolide derivatives are used primarily to treat respiratory infections and macrolide-resistant bacteria. The macrolides that contain a 15-membered ring include azithromycin which is a semi-synthetic derivative of erythromycin. Azithromycin exhibits a similar spectrum to that of erythromycin, with increased activity against Gram-negative bacteria. The macrolides that contain a 16-membered ring include josamycin, midecamycin, spiramycin, and tylosin. However, it should be noted that none of these 16-membered ring macrolides are approved for use in the United States. Another important macrolide that is not used as an antibiotic is tacrolimus. This drug is a 23-membered ring macrolide isolated from *Streptomyces tsukubaensis* that is used as an immunosuppressant, principally following allogenic organ transplantation. Tacrolimus is also known as FK-506 or fujimycin.

Lincosamides: The lincosamides have some structural similarities to the macrolides but do not contain the lactone ring. This class of antibiotic consists of lincomycin and its more robust semi-synthetic derivative, clindamycin. Lincomycin was originally isolated from *Streptomyces lincolnensis*. The lincosamides are effective against Gram-positive bacteria including Streptococci, Staphylococci, and Mycoplasma. In addition, the lincosamides are effective against Actinomyces, some species of Plasmodium, and against the protozoan Toxoplama gondii. Due to the toxicity spectrum associated with lincomycin use, clindamycin is currently the only lincosamide routinely prescribed. Clindamycin is effective in patients with infections caused by anaerobic bacteria, in some malaria patients, and in the treatment of methicillin-resistant *Staphylococcus aureus* (MRSA) infections. Lincomycin is only utilized to treat patients that are allergic to penicillin or who have contracted an infection by an antibiotic-resistant strain of Gram-positive bacteria.

CLINICAL BOX 24–3 (CONTINUED)

Streptogramins: The streptogramin family of antibiotics are natural antibiotics produced by various strains of Streptomyces. The streptogramin antibiotics are classified into two distinct groups: streptogramin A and streptogramin B. The first isolated mixture of streptogramins came from *Streptomyces graminofaciens* found in a soil sample in Texas, hence the derived name of these antibiotics. Although most streptogramins are produced by Streptomyces, other bacterial strains such as Actinoplanes, Actinomadura, and Micromonospora are known to produce streptogramins. Very few streptogramins are utilized as human antibiotics, most are utilized as growth promoters in animal husbandry. The streptogramins function as antibiotics by binding to the 23*S* rRNA close to the peptidyltransferase center of the 50*S* subunit. In so doing, these antibiotics block extension of the peptide chain and lead to dissociation of peptidyl-tRNA. The group A streptogramins are members of the polyketide family synthesized by the bacteria *Streptomyces virginiae*. Each of the group A streptogramins are composed of a 23-membered polyunsaturated macrolactone ring with peptide bonds. The group B streptogramins are cyclic hexadepsipeptides of the non-ribosomal peptide antibiotic family. The major streptogramins of the group A class are virginiamycin M, pristinamycin IIA, and dalfopristin. Those of the group B class include pristinamycin IA, quinupristin, and virginiamycin S. Although the two classes of streptogramin are structurally different, they act synergistically, allowing them to exert greater antibiotic activity than the either class do separately. The pristinamycins are close structural relatives of the virginiamycins and they are highly effective human antibiotics. Pristinamycins are highly active against a wide range of Gram-positive bacteria, including methicillin-resistant Staphylococcus aureus (MRSA), vancomycin-resistant Staphylococcus aureus (VRSA), vancomycin-resistant strains of *Enterococcus faecium* (VREF), and drug resistant *Streptococcus pneumoniae*. In addition to these Gram-positive bacteria, pristinamycin is effective against a few Gram-negative bacteria, such as *Haemophilus influenzae* and *Haemophilus parainfluenzae* as well as other pathogens that cause atypical pneumonia such as *Mycoplasma pneumoniae*, *Chlamydophila pneumoniae*, and *Legionella pneumophila*.

Amphenicols: The amphenicols are a class of antibiotics with a phenylpropanoid structure that function by blocking prokaryotic peptidyltransferase in the 50*S* ribosome. Amphenicols are effective against a wide variety of Gram-positive and Gram-negative bacteria, including most anaerobic organisms. Their activity profile classifies the amphenicols as broad-spectrum antibiotics. Chloramphenicol was the first isolated amphenicol and was obtained from *Streptomyces venezuelae*. Chloramphenicol, and its derivatives thiamphenicol and florfenicol, are now chemically synthesized. Due to bone marrow toxicity, chloramphenicol is now very rarely used except for the treatment of brain abscesses and eye infections, or in developing countries because it is inexpensive. The advantage of thiamphenicol is that, despite its inhibitory effect on the red cell count, it has never been associated with aplastic anemia, whereas, florfenicol does carry a risk for development of aplastic anemia. Bacterial resistance to chloramphenicol (and thiamphenicol) is the result of enzymatic modification by chloramphenicol acetyltransferases (CAT). These enzymes covalently link an acetyl group from acetyl-CoA to chloramphenicol, preventing it from binding to the ribosomes. The CAT enzymes do not confer resistance to florfenicol.

Linezolid: Linezolid is a member of a class of drug referred to as the oxazolidinone class. Linezolid is active against most Gram-positive bacteria and is used to treat infections such as pneumonia (especially in a hospital setting), and infections of the skin and blood. Linezolid is used principally to treat vancomycin-resistant strains of Enterococcus (VRE) and methicillin-resistant *Staphylococcus aureas* (MRSA). Enterococci are Gram-positive lactic acid bacteria that belong to the Phylum Firmicutes. The most significant negative side-effect associated with the use of Linezolid is myelosuppression, which includes anemia, leukopenia, pancytopenia, and thrombocytopenia. The discontinuance of Linezolid results in a return to normal hematological parameters. Therefore, it is highly recommended that patients taking this drug for more than 2 weeks have their blood counts monitored on a weekly basis.

Aminoglycosides: The aminoglycosides are antibiotics that have been isolated from various strains of *Streptomyces* or *Micromonospora*. The names of the drugs isolated from *Streptomyces* all contain the suffix –mycin, whereas those isolated from *Micromonospora* all contain the suffix –micin. The aminoglycosides are composed of a 6-carbon aminocyclitol ring (2-deoxystreptamin in many instances) linked by glycosidic bonds to one or more sugar derivatives. The initially characterized aminoglycoside was streptomycin isolated from the actinobacterium Streptomyces griseus. Streptomycin was the first drug found to be effective against tuberculosis. The aminoglycosides exert bactericidal activity against Gram-negative bacteria and some facultative anaerobic bacilli. These drugs generally are not effective against Gram-positive bacteria nor anaerobic Gram-negative bacteria. In order to gain access to the ribosome, the aminoglycosides must first cross the lipopolysaccharide (LPS) covering (Gram-negative organisms), the bacterial cell wall, and finally the cell membrane. Because of their polarity a specialized active transport process is required for their entry into the bacterium. Amikacin (synthesized from kanamycin), gentamicin and tobramycin are the major aminoglycosides used in human clinical settings. In addition to these three aminoglycosides, sisomicin, and netilmicin all exert effects across a wide spectrum that includes *Pseudomonas aeruginosa*. The additional aminoglycosides, neomycin, framycetin (neomycin B), paromomycin (aminosidine), and kanamycin have broader bactericidal spectra than streptomycin that includes several Gram-positive as well as many Gram-negative aerobic bacteria. The major toxicities reported with the use of the aminoglycosides are nephrotoxicity and ototoxicity. A number of therapeutic drugs, such as the aminoglycosides, are toxic to functions of the kidney proximal tubule resulting in renal failure due to acute tubular necrosis with secondary interstitial damage (referred to as renal Fanconi syndrome). In addition to the aminoglycosides, the anticancer drugs cisplatin and ifosfamide, the antiretroviral drug tenofovir, and the anticonvulsant sodium valproate can cause renal Fanconi syndrome. The average frequencies of nephrotoxicity for gentamicin and tobramycin are higher than that for amikacin. The average frequency of

CLINICAL BOX 24-3 (CONTINUED)

ototoxicity is highest for amikacin. Due to the associated nephrotoxicity, renal function should be monitored during therapeutic use of any aminoglycoside. Polyuria, decreased urine osmolality, enzymuria, proteinuria, cylindruria (urinary casts), and increased fractional sodium excretion are indicative of aminoglycoside nephrotoxicity. Aminoglycoside-mediated ototoxicity usually manifests as either auditory or vestibular dysfunction. Vestibular injury leads to nystagmus, incoordination, and loss of the righting reflex. These effects of aminoglycosides are most often irreversible. In addition to nephro- and ototoxicity, all aminoglycosides, when administered in doses that result in high plasma concentrations, have been associated with muscle weakness and respiratory arrest attributable to neuromuscular blockade. This blockade is due to the chelation of calcium and competitive inhibition of the release of acetylcholine from presynaptic neurons.

Tetracyclines: The tetracyclines are a family of structurally related compounds derived from the polyketide synthesis pathway functioning in various strains of Streptomyces. The name tetracycline is derived from the four-ring carbocyclic skeleton of their structure. The tetracyclines exhibit a broad spectrum of activity, including Gram-positive and Gram-negative bacteria. Tetracycline was an important antibiotic used historically in the treatment of cholera. Today tetracycline is used in humans primarily to treat acne and rosacea. Tetracyclines function as antibiotics by inhibiting the stable binding of aminoacyl-transfer (t) RNA to the bacterial ribosomal A-site resulting in termination of protein synthesis.

CLINICAL BOX 24-4 BACTERIAL TOXINS

Shiga and Shiga-Like Toxins: The Shiga toxins are a family of structurally and functionally related exotoxins whose principal effects are exerted at the level of protein synthesis but are not exclusive to this biochemical pathway. There are numerous related terms that describe these toxin family members. This toxin family includes Shiga toxin from *Shigella dysenteriae* serotype 1 and the Shiga toxins (Stx) that are produced by enterohemorrhagic strains of *Escherichia coli* (EHEC). The Shiga toxins in *S. dysenteriae* and Shiga-like toxin-producing *E. coli* (STEC) are encoded by a diverse group of lambda bacteriophages. There are seven identified toxins produced in the various strains of STEC. In 1897 the Japanese microbiologist Kiyoshi Shiga characterized that the bacterium, *S. dysenteriae* was a major cause of the potentially lethal disorder referred to as dysentery. Dysentery is a form of inflammatory gastroenteritis that can result from bacterial, viral, protozoal, or parasitic worm infection. In 1977, a group of *E. coli* were identified that produced a toxin whose activity was tested on Vero cells in culture. The toxin killed the Vero cells and so it was termed verotoxin, and the bacteria were termed verotoxin-producing *E. coli* (VTEC). Several strains of *E. coli* were identified in the 1980s that produced toxins that were related to Shiga toxin and therefore, these bacteria were named Shiga-like toxin-producing *E. coli* (STEC). The toxins produced by VTEC and STEC strains of *E. coli* are now identified with the abbreviation: Stx. Shiga toxin from *S. dysenteriae* and the *E. coli*-produced Shiga toxin 1 (Stx1) differ only by a single amino acid. There are two distinct families of *E. coli* Stx toxins identified as the Stx1 and Stx2 families. The Stx1 family is composed of Stx1 and Stx1c, while the Stx2 family is composed of Stx2, Stx2c, Stx2d, Stx2e, and Stx2f. The most common strain of STEC causing hemorrhagic colitis in humans is the serotype O157:H7. The O and H designations for strains of *E. coli* define the O-antigens and the H-antigens, immunologic determinants on the surface of the bacteria. The O-antigens are determined by portions of the lipopolysaccharide (LPS) component of the outer membrane. There are several hundred characterized O-antigens. The H-antigens are determined by the bacterial flagella. Up to 15% of patients with hemolytic colitis, due to ingestion of the O157:H7 strain, go on to develop hemolytic-uremic syndrome (HUS). HUS is characterized by hemolytic anemia, acute renal failure (uremia), and a low platelet count (thrombocytopenia). Shiga toxin and all of the Stx toxins gain entry into host cells via attachment to the cell surface glycosphingolipid, globotriaosylceramide (Gb3; also known as CD77 or the Pk blood group antigen). Following attachment, the toxin is subsequently internalized. The toxin, Stx2e, can also bind to the cell surface glycosphingolipid, globotetraosylceramide (Gb4). Following the binding to Gb3 (or Gb4) receptor molecules, Shiga toxin and the Stx family toxins are internalized by endocytosis from clathrin-coated pits. Although the primary uptake mechanism involves clathrin-coated pits, when clathrin-dependent endocytosis is inhibited, Shiga toxin is still efficiently internalized. Following uptake, Shiga toxins localize to the endosomes and are then transferred to the trans-Golgi network, then to the ER. During membrane transfer host furin endoproteases cleave the toxins into their active forms similar to the process described below for the ADP-ribosylating toxins. Finally, the host cell machinery translocates the catalytic A subunit to the cytosol. Shiga toxin and the Stx toxins possess a highly specific RNA N-glycosidase activity that cleaves an adenine base in the 28S rRNA in the large (60S) ribosomal subunit. The 3′ end of the 28S rRNA functions in aminoacyl-tRNA binding, peptidyltransferase activity and ribosomal translation. The result of toxin modification of the 28S rRNA is inhibition of elongation factor-dependent aminoacyl-tRNA binding and subsequent peptide elongation resulting in cell death. Although Shiga toxins are extremely potent ribosome-modifying enzymes, their effects within the host cell are not limited to the inhibition of protein synthesis. These toxins exert several different cellular effects, including the induction of cytokine expression by macrophages and the activation of what is referred to as the ribotoxic stress response due to the modification of ribosomes. Following Shiga toxin modification of the 28S rRNA, JUN N-terminal kinase (JNK) proteins and p38 family mitogen-activated protein kinases (MAPK) are activated and the signaling exerted by extracellular signal-regulated kinase 1 (ERK1; also known as MAPK3) and ERK2 (also known as MAPK1) are disrupted.

CLINICAL BOX 24–4 (CONTINUED)

ADP-Ribosylating Pathogens: Bacterial ADP-ribosyltransferase toxins (bARTT: also called bacterial ADP-ribosylating exotoxins, bARE) are encoded by a range of bacteria, including the human pathogens, *Corynebacterium diphtheriae*, *Vibrio cholerae*, *Bordetella pertussis*, *Pseudomonas aeruginosa*, *Clostridium botulinum*, and *Streptococcus pyogenes*, as well as certain strains of *Escherichia coli*. The bARTT enzymes are encoded by genes that belong to the family of ADP-ribosyltransferase (ADPRT) encoding genes found in both prokaryotes and eukaryotes. Like all members of the ADPRT family of enzymes the bARTT enzymes use a nicotinamide adenine dinucleotide (NAD^+) donor molecule to catalyze the transfer of the ADP-ribose moiety to a given substrate. The acceptor for these ADP-ribosylation reactions can be an Arg, Asn, Thr, Cys, or Gln residue, depending on the individual toxin. Members of the bARTT family catalyze the addition of ADP-ribose on various eukaryotic substrates, including monomeric G-proteins of the RHO family (eg, *Clostridium botulinum* toxin), heterotrimeric G-proteins (*Vibrio cholerae* and *Bordetella pertussis* toxins), and actin (*Clostridium botulinum* toxin). The toxins produced by *Corynebacterium diphtheriae* and *Pseudomonas aeruginosa* induce the ADP-ribosylation of the critical protein synthesis elongation factor, eEF-2.

Cholera Toxin: The well-characterized toxin produced by *Vibrio cholerae* (identified as CT or CTx) is known to induce the ADP-ribosylation of a specific Arg residue in the α-subunit of a heterotrimeric Gs-type G-protein in intestinal enterocytes resulting in the classic "rice water" diarrhea that is associated with cholera. The major strains of *V. cholerae* that are the causes of cholera are the O1 and O139 strains. However, an additional toxin produced by several clinical strains of *V. cholerae*, identified as ChxA-I (encoded by the *CHX* gene), has been characterized that also induces ADP-ribosylation of eEF-2. The ChxA-I toxin is not produced by the O1 nor the O139 strains of *V. cholerae*.

Pertussis Toxin: *Bordetella pertussis* exerts its pathologic effects in several functionally distinct ways. The bacterium binds to sulfatides on the surface of airway epithelial cells which stimulates the production of a toxin called tracheal cytotoxin (TCT). The action of TCT stops the beating of cilia and prevents the clearing of debris from the lungs. This effect of TCT is what causes the coughing associated with *B. pertussis* infection. Another toxin produced by *B. pertussis* (identified as PTx) is known to induce the ADP-ribosylation of the α-subunit of a heterotrimeric G_i-type G-protein in phagocytes that infiltrate infection site. The effect of PTx is inhibition of the immune response to *B. pertussis* infection. The PTx-medicated inhibition of the inhibitory action of G_i-type G-proteins on adenylate cyclase causes the phagocytes to produce too much cAMP. The elevated cAMP levels disturb the normal signal transduction processes of the phagocytes required for normal immune responses to infection. *B. pertussis* produces another toxin identified as adenylate cyclase toxin that possesses intrinsic adenylate cyclase activity. Coupled with the effects of PTx there is a dramatic increase in cAMP within the phagocytes furthering the degradation of cellular signaling needed to mount a proper immune response.

Diphtheria Toxin: Diphtheria toxin (DT) is encoded on a lysogenic bacteriophage in *C. diphtheriae* that colonizes the upper respiratory tract epithelium. Following bacteriophage lysogeny, *C. diphtheriae* release DT, which then disseminates throughout the body. DT targets many different tissues through its ability to bind to the ubiquitous heparin-binding epidermal growth factor-like growth factor (HB-EGF) receptor. After receptor binding, the DT-receptor complex undergoes clathrin-mediated endocytosis and traffics to an early endosome. Once internalized, DT is processed by host proteases, which results in the formation of a disulfide-bonded dipeptide consisting of an A subunit and a B subunit (A-B toxin). Endosomal acidification promotes the insertion of the B subunit into the membrane to deliver the A domain across the endosomal membrane, where reduction of the disulfide bond releases the A domain into the cytosol. The A subunit then catalyzes the ADP-ribosylation of eEF-2 resulting in the inhibition of the function of eEF-2 and consequent inhibition of protein synthesis. The site of toxin-induced ADP-ribosylation of eEF-2 was originally discovered from work with *C. diphtheriae* and shown to be a His residue (715) in eEF-2 that contains a modification that was subsequently termed a diphthamide residue. The precise purpose for the diphthamide residue, in the function of eEF-2, remains elusive. In eukaryotes, there are seven genes that have been identified in the diphthamide synthesis pathway. These genes are identified as DPH1 through DPH7. The first step in diphthamide residue synthesis requires the *DPH1* through *DPH4* genes, while the second step requires the *DPH5* gene. The terminal steps in diphthamide synthesis involves the *DPH6* and *DPH7* genes. The *DPH1* gene has been found to be frequently deleted in ovarian and breast cancer, therefore, this gene is also identified as the *OVCA1* (ovarian cancer gene 1) gene. Deletion of the *DPH3* gene leads to embryonic death and DPH4 mutants are associated with retarded growth and development. Thus, there is clear evidence for the biological significance of this modification of eEF-2. The diphthamide residue has also been shown to be important in maintaining translational fidelity since a loss of the modification is associated with elevated frameshifting during protein synthesis. Strains of *Escherichia coli* also produce an ADP-ribosylating toxin, termed the heat-labile enterotoxin, that catalyzes the ADP-ribosylation of the same Arg residue in the G_s-type G-protein in the gut as does CT. The consequences of the *E. coli* toxin are often referred to as "traveler's diarrhea."

Pseudomonas Toxin: The toxin produced by *Pseudomonas aeruginosa* is an A-B toxin of 613 amino acids that is closely related to DT. This toxin is referred to as *Pseudomonas aeruginosa* exotoxin (PE, encoded by the *TOXA* gene). Despite limited primary amino acid homology, the A domains of PE and DT are structurally related. PE uses low-density lipoprotein receptor-related protein 1 (LRP1) as a host receptor. Like DT, PE is cleaved by a cellular protease and is internalized via clathrin-mediated endocytosis. However, unlike the mechanism for delivery of the A subunit of CT to the cytosol, PE undergoes retrograde trafficking through the Golgi to the ER. Within the ER, reduction of the disulfide bond and use of the cellular ER-associated degradation (ERAD) system enables the A domain to traverse the ER membrane into the cytosol. Once in the cytosol, the PE A subunit catalyzes the same mechanism as DT, ADP-ribosylation of the diphthamide residue of eEF-2.

PROTEIN MODIFICATIONS

The process of protein synthesis does not directly result in the generation of functional protein. Many proteins must undergo one or more forms of modification that can occur either cotranslationally and/or posttranslationally. Many of the modifications that occur to proteins are not only necessary for their function but also for their correct subcellular localization. In addition, as outlined in the previous section, proteins undergo a folding process resulting in a defined three-dimensional structure. The types of protein modification are many with the most common including methylation, phosphorylation, acetylation, lipid attachment, ADP-ribosylation, sulfation, carboxylation, and hydroxylation.

Posttranslational methylation of proteins occurs on nitrogens and oxygens. The activated methyl donor for these reactions is S-adenosylmethionine (SAM). The most common methylations are on the ε-amine of the R-group of lysine residues and the guanidino moiety of the R-group of arginine. Methylation of lysine residues in histones in the nucleosome is an important regulator of chromatin structure and consequently of transcriptional activity. Humans express 27 lysine (K) methyltransferases (identified as KMT family enzymes) and nine arginine methyltransferases. The latter family of enzymes is identified as the protein arginine (R) methyltransferase (PRMT) family.

Posttranslational acetylation of proteins occurs on the ε-amine of lysine residues same as for the methylation of lysines in proteins. In addition, a large number of proteins (more than 80% of human proteins) are acetylated on the N-terminal amino acid. The enzymes that catalyze protein acetylation of lysine residues are classified as lysine (K) acetyltransferases and denoted by the nomenclature KAT. Humans express 17 genes encoding KAT enzymes. The activated acetyl donor for the KAT enzymes is acetyl-CoA.

Posttranslational phosphorylation is one of the most common reversible protein modifications that occurs in animal cells. Most of the protein phosphorylation events occurs on the hydroxyl oxygen of the R-group of the amino acids serine, threonine, and tyrosine. The amino acid histidine is also an important site for phosphorylation. A metabolically relevant His phosphorylation occurs in the glycolytic enzyme, phosphoglycerate mutase 1 (see Chapter 5).

Protein lipid acylation at the N-terminus most often involves attachment of the 14-carbon fatty acid, myristic acid to an N-terminal glycine residue, referred to as N-myristoylation. Another common fatty acylation of proteins utilizes the 16-carbon fatty acid palmitic acid which is attached to the sulfhydryl group of internal and N-terminal cysteine residues and is, therefore, referred to as S-palmitoylation.

Another important lipid modification of proteins is termed prenylation. Prenylation refers to the addition of the 15-carbon farnesyl group or the 20-carbon geranylgeranyl group to acceptor proteins, both of which are isoprenoid compounds derived from the cholesterol biosynthetic pathway (see Chapter 15). The isoprenoid groups are attached to cysteine residues at the carboxy terminus of proteins in a thioether linkage (C–S–C). A common consensus sequence at the C-terminus of prenylated proteins has been identified and is composed of CAAX, where C is cysteine, A is any aliphatic amino acid (except alanine), and X is the C-terminal amino acid. More than 120 human proteins have been identified that are modified by the addition of a prenyl group.

Protein ADP-ribosylation is a form of posttranslational modification that was originally identified on eukaryotic elongation factor 2 (eEF-2) as a consequence of infection by *Corynebacterium diphtheriae* (Clinical Box 24–4). Numerous proteins have been identified that undergo ADP-ribosylation as a natural mechanism of regulating their function. The process of protein ADP-ribosylation is a reversible posttranslational modification that results in the covalent attachment of either a single ADP-ribose unit (monoADP-ribose: MAR) or polymers of ADP-ribose units (polyADP-ribose: PAR) on the side chain of asparagine, aspartic acid, glutamic acid, arginine, lysine or cysteine resides within target proteins. Protein ADP-ribosylation is catalyzed by a diverse group of ADP ribosyl transferase (ADPRT) enzymes that use ADP-ribose units derived from NAD^+ to catalyze the ADP-ribosylation reaction.

Sulfate modification of proteins occurs at tyrosine residues. As many as 1% of all tyrosine residues present in the eukaryotic proteome are modified by sulfate addition making this the most common tyrosine modification. Tyrosine sulfation is accomplished via the activity of tyrosylprotein sulfotransferases (TPST) which are membrane-associated enzymes of the *trans*-Golgi network. At least 34 human proteins have been identified that are tyrosine sulfated although the total number that is predicted is much higher.

Modifications of proteins that depend upon vitamin C (see Chapter 3) as a cofactor include proline and lysine hydroxylations and carboxy terminal amidation of neuroendocrine peptides. The hydroxylating enzymes are identified as prolyl hydroxylases and lysyl hydroxylases. Some of the most important hydroxylated proteins are the collagens.

Vitamin K (see Chapter 3) is a cofactor in the carboxylation of glutamic acid residues catalyzed by the enzyme gamma-glutamyl carboxylase (γ-glutamyl carboxylase). The result of this type of reaction is the formation of a γ-carboxyglutamate (gamma-carboxyglutamate), referred to as a *gla* residue. The gene encoding γ-glutamyl carboxylase is identified as *GGCX*. The critical gla residue containing proteins function in the process of blood coagulation (see Chapter 33) and include prothrombin, factors VII, IX, X, factor C, and factor S.

SECRETED AND MEMBRANE-ASSOCIATED PROTEINS

Proteins that are membrane bound or are destined for excretion are synthesized by ribosomes associated with the membranes of the ER (Figure 24–10). The ER associated with ribosomes is termed rough ER (RER). This class of protein all contains an N-terminus termed a **signal sequence** or **signal peptide**. The signal peptide is usually 13-36 predominantly hydrophobic residues. The signal peptide is recognized by a multiprotein complex termed the signal recognition particle (SRP). This signal peptide

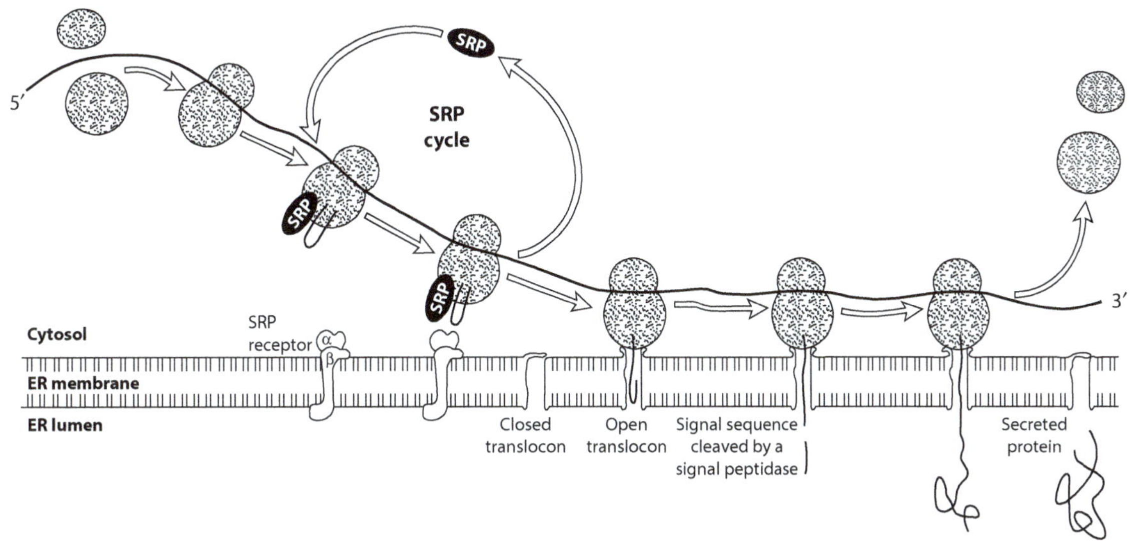

FIGURE 24–10 Mechanism of synthesis of membrane bound or secreted proteins. Ribosomes engage the ER membrane through interaction of the signal recognition particle (SRP) in the ribosome with the SRP receptor in the ER membrane. As the protein is synthesized the signal sequence is passed through the ER membrane into the lumen of the ER. After sufficient synthesis the signal peptide is removed by the action of signal peptidase. Synthesis will continue and if the protein is secreted it will end up completely in the lumen of the ER. If the protein is membrane associated a stop transfer motif in the protein will stop the transfer of the protein through the ER membrane. This will become the membrane-spanning domain of the protein. (Reproduced with permission from themedicalbiochemistrypage, LLC.)

is removed following passage through the ER membrane. The removal of the signal peptide is catalyzed by signal peptidase. Proteins that contain a signal peptide are called preproteins to distinguish them from proproteins. However, some proteins that are destined for secretion are also further proteolyzed following secretion and, therefore contain pro sequences. This class of proteins is termed preproproteins.

ORGANELLE TARGETING OF PROTEINS

Many proteins exert their functions in specific subcellular organelles and, as such, need to be targeted to those locations following their synthesis. Further processing of organelle-targeted proteins can occur once the protein is appropriately localized. The process of organelle targeting involves both direct amino acid sequences in the proteins and proteins involved in the recognition and transport of organellar-specific proteins.

The nucleus is in contact with the lumen of the ER via connections between the outer nuclear membrane and the ER membranes. The inner and outer nuclear membranes are also connected at thousands of locations via multiprotein complexes that generate pores in the nuclear membrane called nuclear pore complexes, NPC. The import and export of nuclear macromolecules through the NPC involves proteins identified as importins and exportins and the monomeric G-protein Ran (with bound GTP; RanGTP). Targeting proteins to the nucleus involves the recognition of a specific nuclear localization sequence, NLS in the target protein. The prototypical monopartite NLS is K-K/R-X-K/R, where K is Lys, R is Arg, and X represents any amino acid.

The mitochondrial proteins that are encoded by the nuclear genome are translated in the cytoplasm and then these proteins are imported into the mitochondria by specialized recognition and transport proteins and complexes. Mitochondrial protein import and localization is controlled by specific amino acid sequences in the precursor proteins. These sequences not only target the proteins to the mitochondria but also ensure that individual proteins are properly distributed into the four mitochondrial compartments: outer mitochondrial membrane (OMM), intermembrane space (IMS), inner mitochondrial membrane (IMM), and matrix.

The biogenesis of peroxisomes is directly tied to the ER with the lipids of the membranes of the peroxisomes being derived from the ER and most peroxisomal membrane proteins (PMP) being synthesized in, and trafficking through, the ER. Enzymes that are targeted to the peroxisomes contain either of two amino acid consensus elements called peroxisome targeting sequences (PTS). The PTS1 is found at the C-terminal end while the PTS2 is found at the N-terminal end of the targeted proteins.

UBIQUITIN AND TARGETED PROTEIN DEGRADATION

One of the major mechanisms for the turnover of cellular proteins, mostly with damaged or misfolded proteins, involves a complex structure referred to as the proteasome. Degradation of proteins in the proteasome occurs via an ATP-dependent mechanism. Proteins that are to be degraded by the proteasome are first tagged by attachment of multimers of the 76 amino acid

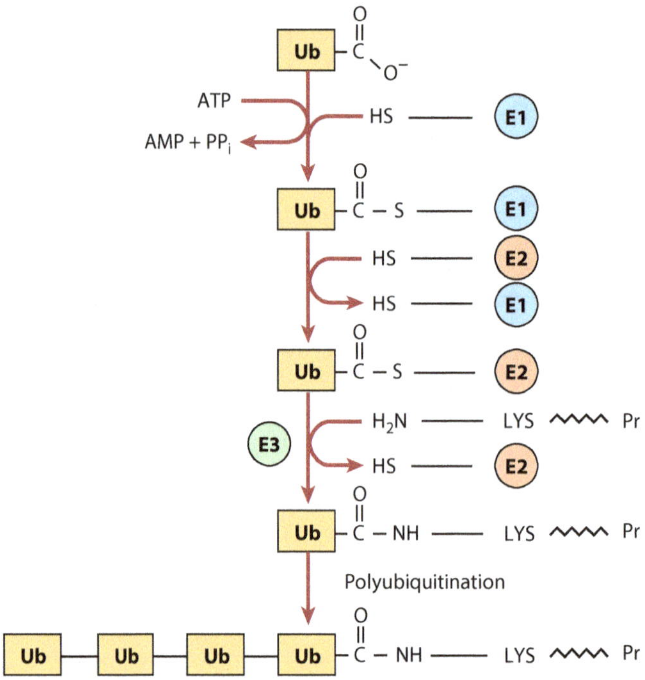

FIGURE 24–11 Reactions involved in the attachment of ubiquitin (Ub) to proteins. Three enzymes are involved. E1 is an activating enzyme, E2 a ligase, and E3 a transferase. While depicted as single entities, there are several types of E1, and more than 500 types of E2. The terminal COOH of ubiquitin first forms a thioester. The coupled hydrolysis of PPi by pyrophosphatase ensures that the reaction will proceed readily. A thioester exchange reaction now transfers activated ubiquitin to E2. E3 then catalyzes the transfer of ubiquitin to the ε-amino group of a lysyl residue of the target protein. Additional rounds of ubiquitination result in subsequent polyubiquitination. (Reproduced with permission from Rodwell VW, Bender DA, Botham KM, et al: *Harper's Illustrated Biochemistry*, 31st ed. New York, NY: McGraw Hill; 2018.)

polypeptide ubiquitin (Figure 24–11). The protein ubiquitin is the founding member of a family of proteins that includes at least 20 members all of which are involved in posttranslational modifications of numerous substrate proteins. Of clinical significance is the fact that deregulation of the functions of the proteasome can contribute to the pathogenesis of various human diseases such as cancer, myeloproliferative diseases, and neurodegenerative diseases.

CHECKLIST

- ☑ Protein synthesis is the process whereby the genetic information, transferred from the DNA of the genes to the mRNAs, is translated into the correct order of amino acids in a protein.
- ☑ The genetic information in the mRNA is decoded in the tandem array of triplet nucleotide codons. Multiple different codons can encode the same amino acid and this phenomenon is referred to as the degeneracy of the genetic code.
- ☑ The process of protein synthesis occurs through the concerted actions of numerous proteins, tRNAs and rRNA that form a functional ribosome. The ribosomal machinery travels down the template mRNA from the 5′-end where it will encounter a start codon (AUG) within the correct sequence context, proceed toward the 3′-end until it encounters a translational stop codon, synthesizing a protein from the N-terminal end to the C-terminal end.
- ☑ Translation consists of three highly ordered steps beginning with initiation, then elongation, followed by termination. Initiation is the most complex of the three processes and involves the largest number of translation factors.
- ☑ Several specialized enzymes involved in red-ox reactions require the incorporation of a modified amino acid, selenocysteine. These enzymes are called selenoproteins and their synthesis requires a dedicated selenocysteinyl-tRNA and a stem-loop structure in the mRNA that directs the incorporation of the modified amino acid at a codon that is normally a stop codon (UGA).
- ☑ Numerous antibiotics function through inhibition of various processes of protein synthesis.
- ☑ Numerous ribosomes can engage a single mRNA at the same time forming what are called polyribosomes, or polysomes. Polysomes associated with the endoplasmic reticulum (ER) form what is called the rough ER.

- ☑ All secreted and membrane-bound proteins are synthesized on rough ER. These proteins all have a signal sequenced recognized by a protein complex that directs the ribosomes to the ER.
- ☑ Many proteins undergo posttranslational modification. These modifications include cleavage, acetylation, methylation, lipid attachment (prenylation or acylation), phosphorylation, sulfation, hydroxylation, carboxylation, and glycosylation. Each of these modifications is necessary for any given protein to be targeted to its site of action and/or for its biochemical function.
- ☑ All proteins have a normal tertiary or quaternary structure for function, and all have a variable life span before being turned over. Proteins that are misfolded and proteins that are destined for turnover are most often "tagged" by incorporation of polymers of the 76-amino acid peptide, ubiquitin. Ubiquitination targets the protein for degradation in the proteasome.

GLYCOPROTEINS

Most proteins that are secreted, or bound to the plasma membrane, are modified by carbohydrate attachment. The posttranslational attachment of carbohydrate to proteins plays a critical role in overall biochemical complexity in humans. The importance of this protein modification can be emphasized by the fact that approximately 50% of all human proteins are known to be glycosylated and at least 1% of the human genome is represented by genes involved in glycan synthesis, processing, and homeostasis.

The glycan biosynthetic gene superfamily represents the enzymes referred to as glycosyltransferases. The glycosyltransferase superfamily is composed of 26 subfamilies in humans, including for example, the UDP glucuronosyltransferase family, members of which are responsible for hepatic bilirubin metabolism (see Chapter 21, and the glycogen phosphorylases (see Chapter 7). Many glycosyltransferases are specific for glycan attachment and modification of proteins while others are specific to the synthesis of glycosaminoglycans (GAG) and GAG modifications in proteoglycans.

In addition to their critical roles in normal biochemical and physiologic processes, the carbohydrate structures of many glycoproteins have been hijacked by pathogens (viruses, bacteria, and parasites) and used as attachment sites for entry into host cells.

The predominant sugars found in glycoproteins are glucose (Glc), galactose (Gal), mannose (Man), fucose (Fuc), *N*-acetylgalactosamine (GalNAc), *N*-acetylglucosamine (GlcNAc), and *N*-acetylneuraminic acid (NANA; also called sialic acid) (Table 24–3). The distinction

TABLE 24–3 The principal sugars found in human glycoproteins.

Sugar	Type	Abbreviation	Nucleotide Sugar	Comments
Galactose	Hexose	Gal	UDP-Gal	Often found subterminal to NeuAc in *N*-linked glycoproteins. Also found in the core trisaccharide of proteoglycans.
Glucose	Hexose	Glc	UDP Glc	Present during the biosynthesis of *N*-linked glycoproteins but not usually present in mature glycoproteins. Present in some clotting factors.
Mannose	Hexose	Man	GDP-Man	Common sugar in *N*-linked glycoproteins
N-Acetylneuraminic acid	Sialic acid (nine C atoms)	NeuAc	CMP-NeuAc	Often the terminal sugar in both *N*- and *O*-linked glycoproteins. Other types of sialic acid are also found, but NeuAc is the major species found in humans. Acetyl groups may also occur as *O*-acetyl species as well as *N*-acetyl.
Fucose	Deoxyhexose	Fuc	GDP-Fuc	May be external in both *N*- and *O*-linked glycoproteins or internal, linked to the GlcNAc residue attached to Asn in *N*-linked species. Can also occur internally attached to the OH of Ser (eg, in t-PA and certain clotting factors).
N-Acetylgalactosamine	Aminohexose	GalNAc	UDP-GalNAc	Present in both *N*- and *O*-linked glycoproteins.
N-Acetylglucosamine	Aminohexose	GlcNAc	UDP-GlcNAc	The sugar attached to the polypeptide chain via Asn in *N*-linked glycoproteins; also found at other sites in the oligosaccharides of these proteins. Many nuclear proteins have GlcNAc attached to the OH of Ser or Thr as a single sugar.
Xylose	Pentose	Xyl	UDP-Xyl	Xyl is attached to the OH of Ser in many proteoglycans. Xyl in turn is attached to two Gal residues, forming a link trisaccharide. Xyl is also found in t-PA and certain clotting factors.

Reproduced with permission from Rodwell VW, Bender DA, Botham KM, et al: *Harper's Illustrated Biochemistry*, 31st ed. New York, NY: McGraw Hill; 2018.

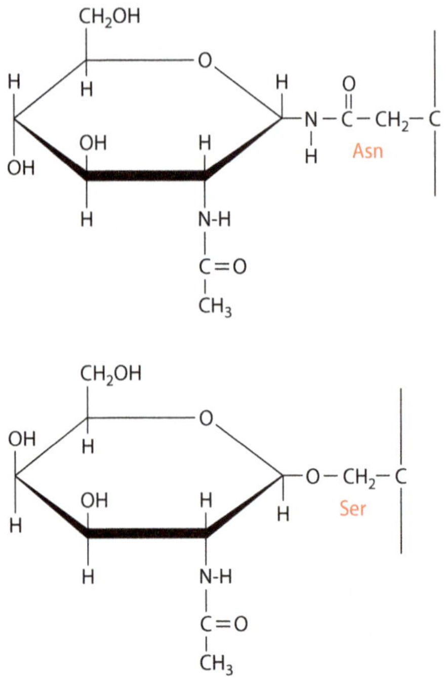

FIGURE 24–12 Representation of the *N*-glycosidic linkage of *N*-acetylglucosamine (GlcNAc) and the *O*-glycosidic linkage of *N*-acetylgalactosamine (GalNAc) to proteins. (Reproduced with permission from themedicalbiochemistrypage, LLC.)

between proteoglycans (see Chapter 25) and glycoproteins resides in the level and types of carbohydrate modification.

The carbohydrates of glycoproteins are linked to the protein component through either *O*-glycosidic or *N*-glycosidic bonds (Figure 24–12). The *N*-glycosidic linkage is through the amide group of asparagine (N). In *N*-linked glycoproteins the sugar attached to the N residue is always GlcNAc. The site of carbohydrate attachment to *N*-linked glycoproteins is found within a consensus sequence of amino acids, N-X-S/T (Asn-X-Ser/Thr), where X is any amino acid except Pro (P), Asp (D), or Glu (E). The *O*-glycosidic linkage is to the hydroxyl of serine (S), threonine (T) or hydroxylysine (hLys). The linkage of carbohydrate to hLys is generally found only in the collagens. When attached to S or T, the sugar of *O*-linked glycoproteins is most often GalNAc. This most common *O*-glycoprotein type is also commonly referred to as a mucin-type glycan.

The protein component of all glycoproteins is synthesized from polyribosomes that are bound to the ER. The processing of the sugar groups occurs co- and posttranslationally in the lumen of the ER and continues in the Golgi apparatus for *N*-linked glycoproteins. Attachment of sugars in *O*-linked glycoproteins occurs predominantly posttranslationally in the Golgi apparatus. Another critical *O*-linkage is GlcNAc (referred to as *O*-GlcNAcylation) that occurs within the cytosol and the nucleus. *O*-GlcNAcylation is a reversible process very similar to that of phosphorylation/dephosphorylation.

The sugars that are added to proteins are first activated by attachment to nucleotides. The synthesis of nearly all nucleotide-activated sugars occurs in the cytosol. The exception to this is the synthesis of CMP-activated NANA which takes place in the nucleus.

HIGH-YIELD CONCEPT

The synthesis of nucleotide-activated sugars is under tight regulatory control such that the alteration in production of only a single nucleotide sugar can significantly impair glycosylation with potentially profound effects. That disruption in the processes of nucleotide-activated sugar synthesis can result in severe clinical symptomology is evident from the large number of disorders classified as congenital disorders of glycosylation, CDG (Clinical Box 24–5).

MECHANISM OF *N*-GLYCOSYLATION

Synthesis of carbohydrate portions of *N*-linked glycoproteins requires a lipid intermediate, dolichol phosphate (Figure 24–13). The function of dolichol phosphate is to serve as the foundation for the synthesis of the precursor carbohydrate structure, termed the lipid-linked oligosaccharide, LLO (also referred to as the *en bloc* oligosaccharide), required for the attachment of carbohydrate to Asp residues in *N*-linked glycoproteins. Synthesis of the LLO unit begins on the cytoplasmic face of the ER membrane and prior to transfer to the protein, the structure "flips" to the luminal side (Figure 24–14).

Immediately following transfer of the LLO unit to the protein, processing and alteration of the composition of the oligosaccharide ensues and continues as the protein passes through the ER then into and through the Golgi apparatus. The action of the various glucosidases and mannosidases leaves *N*-linked glycoproteins containing a common core of carbohydrate consisting of three mannose residues and two GlcNAc. Through the action of a wide range of glycosyltransferases and glycosidases a variety of other sugars are attached to this core as the protein progresses through the Golgi ultimately generating three major families of *N*-linked glycoproteins (Figure 24–15). A summary of the steps of *N*-glycosylation are presented in Table 24–4.

O-GLYCOSYLATION AND MUCIN-TYPE *O*-GLYCANS

The attachment of carbohydrate to the hydroxyl group of serine (Ser, S) or threonine (Thr, T) residues in proteins, as well as hydroxylysine (hLys) in collagens, constitutes the bulk of *O*-linked glycans (*O*-glycans) found in humans. Carbohydrate addition in *O*-glycans occurs via the stepwise addition of nucleotide-activated sugars as the modified proteins traverse the ER and the Golgi network. The major types of *O*-glycans in humans are outlined in Table 24–5.

CLINICAL BOX 24–5 CONGENITAL DISORDERS OF GLYCOSYLATION

Congenital disorders of glycosylation (CDG) represent a constellation of diseases that result from defects in the synthesis of carbohydrate structures (glycans) and in the attachment of glycans to other compounds. At least 130 classified inherited disorders are known to be caused by mutations in genes encoding proteins involved in the synthesis of glycoconjugates with most of these disorders being of the CDG family. The CDG encompassing *N*-glycosylation defects are clustered into two broad categories. Group I CDG diseases are characterized by alterations/deficiencies in the synthesis and/or transfer of the Dol-PP-oligosaccharide precursor (termed the lipid-linked oligosaccharide, LLO) to Asn residues in substrate proteins. Group II CDG diseases are characterized as those that result from defects in subsequent *N*-linked glycan processing. The defective processes resulting in CDG involve the *N*-linked and *O*-linked glycosylation pathways, GPI-linkage, biosynthesis of proteoglycans as well as lipid glycosylation pathways. The majority of CDG are inherited as autosomal recessive disorders with few being autosomal dominant or X-linked. Congenital disorder of glycosylation IIc is more commonly referred to as leukocyte adhesion deficiency syndrome II (LAD II). LAD II belongs to the class of disorders referred to as primary immunodeficiency syndromes as the symptoms of the disease manifest due to defects in leukocyte function. Symptoms of LAD II are characterized by unique facial features, recurrent infections, persistent leukocytosis, defective neutrophil chemotaxis, and severe growth and mental retardation. The genetic defect resulting in LAD II is in the pathway of fucose utilization leading to loss of fucosylated glycans on the cell surface. An additional feature of LAD II is that individuals harbor the rare Bombay (hh) blood type at the ABO locus as well as lack the Lewis blood group antigens. The Bombay blood type is characterized by a deficiency in the H (referred to as the O-type), A and B antigens due to loss of the fucose residue. Each of these blood group antigens contains a Fuc-α-1,2-Gal modification that is the final carbohydrate addition to these antigens. These fucosylation reactions are catalyzed by α-1,2-fucosyltransferase which is encoded by the *H* and *Se* loci (the *Se* locus is the secretor locus). The defective neutrophil chemotaxis is due to the loss of a specific ligand on these cells that is recognized by the selectins. This ligand is the sialylated Lewis X antigen. The recurrent infections seen in LAD II patients are the result of the defective neutrophil function. Neutrophils are involved in innate immunity responses to bacterial infection. To carry out their role in host defense mechanisms, neutrophils must adhere to the surface of the endothelium at the site of inflammation which is an event mediated by cell surface adhesion molecules. Once neutrophils adhere and roll along the surface of the endothelium the integrin family of adhesion molecules allow for firm adherence followed by tissue penetration. The pathways to GDP-fucose synthesis or utilization by the fucosyltransferases in the Golgi are deficient in LAD II. The major defect causing LAD II is an impairment in the transport of GDP-fucose into the Golgi catalyzed by the GDP-fucose transporter encoded by the *FUCT1* gene (also identified as solute carrier family 35, member C1: SCL35C1).

Numerous glycosyltransferases carry out the processes of modification of the carbohydrate structures resulting in the fully modified *O*-glycan. A summary of the steps of *O*-glycosylation are presented in Table 24–6.

The attachment of carbohydrates to proteins forming *O*-glycans serves multiple critical functions with respect to the structure and activity of the modified proteins. *O*-linked glycans are important for protein stability, modulation of enzyme activity, receptor-mediated signaling, immune function and immunity, protein-protein interactions, as well as many other functions. Mucin-type *O*-glycans are also important for binding water and are often found on the outer surfaces of tissues such as the gastrointestinal, urogenital, and respiratory systems.

O-MANNOSYLATION

Incorporation of mannose into target proteins by attachment to Ser and/or Thr, referred to as *O*-mannosylation, serves a critical function in humans. *O*-mannosylation has been identified on α-dystroglycan (α-DG), chondroitin sulfate proteoglycans, total glycopeptides from brain tissue, and also on neuron-specific protein tyrosine phosphatase, receptor type, zeta 1 (PTPRZ1, also known as RPTPβ). Alpha-dystroglycan is a component of the large dystrophin-glycoprotein complex (DGC) that functions as a multi-subunit complex within and across the membranes of cardiac and skeletal muscle cells as well as vascular smooth muscle cells.

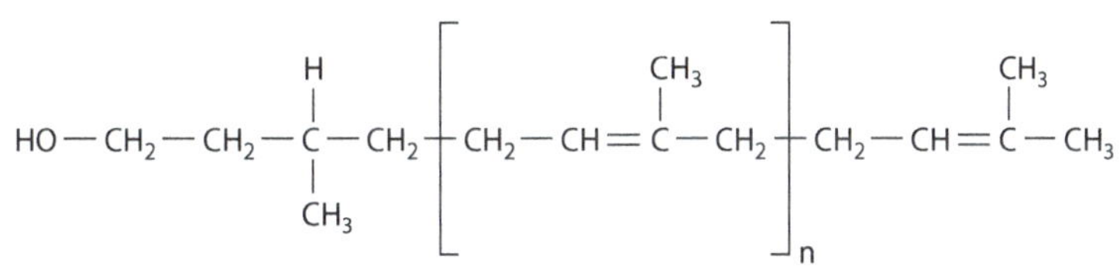

FIGURE 24–13 The structure of dolichol. The phosphate in dolichol phosphate is attached to the primary alcohol group at the left-hand end of the molecule. The group within the brackets is an isoprene unit (n = 17-20 isoprenoid units). (Reproduced with permission from themedicalbiochemistrypage, LLC.)

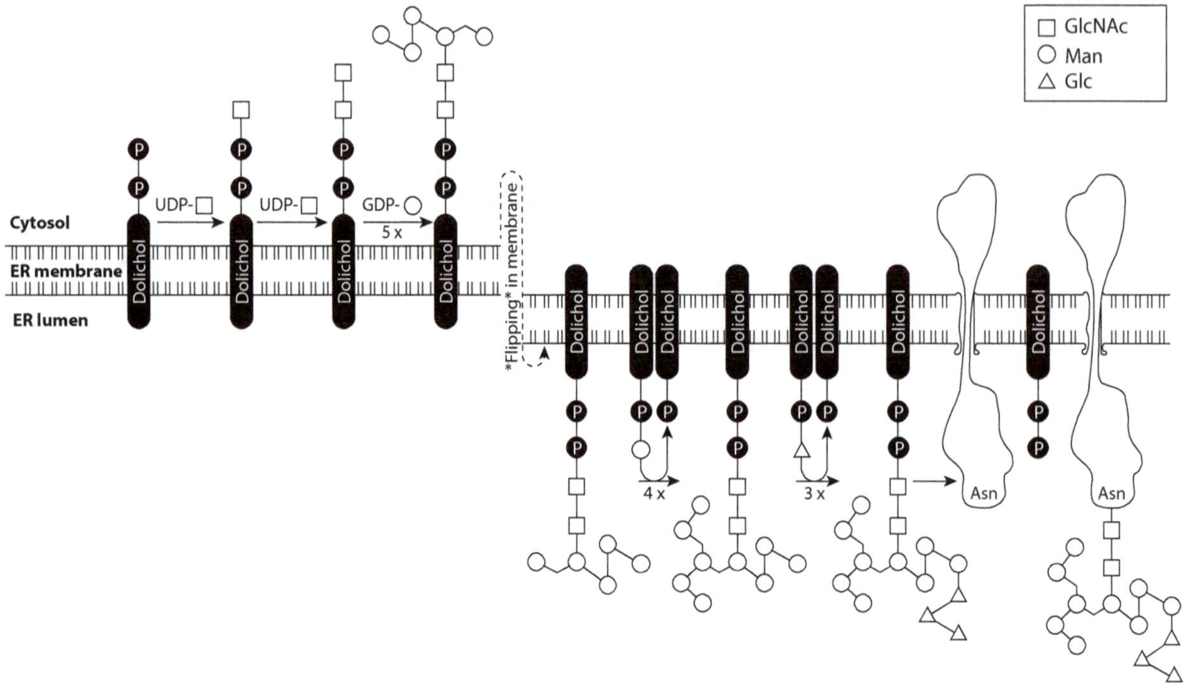

FIGURE 24–14 Synthesis and transfer of the LLO unit to a protein within the ER. The synthesis of the dolichol-coupled oligosaccharide complex (the lipid-linked oligosaccharide, LLO) begins on the cytosolic face of the ER membrane. When the dolichol-sugar complex contains the initial 2 GlcNAc residues and several mannose residues it is flipped such that the carbohydrate portion is moved to the luminal side of the ER membrane. Several more sugars are added to form the complete LLO. The sugars portion of the LLO is then transferred to an appropriate Asn residue in an acceptor protein, leaving the dolichol within the membrane. (Reproduced with permission from themedicalbiochemistrypage, LLC.)

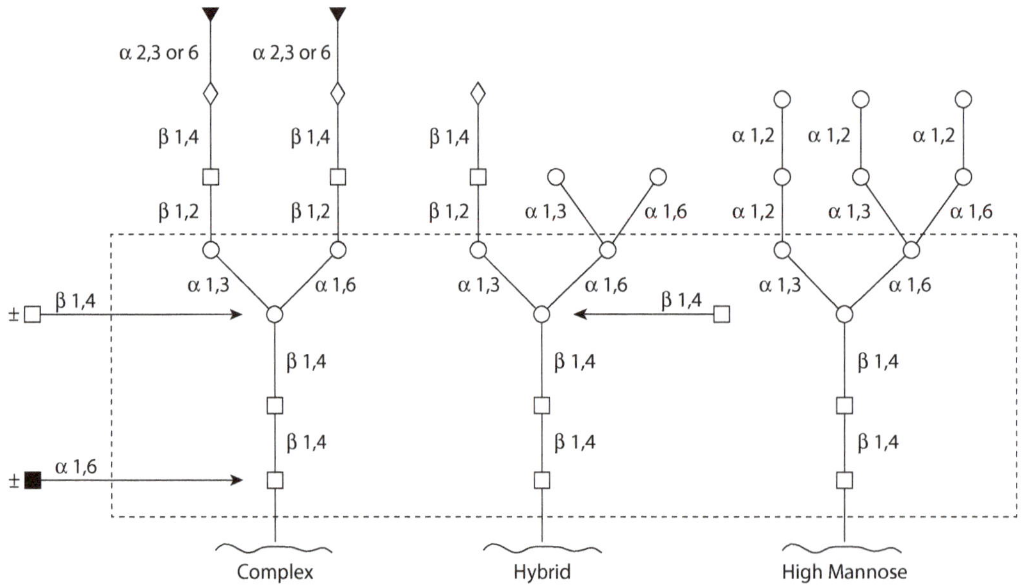

FIGURE 24–15 Structures of oligosaccharides found on the three major classes of *N*-glycoprotein. Open squares: GlcNAc; open circles: mannose; open diamonds: galactose; filled squares: fucose; filled triangles: sialic acid. (Reproduced with permission from themedicalbiochemistrypage, LLC.)

TABLE 24–4 Summary of main features of *N*-glycosylation.

- The oligosaccharide $Glc_3Man_9(GlcNAc)_2$ is transferred from dolichol-P-P-oligosaccharide in a reaction catalyzed by oligosaccharide:protein transferase, which is inhibited by tunicamycin.
- Transfer occurs to specific Asn residues in the sequence AsnX-Ser/Thr, where X is any residue except Pro, Asp, or Glu.
- Transfer can occur cotranslationally in the endoplasmic reticulum.
- The protein-bound oligosaccharide is then partially processed by glucosidases and mannosidases; if no additional sugars are added, this results in a high-mannose chain.
- If processing occurs down to the core heptasaccharide ($Man_5[GlcNAc]_2$), complex chains are synthesized by the addition of GlcNAc, removal of two Man, and the stepwise addition of individual sugars in reactions catalyzed by specific transferases (eg, GlcNAc, Gal, NeuAc transferases) that employ appropriate nucleotide sugars.

Reproduced with permission from Murray RK, Bender DA, Botham KM, et al: *Harper's Illustrated Biochemistry*, 29th ed. New York, NY: McGraw Hill; 2012.

TABLE 24–5 Description of the seven major types of *O*-glycans[1].

O-Glycan Type	Structure of Linkage	Glycoprotein Characteristics
O-linked GlcNAc	GlcNAc-β_1—Ser/Thr	Nuclear and cytoplasmic
Mucin-type	(R)-GalNAc-α_1—Ser/Thr	Plasma membrane-bound and secreted
O-linked mannose	NANA-α_2—3Gal-β_1—4GlcNAc-β_1—2Man-α_1—Ser/Thr	α-Dystroglycan
O-linked fucose	NANA-α_2—6Gal-β_1—4GlcNAc-β_1—3±Fuc-α_1-Ser/Thr[2]	EGF domains; this particular *O*-fucosylation is critical in the function of the receptor protein Notch
O-linked fucose	Glc-β_1—3Fuc-α_1—Ser/Thr	Thrombospondin 1 repeats (TSR)
O-linked glucose	Xyl-α_1—3Xyl-α_1—3±Glc-β_1—Ser	EGF domains
O-linked galactose	Glc-α_1—2±Gal-β_1-O—Lys	Collagens
Glycosaminoglycan (GAG)	(R)-GlcA-β_1—3Gal-β_1—4Xyl-β_1—Ser	Proteoglycans

Abbreviation: Xyl, xylulose.

[1]The (R)- symbol represents the fact that a broad array of additional carbohydrates can be found attached to these basic glycan structures.

[2]The ± symbol indicates that the additional carbohydrate structure is found in some but not all species of that particular *O*-glycan type.

Reproduced with permission from King MW: *Integrative Medical Biochemistry Examination and Board Review*. New York, NY: McGraw Hill; 2014.

TABLE 24–6 Summary of main features of *O*-glycosylation.

- Involves a battery of membrane-bound glycoprotein glycosyltransferases acting in a stepwise manner; each transferase is generally specific for a particular type of linkage.
- The enzymes involved are located in various subcompartments of the Golgi apparatus.
- Each glycosylation reaction involves the appropriate nucleotide sugar.
- Dolichol-P-P-oligosaccharide is not involved, nor are glycosidases; and the reactions are not inhibited by tunicamycin.
- *O*-Glycosylation occurs posttranslationally at certain Ser and Thr residues.

Reproduced with permission from Murray RK, Bender DA, Botham KM, et al: *Harper's Illustrated Biochemistry*, 29th ed. New York, NY: McGraw Hill; 2012.

Highlighting the significance of *O*-mannosylated α-DG is the fact that most of the defects associated with impaired *O*-mannosylation can be explained by reduced function of α-DG. In humans, several disorders are known that result from defects in the *O*-mannosylation of the α-dystroglycan protein of the dystrophin-glycoprotein complex (DGC). These disorders are referred to as muscular dystrophy-dystroglycanopathies (MDDG). The MDDG are also referred to as secondary α-dystroglycanopathies since their common pathological feature is the reduced *O*-mannosylation of α-DG. Several related disorders that result from defects in *O*-mannosylation were originally classified as Walker-Warburg syndrome (WWS; most severe forms) and the muscle-eye-brain diseases (MEB; less severe forms).

HEXOSAMINE BIOSYNTHESIS PATHWAY: HBP

Multiple nuclear and cytoplasmic proteins, including transcription factors, cytoskeletal proteins, oncogenes, and kinases, are posttranslationally modified on serine and threonine residues with β-*N*-acetylglucosamine (*O*-GlcNAc) in a process referred to as *O*-GlcNAcylation. Thus far, more than 600 proteins have been shown to be *O*-GlcNAcylated.

The synthesis of *O*-GlcNAc, which initiates with glucose, occurs via the metabolic pathway called the hexosamine biosynthesis pathway, HBP (Figure 24–16). Upon entering cells most of the glucose is utilized for glycolysis, or glycogen synthesis or in the pentose phosphate pathway; however, 2–5% will enter the HBP to generate UDP-GlcNAc, the end-product of the HBP.

Whereas there are hundreds of different kinases and phosphatases that add and remove phosphate, respectively, from serine and threonine residues in various target proteins, the process of *O*-GlcNAc cycling is maintained by the action of only two enzymes. Addition of GlcNAc (*O*-GlcNAcylation) is catalyzed by the enzyme UDP-*N*-acetylglucosamine:polypeptide

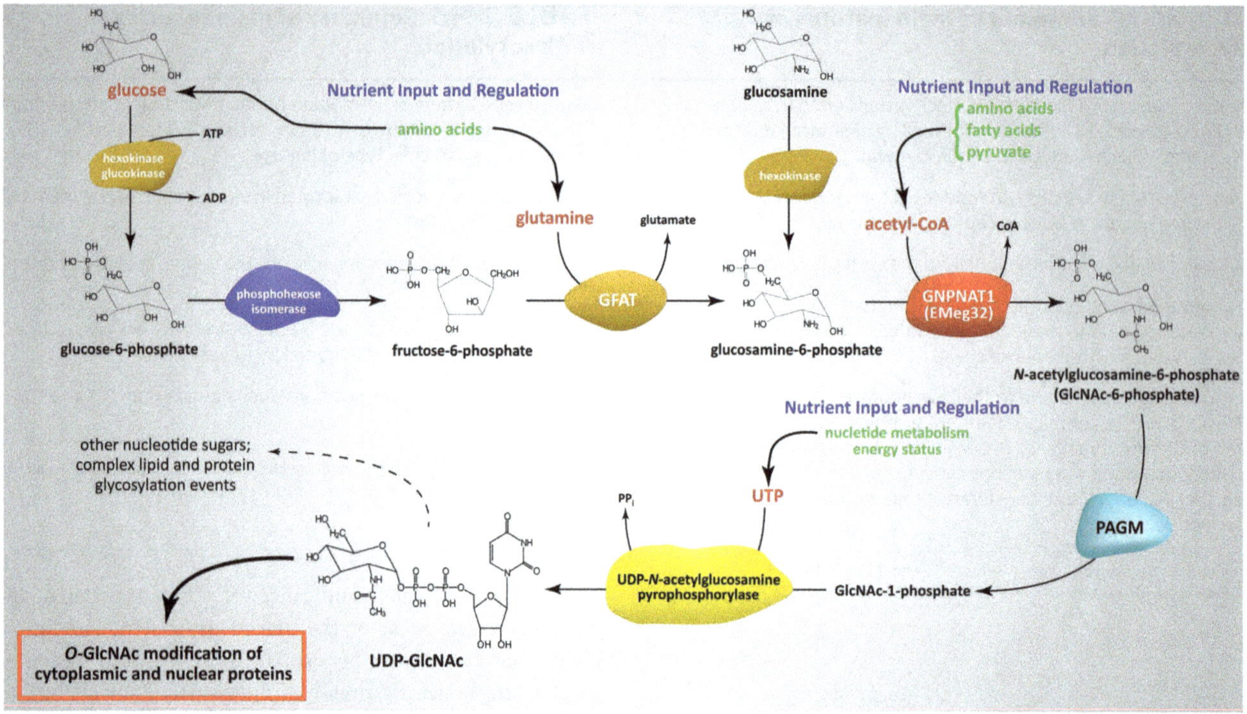

FIGURE 24–16 The hexosamine biosynthesis pathway (HBP). The HBP can serve as a glucose sensor since the synthesis of UDP-GlcNAc relies on the incorporation of products from glucose, amino acid (glutamine), fatty acid (acetyl-CoA), and nucleotide (uridine) metabolism. Although the majority of the glucose taken up by the cell is committed to glycolysis, glycogen synthesis, and the pentose phosphate pathway, in general about 2–5% of it enters the HBP for the formation of UDP-GlcNAc. The UDP-GlcNAc then serves as the substrate for a wide array of glycosylations, including *O*-GlcNAc modification. The first and rate-limiting enzyme in the HBP is glutamine:fructose-6-phosphate aminotransferase 1 (GFAT; also abbreviated GFPT1). Like other metabolic rate-limiting enzymes, GFAT is negatively regulated by the end product of the pathway, UDP-GlcNAc. EMeg32 is glucosamine-6-phosphate *N*-acetyltransferase (also abbreviated GNPNAT1). The derivation EMeg32 is from the fact that the gene was originally isolated from a screen for genes specific for precursors of Erythroid and Megakaryocytic lineages and was clone 32. PHI: phosphohexose isomerase. PAGM: phosphoacetylglucosamine mutase. (Reproduced with permission from themedicalbiochemistrypage, LLC.)

β-*N*-acetylglucosaminyltransferase or more commonly just *O*-GlcNAc transferase, OGT. Removal of the *O*-GlcNAc modification is catalyzed by β-*N*-acetylglucosamindase or more commonly *O*-GlcNAcase, OGA.

HIGH-YIELD CONCEPT

Unlike all other sugar modification of proteins, *O*-GlcNAc modification at serine and threonine residues cycles between addition and removal throughout the life of a target protein. In this respect *O*-GlcNAcylation is a modification akin to protein phosphorylation and dephosphorylation.

The HBP integrates the nutrient status of the cell by utilizing glucose, acetyl-CoA, glutamine, and UTP to produce UDP-GlcNAc. In turn, OGT will transmit this nutrient information throughout the cell changing the level of GlcNAcylated target proteins. This means that the cycling of *O*-GlcNAc is a nutrient-responsive, posttranslational modification that, like phosphorylation, impacts target protein activity. Additionally, disruption of the HBP has a profound impact on diseases of nutrient sensing, such as type 2 diabetes.

LYSOSOMAL TARGETING OF ENZYMES

Enzymes that are destined for the lysosomes (lysosomal enzymes) are directed there by a specific carbohydrate modification (Figure 24–17). During transit through the Golgi apparatus, a residue of GlcNAc-1-phosphate (GlcNAc-1-P) is added to the carbon-6 hydroxyl group of one or more specific mannose residues that have been added to these enzymes.

The GlcNAc is transferred by UDP-GlcNAc:lysosomal enzyme GlcNAc-1-phosphotransferase (often simply referred to as phosphotransferase), yielding a phosphodiester intermediate: GlcNAc-1-P-6-Man-protein. The phosphotransferase complex is a heterohexameric complex composed of two α-, two β-, and two γ-subunits. The α- and β-subunits are both derived from the same gene (*GNTAB*) and the g-subunit is encoded by the *GNPTG* gene. The second reaction is catalyzed by

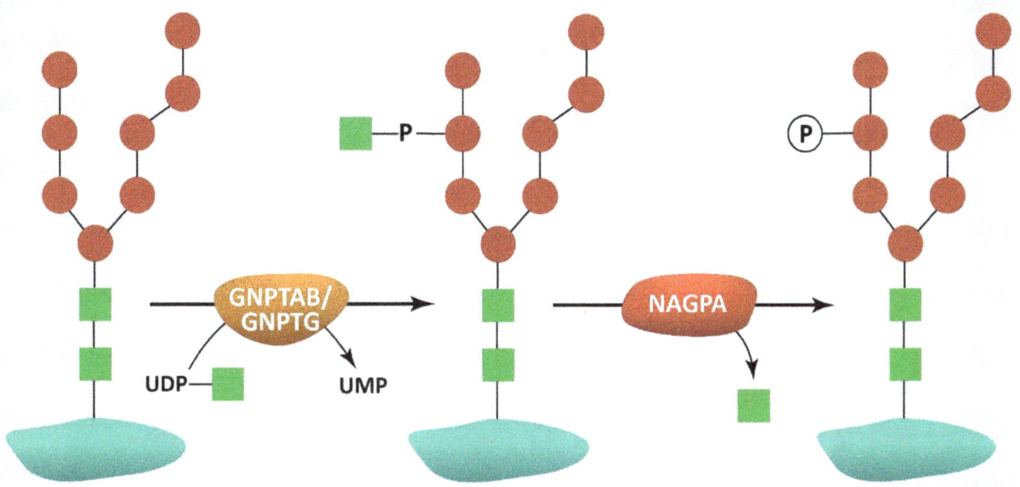

FIGURE 24–17 Mannose-6-phosphorylation of lysosomal enzymes. The majority of the lysosomal hydrolases are targeted to the lysosomes via the modification of mannose residues to mannose-6-phosphate while the proteins are being processed in the Golgi apparatus. The incorporation of the phosphate is catalyzed by the heterohexameric enzyme encoded by the *GNPTAB* and *GNPTG* genes. The substrate for this enzyme complex is UDP-GlcNAc. The *GNPTAB* gene encodes both the α- and β-subunits and the *GNPTG* gene encodes the γ-subunit of the enzyme complex commonly referred to as GlcNAc phosphotransferase. The GlcNAc is removed, leaving the mannose-6-phosphate residue, by the enzyme encoded by the *NAGPA* gene (*N*-acetylglucosamine-1-phosphodiester α-*N*-acetylglucosaminidase). This latter enzyme is commonly called the uncovering enzyme, UCE. The green boxes represent *N*-acetylglucosamine (GlcNAc) residues. The red circles represent mannose residues. (Reproduced with permission from themedicalbiochemistrypage, LLC.)

GlcNAc 1-phosphodiester-*N*-acetylglucosaminidase (encoded by the *NAGPA* gene) that removes the GlcNAc leaving mannose residues phosphorylated in the 6 position, identified as Man-6-P-protein. A specific Man-6-P receptor (MPR) is present in the membranes of the Golgi apparatus. Binding of Man-6-P to this receptor targets proteins to the lysosomes.

Mutations in the *GNPTAB* gene result in the lethal lysosomal storage disease identified as I-cell disease (Clinical Box 24–6). I-cell disease is also known as mucolipidosis II or mucolipidosis II alpha/beta). A related, less severe disease resulting from mutations in the *GNTAB* gene is pseudo-Hurler polydystrophy (mucolipidosis IIIA; also known as mucolipidosis III alpha/beta).

CLINICAL BOX 24–6 I-CELL DISEASE

I-cell disease (also called mucolipidosis IIA, or mucolipidosis II alpha/beta: ML-IIα/β) is an autosomal recessive disorder that results as a consequence of defective targeting of lysosomal hydrolases to the lysosomes. The disorder is so called because fibroblasts from afflicted patients contain numerous phase-dense inclusion bodies in the cytosol. I-cell disease was first described in 1967 and was originally thought to be a variant of Hurler syndrome. However, I-cell disease patients present with symptoms earlier than do Hurler syndrome patients and in addition, I-cell patients do not exhibit mucopolysacchariduria. The inclusion bodies seen in I-cell disease are also observed in another condition called pseudo-Hurler polydystrophy (also called mucolipidosis III alpha/beta; ML-IIIα/β) that presents later and with milder symptoms compared to I-cell disease. The use of the term mucolipidosis for these related disorders is to denote diseases whose combined clinical manifestations are common to both the mucopolysaccharidoses and the sphingolipidoses. I-cell disease is characterized by severe psychomotor retardation that rapidly progresses leading to death between 5 and 8 years of age. Although there are similar signs and symptoms, the earlier onset of symptoms and the lack of mucopolysacchariduria distinguish I-cell disease from Hurler syndrome. I-cell patients exhibit coarse facial features, craniofacial abnormalities, and severe skeletal abnormalities. These skeletal abnormalities include kyphoscoliosis (an abnormal curvature of the spine in both the coronal and sagittal planes), widening of the ribs, lumbar gibbus deformity (refers to a hump or swelling or enlargement on one side of a body surface), anterior beaking and wedging of the vertebral bodies, and proximal pointing of the metacarpals. A clinically unique feature seen in I-cell disease patients that allows easy distinction from Hurler syndrome is a striking gingival hyperplasia. In addition, due to the loss of proper targeting of lysosomal enzymes, I-cell disease patients have measurable levels of numerous lysosomal enzymes in the blood and urine, a feature not shared with any other lysosomal storage diseases. Additional clinical symptoms of I-cell disease include hepatomegaly, cardiomegaly, umbilical hernias, and recurrent upper respiratory infections. The disease progresses rapidly with developmental delay and failure to thrive. Psychomotor retardation is evident in almost all patients by 6 months of age.

More than 70 mutations in the *GNPTAB* gene have been found in I-cell disease patients with the most common (40%) being a nonsense mutation: R1189X. Mutations in the *GNPTG* gene are associated with a disease referred to as mucolipidosis IIIC (also called mucolipidosis III gamma).

GLYCOSYLPHOSPHATIDYLINOSITOL ANCHORED PROTEINS (GPI-LINKAGE)

Many membrane-associated glycoproteins are tethered to the outer leaflet of the plasma membrane via a glycosylphosphatidylinositol (GPI) linkage to their C-termini (Figure 24–18). These types of glycoproteins are termed **glypiated** proteins. At least 150 human proteins are known to be anchored to the plasma membrane via the GPI linkage.

Two clinically important glypiated proteins are the erythrocyte surface glycoproteins, decay-accelerating factor, (DAF; also known as CD55: cluster of differentiation protein 55) and CD59. Both DAF and CD59 prevent erythrocyte lysis by the complement system of immune surveillance involved in responses to pathogen invasion. Other important GPI linked proteins include the ferroxidase, ceruloplasmin, the acetylcholinesterases, the cell adhesion molecule N-CAM-120 (neural cell adhesion molecule-120), and the T-cell markers Thy-1 and LFA-3 (lymphocyte function associated antigen-3).

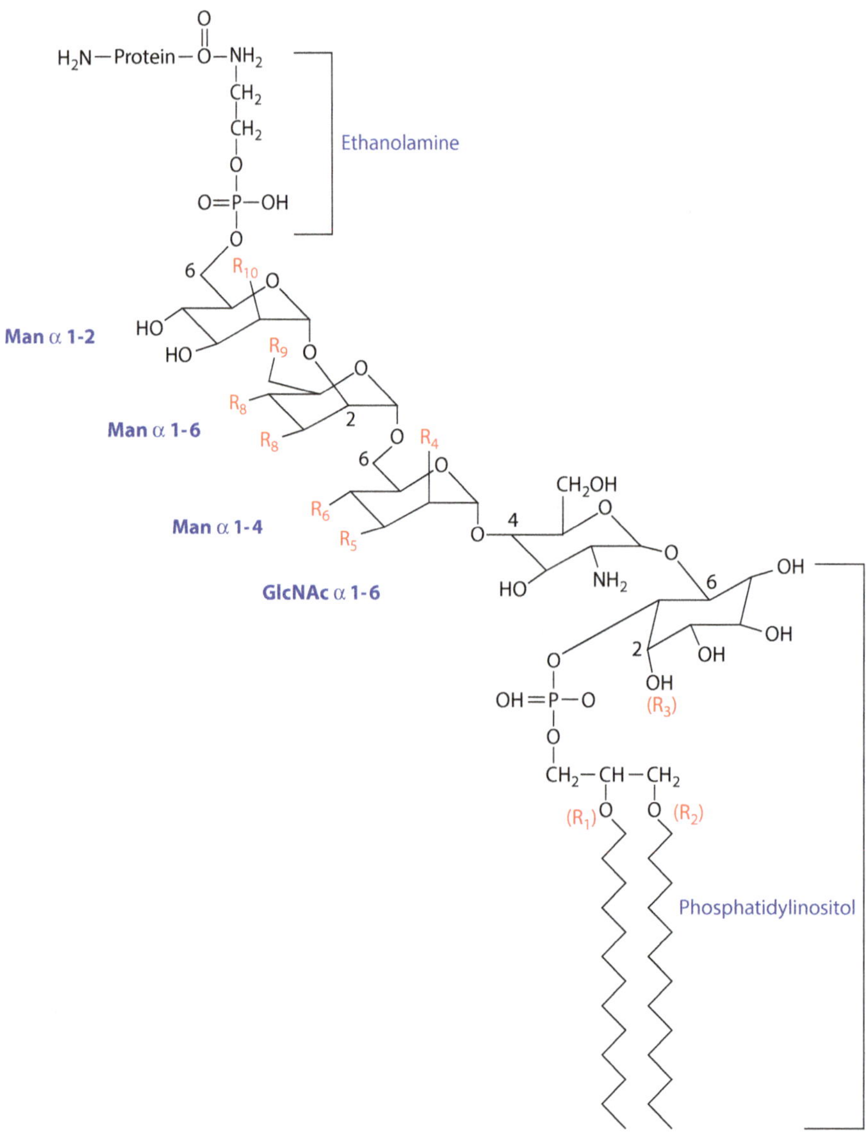

FIGURE 24–18 General structure of the GPI anchor. R1 is most often an unsaturated fatty acid but can be just –OH; R2 is either a fatty acid, alkyl or alkenyl group, can also be ceramide instead of glycerolipid, can also just be –OH; R3 is most often palmitic acid attached to the C-2 carbon of inositol; R4, R9 are ethanolamine phosphate or –OH; R5, R6, R7, R8, R10 are carbohydrate substituents or –OH. (Reproduced with permission from themedicalbiochemistrypage, LLC.)

GLYCOPROTEIN DEGRADATION

Degradation of glycoproteins occurs within lysosomes and requires specific lysosomal hydrolases, termed glycosidases. Several inherited disorders involving the abnormal storage of glycoprotein degradation products have been identified in humans (Table 24–7). As a general class, such disorders are known as lysosomal storage diseases. Numerous proteins and sphingolipids harbor similar carbohydrate modifications. The enzymes that remove these sugar residues are the same for both glycoproteins and glycolipids and as such there is often overlapping phenotypes in diseases that were originally identified as being caused by defects in glycoprotein degradation or glycolipid degradation.

CARBOHYDRATE RECOGNITION: LECTINS

The ability of certain proteins to recognize and bind to specific carbohydrate structures is of critical importance in overall cellular homeostasis. Proteins that recognize specific types of carbohydrates displayed on other proteins and/or lipids are referred to as lectins (Table 24–8). All lectins contain a carbohydrate recognition domain, CRD. The lectin family of proteins does not include the immunoglobulins which by themselves constitute a specialized class of carbohydrate recognizing proteins. The clinical laboratory definition of lectins describes non-immunoglobulins that are capable of differential agglutinization (clumping: Latin for "to glue to") of erythrocytes.

TABLE 24–7 Disorders resulting from defects in glycoprotein degradation.

Disease	Enzyme Deficiency	Symptoms
Aspartylglucosaminuria	Aspartylglycosaminidase (*N*-aspartyl-β-glucosaminidase)	Hallmark symptom is a global delay in psychomotor development that begins between 2 and 4 years of age, progressive severe intellectual impairment, delayed speech and motor development, coarse facial features
α-Mannosidosis	α-Mannosidase	Type I disease is more severe and is the infantile disease presenting between 3 and 12 months of age, rapid mental deterioration and pronounced hepatosplenomegaly lead to fatality between 3 and 8 years of age; Type II disease is the juvenile form; both types of disease exhibit intellectual impairment, coarse facial features, corneal opacities, enlarged skull, thickened calvarium, premature closure of lambdoid and sagittal sutures, shallow orbits, anterior hypoplasia of the lumbar vertebrae, poorly formed pelvis, short clavicles; analysis for the presence of vacuolated lymphocytes is a useful diagnostic finding in α-mannosidosis patients
β-Mannosidosis	β-Mannosidase	Intellectual impairment, hearing loss, and respiratory infections, no corneal opacities, hepatosplenomegaly, or skeletal defects, definitive diagnosis by the measurement of β-mannosidase activity in leukocytes or fibroblasts
G_{M1} Gangliosidosis	β-Galactosidase	Type 1: arrest or delay in developmental milestones beginning between 3 and 6 months of age, severe psycho-motor retardation, frequent seizures, skeletal dysplasia, large low-set ears and hair on the forehead, death within a few years of onset; Type 2: symptoms as seen in type 1 disease absent or greatly reduced in severity, progressive deterioration occurring between 12 and 18 months; Type 3: symptoms not generally evident until at least 3 years of age but often not until the second decade, dystonia is the major neurological finding
Sandhoff disease	β-Hexosaminidases A and B	Infantile forms of Sandhoff disease indistinguishable from Tay-Sachs disease (See Clinical Box 21–4), discrimination accomplished by enzyme assay
Sialidosis (also identified as mucolipidosis I)	Neuraminidase (sialidase)	Type I: walking difficulties and/or the loss of visual acuity; Type II: more severe and presents much earlier than type I; divided into congenital, infantile, and juvenile forms; congenital form is evident in utero, infantile form manifests between birth and 12 months of age, juvenile form manifests after 2 years of age, congenital form associated with hydrops fetalis and afflicted fetuses are stillborn, all patients with type II will develop a progressive severe phenotype including intellectual impairment and a constellation of skeletal abnormalities
Fucosidosis	α-Fucosidase	Type I: more severe infantile form, manifests between 3 and 18 months of age; Type II: milder form, manifests between 1 and 2 years of age, both forms are associated with intellectual impairment and coarse facial features, the major clinical symptom that distinguishes type II from type I is the presence of angiokeratoma corporis diffusum (hyperkeratinized deep red to blue-black skin lesions)

TABLE 24–8 Lectin families and their carbohydrate specificities.

Lectin Family	Characteristics	Binding Specificity
C-type (seven subfamilies)	Require Ca^{2+} for activity	Variable
Collectins (C-type subfamily III)	C-type CRD with collagen-like domains	Variable, mannose
Galectins (S-type lectins)	Sulfhydryl-dependent or β-galactosidase binding	Strict for β-galactosides
Siglecs (I-type lectins)	Contain immunoglobulin-like domains	Sialic acid
Phosphomannosyl receptors (P-type lectins)	Recognize mannose-6-phosphate	Mannose-6-phosphate
Pentraxins	Quaternary structure composed of five identical polypeptides that form a ring with a central hole	Variable and can be noncarbohydrate
Calnexin and calreticulin	Recognition of properly folded glycoproteins in the ER	Glucose
Ficolins	Contain fibrinogen-like homology domain	Variable
Tachylectins	Distinct CRD but also contain fibrinogen-like domain	GlcNAc/GalNAc

Reproduced with permission from King MW: *Integrative Medical Biochemistry Examination and Board Review*. New York, NY: McGraw Hill; 2014.

CHECKLIST

- ☑ Glycoproteins represent a diverse family of widely distributed proteins that contain from one to many covalently linked carbohydrate structures. Essentially all plasma proteins, secreted proteins, and membrane-attached proteins are modified with carbohydrate attachment.
- ☑ Approximately 50% of all human proteins are known to be glycosylated and at least 1% of the human genome is represented by genes involved in glycan processing.
- ☑ There are two broad categories of glycoprotein: those that have carbohydrate attached to asparagine residues (*N*-linked glycoproteins) and those with carbohydrate attached to the hydroxyl of serine, threonine, or hydroxylysine (*O*-linked glycoproteins).
- ☑ Glycoproteins are synthesized as they transit the ER and the Golgi apparatus.
- ☑ Sugars attached to glycoproteins are all activated by nucleotide addition prior to incorporation into proteins via the actions of a family of glycosyltransferases.
- ☑ Glycosidases are responsible for removal of carbohydrates and are involved in the remodeling of the sugar composition of glycoproteins.
- ☑ Synthesis of *N*-linked glycoproteins involves the initial attachment of a core glycan structure to the lipid dolichol pyrophosphate, followed by transfer to the acceptor protein.
- ☑ *N*-linked glycoproteins are represented by three distinct families termed high mannose, complex, and hybrid each of which is determined by the glycan composition of the functional protein.
- ☑ Most lysosomal hydrolases are modified with mannose-6-phosphate which is recognized by a specific receptor in the membranes of the lysosome. Defective production of this modification results in defective lysosome function resulting in a family of disorders termed lysosomal storage disease, many of which have devastating clinical consequences.
- ☑ Synthesis of *O*-linked glycoproteins involves direct attachment of the sugar from a nucleotide-activated intermediate through the action of glycosyltransferases.
- ☑ The most common family of *O*-linked glycoproteins is the mucins. These high molecular weight, heavily glycosylated proteins form gels that lubricate and form chemical barriers on the surfaces of epithelial cells in the gastrointestinal, respiratory, and reproductive systems.
- ☑ Mannosylation is a specialized form of *O*-linkage that is clinically most significant with respect to modification of α-dystroglycan, as evidenced by the fact that the major symptoms associated with defects in *O*-mannosylation are reflective of α-dystroglycan dysfunction.

- ☑ The hexosamine biosynthesis pathway is responsible for the synthesis of *O*-GlcNAc which is an important glycan modification of cytoplasmic and nuclear proteins. Numerous proteins involved in the regulation of insulin function and glucose homeostasis are *O*-GlcNAcylated. Defects in regulation of *O*-GlcNAcylation can lead to insulin resistance with consequent disruption in glucose homeostasis.
- ☑ A number of important proteins are tethered to the plasma membrane via a unique glycan attachment to membrane phospholipid: a glycophosphatidylinositol (GPI) linkage. These proteins are termed glypiated proteins.
- ☑ Many viruses and pathogens gain entry into human cells by recognition of the carbohydrate structures on membrane proteins.
- ☑ Lectins are a family of proteins that all contain a carbohydrate recognition domain.
- ☑ Inherited deficiencies in many of the enzymes responsible for *N*-linkage and *O*-linkage can result in clinically severe disorders. This family of diseases is called the congenital disorders of glycosylation, CDG. Leukocyte adhesion deficiency syndrome II (LAD II) is a primary immunodeficiency resulting from a defect in fucosylation of critical proteins involved in immune homeostasis.

REVIEW QUESTIONS

1. A male infant, delivered at 38 weeks gestation, presents with severe bowing of long bones and craniotabes at birth. Radiographs show severe generalized osteoporosis, broad and crumpled long bones, beading ribs, and a poorly mineralized skull. Ophthalmic examination indicates clearly visible choroidal veins. The symptoms observed in the infant are most characteristic of a defect in which of the following processes?

(A) Basal lamina deposition
(B) Collagen synthesis
(C) Fibrillin synthesis
(D) Glutamate carboxylation
(E) Lysine oxidation

2. A 29-year-old woman is being examined by her physician with complaints of abdominal pain for the past week. History reveals that the patient has frequent and mildly painful urination. The physician makes a diagnosis and prescribes an appropriate pharmacologic intervention with a request to return in 10 days. The patient returns 10 days later with complaints of dizziness and balance difficulties. Given the previous signs and symptoms and the current complaints, which of the following most likely represents the class of drug prescribed by the physician?

(A) Aminoglycoside
(B) Fluoroquinolone
(C) Lincosamide
(D) Macrolide
(E) Tetracycline

3. An 8-year-old girl is undergoing molecular studies to determine the cause of her constrictive pericarditis and flexion contracture of the fingers. These studies have identified a candidate gene that is found to harbor a 77-nucleotide deletion in the coding region. The deletion corresponds to a domain of the wild-type protein that is normally *O*-glycosylated. The deletion is, therefore, most likely to prevent the modification of the encoded protein that would normally occur in which of the following subcellular locations?

(A) Cytosol
(B) Golgi complex
(C) Lysosome
(D) Mitochondria
(E) Plasma membrane
(F) Rough endoplasmic reticulum
(G) Secretory granules
(H) Smooth endoplasmic reticulum

4. Studies are being conducted on the function of a growth factor receptor-associated protein in a breast cancer cell line and comparing its activity to that of the protein in normal breast tissue cells. These studies indicate that the protein is synthesized in both cell types and that the sequences of the two proteins are identical. However, when the membrane fractions are analyzed, it is discovered that the normal cell protein co-immunoprecipitates with the receptor but that the protein from the breast cancer cells do not. This indicates that the cancer cell protein does not properly localize to the receptor site in the membrane. A loss of which of the following modifications would most likely explain the observations?

(A) Acetylation
(B) Methylation
(C) Phosphorylation
(D) Prenylation
(E) Sulfation

5. A 6-year-old girl living in Haiti is brought to a local clinic suffering with a 4-day history of fever and a swollen and sore throat. Physical examination shows gray-white membranes on the tonsils and the pharyngeal wall and larynx. A swab of the throat is taken for culture studies. Based upon the physical signs and symptoms in this patient, which of the following metabolic processes is most likely impaired in this child?

(A) Chloride ion transport by epithelial tissues
(B) Elongation during protein synthesis
(C) Lysosomal degradation of glycosaminoglycans
(D) *N*-Glycosylation of mucus protein
(E) Peptidyl transferase function of ribosomes
(F) Synthesis of mucin-type proteoglycans

6. A 5-year-old girl is brought to the clinic in Haiti suffering from severe dehydration brought about due to vomiting and diarrhea. The child complains of muscle cramping, dry eyes, and dry mouth. Physical examination finds blood pressure is 80/55 mm Hg, pallor, and dry cold skin. Plasma glucose was determined to be 53 mg/dL (N = 60–110 mg/dL). Given these

signs and symptoms, the activity of which of the following proteins is most likely to be abnormal?
(A) Cardiac α_1-adrenergic receptor
(B) Glucagon receptor
(C) Hepatic Cu^{2+} transporter
(D) Insulin receptor
(E) Plasma membrane chloride channel

7. A 4-year-old girl is being examined as a means to determine the cause of her rapidly developing severe psychomotor retardation. Physical examination finds corneal clouding, coarse facies, and a constellation of skeletal abnormalities termed dystosis multiplex. Oral examination reveals the pathology shown in the accompanying image. The symptoms observed in this patient are most likely due to a defect in which of the following?

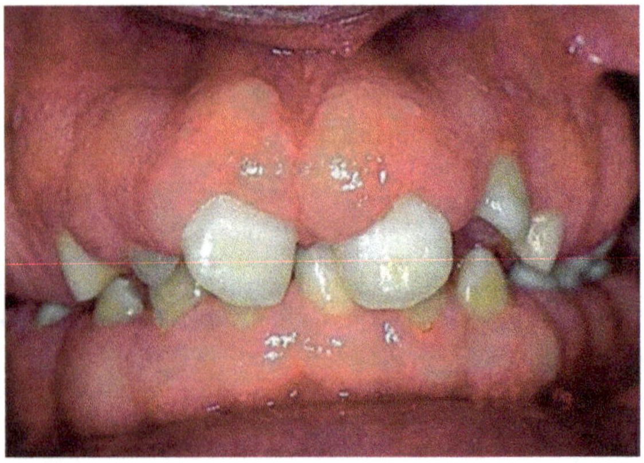

(A) Production of mannose-6-phosphate modifications in lysosomal enzymes
(B) Recycling the lysosomal receptor for mannose-6-phosphate present on lysosomal enzymes
(C) Removing mannose-6-phosphates from lysosomal enzymes prior to their transport to the lysosomes
(D) Synthesizing the mannose-6-phosphate receptor found in lysosomes
(E) Transporting mannose-6-phosphate receptors to lysosomes

8. The mutational changes that occurred in a breast cancer cell line are being studied. The results of these experiments indicate that there is a mutation in the gene encoding an enzyme involved in the incorporation of selenium into proteins. Which of the following is most likely occurring in these cells as a result of this mutation?
(A) Decreased bile acid synthesis
(B) Decreased glycogen synthesis
(C) Decreased rate of hydrogen peroxide reduction
(D) Increased fatty acid incorporation into triglycerides
(E) Increased rate of reactive oxygen species generation
(F) Increased turnover of lysosomal hydrolases

9. A 22-year-old primigravid woman comes to her physician for her first prenatal examination. The woman suffers from epilepsy and is currently taking phenytoin to control her seizures. The physician recommends that she switch to lamotrigine. If the patient fails to comply with this recommendation, which of the following processes will most likely be deficient in her newborn?
(A) Blood coagulation
(B) Collagen processing
(C) Gluconeogenesis
(D) Heme biosynthesis
(E) Synthesis of GABA

10. Experiments are being conducted to characterize the effects of a novel drug on the process of protein synthesis in a cell culture system. When the drug is added to the cells there is a significant reduction in the identification of rough endoplasmic reticulum (ER) with a simultaneous increase in smooth ER. Which of the following is the most likely consequence of the actions of this drug in the treated cells?
(A) Decrease in translation of nearly all proteins
(B) Decrease in translation of peroxisomal proteins
(C) Increase in lysosomal enzyme synthesis
(D) Increase in protein exocytosis
(E) Selective decrease in secretion of glycoproteins
(F) Selective increase in secretion of glycoproteins

11. The function of a specific membrane-localized protein, isolated from a lung tumor cell line, is being compared to the same protein from normal lung tissue. It is discovered that the protein derived from the cancer cells does not carry out its correct function and this is likely due to a structural change resulting in the loss of a critical α-helical domain in the protein. A defect in which of the following would most likely contribute to the observed changes in the protein in this study?
(A) Chaperone function
(B) Lysozyme activity
(C) Mitochondrial localization
(D) Ribosomal protein binding
(E) Zymogen processing

12. A novel compound has been developed as a potential antibiotic. Studies are being carried out to determine the effects of the compound on overall protein synthesis using a cell culture system. Addition of the compound results in premature termination of global protein synthesis through blockage of the A site of the large ribosomal subunit. This novel compound is most likely to be structurally similar to which of the following protein synthesis inhibitors?
(A) Erythromycin
(B) Puromycin
(C) Ricin
(D) Streptomycin
(E) Tetracycline

13. Experiments are being conducted on cells in culture to determine the efficacy potential novel anti-cancer compounds. The experiments find that addition of one compound results in significant reduction in the generation of the GTP-bound form of the translation initiation factor, eIF-2. Which of the following proteins is the most likely target of this compound?
(A) eIF-1
(B) eIF-2B
(C) eIF-4A
(D) eIF-4E
(E) eIF-4G

14. An 8-month-old infant is brought to the emergency department by her parents because of the onset of seizures. Physical examination indicates microcephaly, microphthalmia with retinal detachment, and severe intellectual impairment. Suspecting that these symptoms are associated with a specific

gene defect, the physician orders a test for the presence of mutations in the gene encoding α-dystroglycan. Test results are positive. A defect in which of the following processes is most likely in this patient?
(A) *N*-glycosylation
(B) *O*-GlcNAcylation
(C) *O*-glycosylation mucin-type
(D) *O*-mannosylation
(E) Prenylation

15. A 5-year-old boy is being examined by his pediatrician. The boy was born with a low birth weight and exhibited coarse facial features. Clear psychomotor retardation is apparent on physical examination. Oral findings include severe gingival hyperplasia. Urinalysis detected lysosomal hydrolase activity against gangliosides. Given the findings in this child, which of the following post-translational modifications is most likely to be deficient?
(A) Carboxylation of glutamate
(B) Carboxylation of lysine
(C) Carboxylation of proline
(D) Phosphorylation of galactose
(E) Phosphorylation of glucose
(F) Phosphorylation of mannose

16. Experiments are being conducted on a potential anti-cancer compound that exerts its effects on the process of translation. When the compound is added to cultures of squamous cell carcinoma-derived cells the ability of eEF-2 to hydrolyze GTP is inhibited. Which of the following is most likely to also be inhibited as a result of the addition of this compound?
(A) Amino acid activation by attachment to a tRNA
(B) Formation of peptide bonds
(C) Reactivation of eIF-2
(D) Ribosomal peptidyltransferase activity
(E) Translocation of the ribosome

17. Experiments are being conducted using an *in vitro* eukaryotic system that couples transcription and translation. The temple strand of DNA used in these studies is shown, as is a partial genetic code. Which of the following is the most likely peptide to be produced in this system?

Template strand of DNA: 5′-CATTCCATAGCATGT-3′

Codon	Amino Acid	Codon	Amino Acid
ACA	Thr	CAU	His
ACG	Thr	CUA	Leu
AUG	Met	CGU	Arg
AAU	Asn	CCU	Pro
AGG	Arg	UGC	Cys
AUA	Ile	UGU	Cys
GGA	Gly	UAU	Tyr
GUA	Val	UAC	Tyr
GCA	Ala	UCC	Ser
UGG	Trp		

(A) CysThrIleProTyr
(B) HisSerIleAlaCys
(C) MetLeuTrpAsn
(D) ThrCysTyrGlyMet
(E) ValArgTyrArgThr

18. Experiments are being conducted on a potential anti-cancer compound that exerts its effects on the process of translation. When the compound is added to cultures of squamous cell carcinoma-derived cells there is a failure in the normal interactions with the 5′ cap structure of mRNAs. Which of the following proteins is most likely being inhibited by the actions of the compound?
(A) eIF-2
(B) eIF-2B
(C) eIF-4A
(D) eIF-4E
(E) eIF-4G

19. Experiments are being carried out with a novel compound to examine its effects on erythroid progenitor cell metabolism. The compound has been shown to tightly bind pyridoxal phosphate preventing its use by dependent enzymes. When this compound is added to the cells the rate of synthesis of globin protein significantly declines. Which of the following best explains these observations?
(A) Cap-binding factor becomes dephosphorylated preventing recognition of globin mRNA by the ribosomes
(B) Cap-binding factor becomes phosphorylated preventing recognition of globin mRNA by the ribosomes
(C) RNA polymerase cannot bind to globin mRNA
(D) RNA polymerase is phosphorylated depressing its activity
(E) The initiation factor eIF-2 becomes dephosphorylated, reducing its level of activity
(F) The initiation factor eIF-2 becomes phosphorylated, reducing its level of activity

20. A 23-year-old woman is being examined by her physician with complaints of extreme fatigue and dizziness. Physical examination finds pallor and that her tongue is slightly swollen with a smooth appearance. Blood work shows an MCV of 76 fL (N = 82–98 fL), hematocrit of 30% (N = 36–44%), and hemoglobin of 10.3 g/dL (N = 12–15 g/dL). Given the symptoms and clinical findings in this patient, which of the following is most likely to be impaired?
(A) Binding of eIF-4E to globin mRNA
(B) Elongation of proteins
(C) Initiation of protein synthesis
(D) Phosphorylation of RNA polymerase II
(E) Translocation of ribosomes

21. A 6-year-old girl living in Haiti is brought to a local clinic suffering with a 4-day history of fever and a swollen and sore throat. Physical examination shows gray-white membranes on the tonsils and the pharyngeal wall and larynx. A swab of the throat is taken for culture studies. Given the signs and symptoms in this patient, which of the following activities is most likely inhibited?
(A) Aminoacyl-tRNA synthetase
(B) eEF-2
(C) eIF-2
(D) Peptidyltransferase
(E) Signal recognition particle

22. Experiments are being conducted on cultures of squamous cell carcinoma-derived cells. Molecular studies determine that the gene encoding ferritin has sustained a deletion in the area that forms the iron response element in the ferritin mRNA. Which of the following is the most likely effect of this deletion?
(A) Decreased stability of the mRNA
(B) Decreased translation of the mRNA in the presence of high iron
(C) Decreased translation of the mRNA when iron is low
(D) Increased stability of the mRNA
(E) Increased translation of the mRNA in the presence of high iron
(F) Increased translation of the mRNA when iron is low

23. Experiments are being conducted on the effects of mutations in tRNA genes on the process of protein synthesis. One characterized mutation shows that the anticodon of the $tRNA^{Trp}$ has been changed from CCA to GCA. Which of the following is the most likely result of this mutation?
(A) Frameshift in the reading frame
(B) Increased translation rate
(C) Substitution of one amino acid
(D) Synthesis of a longer protein
(E) Synthesis of a shorter protein

24. Insulin binding to its receptor on hepatocytes results in altered metabolism as well as altered growth properties. The altered growth properties are the downstream effects of the insulin-mediated activation of the kinase identified as AKT (also known as PKB). Which of the following is the most likely consequence of this activation with respect to the process of translation?
(A) Decreased rate of ribosome dissociation
(B) Decreased rate of termination
(C) Enhanced aminoacyl-tRNA binding to the A site of the ribosome
(D) Increased rate of initiation
(E) Increased rate of peptide bond formation

25. Experiments are being conducted on cultures of squamous cell carcinoma-derived cells. Molecular studies determine that the gene encoding a membrane-localized protein has sustained a deletion and the encoded protein is now found in the media of the cultured cells. Which of the following is most likely missing from the protein?
(A) *N*-Glycosylation sites
(B) *O*-Glycosylation sites
(C) Signal sequence
(D) Stop transfer sequence
(E) Zinc binding domain

26. Experiments are being conducted on cultures of squamous cell carcinoma-derived cells. Molecular studies determine that the gene encoding a subunit of the signal recognition particle has sustained a deletion such that functional protein is not produced. Which of the following is most likely to be defective in these cells?
(A) Anchoring the ribosomes to the Golgi membrane
(B) Interaction of glycosyltransferases within the endoplasmic reticulum
(C) Interaction of the N-terminus of nascent polypeptides with the endoplasmic reticulum
(D) Synthesis of nuclear localized proteins
(E) Synthesis of peroxisome-localized proteins

27. Experiments are being conducted on the responses of adipocytes in culture to insulin following addition of a test compound. In the absence of the compound, addition of insulin to the culture system results in increased glucose uptake. However, following addition of the test compound, the effects of insulin on glucose uptake are severely impaired. This impaired glucose transport correlates to increases in the rate of protein *O*-GlcNAcylation. Given these results it is most likely that the compound is functionally related to which of the following?
(A) Fructose
(B) Galactose
(C) Glucosamine
(D) Mannose-6-phosphate
(E) *N*-acetylgalactosamine

28. A 3-month-old infant has been diagnosed with early-onset non-autoimmune insulin-requiring diabetes. The infant also exhibits growth retardation and skeletal dysplasis. Molecular and biochemical analysis of fibroblasts from the infant finds enhanced apoptosis as a result of the accumulation of improperly folded proteins in the endoplasmic reticulum. These findings most likely indicate that the infant is suffering from which of the following disorders?
(A) I-cell disease
(B) Leukocyte adhesion deficiency syndrome II (LAD II)
(C) Tay-Sachs disease
(D) Wolcott-Rallison syndrome
(E) Vanishing white matter leukodystrophy

29. Paroxysmal nocturnal hemoglobinuria (PNH) is associated with intravascular hemolysis typified by reticulocytosis, abnormally high concentration of serum lactate dehydrogenase, indirect bilirubin, and abnormally low concentration of serum haptoglobin. A defect in which of the following is most likely to account for the pathology of this disorder?
(A) Endoplasmic reticulum associated *N*-linked glycosylation
(B) Glycosylphosphatidylinositol anchoring of membrane proteins
(C) Golgi-associated mannose-6-phosporylation
(D) Peroxisomal localization of hydrolytic enzymes
(E) Protein prenylation

30. A 4-year-old boy is being examined to determine the cause of his persistent infections. Physical examination identifies severe growth and intellectual impairment. Blood analysis finds that the patient harbors the rare Bombay (hh) blood type. These findings are most likely indicative of the child suffering from which of the following disorders?
(A) Aspartylglucosaminuria
(B) I-cell disease
(C) Leukocyte adhesion deficiency syndrome II (LAD II)
(D) Tay-Sachs disease
(E) Vanishing white matter leukodystrophy

31. A 27-year-old man is being examined in the Emergency Department with complaints of bloody diarrhea and severe abdominal cramps. History reveals that he has just returned to the United States following 6-month mission trip to Bangladesh. Cultures obtained from a sample of the patient's stool show the presence of *Shigella dysenteriae*. Given these findings, which of the following is inhibited in the intestinal epithelia of this patient?
(A) eEF-2
(B) eIF-2

(C) Peptidyltransferase
(D) Protein *N*-glycosylation
(E) Signal recognition particle

32. Experiments are being conducted on the process of glycoprotein synthesis in cultures of cells derived from a hepatoma. Results from these experiments show that the level of *N*-glycosylation is significantly reduced when compared to normal hepatocytes. These findings are most likely due to a deficiency in the synthesis of which of the following?
(A) Arachidonic acid
(B) 7-Dehydrocholesterol
(C) Dolichol pyrophosphate
(D) Glycosylphosphatidylinositol
(E) *N*-Acetylglucosamine

33. A 29-year-old woman is being examined by her physician with complaints of a chronic cough which constantly yields mucus. The patient also complains of a lack of appetite and notes that she has been losing weight continuously for the past several weeks. Physical examination shows the patient is tachypneic with a temperature of 38.9°C. Auscultation finds rales and dullness to percussion. The physician makes a diagnosis and prescribes an appropriate pharmacologic intervention. Which of the following most likely represents the class of drug prescribed by the physician?
(A) Aminoglycoside
(B) Fluoroquinolone
(C) Lincosamide
(D) Macrolide
(E) Tetracycline

34. Experiments are being conducted to determine the molecular mechanism responsible for the appearance of achondroplasia in a family with no history of the disease. Analysis of the novel mutation finds that it results in premature termination of translation as a result of a single nucleotide change in the codon for amino acid 37 from AAG to UAG. Which of the following is the most likely type of mutation identified in these experiments?
(A) Frameshift mutation
(B) Missense mutation
(C) Nonsense mutation
(D) Silent mutation
(E) Splice-site mutation

35. A 65-year-old, hospitalized for the past week following cardiac bypass surgery, is being prepped for discharge. He complains to the nurse that he has an intense burning sensation in his groin. Upon checking his urine collection bag, it is noted that his urine appears cloudy. A sample is sent to pathology for testing which finds the presence of *Escherichia coli*. His cardiologist prescribes an appropriate antibiotic and stresses the patient to continue the medication, as prescribed, all pills have been taken. The patient is told to return to his cardiologist for a follow-up examination in 5 days. During the follow-up examination the patient complains that over the past 24 hours he has had frequent dizziness and tinnitus in his right ear. Which of the following represents the most likely bacterial process targeted by the prescribed antibiotic?
(A) Cell wall proteoglycan synthesis
(B) DNA replication
(C) Folate synthesis
(D) Protein synthesis
(E) RNA synthesis

ANSWERS

1. Correct answer is **B.** The infant is most likely exhibiting the signs and symptoms of osteogenesis imperfecta. Osteogenesis imperfecta (OI, meaning imperfect bone formation) represents a heterogeneous group of disorders, the majority of which are the result of mutations that affect the structure and function of type I collagens. The most common causes and cases of OI are inherited as autosomal dominant diseases, those being OI types I-IV. Individuals with OI are characterized phenotypically with bone fragility and low bone mass. In addition, patients have soft tissue dysplasia, dentinogenesis imperfecta (abnormalities in the teeth), loss of hearing and alterations in the coloration of the sclera. Although the collagens do play a role in the production of the basal lamina (choice A) the primary defects in OI are at the level of collagen synthesis. Defects in fibrillin synthesis (choice C) are the cause of Marfan syndrome. Any defect, either genetic or nutritional, that interferes with glutamate carboxylation (choice D) would lead to bleeding dysfunction since production of functional prothrombin, factors VII, IX, and X, and protein C and protein S would be impaired. Defective lysine oxidation (choice E) would be associated with the potential inability to generate functional collagen. Although this could theoretically be associated with the manifestation of OI, there are no known mutations in any of the lysyl oxidases associated with the genesis of OI. A disorder of extracellular matrix synthesis is known to result from mutations in one of the lysyl oxidase genes. This is a form of Ehlers-Danlos syndrome (EDS) referred to as kyphoscoliosis EDS.

2. Correct answer is **A.** The patient most likely has a urinary tract infection for which the physician prescribed an aminoglycoside antibiotic, such as neomycin or tobramycin. The aminoglycosides exert their bactericidal effects via the inhibition of prokaryotic 30*S* ribosomal subunit functions. Toxicities associated with aminoglycoside therapy can include nephrotoxicity and ototoxicity. The earliest onset of abnormal side effects with aminoglycosides is noticed by vertigo or balance issues due to vestibular dysfunction. Fluoroquinolones (choice B) are used to treat a number of different types of bacterial infections including bacterial bronchitis, pneumonia, sinusitis, septicemia, and intraabdominal infections. Lincosamides (choice C) are commonly used to treat penicillin-resistant infections such as abdominal infections. Macrolides (choice D) are very commonly prescribed for the treatment of pneumonia. The tetracyclines (choice E) are commonly used in the treatment of pneumonia and other respiratory infections.

3. Correct answer is **B.** The vast majority of proteins that contain carbohydrate attached to serine and threonine hydroxyl groups, termed *O*-glycosylation, have these sugars attached as the protein transits the Golgi complex. Therefore, the deletion of the portion of the coding region of the protein identified in this patient would prevent the normal Golgi complex mediated *O*-glycosylation. There are several proteins that undergo a specialized form of *O*-glycosylation, termed *O*-GlcNAcylation because of the attachment of *N*-acetylglucosamine (GlcNAc), and this modification occurs in both the cytosol (choice A) and the nucleus. However, it is much more likely that the deletion found in the patient's protein is related to *O*-glycosylation occurring in the Golgi complex. Proteins also undergo carbohydrate attachment to asparagine residues, referred to as *N*-glycosylation.

N-glycosylation occurs while protein synthesis is taking place in the rough endoplasmic reticulum (choice F). None of the other subcellular locations (choices C, D, E, G, and H) correspond to normal sites of protein *O*-glycosylation.

4. Correct answer is **D.** Proteins routinely undergo both permanent and reversible posttranslational modifications. Proteins that are targeted to membranes, such as the plasma membrane, are effectively directed to these locations as a result of being modified by lipid attachment. The term prenylation refers to the attachment of isoprenoid molecules, farnesyl and geranyl that are synthesized in the mevalonate pathway portion of endogenous cholesterol biosynthesis, to the carboxy terminus of membrane targeted proteins. The lack of membrane association of the protein characterized in the cancer cells most likely suggests a loss of normal prenylation. None of the other modifications (choices A, B, C, and E) would be directly correlated to loss of membrane association of the growth factor-associated protein characterized in the cancer cells.

5. Correct answer is **B.** The patient has most likely been infected with *Corynebacterium diphtheria* which is associated with fever, weakness, and the accumulation of a thick greyish "pseudomembrane" over the tonsils, nasal tissues, pharynx, and larynx. The bacterium secretes a toxin that is a member of the ADP-ribosylating toxin family. The target of the toxin is the eukaryotic elongation factor eEF-2 that is responsible for the process of ribosomal translocation following peptide bond formation during protein elongation. The bacterium that produces a toxin that alters the activity of the cystic fibrosis transmembrane conductance regulator (CFTR) chloride transporter (choice A) is *Vibrio cholerae.* Impairment in the processes of lysosomal glycosaminoglycan degradation (choice C), protein *N*-glycosylation (choice D), and proteoglycan synthesis (choice F) would not result in the signs and symptoms in this patient. *Shigella dysenteriae* produces a toxin that is an RNA hydrolase whose activity results in the degradation of the 28*S* rRNA in the eukaryotic large ribosome subunit. This rRNA is a ribozyme that catalyzes the peptidyltransferase activity of protein synthesis (choice E).

6. Correct answer is **E.** The patient is most likely infected with *Vibrio cholerae* which cause diarrhea, hypovolemia, and hypoglycemia, due to overactivation of the intestinal epithelial cell chloride channel encoded by the *CFTR* (cystic fibrosis transmembrane conductance regulator) gene. The toxin produced by *V. cholerae* encodes an ADP-ribosylating enzyme that modifies a G_s-type G-protein in intestinal epithelial cells rendering it consecutively active. This active G_s-type G-protein results in elevated activation of adenylate cyclase and a consequent increase in cAMP production. The increased cAMP leads to high levels of activated PKA. One of the targets of PKA is the CFTR protein. Phosphorylation of CFTR results in significant transport of chloride out of the intestinal epithelial cell into the lumen of the intestine. Intestinal enterocytes try to compensate for the lost chloride through the action of a Cl^-/HCO_3^- anion exchanger which transports HCO_3^- into the intestinal lumen in exchange for Cl^-. In addition, the Na^+/H^+ cation exchanger (NHE1) resorbs Na^+ while excreting H^+. The increased H^+ and HCO_3^- in the intestinal lumen forms H_2O resulting in the classic watery diarrhea of *V. cholerae* infection. None of the other proteins (choices A, B, C, and D) are abnormal as a result of *V. cholerae* infestation.

7. Correct answer is **A.** The patient is most likely exhibiting the signs and symptoms of the lysosomal storage disease identified as I-cell disease. I-cell disease (also called mucolipidosis IIA, or mucolipidosis II alpha/beta: ML-IIα/β) is an autosomal recessive disorder that results as a consequence of defective targeting of lysosomal hydrolases to the lysosomes. The targeting of most lysosomal enzymes to lysosomes is mediated by receptors that bind mannose-6-phosphate recognition markers on the enzymes. The recognition marker is synthesized in a two-step reaction in the Golgi complex. The enzyme that catalyzes the first step in this process is UDP-*N*-acetylglucosamine:lysosomal-enzyme *N*-acetylglucosaminyl-1-phosphotransferase (GlcNAc-phosphotransferase). GlcNAc-phosphotransferase is a hexameric ($\alpha_2\beta_2\gamma_2$) complex whose protein subunits are encoded by two genes. The α- and β-subunits of the phosphotransferase are encoded by the *GNPTAB* gene, and the γ-subunits are encoded by the *GNPTG* gene. I-cell disease results from defects in the *GNPTAB* gene. None of the other processes (choices B, C, D, and E) correctly correlates with the cause of I-cell disease.

8. Correct answer is **C.** Selenium is a trace element and is found as a component of several enzymes that are involved in redox reactions. The selenium in these selenoproteins is incorporated as a unique amino acid, selenocysteine (Sec), during translation. Humans express several genes whose encoded proteins contain a selenocysteine residue. A particularly important group of eukaryotic selenoenzymes are the glutathione peroxidases (GPx) which are critically important antioxidant enzymes. The GPx enzymes utilize glutathione in the context of the reduction of hydrogen peroxide (H_2O_2) and other organic hydroperoxides, thereby detoxifying reactive oxygen species, ROS. A loss in the ability to incorporate selenium into the selenocysteine residues in enzymes such as glutathione peroxidase would result in a decrease in the rate at which hydrogen peroxide could be reduced. None of the other options (choices A, B, D, E, and F) are related to the function of selenocysteine containing enzymes.

9. Correct answer is **A.** The hydantoin class (includes phenytoin) of antiseizure medications interfere with the activity of vitamin K in the function of the enzyme γ-glutamyl carboxylase (GGC). Reduced activity of vitamin K-dependent GGC leads to reduced hepatic γ-carboxylation of glutamate residues in the coagulation factors, prothrombin, factor VII, IX, X, and protein C and protein S. The net effect is a defective, potentially fatal, bleeding disorder in a neonate. None of the other processes (choices B, C, D, and E) are significantly affected by the administration of hydantoin class of antiseizure medications.

10. Correct answer is **E.** The majority of proteins that are destined for the plasma membrane, are destined for secretion from the cell, or are modified by carbohydrate addition, are synthesized in the endoplasmic reticulum (ER) and Golgi complex. The signal sequence at the N-terminus of these types of proteins is recognized by the signal recognition particle (SRP) which then attaches the newly synthesized protein to the SRP receptor on the ER membrane. Failure of the ribosomes to attach to the ER would, therefore, lead to a reduced capacity, not increased (choice F), to synthesize secreted proteins, membrane-bound proteins, and glycosylated proteins. Numerous proteins are synthesized without association with the ER and, therefore, there would not be a decrease in translation of nearly all proteins (choice A). Synthesis of peroxisomal proteins (choice B) begins in the cytosol so there would be no decrease in their synthesis under these experimental conditions. Almost all

lysosomal enzymes (choice C) require attachment of phosphate to the 6 position of mannose residues meaning these proteins are synthesized via the ER and Golgi complex pathways. Protein exocytosis (choice D) would decrease, not increase, under these experimental conditions.

11. Correct answer is **A.** The majority of proteins that are destined for the plasma membrane are synthesized in the endoplasmic reticulum (ER) and Golgi complex. As these proteins are synthesized, there are accessory proteins of the ER that aid in the correct folding of the protein into its functional three-dimensional state. Improper folding and protein aggregation can lead to the formation of potentially toxic species. To reduce and prevent these negative outcomes, cells harbor a complex network of molecular chaperones whose functions are to promote efficient folding and to prevent protein aggregation. The structure of proteins within the cell is in a highly dynamic state and, therefore, constant molecular chaperone surveillance is required to ensure protein homeostasis. Defects in none of the other processes (choices B, C, D, and E) would be related to abnormal α-helical domain structures being formed in a membrane-associated protein.

12. Correct answer is **B.** Puromycin has a chemical structure that resembles an aminoacyl-tRNA and it interferes with peptide transfer resulting in premature termination of protein synthesis in both prokaryotes and eukaryotes. Erythromycin (choice A) is a member of the macrolide family of antibiotics that function through inhibition of the transfer of the tRNA bound at the A site of the ribosome to the P site. Ricin (choice C) is a toxin produced by the castor oil plant, Ricinus communis. The toxin possesses rRNA *N*-glycosylase activity that is responsible for the cleavage of a glycosidic bond within the 28S rRNA of the large subunit of eukaryotic ribosomes. The effect of ricin is, therefore, inhibition of eukaryotic peptide bond formation. Streptomycin (choice D) is a member of the aminoglycoside family of antibiotics that function through inhibition of binding of the initiator aminoacyl-tRNA (formyl-methionyl-tRNA) to the prokaryotic small ribosomal subunit. The tetracyclines (choice E) exert their antibiotic function by binding to the small ribosomal subunit and blocking codon-anticodon pairing.

13. Correct answer is **B.** In order for protein synthesis to begin the mRNA, small (40*S*) ribosomal subunit, and the initiator methionyl-tRNA need to come together to form a pre-initiation complex. The formation of this complex requires the activity of the initiation factor, eIF-2, which is a heterotrimeric G-protein composed of α, β, and γ subunits. The precise function of eIF-2 is to facilitate the AUG-dependent met-$tRNA_i^{met}$ binding to the 40*S* ribosome. The formation of this complex involves the energy of GTP hydrolysis by eIF-2 leaving the GDP bound to eIF-2. In order for eIF-2 to be functional to initiate more rounds of translational initiation, the GDP must be exchanged for GTP. This exchange process is referred to as the eIF-2 cycle and is catalyzed by eIF-2B. The most likely effect of the novel compound, resulting in lack of GTP bound eIF-2, is the inhibition of the function of eIF-2B. The initiation factor, eIF-1 (choice A) binds to the 40*S* ribosomal subunit maintaining it in an open state to ensure accessibility of the mRNA and the ternary complex composed of eIF-2, GTP, and the initiator met-$tRNA_i^{met}$. The initiation factors eIF-4A (choice C), eIF-4E (choice D), and eIF-4G (choice E) compose a complex that is responsible for binding to the cap structure of mRNA and unwinding any three-dimensional structure in the mRNA allowing for translational initiation to occur.

14. Correct answer is **D.** The infant is most likely exhibiting the symptoms of Warburg-Walker syndrome (WWS). It is a severe form of congenital muscular dystrophy associated with brain and eye abnormalities. Signs and symptoms are typically present at birth and include hypotonia, muscle weakness, developmental delay, intellectual disability, and occasional seizures. Incorporation of mannose into target proteins by attachment to Ser and/or Thr, is referred to as *O*-mannosylation. The best-studied *O*-mannosylated protein in humans is α-dystroglycan (α-DG). α-DG is an essential component of the dystrophin-glycoprotein complex (DGC) in skeletal muscle. Highlighting the significance of *O*-mannosylated α-DG is the fact that most of the defects associated with impaired *O*-mannosylation can be explained by reduced function of α-DG. Defective *O*-mannosylation is associated with a group of autosomal recessive muscular dystrophies termed congenital muscular dystrophies (CMD) and also referred to as muscular dystrophy-dystroglycanopathies (MDDG). Several of these related disorders resulting from defects in *O*-mannosylation were originally classified as Walker-Warburg syndrome (WWS; most severe forms) and the muscle-eye-brain diseases (MEB; less severe forms). The WWS disorders are associated with multiple malformations and these patients often die within the first year of life. Defects in none of the other processes (choices A, B, C, and E) would be associated with the signs and symptoms presenting in this infant.

15. Correct answer is **F.** The patient is most likely exhibiting the signs and symptoms of the lysosomal storage disease identified as I-cell disease. I-cell disease (also called mucolipidosis IIA, or mucolipidosis II alpha/beta: ML-IIα/β) is an autosomal recessive disorder that results as a consequence of defective targeting of lysosomal hydrolases to the lysosomes. The targeting of most lysosomal enzymes to lysosomes is mediated by receptors that bind mannose-6-phosphate recognition markers on the enzymes. The recognition marker is synthesized in a two-step reaction in the Golgi complex. The enzyme that catalyzes the first step in this process is UDP-*N*-acetylglucosamine:lysosomal-enzyme *N*-acetylglucosaminyl-1-phosphotransferase (GlcNAc-phosphotransferase). GlcNAc-phosphotransferase is a hexameric ($\alpha_2\beta_2\gamma_2$) complex whose protein subunits are encoded by two genes. The α- and β-subunits of the phosphotransferase are encoded by the *GNPTAB* gene, and the γ-subunits are encoded by the *GNPTG* gene. I-cell disease result from defects in the *GNPTAB* gene. A characteristic of I-cell disease is in increased levels of lysosomal enzymes in the blood and urine. Defects in none of the other processes (choices A, B, C, D, and E) correctly correlates with the cause of I-cell disease.

16. Correct answer is **E.** The process of moving the peptidyl-tRNA from the A site to the P site of the large ribosomal subunit is termed translocation. Translocation is catalyzed by eEF-2 coupled to GTP hydrolysis. In the process of translocation, the ribosome is moved along the mRNA such that the next codon of the mRNA resides under the A site of the ribosome. Following translocation eEF-2 is released from the ribosome allowing for the cycle of translocation to be repeated over and over. Inhibition of none of the other processes (choices A, B, C, and D) correctly correlates to the function of the novel compound at the level of eEF-2 function.

17. Correct answer is **C.** Transcription of the synthetic template strand of DNA would result in the generation of an antiparallel complimentary strand of RNA where U would be inserted into the RNA at each location in the template DNA where there was an A. Translation in eukaryotic cells begins with methionine, therefore, translation of the synthetic RNA in this study would begin at the first AUG codon encountered. The RNA resulting from the DNA would have the sequence 5′-ACAUGCUAUGGAAUG-3′. The first AUG in this RNA begins two nucleotides from the 5′-end. The only correct peptide is the one beginning with methionine. None of the other peptides (choices A, B, D, and E) begin with methionine and are, therefore, not likely to be generated in this *in vitro* system.

18. Correct answer is **D.** The specialized cap structure found on the 5′-end of the majority of eukaryotic mRNAs is bound by specific initiation factors prior to association with the pre-initiation complex composed of the 40*S* ribosome and the ternary complex of eIF-2, GTP, and the initiator methionyl-tRNA. Cap binding is accomplished by the initiation factor complex identified as eIF-4F. This complex is composed of three proteins, eIF-4E, eIF-4A, and eIF-4G. The protein, eIF-4E, is the protein of the eIF-4F complex which physically recognizes and binds to the cap structure. Although eIF-4A (choice C) and eIF-4G (choice E) are components of the complex that recognizes the cap structure of mRNA, it is eIF-4E that is the critical component that physically recognizes and binds the cap structure of the mRNA. eIF-2 (choice A) and eIF-2B (choice B) are involved in the process of forming the preinitiation complex of mRNA and small (40*S*) ribosomal subunit.

19. Correct answer is **F.** Protein synthesis in erythroid progenitor cells is regulated by the level of heme. Heme synthesis is critically regulated at the rate-limiting step catalyzed by δ-aminolevulinic acid synthase, ALAS. The activity of ALAS requires pyridoxal phosphate as a cofactor, therefore, the addition of the compound would prevent ALAS from acquiring pyridoxal phosphate. In the absence of heme synthesis, the heme-controlled inhibitor (HCI), which is a member of the eIF-2α kinase family, would be active. Active HCI phosphorylates the α-subunit of the heterotrimeric G-protein, eIF-2. The energy of GTP hydrolysis is used by eIF-2 during translational initiation resulting in generation of the GDP-bound form of eIF-2. In order to reactivate eIF-2, the GDP must be exchanged for GTP. This requires the function of eIF-2B. When eIF-2α is phosphorylated the GDP-bound complex is stabilized and exchange for GTP is inhibited. None of the other options (choices A, B, C, D, and E) require the vitamin-derived cofactor, pyridoxal phosphate.

20. Correct answer is **C.** The patient is most likely exhibiting the signs and symptoms associated with a microcytic anemia as evidenced by the MCV value. One of the most common causes of anemia, particularly microcytic anemia, is iron deficiency. In the absence of sufficient iron, erythroid progenitor cells cannot produce heme from protoporphyrin IX. The reduced level of heme production allows for the heme regulated inhibitor, an eIF-2α kinase, to be active at phosphorylating, and thereby inhibiting, the activity of eIF-2. The loss of eIF-2 activity results in reduced initiation of protein synthesis. This process allows erythroid progenitor cells to shift energy consumption away from protein synthesis and into heme biosynthesis. Impairment in none of the other processes (choices A, B, D, and E) would be correlated with the microcytic anemia apparent in this patient.

21. Correct answer is **B.** The patient has most likely been infected with *Corynebacterium diphtheriae* which is associated with fever, weakness, and the accumulation of a thick greyish "pseudomembrane" over the tonsils, nasal tissues, pharynx, and larynx. The bacterium secretes a toxin that is a member of the ADP-ribosylating toxin family. The target of the toxin is the eukaryotic elongation factor eEF-2 that is responsible for the process of ribosomal translocation following peptide bond formation during protein elongation. None of the other activities (choices A, C, D, and E) are targets of the diphtheria toxin.

22. Correct answer is **F.** Ferritin is an iron-binding protein that prevents toxic levels of ferrous iron (Fe^{2+}) from building up in cells. The level of ferritin protein is controlled by the level of iron and its effects on the translatability of the ferritin mRNA. The ferritin mRNA possesses a structure in the 5′ untranslated region (5′-UTR) referred to as an iron response element, IRE. The structure of the IRE can be bound by a protein termed the iron response element-binding protein, IRBP. The activity of IRBP is controlled by its binding of iron. When iron levels are high the IRBP binds the iron which prevents it from binding to the IRE in the 5′-UTR of the ferritin mRNA. This allows the ferritin mRNA to be translated. Conversely, when iron levels are low, the IRBP binds to the IRE in the ferritin mRNA preventing its translation. Therefore, loss of the IRE in the ferritin mRNA would result in increased translation even when iron levels were low since the IRBP would have nothing to which to bind. None of the other options (choices A, B, C, D, and E) correctly correspond to the effects of loss of the IRE in the ferritin mRNA.

23. Correct answer is **C.** During the process of protein synthesis the correct aminoacyl-tRNA is utilized at the correct codon by the hydrogen bonding between the three nucleotides of the codon in the mRNA and the three nucleotides of the anticodon in the tRNA. Although the aminoacyl-tRNA synthetases that catalyze the attachment of the correct amino acid to the correspondingly correct tRNA recognize, in part, the anticodon sequence of a given tRNA, a change in the anticodon sequences of a tRNA could result in an amino acid substitution due to the altered codon-anticodon interactions. The amino acid normally attached to the CAU-containing tRNA could now be incorporated at the codon (AAC) that the mutated anticodon now recognizes. None of the other effects (choices A, B, D, and E) could result as a consequence of a mutation in the anticodon sequence of a tRNA.

24. Correct answer is **D.** One of the major growth factor effects of insulin is increased protein synthesis and this effect is elicited, in part, via activation of the kinase complex identified as mechanistic target of rapamycin complex 1, mTORC1. When activated by insulin receptor signaling, AKT phosphorylates one of the protein components of the mTORC1 resulting in activation of the kinase activity of the complex. Several mTORC1 targets are proteins that regulate protein synthesis at the level of initiation and elongation. With respect to translation initiation mTORC1 phosphorylates the protein that binds to eIF-4E inhibiting the ability of eIF-4E to engage the cap structure of mRNAs. This eIF-4E interacting protein is referred to as eIF-4E binding protein, 4EBP. When phosphorylated, 4EBP will no longer interact with eIF-4E allowing for enhanced cap structure binding, the consequences of which are increased translational initiation. None of the other processes (choices A, B, C, and E) correctly reflect the effects of insulin-mediated activation of AKT.

25. Correct answer is **D.** The majority of proteins that are destined for the plasma membrane, are destined for secretion from the cell, or are modified by carbohydrate addition, are synthesized in the endoplasmic reticulum (ER) and Golgi complex. The signal sequence at the N-terminus of these types of proteins recognized by the signal recognition particle (SRP) which then attaches the newly synthesized protein to the SRP receptor on the ER membrane. Proteins that are destined to be membrane bound contain a stretch (5 or more) of hydrophobic amino acids that constitutes the transmembrane domain. These hydrophobic amino acids stop the transfer of the protein into the ER lumen and are referred to as anchor sequences or stop-transfer sequences. Loss of the signal sequence (choice C) would prevent association of the newly synthesized protein with the ER and would, therefore, prevent the protein from appearing in the media of the cultured cells. Loss of none of the other sites (choices A, B, and E) would be associated with a normally membrane-bound protein ending up being secreted.

26. Correct answer is **C.** The majority of proteins that are destined for the plasma membrane, are destined for secretion from the cell, or are modified by carbohydrate addition, are synthesized in the endoplasmic reticulum (ER) and Golgi complex. The signal sequence at the N-terminus of these types of proteins is recognized by the signal recognition particle (SRP) which then attaches the newly synthesized protein to the SRP receptor on the ER membrane. Loss of the function of one of the protein subunits of the SRP would result in the inability of the signal sequence of newly synthesized proteins being able to interact with the ER. None of the other processes (choices A, B, D, and E) would be affected by the loss of function of the SRP.

27. Correct answer is **C.** The synthesis of the activated form of *N*-acetylglucosamine (GlcNAc), UDP-GlcNAc, occurs via the process referred to as the hexosamine biosynthesis pathway, HBP. The HBP begins with the input of glucose and its conversion to glucosamine-6-phosphate. However, glucosamine itself can be phosphorylated to glucosamine-6-phosphate via the action of hexokinases. UDP-GlcNAc is utilized by the enzyme *O*-GlcNAc transferase (OGT) to attach GlcNAc to the hydroxyl groups of Ser and Thr residues in both cytoplasmic and nuclear proteins in a process termed *O*-GlcNAcylation. Numerous proteins involved in insulin signaling and the downstream targets of these signaling cascades have been shown to be *O*-GlcNAcylated, the consequences of which are reduced activity of the modified proteins. With respect to insulin receptor signaling proteins, IRS-1, PI3K, AKT, PDK1, and GSK3β are all known to be *O*-GlcNAcylated. These modifications have all been observed in adipocytes which are a major target for the actions of insulin. The inhibition of PDK1 and AKT in adipocytes via *O*-GlcNAcylation results in reduced mobilization of GLUT4 containing vesicles to the plasma membrane with the consequences being the observed reductions in glucose uptake. None of the other carbohydrates (choices A, B, D, and E) function in the context of the hexosamine biosynthesis pathway and the generation of UDP-GlcNAc.

28. Correct answer is **D.** The infant is most likely experiencing the signs and symptoms of Wolcott-Rallison syndrome (WRS). It is a rare autosomal recessive disease, characterized by neonatal-onset of non-autoimmune insulin-requiring diabetes associated with skeletal dysplasia and growth retardation. WRS is caused by mutations in the gene encoding one of the kinases of the eIF-2α kinase family. Specifically, the kinase is PKR-like endoplasmic reticulum kinase (PERK). PERK is an endoplasmic reticulum (ER) transmembrane protein, which plays a key role in translation control during the unfolded protein response. ER dysfunction is central to the disease processes identified in this patient. I-cell disease (choice A) is a lysosomal storage disease resulting from loss of function of the enzyme (phosphotransferase) responsible for incorporating phosphate into mannose residues in lysosomal hydrolases. Leukocyte adhesion deficiency syndrome II, LAD II (choice B), is a form of congenital disorder of glycosylation (CDG) resulting from mutations in the gene encoding α-1,2-fucosyltransferase. Symptoms of LAD II are characterized by unique facial features, recurrent infections, persistent leukocytosis, defective neutrophil chemotaxis and severe growth and intellectual impairment. Tay-Sachs disease (choice C) is a lysosomal storage disease resulting from mutations in the lysosomal hydrolase, hexosaminidase A. Infants with Tay-Sachs disease appear normal at birth but by 6–10 months of age they will begin to show regression of prior acquired motor and mental skills, eventually resulting in death by 2–3 years of age. Vanishing white matter leukodystrophy, VWM, (choice E) results from mutations in any one of the genes encoding the five subunits of the translation factor, eIF-2B. VMW (also called leukoencephalopathy with vanishing white matter) is a progressive disorder that mainly affects the brain and spinal cord. Afflicted individuals show no signs at birth but will eventually show a slightly delayed development of motor skills such as crawling or walking. During early childhood, most affected individuals begin to develop motor symptoms, including spasticity and difficulty with coordinating movements.

29. Correct answer is **B.** Many membrane-associated glycoproteins belong to neither the peripheral nor the transmembrane class. These glycoproteins are tethered to the outer leaflet of the plasma membrane via a glycosylphosphatidylinositol (GPI) linkage to their C-termini. Glycoproteins attached to the membrane in this way are termed glypiated proteins. Paroxysmal nocturnal hemoglobinuria (PNH) is an acquired (due to somatic mutations in bone marrow cells) hematopoietic disorder where the cells lack GPI-anchored proteins. This disorder is characterized by intravascular hemolysis of erythrocytes by their own complement system proteins. This phenotype is principally due to the lack of the complement inhibitor proteins CD55 and CD59, which are GPI-anchored, on the surface of erythrocytes. PNH has been shown to be the result of somatic mutations in the *PIGA* gene whose encoded protein (phosphatidylinositol glycan anchor biosynthesis class A) catalyzes the first reaction in the synthesis of the GPI anchor. Defects in the none of the other processes (choices A, C, D, and E) are associated with the development of paroxysmal nocturnal hemoglobinuria.

30. Correct answer is **C.** The child is most likely exhibiting the signs and symptoms of leukocyte adhesion deficiency syndrome II (LAD II). LAD II is a disease that belongs to the class of disorders referred to as primary immunodeficiency syndromes. Symptoms of LAD II are characterized by unique facial features, recurrent infections, persistent leukocytosis, defective neutrophil chemotaxis, severe growth impairment, and intellectual impairment. The genetic defect resulting in LAD II is in the pathway of fucose incorporation into glycoproteins leading to loss of fucosylated glycans on the cell surface. The affected gene (*SLC35C1*) encodes a fucose transporter located in the Golgi complex. An additional feature of LAD II is that individuals harbor the rare Bombay (hh) blood type at the ABO locus as well as lack the Lewis blood group antigens. The recurrent infections seen in LAD II patients are the result of the defective neutrophil function. Neutrophils are involved in innate immunity responses to bacterial infection. To carry out their role in host defense mechanisms, neutrophils must adhere to the surface of the endothelium at the site of inflammation which is an event mediated by cell surface adhesion molecules. The selectin family (E-, L-, and P-selectins) of animal lectins are necessary to mediate the initial process of neutrophil adherence to the endothelium. The selectins recognize sialylated fucosylated lactosamines typified by the sialyl-Lewis X antigen. Aspartylglucosaminuria (choice A) is a lysosomal storage disease resulting from mutations in the gene encoding *N*-aspartyl-β-glucosaminidase. The hallmark symptom of aspartylglucosaminuria is a global delay in psychomotor development that begins between 2 and 4 years of age. Almost all patients will only reach the mental and developmental age of a 5- to 6-year-old by the time of puberty. Thereafter, there will be a slow deterioration such that in adulthood patients suffer severe intellectual impairment. I-cell disease (choice B) is a lysosomal storage disease resulting from loss of function of the enzyme (phosphotransferase) responsible for incorporating phosphate into mannose residues in lysosomal hydrolases. Tay-Sachs disease (choice D) is a lysosomal storage disease resulting from mutations in the lysosomal hydrolase, hexosaminidase A. Infants with Tay-Sachs disease appear normal at birth but by 6–10 months of age they will begin to show regression of prior acquired motor and mental skills, eventually resulting in death by 2–3 years of age. Vanishing white matter leukodystrophy, VWM, (choice E) results from mutations in any one of the genes encoding the five subunits of the translation factor, eIF-2B. VMW (also called leukoencephalopathy with vanishing white matter) is a progressive disorder that mainly affects the brain and spinal cord. Afflicted individuals show no signs at birth but will eventually show a slightly delayed development of motor skills such as crawling or walking. During early childhood, most affected individuals begin to develop motor symptoms, including spasticity and difficulty with coordinating movements.

31. Correct answer is **C.** *Shigella dysenteriae* serotype 1 exerts its effect through the release of a toxin termed Shiga toxin. Shiga toxin possess a highly specific RNA *N*-glycosidase activity that cleaves an adenine base in the 28*S* rRNA in the eukaryotic large (60*S*) ribosomal subunit. The 3′ end of the 28*S* rRNA functions in aminoacyl-tRNA binding, peptidyltransferase activity, and ribosomal translation. The result of toxin modification of the 28*S* rRNA is inhibition of elongation factor-dependent aminoacyl-tRNA binding and subsequent peptide elongation resulting in cell death. *Shigella dysenteriae* does not inhibit the activity of any of the other proteins or processes (choices A, B, D, and E).

32. Correct answer is **C.** *N*-linked glycoprotein synthesis requires a lipid intermediate, dolichol phosphate. Dolichol phosphate is a polyisoprenoid compound synthesized from the isoprenoid intermediates of the *de novo* cholesterol biosynthesis pathway. The function of dolichol phosphate is to serve as the foundation for the synthesis of the precursor carbohydrate structure, termed the lipid-linked oligosaccharide, LLO (also referred to as the *en bloc* oligosaccharide), required for the attachment of carbohydrate to asparagine residues in *N*-linked glycoproteins. Deficiency in the synthesis of none of the other compounds (choices A, B, D, and E) would have a negative impact on protein *N*-glycosylation.

33. Correct answer is **D.** The patient most likely has pneumonia as evidenced by the fever and the lung sounds. The macrolide class of antibiotics, such as azithromycin and erythromycin, are most commonly used to treat pneumonia. The aminoglycosides (choice A) are commonly used to treat urinary tract infections. Fluoroquinolones (choice B) are used to treat a number of different types of bacterial infections including bacterial bronchitis, pneumonia, sinusitis, septicemia, and intraabdominal infections. Lincosamides (choice C) are commonly used to treat penicillin-resistant infections such as abdominal infections. The tetracyclines (choice E) are used in the treatment of pneumonia and other respiratory infections but not as commonly as the macrolides.

34. Correct answer is **D.** Achondroplasia is a disorder of bone development resulting from mutations in the *FGFR3* gene, and it is the most common type of disproportionate dwarfism. Achondroplasia is inherited as an autosomal dominant disorder, yet over 80% of afflicted individuals acquired the disorder as a result of a new mutation, not from the inheritance of a mutant allele from one of their parents. The mutation of an amino acid codon, such as AAG, to a translation termination codon, such as UAG, is referred to as a nonsense mutation. Frameshift mutations (choice A) result from the insertion or deletion of any number of nucleotides, that do not equal a multiple of three, causing the reading frame of the mRNA to be shifted. Although these types of mutations often result in premature termination of translation due to the introduction of a novel stop codon, this is not the situation identified in these experiments. Missense mutations (choice B) alter the coding capacity of a codon from one amino acid to another. Silent mutations (choice D) are mutations at the wobble position of a codon and thus do not change the encoded amino acid. Since UAG is a stop codon, neither missense nor silent mutations were identified in these experiments. Splice-site mutations (choice E) result in loss of proper pre-mRNA splicing. These types of mutations can occur in the coding region of genes, but in these experiments the identified mutation, UAG, is a stop codon, not a novel splice site recognition sequence.

35. Correct answer is **D.** The patient was most likely prescribed an antibiotic in the aminoglycoside family to treat his urinary tract infection. The aminoglycosides exert their bactericidal effects by inhibiting the functions of the prokaryotic small ribosomal subunit (30*S*) of the translational machinery. The major toxicities reported with the use of the aminoglycosides are nephrotoxicity and ototoxicity. Aminoglycoside-mediated ototoxicity usually manifests as either auditory or vestibular dysfunction. Vestibular injury leads to nystagmus, dizziness, incoordination, and loss of the righting reflex. These effects of aminoglycosides are most often irreversible. The aminoglycosides do not target any of the other prokaryotic processes (choices A, B, C, and E).

CHAPTER

25

Cellular Structure and Organization

High-Yield Terms

Cystic fibrosis transmembrane conductance regulator (CFTR)	Cystic fibrosis transmembrane conductance regulator; chloride channel mutated in cystic fibrosis
Endoplasmic reticulum (ER)	The ER functions as a packaging system working in concert with the Golgi apparatus to create a network of membranes found throughout the whole cell
Golgi apparatus	The Golgi apparatus packages proteins inside the cell before they are sent to their destination; it is particularly important in the processing of proteins for secretion
Apical membrane	Is the layer of plasma membrane on the side toward the lumen of the epithelial cells
Basolateral membrane	The fraction of the plasma membrane at the basolateral side of the cell which faces adjacent cells and the underlying connective tissue
Na^+/K^+-ATPases	Membrane transporters that utilize the energy of ATP hydrolysis to transport sodium into, and potassium out of a cell
Basement membrane	A thin sheet of fibers that underlies the epithelium, which lines the cavities and surfaces of organs including skin, or the endothelium lining the interior surface of blood vessels
Basal lamina	One of the layers of the basement membrane
Ground substance	Is the noncellular component of the ECM composed of a complex mixture of GAGs, proteoglycans, and glycoproteins
Glycosaminoglycan	A family of large polymers containing a repeat disaccharide structure, most often attached to a core protein forming a proteoglycan
Mucopolysaccharidosis	Any of a large family of inherited diseases that result from defects in lysosomal hydrolases responsible for the degradation of GAGs

COMPOSITION AND STRUCTURE OF BIOLOGICAL MEMBRANES

Biological membranes are composed of lipid, protein, and carbohydrate that exist in a fluid state. Sphingolipids and glycerophospholipids (see Chapter 12) constitute the largest percentage of the lipid weight of biological membranes. The lipids of biological membranes orient in such a way as to form the typical bilayer structure. In this orientation, the hydrocarbon portion of these lipids orient in the middle of the bilayer and the polar head groups orient toward the aqueous environment.

In addition to the outer membrane that results in the formation of a typical cell (this membrane is often referred to as the plasma membrane), cells contain intracellular membranes that serve distinct functions in the formation of the various intracellular organelles.

The carbohydrates of membranes are attached either to lipid, forming glycolipids of various classes (see Chapter 12), or to proteins forming glycoproteins (see Chapter 24). The lipid and protein compositions of membranes vary from cell type to cell type as well as within the various intracellular compartments that are defined by intracellular membranes. Protein concentrations can range from around 20% to as much as 70% of the total mass of a particular membrane.

Proteins associated with membranes are of two general types: integral and peripheral (Figure 25–1). Integral membrane proteins are tightly bound to the membrane through hydrophobic interactions and are inserted into and/or penetrate the lipid bilayer. In contrast, peripheral membrane proteins are only loosely associated with the membrane either through interactions with the polar head groups of the lipids or through interactions with integral membrane proteins.

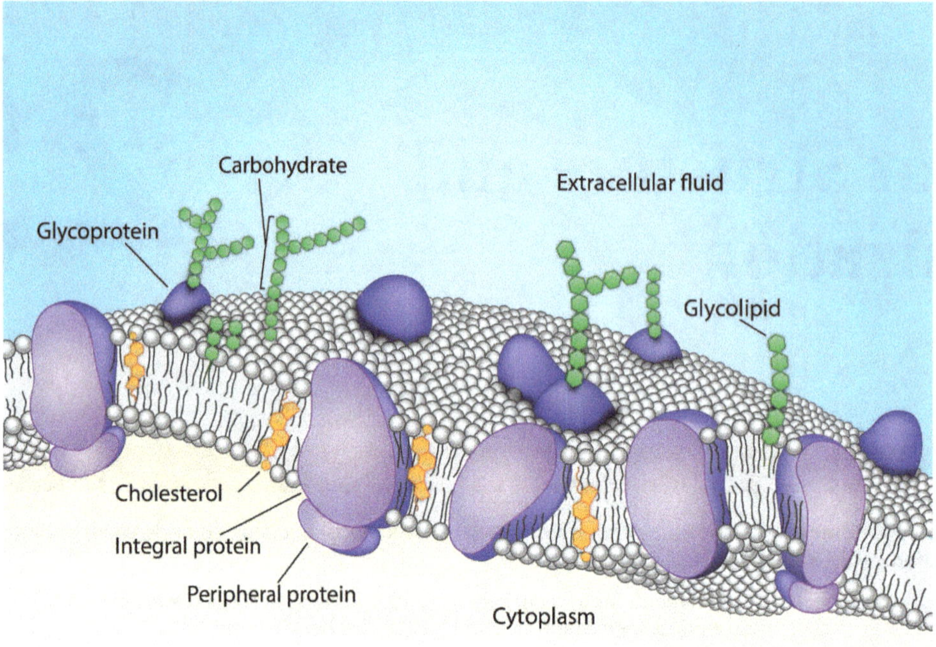

FIGURE 25–1 Structure of the typical lipid bilayer of the plasma membrane. Integral proteins are those that pass through the bilayer. Peripheral proteins are associated with the inner surface of the plasma membrane. Most integral proteins are modified by carbohydrate addition to their extracellular domains. Membranes also contain carbohydrate-modified lipids (glycolipids) in addition to the more common phospholipids and cholesterol that constitute the bulk of the lipid content of the membrane. (Reproduced with permission from themedicalbiochemistrypage, LLC.)

Proteins that are found associated with membranes can also be modified by lipid attachment (see Chapter 24). The lipid allows for the anchoring of the protein to the membrane either through interaction with the lipid bilayer directly or through interactions with integral membrane proteins. Lipoproteins associated with membranes contain one of three types of covalent lipid attachment.

The nucleus and the mitochondria represent unique membrane-enclosed organelles given that both are composed of two lipid bilayers. The nuclear membrane is most often referred to as the nucleolemma and is composed of closely associated inner and outer lipid bilayers. The space between the inner and outer nuclear membranes is in contact with the lumen of the endoplasmic reticulum (ER) via connections between the outer nuclear membrane and the ER membranes.

The mitochondrial inner and outer membranes are separated by a greater distance than those of the nucleus creating the inner membrane space. The two mitochondrial membranes are also functionally very distinct. Whereas the outer mitochondrial membrane is fairly permeable to most small molecules, the inner mitochondrial membrane is essentially impermeable, and transport across the membrane in either direction requires highly specific transporter proteins.

ACTIVITIES OF BIOLOGICAL MEMBRANES

The distribution of lipid and protein between the two different sides of the membrane bilayer is asymmetric. For example, the cytoplasmic side of the plasma membrane (also referred to as the inner leaflet) is enriched in the aminophospholipids phosphatidylserine (PS) and phosphatidylethanolamine (PE), whereas the exoplasmic side (also referred to as the outer leaflet) is enriched in phosphatidylcholine (PC) and sphingomyelin.

The asymmetric distribution of lipids and proteins in membranes results in the generation of highly specialized subdomains within membranes. In addition, certain cells have membrane compositions that are unique to one surface of the cell versus the other. For instance, epithelial cells have a membrane surface that interacts with the luminal cavity of the organ, referred to as the apical membrane, and another that interacts with the interstitial spaces, referred to as the basolateral membrane.

Most eukaryotic cells are in contact with their neighboring cells and these interactions are the basis of the formation of organs. Cells that are touching one another are in metabolic contact which is brought about by specialized tubular particles called junctions. Mammalian cells contain three major types of cell junctions called **gap junctions**, **tight junctions**, and **adherens junctions**.

Gap Junctions

Gap junctions (Figure 25–2) are intercellular channels designed for intercellular communication and their presence allows whole organs to be continuous from within. One major function of gap junctions is to ensure a supply of nutrients to cells of an organ that are not in direct contact with the blood supply. Gap junctions are formed from a type of protein called a connexin (also called gap junction proteins).

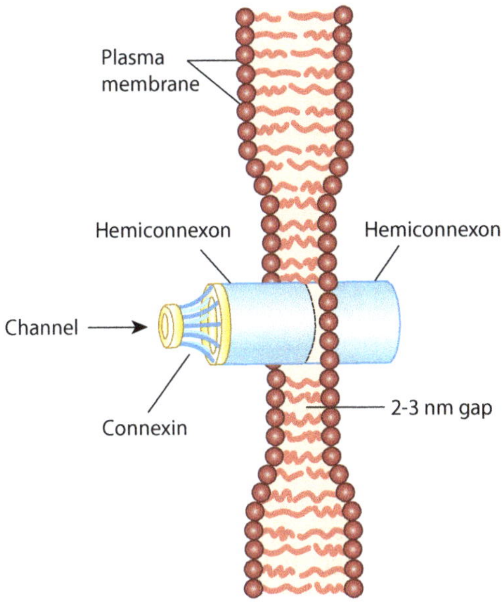

FIGURE 25–2 Schematic diagram of a gap junction. One connexon is made from two hemiconnexons. Each hemiconnexon is made from six connexin molecules. Small solutes are able to diffuse through the central channel, providing a direct mechanism of cell–cell communication. (Reproduced with permission from Murray RK, Bender DA, Botham KM, et al: *Harper's Illustrated Biochemistry*, 29th ed. New York, NY: McGraw Hill; 2012.)

Tight Junctions

Tight junctions (also referred to as occluding junctions) are primarily found in the epithelia and endothelia and are designed for occlusion. Tight junctions act as barriers that regulate the movement of solutes and water between various epithelial and endothelial layers. In addition to forming barrier complexes in the membrane, tight junction proteins also coordinate numerous other signal transduction proteins and intracellular trafficking proteins. The proteins of tight junctions are divided into four major categories; scaffolding, regulatory, transmembrane, and signaling.

Adherens Junctions

Adherens junctions are composed of transmembrane proteins that serve to anchor cells via interactions with the extracellular matrix and intracellular proteins that interact with the actin filaments that control cell movement and shape. The major transmembrane proteins of adherens junctions are members of the cadherin family of Ca^{2+}-dependent adhesion molecules. The intracellular proteins of an adherens junction are the α-catenins, a β-catenin family protein called junction plakoglobin (is also referred to as γ-catenin), and δ-catenins.

MEMBRANE CHANNELS

The movement of ions and molecules across membranes involves several different mechanisms (Figure 25–3) that includes channels and transporters. The definition of a membrane channel (also called a pore) is that of a protein structure that facilitates the translocation of molecules or ions across the membrane through the creation of a central aqueous channel in the protein. Channel proteins do not bind or sequester the molecule or ion that is moving through the channel.

Membrane channels are of three distinct types: α-type channels, β-barrel channels, and the pore-forming toxins. The α-type channels are homo- or hetero-oligomeric structures that in the latter case consist of several different proteins. Molecules move through α-type channels down their concentration gradients and thus require no input of metabolic energy.

HIGH-YIELD CONCEPT

Aquaporins (AQP) are a family of α-type channels responsible for the transport of water across membranes (Figure 25–4).

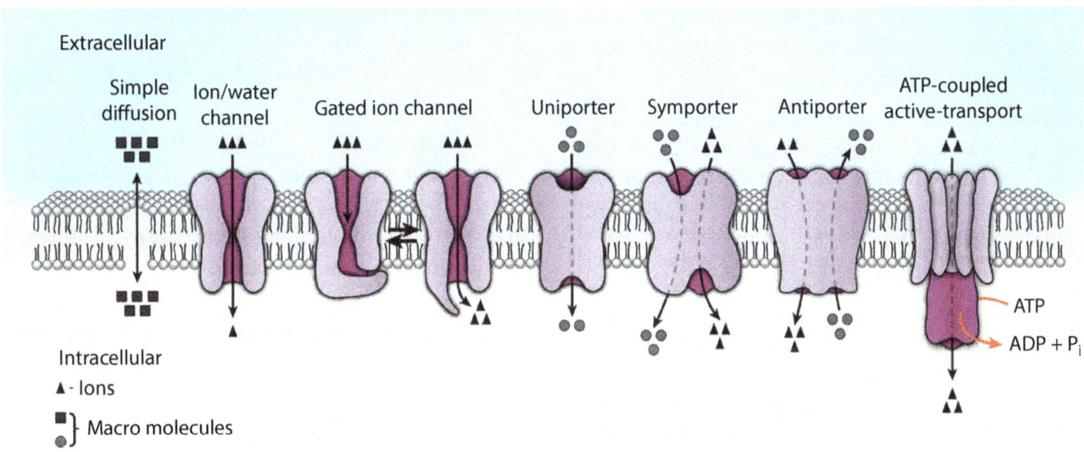

FIGURE 25–3 Representations of the various mechanisms for the passage/transport of ions and molecules across biological membranes. (Reproduced with permission from themedicalbiochemistrypage, LLC.)

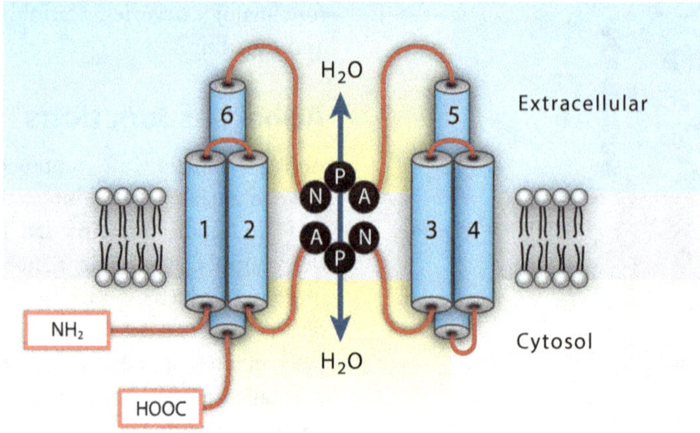

FIGURE 25–4 Diagrammatic representation of the structure of an aquaporin. The pores that form in the aquaporins are composed of two halves referred to as hemipores. Amino acids of the pore that are critical for water transport are the asparagine (N), proline (P), and alanine (A) residues indicated in each hemipore. (Reproduced with permission from themedicalbiochemistrypage, LLC.)

MEMBRANE TRANSPORTERS

Transporters are distinguished from channels because they catalyze (mediate) the movement of ions and molecules by physically binding to and moving the substance across the membrane. Transporters exhibit specificity for the molecule being transported as well as show defined kinetics in the transport process. Transporter activity can be measured by the same kinetic parameters applied to the study of enzyme kinetics. Transporters can also be affected by both competitive and noncompetitive inhibitors.

The action of transporters is divided into two classifications: passive-mediated transport (also called facilitated diffusion) and active transport. Facilitated diffusion involves the transport of specific molecules from an area of high concentration to one of low concentration which results in an equilibration of the concentration gradient. Active transporters transport specific molecules from an area of low concentration to that of high concentration with the input of energy such as ATP hydrolysis or the gradient of another ion.

There are many different classes of transporter that couple the hydrolysis of ATP to the transport of specific molecules. These transporters are referred to as ATPases. There are four different types of ATPases that function in eukaryotes.

1. **E-type ATPases** are cell surface transporters that hydrolyze a range of nucleoside triphosphates that include extracellular ATP. The activity of the E-type ATPases is dependent on Ca^{2+} or Mg^{2+} and it is insensitive to specific inhibitors of P-type, F-type, and V-type ATPases. These transporters derive their nomenclature from the fact that they are involved in extracellular transport.
2. **F-type ATPases** function in the translocation of H^+ in the mitochondria during the process of oxidative phosphorylation. F-type transporters contain rotary motors. Because these transporters transport H^+ they are also referred to as H^+-transporting ATPases. The nomenclature of F-type ATPases derives from phosphorylation factor.
3. **P-type ATPases** are predominantly found in the plasma membrane and are involved in the transport of H^+, K^+, Na^+, Ca^{2+}, Cd^{2+}, Cu^{2+}, and Mg^{2+}. The P-type ATPases are so-called because their activity is modified through phosphorylation. The P-type ATPases contain a core cytoplasmic domain structure that includes a phosphorylation domain (P domain), a nucleotide-binding domain (N domain), and an actuator domain (A domain).
4. **V-type ATPases** are located in acidic vesicles and lysosomes and have homology to the F-type ATPases and also contain rotary motors like F-type ATPases. The V nomenclature is derived from the fact that these transporters are located in vacuoles.

The Na^+/K^+-ATPases

The Na^+/K^+-ATPase family of transporters are critical transporters found in plasma membranes. These transporters move three moles of Na^+ out of cells while simultaneously moving two moles of K^+ into the cell. The difference in ion concentration establishes and maintains an electrochemical gradient across the membrane. This gradient contributes to the excitability of cells such as nerve cells and cardiac muscle cells.

The cardiac Na^+/K^+-ATPases are the site of action of endogenous and exogenous molecules termed cardiotonic steroids (see Clinical Box 25–1).

The Na^+/K^+-ATPases belong to the P_{2C} subclass of P-type ATPases (Figure 25–5). These ATPases are composed of two subunits (α and β) where the α-subunit binds ATP and both Na^+ and K^+ ions and contains the phosphorylation sites typical of the P-type ATPases. The smaller β-subunit is necessary for activity of the transporter by facilitating the plasma membrane localization and activation of the α-subunit.

Many of the Na^+/K^+-ATPases also associate with a family of small single transmembrane-spanning proteins termed the FXYD (*fix-id*) proteins. The founding member of the FXYD proteins was the γ-subunit of the renal Na^+/K^+-ATPase. These proteins get their name from the fact that they all share a signature 35-amino acid domain of homology that contains the conserved four amino acid motif: FXYD (F-phenylalanine, X-any amino acid, Y-tyrosine, D-aspartic acid).

CLINICAL BOX 25–1 CARDIOTONIC STEROIDS

The Na^+/K^+-ATPases are also receptors for the endogenous cardiotonic steroids as well as certain toxins from plants and amphibians. Endogenous cardiotonic steroids (also referred to as cardiac glycosides) are specific inhibitors of Na^+/K^+-ATPases and have been isolated from adrenal glands, heart tissue, the hypothalamus, and cataractous lenses. In addition to inhibition of the Na^+/K^+-ATPases, cardiotonic steroids activate various kinases such as the Src tyrosine kinase and phosphatidylinositol-3-kinase (PI3K). The activation of these kinases results in modulation of cell adhesion and growth. Pregnenolone and progesterone are the precursors in the biosynthesis of endogenous ouabain (also identified as *g*-strophanthin) and endogenous digoxin. Ouabain and digoxin are referred to as cardenolides. Exogenous ouabain is a poisonous compound found in the ripe seeds of the African plant *Strophanthus gratus* and the bark of *Acokanthera ouabaio*. Another class of endogenous cardiotonic steroids is the bufadienolides which include marinobufagenin, marinobufotoxin (the C3-site arginine-suberoyl ester of marinobufagenin), telocinobufagin (the reduced form of marinobufagenin), and 19-norbufalin. There are indications that many more endogenous cardiotonic steroids may exist in mammals. Unlike its role in endogenous oubain synthesis progesterone does not appear to be a precursor of marinobufagenin. However, mevastatin (a statin drug that inhibits HMG-CoA reductase), reduces the biosynthesis of marinobufagenin, indicating that cholesterol is a precursor of bufadienolides in mammals.

When Na^+/K^+-ATPases have ATP bound, they can bind intracellular Na^+ ions. The hydrolysis of the ATP results in the phosphorylation of an Asp residue in the P domain of the α-subunit of all P-type ATPases. The phosphorylation of the pump results in a conformational change which exposes the Na^+ ions to the outside of the cell and they are released. The pump then binds two extracellular K^+ ions which stimulates dephosphorylation of the α-subunit that in turn allows the pump to bind ATP again. In addition to the autophosphorylation site in the P domain of Na^+/K^+-ATPases, these pumps are subject to additional regulatory phosphorylation events catalyzed by PKA and PKC. Adrenergic, cholinergic, and dopaminergic receptor agonists result in PKA-mediated phosphorylation of the pumps.

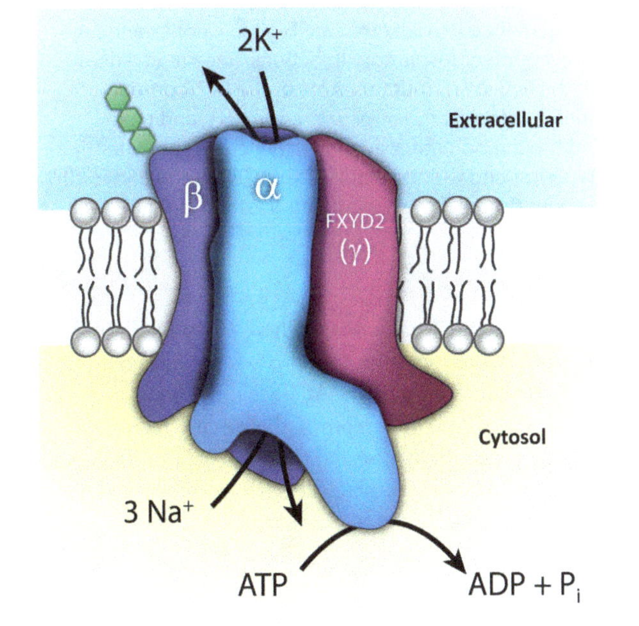

FIGURE 25–5 Functional organization of the α- and β-subunits of Na^+/K^+-ATPases, along with the FXYD2 subunit, in the plasma membrane. The movement of 2 moles of K^+ into the cell as 3 moles of Na^+ are transported out is shown. Associated with ion transport is the hydrolysis of ATP by the α-subunit which provides the energy to drive the process. (Reproduced with permission from themedicalbiochemistrypage, LLC.)

Ion Channels

Ion channels, including those that are ligand- or voltage-gated, are found in all cellular membranes including the plasma membrane and intracellular organelle membranes. The ion channels represent a large class of proteins, and multiprotein complexes, that form pores within membranes that allow the flow of ions across the membrane. The ion channels are broadly classified into six large families of channel proteins or channel complexes. These six families consist of the calcium channels, the chloride channels, the potassium channels, the sodium channels, the gap junction proteins, and the porins (that includes the aquaporins). Within the broad context of the six large families of ion channels, there are numerous distinct subfamilies.

The calcium channel family includes the cation channels sperm associated (CatSper) subfamily, the voltage-gated calcium channels, the IP_3 (inositol-1,4,5-trisphosphate) receptors, the ryanodine receptors, and the two pore segment channels. The chloride channel family includes the calcium-activated chloride channels, the voltage-gated chloride channels, the intracellular chloride channels, and the ATP-gated chloride channel which is most commonly identified as the cystic fibrosis transmembrane conductance regulator (CFTR). Mutations in the *CFTR* gene are the cause of cystic fibrosis (see Clinical Box 25–2).

The gap junction protein channel family includes the connexins and the pannexins. The potassium channel family includes the calcium-activated potassium channels, the voltage-gated potassium channels, the inwardly rectifying potassium subfamily J channels, the sodium-activated potassium subfamily T channels, and the two pore domain potassium subfamily K channels. The porin channel family includes the aquaporins and the voltage-dependent anion channels. The sodium channel family includes the acid-sensing ion channel subunits, the epithelial sodium channels, the sodium leak channels, and the voltage-gated sodium channels.

CLINICAL BOX 25-2 CYSTIC FIBROSIS

Cystic fibrosis (CF) is a disorder that affects numerous organ systems, particularly the pulmonary and the gastrointestinal systems, as a consequence of mutations in the *CFTR* gene which encodes the protein identified as the cystic fibrosis transmembrane conductance regulator. The CFTR protein is a transporter of chloride channel family. Cystic fibrosis is inherited as an autosomal recessive disorder and represents the most common inherited disorder in Caucasians with an incidence rate of 1 in 3500 to 1 in 5000 live births. More than 2000 variants in the *CFTR* gene have been identified with at least 700 of these being identified as disease-causing variants. The most commonly identified mutation in the *CFTR* gene deletes the three nucleotides of codon 508, removing a phenylalanine (F) residue from the protein. This mutation is identified as the ΔF508 (or F508del) mutation. Within the United States, approximately 85% of CF patients harbor the F508del mutation. The various mutations in the *CFTR* gene have been classified based on factors that include translation, processing, expression, and function resulting in six distinct classifications. Class I variants are the result of reduced or absent CFTR protein due to nonsense mutations. Class II variants are the result of CFTR protein misfolding leading to premature degradation. Class III variants are the result of mutations that cause chloride channel gating abnormalities. Class IV variants are the result of mutations that alter the conductance of the chloride channel. Class V variants are the result of mutations that lead to reduced transcription due to promoter mutations or splicing mutations. Class VI variants are the result of mutations that reduce CFTR protein stability leading to increased CFTR protein turnover from the plasma membrane. The normal function of CFTR is the regulation of transepithelial chloride ion transport which in turn regulates water and electrolyte homeostasis in numerous different organ systems. Within sweat glands, CFTR is normally responsible for chloride ion reabsorption such that in the context of CF, affected individuals manifest with salty tasting skin. In tissues such as the intestinal, pancreatic, and airway epithelium, the CFTR protein transports chloride ion out of the cell which in turn promotes bicarbonate secretion as well. In the airway, the normal function of CFTR inhibits the epithelial sodium channel. In the context of CFTR mutations, the impaired chloride and bicarbonate secretions result in thickening of airway secretions, which leads to mucus retention in the airway and persistent bacterial infections, the leading cause of lethality in CF patients. The pancreas of CF patients also has thickened mucus leading to impaired secretion of pancreatic digestive enzymes and fatty infiltration of the organ. The decreased pancreatic enzyme delivery to the small intestine causes impaired digestion of dietary protein and lipid which necessitates pancreatic enzyme replacement therapy for almost all CF patients. The reduced digestion of lipids is associated with steatorrhea and significantly reduced uptake of dietary vitamins. The reduced uptake of vitamin K is most pronounced in comparison to the three other fat-soluble vitamins. A consequence of reduced absorption of vitamin K is an increased potential for bleeding and bruising. This clinical manifestation is the result of impaired vitamin K-dependent γ-carboxylation of several blood coagulation factors (see Chapter 33). In addition, the reduced vitamin K absorption leads to impaired bone homeostasis due to the fact that the normal function of several bone regulatory factors requires vitamin K-dependent γ-carboxylation. The primary therapeutic interventions for CF patients involve nutritional management with diets that are high in calories and fat, replacement of pancreatic enzymes, and aggressive management and prevention of respiratory infections. Recent advances in the treatment of cystic fibrosis include the use of drugs that modulate the activity of mutant forms of the CFTR protein or increase the amount of CFTR mRNA. These drugs are classified as potentiators, stabilizers, correctors, amplifiers, and read-through agents. Currently approved therapies include single, double, and triple modulators, all of which include the potentiator (enhances function) ivacaftor. The double-modulator therapy includes ivacaftor and the corrector (aids CFTR folding and trafficking to the cell surface), tezacaftor. The triple-modulator therapy includes both drugs of the double-modulator therapy as well as the additional corrector, elexacaftor.

Most, but not all, ion channels are voltage gated. For example, the ryanodine receptors and the IP_3 receptors, both of which are Ca^{2+} ion channels, are gated by ligand binding. In the case of the ryanodine receptors the ligand is Ca^{2+} ion, and with the IP_3 receptors the ligand is IP_3.

The ligand-gated ion channel (LGIC) superfamily of ion channels represents a large family of channel proteins/protein complexes that mediate the regulated flow of selected ions across the plasma membrane in response to ligand-specific binding. As the name implies, the LGIC are opened, or gated, by the binding of an appropriate ligand, which is, most often, a neurotransmitter. In addition to gating of the channels in response to ligand binding, there is modulation of the gating process by the binding of endogenous, or exogenous, modulators to allosteric sites.

The large LGIC superfamily of channels that are all activated (gated) by extracellular ligands can be subdivided into 10 families of structurally related channels, several of which are also members of other ion-channel subfamilies. These 10 families are the ionotropic 5-hydroxytryptamine ($5\text{-}HT_3$: serotonin) receptors, nicotinic acetylcholine receptors (nAChR), the ionotropic glutamate receptors, the GABA-A receptors, the glycine receptors (GlyR), the IP_3 receptors, the ATP-gated channel (CFTR), the ryanodine receptors (RYR), the purinergic (P2X) receptors, and the zinc-activated channel (ZAC).

A. Calcium Channels

Much of the membrane transport of Ca^{2+} into and out of cells, and into and out of intracellular organelles is controlled by a large family of voltage-gated calcium channels. In addition, neuronal and striated skeletal muscle excitation involves local depolarization of the plasma membrane (termed the sarcolemma in muscle cells) and the subsequent activation of voltage-gated calcium channels allows Ca^{2+} ion movement across the membrane.

The voltage-gated calcium channels (also called voltage-dependent calcium channels, VDCC) are divided into three distinct families, each with multiple members. These channel families are termed the Cav1.x, Cav2.x, and Cav3.x families. The Cav1.x and Cav2.x families represent the high-voltage activated (HVA) channels while the Cav3.x family represents the low-voltage activated (LVA) family.

Nearly all of the voltage-gated calcium channels are pentameric structures composed of five different protein subunits identified as the α1-, α2-, β-, γ, and δ-subunits. Some voltage-gated calcium channels are composed of only four subunits and lack the γ subunit. These latter four subunit channels are typical of cardiac voltage-gated calcium channels. The α1-subunit is the actual transmembrane channel through which the Ca^{2+} ions flow.

Within striated muscle cells, Ca^{2+} entry across the sarcolemma causes the initiating neural stimulus to spread to the associated T-tubule (transverse tubule) system and deep into the interior of the myofiber. T-tubule depolarization spreads to the sarcoplasmic reticulum (SR: muscle form of the ER), with the effect of the opening of calcium release channels in the SR membranes. These calcium release channels are the ryanodine receptors that belong to the family of ligand-gated ion channels.

Calcium is also critical in the cessation of contractile activity and the accompanying state of relaxation in skeletal and cardiac muscle. When the initiating signal for muscle contraction is removed, the myocytes need to reverse the localization of the activating calcium from the sarcoplasm back into the SR. Sarcoplasmic calcium is pumped back into the lumen of the SR by an extremely active ATP–driven calcium pump, which comprises one of the main proteins of the SR membrane. This SR calcium pump is a member of a family of Ca^{2+}-ATPases identified as sarco/endoplasmic reticulum Ca^{2+}-ATPases (SERCA). Humans express three SERCA encoding genes. For each ATP hydrolyzed by the SR SERCA, two calcium ions are transported into the SR lumen.

B. Potassium Channels

Potassium ions represent approximately 5% of the total electrolyte pool in the human body. The majority of potassium ion in the body is found intracellularly. The average intracellular potassium concentration in around 150 mM, whereas the concentration of potassium in the blood is only around 3.5–5 mM.

Potassium channels constitute a large superfamily of transport proteins and complexes whose functions are critical to numerous biological processes such as the transmission of nerve impulses in the brain and in the control of cardiac muscle and skeletal muscle activity. The Na^+/K^+-ATPases, reviewed earlier, are a good example of critical regulatory channels.

Based on structural features the potassium channels can be divided into four distinct classes. These four classes include those channel proteins that possess two transmembrane (TM) domains and one P region, those that possess four TM domains and two P regions, those that contain six TM domains and one P region, and those that contain seven TM domains and one P region.

The potassium channels that possess two TM domains and a single P region include the inwardly rectifying channels (designated K_{ir} and encoded by the KCNJ family genes) and the ATP-sensitive potassium channels that are also encoded by KCNJ family genes. Within the inwardly rectifying potassium channel family, there are four channels whose activities are regulated by the $\beta\gamma$-subunits of heterotrimeric G-proteins and as such are designated G-protein–coupled inwardly-rectifying potassium channels (GIRK).

The potassium channels that possess four TM domains and two P regions are the two-pore potassium channels that are encoded by genes of the KCNK family. The potassium channels that possess six TM domains and a single P region include the voltage-gated potassium channels (designated Kv and encoded by nine different gene families) and the small/intermediate conductance calcium-activated potassium channels (designated KCa and encoded by members of the KCNN gene family). The potassium channel that possesses seven TM domains and a single P region is the large conductance calcium- and voltage-activated potassium channel (designated KCa1.1 and encoded by the *KCNMA1* gene). The KCNMA1-encoded potassium channel is also known as MaxiK or BK (big potassium). All potassium channels, except the two-pore subfamily, form homotetrameric or heterotetrameric complexes in the membrane. The two-pore subfamily form homodimers.

In addition to the channel proteins themselves, there are 15 human genes that encode potassium channel regulatory subunits. The regulatory subunits are divided into those that are cytosolic and those that are transmembrane. The cytosolic regulatory proteins include the Kvβ proteins (encoded by the *KCNAB1–KCNAB3* genes) and the K^+ channel-interacting proteins (designated KChIP and encoded by the *KCNIP* genes: four genes in family). The transmembrane potassium channel regulators are encoded by the KCNE gene family (six genes).

Along with Na^+ and Ca^{2+} ion channels, K^+ channels are critical to the functions of the heart. Mutations in one gene encoding an inwardly rectifying K^+ channel and in one gene encoding a delayed rectifier K^+ are each associated with forms of long QT syndrome, LQTS (Clinical Box 25–3).

ION CHANNELS AND CARDIAC FUNCTION

The beating (contraction) function of cardiac muscle cells is controlled by electrochemical gradients that are the result of the transport of ions across the cell membrane. Muscle contraction itself is the result of changes in membrane action potentials brought about by transport of ions into, or out of, the muscle cell.

All cardiomyocytes are electrically coupled and therefore contract simultaneously. The electrical communication between cardiomyocytes occurs through gap junctions at points on the cells referred to as nexi. The initiation of an action potential in one cardiomyocyte is rapidly propagated via the nexi to all cells of the heart. This connectivity, referred to as a functional syncytium, effectively serves to allow the heart muscle to act as one large cell.

Cardiomyocyte action potentials are characterized as either fast or slow. Ventricular and atrial cardiomyocytes, as well as those of Purkinje fibers, exhibit fast-response action potentials (Figure 25–6). The cardiomyocytes of the sinoatrial (SA) node and atrioventricular (AV) node exhibit slow-response action potentials (Figure 25–7).

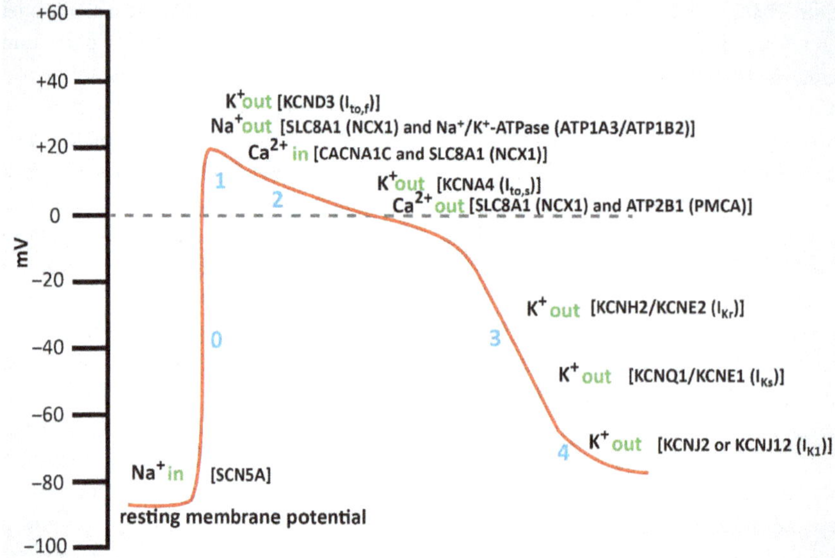

FIGURE 25–6 Representative tracing of the action potential in a single cardiac ventricle muscle cell. The resting membrane potential for cardiac myocytes is approximately −90 mV. On activation there is a rapid depolarization represented by the phase indicated as "0". This is followed by a rapid initiation of repolarization indicated by "1". Phase "0" is mediated by the opening of fast-acting voltage-gated Na^+ channels. These voltage-gated Na^+ channels are composed of an α-subunit and a β-subunit. There are nine α-subunit genes with the cardiac α-subunit being encoded by the *SCN5A* gene. There are four β-subunit genes in humans. Phase "1" is mediated by closure of the voltage-gated Na^+ channels. Simultaneously, Ca^{2+} channels are activated to allow Ca^{2+} influx and K^+ channels are activated to promote K^+ efflux. The uptake of Ca^{2+} occurs through the opening of voltage-gated L-type Ca^{2+} channels (called Cav1.2) that are encoded by the *CACNA1C* gene. In addition, the Na^+/Ca^{2+} exchanger encoded by the *SLC8A1* gene (called the NCX1 channel) functions to transport three Na^+ ions out of the cell in exchange for one Ca^{2+} ion. The NCX1 exchanger functions in this direction when the membrane potential is positive but in the opposite direction when the membrane returns to its negative potential resting state. The efflux of K^+ ions at the start of phase 1 is the function of the voltage-gated K^+ channel encoded by the *KCND3* gene. The KCND3-encoded protein exerts a fast transient outward current and as such is referred to as $I_{to,f}$. The repolarization rate is reduced by the opening of the L-type voltage-gated Ca^{2+} channels (α1-subunit encoded by the *CACNA1C* gene), resulting in the plateau phase indicated by "2". Near the end of the plateau phase the Ca^{2+} channels close and additional voltage-gated K^+ channels open allowing a further continued efflux of K^+. These latter K^+ channels are encoded by the *KCNA4* gene and the channels exert a slow transient outward current movement and as such are referred to as $I_{to,s}$ channels. The activation of the KCNA4 channel initiates the onset of the rapid repolarization of the cell indicated by "3". At the end of phase 2 and the onset of phase 3, as the membrane becomes negative again, the NCX1 exchanger shifts to transporting Ca^{2+} out of the cell. Additionally, Ca^{2+} is transported out of the cell via the action of the ATP-dependent Ca^{2+} transporter encoded by the *ATP2B1* gene. The ATP2B1-encoded transporter is commonly called the plasma membrane Ca^{2+} ATPase, PCMA. The continued efflux of K^+ allows the cardiomyocyte to return to the resting membrane potential indicated by "4". This continuous efflux of K^+ during repolarization is carried out by at least three different transporters. In the early part of phase 3, there is rapid K^+ efflux via the KCNH2 and KCNE2 channel, commonly called I_{Kr}. Later in phase 3 there is activation of the K^+ channel encoded by the *KCNQ1* and *KCNE1* genes, commonly called I_{Ks}. The primary phase 4 K^+ channel is an inwardly rectifying potassium channel can be encoded by either of two genes, *KCNJ2* or *KCNJ12*. This cardiac K^+ channel is commonly called I_{K1} (also identified as $K_{ir}2.1$). The KCNJ2- or KCNJ12-encoded K^+ channel is responsible for the maintenance of the resting membrane potential of ventricular cardiomyocytes as well as that of skeletal muscle. Another member of the $K_{ir}2.x$ family, $K_{ir}2.3$ (encoded by the *KCNJ4* gene) likely also contributes to the inward transport of K^+ that maintains the resting membrane potential of cardiomyocytes. The approximate timing of the influx and efflux of Na^+, Ca^{2+}, and K^+ ions is indicated along the top of the tracing line. The duration of the time from the onset of rapid depolarization to the return to the rested state is on the order of 300 milliseconds (msec) which is around 70 times slower than the action potential of a typical skeletal muscle cell. (Reproduced with permission from themedicalbiochemistrypage, LLC.)

The primary ions controlling the generation, propagation, and termination of cardiomyocyte action potentials are K^+, Na^+, and Ca^{2+}.

THE ABC FAMILY OF TRANSPORTERS

The ABC transporters comprise the ATP-binding cassette transporter superfamily. All members of this superfamily of membrane proteins contain a conserved ATP-binding domain and use the energy of ATP hydrolysis to drive the transport of various molecules across all cell membranes.

There are 48 known members of the ABC transporter superfamily, and they are divided into seven subfamilies based on phylogenetic analyses. These seven subfamilies are designated ABCA (ABC1), ABCB (also called TAP/MDR for transporter, ATP cassette), ABCC (also called MRP for multidrug resistance protein), ABCD (also called ALD for adrenoleukodystrophy),

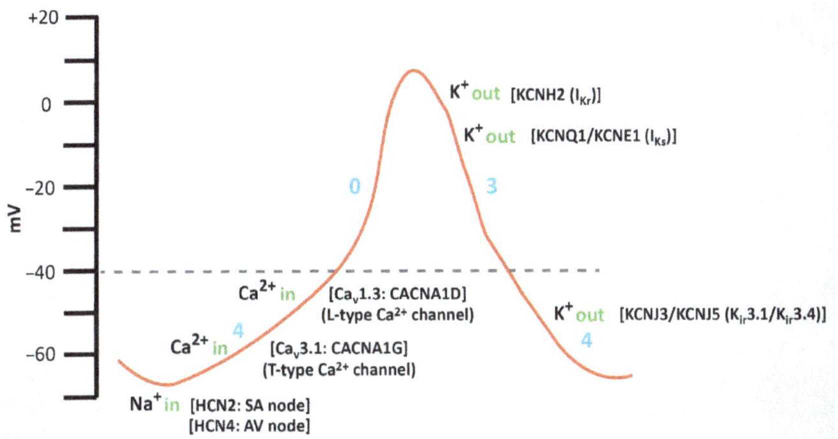

FIGURE 25–7 Representative tracing of the action potential in a single cardiac sinoatrial (SA) node cell. The resting membrane potential for sinoatrial node cells is approximately –60mV. Nodal cell action potential activation involves an initial hyperpolarization event that occurs in the typical phase "4", resting state of the cell. This hyperpolarization results in the activation of slow-acting Na^+ channels. These channels were originally identified as funny current channels. These channels are encoded by genes of the hyperpolarization-activated cyclic nucleotide-gated channel (HCN) gene family. The SA node channel is encoded by the *HCN2* gene and the atrioventricular (AV) node channel is encoded by the *HCN4* gene. The influx of Na^+ begins to depolarize the nodal cells which results in the activation of T-type Ca^{2+} channels (identified as Cav3.1) leading to influx of calcium ions. The α-subunit of Cav3.1 channel is encoded by the *CACNA1G* gene. The slow depolarization of nodal cells, relative to other cardiomyocytes, is due to both the slow acting HCN channels and the slow acting T-type calcium channels. This period of nodal cell depolarization is referred to as phase "0". As the membrane potential approaches around –40 mV, L-type Ca^{2+} channels open. These channels are identified as Cav1.3 and their α-subunit is encoded by the *CACNA1D* gene. As the membrane attains a positive potential, the Ca^{2+} channels close and K^+ channels open to initiate the repolarization. The repolarization of nodal cells is referred to as phase "3". The primary K^+ channels responsible for nodal repolarization are the same as those in other cardiomyocytes, namely I_{Kr} and I_{Ks}. Complete repolarization in nodal cells involves the inwardly rectifying K^+ channels, whose function is the same as the I_{K1} (encoded by the *KCNJ2* gene) channel in ventricular cardiomyocytes. However, in nodal cells these inwardly rectifying K^+ channels are identified as I_{KACh} given that they were originally demonstrated to be activated by muscarinic agonists such as acetylcholine and carbachol. The I_{KACh} channels are composed of proteins identified as $K_{ir}3.1$ (encoded by the *KCNJ3* gene) and $K_{ir}3.4$ (encoded by the *KCNJ5* gene). (Reproduced with permission from themedicalbiochemistrypage, LLC.)

CLINICAL BOX 25–3 LONG QT SYNDROME

Long QT syndrome (LQTS) refers to a condition in which repolarization of the heart after a heartbeat is affected. The syndrome is recognizable during a standard cardiac function examination through the reading of an electrocardiogram (ECG or EKG). The interval between the Q wave and T wave on the ECG is referred to as the QT interval. The QT interval reflects the electrical activity of the ventricles of the heart. LQTS results in an increased risk of an irregular heartbeat which can result in fainting, drowning, seizures, or sudden death. The protein encoded by the *KCNQ1* gene is a member of the delayed rectifying K^+-channel family. The KCNQ1-encoded protein forms a heteromeric complex with the regulatory subunit encoded by the *KCNE1* gene and can also form heteromeric complexes with the KCNE3 regulatory subunit. The KCNQ1/KCNE1 ion channel constitutes the delayed rectifier I_{Ks} current that contributes to the latter part of the repolarization (phase 3) of ventricular cardiomyocyte action potential propagation. Inactivating mutations in the *KCNQ1* gene are associated with long QT syndrome (LQTS) type 1, hence the gene is also known as *KvLQT1*. Gain-of-function mutations in the *KCNQ1* gene are associated with short QT syndrome (SQTS) variant 2. The protein encoded by the *KCNH2* gene is a member of the inwardly rectifying K^+-channel family. The KCNH2 encoded protein forms a heteromeric complex with the regulatory subunit encoded by the *KCNE2* gene to generate the delayed rectifier I_{Kr} current that contributes to the early part of the repolarization (phase 3) of ventricular cardiomyocyte action potential propagation (see Figure 25–6). Inactivating mutations in the *KCNH2* gene are associated with long QT syndrome type 2 (LQTS2). LQTS2 is associated with Torsade de Pointes ventricular arrhythmia and sudden cardiac death. Gain-of-function mutations in the *KCNH2* gene are associated with short QT syndrome (SQTS) variant 1.

ABCE (also called OABP for oligoadenylate-binding protein), ABCF (also called GCN20), and ABCG (also called White). Each member of a given subfamily is distinguished with numbers (eg, ABCA1).

Mutations in several ABC transporter encoding genes have been identified in several inherited disorders (see Clinical Box 25–3).

THE SOLUTE CARRIER FAMILY OF TRANSPORTERS

The solute carrier (SLC) family of transporters includes more than 300 proteins functionally grouped into 52 families. The SLC family of transporters includes facilitative transporters, primary and secondary active transporters, ion channels, and the aquaporins.

Mutations in many SLC transporter-encoding genes have been identified in several inherited disorders (Clinical Boxes 25–4 and 25–5).

THE EXTRACELLULAR MATRIX

A substantial portion of the volume of tissues is extracellular space, which is largely filled by an intricate network of macromolecules constituting the extracellular matrix, ECM. The ECM is composed of three major classes of biomolecules:

1. Structural proteins: for example, the collagens, the fibrillins, and elastin.
2. Specialized proteins: for example, fibronectin, the laminins, and the integrins.
3. Proteoglycans: these are composed of a protein core to which is attached long chains of repeating disaccharide units termed glycosaminoglycans (GAGs) forming extremely complex high molecular weight components of the ECM.

Connective tissue (Figure 25–8) refers to the matrix composed of the ECM, cells (primarily fibroblasts), and **ground substance** that is tasked with holding other tissues and cells together forming

CLINICAL BOX 25–4 TRANSPORTER DEFECTS AND DISEASE

ABCA1 is involved in the transport of cholesterol out of cells when HDLs are bound to their cell surface receptor, SR-B1 (see Chapter 16 for more details). One important consequence of the activity of ABCA1 in macrophages is that the efflux of cholesterol results in a suppression of inflammatory responses triggered by macrophages that have become foam cells due to cholesterol uptake. Defects in ABCA1 result in Tangier disease (see Clinical Box 16–1) which is characterized by two clinical hallmarks; enlarged lipid-laden tonsils and low serum HDL.

ABCG5 and ABCG8 form an obligate heterodimer pair that function to limit plant sterol and cholesterol uptake by the gut and mediate cholesterol efflux from the liver into the bile. Mutations in either ABCG5 or ABCG8 result in a rare genetic disorder identified as sitosterolemia (also called phytosterolemia). This disorder is characterized by unrestricted absorption of plant sterols (such as sitosterol) and cholesterol. Individuals afflicted with this disorder manifest with very high levels of plant sterols in the plasma and develop tendon and tuberous xanthomas, accelerated atherosclerosis, and premature coronary artery disease.

ABCB11 is also known as bile salt export protein (BSEP) which is involved in bile salt transport out of hepatocytes into the bile canaliculi (see Chapter 15). Defects in this gene are associated with progressive familial intrahepatic cholestasis type 2 (PFIC2). The symptoms of PFIC2 usually present in early infancy as failure to thrive, jaundice, and severe pruritus (unpleasant sensation eliciting a desire to scratch). The symptoms of PFIC2 progress continuously, leading ultimately to liver failure and the need for liver transplantation in order to survive.

ABCC2 was first identified as the canalicular multispecific organic anion transporter (CMOAT) and is also called multidrug resistance-associated protein 2 (MRP2). Defects in the gene encoding ABCC2 result in Dubin-Johnson syndrome (see Clinical Box 21–6), which is a form of conjugated hyperbilirubinemia.

ATP7A and ATP7B are copper-transporting ATPases that are related to SLC31A1. Defects in ATP7A result in Menkes disease (Clinical Box 3–12) and defects in ATP7B are associated with Wilson disease (Clinical Box 3–13).

SLC6A19 is also called system B(0) neutral amino acid transporter 1 [B(0)AT1]. This transporter is involved in neutral amino acid transport with highest levels of expression in the kidney and small intestine. Deficiency in SLC6A19 leads to Hartnup disease (see Clinical Box 18–1) which results from impaired transport of neutral amino acids across epithelial cells in renal proximal tubules and intestinal mucosa. Symptoms include transient manifestations of pellagra-like light sensitive rash, cerebellar ataxia, and psychosis.

SLC35C1 is also known as the GDP-fucose transporter (gene symbol = *FUCT1*). Defects in the *FUCT1* gene result in a congenital disorder of glycosylation, CDG (see Clinical Box 24–5). Specifically, the disorder is a type II CDG identified as CDGIIc. Type II CDGs result from defects in the processing of the carbohydrate structures on *N*-linked glycoproteins. CDGIIc is also called leukocyte adhesion deficiency syndrome II (LAD II). LAD II is a primary immunodeficiency syndrome which manifests due to leukocyte dysfunction. Symptoms of LAD II include unique facial features, recurrent infections, persistent leukocytosis, defective neutrophil chemotaxis, and severe growth and mental retardation.

CLINICAL BOX 25-5 CYSTINURIA

As the name implies, cystinuria is a disorder associated with excess cystine in the urine. Cystine is the oxidized disulfide homodimer of two cysteines. Type I cystinuria is an autosomal recessive disorder that results from a failure of the renal proximal tubules to reabsorb cystine that was filtered by the glomerulus. The accumulation of cystine and its formation of crystals within the distal tubules results in the formation of cystine stones in the kidneys (nephrolithiasis). Among the various forms and causes of kidney stones, the presence of cystine stones represents 1–2% of all adult urinary nephrolithiasis patients, but in children 6–8% of patients suffer from cystine stones. The etiology of nephrolithiasis can be complex and includes factors such as diet and fluid intake. The overall prevalence of cystinuria is 1:7,000 with population-specific variation such that in Americans the rate is 1:25,000 and the highest incidence of 1:2,500 being found in Libyan Jews. Cystinuria results from defects in either of the two protein subunits of the cystine transporter which is distinct from the renal cysteine transporter. In addition to excess cystine in the urine, the disorder is associated with increased urinary excretion of the dibasic amino acids arginine, lysine, and ornithine. However, clinical consequences are only associated with the increased urinary cystine and is due to the poor solubility of this homodimeric compound. The two subunits of the cystine transporter are both members of the SLC family of transporter proteins and they are encoded by the *SLC3A1* and *SLC7A9* genes. The SLC3A1-encoded protein is one of the heavy subunits of the heteromeric amino acid transporters. The protein is commonly referred to as the basic amino acid transport protein (rBAT). The functional subunit of the transporter is one of the light chain subunits of the heteromeric amino acid transporters and is encoded by the *SLC7A9* gene. The SLC7A9-encoded protein is a Na^+-independent amino acid transporter most often referred to as $b^{(0,+)}$AT. The "b" refers to broad specificity and the 0 and + signify that the transporter transports both neutral (0) and basic (+) amino acids. The "AT" refers to Amino acid Transporter. Mutations in the *SLC3A1* gene are associated with the autosomal recessive type I cystinurias while mutations in the *SLC7A9* gene are associated with non-type I cystinurias that exhibit broad clinical variability even within the same family. The initial diagnosis of cystinuria is usually precipitated by the finding of kidney stones (renal lithiasis) which show typical cystine crystals. Cystine crystals are long hexagonal translucent crystals that when removed from a patient often appear pink or yellow but turn greenish on exposure to air. Determination as to whether or not a person is suffering from renal lithiasis, due to cystinuria, is accomplished via the sodium cyanide-nitroprusside test. In this assay urine is exposed to the reagent which turns purple within 2–10 minutes. The sodium cyanide reduces the cystine to cysteine which then binds the nitroprusside causing the purple color. The clinical classifications of cystinuria were originally divided into three major types. These types are distinguished by the urinary phenotype of the parents (obligate heterozygotes) of afflicted patients. Type I cystinuria is distinguished by heterozygotes that excrete cystine at normal levels. The original designations of type II and type III cystinuria were defined by heterozygotes that had high or moderately elevated cystine excretion. However, since the genetic mutations that predispose an individual to cystinuria could not be correlated to a type II versus a type III individual, these two designations were changed to the classification of non-type I cystinurias. The distinction of non-type I heterozygotes is that they exhibit variable hyperexcretion of cystine and the dibasic amino acids in their urine. Due to these designations of the phenotype, type I cystinuria mainly exhibits an autosomal-recessive inheritance trait while non-type I cystinuria can be regarded as an autosomal dominant disorder with incomplete penetrance for cystine lithiasis. The diagnosis of cystinuria can be further complicated by the fact that some patients exhibit a mixed cystinuria due to their carrying both type I and non-type I alleles. The majority of cystinuria patients will manifest renal calculi formation sometime within the first two decades of life. However, it is important to note that even within the same family there can be variation in disease phenotype and severity. Males with cystinuria are affected more severely and with a greater frequency than females. In addition, the cystine stones that form in males are often larger than those in female patients. Generally, type I homozygous patients have earlier manifestation of stone formation while non-type I homozygous patients as well as mixed type patients will develop stones later in life. Common treatments for patients with cystinuria are to decrease protein and salt intake as well as to ensure increased hydration as this will dilute the cystine in the urine reducing the potential for crystal formation. In addition, patients are given drugs, such as acetazolamide (a carbonic anhydrase inhibitor principally utilized in the treatment of glaucoma and certain forms of hypertension), which alkalizes the urine thereby reducing the potential for urinary precipitation of cystine. In addition, thiol drugs can be used to compete for the formation of cystine. These drugs include captopril (an angiotensin-converting enzyme [ACE] inhibitor used principally in the treatment of hypertension), D-penicillamine (a chelator drug used in the treatment of Wilson disease, lead poisoning, and rheumatoid arthritis), and alpha-mercaptopropionylglycine, α-MPG (a second-generation chelating drug). The composition of cystine stones makes their removal by extracorporeal lithotripsy difficult. In patients that are diagnosed with large stones, their treatment will require percutaneous nephrostomy placement in order to remove the stones. Due to the fact that patients with cystinuria, in particular type I patients, experience episodic stone symptoms it is necessary for repeated stone removal. This episodic character to cystine stone formation and removal can lead to serious renal damage as well as damage to surrounding organs. In rare cases, where proper interventional therapy is not activated, patient deaths have been reported.

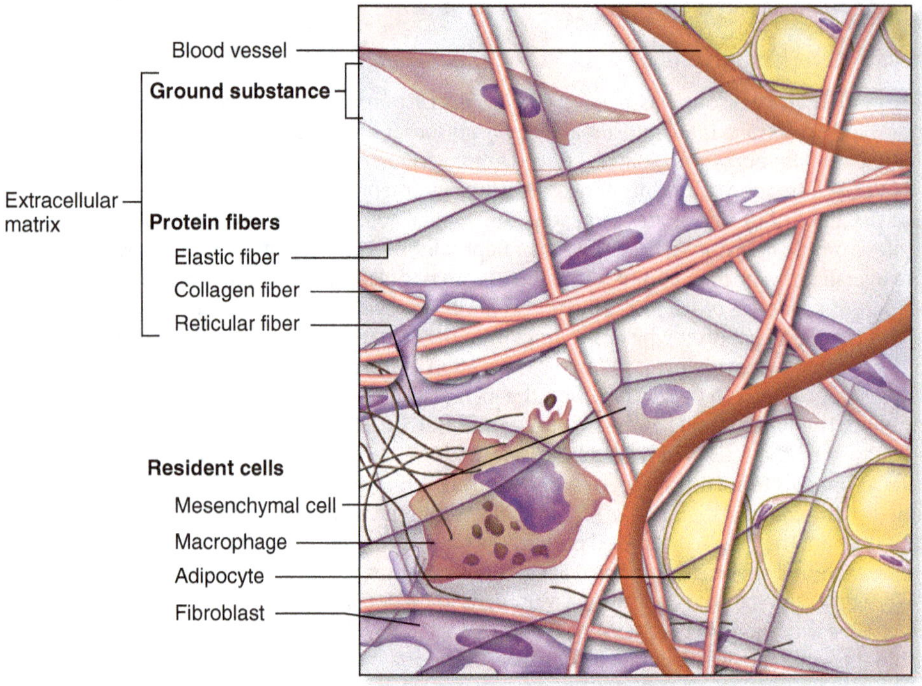

FIGURE 25–8 Components of typical connective tissue. In addition to the extracellular matrix, typical connective tissues contain cells (primarily fibroblasts) all of which is surrounded by ground substance. (Reproduced with permission from Mescher AL. *Junqueira's Basic Histology Text and Atlas*. 16th ed. New York, NY: McGraw Hill; 2021.)

the organs. Ground substance is a complex mixture of GAGs, proteoglycans, and glycoproteins (primarily laminin and fibronectin) but generally does not include the collagens.

COLLAGENS

Collagens are the most abundant proteins found in the animal kingdom. The various collagens constitute the major proteins comprising the ECM. Humans express 44 different collagen genes that encode proteins that combine in a variety of ways to create over 28 different types of collagen fibrils (Figure 25–9).

Collagen proteins have a unique amino acid composition unlike any other protein in the human body. These proteins contain upwards of hundreds of repeats of the sequence Gly-Pro-X or Gly-X-HyP, where X represents any amino acid except glycine or proline and HyP denotes hydroxyproline. As much as 35% of a collagen monomer is composed of glycine with another 20–25% being proline.

Collagen protein monomers (termed α-chains) self-associate into a triple helical structure. The different collagen triple helix types are identified by Roman numeral designation. The nomenclature for collagens involves the chain composition and the numbering of the collagen gene encoding a particular α-chain. For example, type I collagens are encoded by the *COL1A1* and *COL1A2* genes. The triple helix of type I collagen is denoted $[\alpha1(I)]_2[\alpha2(I)]$ where the cardinal numeral designates the specific gene and the Roman numeral designates the fibril as type I.

Types I, II, and III collagens are the most abundant forms of collagen with type I constituting nearly 90% of all the collagen in the human body. Type IV collagen forms a two-dimensional reticulum and is a major component of all basement membrane.

The various collagens are grouped according to the major structures formed through subunit interactions. These groupings consist of the fibril-forming, the sheet-forming, and the anchoring (or linking) collagens. For example, type I collagen, the most abundant collagen, is a member of the fibril-forming group and forms large fibrils that constitute the framework for the dermis, tendons, and organ capsules.

Collagens are synthesized as preproproteins (Figure 25–10) and undergo extensive co- and posttranslational processing. Collagens originate as longer precursor proteins called preprocollagens. Following removal of the signal peptide from the preprocollagen precursor, which occurs in the lumen of the rough ER, the remaining protein is referred to as a procollagen (or tropocollagen). Procollagen proteins contain extra amino acids at the N- and C-termini (pro-domains) that will be removed during the further processing that occurs. The pro-domains are globular and form multiple intrachain disulfide bonds that stabilize the proprotein allowing the triple helical section to form.

Numerous modifications take place to amino acid residues on the procollagen proteins. These modifications include hydroxylations and carbohydrate additions. Specific proline residues are hydroxylated by prolyl hydroxylases and specific lysine residues are hydroxylated by lysyl hydroxylases. The collagen prolyl and lysyl hydroxylases require ascorbic acid (see Chapter 3) as cofactor.

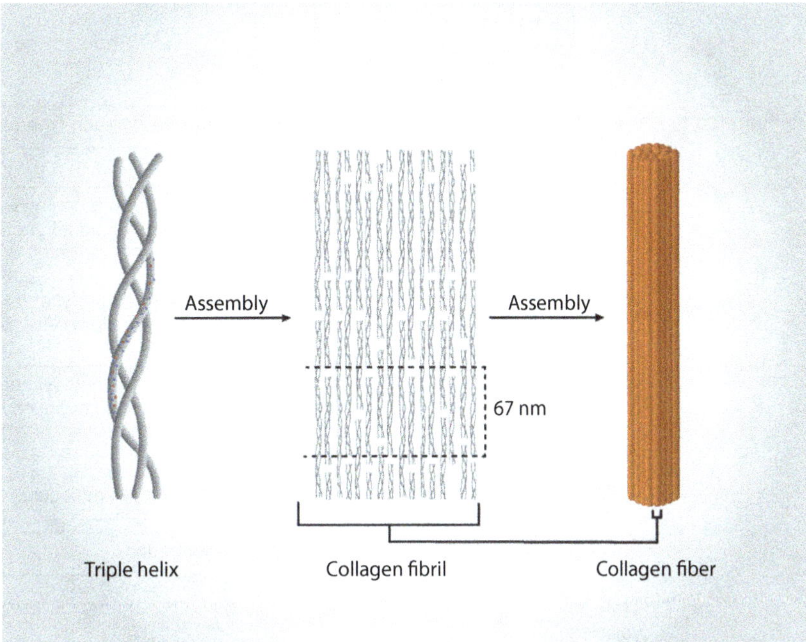

FIGURE 25–9 Higher-order structural features of a typical collagen fibril. Each individual polypeptide chain is twisted into a left-handed triple helix comprising the Gly-X-Y residues. The triple helical structure of processed collagen is formed by right-handed coiling of three polypeptides into a superhelix. (Reproduced with permission from themedicalbiochemistrypage, LLC.)

The collagen proly and lysyl hydroxylases all belong to the large family of 2-oxoglutarate and Fe^{2+}-dependent dioxygenases.

The procollagen proteins are then secreted into the extracellular space. Several reactions take place to a procollagen protein within the extracellular compartment. Proteases remove the globular pro-domains at both the N- and C-termini. The collagen molecules then polymerize to form collagen fibrils. Accompanying fibril formation is the oxidation of certain lysine residues by the extracellular enzyme lysyl oxidase. Lysyl oxidase acts on lysines and hydroxylysines producing aldehyde groups, which will eventually undergo covalent bonding between tropocollagen molecules. Lysyl oxidase is an extracellular Cu^{2+}-dependent enzyme whose function is disrupted in Menkes disease (see Clinical Box 3–12).

Alterations in collagen structure, resulting from abnormal collagen genes or abnormal processing of collagen proteins, result in numerous diseases such as Alport syndrome, Larsen syndrome, and numerous chondrodysplasias as well as the more commonly known clusters of related syndromes of osteogenesis imperfecta (Clinical Box 25–6) and Ehlers-Danlos syndrome (Clinical Box 25–7).

ELASTIN

Elastin is synthesized as the precursor, tropoelastin from the elastin gene (symbol: *ELN*). Tropoelastin has two major types of alternating domains. One domain is hydrophilic and rich in Lys (K) and Ala (A) while the other domain is hydrophobic and rich in Val (V), Pro (P), and Gly (G) where these amino acids are frequently contained in repeats of either VPGVG or VGGVG. The hydrophobic domains of elastin are responsible for its elastic character.

Tropoelastin is translated and then secreted as a mature protein into the ECM and accumulates at the surface of the cell. After secretion and alignment with ECM fibrils, numerous K residues are oxidized by lysyl oxidase, a reaction which initiates cross-linking of elastin monomers. The highly stable cross-linking of elastin is what ultimately imparts the elastic properties to elastic fibers.

Loss of the elastin gene is found associated with the disorder known as Williams-Beuren syndrome (also known as just Williams syndrome) which is, in part, characterized by connective tissue dysfunction that plays a causative role in the supravalvular aortic stenosis (SVAS) typical of this disorder. Williams-Beuren syndrome results from spontaneous deletion of a region of the q arm (q11.23) of one of the two copies of chromosome 7. Defective elastin is also associated with a group of skin disorders called cutis laxa (autosomal dominant form in the case of ELN gene defects). In these disorders the skin has little to no elastic character and hangs in large folds.

FIBRILLINS

Along with elastin, the fibrillins are major proteins in elastic fibers. Humans express three fibrillin genes identified as *FBN1, FBN2,* and *FBN3*. Fibrillin monomers link head to tail in microfibrils which can then form two- and three-dimensional structures. The most abundant fibrillin in elastic fibers is the FBN1-encoded protein, fibrillin 1. FBN1 expression is high in most cell types of mesenchymal origin, particularly bone.

Mutations in fibrillin genes result in connective tissue disorders referred to as fibrillinopathies. These disorders are characterized

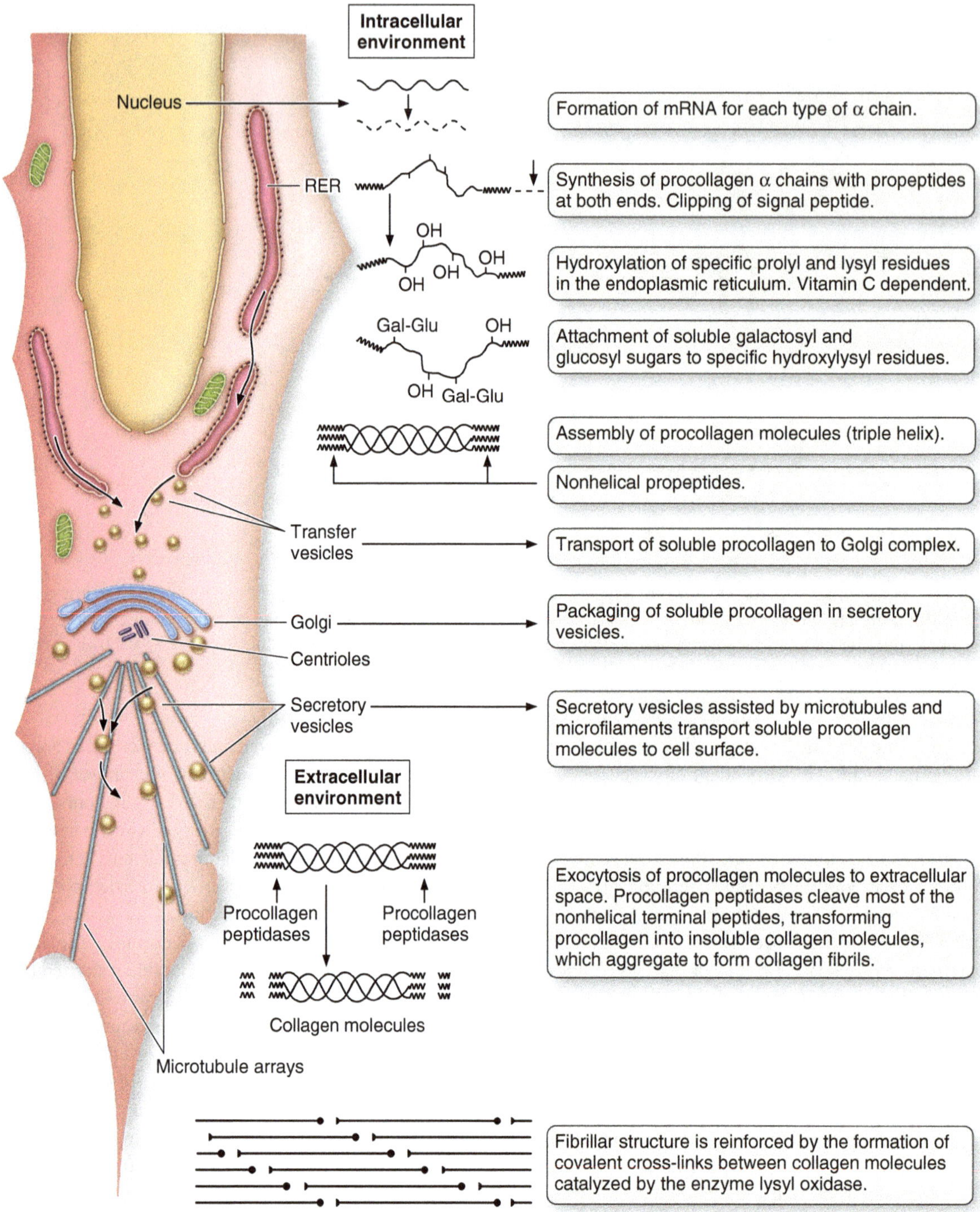

FIGURE 25–10 Synthesis of collagen. Each collagen is composed of a α-chain encoded by 1 of the 30 different α-collagen genes. Synthesis, hydroxylation, and glycosylation of the procollagen protein occurs during transit through the ER. Final assembly into structural fibrils occurs after procollagen is secreted into the ECM. (Reproduced with permission from Mescher AL. *Junqueira's Basic Histology Text and Atlas*. 16th ed. New York, NY: McGraw Hill; 2021.)

by structural failure of the ECM due to the absence or abnormality in fibrillin proteins. The various fibrillinopathies that have been characterized to date resulting from mutations in either the *FBN1* or *FBN2* genes. No diseases are currently known to be associated with the *FBN3* gene in humans. The FBN1-associated fibrillinopathies include Marfan syndrome (MFS: Clinical Box 25–8), familial ectopia lentis, familial aortic aneurysm ascending and dissection, autosomal dominant Weill-Marchesani syndrome type 2 (WMS2), and MASS syndrome (MASS designates the involvement of the mitral valve, aorta, skeleton, and skin). The FBN2-associated fibrillinopathy is congenital contractural arachnodactyly.

CLINICAL BOX 25–6 OSTEOGENESIS IMPERFECTA

OI represents a heterogeneous group of disorders, the majority of which are the result of mutations that affect the structure and function of type I collagens. The most common causes and cases of OI are inherited as autosomal dominant diseases, those being types I-IV. Some individuals with type III OI inherited the disorder as an autosomal recessive trait. Most infants who have the severe forms of type II and type III OI acquired the disorder as a result of the appearance of a new mutation. Individuals with OI are characterized phenotypically with bone fragility and low bone mass. In addition, patients have soft tissue dysplasia, dentinogenesis imperfecta (abnormalities in the teeth), loss of hearing, and alterations in the coloration of the sclera. Because of the heterogeneity of OI disorders, this syndrome has been divided into 15 types with types I–IV being the result of mutations in specific collagen genes.

Type I OI is an autosomal dominant disease that is referred to as the mild type. Type I OI results from null mutations (no functional protein) in the *COL1A1* gene. The classic features of type I OI include bone fragility and bluish sclera. In a patient with type I OI, the appearance of abnormal coloration of the sclera is most often seen on ophthalmic examination. The bluish-gray coloration results from the thinning of the sclera due to loss of type I collagen deposition and a resultant ability to visualize the underlying choroid veins. The prevalence of type I OI is approximately 1 in 10,000 to 1 in 25,000. Diagnosis of type I OI is done by analysis of the production of type I procollagen in dermal fibroblasts in culture.

Type II OI is an autosomal dominant disease that is referred to as the perinatal lethal type. Type II OI results from mutations in the *COL1A1* and *COL1A2* genes. The mutations result in exon skipping and C-terminal proprotein mutants that interfere with collagen chain associations. Type II is characterized by severe bone fragility, absent calvarial mineralization and dark sclera. The frequency of type II OI is between 1 in 20,000 and 1 in 60,000. Affected infants are usually born premature and with low birth weight. Infants have characteristic facial features that include dark sclera, a beaked nose and an extremely soft calvarium. The outlook for type II OI patients is grim as this is a lethal disorder with life spans of only minutes to a few months. Death is usually the result of congestive heart failure, pulmonary insufficiency or infection.

Type III OI is an autosomal dominant form that is referred to as the deforming type and is the result of exon skipping mutations in the *COL1A1* and *COL1A2* genes. The disorder is characterized by short stature, dentinogenesis imperfecta, light sclera, and bone fragility leading to progressive deformities.

Type IV OI is an autosomal dominant form that is called the mild deforming type and is the result of mutations in the *COL1A1* and *COL1A2* genes that result in exon skipping as well as the result of partial gene deletion mutants. The symptoms of type IV are similar to those of type III with individuals having mild short stature, dentinogenesis imperfecta, and grayish sclera.

CLINICAL BOX 25–7 EHLERS-DANLOS SYNDROME

EDS represents a heterogeneous group of generalized connective tissue disorders. The predominant forms of EDS result from defects in collagen synthesis and or processing as well as several forms resulting from mutations in genes encoding enzymes in glycosaminoglycan processing or in the complement pathway of the immune system. The major manifestations of the EDS family of disorders are skin fragility, skin hyperextensibility, and joint hypermobility. Original designations for the various forms of EDS used Roman numerals (eg, type I, II, III, etc.). However, in 1997 the Villefranche nomenclature was adopted which uses descriptive designations, for example, EDS type I now being referred to as classical EDS. As of 2017 a total of 13 distinct forms of EDS had been characterized. Many of the EDS forms have significant overlapping clinical pathology. The predominant forms of EDS are classical EDS, vascular EDS, and hypermobile EDS. The other 10 recognized forms of EDS are considered rare and are classic-like EDS, kyphoscoliosis EDS, arthrochalasia EDS, dermatosparaxis EDS, periodontal EDS, brittle cornea syndrome EDS, musculocontractural EDS, spondylodysplastic EDS, myopathic EDS, and cardiac valvular EDS.

Classical EDS: The originally identified EDS types I and II are now referred to as classical EDS. Classical EDS is the result of mutations in the collagen genes, *COL5A1* and *COL5A2*. Classical EDS is inherited as an autosomal dominant disease. The characteristic clinical features of classical EDS are soft, velvety, and hyperextensible skin and easy bruising. The joints are quite hypermobile. Many patients with classical EDS have mitral valve prolapse. Trauma to the skin usually results in large gaping wounds that bleed less than expected. Repeated trauma to the knees, elbows, and shins leads to pigmented scarring. In addition, the skin develops thin "cigarette-paper" scars as a result of trauma.

Vascular EDS (formerly type IV) is the arterial type of the disease. Vascular EDS is inherited as an autosomal dominant disease and is the result of mutations in the *COL3A1* genes. The mutations alter the synthesis, structure, and secretion of type III collagen. The characteristic features of vascular EDS are thin, translucent skin with visible veins which causes marked bruising. Patients with vascular EDS are subject to arterial, uterine, and bowel rupture.

Hypermobile EDS (formerly type III) is characterized by marked hypermobility of both the large and small joints. The skin is soft, smooth, velvety, and bruises easily but doesn't scar like in classical EDS. A clear genetic mutation (or mutations) has not yet been characterized as being associated with the generation of hypermobile EDS. Within one family, characterized to have several members with hypermobile EDS, a mutation in the *COL3A1* gene was identified. However, COL3A1 mutations are characteristic of vascular EDS and thus, it is likely that this family was incorrectly diagnosed.

CLINICAL BOX 25-8 MARFAN SYNDROME

Marfan syndrome (MFS) is an autosomal dominant disorder affecting the connective tissue. The symptoms of MFS are the result of inherited defects in the extracellular matrix glycoprotein fibrillin 1. The cardinal manifestations of MFS are tall stature with dolichostenomelia (condition of unusually long and thin extremities) and arachnodactyly (abnormally long and slender fingers and toes), joint hypermobility and contracture, deformity of the spine and anterior chest, mitral valve prolapse, dilatation and dissection of the ascending aorta, pneumothorax and ectopia lentis (displacement of the crystalline lens of the eye). Correct diagnosis of MFS relies on the presence of a combination of manifestations in several organ systems. Individuals with MFS are taller at all ages than would be predicted based on their kinship. The tall stature is the result of overgrowth of the long bones which leads to the characteristic features of MFS such as disproportionately long legs, arms, and digits. This phenotype is called dolichostenomelia where one diagnostic feature is that the arm span will exceed the body height. The overgrowth of the tubular bones leads to deformity of the anterior chest. This can result in the ribs pushing either in (pectus excavatum) or out (pectus carinatum) or in on one side and out on the other. The skull is often elongated (termed dolichocephaly), the mandible underdeveloped with the palate narrow and highly arched, and the face is long and narrow. Because of ligament laxity the joints are hypermobile and there is often joint pain. Persons with MFS are now living longer due to clinical interventions in the cardiovascular abnormalities but this leads to an increased occurrence of degenerative skeletal problems such as osteoarthritis. Mitral valve prolapse (MVP) is the most common finding in children with MFS. The prolapse is due to redundancy of the valve tissue, elongation of the valve annulus (valve ring) and elongation of the chordae tendineae (these are the tendons that connect the papillary muscles to the tricuspid and mitral valves). MVP will progress to severe mitral regurgitation which requires surgical intervention usually before 10 years of age. Progressive dilation of the proximal portions of both the aorta and main pulmonary arteries occurs in MFS and are highly important diagnostic and prognostic indicators. The combination of the deformity of the anterior chest and pectus excavatum results in a reduction in lung volume which can lead to severe restrictive pulmonary deficits. Spontaneous pneumothorax occurs in 4–5% of MFS patients. Due to laxity of the hypopharyngeal tissue obstructive sleep apnea is a common symptom in MFS. The ocular hallmark of MFS is displacement of the lens from the center of the pupil (ectopia lentis). Because of the presence of this symptom in a high percentage of MFS patients, displacement of the lens in the absence of any traumatic event should lead to a consideration of MFS. The cornea of MFS patients is often flatter than normal. Detection of the corneal abnormality and surgical correction are necessary at an early age to prevent persistent amblyopia (lazy eye). Later in life many MFS patients will suffer from cataracts and/or glaucoma.

FIBRONECTIN

Fibronectin is a major fibrillar glycoprotein of the ECM where its role is to attach cells to a variety of ECM types (Figure 25–11). Fibronectin is functional as a dimer of two similar peptide chains. At least 11 different fibronectin proteins have been identified that arise by alternative RNA splicing of the primary transcript from a single fibronectin gene (symbol: ***FN1***). Fibronectin attaches cells to all extracellular matrices except type IV. Type IV matrices involve laminins as the adhesive proteins.

Fibronectin consists of a multimodular structure composed predominantly of three different amino acid repeat domains termed modules. These repeat domains are termed FN-I, FN-II, and FN-III. The three fibronectin repeat domains are each composed of two antiparallel β-sheets. Each of the two fibronectin subunits in a functional fibronectin dimer consists of twelve FN-I, two FN-II, and 15–17 FN-III modules, respectively. These functional modules are responsible for fibronectin binding to fibrin, collagen, heparan sulfate proteoglycans (HSPG), DNA, and the integrins in plasma membranes. The primary amino acid sequence motif in fibronectin that binds to an integrin is a tripeptide, Arg-Gly-Asp (RGD).

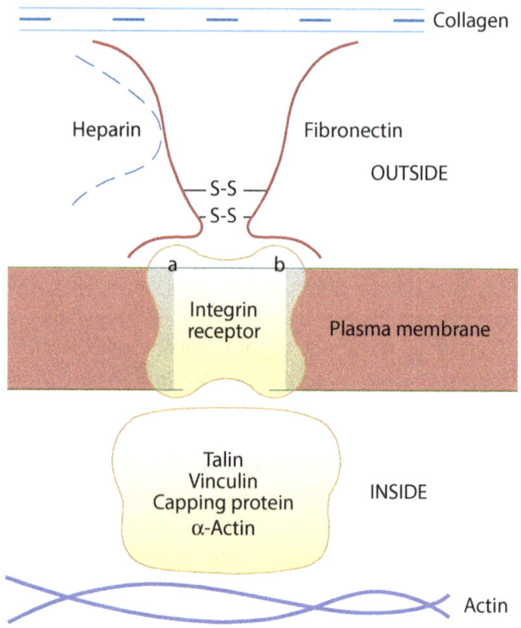

FIGURE 25–11 Representation of fibronectin interaction with an integrin receptor. Extracellular fibronectin interacts with an integrin present in the plasma membrane. The interaction of fibronectin with an integrin triggers activation of intracellular protein complexes that are associated with the actin microfilaments that control cell shape and movement. (Reproduced with permission from Rodwell VW, Bender DA, Botham KM, et al: *Harper's Illustrated Biochemistry*, 31st ed. New York, NY: McGraw Hill; 2018.)

LAMININ

All basal lamina contain a common set of proteins, GAGs, and proteoglycans. These include type IV collagen, heparan sulfate proteoglycans (HSPGs), nidogens (entactins), and laminins. Because of the presence of type IV collagens, the basal lamina is often referred to as the type IV ECM. Laminins anchor cell surfaces to the basal lamina.

Laminins are heterotrimeric proteins that contain an α-chain, a β-chain, and a γ-chain. The historical designations for these three protein chains were A, B1, and B2, respectively. Humans express five genes encoding the α-chains, four encoding the β-chains, and three encoding the γ-chains. The different laminin proteins have been found to form at least 15 different types of heterotrimers. The nomenclature for a laminin molecule relates to the peptide chain composition. For example, the laminin molecule identified as laminin-111 (originally identified as laminin-1) is composed of the α1, β1, and γ1 gene encoded proteins (α1β1γ1 composition), and laminin-211 (formerly laminin-2) has the composition, α2β1γ1. Laminins contain common structural features that include a tandem distribution of globular, rod-like and coiled-coil domains. The coiled-coil domains are responsible for joining the three chains into a characteristic heterotrimeric structure.

Laminins are critical components of the ECM that bind to the integrins, the dystroglycans, and numerous other receptors. These laminin interactions are critical for cell differentiation, cell movement, cell shape, and the promotion of cell survival. Given this broad range of contributions to tissue formation and survival, it is not surprising that loss of functional laminin genes can result in potentially devastating disorders such as certain forms of epidermolysis bullosa, EB. The junctional form of EB can be caused by mutations in either an integrin gene or a laminin gene. A form of congenital muscular dystrophy is caused by defective laminin-211 production due to defects in the *LAMA2* gene.

INTEGRINS

The term integrin was derived from the observations that these cell-surface proteins (the integrins) served as transmembrane linkers (integrators) whose functions were to mediate the interactions between the ECM and the intracellular cytoskeleton (see Figure 25–11).

Integrins function as heterodimeric glycoproteins, composed of an α- and a β-subunit. Humans express 18 integrin α-subunit genes and 8 integrin β-subunit genes. Both subunits of an integrin are single-pass transmembrane proteins, which bind components of the ECM or counter-receptors expressed on other cells. Several different matrix proteins are bound by integrins, such as laminins and fibronectin. Many ligands for the integrins bind only in the presence of the divalent cations, Ca^{2+} or Mg^{2+}.

Integrins provide a link between ligand and the actin cytoskeleton via short intracellular domains. This linkage between the outside (extracellular matrix) and inside (cytoskeleton) of cells, mediated by integrin-ligand interactions, allows for both outside-in and inside-out signal transduction. Integrin-ligand interactions can trigger certain intracellular signal transduction pathways via the regulation of the activity of certain protein kinases. These kinases include focal adhesion kinase (FAK) and integrin-linked kinase (ILK).

THROMBOSPONDINS

Thrombospondin is the term that was used to define a "thrombin-sensitive protein" first isolated from platelets that had been stimulated with thrombin. The initially characterized protein is now called thrombospondin 1 (TSP1). Several additional thrombospondins have been identified and the human thrombospondin family now consists of five proteins identified as TSP1, TSP2, TSP3, TSP4, and COMP (cartilage oligomeric matrix protein; also referred to as TSP5).

The five thrombospondin proteins are divided into two subgroups determined by their domain structure. Subgroup A includes TSP1 and TSP2, while subgroup B includes TSP3, TSP4, and COMP (TSP5). The subgroup A thrombospondins assemble into trimeric structures while the subgroup B thrombospondins function as pentamers.

The thrombospondins are secreted extracellular multisubunit glycoproteins that belong to the larger family of proteins termed matricellular proteins. Matricellular proteins are present in the ECM, however, they do not contribute to the primary structural functions of the ECM. Thrombospondins, like other matricellular proteins, integrate functions of the ECM with cells physically embedded in the ECM.

The thrombospondins interact with a number of cell surface receptors as well as with many other ECM structural proteins such as the collagens. Indeed, TSP1 has been shown to interact with at least 12 different cell adhesion molecules, several growth factors, as well as with numerous proteases. The numerous roles for the thrombospondins include, but are not limited to, the regulation of endothelial cell apoptosis exerting anti-angiogenesis effects, promotion of smooth muscle cell adhesion, proliferation and migration, antagonism of nitric oxide (NO) signaling, maintenance of cardiac function and integrity, promotion of neurogenesis, regulation of bone mineralization/demineralization processes, regulation and modulation of immune functions, and processes of wound repair via regulation of fibrosis.

GLYCOSAMINOGLYCANS

The most abundant heteropolysaccharides in the body are the glycosaminoglycans (GAGs). The GAGs are historically referred to as the mucopolysaccharides given that they were originally characterized in mucus membranes and mucosal exudates. The GAG molecules are long unbranched polysaccharides containing a repeating disaccharide unit. The disaccharide units contain either of two hexosamines, *N*-acetylgalactosamine (GalNAc) or *N*-acetylglucosamine (GlcNAc), and a uronic acid such as glucuronate (GlcA) or iduronate (IdoA) or a galactose residue. GAGs are highly negatively charged molecules, with extended conformation that imparts high viscosity to the solution in which they reside. As such, the GAGs are located primarily on the surface of cells or in the ECM but are also found in secretory vesicles in some types of cells.

Along with the high viscosity of GAGs is low compressibility, which makes these molecules ideal for a lubricating fluid in the joints. At the same time, their rigidity provides structural integrity to cells and provides passageways between cells, allowing for cell migration. The specific GAGs of physiologic significance are hyaluronic acid, dermatan sulfate, chondroitin sulfate, heparin, heparan sulfate, and keratan sulfate. Although each of these GAGs has a predominant disaccharide component (Table 25–1), heterogeneity does exist in the sugars present in the make-up of any given class of GAG.

TABLE 25–1 Composition of the disaccharide units of the major glycosaminoglycans.

Structure	Description
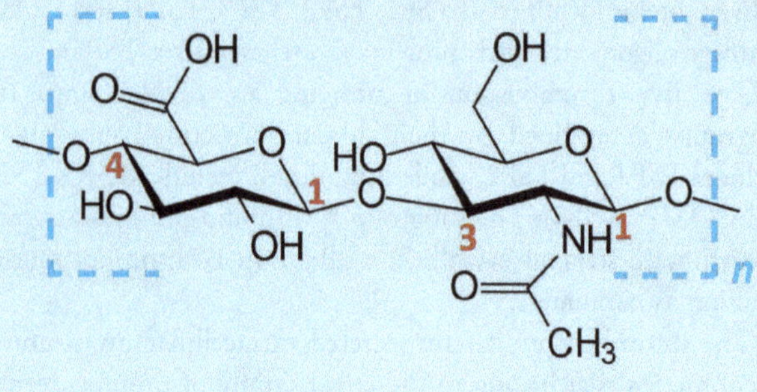 D-glucuronate (GlcA) GlcNAc	**Hyaluronates:** Composed of D-glucuronate (GlcA) plus GlcNAc; linkage is β(1,3)
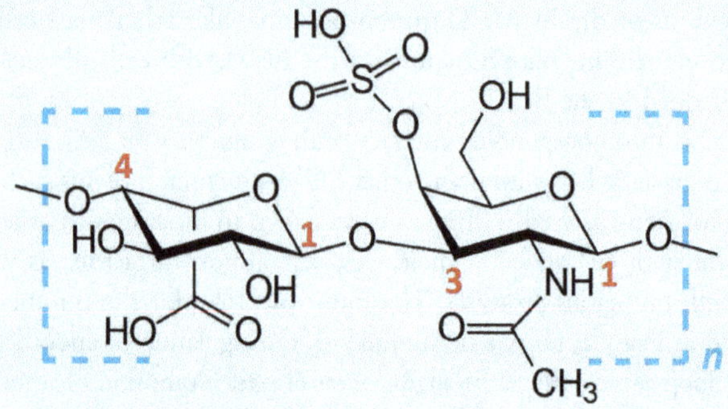 L-iduronate (IdoA) GalNAc-4-Sulfate	**Dermatan sulfates:** Composed of L-iduronate (IdoA) or D-glucuronate (GlcA) plus GalNAc-4-sulfate; GlcA and IdoA sulfated; linkages is β(1,3) if GlcA, α(1,3) if IdoA
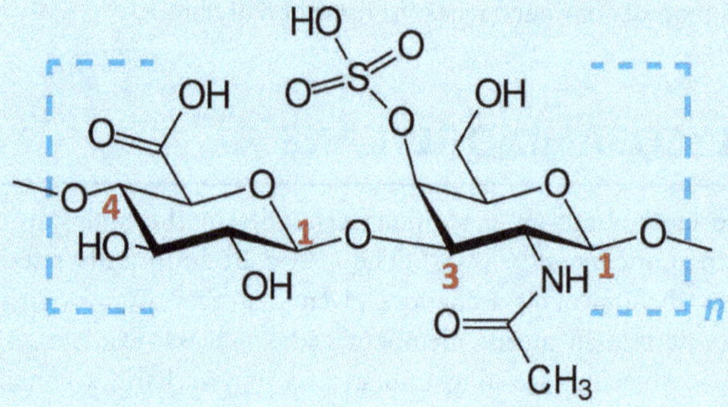 D-glucuronate (GlcA) GalNAc-4-Sulfate	**Chondroitin 4- and 6-sulfates:** Composed of D-glucuronate (GlcA) and GalNAc-4- or 6-sulfate; linkage is β(1,3); this figure contains GalNAc-4-sulfate
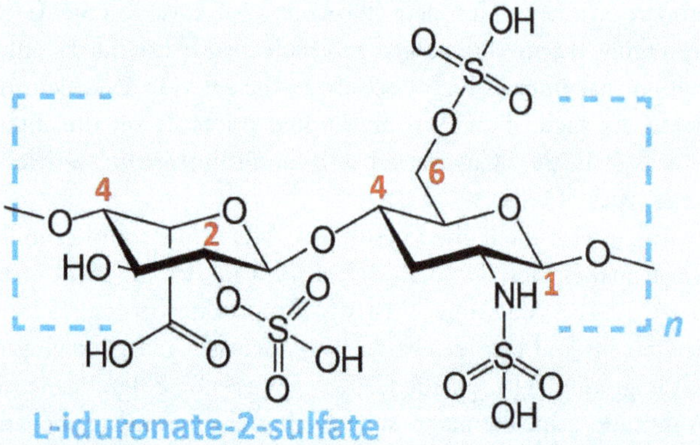 L-iduronate-2-sulfate N-sulfo-GlcNAc-6-sulfate	**Heparin and heparan sulfates:** Composed of L-iduronate (IdoA: many with 2-sulfate) or D-glucuronate (GlcA: many with 2-sulfate) and *N*-sulfo-D-glucosamine-6-sulfate; linkage is α(1,4) if IdoA, β(1,4) if GlcA: heparans have less overall sulfate than heparins

TABLE 25–1 Composition of the disaccharide units of the major glycosaminoglycans. (*Continued*)

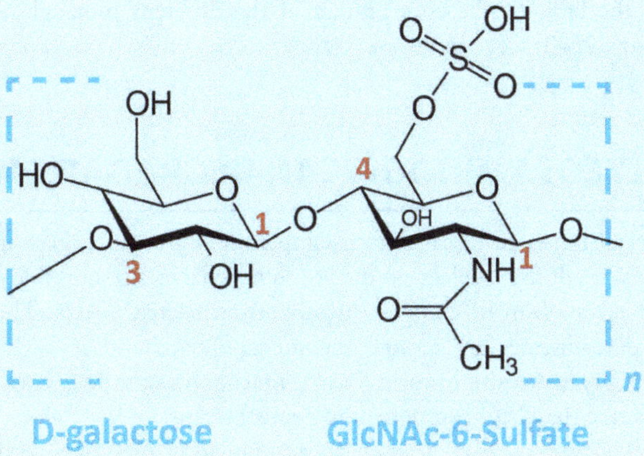

Keratan sulfates: Composed of galactose plus GlcNAc-6-sulfate; linkage is β(1,4)

Hyaluronic acid (also called hyaluronan) is unique among the GAGs in that it does not contain any sulfate and is not found covalently attached to proteins as a proteoglycan. It is, however, a component of noncovalently formed complexes with proteoglycans in the ECM (see Figure 25–13). Hyaluronic acid polymers are very large and can displace a large volume of water. This property makes them excellent lubricators and shock absorbers.

Each of the GAGs serves a distinct function in the formation of the various types of ECM (Table 25–2). One well-defined function of the GAG heparin is its role in preventing coagulation

TABLE 25–2 Characteristics of the various glycosaminoglycans.

GAG	Localization	Characteristics
Hyaluronate	Synovial fluid, articular cartilage, skin, vitreous humor, ECM of loose connective tissue	Large polymers, molecular weight can reach 1 million Daltons; high shock absorbing character; average person has 15 g in body, 30% turned over every day; synthesized in plasma membrane by three hyaluronan synthases: HAS1, HAS2, and HAS3
Chondroitin sulfate	Cartilage, bone, heart valves	Most abundant GAG; principally associated with protein to form proteoglycans; the sulfation of chondroitin sulfates occurs on the C-2 position of the uronic acid residues and the C-4 and/or C-6 positions of GalNAc residues; the chondroitin sulfate proteoglycans form a family of molecules called lecticans and includes aggrecan, versican, brevican, and neurcan; major component of the ECM; loss of chondroitin sulfate from cartilage is a major cause of osteoarthritis
Heparan sulfate	Basement membranes, components of cell surfaces	Contains higher acetylated glucosamine than heparin; found associated with protein forming heparan sulfate proteoglycans (HSPG); major HSPG forms are the syndecans and GPI-linked glypicans; HSPG binds numerous ligands such as fibroblast growth factors (FGFs), vascular endothelial growth factor (VEGF), and hepatocyte growth factor (HGF); HSPG also binds chylomicron remnants at the surface of hepatocytes; HSPG derived from endothelial cells act as anti-coagulant molecules
Heparin	Component of intracellular granules of mast cells, lining the arteries of the lungs, liver, and skin	More sulfated than heparan sulfates; clinically useful as an injectable anticoagulant although the precise role *in vivo* is likely defense against invading bacteria and foreign substances
Dermatan sulfate	Skin, blood vessels, heart valves, tendons, lung	Was originally referred to as chondroitin sulfate B which is a term no longer used; the sulfation of dermatan sulfates occurs on the C-2 position of the uronic acid residues and the C-4 and/or C-6 positions of GalNAc residues; may function in coagulation, wound repair, fibrosis, and infection; excess accumulation in the mitral valve can result in mitral valve prolapse
Keratan sulfate	Cornea, bone, cartilage aggregated with chondroitin sulfates	Usually associated with protein-forming proteoglycans; keratan sulfate proteoglycans include lumican, keratocan, fibromodulin, aggrecan, osteoadherin, and prolargin

of the blood. Heparin is abundant in granules of mast cells that line blood vessels. The release of heparin from these granules, in response to injury, and its subsequent entry into the serum, leads to an inhibition of blood clotting. Free heparin complexes with, and activates, antithrombin III which in turn inhibits all the serine proteases of the coagulation cascade (see Chapter 33). This phenomenon has been clinically exploited in the use of heparin injection for anticoagulation therapies.

PROTEOGLYCANS

The majority of GAGs in the body are linked to core proteins, forming proteoglycans. The GAGs extend perpendicularly from the core in a brush-like structure. The linkage of GAGs to the protein core, in most but not all proteoglycans, involves a specific tetrasaccharide linker composed of a glucuronic acid (GlcA) residue, two galactose (Gal) residues, and a xylose (Xyl) residue (Figure 25–12).

The tetrasaccharide linker is coupled to the protein core through an *O*-glycosidic bond to a Ser residue in the protein. In the case of the keratan sulfates, attachment of the sugar linker to the core protein can occur via *O*-linkage or via *N*-linkage. There are two major types of keratan sulfates (KSI and KSII) where KSI containing proteoglycans are formed via *N*-linkage and KSII containing proteoglycans are formed via *O*-linkage.

Different types of proteoglycans are classified based not only on the type(s) of GAG attached to the protein core but also on the basis of the core protein of the different proteoglycans (Table 25–3).

GLYCOSAMINOGLYCAN DEGRADATION

Several inherited diseases, for example the lysosomal storage diseases, result from defects in the lysosomal enzymes responsible for the metabolism of complex membrane-associated GAGs. These specific diseases are termed the mucopolysaccharidoses (MPS) in reference to the historical term, mucopolysaccharide, used to describe the GAG component of proteoglycans.

The various MPS lead to an accumulation of GAGs within lysosomes of affected cells. There are at least 14 known types of lysosomal storage diseases that affect GAG catabolism. Some of the more commonly encountered mucopolysaccharidoses are Hurler syndrome (Clinical Box 25–9) and Hunter syndrome (Clinical Box 25–10).

All of the MPS diseases are chronic, progressively debilitating disorders that in many instances lead to severe psychomotor retardation and premature death. In addition, the clinical spectrum of these disorders can vary widely due to the differing effects of different mutations in the same gene.

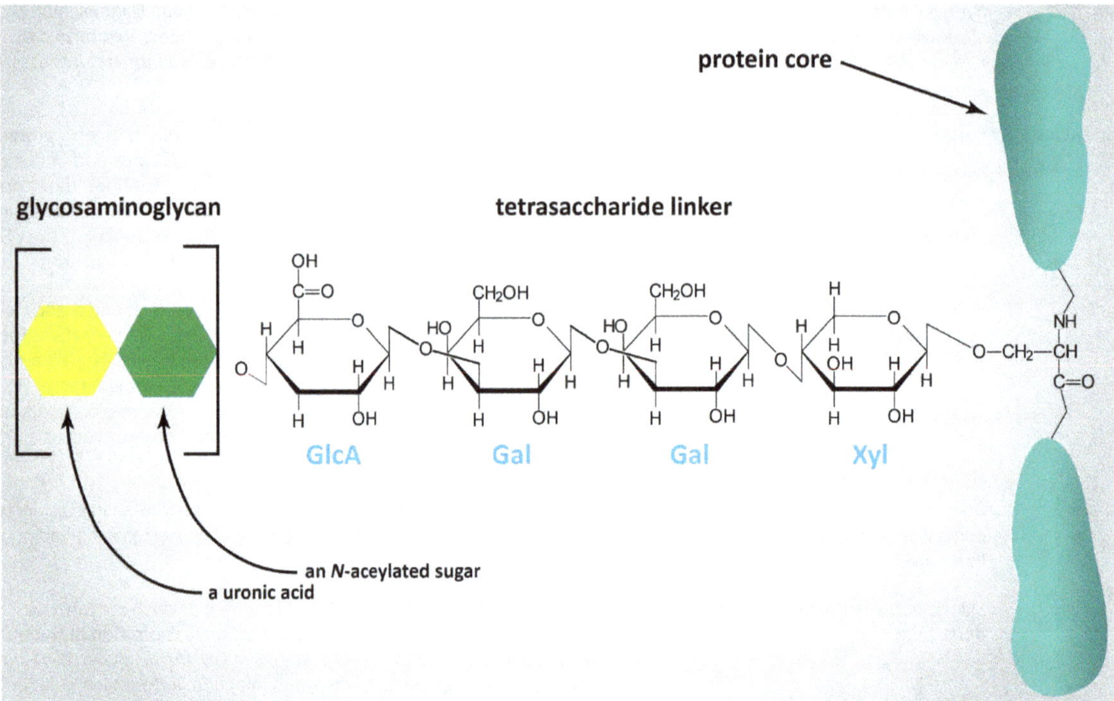

FIGURE 25–12 Structure of the GAG linkage to protein in proteoglycans. The majority of GAGs linked to protein to form a proteoglycan are attached via a tetrasaccharide linker that consist of GlcA–Gal–Gal–Xyl–Ser residue in the protein core. This is true for most, but not all, heparin, heparan sulfate, chondroitin sulfate, and dermatan sulfate polymers attached to proteins in proteoglycans. (Reproduced with permission from themedicalbiochemistrypage, LLC.)

TABLE 25–3 Representative mammalian proteoglycan types.

Proteoglycan	Comments
Aggrecan (Figure 25–13)	Belongs to the lectican family; a chondroitin sulfate proteoglycan (CSPG); protein core encoded by the *ACAN* gene; forms a complex with hyaluronan; major component of articular cartilage
Brevican	Belongs to the lectican family; a chondroitin sulfate proteoglycan (CSPG); protein core encoded by the *BCAN* gene; predominantly expressed in the central nervous system; brevican protein devoid of glycosaminoglycan chains is also found within the brain
Decorin	Is a member of the small leucine-rich proteoglycan (SLRP) family; protein core encoded by the *DCN* gene; binds to type I collagen fibrils; also interacts with fibronectin, thrombospondin, the epidermal growth factor receptor (EGFR) and transforming growth factor-beta (TGF-β); may play a role in epithelial/mesenchymal interactions during organ development
Keratocan	A keratan sulfate proteoglycan (KSPG); protein core encoded by the *KERA* gene; is a member of the small leucine-rich proteoglycan (SLRP) family; important to the transparency of the cornea
Lumican	Major keratan sulfate proteoglycan (KSPG); the protein core encoded by the *LUM* gene; is a member of the small leucine-rich proteoglycan (SLRP) family, also referred to as the small interstitial proteoglycan gene (SIPG) family; present in large quantities in the corneal stroma and in interstitial collagenous matrices of the heart, aorta, skeletal muscle, skin, and intervertebral discs; interacts with collagen fibrils; may regulate collagen fibril organization, corneal transparency, and epithelial cell migration and tissue repair
Neurocan	Belongs to the lectican family; a chondroitin sulfate proteoglycan (CSPG); a nervous system proteoglycan; protein core encoded by the *NCAN* gene; is a susceptibility factor for bipolar disorder, absence of the *NANC* gene in mice results in a variety of manic-like behaviors which can be normalized by administration of lithium
Perlecan	More commonly called heparan sulfate proteoglycan (HSPG) of basement membrane; protein core encoded by the *HSPG2* gene; possesses angiogenic and growth-promoting properties primarily by acting as a coreceptor for fibroblast growth factor 2 (FGF2)
Syndecans	A family of cell surface heparan sulfate proteoglycans (HSPGs) that act as transmembrane cell surface receptors; consists of four members: syndecan-1, -2, -3, and -4; aberrant syndecan regulation plays a critical role postnatal tissue repair, inflammation and tumor progression; syndecan-1 expression is prevalent in differentiating plasma cells and its expression can serve as a marker for cells that are secreting immunoglobulin; syndecan-2 (also referred to as the original HSPG) prevalent on endothelial cells; strong expression of syndecan-3 found in many regions of the brain; syndecan-4 prevalently expressed in epithelial and fibroblastic cells; protein core of syndecan-1 encoded by the *SDC1* gene; syndecan-2 protein core encoded by the *SDC2* gene; protein core of syndecan-3 encoded by the *SDC3* gene; protein core of syndecan-4 encoded by the *SDC4* gene
Versican	Belongs to the lectican family; a chondroitin sulfate proteoglycan (CSPG); protein core encoded by the *VCAN* gene; alternative splicing generates three versican species designated V0, V1, and V2 that differ in the length of the attached glycosaminoglycans; one of the main components of the ECM; significant proteoglycan in vitreous body of the eye; participates in cell adhesion, proliferation, migration, and angiogenesis; contributes to the development of atherosclerotic vascular diseases, cancer, tendon remodeling, hair follicle cycling, central nervous system injury, and neurite outgrowth; Wagner syndrome is caused by mutation in the *VCAN* gene, causes vitreoretinal degeneration

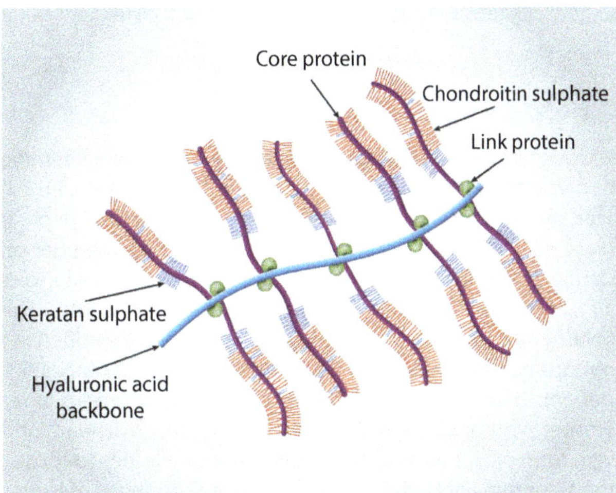

FIGURE 25–13 Structure of typical hyaluronic acid-based proteoglycan. (Reproduced with permission from themedicalbiochemistrypage, LLC.)

CLINICAL BOX 25–9 HURLER AND SCHEIE SYNDROMES

Hurler and Scheie syndromes are autosomal recessive disorders that belong to a family of disorders identified as lysosomal storage diseases, and historically as the mucopolysaccharidoses (MPS). Due to the association with the term MPS the Hurler and Scheie syndromes are collectively identified as MPS I (or MPS1). The MPS I disorders are characterized by the lysosomal accumulation of dermatan and heparan sulfates as a consequence of defects in the lysosomal hydrolase, α-L-iduronidase. This enzyme hydrolyzes terminal α-L-iduronic acid residues from the two classes (dermatan and heparan sulfates) of glycosaminoglycans. Numerous mutations have been identified in the *IDUA* gene resulting in Hurler and Scheie diseases. The most commonly occurring mutations seen in the Caucasian population are two that cause truncation of the functional enzyme. One mutation truncates the protein at amino acid 402 following a tryptophan residue (the mutation is designated as: W402X) and the other at amino acid 70 following a glutamine residue (the mutation is designated as: Q70X). Deficiencies in α-L-iduronidase results in a wide spectrum of clinical manifestations that are classified into three clinical diseases. Hurler disease represents the most severe end of the spectrum and Scheie the least severe with the Hurler-Scheie syndrome representing the phenotype that is intermediate between the other two. Hurler syndrome is a progressive disorder manifesting with multiple organ and tissue involvement leading to death in early childhood. Most Hurler infants succumb to cardiomyopathy. Diagnosis of Hurler syndrome is usually made between 4 and 18 months of age in infants that appeared normal at birth. Early symptoms that prompt medical attention are hepatosplenomegaly, coarse facial features and an enlarged tongue. Developmental delay is apparent by 12 months with maximum attainment of a functional age of 2–4 years. Progressive deterioration is seen as the disease progresses. Hearing loss is also typical in Hurler syndrome. As the disease progresses there is an increase in the degree of corneal clouding. Most patients have recurrent ear and upper respiratory tract infections, persistent nasal discharge, and noisy breathing. Typical of other mucopolysaccharidoses, Hurler patients exhibit the constellation of skeletal abnormalities referred to dystosis multiplex. Dystosis multiplex is characterized by an enlarged skull, thickened calvarium, premature closure of lamboid and sagittal sutures, shallow orbits, enlarged J-shaped sella turcica (a saddle-shaped skull structure into which sits the bottom of the pituitary gland), and abnormal spacing of the teeth with dentigerous cysts. There is anterior hypoplasia of the lumbar vertebrae, the long bone diaphyses are enlarged and an irregular appearance of the metaphyses. The epiphyseal centers are not well developed, the pelvis is poorly formed with small femoral heads and coxa valga. The clavicles are short, thick, and irregular and the ribs are oar shaped. Phalanges are shortened and trapezoidal in shape. Hurler patients have a short neck and odontoid hypoplasia (decreased ossification of the odontoid bone which is the anterior process of the second vertebra). This latter symptom can result in atlantoaxial subluxation which is a misalignment between the first and second cervical vertebrae. The clinical phenotype associated with Hurler-Scheie syndrome is intermediate between that of Hurler and Scheie syndromes. This form of the disease is characterized by progressive dystosis multiplex with no deficit in intellect. The onset of symptoms is usually observed between the ages of 3 and 8 years. Patients with Hurler-Scheie syndrome often survive into adulthood. In addition to the skeletal abnormalities, patients exhibit progressive corneal clouding, deafness, aortic valve abnormalities and joint stiffness. Scheie syndrome is the mild form of mucopolysaccharidosis type I. This form of the disease is characterized by corneal clouding, aortic valve abnormalities, and joint stiffness with few of the other features seen in the more severe forms of the disease. The onset of symptoms in Scheie syndrome does not usually occur until after the age of 5. Diagnosis is often made only when a patient is between 10 and 20 years of age. Enzyme replacement therapy (ERT), bone marrow transplantation, hematopoietic stem cell transplant, and gene transfer to patient bone marrow have all had a level of success in treating several patients suffering from MPS I. A current clinically approved ERT for Hurler syndrome is the Sanofi drug Aldurazyme (iaronidase).

CLINICAL BOX 25–10 HUNTER SYNDROME

Hunter syndrome is an X-linked recessive disorder that belongs to a family of disorders identified as lysosomal storage diseases, and historically as one of the mucopolysaccharidoses. Hunter syndrome is the only one of the mucopolysaccharidoses that is X-linked. This disorder is characterized by the lysosomal accumulation of dermatan and heparan sulfates as a consequence of deficiencies in the lysosomal hydrolase, iduronate sulfatase. Iduronate sulfatase is a member of a family of sulfatases, many of which are necessary for the degradation of the glycosaminoglycans. Iduronate sulfatase (also called iduronate 2-sulfatase) hydrolyzes sulfates from the 2- position of L-iduronate present in dermatan and heparan sulfates. The enzyme was originally referred to as the "Hunter corrective factor." Numerous mutations and deletions have been identified in the *IDS* gene resulting in Hunter syndrome. The majority of Hunter syndrome mutations are missense, nonsense, and frameshift mutations with several small deletions or insertions as well. All patients harboring mutations caused by large deletions or rearrangements in the *IDS* gene manifest with the severe forms of Hunter syndrome. Clinically, Hunter syndrome is divided into severe and mild classifications. The clinical presentation of the severe form of Hunter syndrome has many similarities to those seen in Hurler syndrome without the corneal clouding. In addition, the symptoms of Hunter progress slower than those of Hurler syndrome. The mild form of Hunter syndrome is similar to the Hurler-Scheie syndrome and Scheie syndrome. Hunter syndrome is inherited as an X-linked

CLINICAL BOX 25–10 (CONTINUED)

recessive disorder and affected males do not reproduce. This latter fact precludes the presentation of affected females. Patients with the severe form of Hunter syndrome present with characteristic clinical features. These include short stature, skeletal deformities, joint stiffness, coarse facial features, and intellectual impairment. Onset of symptoms of the severe form are usually seen between 2 and 4 years of age. As a consequence of autonomic nervous system involvement many patients suffer from chronic diarrhea. Extensive neurologic degeneration precedes death in patients with the severe form of Hunter syndrome with death occurring between 10 and 15 years of age. Patients with the mild form of Hunter syndrome generally have normal intelligence and survive into adulthood. Some of the symptoms in mild form patients can be as severe as those in the severe form but the progression of deterioration is much slower. Although some patients with the mild form of Hunter can survive into their 50s or 60s, death often occurs in early adulthood as a consequence of cardiac failure and pulmonary obstruction.

CHECKLIST

- ☑ Biological membranes consist of phospholipids, cholesterol, proteins, and carbohydrates.
- ☑ Biological membranes are composed of a lipid bilayer formed by two sheets of phospholipids whose hydrophobic tails interact and their polar head groups are presented on the outer surfaces where they interact with the aqueous environment.
- ☑ The structure of membranes is dynamic with lateral diffusion of lipids and proteins. In addition, lipids can flip-flop between the two faces of the membrane.
- ☑ Proteins that are associated with membranes can interact with the outer or inner surfaces or they can be embedded in, or through, the membrane. Integral membrane proteins are those that are firmly embedded in the membrane whereas, those that are attached by simple interaction are peripheral proteins.
- ☑ The various membranes of a cell have different compositions which in turn, defines the functional characteristics of the particular membrane. Within a given membrane, such as the plasma membrane, there can be highly specialized localized environments.
- ☑ Ions and molecules can move across membranes either by passive or active means. Ions are generally transported across membranes via the action of ligand-gated channels, whereas, various types of transporter proteins are used to move solutes and other larger molecules across membranes.
- ☑ Membrane transporter classes are defined by the overall process of transport and also by whether or not energy is required for the process.
- ☑ There are several classes of ATP-driven membrane transporters including the ATP-binding cassette family (ABC), and the P-type (phosphorylated), F-type (energy factor), E-type (extracellular), and V-type (vacuolar).
- ☑ Numerous types of transporters are present in the membrane involved in transport of various solutes and are referred to as the solute carrier (SLC) family.
- ☑ Mutations that affect the structure and function of membrane proteins such as transporters, receptors, ion channels, can have profound effects leading to disease and disability.
- ☑ The extracellular matrix (ECM) provides the structural support that holds cells together to form the various tissues.
- ☑ The ECM is composed of structural proteins (primarily collagens and elastin), specialized proteins (such as fibronectin and laminin), and a variety of proteoglycans.
- ☑ Collagen is the most abundant protein in the human body. There are 28 different types of collagen all derived from 30 different α-collagen genes. Functional collagens comprise three polypeptides wound around each other to form a triple helix. The collagen monomers in the triple helix are held together by cross-linking between the chains. Each collagen protein contains a highly repeating sequence of $(Gly\text{-}X\text{-}Y)_n$.
- ☑ Numerous disorders in collagen synthesis and processing are known and include the various types of osteogenesis imperfect and Ehlers-Danlos syndrome.
- ☑ Elastin forms cross-linked fibers via a mechanism similar to that in collagen but is unique in that three lysine-derived aldehydes (allysyl) cross-link with an unmodified lysine forming a tetrafunctional structure called a desmosine. The highly stable cross-linking of elastin is what ultimately imparts its elastic properties.
- ☑ Fibrillin is found interspersed in cross-linked elastin fibers and plays a role in the elastic character of elastic fibers; deficiencies in fibrillin result in the connective tissue disorder called Marfan syndrome.

- ☑ Fibronectin is a major ECM glycoprotein that interacts with cell surface receptors of the integrin family, connecting the ECM to intracellular signaling pathways.
- ☑ Laminin are heterotrimeric ECM proteins that are quite large, ranging from under 500,000 to nearly a 1,000,000 Da in mass. Laminins contain common structural features that include a tandem distribution of globular, rod-like, and coiled-coil domains. The coiled-coil domains are responsible for joining the three chains into the characteristic heterotrimeric structure called merosin.
- ☑ Glycosaminoglycans (GAGs) are composed of various repeating disaccharides that consist of a uronic acid (glucuronic or iduronic acid) and a hexose or hexosamine (galactose, galactosamine, or glucosamine). Many GAGs also have varying degrees of sulfate addition.
- ☑ The major GAGs in human tissues are hyaluronic acid, chondroitin sulfate, keratin sulfate, dermatan sulfate, heparin, and heparan sulfate.
- ☑ Proteoglycans are heavily glycosylated ECM proteins composed of one or more GAGs attached to serine residues. The GAGs extend perpendicularly from the core protein forming a brush-like structure. Proteoglycans are extremely large and confer lubricating and shock-absorbing properties to the tissues.
- ☑ Inherited deficiencies in the enzymes responsible for lysosomal degradation of GAGs result in a class of lysosomal storage diseases commonly referred to as the mucopolysaccharidoses.

REVIEW QUESTIONS

1. A 7-month-old infant is being examined due to progressive neurodegeneration and connective tissue abnormalities. X-rays show demonstrable osteoporosis and metaphyseal dysplasia. Molecular analysis finds a deletion in the coding region of a gene encoding a copper transporter. Which of the following additional symptoms is most likely to be seen in this infant?

(A) Cholestatic liver disease
(B) Hemochromatosis
(C) Polydipsia and polyuria
(D) Prolonged bleeding time
(E) Recurrent infections

2. A 28-year-old man sees his physician on a regular basis because he has suffered from bronchiectasis, chronic sinusitis, rhinitis, and secretory otitis media since childhood. He is currently being evaluated for infertility because he and his wife have been unable to conceive. His wife has been evaluated, and no abnormalities were found. The volume of his ejaculate and his sperm count are within reference ranges. Given his history and current findings his infertility could best be explained by defective or absent activity of which of the following cell structures?

(A) Golgi complex
(B) Microtubules
(C) Mitochondria
(D) Peroxisomes
(E) Ribosomes

3. Experiments are being conducted on cultures of pancreatic endocrine cells. The cells are treated with a novel compound that is structurally related to colchicine. Which of the following is the most likely effect of the addition of this compound to these cell cultures?

(A) Induction of lamellipodia
(B) Induction of nerve cell action potentials
(C) Inhibition of adenylate cyclase
(D) Inhibition of hormone secretion
(E) Stimulation of Ca^{2+} transport
(F) Stimulation of Na^+-K^+ transport

4. An 87-year-old man, suspected of suffering from Alzheimer disease, has died. Postmortem histopathologic analysis of liver sections finds hepatocytes that contain numerous golden-brown cytoplasmic granules. Which of the following represents the cellular organelles most typically associated with these histopathological results?

(A) Endosomes
(B) Golgi apparatus
(C) Lysosomes
(D) Peroxisomes
(E) Vacuoles

5. A 57-year-old woman is being examined by her physician following her discovery of a lump in her right breast. Her physician takes a biopsy sample for histological analysis which indicates the tissue is ductal carcinoma. Immunohistochemical staining, of isolated carcinoma cells, would show that these cells are most likely to have significantly reduced levels of which of the following cell adhesion proteins?

(A) Cadherins
(B) Fibronectins
(C) Integrins
(D) Laminins
(E) Selectins

6. A 3-year-old girl is being examined by her pediatrician due to concerns by her parents that she bruises very easily. Upon examination it is noted that her skin is highly pliable and that her joints are loose and hyperextensible. A defect in the synthesis of which of the following is most likely to explain the observations in this patient?

(A) Actin
(B) Collagen
(C) Elastin
(D) Fibrillin
(E) Myosin

7. A 14-year-old girl is being examined by an ophthalmologist with complaints of blurred vision and nearsightedness. These visual problems have gotten progressively worse over the past year. Physical examination shows the patient is 5 ft 10 in tall and weighs 137 lb with a BMI of 20 kg/m^2. The patient also has an increased arm span-to-height ratio, decreased upper-to-lower segment ratio, and positive thumb and wrist signs. Ophthalmoscopic examination shows demonstrable ectopia lentis in both eyes. A mutation in the gene encoding which of the following is the most likely cause of the signs and symptoms in this patient?
(A) Collagen
(B) Elastin
(C) Fibrillin
(D) Fibronectin
(E) Laminin

8. A 2-month-old infant is being examined by a pediatrician due to concerns about his coarse facial features. Physical examination finds hypotonia and a persistent head lag. Blood works finds significantly elevated levels of acid sphingomyelinase and β-hexosaminidase A activity. Histopathological examination of skin fibroblasts shows inclusion bodies. A defect in which of the following processes is the most likely cause of the infant's pathology?
(A) Synthesis of lysosomal proteins
(B) Synthesis of lysosomes
(C) Synthesis of peroxisomal proteins
(D) Targeting of lysosomal lipids
(E) Targeting of lysosomal proteins
(F) Targeting of peroxisomal proteins

9. The parents of a 7-month-old infant bring their son to the pediatrician because they have noticed that their child has a dull response to outside stimuli. In addition, they note that their child exhibits exaggerated arm and leg extension in response to sharp sounds and that he seems to be losing previously acquired motor and mental skills. The signs and symptoms observed in this infant are most likely to be due to a defect in which of the following metabolic processes?
(A) Branched-chain amino acid catabolism
(B) Cardiac glycogen breakdown
(C) Glycosphingolipid metabolism
(D) Hepatic urea synthesis
(E) Peroxisomal fatty acid α-oxidation

10. A 28-year-old woman is being examined by her physician with complaints of severe bone pain, weakness, and frequent nose bleeds. Physical examination reveals hepatosplenomegaly and numerous ichthyosis-like skin lesions. Serum studies demonstrate an anemia with the presence of enlarged cells that contain a large amount of a course fibrillary looking substance. Given the signs and symptoms in this patient, which of the following would most likely represent the metabolic defect causing the pathology?
(A) Bone marrow glycolipid metabolism
(B) Cardiac lysosomal carbohydrate metabolism
(C) Erythrocyte glucose metabolism
(D) Hepatic glycogen metabolism
(E) Peroxisomal complex lipid metabolism
(F) Skeletal muscle fatty acid metabolism

11. A 4-month-old infant, who appeared normal at birth, now presents with coarse facial features and macroglossia. Physical examination shows hepatosplenomegaly, nasal discharge, difficulty breathing, corneal opacities, and joint contractures. Laboratory studies demonstrate the accumulation of heparan sulfates in the urine. The child's physical symptoms and laboratory results are most likely to be associated with which of the following modes of inheritance?
(A) Autosomal dominant
(B) Autosomal recessive
(C) X-linked dominant
(D) X-linked recessive
(E) Mitochondrial

12. The parents of 6-month-old are alarmed at the apparent regression of their child's psychomotor skills. The infant has had difficulty in feeding accompanied by recurrent vomiting. Examination reveals a protuberant abdomen with clear hepatosplenomegaly and thin emaciated extremities. Histochemical examination of the monocytic fraction of the plasma demonstrates the presence of cells containing an unusual myelin-like membranous substance. Given the findings in this child, which of the following represents the most likely metabolic defect?
(A) Membrane phospholipid metabolism
(B) Neuronal iron homeostasis
(C) Neutral amino acid absorption
(D) Peroxisomal lipid metabolism
(E) Protein glycosylation

13. A 12-year-old girl is being examined to determine the cause of her intense and uncontrollable thirst with a strong craving for ice water. The patient produces large amounts of urine (8–10 L per day). Additional symptoms include fatigue, headache, irritability, and muscle pains. Molecular studies determine that the gene (*AVPR2*) encoding the arginine vasopressin receptor 2 is intact. A mutation in a gene encoding which of the following would most likely be responsible for the patient's symptoms?
(A) Aquaporin 2
(B) Cystine transporter
(C) Divalent metal transporter 1
(D) Multidrug-resistance associated protein 2
(E) Neutral amino acid transporter

14. A 1-year-old infant presents with unique facial features, recurrent infections, persistent leukocytosis, defective neutrophil chemotaxis, and severe growth and intellectual impairment. A defect in which of the following transport systems would most likely account for the signs and symptoms in this infant?
(A) Aquaporin 2
(B) Divalent metal transporter 1
(C) Ferroportin
(D) GDP-fucose transporter
(E) Na^+/K^+-ATPase

15. A 35-year-old woman is being examined by her physician with complaints of resting tremors and diminished facial expressions. Physical examination finds choreoathetoid movements. Biochemical studies on liver biopsy-derived cells find a defect in the activity of a metal transporter. Which of the following additional findings would most likely be found in this patient?
(A) Bronze diabetes
(B) Heinz bodies in erythrocytes
(C) Kayser-Fleischer rings
(D) Port wine colored urine
(E) Trinucleotide repeat expansion

16. Experiments are being undertaken to examine the effects of a compound on the movement of ions across cell membranes using a cell culture system. These experiments find that the compound interferes with ion and small molecule movement from the cytosol of one cell to another. These results suggest that the compound most likely interferes with the function of which of the following?
(A) ABC family transporters
(B) Adherens junctions
(C) Aquaporins
(D) Gap junctions
(E) Na^+-K^+-ATPases
(F) Tight junctions

17. A 17-year-old girl comes to the physician because of decreased range of motion, redness, and swelling of the joints due to arthritis. Physical examination shows xanthomas of the Achilles tendon and extensor tendons of the hand, and splenomegaly. Laboratory studies show very high serum levels of sitosterol, campesterol, stigmasterol, and avenosterol. This patient most likely has a defect in a gene encoding which of the following class of protein?
(A) ATP-binding cassette (ABC) transporters
(B) Aquaporins
(C) Gap junctions
(D) Na^+/K^+-ATPases
(E) Solute carrier (SLC) transporters

18. A male infant, delivered at 38 weeks' gestation, presents with severe bowing of long bones and craniotabes at birth. Radiographs show severe generalized osteoporosis, broad and crumpled long bones, beading ribs, and a poorly mineralized skull. Ophthalmic examination indicates clearly visible choroidal veins. The symptoms observed in the infant are most characteristic of a defect in which of the following processes?
(A) Basal lamina deposition
(B) Collagen synthesis
(C) Fibrillin synthesis
(D) Glutamate carboxylation
(E) Lysine oxidation

19. A 37-year-old man is being examined by his physician with complaints chronic pain in his stomach area. Physical examination shows the patient to be mildly jaundiced. Palpation of his abdomen elicits a sharp pain response and indicates hepatosplenomegaly. Histological examination of a blood smear from the patient shows foamy fat-laden cells of the granulocyte-macrophage lineage. The appearance of which of the following in the blood and/or urine would be most useful in making a correct diagnosis in this patient?
(A) Ceramides
(B) Glucocerebrosides
(C) G_{M2} gangliosides
(D) Sphingomyelins
(E) Sulfatides

20. An 8-month-old infant is being examined by his pediatrician due to concerns by his parents about deteriorating motor skills. The child was normal at birth, but the deteriorating signs began about 1 month ago. Ophthalmoscopic examination identifies a milky halo surrounding the fovea centralis. The enzyme, whose deficiency is resulting in the observed signs and symptoms in this child, is most likely responsible for which of the following functions?
(A) Degradation of glycolipids in skeletal muscle
(B) Degradation of glycolipids in the brain
(C) Degradation of glycolipids in the bone marrow
(D) Synthesis of glycolipids in smooth muscle
(E) Synthesis of glycolipids in the brain
(F) Synthesis of glycolipids in the liver

21. Experiments are being carried out using a novel compound designed to exert a positive inotropic effect on the hearts of human test subjects. The compound is structurally related to digoxin. The activity of which of the following is most likely to be affected in ventricular cardiomyocytes of patients to whom this compound is administered?
(A) Calcium-activated potassium channels
(B) Epithelial sodium channels
(C) Inositol-1,4,5-trisphosphate (IP_3) receptors
(D) Na^+/Ca^{2+} exchange protein 1 (NCX1)
(E) T-type calcium channels

22. A 3-day-old male infant is diagnosed with meconium ileus. Which of the following disorders is most likely to be associated with this condition in neonates?
(A) Cystic fibrosis
(B) Hartnup disease
(C) Menkes disease
(D) Sitosterolemia
(E) Tangier disease

23. A 20-month-old child presents with coarse facial features, corneal clouding, and hepatosplenomegaly. The child has a persistent nasal discharge and a noisy breathing pattern. Radiographic analysis indicates enlargement of the diaphyses of the long bones. Biochemical studies discovered cellular accumulation of heparan sulfate. The signs and symptoms in this patient are most likely due to a defect in which of the following processes?
(A) Collagen maturation
(B) Glycosaminoglycan metabolism
(C) Protein *N*-glycosylation
(D) Protein *O*-glycosylation
(E) Proteoglycan synthesis

24. A 3-year-old girl is undergoing an examination to determine the cause of her severe developmental delay. Physical examination shows macrocephaly, dysmorphic facies, clear corneas, hypotonia, and hepatosplenomegaly. There is also a pebbly ivory-colored lesion over the infant's back. This infant is most likely suffering from the consequences of which of the following disorders?
(A) Ehlers-Danlos syndrome
(B) Hunter syndrome
(C) Hurler syndrome
(D) Marfan syndrome
(E) Sly syndrome

25. A 6-year-old girl is being examined to determine the cause of her severe psychomotor retardation. Physical examination shows distinct hepatosplenomegaly, corneal clouding, coarse facial features, and short stature. Analysis of a skin biopsy finds lysosomal accumulation of dermatan sulfate. The signs and symptoms in this patient are most likely due to a defect in which of the following processes?
(A) Collagen maturation
(B) Glycosaminoglycan metabolism
(C) Protein *N*-glycosylation
(D) Protein *O*-glycosylation
(E) Proteoglycan synthesis

26. A female infant, delivered at 37 weeks gestation, presents with severe bowing of long bones. X-rays show broad and crumpled long bones. Ophthalmoscopic examination finds demonstrably visible choroid veins. The signs and symptoms in this patient are most likely due to a defect in which of the following processes?
(A) Collagen maturation
(B) Glycosaminoglycan metabolism
(C) Protein *N*-glycosylation
(D) Protein *O*-glycosylation
(E) Proteoglycan synthesis

27. A 3-year-old girl is undergoing an examination to determine the cause of her severe developmental delay. Physical examination shows macrocephaly, dysmorphic facies, clear corneas, hypotonia, and hepatosplenomegaly. There is also a pebbly ivory-colored lesion over the infant's back. Which of the following is most likely to be found at high levels in fibroblasts from a skin biopsy from this patient?
(A) Chondroitin sulfates
(B) Dermatan sulfates
(C) Glucocerebrosides
(D) Glycogen
(E) G_{M2} gangliosides
(F) Phytanic acid

28. A 10-month-old boy is referred for further evaluation because of apparent delayed development. Physical examination shows coarse facial features, macroglossia, and hepatomegaly. Molecular studies find the presence of a missense mutation in the iduronate sulfatase gene. Lysosomal metabolism of which of the following substances is most likely defective in this child?
(A) Glycogen
(B) Glycosaminoglycans
(C) Glycosphingolipids
(D) G_{M2} gangliosides
(E) Sphingomyelins

29. A 26-month-old girl has suffered numerous fractures. Physical examination finds demonstrably visible choroid veins, misshapen teeth, and hearing difficulty. Which of the following is the most likely cause of these findings?
(A) An inability to synthesize calcitriol
(B) Excessive renal phosphate loss
(C) Inadequate mineralization of bone matrix
(D) Lysosomal accumulation of dermatan sulfates
(E) Synthesis of abnormal type I collagen

30. An 18-month-old girl is brought to the physician because of apparent intellectual impairment and loss of vision. The infant exhibits a demonstrable startle reflex. Ophthalmoscopic examination finds a milky appearance around the fovea centralis. These signs and symptoms are most likely associated with intracellular accumulation of which of the following?
(A) Chondroitin sulfates
(B) Dermatan sulfates
(C) Galactocerebrosides
(D) Glucocerebrosides
(E) G_{M2} gangliosides
(F) Sphingomyelins

31. A 12-year-old boy has suffered from chronic sinopulmonary disease including persistent infection of the airway with *Pseudomonas aeruginosa*. He has constant and chronic sputum production as a result of the airway infection. Additionally, he suffers from gastrointestinal and nutritional abnormalities that include biliary cirrhosis and pancreatic insufficiency. The symptoms are most likely associated with a defect in the transport of which of the following?
(A) Chloride
(B) Copper
(C) GDP-fucose
(D) Iron
(E) Neutral amino acids
(F) Sitosterol

32. A 19-year-old man is being examined in the Emergency Department following a fainting spell. The patient reports that he has had periods of dizziness, lightheadedness, and a pounding heartbeat and that these symptoms have been occurring more frequently of late and most often following his workouts. When questioned, he states that he has fainted twice in the past month during these episodes. The attending physician orders an EKG, during which the patient's QT interval is found to be 0.53 msec (N = 0.39–0.45 msec). History reveals that his father died from a heart attack at the age of 47 and that his maternal grandfather also succumbed to a heart attack. Given the signs and symptoms in this patient, he is most likely affected by a mutation in a transporter that is responsible for which phase of the typical ventricular myocyte action potential shown in the figure below?
(A) Phase 0
(B) Phase 1
(C) Phase 2
(D) Phase 3
(E) Phase 4

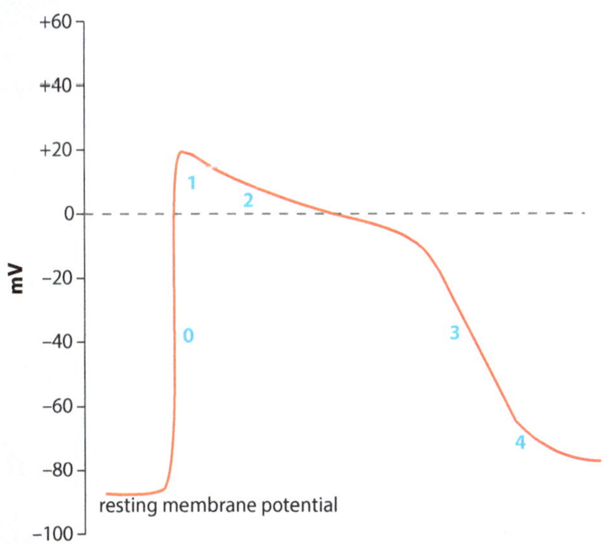

33. A 23-year-old man has admitted himself to the Emergency Department with a complaint of sudden-onset stabbing chest pain that is radiating to his upper back. He reports that the pain was sudden in onset and that he was not exercising at the time. Physical examination shows a patient who is tall with long arms and arachnodactyly. Examination of his chest shows pectus carinatum. Eye examination finds ectopia lentis. Given the signs and symptoms in this patient, which of the following is most likely to be found to be defective?

(A) Cellular attachment to the extracellular matrix
(B) Cytoskeletal integration to the extracellular matrix
(C) Elastic fiber scaffolding
(D) Formation of basal lamina
(E) Tissue contraction following stretch

34. A 3-year-old girl is being attended to in the Emergency Department for broken arm that her mother states was the result of a fall from a dining room chair. An x-ray of the patient's arm shows a greenstick-type fracture of the right radius. On physical examination, it is noted that the girl's teeth appear opalescent and there are visible choroid veins in both eyes. A deficiency in which of the following is the most likely cause of the signs and symptoms in this patient?
(A) Fibrillin 1 synthesis
(B) Fucosylation of cell surface glycans
(C) Targeting of lysosomal enzymes
(D) Type I collagen synthesis
(E) Type 5 collagen synthesis

35. An 18-year-old woman is brought to the Emergency Department by her father complaining of severe abdominal and right flank pain. The patient informs the attending physician that the pain has been varying in intensity all day and that she noted blood in her urine in the morning. Physical examination finds a normal, otherwise healthy and afebrile female. Urinalysis confirms hematuria and the presence of yellowish-pink hexagonal crystals. A deficiency in which of the following renal processes is most likely to account for the signs and symptoms in this patient?
(A) Cystine excretion
(B) Cystine reabsorption
(C) Neutral amino acid excretion
(D) Neutral amino acid reabsorption
(E) Uric acid excretion
(F) Uric acid reabsorption

36. A 5-year-old boy is being examined by his pediatrician because his parents are concerned that he seems to have a constantly runny nose, breathes through his mouth, and also has frequent nosebleeds. The parents note that their son also seems to bruise more easily than their other son, who is 8 years old, and that his stools are often foul-smelling and appear very oily as they often float in the toilet. History reveals that the patient has had two episodes of bacterial pneumonia in the past 18 months. Given the bruising and frequent epistaxis the pediatrician orders blood coagulation tests to be performed with the results showing a prothrombin time (PT) of 18 seconds (N = 11.0–12.5 seconds), bleeding time of 4 minutes (N = 3–8 minutes), and an activated partial thromboplastin time (aPTT) of 44 seconds (N = 30–40 seconds). Given the presentation in this patient, he is most likely to be treated by which of the following interventions?
(A) Bone marrow transplantation
(B) Fructose-restricted diet
(C) Liver transplantation
(D) Pancreatic enzyme supplementation
(E) Recombinant factor VIII

37. Experiments are being conducted on cardiac nodal myocytes in culture to identify and characterize novel cardiac output-regulating compounds. Preliminary characterization has shown that when these cells are stimulated, they contract and conduct action potentials to adjacent cells as expected for nodal cardiomyocytes. The first drug to be tested has been shown, in other cell types, to inhibit T-type calcium channels. If this novel drug exerts effects as expected, where on the typical nodal cardiomyocyte action potential, shown in the accompanying figure, would the effects be most pronounced?
(A) First Phase 4
(B) Phase 0
(C) Phase 3
(D) Second Phase 4

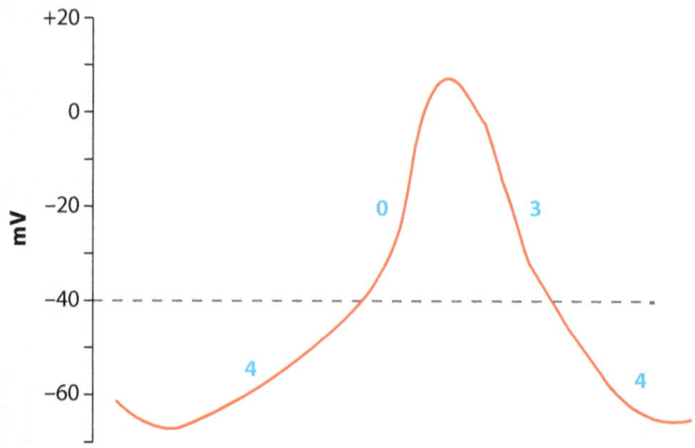

38. An 18-month-old infant was admitted to the hospital following an examination by his pediatrician who diagnosed complications of ischemic cardiomyopathy. The infant appeared normal at birth, but now presents with coarse facial features and macroglossia. Physical examination shows coarse facial features, macroglossia, hepatosplenomegaly, nasal discharge, difficulty breathing, corneal opacities, and joint contractures. Despite being under continuous care, the infant died 5 days after admission. Examination of the heart at autopsy found cardiomegaly and accumulation of dermatan and heparan sulfate. A deficiency in which of the following most likely accounts for the outcome in this infant?
(A) Galactosylceramidase
(B) β-Hexosaminidase A
(C) Iduronate 2-sulfatase
(D) α-L-Iduronidase
(E) Sphingomyelinase

39. A 3-year-old boy is being examined by his pediatrician because his parents are concerned about his persistent cough and the fact that the cough is associated with, what they perceive as bloody sputum. History indicates that the parents adopted their son, but that his medical history was not made available to them. At the time of the adoption, the parents were told that he had an older brother who had persistent lung problems and ultimately succumbed to a severe infection. There is additional history showing that the patient has experienced several respiratory infections over the past 12 months that have required antibiotic treatment. Auscultation reveals rales and rhonchi. Physical examination shows nasal polyps bilaterally with mild mucosal edema. A sweat chloride test finds the level to be 64 mmol/L (N = <29 mmol/L). Which of the following is the most likely additional complication to be observed in this patient?
(A) Combined immunodeficiency
(B) Corneal clouding
(C) Frequent epistaxis
(D) Intellectual impairment
(E) Renal lithiasis

40. Experiments are being conducted on cardiac ventricular myocytes in culture to identify and characterize novel blood pressure medications that can exert effects on cardiac function. Preliminary characterization has shown that when these cells are stimulated, they contract and conduct action potentials to adjacent cells. The first drug to be tested has been shown, in other cell types, to inhibit L-type calcium channels. If this novel drug exerts effects as expected, where on the typical ventricular cardiomyocyte action potential, shown in the accompanying figure, would the effects be most pronounced?

(A) Phase 0
(B) Phase 1
(C) Phase 2
(D) Phase 3
(E) Phase 4

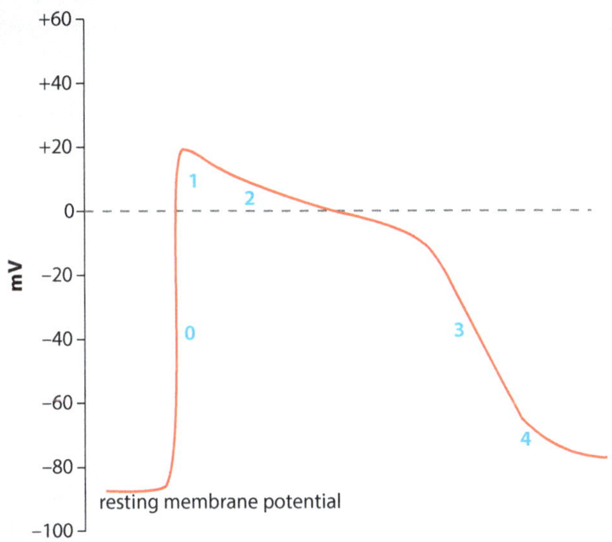

ANSWERS

1. Correct answer is **D.** The infant is most likely suffering the symptoms of Menkes disease. Menkes disease is the result of defects in the P-type ATPase protein (ATP7A) that is responsible for the translocation of copper across the intestinal basolateral membrane into the blood, thus allowing for uptake of dietary copper, as well as for uptake of copper from the blood into most tissues. The clinical spectrum associated with Menkes disease is due in large part to the reduced activity of cytochrome c oxidase, dopamine β-hydroxylase, ceruloplasmin, and lysyl oxidase, all of which are critical copper-dependent enzymes. Lysyl oxidase is an important copper-requiring enzyme necessary for extracellular collagen processing. Defective collagen processing, in addition to resulting in connective tissue and skeletal anomalies, also results in impaired platelet adhesion to exposed subendothelial extracellular matrices. The loss of effective platelet adhesion leads to impaired platelet activation at sites of vessel injury which in turn leads to dramatically prolonged bleeding times in Menkes patients. None of the other symptoms (choices A, B, C, and E) would be expected to be present in an infant suffering from Menkes disease.

2. Correct answer is **B.** The patient is most likely manifesting the signs and symptoms Kartagener syndrome, also referred to as primary ciliary dyskinesia. Kartagener syndrome is most often associated with ultrastructural defects of the axoneme, the skeleton of cilia and flagella, and can result from mutations in several different genes including dyneins, kinesins, and microtubule-associated proteins. All of these proteins are associated with or direct contributors to the function of the microtubule machinery of the seller. Defects in none of the other cell structures (choices A, C, D, and E) are related to the manifestation of symptoms in Kartagener syndrome.

3. Correct answer is **D.** Colchicine inhibits microtubule polymerization by binding to its constitutive protein, tubulin. Microtubules are required for movement of secretory vesicles to the plasma membrane and so inhibition of the function of microtubules would inhibit secretory processes such as hormone secretion. Microtubules grow, through polymerization, from the center of the cell to its periphery, where their plus ends interact with several sites that help to coordinate the formation of lamellipodia. Therefore, inhibition of microtubule functions would inhibit, not induce (choice A) the formation of lamellipodia. Colchicine addition to pancreatic endocrine cells would not result in any of the other activities (choices B, C, E, and F).

4. Correct answer is **C.** Excess accumulation of iron, particularly in macrophages and macrophage-related cells such as the Kupffer cells of the liver, results in the precipitation of the iron storage protein ferritin and its partial digestion by the lysosomes producing what is termed, hemosiderin. Hemosiderin accumulation in lysosomes leads to golden-brown refractile granules being visible in histopathology sections stained with hematoxylin and eosin. None of the other organelles (choices A, B, D, and E) give rise to the typical hematoxylin and eosin visible coloration in histopathology.

5. Correct answer is **A.** Cadherins are a family of calcium-dependent adhesion molecules that form anchoring junctions at the cell surface. These proteins mediate not only cell-cell adhesion but also transmembrane signaling. Loss of one specific cadherin family member, E-cadherin, has been shown to be directly correlated with metastatic potential of certain types of cancers, particularly carcinomas. Fibronectins (choice B), integrins (choice C), laminins (choice D), and selectins (choice E) all contribute to tumorigenesis, and for fibronectins and integrins there is a contribution to cancer metastasis; however, the correlation with all of these proteins is with enhanced expression, not reduced expression.

6. Correct answer is **B.** The child is most likely suffering from a form of Ehlers-Danlos syndrome. Ehlers-Danlos syndrome (EDS) represents a heterogeneous group of generalized connective tissue disorders. The predominant forms of EDS result from defects in collagen synthesis and or processing as well as several forms resulting from mutations in genes encoding enzymes in glycosaminoglycan processing or in the complement pathway of the immune system. Classical EDS is the result of mutations in the collagen genes, *COL5A1* and *COL5A2*. Classical EDS is inherited as an autosomal dominant disease. The characteristic clinical features of classical EDS are soft, velvety, and hyperextensible skin and easy bruising. The joints are quite hypermobile. Many patients with classical EDS have mitral valve prolapse. Trauma to the skin usually results in large gaping wounds that bleed less than expected. Repeated trauma to the knees, elbows and shins leads to pigmented scarring. In addition, the skin develops thin "cigarette-paper" scars as a result of trauma. Mutations in the gene encoding fibrillin (choice D) result in the

connective tissue disorder known as Marfan syndrome. The cardinal manifestations of Marfan syndrome are tall stature with dolichostenomelia (condition of unusually long and thin extremities) and arachnodactyly (abnormally long and slender fingers and toes), joint hypermobility and contracture, deformity of the spine and anterior chest, mitral valve prolapse, dilatation and dissection of the ascending aorta, pneumothorax, and ectopia lentis (lens dislocation). Defects in none of the other proteins (choices A, C, and E) are associated with the symptoms of Ehlers-Danlos syndrome.

7. Correct answer is **C.** The patient is most likely exhibiting the signs and symptoms of the connective tissue disorder known as Marfan syndrome. The symptoms of Marfan syndrome are the result of inherited defects in the extracellular matrix glycoprotein, fibrillin 1. The cardinal manifestations of Marfan syndrome are tall stature with dolichostenomelia (condition of unusually long and thin extremities) and arachnodactyly (abnormally long and slender fingers and toes), joint hypermobility and contracture, deformity of the spine and anterior chest, mitral valve prolapse, dilatation and dissection of the ascending aorta, pneumothorax, and ectopia lentis (lens dislocation). Mutations in genes encoding none of the other proteins (choices A, B, D, and E) are associated with the signs and symptoms exhibited by this patient.

8. Correct answer is **E.** The infant is most likely suffering from the lysosomal storage disease identified as I-cell disease. I-cell disease results from the loss of correct targeting of lysosomal enzymes to the lysosomes. The disorder is characterized by severe psychomotor retardation that rapidly progresses leading to death between 5 and 8 years of age. I-cell disease patients exhibit coarse facial features, craniofacial abnormalities, severe skeletal abnormalities, and striking gingival hyperplasia. The targeting of lysosomal enzymes to lysosomes is mediated by receptors that bind mannose-6-phosphate recognition markers on the enzymes. The recognition marker is synthesized in a two-step reaction in the Golgi complex. The enzyme that catalyzes the first step in this process is UDP-*N*-acetylglucosamine:lysosomal-enzyme *N*-acetylglucosaminyl-1-phosphotransferase (GlcNAc-phosphotransferase). GlcNAc-phosphotransferase is an $\alpha_2\beta_2\gamma_2$ hexameric complex whose protein subunits are encoded by two genes. The α- and β-subunits of the phosphotransferase are encoded by the *GNPTAB* gene, and the γ-subunits are encoded by the *GNPTG* gene. I-cell disease result from mutations in the *GNPTAB* gene. Defects in none of the other processes (choices A, B, C, D, and F) correlate with the causation of the pathology of I-cell disease.

9. Correct answer is **C.** The infant is most likely suffering from the lysosomal storage disease, Tay-Sachs disease. Tay-Sachs disease results from defects in the *HEXA* gene encoding the α-subunit of the lysosomal hydrolase, β-hexosaminidase A. Infants with Tay-Sachs disease appear normal at birth. Symptoms usually begin with mild motor weakness by 3–5 months of age. Another early symptom is an exaggerated startle response to sharp sounds. By 6–10 months of age infants will begin to show regression of prior acquired motor and mental skills. It is the loss of these activities that will normally prompt parents to seek a medical opinion. A progressive loss in visual attentiveness may lead to an ophthalmological consultation which will reveal macular pallor and the presence of the characteristic "cherry-red spot" in area of the fovea centralis of the eye. At around 8–10 months of age the symptoms of Tay-Sachs disease begin to progress rapidly. Seizures become progressively more severe and are very frequent by the end of the first year. Psycho-motor deterioration increases by the second year and invariably leads to decerebrate posturing. Ultimately, the patient will progress to an unresponsive vegetative state with death resulting from bronchopneumonia resulting from aspiration in conjunction with a depressed cough. Deficiency in branched-chain amino acid catabolism (choice A) is the cause of maple syrup urine disease. Defective lysosomal cardiac glycogen breakdown (choice B) results in the lethal glycogen storage disease known as Pompe disease. Deficiency in hepatic urea synthesis (choice D) results from mutations in any one of the genes encoding enzymes of the urea cycle. The most severe urea cycle disorders result from deficiencies in carbamoyl phosphate synthetase 1 (CPS1) and deficiencies in ornithine transcarbamylase. Deficiencies in peroxisomal fatty acid oxidation (choice E) results in the disorder called Refsum disease.

10. Correct answer is **A.** The patient is most likely exhibiting the signs and symptoms of the most prevalent form of Gaucher disease. Gaucher disease is an autosomal recessive disorder that is characterized by the lysosomal accumulation of glucosylceramide (glucocerebroside) which is a normal intermediate in the catabolism of globosides and gangliosides. Gaucher disease results from defects in the gene encoding the lysosomal hydrolase, glucosylceramidase beta, also called acid β-glucosidase or glucocerebrosidase. The hallmark of Gaucher disease is the accumulation of lipid-engorged cells of the monocyte/macrophage lineage with a characteristic appearance in a variety of tissues. The primarily affected tissues are bone, bone marrow, spleen, and liver. These distinctive cells contain one or more small nuclei, and their cytoplasm contains a coarse fibrillary material that forms a striated tubular pattern often described as "wrinkled tissue paper." Defective cardiac carbohydrate metabolism (choice B) results in the lethal glycogen storage disease known as Pompe disease. Defective erythrocyte glucose metabolism (choice C) is the basis of the inherited hemolytic anemia, erythrocyte pyruvate kinase deficiency, that results from mutations in the *PKLR* gene. Numerous disorders are the result of defects in hepatic glycogen metabolism (choice D) with the major disorders, Anderson disease, McArdle disease, and Cori disease manifesting in infancy or adolescence. Deficiencies in peroxisomal complex lipid metabolism (choice E) would most likely be Refsum disease which is caused by mutations in the gene-encoding phytanoyl-CoA hydroxylase. Deficiencies in skeletal muscle fatty acid metabolism (choice F) most likely represent the disorder known as adult myopathic carnitine palmitoyltransferase deficiency whose symptoms manifest in young children or adolescents.

11. Correct answer is **B.** The infant is most likely manifesting the symptoms of the mucopolysaccharidotic disorder known as Hurler syndrome. Hurler syndrome is characterized by the lysosomal accumulation of dermatan and heparan sulfates as a consequence of defects in the lysosomal hydrolase, α-L-iduronidase. Hurler syndrome is a progressive disorder manifesting with multiple organ and tissue involvement leading to death in early childhood. Most Hurler infants succumb to cardiomyopathy. Diagnosis of Hurler syndrome is usually made between 4 and 18 months of age in infants that appeared normal at birth. Early symptoms that prompt medical attention are hepatosplenomegaly, coarse facial features, and an enlarged tongue. Developmental delay is apparent by 12 months with maximum attainment of a functional age of 2–4 years. Progressive deterioration is seen as the disease progresses. Hurler syndrome is inherited as an autosomal

recessive disorder. None of the other modes of inheritance (choices A, C, D, and E) represent the inheritance of Hurler syndrome.

12. Correct answer is **A.** The infant is most likely exhibiting the hallmark symptoms of Niemann-Pick disease type A (NPA). There are two distinct sub-families of Niemann-Pick diseases. Niemann-Pick type A (NPA) and type B (NPB) diseases are caused by defects in the acid sphingomyelinase gene (*ASM*) whose encoded enzyme is responsible for lysosomal degradation of sphingomyelins. Sphingomyelins are sphingolipids that are also phospholipids due to the presence of phosphocholine. Niemann-Pick type C1 (NPC1) disease is caused by defects in a gene involved in LDL-cholesterol homeostasis identified as the *NPC1* gene. Type A Niemann-Pick disease is associated with a rapidly progressing neurodegeneration leading to death by 2–3 years of age. The course of type A Niemann-Pick disease is rapid. Infants are born following a typically normal pregnancy and delivery. Within 4–6 months the abdomen protrudes, and hepatosplenomegaly will be diagnosed. The early neurological manifestations include hypotonia, muscular weakness and difficulty feeding. As a consequence of the feeding difficulties and the swollen spleen, infants will exhibit a decrease in growth and body weight. By the time afflicted infants reach 6 months of age the signs of psycho-motor deterioration become evident. Defects in none of the other metabolic processes (choices B, C, D, and E) manifest with the characteristic symptoms of Niemann-Pick disease type A.

13. Correct answer is **A.** The patient is most likely manifesting the symptoms of a defect in renal water homeostasis. The disorder in this patient is most likely the inherited disorder referred to as nephrogenic diabetes insipidus, NDI. NDI is a disorder in which a defect in the tubules in the kidneys causes a person to pass a large amount of dilute urine. This disorder is caused by an improper response of the kidney to antidiuretic hormone (ADH, also called vasopressin), leading to a decrease in the ability of the kidney to concentrate the urine by removing free water. Nephrogenic diabetes insipidus can be either acquired or hereditary. The acquired form is brought on by certain drugs and chronic diseases and can occur at any time during life. The hereditary form of NDI is caused by mutations in the gene (*AVPR2*) encoding arginine vasopressin receptor 2 or in the gene (*AQP2*) encoding aquaporin 2. Mutations in the *AVPR2* gene account for 90% of the inherited forms of NDI, while mutations in the *AQP2* gene account for 10% of cases. Mutations in the gene encoding the cystine transporter (choice B) result in a form of renal lithiasis due to cystine crystal formation in the nephron. Mutations in the gene encoding divalent metal transporter 1 (choice C) have only recently been identified and are associated with a rare form of late onset neural degeneration. Mutations in the gene (*ABCC2*) encoding multidrug resistance-associated protein 2 (choice D) are the cause of Dubin-Johnson syndrome. Mutations in the gene encoding a neutral amino acid transporter (choice E) are the cause of Hartnup disease, a disease whose symptoms are similar to those of niacin deficiency.

14. Correct answer is **D.** The patient is most likely exhibiting the symptoms associated with the disorder known as leukocyte adhesion deficiency syndrome II (LAD II). LAD II belongs to the class of disorders referred to as primary immunodeficiency syndromes as the symptoms of the disease manifest due to defects in leukocyte function. Symptoms of LAD II are characterized by unique facial features, recurrent infections, persistent leukocytosis, defective neutrophil chemotaxis, and severe growth and intellectual impairment. The genetic defect resulting in LAD II is in the pathway of fucose utilization leading to loss of fucosylated glycans on the cell surface. Specifically, LAD II patients harbor mutations in the gene (*SLC35C1*) encoding a GDP-fucose transporter. A defect in the function of aquaporin 2 (choice A) is one of the causes of inherited nephrogenic diabetes insipidus. Defects in the function of divalent metal transporter 1 (choice B) have only recently been identified and are associated with a rare form of late onset neural degeneration. Defects in the function of ferroportin (choice C) resulting in a form of hemochromatosis known as type 4 hemochromatosis. Defects in the function of one of the Na^+/K^+-ATPases (choice E) have only recently been identified and affect both the brain and the kidney and results in excessive potassium excretion triggering epileptic seizures.

15. Correct answer is **C.** The patient is most likely exhibiting the signs and symptoms of the copper transport defect disease known as Wilson disease. Wilson disease is the result of defects in the P-type ATPase protein that is primarily responsible for copper homeostasis mediated by the liver. The most significant sign in the diagnosis of Wilson disease results from the deposition of copper in Descemet's membrane of the cornea. These golden-brown deposits can be seen with a slit-lamp and are referred to as Kayser-Fleischer rings. Bronze diabetes (choice A) is associated with primary hemochromatosis. Heinz bodies in erythrocytes (choice B) is a histopathological finding in patients with the inherited hemolytic anemia resulting from mutations in the gene encoding glucose-6-phosphate dehydrogenase. Port wine colored urine (choice D) is a feature of the two most common porphyrias, acute intermittent porphyria and porphyria cutanea tarda. Numerous disorders are associated with trinucleotide repeat expansion (choice E) such as Huntington disease, myotonic dystrophy type 1, and fragile X syndrome.

16. Correct answer is **D.** Given the findings in this experiment the compound is most likely inhibiting the function of gap junctions. Gap junctions are intercellular channels designed for intercellular communication and their presence allows whole organs to be continuous from within. One major function of gap junctions is to ensure a supply of nutrients to cells of an organ that are not in direct contact with the blood supply. Gap junctions are formed from a type of protein called a connexin. The ABC family transporters (choice A) comprise the ATP-binding cassette transporter superfamily. All members of this superfamily of membrane proteins contain a conserved ATP-binding domain and use the energy of ATP hydrolysis to drive the transport of various molecules across all cell membranes. Adherens junctions (choice B) are composed of transmembrane proteins that serve to anchor cells via interactions with the extracellular matrix and intracellular proteins that interact with the actin filaments that control cell movement and shape. Aquaporins (choice C) are a family of α-type channels responsible for the transport of water across membranes. Na^+/K^+-ATPases (choice E) are transporters involved in the transport of Na^+ out of, and K^+ into, cells. Tight junctions (choice F), also referred to as occluding junctions, are primarily found in the epithelia and endothelia and are designed for occlusion. Tight junctions act as barriers that regulate the movement of solutes and water between various epithelial and endothelial layers.

17. Correct answer is **A.** The patient is most likely experiencing the signs and symptoms of a disorder that results from a disturbance in lipid transport known as sitosterolemia. Sitosterolemia is a rare autosomal recessively inherited disorder characterized by hyperabsorption, and decreased biliary excretion, of dietary sterols leading to hypercholesterolemia, tendon and tuberous xanthomas, premature development of atherosclerosis, and abnormal hematologic and liver function test results. The disorder is caused by mutations in either of the two ABC transporter proteins of the obligate heterodimer composed of ABCG5 and ABCG8. This transporter complex is expressed in intestinal enterocytes and hepatocytes where it functions to limit plant sterol and cholesterol absorption from the diet by facilitating efflux out of enterocytes into the intestinal lumen and out of hepatocytes into the bile canaliculi. Defects in none of the other protein classes (choices B, C, D, and E) would result in the symptoms observed in this patient.

18. Correct answer is **B.** The infant is most likely manifesting the signs and symptoms of osteogenesis imperfecta (OI) type I. The classic features of type I OI include bone fragility and bluish sclera. In a patient with type I OI, the appearance of abnormal coloration of the sclera is most often seen upon ophthalmic examination. The bluish-gray coloration results from the thinning of the sclera due to loss of type I collagen deposition and a resultant ability to visualize the underlying choroid veins. Osteogenesis imperfecta consists of a group of at fifteen related disorders resulting from mutations in several different genes. The four most common forms of OI arise due to defects in two collagen genes, the *COL1A1* and *COL1A2* genes. The mutations lead to decreased expression of collagen or abnormal type 1 collagen proteins. The abnormal proteins associate with normal collagen subunits, which prevents the triple helical structure of normal collagen to form. The result is degradation of all the collagen proteins, both normal and abnormal. Several different disorders have been identified that have, as a basis of their pathology, defective basal lamina production and deposition (choice A). However, none of these disorders manifest with symptoms seen in this patient. Defects in fibrillin synthesis (choice C) result in the connective tissue disorder called Marfan syndrome. Defects in glutamate carboxylation (choice D) would result in abnormal blood coagulation as a consequence the lack of the necessary *gla* residues in the coagulation proteins, prothrombin, factors VII, IX, and X, and protein C and protein S. Defective lysine oxidation (choice E) would be associated with connective tissue pathology due to defective collagen processing and is most likely represented by one of the forms of Ehlers-Danlos syndrome.

19. Correct answer is **B.** The patient is most likely exhibiting the signs and symptoms of the most prevalent form of Gaucher disease. Gaucher disease is an autosomal recessive disorder that is characterized by the lysosomal accumulation of glucocerebrosides which are a normal intermediate in the catabolism of globosides and gangliosides. Finding glucocerebrosides in the blood and urine of a patient would be highly diagnostic for Gaucher disease. Gaucher disease results from defects in the gene encoding the lysosomal hydrolase, glucosylceramidase beta, also called acid β-glucosidase or glucocerebrosidase. The hallmark of Gaucher disease is the accumulation of lipid-engorged cells of the monocyte/macrophage lineage with a characteristic appearance in a variety of tissues. The primarily affected tissues are bone, bone marrow, spleen, and liver. These distinctive cells contain one or more small nuclei, and their cytoplasm contains a coarse fibrillary material that forms a striated tubular pattern often described as "wrinkled tissue paper." An analysis of the blood and urine for none of the other lipids (choice A, C, D, and E) would aid in a diagnosis of Gaucher disease.

20. Correct answer is **B.** The infant is most likely suffering from the lysosomal storage disease, Tay-Sachs disease. Tay-Sachs disease results from defects in the HEXA gene encoding the α-subunit of the lysosomal hydrolase, β-hexosaminidase A. The normal function of β-hexosamindase A is the lysosomal degradation of glycolipids of the G_{M2} ganglioside class. Infants with Tay-Sachs disease appear normal at birth. Symptoms usually begin with mild motor weakness by 3–5 months of age. Another early symptom is an exaggerated startle response to sharp sounds. A progressive loss in visual attentiveness may lead to an ophthalmological consultation which will reveal macular pallor and the presence of the characteristic "cherry-red spot" in area of the fovea centralis of the eye. Deficiency in none of the other processes (choices A, C, D, E, and F) are associated with the signs and symptoms manifesting in this infant.

21. Correct answer is **D.** Digoxin is a cardiac glycoside that exerts a positive inotropic effect on the heart. Cardiac inotropy refers to the force of the contractions of the atria and ventricles of the heart. Digoxin exerts these effects by inhibiting the cardiac Na^+/K^+-ATPase preventing the transport of sodium from the intracellular to the extracellular space. Due to increased intracellular sodium concentration, the Na^+/Ca^{2+} exchange protein 1 (NCX1) can transfer less calcium from inside the cell and the intracellular concentration of calcium will increase. This increases cardiac inotropy since contractile force is dependent on intracellular calcium. Although calcium influx into ventricular cardiomyocytes through T-type calcium channels (choice E) is also an important source of calcium involved in the regulation of ventricular contraction, these channels are not regulated by the actions of digoxin. None of the other channels or receptors (choices A, B, and C) participate in the inotropic effects exerted by digoxin or digoxin-related molecules.

22. Correct answer is **A.** Meconium ileus is a bowel obstruction that occurs when the meconium in the fetal intestine is thicker and stickier than normal meconium which results in a blockage in the terminal ileum. Meconium ileus is a very common early clinical manifestation of the pathology associated with cystic fibrosis. Cystic fibrosis is caused by mutations in the gene (*CFTR*) that encodes the cystic fibrosis transmembrane conductance regulator (CFTR). CFTR is a member of the ATP-binding cassette (ABC) family of membrane transporters. CFTR is a chloride channel expressed in numerous epithelial cell membranes. One of the normal functions of CFTR is to transport chloride ions out of the cell into the thick mucus of the digestive and respiratory tracts. This results in water movement into the mucus making it less viscous. In cystic fibrosis, CFTR function is impaired resulting in chloride trapping inside the cell which in turn prevents water from thinning out the mucus secretions. As a result, the mucus is unusually thick and sticky. This mucus builds up and obstructs the organs where it is secreted such as in the intestine resulting in meconium ileus in the fetus. Hartnup disease (choice B) is associated with symptoms similar to niacin (nicotinic acid) deficiency resulting from mutations in a neutral amino acid transporter. The defective transporter leads to deficiency in tryptophan. Tryptophan metabolism is used to contribute to the pool of NAD^+ (see Figure 18–12), the cofactor active form of nicotinic acid. Menkes disease (choice C) is a disorder of copper homeostasis resulting in progressive and lethal neural degeneration. Sitosterolemia (choice D) results from deficiency in the transport of plant steroids and cholesterol from the liver into the bile. Tangier disease (choice E) is a disorder of cholesterol homeostasis resulting from lack of HDL synthesis.

23. Correct answer is **B.** The patient is most likely manifesting the signs and symptoms of Hurler syndrome. Hurler syndrome is an autosomal recessive disorder that belongs to a family of disorders identified as lysosomal storage diseases, and historically as the mucopolysaccharidoses (MPS). Hurler syndrome is characterized by the lysosomal accumulation of dermatan and heparan sulfates as a consequence of defects in the lysosomal hydrolase, α-L-iduronidase that hydrolyzes terminal α-L-iduronic acid residues from the glycosaminoglycans, dermatan and heparan sulfates. Hurler syndrome is a progressive disorder manifesting with multiple organ and tissue involvement leading to death in early childhood. As the disease progresses there is an increase in the degree of corneal clouding. Most patients have recurrent ear and upper respiratory tract infections, persistent nasal discharge, and noisy breathing. Most Hurler infants succumb to cardiomyopathy. Defects in none of the other processes (choices A, C, D, and E) result in the symptoms observed in this patient.

24. Correct answer is **B.** The patient is most likely exhibiting the symptoms of Hunter syndrome. Hunter syndrome is an X-linked disorder that belongs to a family of disorders identified as lysosomal storage diseases, and historically as one of the mucopolysaccharidoses. Hunter syndrome results from a defect in the activity of the lysosomal hydrolase, iduronate sulfatase that results in the lysosomal accumulation of dermatan and heparan sulfates. Patients with the severe form of Hunter syndrome present with characteristic clinical features. These include short stature, skeletal deformities, joint stiffness, coarse facial features, and intellectual impairment. Onset of symptoms of the severe form are usually seen between 2 and 4 years of age. As a consequence of autonomic nervous system involvement many patients suffer from chronic diarrhea. Extensive neurological degeneration precedes death in patients with the severe form of Hunter syndrome with death occurring between 10 and 15 years of age. Although the symptoms and lysosomal accumulations are very similar to those of Hurler syndrome (choice C), Hunter syndrome is not associated with corneal opacities as is typical in Hurler syndrome. None of the other disorders (choices A, D, and E) manifest with symptoms similar to those observed in this patient.

25. Correct answer is **B.** The patient is most likely manifesting the signs and symptoms of Maroteaux-Lamy syndrome. Maroteaux-Lamy syndrome (mucopolysaccharidosis type VI; MPS VI) is an autosomal recessive disorder that belongs to a family of disorders identified as lysosomal storage diseases, and historically as the mucopolysaccharidoses. This disorder is characterized by the lysosomal accumulation of dermatan sulfates as a consequence of deficiencies in the lysosomal hydrolase *N*-acetylgalactosamine 4-sulfatase (arylsulfatase B). Arylsulfatase B is a member of a family of sulfatases, many of which are necessary for the degradation of the glycosaminoglycans. Although mental development proceeds normally in Maroteaux-Lamy patients, the progression of physical and visual impairments ultimately impedes psychomotor abilities. The clinical features and severity in Maroteaux-Lamy patients is variable, but usually include short stature, hepatosplenomegaly, stiff joints, corneal clouding, cardiac abnormalities, facial dysmorphism, and dystosis multiplex. Hepatosplenomegaly is always present in Maroteaux-Lamy patients after the age of 6. In patients with the most severe forms of the disease there is a shortened trunk, protuberant abdomen, and prominent lumbar lordosis. Defects in none of the other processes (choices A, C, D, and E) result in the symptoms typically found in Maroteaux-Lamy syndrome.

26. Correct answer is **A.** The infant is most likely manifesting the signs and symptoms of osteogenesis imperfecta (OI) type I. The classic features of type I OI include bone fragility and bluish sclera. In a patient with type I OI, the appearance of abnormal coloration of the sclera is most often seen upon ophthalmic examination. The bluish-gray coloration results from the thinning of the sclera due to loss of type I collagen deposition and a resultant ability to visualize the underlying choroid veins. Osteogenesis imperfecta consists of a group of at fifteen related disorders resulting from mutations in several different genes. The four most common forms of OI arise due to defects in two collagen genes, the *COL1A1* and *COL1A2* genes. The mutations lead to decreased expression of collagen or abnormal type 1 collagen proteins. The abnormal proteins associate with normal collagen subunits, which prevents the triple helical structure of normal collagen to form. The result is degradation of all the collagen proteins, both normal and abnormal. Defects in none of the other processes (choices B, C, D, and E) would manifest with the symptoms observed in this patient.

27. Correct answer is **B.** The patient is most likely exhibiting the symptoms of Hunter syndrome. Hunter syndrome is an X-linked disorder that belongs to a family of disorders identified as lysosomal storage diseases, and historically as one of the mucopolysaccharidoses. Hunter syndrome results from a defect in the activity of the lysosomal hydrolase, iduronate sulfatase that results in the lysosomal accumulation of dermatan and heparan sulfates. Chondroitin sulfates (choice A) would be found accumulating in the lysosomes of patients with Morquio syndrome type A. Glucocerebrosides (choice C) accumulate in the lysosomes of bone marrow-derived cells in Gaucher disease. Glycogen accumulation (choice D) would be found in the liver (eg, Andersen disease) or skeletal muscle (eg, McArdle disease) in different glycogen storage diseases. G_{M2} gangliosides (choice E) accumulate in lysosomes, predominantly in the nervous system, of patients with Tay-Sachs disease. Phytanic acid (choice F) accumulates in patients with Refsum disease.

28. Correct answer is **B.** The child is most likely suffering from Hunter syndrome. Hunter syndrome is an X-linked recessive disorder that belongs to a family of disorders identified as lysosomal storage diseases, and historically as one of the mucopolysaccharidoses. Hunter syndrome is characterized by the lysosomal accumulation of dermatan and heparan sulfates as a consequence of deficiencies in the lysosomal hydrolase iduronate sulfatase. Iduronate sulfatase is a member of a family of sulfatases, many of which are necessary for the degradation of the glycosaminoglycans. Defective lysosomal metabolism of glycogen (choice A) results in Pompe disease. Defective lysosomal metabolism of glycosphingolipids (choice C) is the basis for several different lysosomal storage diseases such as Gaucher disease, Krabbe disease, and Fabry disease. Defective lysosomal metabolism of G_{M2} gangliosides (choice D) results in Tay-Sachs disease. Defective lysosomal metabolism of sphingomyelins (choice E) is the cause of Niemann-Pick disease.

29. Correct answer is **E.** The infant is most likely manifesting the signs and symptoms of osteogenesis imperfecta (OI) type I. The classic features of type I OI include bone fragility and bluish sclera. In a patient with type I OI, the appearance of abnormal coloration of the sclera is most often seen upon ophthalmic examination. The bluish-gray coloration results from the thinning of the sclera due to loss of type I collagen deposition and a resultant ability to visualize the underlying choroid veins. Osteogenesis imperfecta consists of a group of at least fifteen related disorders resulting from mutations in several different genes. The four most common forms of OI arise due to defects in two collagen genes, the *COL1A1* and *COL1A2* genes encoding type I collagens. None of the other options (choices A, B, C, and D) correlate with the symptoms of osteogenesis imperfecta observed in this patient.

30. Correct answer is **E.** The infant is most likely suffering from the lysosomal storage disease, Tay-Sachs disease. Tay-Sachs disease results from defects in the *HEXA* gene encoding the α-subunit of the lysosomal hydrolase, β-hexosaminidase A. β-Hexosaminidase A is responsible for the lysosomal degradation of G_{M2} gangliosides. Infants with Tay-Sachs disease appear normal at birth. Symptoms usually begin with mild motor weakness by 3–5 months of age. Another early symptom is an exaggerated startle response to sharp sounds. By 6–10 months of age infants will begin to show regression of prior acquired motor and mental skills. It is the loss of these activities that will normally prompt parents to seek a medical opinion. A progressive loss in visual attentiveness may lead to an ophthalmological consultation which will reveal macular pallor and the presence of the characteristic "cherry-red spot" in area of the fovea centralis of the eye. At around 8–10 months of age the symptoms of Tay-Sachs disease begin to progress rapidly. Intracellular accumulation of chondroitin sulfates (choice A) would be found in patients with Morquio syndrome type A. Intracellular accumulation of dermatan sulfates (choice B) is found in patients with Hunter syndrome and Hurler syndrome. Intracellular accumulation of galactocerebrosides (choice C) is associated with Krabbe disease. Intracellular accumulation of glucocerebrosides (choice D) is found in patients with Gaucher disease. Intracellular accumulation of sphingomyelins (choice F) is found in patients with Niemann-Pick disease.

31. Correct answer is **A.** The patient is most likely manifesting the signs and symptoms associated with cystic fibrosis. Cystic fibrosis is caused by mutations in the gene (*CFTR*) that encodes the cystic fibrosis transmembrane conductance regulator (CFTR). CFTR is a member of the ATP-binding cassette (ABC) family of membrane transporters. CFTR is a chloride channel expressed in numerous epithelial cell membranes. One of the normal functions of CFTR is to transport chloride ions out of the cell into the thick mucus of the digestive and respiratory tracts. This results in water movement into the mucus making it less viscous. As a result of the abnormal transport of chloride and sodium across an epithelium, CF patients have thick, viscous mucus secretions. This mucus builds up in the breathing passages of the lungs, as well as in the pancreas and intestines. Difficulty clearing the alveoli in the lungs is the most serious symptom and results in frequent lung infections, particularly with *Pseudomonas aeruginosa*. The secretions in the pancreas block the exocrine movement of the digestive enzymes into the duodenum and result in irreversible damage to the pancreas. The lack of digestive enzymes leads to difficulty absorbing nutrients with their subsequent excretion in the feces resulting in a malabsorption disorder. Defective transport of none of the other ions or substances (choices B, C, D, E, and F) relates to the symptoms associated with cystic fibrosis.

32. Correct answer is **D.** The patient is most likely exhibiting the consequences of inherited long QT syndrome, LQTS. LQTS refers to a condition in which repolarization of cardiomyocytes of the heart, following an action potential leading to a heartbeat, is affected. The syndrome is recognizable during a standard cardiac function examination through the reading of an electrocardiogram (ECG or EKG). The interval between the Q wave and T wave on the ECG is referred to as the QT interval. The QT interval reflects the electrical activity of the ventricles of the heart. LQTS results in an increased risk of an irregular heartbeat which can result in fainting, drowning, seizures, or sudden death. The inherited forms of LQTS are autosomal dominant, and the most common form, LQTS type 1, results from inherited mutations in the *KCNQ1* gene. The protein encoded by the *KCNQ1* gene forms the core of a heteromeric complex generating the potassium channel responsible for the delayed rectifier current (I_{Ks}) that contributes to phase 3 of ventricular cardiomyocyte action potentials. Phase 0 (choice A) of a typical ventricular cardiomyocyte action potential represents the initial rapid depolarization initiated by the opening of fast-acting voltage-gated Na^+ channels. Phase 1 (choice B) of a typical ventricular cardiomyocyte action potential represents the closure of the Na^+ channels and the opening of Ca^{2+} and K^+ channels. Phase 2 (choice C) of a typical ventricular cardiomyocyte action potential represents the plateau phase which is a slowing of the repolarization due to the opening of L-type Ca^{2+} channels. Phase 4 (choice E) of a typical ventricular cardiomyocyte action potential represents the final stage of repolarization that occurs through the efflux of K^+ ions via the action of inwardly rectifying potassium channels.

33. Correct answer is **C.** The patient is most likely exhibiting the characteristic features of Marfan syndrome, MFS. The cardinal manifestations of MFS are tall stature with dolichostenomelia (condition of unusually long and thin extremities) and arachnodactyly (abnormally long and slender fingers and toes), joint hypermobility and contracture, deformity of the spine and anterior chest, mitral valve prolapse, dilatation and dissection of the ascending aorta, pneumothorax and ectopia lentis (displacement of the crystalline lens of the eye). The symptoms of MFS are the result of inherited defects in the gene encoding the extracellular matrix glycoprotein, fibrillin 1 which is encoded by the *FBN1* gene. Humans express three fibrillin genes identified as *FBN1*, *FBN2*, and *FBN3*. Fibrillin 1 serves as the scaffold in elastic fibers upon which cross-linked elastin is deposited. Cellular attachment to the extracellular matrix (choice A) is the function of fibronectin. Fibronectin is a major fibrillar glycoprotein of the ECM where its role is to attach cells to a variety of ECM types. Cytoskeletal integration to the extracellular matrix (choice B) is the function of proteins of the integrin family. Integrins serve as transmembrane linkers (integrators) whose functions mediate the interactions between the extracellular matrix and the intracellular cytoskeleton. Formation of the basal lamina (choice D) is the function of proteins of the laminin family. All basal lamina contain a common set of proteins, glycosaminoglycans (GAG), and proteoglycans. Laminins anchor cell surfaces to the basal lamina. Tissue contraction following stretch (choice E) involved proteins of the fibulin family. Fibulins (pronounced FIE byoo lins) are calcium-binding glycoproteins that serve as major components of elastic fibers in the ECM. The fibulins function to allow tissues the ability to contract after stretching, a property referred to as elastogenesis.

34. Correct answer is **D.** The child is most likely exhibiting the signs of type I osteogenesis imperfecta, OI. Type I OI is an autosomal dominant disease that is referred to as the mild type. Type I OI results from null mutations (no functional protein) in the *COL1A1* gene. The classic features of type I OI include bone fragility and bluish sclera. In a patient with type I OI, the appearance of abnormal coloration of the sclera is most often seen upon ophthalmic examination. The bluish-gray coloration results from the thinning of the sclera due to loss of type I collagen deposition and a resultant ability to visualize the underlying choroid veins. Deficiency in fibrillin 1 synthesis (choice A) is the cause of Marfan syndrome. Deficiency in glycan fucosylation (choice B) is the cause of the disorder of glycosylation identified as leukocyte adhesion deficiency syndrome II, LAD II. LAD II belongs to the class of disorders referred to as primary immunodeficiency syndromes, as the symptoms of the disease manifest due to defects in leukocyte function. Symptoms of LAD II are characterized by unique facial features, recurrent infections, persistent leukocytosis, defective neutrophil chemotaxis, and severe growth and intellectual impairment. Deficiency in the correct targeting of lysosomal enzymes (choice C), due to loss of mannose-6 phosphorylation, is the cause of I-cell disease. I-cell disease is characterized by severe psychomotor impairment that rapidly progresses, leading to death between 5 and 8 years of age. Deficiency in type 5 collagen synthesis (choice E) is the cause of the classical form of Ehlers-Danlos syndrome, EDS. The characteristic clinical features of classical EDS are soft, velvety, and hyperextensible skin and easy bruising. The joints are quite hypermobile. Many patients with classical EDS have mitral valve prolapse.

35. Correct answer is **B.** The patient is most likely manifesting the symptoms of cystinuria, a disorder associated with excess cystine in the urine. The initial diagnosis of cystinuria is usually precipitated by the finding of kidney stones (renal lithiasis) which show typical cystine crystals. Cystine crystals are long hexagonal translucent crystals that when removed from a patient often appear pink or yellow but turn greenish upon exposure to air. Cystinuria results from defects in either of the two protein subunits of the cystine reuptake transporter which is distinct from the renal cysteine transporter. In addition to excess cystine in the urine, the disorder is associated with increased urinary excretion of the dibasic amino acids, arginine, lysine, and ornithine. However, clinical consequences are only associated with the increased urinary cystine and are due to the poor solubility of this homodimeric compound. The majority of cystinuria patients will manifest renal calculi formation sometime within the first two decades of life. Cystinuria is not the result of defects in renal cystine excretion (choice A). Defects in the excretion or reabsorption of neutral amino acids (choices C and D) or uric acid (choices E and F) do not manifest with the formation of the typical hexagonal, yellow-pink crystals associated with cystinuria.

36. Correct answer is **D.** The patient is most likely exhibiting the signs and symptoms of cystic fibrosis, CF. CF is an autosomal recessive disorder that is associated with the production of abnormally thick and sticky mucus, leading to lung and digestive problems. CF is caused by mutations in the *CFTR* (cystic fibrosis transmembrane conductance regulator) gene. The normal function of CFTR is the regulation of transepithelial chloride ion transport which in turn regulates water and electrolyte homeostasis in numerous different organ systems. Within sweat glands CFTR is normally responsible for chloride ion reabsorption such that in the context of CF, affected individuals manifest with salty tasting skin. In tissues such as the intestinal, pancreatic, and airway epithelium the CFTR protein transports chloride ion out of the cell which in turn promotes bicarbonate secretion as well. In the airway, the normal function of CFTR inhibits the epithelial sodium channel. In the context of CFTR mutations, the impaired chloride and bicarbonate secretions result in thickening of airway secretions, which leads to mucus retention in the airway and persistent bacterial infections, the leading cause of lethality in CF patients. The pancreas of CF patients also has thickened mucus leading to impaired secretion of pancreatic digestive enzymes and fatty infiltration of the organ. The decreased pancreatic enzyme delivery to the small intestine causes impaired digestion of dietary protein and lipid which necessitates pancreatic enzyme replacement therapy for almost all CF patients. The reduced digestion of lipids is associated with steatorrhea and significantly reduced uptake of dietary vitamins. The reduced uptake of vitamin K is most pronounced in comparison to the three other fat-soluble vitamins. A consequence of reduced absorption of vitamin K is an increased potential for bleeding and bruising. The primary therapeutic interventions for CF patients involve nutritional management with diets that are high in calories and fat, replacement of pancreatic enzymes, and aggressive management and prevention of respiratory infections. Bone marrow transplantation (choice A) nor liver transplantation (choice C) would be of any benefit to CF patients. Dietary fructose restriction (choice B) is recommended for patients with hereditary fructose intolerance. Recombinant factor VIII (choice E) is the treatment used in patients with hemophilia A.

37. Correct answer is **B.** Since the experimental drug being tested has been shown to function as an inhibitor of T-type calcium channels the effects are being exerted during the slow depolarization stage of the action potential for nodal cardiomyocytes. The slow-acting T-type calcium channels, encoded by the *CACNA1G* gene that forms the α-subunit of the $Ca_v3.1$ channel, open during the initial depolarization event that is referred to as phase 0. Phase 0 also involves the opening of L-type Ca^{2+} channels when an action potential reaches around −40 mV. Nodal cell activation involves an initial hyperpolarization event, the first phase 4 (choice A) that involves slow-acting Na^+ channels of the hyperpolarization-activated cyclic nucleotide-gated channel (HCN) family. These HCN channels are often referred to as "funny" current channels. The second phase 4 (choice D), representing the return to the resting state, involves the efflux of K^+ ions via the opening of inwardly rectifying potassium channels. These potassium channels were originally identified by their sensitivity to acetylcholine and carbachol and as such are identified as I_{KACh} channels. Phase 3 (choice C) of nodal action potentials, the initial repolarization phase, involves the efflux of K^+ ions through inwardly rectifying potassium channels that are the same as those responsible for phase 3 of ventricular cardiomyocyte action potentials, the I_{Kr} and I_{Ks} channels.

38. Correct answer is **D.** The patient is most likely manifesting the signs and symptoms of Hurler syndrome. Hurler syndrome is an autosomal recessive disorder that belongs to a family of disorders identified as lysosomal storage diseases, and historically as the mucopolysaccharidoses (MPS). Hurler syndrome is characterized by the lysosomal accumulation of dermatan and heparan sulfates as a consequence of defects in the lysosomal hydrolase, α-L-iduronidase that hydrolyzes terminal α-L-iduronic acid residues from the glycosaminoglycans, dermatan and heparan sulfates. Hurler syndrome is a progressive disorder manifesting with multiple organ and tissue involvement leading to death in early childhood. As the disease progresses, there is an increase in the degree of corneal clouding. Most patients have recurrent ear and upper respiratory tract infections, persistent nasal discharge, and noisy breathing. Most Hurler infants succumb to cardiomyopathy. Deficiency in galactosylceramidase (choice A) results in Krabbe disease. The characteristic feature of Krabbe disease is the accumulation of multinucleated globoid cells in the white matter of the brain, such that the disease is also known as infantile globoid cell leukodystrophy (GLD). Deficiency in β-hexosaminidase A (choice B) results in Tay-Sachs disease. Infants with Tay-Sachs disease appear normal at birth with symptoms of mild motor weakness appearing by 3 to 5 months of age. Another early symptom is an exaggerated startle response (sudden extension of arms and legs) to sharp sounds. By 6 to 10 months of age infants will begin to show regression of prior acquired motor and mental skills. Deficiency in iduronate 2-sulfatase (choice C) results in Hunter syndrome. The clinical presentation of the severe form of Hunter syndrome has many similarities to those seen in Hurler syndrome without the corneal clouding. Patients with the severe form of Hunter syndrome present with characteristic clinical features. These include short stature, skeletal deformities, hydrocephalus, joint stiffness, coarse facial features, and intellectual impairment. The onset of symptoms of the severe form usually occurs between 2 and 4 years of age. Typical symptoms include macroglossia, a broad nose, full lips, and large rounded cheeks. As a result of vocal cord enlargement, a hoarse, deep voice results. Patients with the severe form of Hunter syndrome develop hepatosplenomegaly, macrocephaly, umbilical hernia, inguinal hernia, hearing loss, and recurrent respiratory infections. Deficiency in sphingomyelinase (choice E) results in Niemann-Pick disease types A and B. The course of type A Niemann-Pick disease is rapid. Infants are born following a typically normal pregnancy and delivery. Within 4–6 months the abdomen protrudes, and hepatosplenomegaly will be diagnosed. The early neurological manifestations include hypotonia, muscular weakness, and difficulty feeding. As a consequence of the feeding difficulties and the swollen spleen, infants will exhibit a decrease in growth and body weight. By the time afflicted infants reach 6 months of age, the signs of psychomotor deterioration become evident. Affected infants become weaker and progressively hypotonic.

39. Correct answer is **C.** The patient is most likely exhibiting the signs and symptoms of cystic fibrosis (CF), one of which is frequent nose bleeds (epistaxis). CF is an autosomal recessive disorder that is associated with the production of abnormally thick and sticky mucus, leading to lung and digestive problems. CF is caused by mutations in the *CFTR* (cystic fibrosis transmembrane conductance regulator) gene. The normal function of CFTR is the regulation of transepithelial chloride ion transport which in turn regulates water and electrolyte homeostasis in numerous different organ systems. Within sweat glands CFTR is normally responsible for chloride ion reabsorption such that in the context of CF, affected individuals manifest with salty tasting skin. In tissues such as the intestinal, pancreatic, and airway epithelium the CFTR protein transports chloride ion out of the cell which in turn promotes bicarbonate secretion as well. In the airway, the normal function of CFTR inhibits the epithelial sodium channel. In the context of CFTR mutations, the impaired chloride and bicarbonate secretions result in thickening of airway secretions, which leads to mucus retention in the airway and persistent bacterial infections, the leading cause of lethality in CF patients. The pancreas of CF patients also has thickened mucus leading to impaired secretion of pancreatic digestive enzymes and fatty infiltration of the organ. The decreased pancreatic enzyme delivery to the small intestine causes impaired digestion of dietary protein and lipid which necessitates pancreatic enzyme replacement therapy for almost all CF patients. The reduced digestion of lipids is associated with steatorrhea and significantly reduced uptake of dietary vitamins. The reduced uptake of vitamin K is most pronounced in comparison to the three other fat-soluble vitamins. A consequence of reduced absorption of vitamin K is an increased potential for bleeding and bruising. In addition to coagulation dysfunction in CF patients, frequent epistaxis can result from the chronic sinusitis and the development of nasal polyps that are typical in these individuals. The primary therapeutic interventions for CF patients involve nutritional management with diets that are high in calories and fat, replacement of pancreatic enzymes, and aggressive management and prevention of respiratory infections. None of the other pathologies (choices A, B, D, and E) is typically associated with cystic fibrosis.

40. Correct answer is **C.** Since the experimental drug being tested has been shown to function as a calcium channel blocker it is most likely going to affect the L-type calcium channel, encoded by the *CACNA1C* gene that forms the core of the voltage-gated $Ca_v1.2$ channel that opens during phase 2 of the typical ventricular cardiomyocyte action potential allowing Ca^{2+} to enter the cardiomyocyte. The opening of these Ca^{2+} channels reduces the repolarization of ventricular cardiomyocytes and represents the plateau phase of the action potential. Phase 0 (choice A) represents the rapid depolarization stage of ventricular cardiomyocyte action potentials and is the result of the opening of fast-acting Na^+ channels. Phase 1 (choice B) of ventricular cardiomyocyte action potentials results from the closure of the fast-acting Na^+ channels and the efflux of K^+ ions through voltage-gated potassium channels encoded by the *KCND3* gene. Phase 3 (choice D) of ventricular cardiomyocyte action potentials represents the rapid repolarization phase that is the result of efflux of both Ca^{2+} and K^+ ions. The Ca^{2+} efflux is mediated by the NCX1 (Na^+/Ca^{2+} exchanger) and PMCA (plasma membrane Ca^{2+} ATPase) channels. Phase 4 (choice E) of a typical ventricular cardiomyocyte action potential represents the final stage of repolarization that occurs through the efflux of K^+ ions via the action of inwardly rectifying potassium channels.

CHAPTER

26

Mechanisms of Signal Transduction

High-Yield Terms

Signal transduction	Refers to the movement of signals from outside the cell to inside, resulting in a change in the "state" of the cell
Growth factor	Any of a family of proteins that bind to receptors with the primary result of activating cellular proliferation and/or differentiation
Cytokine	Any of unique family of growth factor proteins primarily secreted from leukocytes
Chemokine	A subfamily of cytokines (**chemo**tactic cyto**kines**) that is capable of inducing chemotaxis
Interleukin	Any of a family of multifunctional cytokines that are produced by a variety of lymphoid and nonlymphoid cells
G-protein	Any of a large family of proteins that bind and hydrolyze GTP in the act of transmitting signals; includes the heterotrimeric and the monomeric G-protein families
G-protein–coupled receptors	Receptors that are coupled, inside the cell, to GTP-binding and hydrolyzing proteins (termed G-proteins)
Nuclear receptors	Intracellular receptors that bind lipophilic ligands and then bind to specific DNA sequences in target genes regulating their expression

SIGNALING MOLECULES

Signal transduction, at the cellular level, refers to the process by which a chemical or macromolecule signals, from outside the cell to inside resulting in a series of molecular events. These molecular events can be an alteration in cellular activity, altered metabolism, and/or changes in the program of genes expressed within the responding cells.

The range of molecules that can elicit signals through their interaction with proteins is vast and can include ions, small organic compounds, and peptides or proteins (Table 26–1). The mechanisms by which these signaling molecules exert their effects involve the interaction with different types of receptors. These receptors are proteins that can span the plasma membrane, reside in intracellular membranes, be present in the cytosol, or reside in the nucleus.

The majority of signal transduction pathways involve the coupling of ligands to plasma membrane receptors triggering many intracellular events. These events generally include phosphorylation by tyrosine kinases and/or serine/threonine kinases. Protein phosphorylation changes enzyme activities and protein conformations leading to the transmission of the signal.

GROWTH FACTORS AND CYTOKINES

Growth factors are classified as substances that bind to receptors with the primary result of activating cellular proliferation and/or differentiation. The vast majority of growth factors are proteins that bind to extracellular ligand-binding domains (LBDs) of transmembrane receptors. However, some steroid hormones (see Chapter 32) have growth factor activity. Many growth factors are quite versatile, stimulating cellular division in numerous different cell types; while others are specific to a particular cell-type. Individual growth factor proteins tend to occur as members of larger families of structurally and evolutionarily related proteins.

Cytokines are a unique family of growth factors that are primarily secreted from leukocytes. Cytokines that are secreted from lymphocytes are termed **lymphokines**, whereas those secreted by monocytes or macrophages are termed **monokines**. Many of the lymphokines are more commonly known as **interleukins (IL)**, since they are not only secreted by leukocytes but are also able to affect the cellular responses of leukocytes. Specifically, interleukins are growth factors targeted to cells of hematopoietic origin. Chemokines represent a subfamily of cytokines whose name is derived from **chemo**tactic cyto**kines**. These proteins are capable of inducing chemotaxis in nearby responsive cells.

TABLE 26–1 Examples of signal-transducing molecules.

Signaling Molecule Type	Example	Receptor(s)	Signaling Events
Ion	Calcium (Ca^{2+})	Calcium-sensing receptor, CaSR	CaSR is a member of the G-protein–coupled receptor (GPCR; metabotropic receptors) superfamily; CaSR is coupled to G_i, G_q, and G_{12}-type G-proteins; Ca^{2+} binding triggers signal cascade leading to increased proteolysis of parathyroid hormone (PTH) in the parathyroid gland
Gas	Nitric oxide, NO	Soluble guanylate cyclase	NO receptor is intracellular residing in the cytosol of smooth muscle cells; on NO binding to the heme moiety of the guanylate cyclase the enzyme is activated producing cGMP; the cGMP itself, and through activation of protein kinase G (PKG) triggers signaling events resulting in smooth muscle cell relaxation
Small organic molecule	Cortisol	Glucocorticoid receptor (GR)	Cortisol is derived from cholesterol; GR is member of steroid/thyroid hormone superfamily of nuclear receptors; on ligand binding GR in the cytosol the complex migrates to nucleus and interacts with sequences in target genes termed glucocorticoid response elements (GRE); interaction of GR with GRE leads to increased transcription of target genes
Small organic molecule	Acetylcholine (ACh)	Two different receptor types	ACh is derived from acetyl-CoA; ACh receptors are ion channels (ionotropic nicotinic ACh receptors) and members of the GPCR superfamily (muscarinic metabotropic ACh receptors); ACh is the neurotransmitter of both sympathetic and parasympathetic preganglionic neurons; ACh exerts effects in both the CNS and in the periphery
Amino acid	Glutamate	Five different receptor types	Glutamate binds to four different receptor types that are ion channels (ionotropic receptors) and a fifth receptor class that are members of the GPCR (metabotropic) superfamily; glutamate binding to receptors triggers neuronal cell activity within the CNS and numerous effects in the periphery
Amino acid derivative	Epinephrine	Two different classes of receptor	Epinephrine is derived from tyrosine; Epinephrine binds to the α- and β-adrenergic receptors; all of the adrenergic receptors are members of the GPCR superfamily; epinephrine functions as a neurotransmitter and as a hormone
Peptide	Angiotensin II	Two receptors	Angiotensin II is an octapeptide; receptors are both members of the GPCR superfamily; primary response to receptor activation in the periphery is vasoconstriction
Protein	Insulin	Insulin receptors	Insulin receptor is member of the receptor tyrosine kinase (RTK) family of receptors; insulin binding triggers metabolic effects as well as growth-stimulating effects

CLASSIFICATIONS OF SIGNAL-TRANSDUCING RECEPTORS

Signal-transducing receptors are of three general classes:

1. Receptors that penetrate the plasma membrane and have intrinsic enzymatic activity. Receptors that have intrinsic enzymatic activities include those that are tyrosine kinases (RTK), serine/threonine kinases (RSK), tyrosine phosphatases, and guanylate cyclases. Receptors with intrinsic tyrosine kinase activity are capable of autophosphorylation as well as phosphorylation of other substrates. Additionally, several families of receptors lack intrinsic enzyme activity, yet are coupled to intracellular tyrosine kinases by direct protein-protein interactions.
2. Receptors that are coupled, inside the cell, to GTP-binding and hydrolyzing proteins (termed G-proteins) are termed G-protein–coupled receptors (GPCR). Because many GPCR activate signal transduction cascades that alter metabolic processes, this large superfamily of receptors are classified as **metabotropic** receptors. Examples of this class are the adrenergic receptors, odorant receptors, and certain hormone receptors (eg, glucagon, angiotensin, vasopressin, and bradykinin).
3. Receptors that are found intracellularly and on ligand binding migrate to the nucleus where the ligand-receptor complex directly affects gene transcription. Because this class of receptors is intracellular and functions in the nucleus as transcription factors, they are commonly referred to as the **nuclear receptors**. Receptors of this class include the large family of steroid and thyroid hormone receptors. Receptors in this class have a LBD, a DNA-binding domain, and a transcriptional regulatory domain.

RECEPTOR TYROSINE KINASES

The receptor tyrosine kinase (RTK) family of transmembrane ligand-binding proteins is comprised of 58 members in the human genome. Each of the RTK exhibit similar structural and functional characteristics (Figure 26–1). Most RTK are monomers, and their domain structure includes an extracellular LBD, a transmembrane domain, and an intracellular domain possessing the tyrosine kinase activity. The insulin and insulin-like growth factor receptors are the most complex in the RTK family being disulfide linked heterotetramers.

The amino acid sequences of the tyrosine kinase domains of RTK are highly conserved with those of cAMP-dependent protein kinase (PKA) within the ATP-binding and substrate-binding regions. RTK proteins are classified into families based on structural features in their extracellular portions as well as the presence or absence of a kinase domain insert. Based on the presence of various extracellular domains, the RTK have been subdivided into at least 20 different subfamilies identified as classes (Table 26–2).

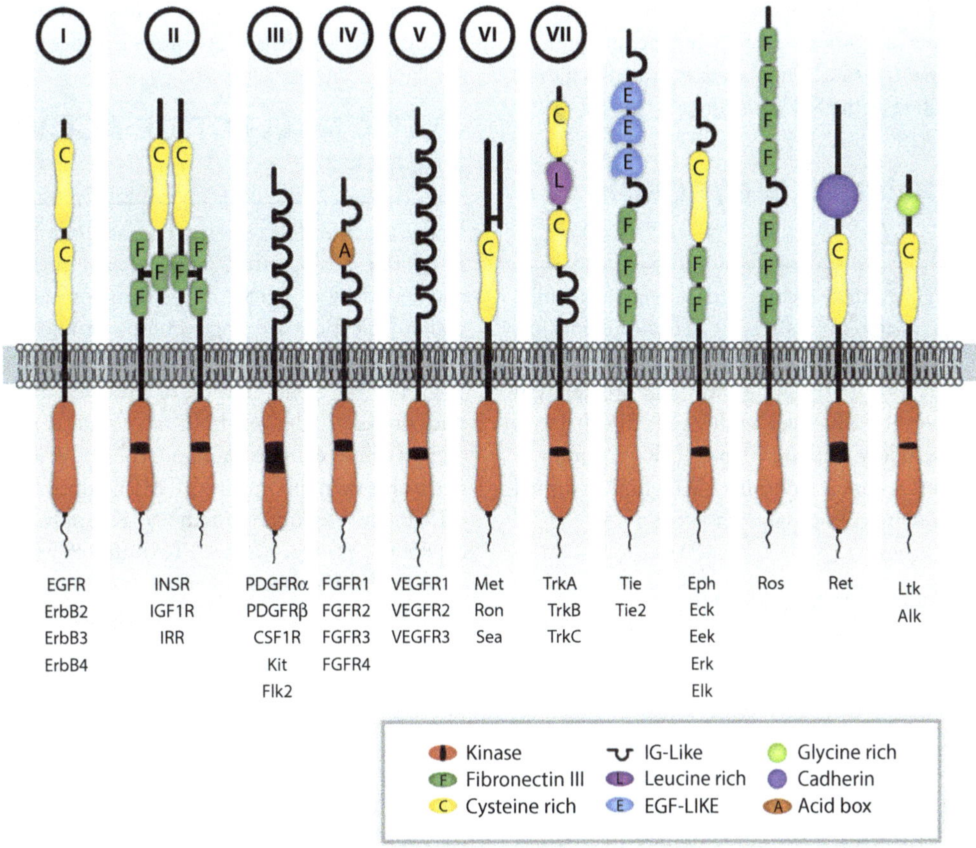

FIGURE 26–1 A diagrammatic representation of several members of the receptor tyrosine kinase (RTK) family. Several members of each receptor subfamily are indicated below each representative. The Roman numerals above the first seven subtypes correspond to those subtypes described in Table 26–2. These RTK subtypes do not represent the entire RTK family. (Reproduced with permission from themedicalbiochemistrypage, LLC.)

Many receptors that have intrinsic tyrosine kinase activity, as well as the tyrosine kinases that are associated with cell surface receptors, contain tyrosine residues, that on phosphorylation, interact with other proteins of the signaling cascade. These other proteins contain a domain of amino acid sequences that are homologous to a domain first identified in the kinase encoded by the SRC proto-oncogene. These domains are termed SH2 domains (SRC homology domain 2). Several SH2 domain

TABLE 26–2 Characteristics of the common classes of RTK.

Class	Family Name	Examples	Structural Features of Class
I	ErbB receptor family	Epidermal growth factor (EGF) receptor (ERBB1); NEU/HER2 (ERBB2); HER3 (ERBB3); HER4 (ERBB4)	Cysteine-rich sequences; receptors dimerize in response to ligand binding; numerous ligands bind and activate the EGFR (ERBB1) including EGF, TGF-α, and amphiregulin
II	Insulin receptor family	Insulin receptor (InsR); IGF-1 receptor (IGF1R); insulin receptor-related receptor (IRR)	Cysteine-rich sequences; characterized by disulfide-linked heterotetramers
III	PDGF receptor family	Platelet-derived growth factor (PDGF) receptors (PDGFα and PDGFβ); c-Kit, CSF-1 receptor (CSFR); fms-related tyrosine kinase 3 (FLT3)	Contains five immunoglobulin-like domains; contains the kinase insert
IV	VEGF receptor family	Vascular endothelial cell growth factor (VEGF) receptor-1 (VEGFR-1; also known as fms-related tyrosine kinase-1 (FLT1); kinase insert domain receptor (VEGFR-2); fms-related tyrosine kinase 4 (VEGFR-3)	Contains seven immunoglobulin-like domains as well as the kinase insert domain
V	FGF receptor family	Fibroblast growth factor receptor 1 (FGFR1); FGFR2; FGFR3; FGFR4	Contain three immunoglobulin-like domains as well as the kinase insert; acidic domain

containing proteins that have intrinsic enzymatic activity include phospholipase Cγ (PLCγ) and phosphatidylinositol-3-kinase (PI3K). Another conserved protein-protein interaction domain identified in many signal transduction proteins is related to a third domain in SRC identified as the SH3 domain.

NONRECEPTOR PROTEIN TYROSINE KINASES

Humans express 32 genes that encode intracellular (cytosolic) nonreceptor protein tyrosine kinases (PTK) that are responsible for phosphorylating a variety of intracellular proteins on tyrosine residues following activation of cellular growth and proliferation signals. The proteins in the PTK superfamily can be divided into 10 distinct subgroups where the archetypal PTK subgroup is related to the SRC protein that is a tyrosine kinase first identified as the transforming protein in Rous sarcoma virus.

RECEPTOR SERINE/THREONINE KINASES

At least 12 receptor serine/threonine kinases (RSK) encoding genes are expressed in humans. These receptors can be divided into two subfamilies identified as the type I and type II receptors. The type I RSK are also known as activin receptors or activin receptor-like kinases, ALK. Ligands first bind to the type II receptors which then leads to interaction with the type I receptors. The type II protein phosphorylates the kinase domain of the type I partner leading to displacement of proteins called subunit (or protein) partners.

NONRECEPTOR SERINE/THREONINE KINASES

There are at least 125 genes in humans that encode members of the nonreceptor serine/threonine kinases (STK) family that includes the 12 RSK genes. In the context of metabolic biochemistry, cAMP-dependent protein kinase (PKA) and the protein kinase C (PKC) subfamily are some of the most important members of the STK superfamily. Humans express 10 genes of the PKC family divided into the conventional (four genes), novel (four genes), and atypical (two genes) PKC subfamilies.

A family of STK that are critical in regulating growth and proliferation signal transduction events is the mitogen-activated kinase (MAPK) family. MAP kinases are also called ERK for extracellular signal-regulated kinases. The MAPK family is composed of 13 genes whose encoded proteins are divided into four distinct MAPK cascades. These four MAPK cascades are the extracellular signal-regulated kinase 1/2 (ERK1/2), the c-Jun N-terminal kinase (JNK), the p38, and the ERK5 cascades. Each of these four cascades is in turn comprised of a core component that consists of three tiers of protein kinases termed MAPK, MAPKK (MAP kinase kinase), and MAP3K (MAP kinase kinase kinase: MAPKKK). In several cases, the cascade contains two additional tiers consisting of an upstream MAP4K and a downstream MAPKAPK (MAP kinase-activated kinase; MAPKAPK).

CYCLIC NUCLEOTIDE-ACTIVATED KINASES

Cyclic nucleotides represent a family of naturally occurring nucleotide analogs that act as second messengers in hormone and ion-channel signal transduction processes. Structurally, the cyclic nucleotides are single phosphate nucleotides that harbor a "cyclic" bond between the phosphate and both the 3′-OH and the 5′-OH of the ribose portion of the nucleotide. The major cyclic nucleotides are derived from adenosine and guanosine forming 3′,5′-cyclic adenosine monophosphate (cAMP) and 3′,5′-cyclic guanosine monophosphate (cGMP), respectively. Both cAMP and cGMP activate kinases of the STK family identified as cAMP-dependent protein kinase (PKA) and cGMP-dependent protein kinase (PKG), respectively.

The formation of cAMP is catalyzed by a family of adenylate cyclases, while the formation of cGMP is catalyzed by a family of guanylate cyclases. The human adenylate cyclases are divided into two distinct subtypes, the transmembrane adenylate cyclases (tmAC) and the soluble adenylate cyclase (sAC). Humans express 10 adenylate cyclase genes with nine of the genes encoding tmAC isoforms and one gene encoding a sAC isoform. Similarly, there are two distinct types of guanylate cyclases expressed in humans, the soluble enzymes (sGC) and the single transmembrane-spanning guanylate cyclases.

The sAC is not localized to the cytosol but is actually distributed within discrete subdomains within the cell such as the nucleus, mitochondria, mitotic spindle, and cilia. The discrete localization allows for what are referred to as, microdomains of cAMP production and action to be established. Soluble AC is tethered to these sites by being anchored to PKA or scaffold proteins called A-kinase anchoring proteins (AKAP).

The guanylate cyclases are regulated by a broad spectrum of agents that includes nitric oxide (NO), bicarbonate ion (HCO_3^-), the natriuretic peptides (see Chapter 31), and the guanylyl cyclase activating proteins (GCAP). The sGC family members function as heterodimers and contain a heme moiety. It is the heme to which NO binds resulting in activation of the enzyme.

CYCLIC NUCLEOTIDE PHOSPHODIESTERASES

Phosphodiesterases (PDE) catalyze the hydrolysis of a phosphodiester bond. Humans express a large number of PDE, with the cyclic nucleotide PDE being the class of enzymes most commonly associated with the term, phosphodiesterase. The PDE expressed in human tissues hydrolyze cAMP to AMP and/or cGMP to GMP. Certain members of the human PDE family are specific for one cyclic nucleotide or the other, while some do not exhibit substrate specificity and can hydrolyze either cAMP or cGMP.

Humans express 12 PDE gene families. Within each gene family there may be several distinct genes and many of these genes generate alternatively spliced mRNAs encoding variant isoforms of the enzyme.

HIGH-YIELD CONCEPT

The *PDE5* gene generates several protein variants that are critical enzymes involved in smooth muscle cell relaxation in the cardiovascular system. The PDE5-encoded enzymes are the target of inhibitory drugs (eg, sildenafil, tadalafil, and vardenafil) used to treat erectile dysfunction (ED) and pulmonary hypertension.

G-PROTEINS

G-proteins are so-called because their activities are regulated by binding and hydrolyzing GTP. When a G-protein has GTP bound it is in the active state and when the GTP is hydrolyzed to GDP the protein is in the inactive state. The hydrolysis of GTP by G-proteins provides the energy for the activation of the next protein in a signaling cascade.

There are two major classes of G-protein: the heterotrimeric family that are composed of three distinct subunits (α, β, and γ), and the monomeric class that are related to the archetypal member RAS (originally identified as the **ra**t **s**arcoma oncogene). The monomeric family of G-proteins is also referred to as the RAS superfamily. The structure and function of the monomeric G-proteins are similar to those of the α-subunits of the heterotrimeric G-proteins.

Heterotrimeric G-Proteins

All known cell surface receptors that are of the GPCR class interact with heterotrimeric G-proteins. The α-subunit of the heterotrimeric class of G-proteins is responsible for the binding of GDP or GTP. When either heterotrimeric or monomeric G-protein are activated by receptors, or intracellular effector proteins, there is an exchange of GDP for GTP turning on the G-protein which enables it to transmit the original activating signal to downstream effector proteins.

In the heterotrimeric class of G-protein, when the associated GPCR is activated by ligand binding there is stimulation of GDP for GTP exchange in the α-subunit. Following this exchange the protein complex dissociates into separate α- and βγ-activated complexes (Figure 26–2). The released and activated βγ complex serves as a docking site for interaction with downstream effectors of the signal transduction cascade. Once the α-subunit hydrolyzes the bound GTP to GDP it reassociates with the βγ complex, thereby terminating its activity.

The GTPase activity of G-proteins is augmented by GTPase-activating proteins (GAP) and the GDP for GTP exchange reaction is catalyzed by guanine nucleotide exchange factors (GEF). Within the small GTPase family (Ras family) of G-proteins, there are guanosine nucleotide dissociation inhibitors (GDI) that maintain the G-protein in its inactive state.

A. G_α Subunits and Functions

The Gα subunits are a family of 39–52 kDa proteins that share 45–80% amino acid similarity. There are at least 16 Gα subunit genes in the human genome, with several genes expressing splice variants. The distinction of the different types of α-subunits found in heterotrimeric G-proteins is based on the downstream signaling responses activated or inhibited as a result of G-protein activation.

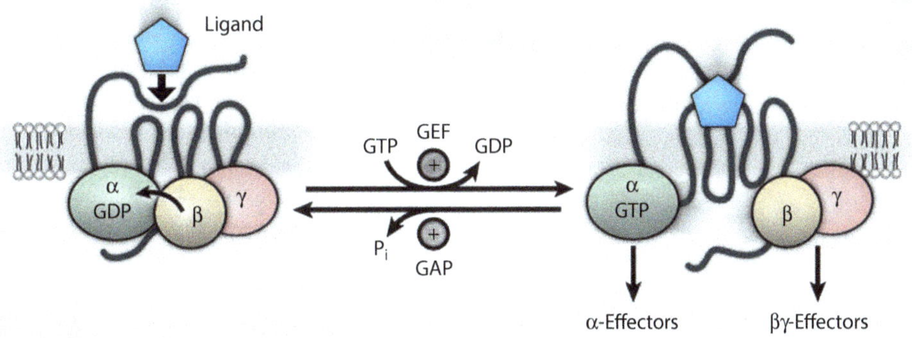

FIGURE 26–2 A diagrammatic representation of the activation of trimeric G-proteins on ligand binding to typical G-protein–coupled receptors. On ligand binding to a GPCR, there is an activated exchange of GDP bound to the α-subunit for GTP catalyzed by an associated guanine nucleotide exchange factor (GEF). The resultant GTP-associated α-subunit can then activate downstream effector proteins. In some cases, G-protein βγ-subunits also regulate the activity of downstream effectors. Hydrolysis of GTP to GDP during the G-protein activation of effectors as a result of the action of GTPase-activating proteins (GAPs) results in termination of the activity of the α-subunit. (Reproduced with permission from themedicalbiochemistrypage, LLC.)

TABLE 26–3 Families of G-proteins defined by α-subunits.

Gα Type	Members	Activities
$G_{\alpha s}$ (G_s)	$G_{\alpha s}$ and $G_{\alpha olf}$	Stimulates the activity of adenylate cyclase resulting in increased production of cAMP which then results in the activation of PKA; $G_{\alpha olf}$ was originally identified as being involved in olfaction; the $G_{\alpha s}$ proteins are encoded by the GNAS locus; the GNAS locus exhibits a complex pattern of expression being controlled by imprinting and four alternative promoters; the GNAS locus controls maternally, paternally, and biallelically derived mRNAs and also exerts added complexity via alternative splicing such that 10 different protein isoforms result.
$G_{\alpha i}$ (G_i)	$G_{\alpha i}$, $G_{\alpha o}$, $G_{\alpha z}$, $G_{\alpha t}$, and $G_{\alpha gust}$	α-Subunits either inhibit adenylate cyclase thereby, inhibiting the production of cAMP ($G_{\alpha i}$, $G_{\alpha o}$, $G_{\alpha z}$) or activate phosphodiesterase leading to increased hydrolysis of cGMP ($G_{\alpha t}$) or cAMP ($G_{\alpha gust}$); the βγ subunits that are associated with $G_{\alpha i}$ and $G_{\alpha o}$ function to open inwardly rectifying K^+ channels; $G_{\alpha t}$ is the α-subunit of transducin (see Chapter 3); $G_{\alpha gust}$ is the α-subunit in gustducin which is involved in the gustatory system which is the sensory system for taste; humans express three $G_{\alpha i}$ genes (*GNAI1, GNAI2,* and *GNAI3*), one $G_{\alpha o}$ gene (*GNAO1*), three $G_{\alpha t}$ genes (*GNAT1, GNAT2,* and *GNAT3*), and one $G_{\alpha z}$ gene (*GNAZ*).
$G_{\alpha q}$ (G_q)	$G_{\alpha q}$, $G_{\alpha 11}$, $G_{\alpha 14}$, and $G_{\alpha 15}$	Activates membrane-associated PLCβ resulting in increased production of the intracellular messengers IP_3 and DAG; there are four α-subunit encoding genes in this family: *GNAQ, GNA11, GNA14,* and *GNA15.*
$G_{\alpha 12}$ (G_{12})	$G_{\alpha 12}$ and $G_{\alpha 13}$	Involved in the activation of the Rho family of monomeric G-proteins; there are two α-subunit encoding genes in this family: *GNA12* and *GNA13.*

These classifications allow the Gα subunits to be divided into four subtypes including G_s, G_i, G_q, and G_{12} (Table 26–3). Since it is the α-subunit, these designations are to be written $G\alpha_s$ and so on.

B. $G_{\beta\gamma}$ Subunits and Functions

A total of five Gβ genes and twelve Gγ are genes expressed in humans. The primary function that was originally proposed for the βγ-subunits (Gβγ dimer) was solely that of an inactivator of Gα subunits. However, research demonstrated that Gβγ dimers were able to activate a cardiac inwardly rectifying K^+ channel normally activated by acetylcholine. Subsequently, Gβγ subunits were shown to modulate many other effectors via direct interactions. Indeed, many of the effectors are those that are also regulated by Gα subunits such as phospholipase Cβ (PLCβ), several adenylate cyclase (AC) isoforms, phosphoinositide-3 kinases (PI3K), and voltage-gated calcium channels.

In addition to these membrane-associated targets activated by Gβγ subunits, the dimers have also been shown to effect modulation of numerous other proteins located throughout the cell. These include proteins in the cytosol, nucleus, endosomes, mitochondria, ER, Golgi apparatus, and cytoskeleton.

Monomeric G-Proteins

The RAS superfamily of small monomeric G-proteins comprises well over 100 different proteins. This superfamily is divided into several main families with some families being comprised of subfamilies. The major families are RAS, RHO, MIRO (mitochondrial RHO), RAB, RAN, RAB-like, RAS-related, and ARF.

The RAS family proteins are primarily responsible for regulation of events of cell proliferation. The RHO family proteins are involved in the regulation of cell morphology through control of cytoskeletal dynamics. The RAB family proteins are involved in membrane trafficking events. The RAN family is composed of a single protein that is involved in the regulation of nuclear transport. The ARF family is involved in intracellular vesicle transport.

G-PROTEIN REGULATORS

The activity state of G-proteins is regulated both by the rate of GTP exchange for GDP and by the rate at which the GTP is hydrolyzed to GDP. The former process is catalyzed by GEF that in the case of GPCR is the receptor itself. The activity of G-proteins, with respect to GTP hydrolysis, is regulated by a family of proteins termed GTPase-activating proteins (GAP). Both of these regulatory protein classes are termed regulators of G-protein signaling (RGS). Humans express a total of 21 genes in the RGS family.

Two clinically relevant examples of the GAP family of proteins are encoded by the neurofibromatosis type-1 (NF1) susceptibility locus and the BCR locus (break-point cluster region gene). The NF1 gene is a tumor-suppressor gene and the encoded protein is called neurofibromin. The BCR locus is rearranged in chronic myelogenous leukemias (CML) harboring the Philadelphia positive (Ph^+) chromosome. The Ph^+ chromosome is the result of a translocation between chromosomes 9 and 22 that fuses the *BCR* gene on chromosome 22 with the Abelson tyrosine kinase (ABL) on chromosome 9.

G-PROTEIN–COUPLED RECEPTORS

All GPCR are composed of a similar structure that includes seven membrane-spanning helices connected by three intracellular loops and three extracellular loops with an extracellular amino terminus and an intracellular carboxy terminus (Figure 26–3). There are at least 1409 identified *GPCR* genes in the human genome, although not all are protein coding as several hundred are pseudogenes.

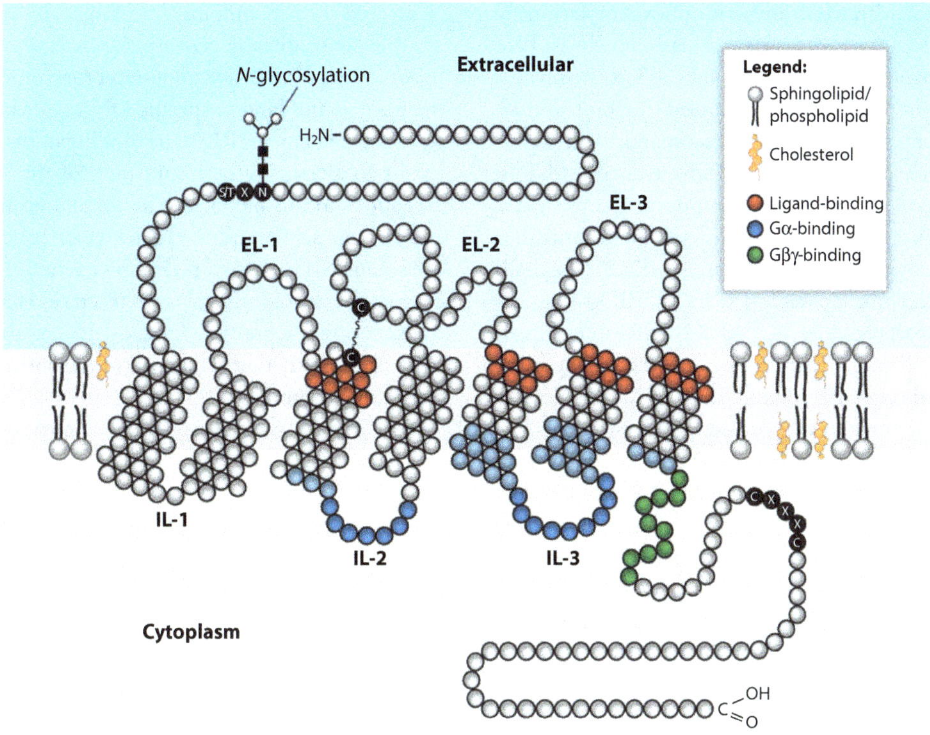

FIGURE 26–3 A diagrammatic representation of a typical member of the serpentine class of G-protein–coupled receptor. White, red, blue, and green spheres represent amino acids. Serpentine receptors are so called because they pass through the plasma membrane seven times. Structural characteristics include the three extracellular loops (EL-1, EL-2, EL-3) and three intracellular loops (IL-1, IL-2, IL-3). Most GPCRs are modified by carbohydrate attachment to the extracellular portion of the protein. Shown is typical *N*-linked carbohydrate attachment. The different-colored spheres are involved in ligand binding and associated G-protein binding as indicated in the legend. (Reproduced with permission from themedicalbiochemistrypage, LLC.)

In addition, many of the protein-coding GPCR genes encode proteins for whom the ligand(s) is unknown and are, therefore, referred to as orphan GPCR.

The GPCR superfamily consists of seven defined families or classes. These seven families are the class A rhodopsin-like receptors, the class B secretin-like receptors, the class C metabotropic glutamate/pheromone receptors, the class F frizzled receptors, the taste receptors, the vomeronasal receptors, and the 7-transmembrane (7TM) orphan receptors. There are several orphan receptors in the class A and class C families, but the 7TM orphan receptors represent a separate distinct family of orphan receptors.

Class A family: The class A GPCR superfamily is referred to as the rhodopsin-like family. Class A contains the largest number of members compiled into at least 21 classes (families). Class A GPCR include opsins, the vast majority of the odorant (olfactory) receptors, and receptors for monoamines, purines, opioids, chemokines, some small peptide hormones, and the large glycoprotein hormones that consist of thyroid-stimulating hormone (TSH), luteinizing hormone (LH), and follicle-stimulating hormone (FSH). Currently there are 78 orphan receptor genes in the class A family.

Class B family: The class B GPCR superfamily is referred to as the secretin-like receptor class. Class B is comprised of six classes (families) that include the receptors for calcitonin, parathyroid hormone, corticotropin-releasing hormone, glucagon, and vasoactive intestinal peptide in addition to the large adhesion receptors family.

Class C family: The class C superfamily is referred to as the metabotropic glutamate/pheromone receptor family. Class C is comprised of four classes (families) that include the metabotropic glutamate receptors (mGluR), extracellular Ca^{2+}-sensing receptors, the GABA-B type receptors, as well as the eight class C orphan receptors.

GPCR DESENSITIZATION

A characteristic feature of GPCR activity following ligand binding is a progressive loss of receptor-mediated signal transduction. This process is referred to as **desensitization** or **adaptation**. The primary mechanism accounting for GPCR desensitization is phosphorylation and is a short-term form of desensitization. Desensitization of this type is divided into homologous and heterologous mechanisms.

Short-term desensitization is augmented by receptor downregulation which involves the loss of membrane-associated receptor through a combination of protein degradation as well as transcriptional and posttranscriptional mechanisms.

Heterologous desensitization involves phosphorylation of GPCR by second messenger-dependent kinases, such as PKA and PKC. Homologous desensitization of GPCR involves a family of kinases termed G-protein–coupled receptor kinases (GRK). The GRK constitute a family of six mammalian serine/threonine kinases that phosphorylate ligand-activated GPCR as their primary substrates, hence the designation of the process as homologous desensitization. These six kinases are identified as GRK1 (originally called rhodopsin kinase), GRK2 (originally called β-adrenergic receptor kinase-1, βARK1), GRK3 (originally called β-adrenergic receptor kinase-2, βARK2), GRK4 (originally called IT-11), GRK5, and GRK6. These kinases preferentially phosphorylate ligand (agonist) bound and activated receptor rather than inactive or antagonist-occupied GPCR substrates.

On receptor phosphorylation by a GRK there is binding to one of a family of cytoplasmic inhibitory proteins called the arrestins. In the rhodopsin system this inhibitory protein is referred to as arrestin. In nonretinal tissues there are two related inhibitory proteins known as β-arrestin-1 and β-arrestin-2. As a result of arrestin or β-arrestin binding, the GPCR is prevented from activating its G-protein and, therefore, its downstream effector(s).

INTRACELLULAR HORMONE RECEPTORS (NUCLEAR RECEPTORS)

The steroid and thyroid hormone receptor superfamily (eg, glucocorticoid receptor [GR]) is a class of proteins that reside in the cytoplasm, or the nucleus, and bind their lipophilic hormone ligands in these locations since the hormones are capable of freely penetrating the hydrophobic plasma membrane. Because these receptors bind ligand intracellularly and then interact with DNA directly, they are more commonly called the nuclear receptors (NR). All the NR contain a ligand-binding domain (LBD), a DNA-binding domain (DBD), and two activation function domains, AF-1 and AF-2 (Figure 26–4).

In addition to binding hormone, all receptors of this class are capable of directly activating gene transcription. On binding ligand, cytoplasmic hormone-receptor complexes translocate to the nucleus and bind to specific DNA sequences termed hormone response elements (HRE). The binding of the complex to an HRE results in altered transcription rates of the associated gene. The exceptions to this model are the thyroid hormone receptors (TR) and retinoic acid receptors (RAR) which are constitutively present in the nucleus bound to their target genes in the absence of their cognate hormones. These two receptor families exhibit potent transcriptional repression function in the absence of ligand and the repressor function is mapped to the domain that is responsible for binding ligand.

The human genome contains 48 nuclear receptor genes that can be classified into seven defined subfamilies. Many of these genes are capable of yielding more than one receptor isoform. Some members of the NR family bind to DNA as homodimers such as the estrogen receptor (ER), mineralocorticoid receptor (MR), progesterone receptor (PR), androgen receptor (AR), and the glucocorticoid receptor (GR). Other family members bind to DNA as heterodimers through interactions with the retinoid X receptors (RXR).

In addition to the steroid hormone and thyroid hormone receptors there are numerous additional family members that bind lipophilic ligands. These include the retinoid X receptors (RXR), the liver X receptors (LXR), the farnesoid X receptors (FXR), and the peroxisome proliferator-activated receptors (PPAR).

Although all members of the NR family possess activation function domains that are responsible for the regulation of transcription of target genes, the regulation of transcription is much more complex due to the association of numerous coregulatory proteins. These coregulatory proteins are of two distinct classes: those that function to coactivate the NR and those that function to co-repress the receptor complex. Coactivators are found to be associated with ligand-bound NR and thereby induce

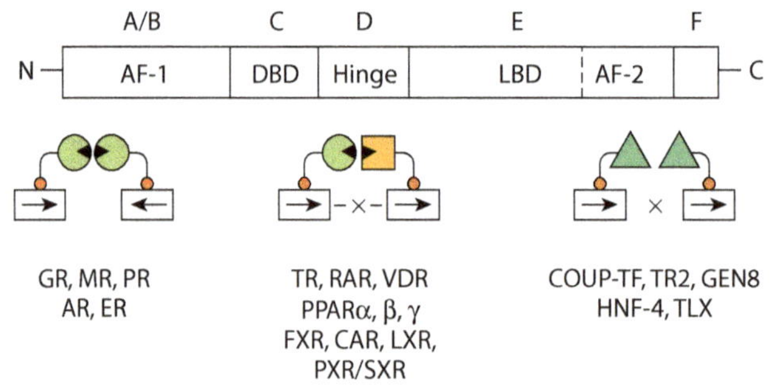

Receptors:	Steroid class	RXR partnered	Orphans
Binding:	Homodimers	Heterodimers	Homodimers
Ligand:	Steroids	9-*Cis* RA + (x)	?
DNA element:	Inverted repeat	Direct repeats	Direct repeats

FIGURE 26–4 Structure of the nuclear receptor superfamily. Top: The six structural domains described in the text are indicated. Several classes of nuclear receptor are indicated (abbreviations are described in the text) along with ligand type, binding characteristics, and type of DNA element bound. Orphan nuclear receptors are so called because the ligand or ligands that are specific to those receptors have not yet been fully characterized. (Reproduced with permission from Rodwell VW, Bender DA, Botham KM, et al: *Harper's Illustrated Biochemistry*, 31st ed. New York, NY: McGraw Hill; 2018.)

gene expression. Co-repressors selectively repress gene expression through interaction with NR that are ligand-free or bound to antagonists.

HIGH-YIELD CONCEPT

The PPAR family is composed of three family members: PPARα, PPARβ/δ, and PPARγ. Each of these receptors forms a heterodimer with the RXR. The first family member identified was PPARα and it was found by virtue of the fibrate class of anti-hyperlipidemic drugs binding to it and resulting in the proliferation of peroxisomes in hepatocytes, hence the derivation of the name of the protein. PPARγ is a master regulator of adipogenesis and is most abundantly expressed in adipose tissue. PPARγ was identified as the target of the thiazolidinedione (TZD) class of drugs used in the treatment of type 2 diabetes (see Chapter 30).

PHOSPHOLIPIDS IN SIGNAL TRANSDUCTION

Phospholipases and phospholipids are involved in the processes of transmitting ligand-receptor induced signals from the plasma membrane to intracellular proteins. The primary enzymes whose activities are modulated as a consequence of plasma membrane receptor activation are the members of the phospholipase C (PLC) family. Once a PLC enzyme is activated, a chain of events occurs leading to subsequent activation of the kinase, PKC. PKC is maximally active in the presence of calcium ion (Ca^{2+}) and diacylglycerol (DAG).

Phospholipase C Family

Activation of PLC enzymes results in the hydrolysis of membrane phospholipids, primarily phosphatidylinositol-4,5-bisphosphate (PIP_2) leading to an increase in intracellular DAG and inositol-1,4,5-trisphosphate (IP_3). The released IP_3 interacts with receptors in the membranes of the ER. The IP_3 receptors are ligand-gated Ca^{2+} channels that on IP_3 binding release stored Ca^{2+} to the cytosol. Together, the increased DAG and intracellular free calcium ion concentrations lead to increased activity of PKC.

A total of 13 PLC genes have been identified in the human genome. The proteins encoded by these 13 genes have been assigned to six subclasses of enzyme defined on the basis of structure and regulatory activation mechanisms. These six subfamilies are referred to as PLC-beta (PLCβ), PLC-gamma (PLCγ), PLC-delta (PLCδ), PLC-epsilon (PLCε), PLC-zeta (PLCζ), and PLC-eta (PLCη).

Activation of the PLCβ family members occurs via association with GPCR that are coupled to the G_q class of G-protein. The PLCγ enzymes contain an SH2 domain that allows them to interact with phosphotyrosine residues present on receptors with intrinsic tyrosine kinase activity or with receptor-associated tyrosine kinases. The PLCε family member is activated by GPCRs that are associated with members of the G_{12} G-protein family or by receptors that activate members of the RAS and RHO family of monomeric G-proteins.

Phospholipase A Family

The phospholipase A (PLA) family of lipases consists of the PLA_1 and PLA_2 subfamilies. The designation of PLA_1 or PLA_2 relates to the target of the enzyme. PLA_1 enzymes catalyze hydrolysis of fatty acids from the sn-1 position of glycerophospholipids generating 2-acyl-lysophospholipids and free fatty acids. Mammals express several different extracellular enzymes that exhibit PLA_1 activity all of which belong to the pancreatic lipase gene family.

PLA_2 enzymes catalyze hydrolysis of the sn-2 position of glycerophospholipids releasing free fatty acids and 1-acyl-lysophospholipids. The mammalian genome contains more than 30 genes encoding PLA_2 and PLA_2-related enzymes. All of these genes are subdivided into several classes that includes the low-molecular-weight secreted PLA_2 enzymes ($sPLA_2$), the Ca^{2+}-dependent cytosolic PLA_2 enzymes ($cPLA_2$), the Ca^{2+}-independent PLA_2 enzymes ($iPLA_2$), the platelet-activating factor acetylhydrolases (PAF-AH), and the lysosomal PLA_2 enzymes.

Phospholipase D Family

Enzymes of the phospholipase D (PLD) family hydrolyze phospholipids such that the polar head group, attached to the phosphate, is released along with phosphatidic acid. Humans express two major PLD isoforms identified as PLD1 and PLD2. Both PLD1 and PLD2 are capable of hydrolyzing PC, PE, PS, lysophosphatidylcholine (LPC), and lysophosphatidylserine (LPS). However, these two enzymes are not capable of hydrolyzing PI, PG, or cardiolipin. There are other genes in the PLD family but not all of the encoded proteins exhibit phospholipid hydrolyzing activity. A related activity termed lysophospholipase D (lysoPLD) hydrolyzes lysoglycerophospholipids (lysoPL) to produce lysophosphatidic acid (LPA) and an amine.

Lysophospholipids

Lysophospholipids (LPL) are minor lipid components compared to the major membrane phospholipids such as phosphatidylcholine (PC), phosphatidylethanolamine (PE), and sphingomyelin. The most biologically significant LPL are lysophosphatidic acid (LPA), lysophosphatidylcholine (LPC), lysophosphatidylinositol (LPI), sphingosine 1-phosphate (S1P), and sphingosylphosphorylcholine (SPC). Each of these LPL functions via interaction with specific GPCR leading to autocrine or paracrine effects. Currently there are 15 characterized LPL receptors.

Activation of the LPA receptors triggers several different downstream signaling cascades. These include activation of MAP kinase (MAPK), activation of PLC, calcium mobilization, release of arachidonic acid, inhibition or activation of adenylate cyclase, and activation of several small GTPases such as RAS, RHO, and RAC. The LPL exert a wide-range of biochemical and physiological responses including platelet activation, smooth muscle contraction, cell growth, and fibroblast proliferation.

Phosphatidylinositol-3-Kinases

A family of kinases is responsible for the phosphorylation of membrane phospholipids on the 3-OH to generate phosphatidylinositol-3,4,5-trisphosphate, PIP_3. These kinases are referred to as the phosphatidylinositol-3-kinases, PI3K. The PI3K enzymes represent a family of both receptor-activated and nonreceptor-activated phosphatidylinositide kinases.

The original PI3K is composed of two protein subunits, one of 85 kDa (p85) and the other of 110 kDa (p110). The p110 subunit possess the kinase activity of the complex. The p85 subunit contains a protein-protein interaction domain of the SRC homology domain 3 (SH3) type and two phosphotyrosine-binding sites of the SRC SH2 type. The presence of the SH3 domain allows p85 and p110 to form a heterodimer and the presence of the SH2 domains allows the heterodimer to bind to phosphorylated tyrosine docking sites on growth factor receptors harboring intrinsic tyrosine kinase activity.

The receptor-activated PI3K members include both RTK and G-protein–coupled receptor (GPCR) activated isoforms. The GPCR activated PI3K enzymes consist of the p110 catalytic subunit and a different regulatory subunit identified as p101. The p101 subunit facilitates interaction of the catalytic p110 subunit with the βγ-subunits that are released from the heterotrimeric G-proteins activated by GPCR stimulation.

PHOSPHATASES IN SIGNAL TRANSDUCTION

Since the activation of many signal transduction events is controlled by addition of phosphate, removal of the incorporated phosphates must be a necessary event in order to modulate the initial signals. There are two classes of kinase, the serine/threonine and the tyrosine kinases. Thus, there are two classes of phosphatase necessary for phosphate removal, the protein serine/threonine phosphatases (PSP) and the protein tyrosine phosphatases (PTP).

Protein Tyrosine Phosphatases

There are two broad classes of protein tyrosine phosphatases (PTP) divided into four families. There are at least 107 genes in the human genome that encode enzymes that belong to one or the other of the broad classes of PTP. One broad class are single-pass transmembrane-spanning (transmembrane receptor-like) enzymes that contain the phosphatase activity domain in the intracellular portion of the protein. The transmembrane PTP are commonly called the receptor (R) class and designated RTP. The other broad class is intracellularly localized enzymes that are referred to as NT PTP (for non-transmembrane protein tyrosine phosphatase).

Protein Serine/Threonine Phosphatases

The PSP are grouped into three major families: phosphoprotein phosphatases (PPP), metal-dependent protein phosphatases (PPM), and the aspartate-based phosphatases represented by FCP/SCP. This latter family name is derived from transcription factor II**F** (TFIIF)-associating component of RNA polymerase II **C**-terminal domain (CTD) **p**hosphatase/**s**mall **C**TD **p**hosphatase.

Protein phosphatase 1 (PP1) is the major PSP and various isoforms of PP1 are expressed in all cells. PP1 plays an important role in a wide range of cellular processes, including protein synthesis, metabolism, regulation of membrane receptors and channels, cell division, apoptosis, and reorganization of the cytoskeletal architecture.

The broad spectrum of activity associated with the members of the PPP family stems from the ability of the catalytic subunits to associate with a large variety of different regulatory/inhibitory subunits. The regulatory/inhibitory subunits are grouped into five subfamilies termed the protein phosphatase (1, 2, 3, 4, and 6) regulatory subunit families. The designations for these regulatory gene families are PPP1R, PPP2R, PPP3R, PPP4R, and PPP6R. The number of PPP regulatory subunit genes is vast with, for example, the PPP1R family being composed of 181 genes in humans. Although there are several PPP regulatory subunit genes involved in the regulation of metabolism, the proteins encoded by the *PPP1R3A* and *PPP1R3B* genes are involved in the regulation of PP1.

CHECKLIST

- Signal transduction refers to the cellular process in which a signal is conveyed to trigger a change in the activity or state of a cell.
- Signal transduction involves cell surface receptors and intracellular receptors, both of which bind specific ligands and become activated by this binding, resulting in a triggering of all of the resultant downstream events.
- Signal-transducing receptors are represented by three broad families, two of which are cell surface receptors and one of which are intracellular receptors.
- Cell surface receptors of one group possess intrinsic enzymatic activity while the other class is coupled to the activation of a family of GTP hydrolyzing proteins termed G-proteins.
- Intracellular receptors bind lipophilic ligands and on ligand binding the complexes binds to specific DNA sequences resulting in regulated transcription of target genes.
- Receptors with intrinsic enzymatic activity generally span the plasma membrane once.

- ☑ The G-protein–coupled receptors (GPCR) span the membrane seven times and are also referred to as the serpentine receptors.
- ☑ GPCR are coupled to a family of heterotrimeric G-proteins composed of α, β, and γ subunits. The α-subunits bind and hydrolyze GTP, a process that regulates the activity of the G-protein.
- ☑ There are four distinct families of G-proteins that are classified based on the subsequent proteins whose activities they influence. This includes G-proteins that activate adenylate cyclase (G_s), those that inhibit adenylate cyclase (G_i), those that activate phospholipase Cγ (G_q), and those that activate a family of monomeric G-proteins (G_{12}).
- ☑ The activity state of G-proteins is regulated by the rate of GTP hydrolysis and the rate of exchange of GDP for GTP. The former involves a family of proteins called GTPase activating proteins (GAP) and the latter is regulated by a family of guanine nucleotide exchange factor (GEF) proteins.
- ☑ The intracellular receptors are all members of the steroid hormone and thyroid hormone-binding receptors. These receptors bind ligand inside the cell via a ligand-binding domain (LBD), possess a DNA-binding domain (DBD), and one or two activation function domains (AF-1, AF-2) that regulate the transcription of target genes.
- ☑ Many signal transduction pathways involve the phosphorylation of proteins and therefore, in order to terminate the signals there are numerous phosphatases that remove the activating phosphates. The phosphorylation events involve both tyrosine kinases and serine/threonine kinases, thus there are tyrosine phosphatases and serine/threonine phosphatase to terminate the signaling.
- ☑ Many plasma membrane receptors signal via the hydrolysis of membrane polyphosphoinositides (eg, phosphatidylinositol-4,5-bisphposphate, PIP_2) and the resultant products of this hydrolysis act as signaling molecules in the cascade.

REVIEW QUESTIONS

1. Experiments are being conducted on the activity of the G-protein RAS in cultures of cells isolated from a colonic carcinoma. Results from these studies reveal that the RAS protein can bind GTP and become activated with the same efficiency as RAS from normal cells. However, the rate at which the cancer cell RAS activity is decreased is 10 times slower than in normal cells. Which of the following proteins is most likely to be defective in the carcinoma cells accounting for these observations?

(A) G_i type G protein
(B) G_q type G-protein
(C) G_s type G-protein
(D) GTPase-activating protein
(E) Guanine nucleotide exchange factor

2. Experiments are being conducted using cultures of cells isolated from biopsy tissue isolated from a patient with non–small-cell lung cancer. Molecular studies have identified that the gene encoding the EGF receptor family member, HER2, has sustained a missense mutation in the transmembrane domain. Which of the following represents the most likely reason for the contribution of this mutation to the development of this cancer?

(A) It interferes with the normal activity of BRCA1
(B) The mutation is a gain-of-function mutation in its activation loop
(C) The protein can be activated by TGFα
(D) The protein constitutively dimerizes with other EGF receptors
(E) The protein now binds the monomeric G-protein RAS

3. Clinical trials are being conducted with a novel member of the selective estrogen receptor antagonist (SERM) family of compounds. Which of the following would most likely indicate that this novel compound was exerting the expected effect?

(A) Failure to recruit coactivator proteins to estrogen response elements
(B) Failure to recruit co-repressor proteins to estrogen response elements
(C) Interference with estrogen receptor dimerization with RXR
(D) Interference with estrogen receptors from entering the nucleus
(E) Preventing displacement of co-repressor proteins from the estrogen receptor
(F) Preventing heat shock proteins from dissociating from receptors

4. Experiments are being conducted to determine the efficacy of a new drug on cardiac function. Injection of the drug into test animals results in the changes in cardiac muscle function as indicated by the line in the Figure denoted by the letter A. Given these results, the activity of which of the following proteins is most likely to be affected in a positive way by the drug in question?

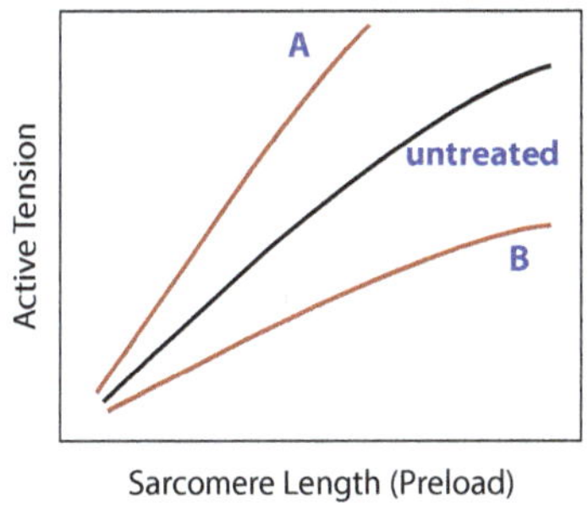

(A) A G_i-type G-protein
(B) A G_s-type G-protein
(C) A G_q-type G-protein
(D) cGMP-dependent protein kinase, PKG
(E) Phosphodiesterase 5, PDE5

5. A 57-year-old man was seen by his physician with complaints of difficulty with starting and stopping urination, frequent urgency, and having to urinate frequently at night. His physician prescribed an appropriate medication and indicated that the patient return in 3 weeks for a follow-up. At this follow-up visit, the patient reports that he has observed no changes in urinary difficulties. Given these results, which of the following proteins is most likely to be dysregulated in the patient's urogenital system accounting for the negative pharmacologic effects?
(A) A G_i-type G-protein
(B) A G_s-type G-protein
(C) A G_q-type G-protein
(D) cAMP-dependent protein kinase, PKA
(E) cGMP-dependent protein kinase, PKG
(F) Phosphodiesterase 5, PDE5

6. Clinical trials are being carried out in patients with invasive ductal carcinoma utilizing a novel compound that is structurally related to tamoxifen. Trial participants who are given the compound would most likely have the action of estrogen modulated by which of the following mechanisms?
(A) Activation of glucocorticoid responsive genes
(B) Activation of the MAP kinase pathway
(C) Binding to a nuclear receptor
(D) Binding to a receptor tyrosine kinase
(E) Dimerization of its receptor in the nuclear membrane
(F) Dimerization of its receptor in the plasma membrane

7. A 33-year-old woman is being examined by her physician with complaints of headaches, sweating, tremors, and confusion over the course of the past 3 months. History reveals that these symptoms are the most severe in the mornings but seem to lessen by eating. Physical examination shows no abnormalities. Fasting blood work shows serum glucose concentration of 37 mg/dL (N = 60 – 110 mg/dL). The hypoglycemia is the result of hormone-receptor interactions that are most likely resulting in the activation of which of the following?
(A) cAMP-dependent protein kinase A (PKA)
(B) Nuclear hormone-receptor-mediated transcription
(C) Phospholipase Cβ PLCβ)
(D) Serine/threonine kinase phosphorylation
(E) Tyrosine kinase phosphorylation

8. Studies are being carried out to examine the responses of cultured human hepatocytes following their exposure to γ-irradiation. In comparison to normal hepatocytes, it is shown that when glucagon is added, the normal cells exhibit reduced synthesis of palmitate, whereas the irradiated cells do not. Binding studies show that both cell populations bind the same amount of glucagon with the same dissociation kinetics. Which of the following proteins is most likely to be defective in the irradiated hepatocytes?
(A) G_i type G-protein
(B) G_q type G-protein
(C) G_s type G-protein
(D) GTPase activating protein
(E) Guanine nucleotide exchange factor
(F) Protein kinase C

9. Experiments are being conducted to determine the efficacy of a new drug on cardiac function. Injection of the drug into test animals results in the changes in cardiac muscle function as indicated by the line in the Figure denoted by the letter A. Given these results, which of the following is the experimental drug most likely to be mimicking?

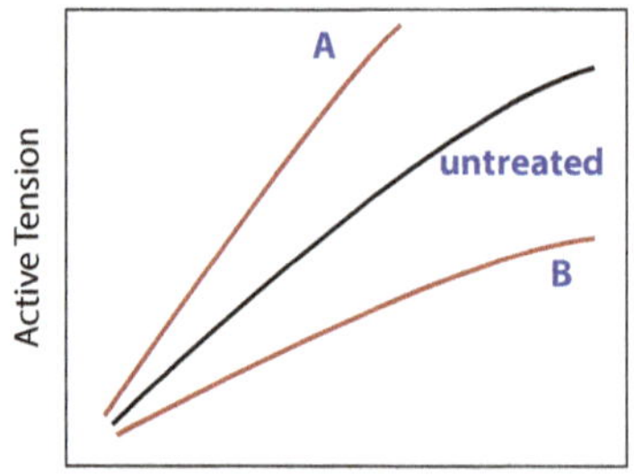

(A) Acetylcholine
(B) Amiodarone
(C) Amlodipine
(D) Norepinephrine
(E) Procainamide
(F) Propranolol

10. Studies are being carried out to examine the metabolic responses of cultured myocytes following their exposure to γ-irradiation. The irradiated cells do not take up glucose following insulin addition as is the case for normal myocytes in culture. Biochemical studies determine that both cell populations bind the same amount of insulin with the same dissociation kinetics indicating the receptors on the irradiated cells are unchanged. Given these results, which of the following proteins is most likely to be defective in the irradiated cells?
(A) A G_i-type G-protein
(B) A G_q type G-protein
(C) A G_s type G-protein
(D) Phosphatidylinositol-3-kinase, PI3K
(E) Protein kinase A, PKA
(F) Protein kinase G, PKG

11. Experiments are being carried out to assess the metabolic effects of a novel compound structurally related to dexamethasone. The compound is being tested using cultures of human hepatocytes. Addition of the compound to these cells is most likely to be associated with activation of which of the following processes?
(A) Activation of DNA replication
(B) Enhanced transcription of specific genes
(C) Enhanced translation of specific mRNAs
(D) Posttranscriptional processing of specific mRNAs
(E) Posttranslational processing of specific proteins

12. In a comparative study of two related cell lines it is discovered that one responds normally to insulin while the other has an impaired response. Analysis of both cell lines shows that they both bind insulin with equal affinity but that the impaired response is manifest in an inability to recruit the insulin response substrate-1 (IRS-1) protein to the receptor. This would most likely be due to which of the following?
(A) Inability of the receptor to phosphorylate the RAS G-protein
(B) Loss of activation of phospholipase C-β (PLCβ)
(C) Mutation in the tyrosine phosphate recognition site of IRS-1
(D) Serine phosphorylation of the insulin receptor preventing IRS-1 binding
(E) Tyrosine phosphorylation of the insulin receptor leading to the loss of the IRS-1 binding site

13. Experiments are being carried out to examine the metabolic processes in cultured cells derived from a human hepatocellular carcinoma. Molecular studies identified a missense mutation in the gene encoding the regulatory subunit of protein kinase A (PKA). Biochemical studies determine that the mutant protein does not bind cAMP. Given these findings, the actions of which of the following hormones is most likely to be impaired?
(A) Calcitriol
(B) Glucagon
(C) Insulin
(D) Prolactin
(E) Thyroxine (T_4)

14. Metabolic studies are being carried out using adipocytes in culture that have been exposed to a carcinogen. When these treated cells are exposed to repeated doses of epinephrine there is no change in the level of activation of hormone sensitive lipase, in contrast to the reduced effects observed with the same treatment in normal adipocytes. A mutation in which of the following genes is most likely to account for these observations?
(A) Adiponectin
(B) α_1-Adrenergic receptor
(C) β-Adrenergic receptor kinase (βARK)
(D) Protein kinase A
(E) Protein kinase C

15. Experiments are being carried out to examine the metabolic processes in cultured cells derived from a human ductal breast carcinoma. Molecular studies identified a missense mutation in the gene encoding phospholipase Cγ (PLCγ). This mutation is associated with a loss of the ability of epidermal growth factor to activate intracellular calcium mobilization from the endoplasmic reticulum. This is most likely loss of function of which of the domains of the mutant PLCγ?
(A) G_s-type G-protein binding
(B) G_q-type G-protein binding
(C) SH2 domains
(D) SH3 domains
(E) Tyrosine kinase

16. Experiments are being conducted to determine the molecular mechanism that has contributed to a novel form of testicular cancer. To carry out the analysis, cells are isolated from the tumor tissue and propagated in cell culture. When different signal transduction pathways are examined, the researchers discover that the tumor cells express a highly active form of an enzyme of the phospholipase C (PLC) family. Given these findings, which of the following is also most likely to be found in the tumor cells, relative to normal cells?
(A) Decreased cAMP
(B) Decreased cGMP
(C) Decreased intracellular calcium
(D) Increased cAMP
(E) Increased cGMP
(F) Increased intracellular calcium

17. Experiments are being carried out on cardiac nodal cardiomyocytes in a cell culture system. These experiments are aimed at identifying novel compounds that inhibit the actions of parasympathetic postganglionic nerve impulses on the sinoatrial (SA) node in human hearts. The successful identification of compounds that are inhibiting these nerve impulses would most likely be associated with reduced levels of activity of which of the following signaling molecules within the cultured cells?
(A) G_i-type G-protein
(B) G_q-type G-protein
(C) G_s-type G-protein
(D) Phosphatidylinositol-4,5-bisphosphate (PIP_2)
(E) Src tyrosine kinase

18. Experiments are being conducted to determine the molecular mechanism that has contributed to a novel form of colorectal carcinoma. To carry out the analysis, cells are isolated from the tumor tissue and propagated in cell culture. When different signal transduction pathways are examined, the researchers discover that the tumor cells express a highly active form of an enzyme of the phospholipase C (PLC) family. Given these findings, which of the following is most likely to be found at increased concentration or activity in the tumor cells, relative to normal cells?
(A) Acetylcholine
(B) AMP-dependent protein kinase (AMPK)
(C) Phosphatidylinositol-1,4,5-bisphosphate (PIP_3)
(D) Phosphatidylinositol 3-kinase (PI3K)
(E) Phosphatidylinositol-4,5-bisphosphate (PIP_2)

19. Experiments are being carried out on cardiac nodal cardiomyocytes in a cell culture system. These experiments are aimed at identifying novel compounds that mimic the actions of parasympathetic postganglionic nerve impulses on the sinoatrial (SA) node in human hearts. The successful identification of compounds that are mimicking these nerve impulses would most likely be associated with reduced levels of which of the following signaling molecules within the cultured cells?
(A) cAMP
(B) cGMP
(C) Inositol-1,3,5-trisphosphate (IP_3)
(D) Phosphatidylinositol-4,5-bisphosphate (PIP_2)
(E) Potassium

20. Experiments are being conducted to determine the metabolic disturbances that have contributed to a novel form of hepatocellular carcinoma. To carry out the analysis, cells are isolated from the tumor tissue and propagated in cell culture. The researchers discovered that the tumor cells express a highly active form of an enzyme of the phospholipase C (PLC) family. Given these findings, which of the following metabolic enzymes is most likely to be found to have decreased activity in the tumor cells, relative to normal cells?
(A) Glucose-6-phosphate dehydrogenase (G6PDH)
(B) Glycogen phosphorylase
(C) Glycogen synthase
(D) Phosphoenolpyruvate carboxykinase (PEPCK)
(E) 6-Phosphofructo-1-kinase (PFK1)

ANSWERS

1. Correct answer is **D.** The proto-oncogenic protein, RAS, is a monomeric G-protein involved in a wide array of cellular processes. When RAS binds GTP, it is in an active conformation which enable it to bind to and activate downstream effectors. The hydrolysis of GTP to GDP inactivates RAS. GTPase-activating proteins (GAP) are responsible for accelerating the intrinsically slow GTPase activity of RAS. Oncogenic RAS mutations render the protein incapable of hydrolyzing GTP allowing it to remain constitutively active. These types of mutations are identified in RAS in 20–30% of human cancers. In addition to the role of GAP proteins in G-protein activity, their activity state is regulated by the rate of GTP exchange for GDP which returns the G-protein from the inactive state to the active state. The GTP for GDP exchange process is catalyzed by guanine nucleotide exchange factor (GEF) activity (choice E). RAS is a monomeric G-protein and as such is not a member of the G_i (choice A), G_q (choice B), or G_s (choice C) families of heterotrimeric G-proteins.

2. Correct answer is **D.** HER2 is a member of the human epidermal growth factor receptor (EGFR) family that includes the human epidermal growth factor receptor (HER1, erbB1), HER2 (erbB2), HER3 (erbB3), and HER4 (erbB4). The extracellular domain of HER2 has no identifiable ligand, unlike the other EGF family receptors. HER2 is present in an active conformation and can undergo ligand-independent dimerization with other members of the EGF receptor family. Mutations in the transmembrane domain of HER2 have been identified in numerous patients with lung cancer. These mutations allow the HER2 protein to heterodimerize with other EGF receptor family members triggering a kinase active conformation of that receptor even in the absence of bound ligand. The HER2 protein is also involved in the development of breast cancer but in this disease the gene encoding the protein is amplified resulting in excess HER2 in these cancer cells. None of the other options (choices A, B, C, and E) represent the mechanism by which transmembrane mutations in the *HER2* gene contribute to the development of lung cancer.

3. Correct answer is **A.** Selective estrogen receptor modulators (SERM) are a class of drugs that exert their effects on the estrogen receptor (ER). SERM can function as agonists in some tissues but can function as antagonists in other tissues, thereby granting the possibility to selectively inhibit or stimulate estrogen-like action in different tissues. The primary reason for these tissue-specific differences is that there are two ER in humans, ERα and ERβ. ERα is the predominant ER in the female reproductive tract and mammary glands while ERβ is primarily in vascular endothelial cells, bone, and male prostate tissue. In addition, the concentrations of ERα and ERβ are different in tissues during development, aging, and in various disease states. Estrogen receptors are members of the nuclear receptor family of ligand-activated DNA-binding transcription factors. All members of the nuclear receptor family are composed of a ligand-binding domain, a DNA-binding domain, and transactivation domains. Within the cell the ER is associated with target genes in a heterodimer with RXR proteins (choice C) in the absence of ligand but in a complex with transcriptional co-repressors (choice B). Binding of ligand results in displacement of the co-repressors with simultaneous recruitment of coactivator proteins. One function of some of the members of the SERM family of drugs is the blocking of the recruitment of coactivators to the ER preventing the receptor from activating transcription of target genes. None of the other options (choices D, E, and F) represent the more correct processes by which SERM interfere with the function of the ER.

4. Correct answer is **B.** The effect of the novel drug is most likely enhancing the inotropic properties of the heart. Cardiac inotropy refers to the force of contraction. When heart muscle contracts, all muscle fibers are activated. There are two mechanisms that can alter force generation, changes in fiber length and changes in inotropy. The influence of inotropic changes in force generation is clearly demonstrated by use of length-tension diagrams such as shown in this question. The increased velocity of fiber shortening that occurs with increased inotropy increases the rate of ventricular pressure development. Increasing inotropy leads to an increase in ventricular stroke volume. The most important physiologic mechanism regulating inotropy is the autonomic nervous system. Sympathetic postganglionic nerves play a prominent role in enhancing ventricular and atrial inotropic regulation, while parasympathetic postganglionic nerves exert a negative inotropic effect in the atria but only a small effect in the ventricles. Most of the signal transduction pathways that stimulate inotropy ultimately involve Ca^{2+}. These effects can be exerted by increasing Ca^{2+} influx into sinoatrial node cardiomyocytes during an action potential via the opening voltage-gated L-type and T-type calcium channels, by increasing the release of sarcoplasmic reticulum (SR) stored Ca^{2+} through the opening of the ryanodine receptors (calcium release channels) that are ligand-gated calcium channels, or by sensitizing troponin C (TnC) to Ca^{2+}. The sympathetic postganglionic neurotransmitter is norepinephrine which binds the β_1-adrenergic receptor on sinoatrial node cardiomyocytes. The β-adrenergic receptors are coupled to G_s-type G-proteins that when activated result in enhanced production of cAMP and increased PKA activity. Increases in cAMP, independent of PKA activation, results in the activation of Ca^{2+}/calmodulin kinase II (CaMK2). When activated, CaMK2 phosphorylates the calcium release channel, ryanodine receptor 2, RYR2, resulting in increased release of Ca^{2+} stored within the SR. Increased free intracellular Ca^{2+} plays a major role in the contractile activity of cardiac muscle cells through, among other effects, the activation of the calmodulin subunit of myosin light-chain kinases. Thus, the stimulated release of Ca^{2+} from the SR contributes to the increased inotropic and chronotropic effects of β_1-adrenergic receptor activation. PKA phosphorylates L-type Ca^{2+} channels in the plasma membrane and it also phosphorylates RYR2 in the SR. The PKA-mediated phosphorylation of plasma membrane L-type Ca^{2+} channels results in increased influx of Ca^{2+} and the phosphorylation of the RYR2 channel results in increased release of Ca^{2+} stored in the SR. Both events lead to increased Ca^{2+} availability for activation of the calmodulin subunit of myosin light-chain kinase, MLCK. The released Ca^{2+} also interacts with troponin C (TnC) resulting in a conformational change to the troponin complex and increased contractile activity ensues. A variety of inotropic drugs are used clinically to stimulate the heart, such as in congestive heart failure, and include digoxin, β-adrenergic receptor agonists, (eg, isoproterenol), and phosphodiesterase inhibitors (eg, milrinone). Enhancement of the activity of the none of the other proteins (choices A, C, D, and E) would result in increased inotropic properties of the heart.

5. Correct answer is **C.** The patient is most likely experiencing the symptoms of benign prostatic hyperplasia, BPH. There are several therapeutic mechanisms to treat BPH including the use of drugs and surgery such as prostate artery embolization (PAE). The initial treatment of BPH is with drugs that are α_1-adrenergic receptor antagonists such as tamsulosin and alfuzosin. Therefore, the most likely medication prescribed by the patient's physician was an α_1-adrenergic receptor blocker. The α_1-adrenergic receptor is coupled to a G_q-type G-protein. The apparent ineffectiveness of the therapeutic intervention in this patient most likely was the result of a G_q-type G-protein that was active (dysregulated) in the absence of normal α_1-adrenergic receptor activation. None of the other proteins (choices A, B, D, E, and F) are directly involved in the signal transduction cascade elicited via the α_1-adrenergic receptor.

6. Correct answer is **C.** Tamoxifen is a drug that is a member of the selective estrogen receptor modulators (SERM). SERM are a class of drugs that exert their effects on the estrogen receptor (ER). SERMs can function as agonists in some tissues but can function as antagonists in other tissues, thereby granting the possibility to selectively inhibit or stimulate estrogen-like action in different tissues. There are two ER in humans, ERα and ERβ. ERα the predominant ER in the female reproductive tract and mammary glands while ERβ is primarily in vascular endothelial cells, bone, and male prostate tissue. Estrogen receptors are members of the nuclear receptor family of ligand-activated DNA-binding transcription factors. None of the other options (choices A, B, D, E, and F) correctly correspond to the function of the nuclear receptor family of transcription factors.

7. Correct answer is **E.** The patient is most likely experiencing the consequences of hypoglycemia induced by inappropriate or unregulated release of insulin from the pancreas. Insulin modifies numerous pathways metabolism in order to enhance storage of excess carbon. Within the liver insulin promotes glucose storage as glycogen and glucose oxidation via gluconeogenesis and the pyruvate dehydrogenase complex (PDHc) such that the resultant acetyl-CoA can be used for the synthesis of fatty acids. Within adipose tissue and skeletal muscle, the actions of insulin lead to increased glucose uptake by these tissues. This latter effect of insulin can significantly contribute to hypoglycemia. Insulin exerts all of these effects by binding to its receptor. The insulin receptor possesses intrinsic tyrosine kinase activity. None of the other signal transduction processes (choices A, B, C, and D) are directly affected by insulin binding to its receptor.

8. Correct answer is **C.** When glucagon binds its receptor it activates an associated G_s-type G-protein. The activated G-protein in turn activates adenylate cyclase which catalyzes the synthesis of cAMP from ATP. The cAMP binds to the regulatory subunits of protein kinase A (PKA) resulting in activation of the catalytic subunits. Once activated, PKA will phosphorylate numerous substrates within hepatocytes. One of the targets of PKA is the rate-limiting enzyme of de novo fatty acid synthesis, acetyl-CoA carboxylase 1 (ACC1). PKA-mediated phosphorylation of ACC1 results in its inhibition resulting in reduced *de novo* fatty acid synthesis. None of the other proteins (choices A, B, D, E, and F), if defective, would be as likely to result in the loss of glucagon-mediated regulation of fatty acid synthesis.

9. Correct answer is **D.** The results demonstrate that the effect of the novel drug is most likely enhancing the inotropic properties of the heart. Cardiac inotropy refers to the force of contraction. When heart muscle contracts, all muscle fibers are activated. There are two mechanisms that can alter force generation, changes in fiber length and changes in inotropy. The influence of inotropic changes in force generation is clearly demonstrated by use of length-tension diagrams such as shown in this question. The most important physiologic mechanism regulating inotropy is the autonomic nervous system. Sympathetic post-ganglionic nerves play a prominent role in enhancing ventricular and atrial inotropic regulation, while parasympathetic postganglionic nerves exert a negative inotropic effect in the atria but only a small effect in the ventricles. Most of the signal transduction pathways that stimulate inotropy ultimately involve Ca^{2+}. These effects can be exerted by increasing Ca^{2+} influx into sinoatrial node cardiomyocytes during an action potential via the opening voltage-gated L-type and T-type calcium channels, by increasing the release of sarcoplasmic reticulum (SR) stored Ca^{2+} through the opening of the ryanodine receptors (calcium release channels) that are ligand-gated calcium channels, or by sensitizing troponin C (TnC) to Ca^{2+}. The sympathetic postganglionic neurotransmitter is norepinephrine which binds the β_1-adrenergic receptor on sinoatrial node cardiomyocytes. The β-adrenergic receptors are coupled to G_s-type G-proteins that when activated result in enhanced production of cAMP and increased PKA activity. Increases in cAMP, independent of PKA activation, results in the activation of Ca^{2+}/calmodulin kinase II (CaMK2). When activated, CaMK2 phosphorylates the calcium release channel, ryanodine receptor 2, RYR2, resulting in increased release of Ca^{2+} stored within the SR. Increased free intracellular Ca^{2+} plays a major role in the contractile activity of cardiac muscle cells through, among other effects, the activation of the calmodulin subunit of myosin light-chain kinases. Thus, the stimulated release of Ca^{2+} from the SR contributes to the increased inotropic and chronotropic effects of β_1-adrenergic receptor activation. PKA phosphorylates L-type Ca^{2+} channels in the plasma membrane and also phosphorylates RYR2 in the SR. The PKA-mediated phosphorylation of plasma membrane L-type Ca^{2+} channels results in increased influx of Ca^{2+} and the phosphorylation of the RYR2 channel results in increased release of Ca^{2+} stored in the SR. Both events lead to increased Ca^{2+} availability for activation of the calmodulin subunit of myosin light-chain kinase, MLCK. The released Ca^{2+} also interacts with troponin C (TnC) resulting in a conformational change to the troponin complex and increased contractile activity ensues. Acetylcholine (choice A) is the neurotransmitter released from postganglionic parasympathetic neurons. The cardiac receptor that binds the ACh released from parasympathetic postganglionic nerves is the M2-type muscarinic acetylcholine receptor. The M2 receptor is coupled to a G_i-type G-protein. Activation of the M2 receptor results in decreased levels of cAMP and decreased activity of PKA, thereby reducing all the positive inotropic effects in the heart exerted by sympathetic outflow. The effects of acetylcholine would result in a decrease, not an increase in the length-tension curve. Amiodarone (choice B) is a K^+ channel blocker which prevents the rapid repolarization of cardiomyocytes. This effect slows down the action potential propagation leading to a negative effect on inotropy. The actions of a drug like this would decrease, not increase the length-tension curve. Amlodipine (choice C) is a Ca^{2+}-channel blocker resulting in less influx of calcium into cardiomyocytes. Since increases in inotropy are due to Ca^{2+}, the actions of a drug like this would decrease, not increase the length-tension curve. Procainamide is a Na^+ channel blocker the effects of which would be slowing of the rapid initial phase of cardiomyocyte action potential propagation leading to a negative effect on inotropy. The actions of a drug like this would decrease, not increase the length-tension curve. Propranolol (choice F) is a non-specific β-blocker which would decrease all the positive inotropic effects in the heart exerted by sympathetic outflow. The effects of propranolol would result in a decrease, not an increase in the length-tension curve.

10. Correct answer is **D.** In adipocytes and skeletal muscle, insulin stimulates an increase in glucose uptake by increasing the number of plasma membrane glucose transporters, specifically GLUT4 in the plasma membrane of the cells in these tissues. When insulin binds its receptor on these cells the signal transduction cascade that is initiated includes the activation of phosphatidylinositol-3-kinase, PI3K. PI3K phosphorylates membrane phospholipids generating phosphatidylinositol-3,4,5-trisphophate (PIP_3) from phosphatidylinositol-4,5-bisphosphate (PIP_2). PIP_3 then activates the kinase, PIP_3-dependent kinase 1 (PDK1) which in turn phosphorylates and activates a protein kinase C isoform (PKCζ) involved in the mobilization of GLUT4 to the plasma membrane. Loss of PI3K activation or activity would, therefore, result in reduced capacity to mobilize GLUT4 containing vesicles to the membrane. The insulin receptor is a member of the receptor family that possess intrinsic tyrosine kinase activity as opposed to a member of the G-protein–coupled receptor family (choices A, B, and C). Insulin-mediated signal transduction does regulate the activity of PKA (choice E); however, this does not involve the role of insulin in the mobilization of GLUT4 to the plasma membrane. The insulin receptor does not mediate any effects through protein kinase G, PKG (choice F).

11. Correct answer is **B.** Dexamethasone is a synthetic glucocorticoid. The glucocorticoids, such as cortisol, exert their effects by binding to a receptor that is a member of the nuclear receptor superfamily. All proteins of the nuclear receptor superfamily are ligand activated transcription factors. These receptors possess a ligand-binding domain, a DNA-binding domain, and a transactivation domain. On ligand binding the glucocorticoid receptor (GR) is released from complexes in the cytosol and it then migrates into the nucleus where it binds to specific target DNA sequences (termed hormone response elements, HRE) in various glucocorticoid-regulated genes. The binding of steroid-receptor complexes to HRE results in an altered rate of transcription of the associated gene(s). The effects of steroid-receptor complexes on specific target genes can be either stimulatory or inhibitory with respect to the rate of transcription. None of the other processes (choices A, C, D, and E) would be directly affected by a novel compound related to dexamethasone.

12. Correct answer is **C.** The insulin receptor belongs to the family of receptors that harbor intrinsic tyrosine kinase activity. Binding of insulin to its receptor triggers activation of this intrinsic tyrosine kinase activity. The initial event that occurs on insulin binding to its receptor is the activation of this intrinsic tyrosine kinase activity which results in the autophosphorylation of the receptor itself. The presence of phosphotyrosine in the insulin receptor serves as a docking site for proteins involved in mediating insulin signal transduction. One of the initial proteins to interact with the insulin receptor, following its activation by binding insulin, is the protein identified as insulin receptor substrate 1, IRS-1. If the gene encoding IRS-1 order to sustain a mutation in the phosphotyrosine recognition motif of IRS-1, the result would be impaired insulin-mediated signaling through IRS-1. The insulin receptor does not phosphorylate RAS (choice A). The insulin receptor does not activate phospholipase Cβ (choice B). Serine phosphorylation of the insulin receptor is not known to interfere with IRS-1 binding (choice D). Tyrosine phosphorylation of the insulin receptor is the mechanism by which IRS-1 can interact with the receptor, it does not prevent IRS-1 binding (choice E).

13. Correct answer is **B.** Hormones that exert their effects through activation of PKA bind to receptors of the G-protein–coupled receptor (GPCR) superfamily, specifically GPCR coupled to G_s-type G-proteins. The glucagon receptor belongs to the GPCR superfamily. When glucagon binds its receptor on cells, such as hepatocytes, it activates the associated G_s-type G-protein. The activated G-protein in turn activates adenylate cyclase which catalyzes the synthesis of cAMP from ATP. The cAMP binds to the regulatory subunits of protein kinase A (PKA) resulting in activation of the catalytic subunits. The activation of PKA leads to the phosphorylation of numerous proteins that are responsible for the normal responses of cells to glucagon. The receptor for calcitriol (choice A) and thyroxine (choice E) are members of the nuclear receptor superfamily of ligand-activated transcription factors. The insulin receptor (choice C) is a member of the receptor tyrosine kinase family of receptors. With respect to insulin the effect of receptor activation is hydrolysis of cAMP and reduced levels of active PKA. The prolactin receptor (choice D) is a member of the class I cytokine receptor family, which includes receptors such as the growth hormone receptor (GHR) and the interleukin-6 (IL-6) receptor.

14. Correct answer is **C.** Epinephrine exerts its effects in adipocytes by binding to the β_3-adrenergic receptor present on these cells. The β-adrenergic receptors are G-protein–coupled receptors (GPCR) that are coupled to a G_s-type G-protein. The activation of the G_s-type G-proteins results in elevated activity of PKA which then phosphorylates and activates hormone sensitive lipase. A characteristic feature of GPCR activity following ligand binding is a progressive loss of receptor-mediated signal transduction. This process is referred to as desensitization or adaptation. In the majority of cases, it is impairment of the receptor's ability to activate its G-protein that accounts for most desensitization, especially within minutes of agonist stimulation. This desensitization process involves phosphorylation of the GPCR on one or more intracellular domains. Heterologous desensitization involves phosphorylation of GPCR by second messenger-dependent kinases, such as PKA and PKC. Homologous desensitization of GPCR involves a family of kinases termed G-protein–coupled receptor kinases (GRK). The GRKs constitute a family of six mammalian serine/threonine kinases that phosphorylate ligand-activated GPCR as their primary substrates, hence the designation of the process as homologous desensitization. These GRK include GRK2 (originally called β-adrenergic receptor kinase-1, βARK1) and GRK3 (originally called β-adrenergic receptor kinase-2, βARK2). These kinases preferentially phosphorylate ligand (agonist) bound and activated receptor rather than inactive or antagonist occupied GPCR substrates. The loss of function of β-adrenergic receptor kinases would result in the ability to repeatedly activated the β3 adrenergic receptor in adipocytes. None of the other proteins (choices A, B, D, and E) are involved in the process of adrenergic receptor desensitization.

15. Correct answer is **C.** The epidermal growth factor (EGF) receptor family consists of receptors with intrinsic tyrosine kinase activity. Upon ligand binding, EGF receptors dimerize, and the kinase domains carry out transphosphorylation of the receptor protein. The resultant phosphotyrosine residues in the receptors serve as docking sites for signal-transducing proteins.

Proteins that interact with phosphotyrosine residues, particularly those in plasma membrane receptors, possess a domain termed an SH2 domain (SRC homology domain 2) that binds the phosphotyrosine. One of the signal-transducing proteins that interacts with growth factor receptors, such as the EGF receptor, is a member of the phospholipase C family, specifically phospholipase Cγ (PLCγ). Activated PLCγ hydrolyzes membrane-localized phosphatidylinositol-4,5-bisphosphate (PIP_2) into diacylglycerol (DAG) and inositol-1,4,5-trisphosphate (IP_3). IP_3 binds to receptors in the endoplasmic reticulum (ER) that are ligand-activated calcium channels. The consequence of IP_3 binding its receptor is release of stored calcium to the cytosol. Mutation of the SH2 domain of PLCγ would result in an inability for the EGF receptor to mobilize calcium from the ER. None of the other protein domains (choices A, B, D, and E) play a part in growth factor receptor-mediated calcium mobilization from the ER.

16. Correct answer is **F.** Enzymes of the PLC family hydrolyze membrane-associated phosphatidylinositol-4,5-bisphosphate (PIP_2; PtdIns-4,5-P2), resulting in the generation of two second messengers, inositol-1,4,5-trisphosphate (IP_3; Ins-1,4,5-P_3) and diacylglycerol (DAG), in response to activation of receptors by hormones, growth factors, and neurotransmitters. Upon its generation, IP_3 binds to one of three IP_3 receptors (IP3R) present in the membranes of the endoplasmic and sarcoplasmic reticulum (ER and SR) which activate the release of stored Ca^{2+}. The released Ca^{2+}, along with DAG, activates kinases of the protein kinase C (PKC) family. None of the other changes (choices A, B, C, D, and E) is seen as a direct or immediate result of the activation of PLC family enzymes.

17. Correct answer is **A.** Within the cardiovascular system, the primary target cells of the heart that receive parasympathetic innervation are the SA node (from the right vagus nerve), the atrioventricular (AV) node (from the left vagus nerve), and atrial cells. The parasympathetic postganglionic neurotransmitter is acetylcholine, and it binds to muscarinic acetylcholine receptors on these cells. The cardiac muscarinic receptor that binds the ACh released from parasympathetic postganglionic nerves is the M2 type receptor. The M2 receptors are coupled to a G_i-type G-protein. Thus, compounds that interfere with the activity of acetylcholine on cardiac nodal cells will be associated with reduced activity of the M2 receptor-associated G_i-type G-protein. None of the other signaling molecules (choices B, C, D, and E) play a direct role in the propagation of acetylcholine activity from parasympathetic postganglionic nerves.

18. Correct answer is **E.** Enzymes of the PLC family hydrolyze membrane-associated phosphatidylinositol-4,5-bisphosphate (PIP_2; PtdIns-4,5-P2) resulting in the generation of two second messengers, inositol-1,4,5-trisphosphate (IP_3; Ins-1,4,5-P_3) and diacylglycerol (DAG), in response to activation of receptors by hormones, growth factors, and neurotransmitters. Upon its generation, IP_3 binds to one of three IP_3 receptors (IP3R) present in the membranes of the endoplasmic and sarcoplasmic reticulum (ER and SR) which activate the release of stored Ca^{2+}. The released Ca^{2+}, along with DAG, activates kinases of the protein kinase C (PKC) family. None of the other enzymes or signaling molecules (choices A, B, C, and D) would be appreciably changed in the context of increased PLC activity.

19. Correct answer is **A.** Within the cardiovascular system the primary target cells of the heart that receive parasympathetic innervation are the SA node (from the right vagus nerve), the atrioventricular (AV) node (from the left vagus nerve), and atrial cells. The parasympathetic postganglionic neurotransmitter is acetylcholine, and it binds to muscarinic acetylcholine receptors on these cells. The cardiac muscarinic receptor that binds the ACh released from parasympathetic postganglionic nerves is the M2 type receptor. The M2 receptors are coupled to a G_i-type G-protein. Activation of the M2 receptor results in decreased levels of cAMP leading to reduced direct effects of cAMP and reduced activation of PKA, all of which result in decreased cardiac conductance and heart rate. None of the other substances or compounds (choices B, C, D, and E) are involved in the propagation of signals from parasympathetic postganglionic nerves that impinge on SA nodal cardiomyocytes.

20. Correct answer is **C.** Enzymes of the PLC family hydrolyze membrane-associated phosphatidylinositol-4,5-bisphosphate (PIP_2; PtdIns-4,5-P2) resulting in the generation of two second messengers, inositol-1,4,5-trisphosphate (IP_3; Ins-1,4,5-P_3) and diacylglycerol (DAG), in response to activation of receptors by hormones, growth factors, and neurotransmitters. Upon its generation, IP_3 binds to one of three IP_3 receptors (IP3R) present in the membranes of the endoplasmic and sarcoplasmic reticulum (ER and SR) which activate the release of stored Ca^{2+}. The increased intracellular Ca^{2+} binds to the calmodulin subunit of phosphorylase kinase (PHK), thereby activating the kinase. PHK phosphorylates numerous substrates including glycogen synthase and glycogen phosphorylase (choice B). The effect of these phosphorylations is decreased glycogen synthase activity and increased glycogen phosphorylase activity. None of the other enzymes (choices A, D, and E) are targets of PHK, nor are their activities appreciably affected by Ca^{2+} ions.

CHAPTER

27

Molecular Biology Tools

High-Yield Terms

Restriction endonuclease	Any of a large family of enzymes that recognize, bind to, and hydrolyze specific nucleic acid sequences in double-stranded DNA
Cloning	In molecular biology this term refers to the production of large quantities of identical DNA molecules
Blotting	In molecular biology this term refers to a method of transferring proteins, DNA or RNA, out of the size-separating gel onto a solid support such as filter paper
DNA sequencing	The process of determining the precise order of nucleotides within a DNA molecule
Microarray	Commonly known as DNA chip, is a collection of microscopic DNA spots attached to a solid surface
Gene chip	Is the solid medium of a microarray containing the DNA spots
Transgenesis	The process of inserting a gene from one source into a living organism that would not normally contain it
Gene therapy	A technique involving the insertion of genes into an individual's cells and tissues to treat a disease, such as a hereditary disease in which a deleterious mutant allele is replaced with a functional one
CRISPR-Cas9	A method for editing genomes that was adapted from a naturally occurring microbial adaptive immune system that utilizes RNA-guided nucleases; term derived from **C**lustered **R**egularly **I**nterspaced **S**hort **P**alindromic **R**epeats and **C**RISPR-**as**sociated protein **9**
RNAi	RNA interference, a method of posttranscriptional gene silencing that involves the use of small antisense RNA to promote mRNA degradation and inhibition of protein synthesis

INTRODUCTION

Molecular medicine encompasses the utilization of many molecular biological techniques in the analysis of disease, disease genes, and disease gene function. The study of disease genes and their function in an unaffected individual has been possible by the development of recombinant DNA and cloning techniques. The basis of the term recombinant DNA refers to the recombining of different segments of DNA. Cloning refers to the process of preparing multiple copies of an individual type of recombinant DNA molecule. The classical mechanisms for producing recombinant molecules involve the insertion of exogenous fragments of DNA into either bacterially derived plasmid (circular double-stranded autonomously replicating DNAs found in bacteria) vectors or bacteriophage- (viruses that infect bacteria) based vectors. The term vector refers to the DNA molecule used to carry or transport DNA of interest into cells.

The technologies of molecular biology are critical to modern medical diagnosis and treatment. For example, cloning allows large quantities of therapeutically beneficial human proteins to be produced in pure form. In addition, the cloning of genes allows for the utilization of the DNA for treatments referred to as gene therapy which involves the introduction of a normal copy of a gene into an individual harboring a defective gene. These molecular biology techniques involve the use of a wide array of different enzymes, many of which are purified from bacteria (Table 27–1).

RESTRICTION ENDONUCLEASES

Restriction endonucleases are enzymes that will recognize, bind to, and hydrolyze specific nucleic acid sequences in double-stranded DNA. The key to the *in vitro* utilization of restriction endonucleases is their strict nucleotide sequence specificity. The different enzymes are identified by being given a name indicating the bacterium from which they were isolated, for example, the enzyme EcoRI, which recognizes the sequences, 5′–GAATTC–3′, was isolated from *Escherichia coli*.

TABLE 27–1 Some of the enzymes used in recombinant DNA research.

Enzyme	Reaction	Primary Use
Phosphatases	Dephosphorylates 5′ ends of RNA and DNA	Removal of 5′-PO_4 groups prior to kinase labeling; also used to prevent self-ligation
DNA ligase	Catalyzes bonds between DNA molecules	Joining of DNA molecules
DNA polymerase I	Synthesizes double-stranded DNA from single-stranded DNA	Synthesis of double-stranded cDNA; DNA labeling and nick translation; generation of blunt ends from sticky ends
Thermostable DNA polymerases	Synthesize DNA at elevated temperatures (60-80°C)	Polymerase chain reaction (DNA synthesis), mutagenesis
DNase I	Under appropriate conditions, produces single-stranded nicks in DNA	Nick translation; mapping of hypersensitive sites; mapping protein-DNA interactions
Exonuclease III	Removes nucleotides from 3′ ends of DNA	DNA sequencing; ChIP-Exo, mapping of DNA-protein interactions
λ Exonuclease	Removes nucleotides from 5′ ends of DNA	DNA sequencing, mapping of DNA-protein interactions
Polynucleotide kinase	Transfers terminal phosphate (γ position) from ATP to 5′-OH groups of DNA or RNA	^{32}P end-labeling of DNA or RNA
Reverse transcriptase	Synthesizes DNA from RNA template	Synthesis of cDNA from mRNA; RNA (5′ end) mapping studies
RNAse H	Degrades the RNA portion of a DNA–RNA hybrid	Synthesis of cDNA from mRNA
S1 nuclease	Degrades single-stranded DNA	Removal of "hairpin" in synthesis of cDNA; RNA mapping studies (both 5′ and 3′ ends)
Terminal transferase	Adds nucleotides to the 3′ ends of DNA	Homopolymer tailing
Recombinases (CRE, INT, FLP)	Catalyze site-specific recombination between DNA containing homologous target sequences	Generation of specific chimeric DNA molecules, work both in vitro and in vivo
CRISPER-Cas9/C2c2	RNA-targeted DNA-, or RNA-directed nuclease	Genome editing and with variations in modulation of gene expression at DNA and RNA levels

Reproduced with permission from Rodwell VW, Bender DA, Botham KM, et al: *Harper's Illustrated Biochemistry*, 31st ed. New York, NY: McGraw Hill; 2018.

One unique feature of restriction enzymes is that the nucleotide sequences they recognize are palindromic, that is, they are the same sequences in the 5′→3′ direction of both strands. Some restriction endonucleases make staggered symmetrical cuts away from the center of their recognition site within the DNA duplex, some make symmetrical cuts in the middle of their recognition site while still others cleave the DNA at a distance from the recognition sequence. Enzymes that make staggered cuts leave the resultant DNA with cohesive or sticky ends (Figure 27–1). Enzymes that cleave the DNA at the center of the recognition sequence leave blunt-ended fragments of DNA.

Any two pieces of DNA containing the same sequences within their sticky ends can anneal together and be covalently ligated together in the presence of DNA ligase. Any two blunt-ended

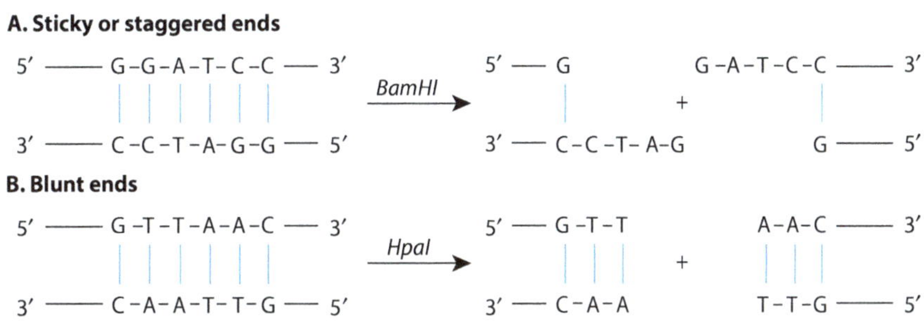

FIGURE 27–1 Results of restriction endonuclease digestion. Digestion with a restriction endonuclease can result in the formation of DNA fragments with sticky or cohesive ends (**A**), or blunt ends (**B**); phosphodiester backbone, black lines; interstrand hydrogen bonds between purine and pyrimidine bases, blue. Generating fragments whose ends have particular structures (ie, blunt, cohesive) is an important consideration in devising cloning strategies. (Reproduced with permission from Rodwell VW, Bender DA, Botham KM, et al: *Harper's Illustrated Biochemistry*, 31st ed. New York, NY: McGraw Hill; 2018.)

fragments of DNA can be ligated together irrespective of the sequences at the ends of the duplexes.

CLONING DNA

Any fragment of DNA can be cloned once it is introduced into a suitable vector. Cloning refers to the production of large quantities of identical DNA molecules and usually involves the use of a bacterial cell as a host for the DNA, although cloning can be done in eukaryotic cells as well. cDNA cloning refers to the production of a library of cloned DNAs that represent all mRNAs present in a particular cell or tissue. Genomic cloning refers to the production of a library of cloned DNAs representing the entire genome of a particular organism. From either of these types of libraries, one can isolate (by a variety of screening protocols) a single cDNA or a single-gene clone.

In order to clone either cDNAs or copies of genes a vector is required to carry the cloned DNA. Vectors used in molecular biology are of two basic classes. One class of vectors is derived from bacterial plasmids (Figure 27–2). Plasmids are circular DNAs found in bacteria that replicate autonomously from the host genome. These DNAs were first identified because they harbored genes that conferred antibiotic resistance to the bacteria. The antibiotic resistance genes found on the original plasmids are used in modern *in vitro* engineered plasmids to allow selection of bacteria that have taken up the plasmids containing the DNAs of interest. Plasmids are limited in that, in general, fragments of DNA less than 10,000 base pairs (bp) can be cloned (Table 27–2).

The second class of vector is derived from the bacteriophage (bacterial virus) lambda. The advantage to lambda-based vectors is that they can carry fragments of DNA up to 25,000 bp. In the analysis of the human genome, even lambda-based vectors are limiting and a yeast artificial chromosome (**YAC**) vector system has been developed for the cloning of DNA fragments from 500,000 bp to 3,000,000 bp.

cDNA Cloning

cDNAs are made from the mRNAs of a cell by any number of related techniques (Figure 27–3). Each technique consists of first reverse transcription of the mRNA followed by synthesis of the second strand of DNA and insertion of the double-stranded cDNA into either a plasmid or lambda vector for cloning. This process creates a library of cloned cDNA representing each mRNA species. Screening of the library for a particular cDNA clone

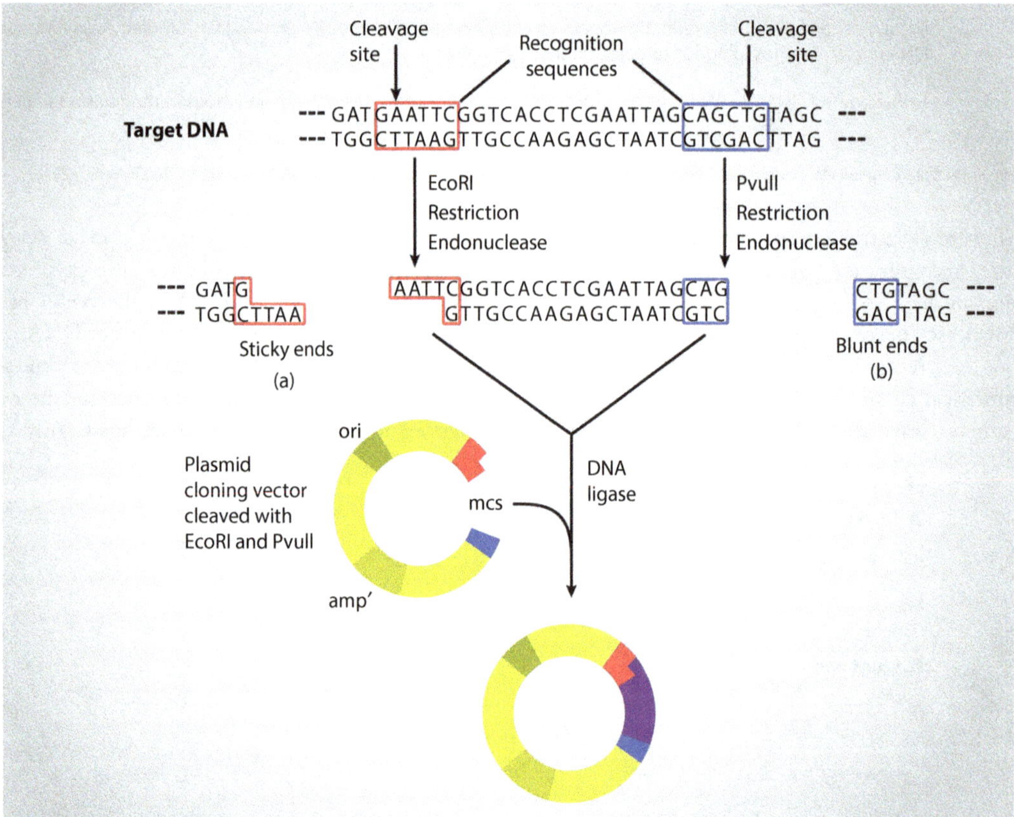

FIGURE 27–2 Typical plasmid vector cloning. A plasmid cloning vector is digested with the same enzymes (EcoRI and PvuII) as the target DNA. Most cloning plasmids have a section of unique restriction endonuclease sites called the multicloning site (MCS). The target DNA is ligated into the plasmid with DNA ligase with the result being a recombinant plasmid that can be used to transfect bacteria. (Reproduced with permission from themedicalbiochemistrypage, LLC.)

TABLE 27–2 Cloning capacities of common cloning vectors.

Vector	DNA Insert Size (kb)
Plasmid pUC19	0.01–10
Lambda charon 4A	10–20
Cosmids	35–50
BAC, P1	50–250
YAC	500–3000

Reproduced with permission from Rodwell VW, Bender DA, Botham KM, et al: *Harper's Illustrated Biochemistry*, 31st ed. New York, NY: McGraw Hill; 2018.

is accomplished using nucleic acid or protein-based (proteins or antibodies) probes. cDNA libraries can also be screened by biological assay of the products produced by the cloned cDNAs. Screening with proteins, antibodies, or by biological assay are mechanisms for analysis of the expression of proteins from cloned cDNAs and is given the term **expression cloning**. Nucleic acid probes can be generated from DNA (including synthetic oligonucleotides, oligos) or RNA. Nucleic acid probes can be radioactively labeled or labeled with modified nucleotides that are recognizable by specific antibodies and detected by colorimetric or chemiluminescent assays.

Genomic Cloning

The majority of genomic cloning utilizes lambda-based vector systems. These vector systems are capable of carrying 15–25,000 bp of DNA. Still larger genomic DNA fragments can be cloned into YAC vectors (Figure 27–4). Genomic DNA can be isolated and cloned from any nucleated cell. The genomic DNA is first partially digested with restriction enzymes to generate fragments in the size range that are optimal for the vector being utilized for cloning. The partially digested DNA is then size selected by a variety of techniques (eg, gel electrophoresis or gradient centrifugation) prior to cloning. Screening of genomic libraries is accomplished primarily with nucleic acid-based probes. However, they can be screened with proteins that are known to bind specific sequences of DNA (eg, transcription factors).

ANALYSIS OF CLONED PRODUCTS

The analysis of cloned cDNAs and genes involves a number of techniques. The initial characterization usually involves mapping of the number and location of different restriction enzyme sites.

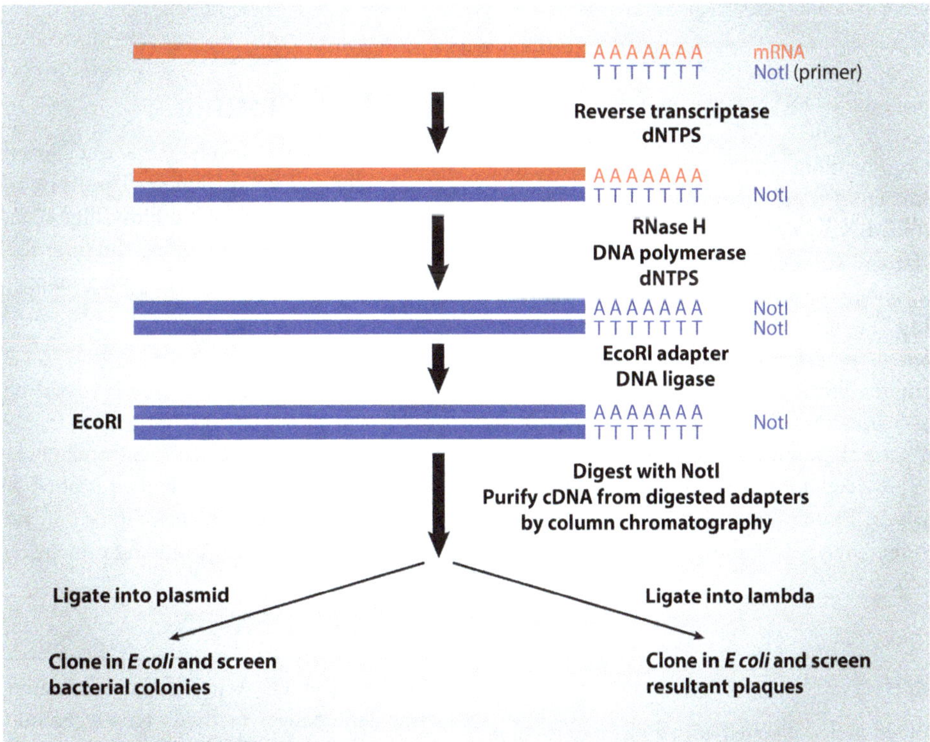

FIGURE 27–3 Typical process for production and cloning of cDNA. This example shows the use of a specific primer-adapter containing the sequences for the restriction enzyme NotI in addition to the poly(T) for annealing to the poly(A) tail of the RNA. It is possible to use only poly(T) or poly(T) with other restriction sites or random primers (a mixture of oligos that contain random sequences) to initiate the first-strand cDNA reaction. In some cases poly(T) priming does not allow for extension of the cDNA to the 5′-end of the RNA; the use of random primers can overcome this problem since they will prime first-strand synthesis all along the mRNA. This technique shows the ligation of EcoRI adapters followed by EcoRI and NotI digestion. This process allows the cDNAs to all be cloned in one direction, termed directional cloning. (Reproduced with permission from themedicalbiochemistrypage, LLC.)

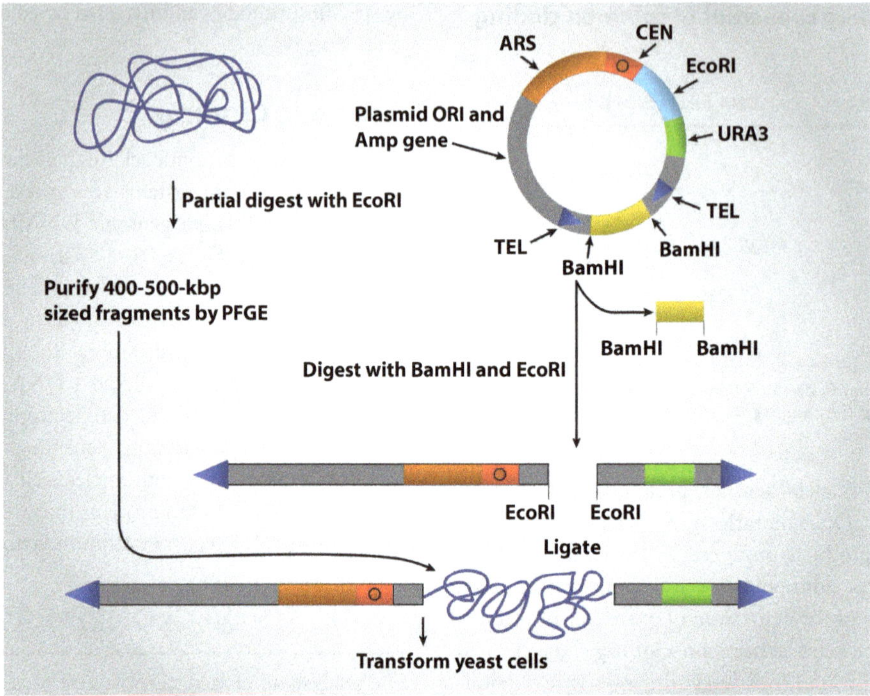

FIGURE 27–4 Diagrammatic representation of a typical YAC vector used to clone genomic DNA. The vector contains yeast telomeres (TEL), a centromere (CEN), a selectable marker (URA3), and autonomously replicating sequences (ARS) as well as bacterial plasmid sequences for antibiotic selection and replication in *E. coli*. PFGE, pulsed-field gel electrophoresis. (Reproduced with permission from themedicalbiochemistrypage, LLC.)

This information is useful for DNA sequencing since it provides a means to digest the clone into specific fragments for subcloning, a process involving the cloning of fragments of a particular cloned DNA. Once the DNA is fully characterized cDNA clones can be used to produce RNA *in vitro* and the RNA translated *in vitro* to characterize the encoded protein. Clones of cDNAs also can be used as probes to analyze the structure of a gene by **Southern blotting** (Figure 27–5) or to analyze the size of the RNA and pattern of its expression by **Northern blotting** (Figure 27–5). Northern blotting is also a useful tool in the analysis of the exon-intron organization of gene clones since only fragments of a gene that contain exons will hybridize to the RNA on the blot, provided it is the pool of mRNAs that have been selected for analysis. Proteins in tissues or those expressed by cloned cDNA can be analyzed by the technique of **Western blotting** (Figure 27–5).

Southern Blotting

The DNA to be analyzed is first digested with a given restriction enzyme, then the resultant DNA fragments are separated in an agarose gel. The DNA is transferred from the gel to a solid support, such as a nylon filter, by either capillary diffusion or under electric current. The DNA is fixed to the filter by baking or ultraviolet light treatment. The filter can then be probed for the presence of a given fragment(s) of DNA by various radioactive or nonradioactive means.

Northern Blotting

Northern blotting involves the analysis of RNA following its attachment to a solid support. The RNA is sized by gel electrophoresis, then transferred to nitrocellulose or nylon filter paper as for Southern blotting. Probing the filter for a particular RNA is done similarly to probing of Southern blots.

Western Blotting

Western blotting involves the analysis of proteins following attachment to a solid support. The proteins are separated by size SDS-PAGE and transferred to nitrocellulose or nylon filters via an electric current. The filter is then probed with antibodies raised against a particular protein or they can be probed with DNA probes if analyzing DNA-binding proteins.

DNA SEQUENCING

Sequencing of DNA utilizes an enzymatic technique originally termed the Sanger method. This technique involves the use of dideoxynucleotides (2′,3′-dideoxy) that terminate DNA synthesis and is, therefore, also called dideoxy chain termination sequencing (Figure 27–6).

High-Throughput Sequencing

High-throughput sequencing, also known as next-generation sequencing (NGS), refers to the rapid sequencing technologies

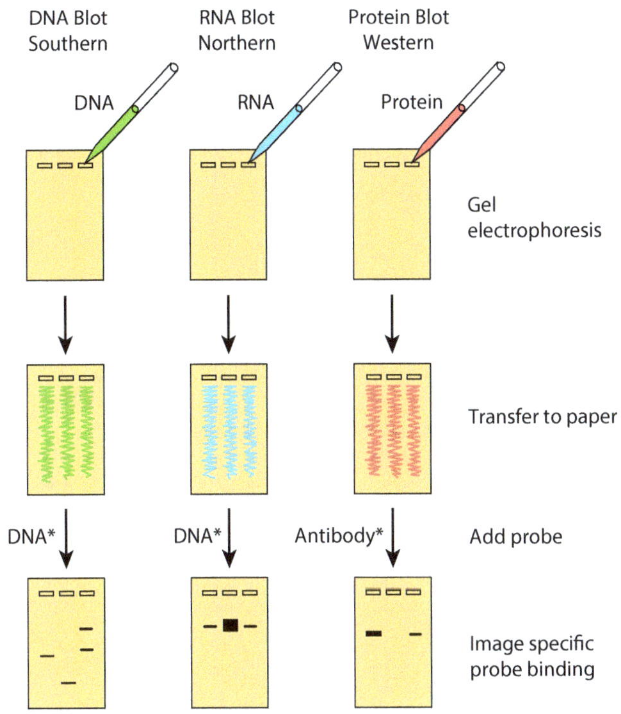

FIGURE 27–5 The blot transfer procedure. In a Southern, or DNA blot transfer, DNA isolated from a cell line or tissue is digested with one or more restriction enzymes. This mixture is pipetted into a well in an agarose or polyacrylamide gel and exposed to a direct electrical current. DNA, being negatively charged, migrates toward the anode; the smaller fragments move the most rapidly. After a suitable time, the DNA within the gel is denatured by exposure to mild alkali and transferred, via capillary action (or electrotransfer—not shown), to nitrocellulose or nylon paper, resulting in an exact replica of the pattern on the gel, using the blotting technique devised by Southern blot. The DNA is bound to the paper by exposure to heat or UV, and the paper is then exposed to the labeled DNA probe, which hybridizes to complementary strands on the filter. After thorough washing, the paper is exposed to x-ray film or an imaging screen, which is developed to reveal several specific bands corresponding to the DNA fragment(s) that were recognized (hybridized to) the sequences in the DNA probe. The RNA, or Northern, blot is conceptually similar. RNA is subjected to electrophoresis before blot transfer. This requires some different steps from those of DNA transfer, primarily to ensure that the RNA remains intact, and is generally somewhat more difficult. In the protein, or Western, blot, proteins are electrophoresed and transferred to special paper that avidly binds proteins and then probed with a specific antibody or other probe molecule. (Asterisks signify labeled probes, either radioactive or fluorescent.) In the case of Southwestern blotting (see the text; not shown), a protein blot similar to that shown above under "Western" is exposed to labeled nucleic acid, and protein–nucleic acid complexes formed are detected by autoradiography or imaging. (Reproduced with permission from Rodwell VW, Bender DA, Botham KM, et al: *Harper's Illustrated Biochemistry*, 31st ed. New York, NY: McGraw Hill; 2018.)

that have been developed in the last 20 years for determining the sequences of DNA and RNA. As recently as 2016 DNA-sequencing technology was at a stage where an entire human genome could be sequenced in 1–2 days. With NGS technologies, it is now possible to obtain an entire genome sequence in several hours.

The power of NGS is that the millions of nucleotide differences (polymorphisms) that exist in the genomes of every individual can rapidly be analyzed. The vast majority of these polymorphisms do not result in disease or dysfunction but nonetheless, define an individual's genetic make-up. A useful example to consider is the fact that many polymorphisms in drug metabolizing genes result in different rates of drug metabolism in different individuals. This means that a particular dose of a drug is likely to have different efficacies in different individuals. The analysis of an individual's genome prior to therapeutic intervention underlies the concept of **pharmacogenomics** and is based on the concept of individual genetic polymorphisms.

RNA-Seq

RNA-Seq is the term that refers to the process of using NGS methods to rapidly identify the transcriptome of a cell, alternatively spliced mRNAs, posttranscriptional modifications, and mutations all at the level of the RNA. RNA-Seq can look at all the RNA types in a cell including mRNA, rRNA, tRNA, as well as short and long noncoding RNAs.

In this technique the RNA is converted to cDNA with the use of reverse transcriptase. Prior to reverse transcription the various RNA populations can be fractionated (eg, polyadenylated mRNAs) or used outright. The power of current NGS techniques allows for direct sequencing of the cDNA molecules, eliminating the need for cloning which itself can introduce biases into the analysis. The RNA-Seq technique has advanced to the state where this technique can be applied to the analysis of single cells.

HIGH-YIELD CONCEPT

The PCR is a powerful technique used to amplify a specific sequence of DNA in a short period of time through a process of repeated replication of a template (Figure 27–7).

DIAGNOSTIC METHODOLOGIES

The Polymerase Chain Reaction

The polymerase chain reaction (PCR) technique utilizes sets of specific *in vitro* synthesized oligonucleotides to prime DNA synthesis. The design of the primers is dependent upon the sequences of the DNA that is desired to be analyzed. The technique is carried out through many cycles (usually 20–50) of melting the DNA template at high temperature, allowing the primers to anneal to complimentary sequences within the template and then replicating the template with DNA polymerase. The PCR has been automated with the use of thermostable DNA polymerases.

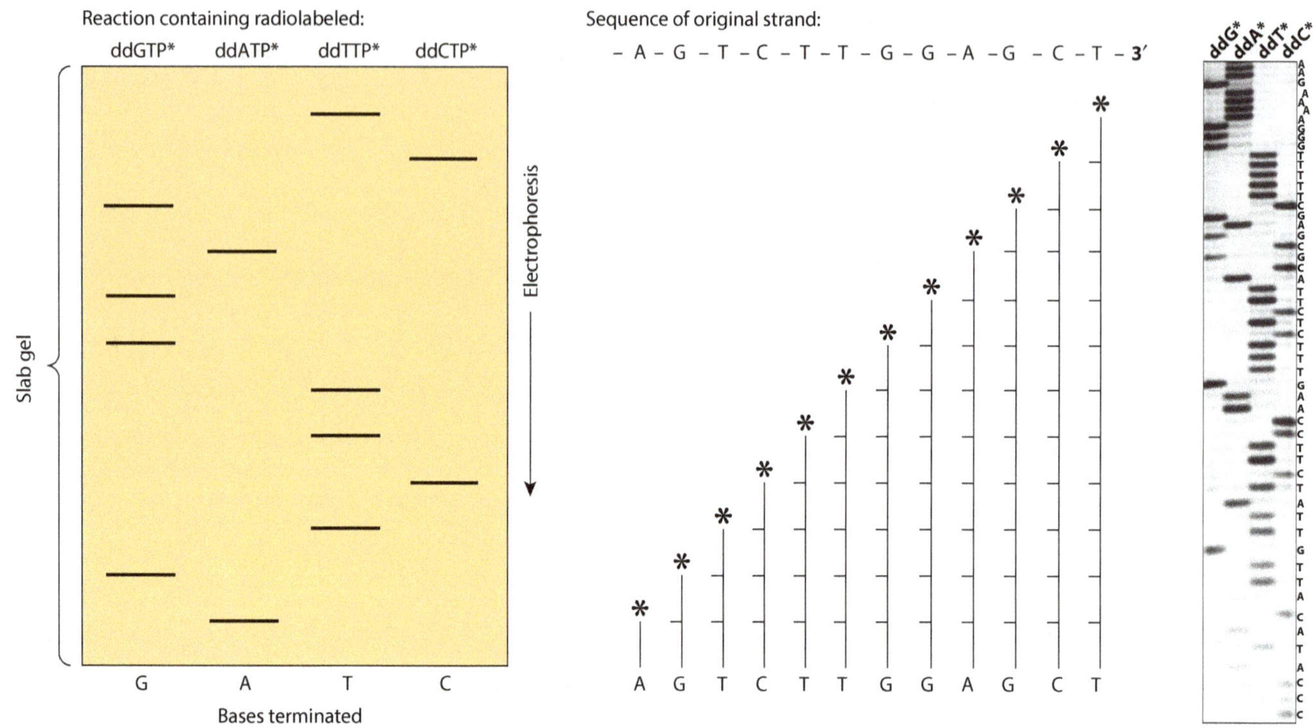

FIGURE 27–6 Sequencing of DNA by the chain termination method devised by Sanger. The ladder-like arrays represent, from bottom to top, all of the successively longer fragments of the original DNA strand. Knowing which specific dideoxynucleotide reaction was conducted to produce each mixture of fragments, one can determine the sequence of nucleotides from the unlabeled end toward the labeled end (*) by reading up the gel. The base-pairing rules of Watson and Crick (A–T, G–C) dictate the sequence of the other (complementary) strand. (Asterisks signify site of radiolabeling.) Schematically shown **(left, middle)** are the terminated synthesis products of a hypothetical fragment of DNA, sequence listed **(middle, top)**. An autoradiogram **(right)** of an actual set of DNA sequencing reactions that utilized the four ^{32}P-labeled dideoxynucleotides indicated at the top of the scanned autoradiogram (ie, dideoxy(dd)G, ddA, ddT, ddC). Electrophoresis was from top to bottom. The deduced DNA sequence is listed on the right side of the gel. Note the log-linear relationship between distance of migration (ie, top to bottom of gel) and DNA fragment length. Current state-of-the-art DNA sequencers no longer utilize gel electrophoresis for fractionation of labeled synthesis products. Moreover, in the majority of NGS sequencing platforms, synthesis is followed by monitoring incorporation of the four fluorescently labeled dXTPs. (Reproduced with permission from Rodwell VW, Bender DA, Botham KM, et al: *Harper's Illustrated Biochemistry*, 31st ed. New York, NY: McGraw Hill; 2018.)

During the first round of replication a single copy of DNA is converted to two copies and so on resulting in an exponential increase in the number of copies of the sequences targeted by the primers. After just 20 cycles, a single copy of DNA is amplified more than 2,000,000-fold. The products of PCR reactions are generally analyzed by separation in agarose gels followed by ethidium bromide staining and visualization with *uv* transillumination or they can be directly sequenced using NGS techniques.

The PCR technique also can be used to identify the level of expression of genes in extremely small samples of material, for example, tissues or cells from the body. This technique is termed **reverse transcription-PCR (RT-PCR)**, because the mRNA is first converted into single-stranded DNA by reverse transcriptase and then the DNA is amplified.

Restriction Fragment Length Polymorphism Analysis

The genetic variability at a particular locus due to even single base changes (single nucleotide polymorphisms [SNP]) can alter the pattern of restriction enzyme digestion fragments that can be generated. Restriction fragment length polymorphism (RFLP) analysis takes advantage of this and utilizes Southern blotting of restriction enzyme digested genomic DNA or more commonly, PCR products, to detect familial patterns of the fragments of a given gene. A classic example of a disease caused by SNP that can be detectable by RFLP is sickle cell anemia (Figure 27–8).

Sickle cell anemia results (at the level of the gene) from a single nucleotide change (A to T) at codon 6 within the β-globin gene. This alteration leads to a glu (G) to val (V) amino acid substitution, while at the same time abolishing a MstII restriction site. As a result, a β-globin gene probe can be used to detect the different MstII restriction fragments. It should be recalled that there are two copies of each gene in all human cells, therefore, RFLP analysis detects both copies: the mutant allele and the wild-type allele.

Size variability in detectable fragments within a family pedigree indicates differences in the pattern of restriction sites within and around the gene being analyzed. RFLP patterns are inherited and segregated in Mendelian fashion, thus allowing their use in genotyping such as in cases of paternity dispute or in criminal investigations.

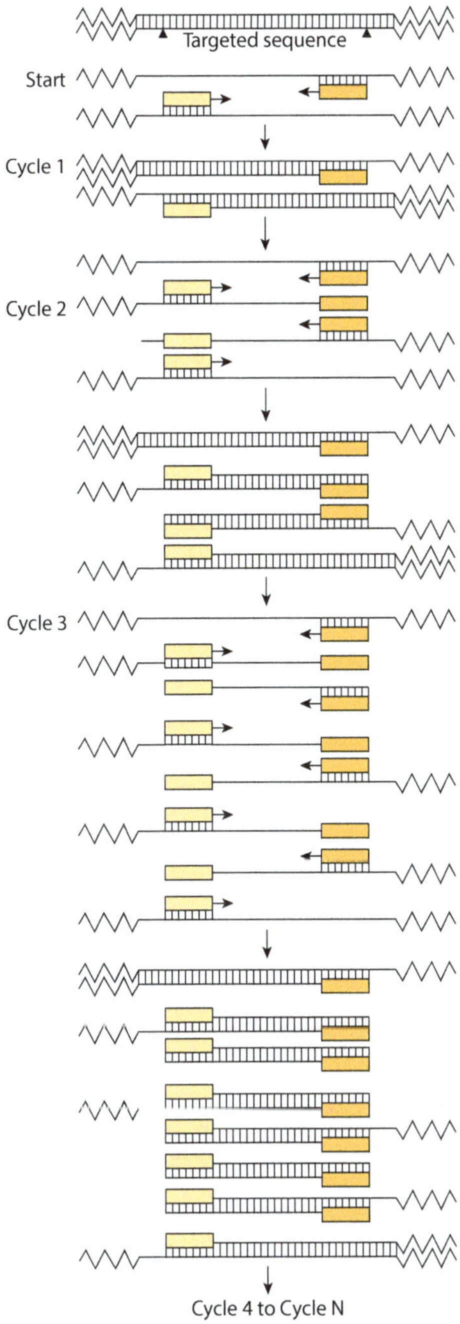

FIGURE 27–7 The polymerase chain reaction technique is used to amplify specific gene sequences. Double-stranded DNA is heated to separate it into individual strands. These bind two distinct primers that are directed at specific sequences on opposite strands and that define the segment to be amplified. DNA polymerase extends the primers in each direction and synthesizes two strands complementary to the original two. This cycle is repeated 30 or more times, giving an amplified product of defined length and sequence. Note that the four dXTPs and the two primers are present in excess to minimize the possibility that these components are limiting for polymerization/amplification. It is important to note though that as cycle number increases incorporation rates can drop, and mutation/error rates can increase. (Reproduced with permission from Rodwell VW, Bender DA, Botham KM, et al: *Harper's Illustrated Biochemistry*, 31st ed. New York, NY: McGraw Hill; 2018.)

HIGH-YIELD CONCEPT

Microarray analysis involves the use of what are commonly called "gene chips" to determine the expression of a large set of genes at the same time in a single experiment.

MICROARRAY ANALYSIS

DNA microarrays are referred to as gene chips. Gene chips can be purchased ready-made or they can be custom prepared. Most gene chips are created through the covalent attachment of synthetic oligonucleotides (oligos) to a small surface. In general, there are 20 or more different oligos on the chip corresponding to different regions of each gene to be analyzed. In addition, a set of oligos that each contain a nucleotide mismatch are included as negative controls for each gene. The technology of creating gene chips is such that there can be tens of thousands of different genes represented on a single chip approximately 2 cm square. Many custom gene arrays are created by robotic spotting of DNA (most often cDNAs) onto glass slides.

Although there are numerous uses for gene chips, the most common experiment involves a comparison of the expression of the genes on the chip between two samples, for example, cancer cells and normal cells. The assay is carried out by preparing RNA from each sample and converting the RNA to cDNA in the presence of fluorescent nucleotides. For example, one RNA sample is converted to cDNA with a green fluorescent nucleotide and the other RNA sample is converted to cDNA in the presence of a red fluorescent nucleotide. These "tagged" cDNA preparations are mixed together and hybridized to the gene chip. When the process is complete, computerized image processing is used to identify the intensity of various colors. Fluorescent color detection can be only green, only red, or a color in between that represents a mix of some red and some green (Figure 27–9). Thus, some spots will be yellow, some will be orange, or degrees of these intermediate combination colors. Spots that are only red indicate that the gene was expressed only in the source of the red-labeled cDNAs and *vice versa* for green spots.

HIGH-YIELD CONCEPT

Transgenesis refers to the process of introducing exogenous genes into the germ line of an organism.

TRANSGENESIS

The first successful transgenesis experiments were carried out in mice. To create a transgenic animal the gene of interest must be passed from generation to generation, that is, it must be inherited in the germ line. To accomplish this with mice or livestock animals, vectors containing the gene of interest with appropriate regulatory elements (eg, the β-lactoglobulin promoter if expression of the

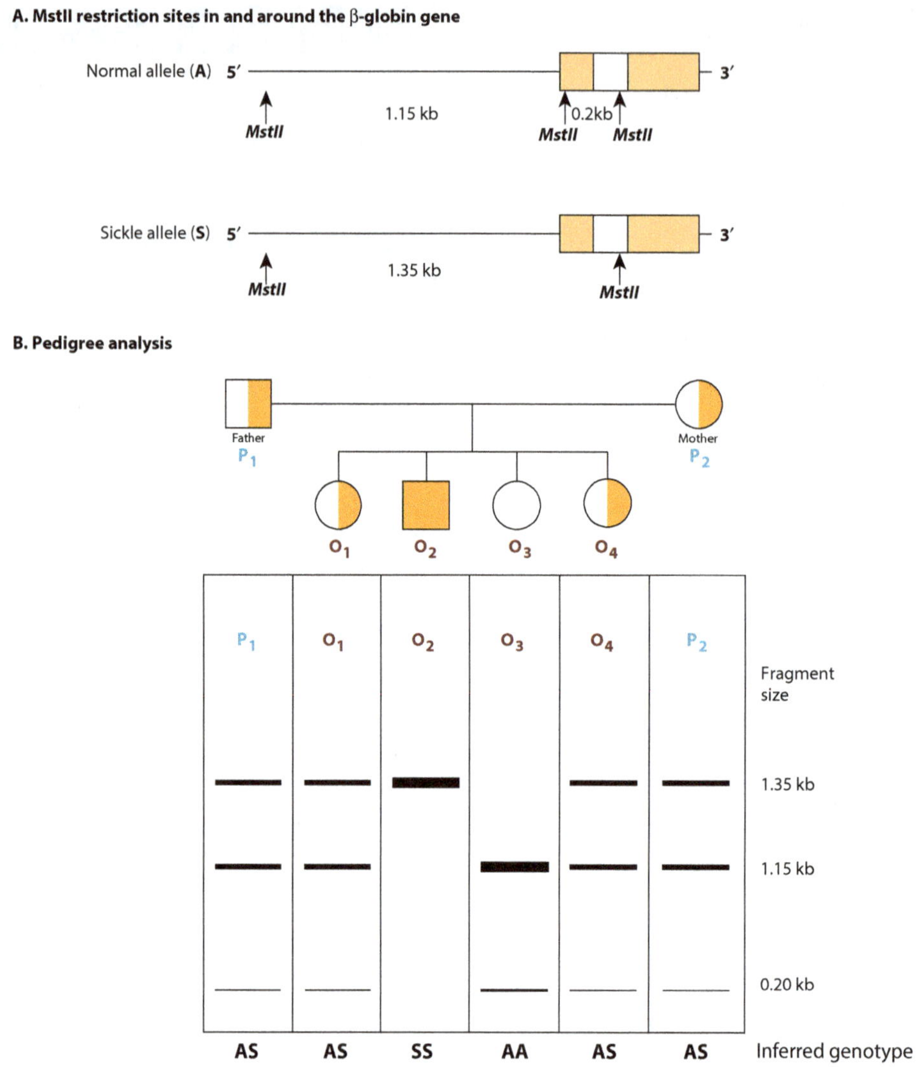

FIGURE 27–8 Pedigree analysis of sickle cell disease. The top part of the figure **(A)** shows the first part of the β-globin gene and the *MstII* restriction enzyme sites in the normal (A) and sickle cell (S) β-globin genes. Digestion with the restriction enzyme *MstII* results in DNA fragments 1.15- and 0.2-kb long in normal individuals. The T-to-A change in individuals with sickle cell disease abolishes one of the three *MstII* sites around the β-globin gene; hence, a single restriction fragment 1.35 kb in length is generated upon cleavage with *MstII*. This size difference is easily detected on a Southern blot. **(B)** Pedigree analysis shows three possibilities for four offspring O_1, O_2, O_3, and O_4, given Parental (P_1, P_2) heterozygous genotypes (**AS**): AA, normal (open circle); AS, heterozygous (half-solid circles, half-solid square); SS, homozygous (solid square). (Reproduced with permission from Rodwell VW, Bender DA, Botham KM, et al: *Harper's Illustrated Biochemistry*, 31st ed. New York, NY: McGraw Hill; 2018.)

transgene in the milk is desired) are injected into the nucleus of fertilized eggs. The eggs are then transplanted into the uterus of receptive females for development of the potential transgenic offspring.

GENE THERAPY

Transgenesis with humans would allow for the elimination of disease genes in a population of offspring, however, technical as well as ethical issues likely will prevent or limit any transgenic experiments to be carried out with human eggs. The current goal of gene therapy in humans is to replace known disease genes with normal copies in the correct somatic cells of afflicted individuals.

Early gene therapy protocols utilized bone marrow-derived cells such as was the case for the treatment of adenosine deaminase deficient SCID patients. With the advent of stem-cell technologies, in particular the use of induced pluripotent stem cells (iPSC), it is possible to generate the correct target cell type *in vitro* and then generate transgenic cells for reimplantation into an afflicted individual. The advantage of the use of iPSC is that the technique involves generation of the iPSC from the individual into which the transgenic cells will be reintroduced. This eliminates the possibility for rejection by the patient's immune system.

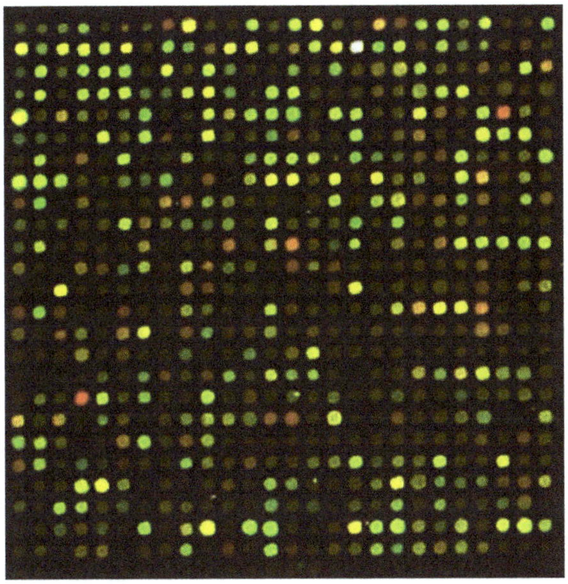

FIGURE 27–9 Example results from a spotted DNA array screen. (Reproduced with permission from themedicalbiochemistrypage, LLC.)

CRISPR-Cas9: Gene Editing

One of the newest techniques with potential for treating diseases caused by gene mutations utilizes a gene editing and regulatory system referred to as CRISPR-Cas9, a term derived from **C**lustered **R**egularly **I**nterspaced **S**hort **P**alindromic **R**epeats and CRISPR-**as**sociated protein **9**. This technique is a method for editing genomes that was adapted from a naturally occurring microbial adaptive immune system that utilizes RNA-guided nucleases (Figure 27–10).

The power and utility of the CRISPR-Cas9 technique is that it can be used to replace mutant genes with wild-type copies directly *in vivo* at any time in development. The technique can also be used to eliminate single genes or even entire chromosomes. The ability of the CRISPR-Cas9 technique to eliminate entire chromosomes at any time during development could theoretically be used to treat disorders associated with abnormal chromosome number such as Down syndrome.

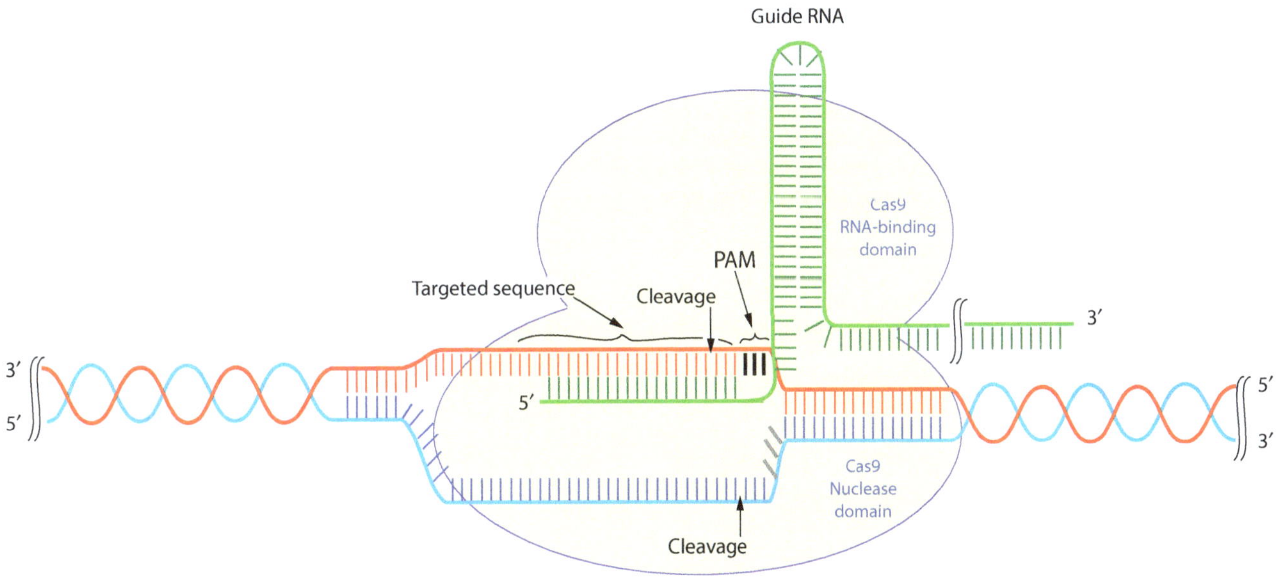

FIGURE 27–10 Overview of the mechanism of CRISPR-Cas9. Shown is the two-domain CRISPR-Cas9 nuclease protein bound to target genomic DNA (red, blue) and specific guide RNA (green), which through base complementarity (20 nts) locates its genomic target, which is adjacent to a short protospacer adjacent motif, or PAM. The guide RNA binding and nuclease domains are labeled. Once specifically localized, the two distinct Cas9 nuclease active centers cleave both strands of the targeted genomic DNA (cleavage; arrows) immediately downstream of the PAM, which results in DNA double-strand break. Subsequent DNA repair by cellular activities (see Chapter 22) can introduce mutations thereby inactivating the targeted gene. Variations on the use of CRISPR-Cas9 are numerous and allow for the sculpting of the structure and expression of genomic DNA. (Reproduced with permission from Rodwell VW, Bender DA, Botham KM, et al: *Harper's Illustrated Biochemistry*, 31st ed. New York, NY: McGraw Hill; 2018.)

CHECKLIST

- ☑ Molecular biology is a technical field that involves the study of genes and the control of their expression in the elaboration of cellular and organismal function.
- ☑ A variety of enzymes, most isolated from bacteria, are utilized in the molecular study of DNA and genes.
- ☑ Cloning refers to the production of large quantities of identical DNA molecules and usually involves the use of a bacterial cell as a host for the DNA, although cloning can be done in eukaryotic cells as well.
- ☑ Reverse transcriptase is an RNA-dependent DNA polymerase that is used to generate complimentary DNA (cDNA) copies of the mRNAs present in a cell or tissue. The resultant cDNAs are generally inserted into an appropriate vector to generate a library of cDNA clones.
- ☑ Genomic cloning refers to the process of digesting the genome of an organism and inserting it into an appropriate vector system for the generation of a library of gene clones.
- ☑ Common means of molecular analysis include Southern blotting (analyzing DNA), Northern blotting (analyzing RNA), and Western blotting (analyzing proteins).
- ☑ Gene therapy is a term used to describe a technique designed to introduce a functional gene into the cells or tissues of an individual in order to treat a disease resulting from an inherited gene defect.
- ☑ CRISPR-Cas9 is a powerful gene editing tools that may revolutionize the treatment of inherited and acquired disorders caused by gene mutations and chromosome abnormalities.

REVIEW QUESTIONS

1. A 2-year-old boy is being examined in the emergency department due to concerns of his parents about his progressive lethargy. Physical examination shows marked pallor, motor skill abnormalities, and clear failure to thrive. Blood work indicates the infant has a microcytic, hypochromic anemia with increased concentrations of target cells and acanthocytes. The attending physician recommends the child be tested for the possibility of a genetic defect resulting in the anemia. Which of the following techniques would be the most useful in identifying the most common cause of the infant's disorder?
(A) Dot blot
(B) Enzyme-linked immunosorbent assay (ELISA)
(C) Northern blot
(D) Southern blot
(E) Western blot

2. A 5-year-old girl, with a history of recurrent vasculo-occlusive episodes, is undergoing an examination by her pediatrician. Her parents report that she complains often of dizziness, severe headaches, and intense pain in her legs. Physical examination shows icteric sclera. Which of the following tests would be most useful in aiding in a correct diagnosis of the cause of the patient's symptoms?
(A) cDNA cloning
(B) Genomic cloning
(C) Northern blotting
(D) Polymerase chain reaction (PCR)
(E) Restriction fragment length polymorphism (RFLP)

3. Molecular studies are being conducted to ascertain the differences between normal colonic epithelial cells and cells isolated from an adenomatous polyp. These experiments are designed to determine any differences in global gene activity between the two cell types. Which of the following is the best technique to use for these studies?
(A) cDNA cloning
(B) Genomic cloning
(C) Polymerase chain reaction, PCR
(D) Southern blotting
(E) Restriction fragment length polymorphism, RFLP

4. A 41-year-old divorced female with four children is suing her ex-husband for child support. The man has made the claim that he is not the biological father to all four children. The court ordered DNA testing of all six individuals. DNAs were analyzed using a single-locus STR probe. The results of the analysis are shown in the accompanying figure. DNA samples are as follows: lane 1 mother, lane 2 father, lane 3 child 1, lane 4 child 3, lane 5 child 3, lane 6 child 4. Based upon these results, which, if any, of the four children can most likely be excluded as being biologic to the tested male?

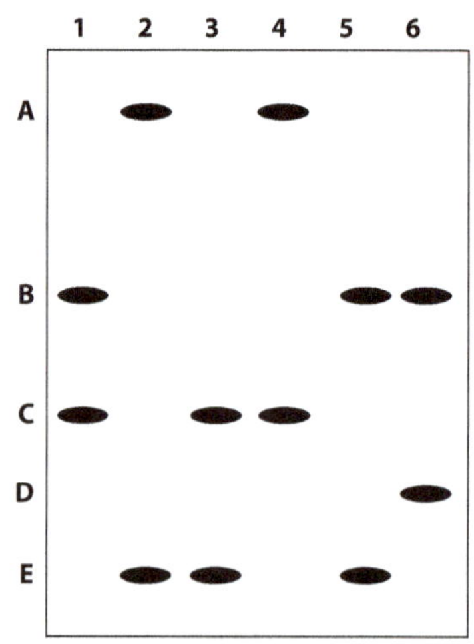

(A) All four children
(B) Child 1
(C) Child 2
(D) Child 3
(E) Child 4
(F) None of the children can be excluded

5. Single-locus STR analysis was performed on DNA from four children and their biological father. During the analysis, the label on the tube of DNA from the father was marred and thus, unreadable. The results of the STR analysis are shown in the figure where the letters A through D correspond to the different alleles of the analyzed STR. Given these results, which of the following STR alleles most likely corresponds to those that would correspond to the biological mother of the four children?

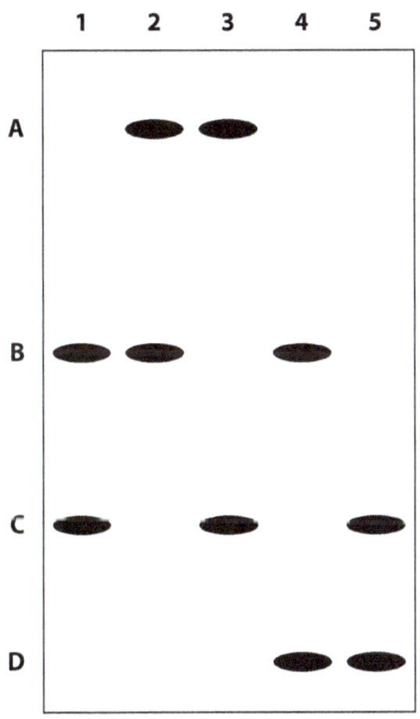

(A) A and B
(B) A and C
(C) A and D
(D) B and C
(E) B and D

6. The parents of four children are expecting their fifth child. Their first child (II-1), a 10-year-old female, has had numerous episodes of mild to moderate splenomegaly, mild chronic hemolysis, and jaundice. These symptoms appear during periods of acute viral infection such as the flu. The parents are concerned that their unborn child might also suffer the same symptoms. The family was tested via RFLP analysis. The accompanying pedigree includes Southern blot RFLP results from a marker exhibiting negligible recombination with the disease gene in this family. Unfortunately, no results could be obtained for either the mother (I-2) or the affected daughter (II-1). The unborn child has also been tested but the disease status of the fetus is unknown at this time. Based upon the available RFLP data, which of the following most likely represents the genotype and expected RFLP banding pattern for the affected child, II-1?

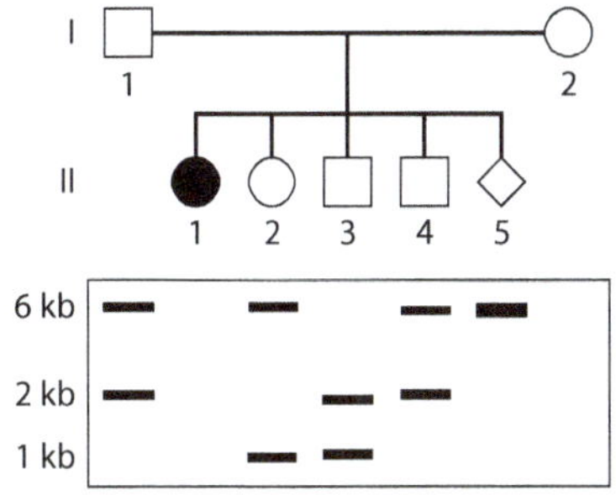

(A) Heterozygous 2 kb/1 kb
(B) Heterozygous 6 kb/1 kb
(C) Heterozygous 6 kb/2 kb
(D) Homozygous 1 kb/1 kb
(E) Homozygous 2 kb/2 kb
(F) Homozygous 6 kb/6 kb

7. A 27-year-old woman, gravida 2, para 1, who is at 10 weeks' gestation is being tested at a molecular genetics clinic. The patient's first child has a transfusion-dependent form of β-thalassemia. The prenatal diagnostic test used to determine if the fetus is affected is based upon the polymerase chain reaction method. Which of the following is most likely necessary to carry out this test?
(A) Chain-terminating dideoxynucleotides
(B) Cloned copies of the child's β-globin genes
(C) DNA ligase
(D) Oligonucleotides complementary to sequences in the β-globin gene
(E) Restriction endonucleases

8. A family has undergone molecular testing to hopefully identify the cause of a disease that is afflicting three family members. DNA was isolated from each individual and subjected to PCR using primers for a gene suspected of being the cause of the disease in this family. Given the results of this assay, which of the following is the most likely mechanism contributing to the manifestation of the disease?

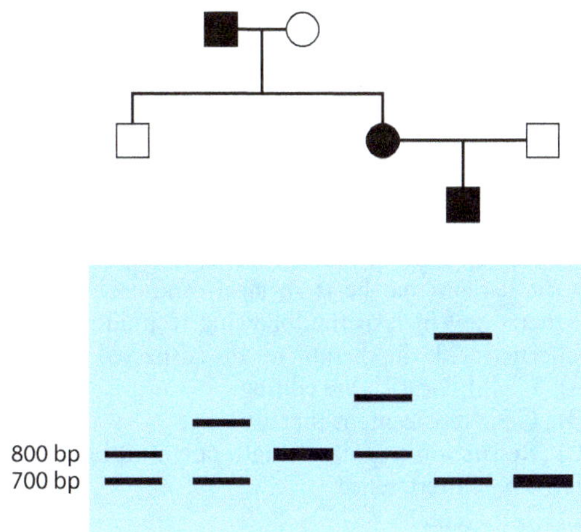

(A) Aberrant imprinting
(B) Exon skipping
(C) Frame-shift mutation
(D) Germ-line mosaicism
(E) Trinucleotide repeat expansion

9. A PCR-based test is being developed in order to test for the presence of a specific disease gene allele in several individuals. Genomic DNA is used as the source of template in this assay and the PCR primers are designed to amplify a region suspected of harboring a restriction fragment length polymorphism (RFLP). Following PCR and restriction enzyme digestion, the products are separated by gel electrophoresis with the results shown. Which of the following lanes most likely corresponds to the results that would be expected in an individual demonstrating heterozygosity at the RFLP?

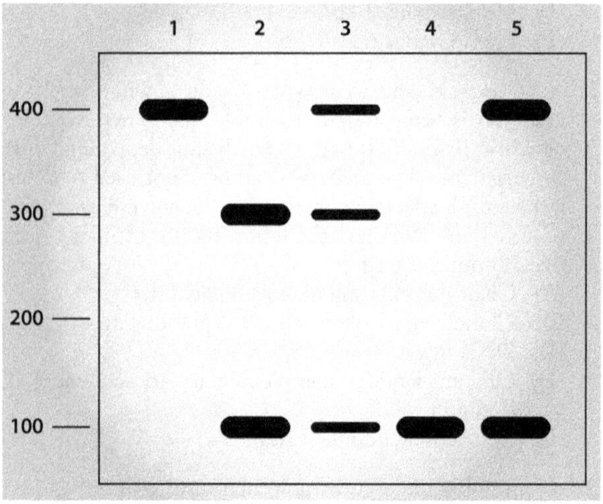

(A) 1
(B) 2
(C) 3
(D) 4
(E) 5

10. A 47-year-old man is being examined by his personal physician because of a progressive dementia, evolving involuntary movements, and changes to his affect. History indicates that the patient noticed frequent uncontrolled spasmodic twitching of his fingers beginning about 1 year ago. Physical examination indicates clumsiness, hyperreflexia, and eye movement disturbances. The physician makes a diagnosis and suggests to the patient that he is an ideal candidate for a new form of therapy. Which of the following techniques is most likely associated with the therapy for the suspected disease?
(A) CRISPR-cas9 gene editing
(B) Gene replacement therapy
(C) Restriction fragment length polymorphism, RFLP
(D) RNA interference
(E) Transgenesis

11. Clinical trials are being carried out to assess the efficacy of a new treatment for age-related macular degeneration. These trials involve the introduction of a vector expressing a short hairpin RNA that targets the vascular endothelial cell growth factor receptor (VEGFR). Which of the following statements most closely describes the characteristics of this form of therapy that make it useful as a therapeutic approach to treatment of this disease?
(A) It activates a phosphodiesterase thus, interfering with the cAMP signaling mediated by VEGFR activation
(B) It prevents an agonist of the VEGFR protein
(C) It produces an antagonist of the VEGFR protein
(D) It specifically targets the VEGFR mRNA for degradation
(E) It triggers the interferon response preventing translation of the VEGFR mRNA

12. Experiments are being carried out to insert fragments of the human genome into an appropriate vector and using the vector to transform bacterial cells. Which of the following is the most likely material to be used to generate these constructs?
(A) DNA complexed with bacterial histones
(B) Human chromosomal fragments
(C) Purified DNA treated with restriction endonucleases
(D) Purified euchromatin treated with restriction endonucleases
(E) Purified heterochromatin treated with restriction endonucleases

13. A 2-year-old boy has been diagnosed with deficiency in glucose-6-phosphate dehydrogenase. There is no family history of the disease. Molecular analysis of the infant's DNA identifies a novel deletion of six nucleotides in exon 12. Which of the following mechanisms best accounts for the symptoms in this infant?
(A) Deletion of two codons
(B) Exon skipping
(C) Frameshift mutation
(D) Missense mutation
(E) Trinucleotide expansion

14. Experiments are being conducted on the regulated expression of genes from the β-globin cluster by studying a known transcription factor. These experiments involve analysis of primary cultures of cells isolated from fetal, neonatal, and adult liver and bone marrow. The analysis will utilize a DNA-based probe containing sequences complimentary to the target transcription factor. Which of the following represents the best technique for determining the tissue culture sample that expresses the gene of interest?
(A) DNA sequencing
(B) Northern blot
(C) Polymerase chain reaction (PCR)
(D) Southern blot
(E) Western blot

15. Experiments are being conducted to determine which genes are differentially expressed in comparison between cells isolated from malignant breast cancer versus those in normal breast tissue. Pools of mRNA are purified from both types of cells and separately converted to cDNA in the presence of fluorescent nucleotides. These cDNA pools are collectively hybridized to a glass slide to which are attached synthetic oligonucleotides representing segments of 20,000 different genes. Which of the following most likely represents the technique being used in these experiments?
(A) CRISPR-mediated gene modification
(B) Fluorescence *in situ* hybridization
(C) Karyotype analysis
(D) Microarray analysis
(E) Southern blotting

16. A 10-year-old boy has suffered from chronic sinopulmonary disease including persistent infection of the airway with *Pseudomonas aeruginosa*. He has constant and chronic sputum production as a result of the persistent airway infection. Additionally, he suffers from gastrointestinal and nutritional abnormalities that include biliary cirrhosis and pancreatic insufficiency. The boy's mother is concerned about the chances of having another child with the same disease. Which of the following tests would be most useful for the determination of the probability of disease in another child?
(A) CRISPR-Cas9
(B) Karyotype analysis
(C) Microarray analysis
(D) Northern blot
(E) Southern blot

17. The postnatal examination of a newborn girl finds significant hypotonia. The infant was born at 35 weeks to a 43-year-old gravida 3 para 1 woman who did not undergo any ultrasonic examination during this latest pregnancy. The infant has a flat facial profile, upward-slanting eyes, and her tongue appears to protrude from her mouth. Given the most likely diagnosis, which of the following molecular testing methods would be the most useful for confirming this diagnosis?
(A) CRISPR-Cas9
(B) Karyotype analysis
(C) Microarray analysis
(D) Northern blot
(E) Southern blot

18. Experiments are being conducted to determine the molecular pathogenesis of colorectal cancer. These experiments aim to determine the level of overexpression and/or downregulation of certain genes in the colorectal tissues when compared to normal tissues. Which of the following laboratory techniques would be the one most likely to be used to best obtain the desired study results?
(A) Enzyme-linked immunosorbent assay (ELISA)
(B) Fluorescence *in situ* hybridization
(C) Karyotyping
(D) Northern blot
(E) Southern blotting

19. Clinical trials are being carried out to assess the efficacy of a new treatment for a form of colorectal carcinoma. These trials involve the use of a vector expressing a double-stranded RNA molecule that is 22 base pairs long and has one strand that is complimentary to region of the mRNA encoding the β-catenin protein. When this vector is introduced into colorectal carcinoma cells in culture, there is observed a significant reduction in the proliferative capacity of the cells. Which of the following best explains the mechanism by which this treatment exerted its effects?
(A) Activation of histone deacetylation
(B) Enhanced proteasome degradation of target proteins
(C) Interference with pre-mRNA splicing
(D) Post-transcriptional gene silencing
(E) Repression of transcription

20. A 4-month-old boy is brought to his pediatrician by his parents because they have noticed that he has developed a progressive lack of response to outside stimuli and that he does not seem to follow their voices with his eyes as he did the previous month. In addition, they say that their son exhibits an exaggerated startle response to sharp sounds and that he seems to be losing previously acquired motor and mental skills. History indicates that the patient's parents are both Hasidic Jews. The pediatrician suspects that the infant has inherited a specific metabolic disease and recommends tissue testing. A biopsy is taken, and the pathology lab prepares the sample for analysis. Which of the following represents the most likely technique that the pathology lab will carry out on the biopsy sample?
(A) CRISPR-Cas9
(B) Fluorescence *in situ* hybridization
(C) Karyotype analysis
(D) Molecular cloning
(E) Western blot

ANSWERS

1. Correct answer is **C.** The patient is most likely experiencing the symptoms of a β-thalassemia. The β-thalassemia result from mutations in the gene (*HBB*) encoding the β-globin protein resulting in reduced production of β-globin protein and accumulation of excess α-globin protein. Afflicted individuals suffer from severe anemia beginning in the first year of life leading to the need for blood transfusions. As a consequence of the anemia the bone marrow dramatically increases its' effort at blood production. The cortex of the bone becomes thinned leading to pathologic fracturing and distortion of the bones in the face and skull. In addition, there is marked hepatosplenomegaly as the liver and spleen act as additional sites of blood production. Without intervention these individuals will die within the decade of life. A characteristic feature of the erythrocytes in β-thalassemia gives them the appearance of a target. The target cell has an area of central density (a hyperchromic "bulls-eye") surrounded by a halo of pallor (hypochromic). Although not exclusive to β-thalassemia, target cells are, nonetheless, considered a characteristic feature of this disease. The most common cause of β-thalassemia is a mutation resulting in abnormal splicing of the mRNA derived from the *HBB* gene. This mutation results in an mRNA that is larger than normal and hence most easily detectable using a Northern blot. A dot blot (choice A) would not allow for the detection of size differences in mRNA or protein; it is only useful to detect the presence or absence of a particular macromolecule and the level of that macromolecule in a sample. The ELISA assay (choice B) could detect differences in amount of β-globin protein but if the antibody used in the assay was detecting an epitope of the β-globin protein that was now missing due to the slicing error, this assay would be of limited benefit. Southern blotting (choice D) would be useful provided the mutation resulting in the slicing error either introduced or removed a known restriction endonuclease recognition site. Western blotting (choice E), like the ELISA assay, is not the best choice for detection of the most common cause of the patient's β-thalassemia.

2. Correct answer is **E.** The patient most likely has sickle cell anemia. Sickle cell anemia is characterized by persistent episodes of hemolytic anemia and the occurrence of acute episodes referred to as sickling crises. The sickling red cells result in clogging of the fine capillary beds. In addition, due to these recurrent vasculo-occlusive episodes there are a series of complications. Because bones are particularly affected by the reduced blood flow, frequent and severe bone pain results. This is the typical symptom during a sickle cell crisis. In long term, the recurrent clogging of the capillary beds leads to damage to the internal organs, in particular the kidneys, heart, and lungs. The continual destruction of the sickled red blood cells leads to chronic anemia and episodes of hyperbilirubinemia. The mutation causing sickle cell anemia is a single nucleotide substitution (A to T) in the codon for amino acid 6. The change converts a glutamic acid codon (GAG) to a valine codon (GTG). The form of hemoglobin in persons with sickle cell anemia is referred to as HbS. The mutation in the *HBB* gene that causes sickle cell anemia results in the loss of a particular restriction endonuclease recognition site (MstII). This change in restriction endonuclease digestion of the *HBB* gene is the basis of the restriction fragment length polymorphism (RFLP) assay. By using cDNA cloning (choice A) one could detect the mutation causing sickle cell anemia, but the process is much longer and less specific than the RFLP assay. Genomic cloning (choice B) would present the same limitations, such as time and specificity, as cDNA cloning. The mutation causing sickle cell anemia is a single nucleotide change, therefore the resulting β-globin mRNA would not be different in size compared to wild-type β-globin mRNA and this mutation would not be detectable by Northern blotting (choice C). The polymerase chain reaction (choice D) is actually the foundation for most RFLP assays but is not exclusive to this assay, and therefore does not represent the most correct assay for diagnosis in this patient.

3. Correct answer is **C.** In order to determine global transcription differences, one needs to first convert all the mRNAs to cDNAs with the use of reverse transcriptase and then utilize quantitative PCR to amplify the resultant cDNAs to determine expression differences. The technique is referred to as RT-qPCR. cDNA cloning (choice A) would not allow for detection of differences in gene activity because the differences in the relative amounts of mRNA would be obscured by the process of converting them to cDNA. Genomic cloning (choice B) would not allow for determination of global expression differences between the two cell types. Southern blotting (choice D) and restriction fragment length polymorphism (choice E) would allow for detection of mutations in genes that might be responsible for the formation of the adenomatous polyp but would not allow for detection of differences in the expression level of the mutant and wild type genes.

4. Correct answer is **E.** All biological children will share alleles in common with their parents. Since each parent contributes only 50% of their alleles to each child, and the distribution is random, the pattern of alleles in children will not be the same as either parent. In this analysis it can be seen that the mother possesses alleles B and C while the father possesses alleles A and E of this particular STR. Therefore, all of their children should have some combination of the A, B, C, and E alleles. Since child 4 has allele B from the mother and a unique allele, D, not found in the father, this child is biologic to the mother but not to the father. Since child 4 is the only child that is not biologic to the father all four of the children (choice A) cannot be excluded. Child 1 (choice B), child 2 (choice C), and child 3 (choice D) are all biologic to the father and thus, cannot be excluded. The data generated in this STR analysis conclusively demonstrate the nonbiologic nature of child 4 so one, not none (choice F), of the children can be excluded.

5. Correct answer is **C.** To interpret this STR result, such that the alleles of the missing mother can be determined, it is first necessary to determine which lane corresponds to the alleles of the father. Each parent contributes one set of alleles to each child therefore, each child will share one band with the mother and one with the father. A process of elimination is used to determine which lane (1 through 5) contains the father's DNA. Once this has been accomplished then the alleles in the children that are not shared with the father must have been contributed by the missing mother. Lane 2 contains the alleles A and B and lane 5 contains alleles C and D and because these two lanes have no bands in common, neither lane can contain the DNA of the father. Similarly, lanes 3 and 4 contain no matching alleles so these lanes also cannot represent the father's DNA. Having ruled lanes 2 through 5 as being representative of the father's DNA this leaves only lane 1. Since biological children will contain at least one allele from the father and one from the mother, the alleles that came from the missing mother must be the A and D alleles. Choices A, B, D, and E all contain one of the father's STR alleles and thus, cannot represent the alleles of the missing mother.

6. Correct answer is **F.** Parents donate 50% of their alleles to their offspring so each child will inherit one allele from their mother and one from their father. From the available RFLP data it is evident that the 1 kb allele present in II-2 and II-3 must have come from the mother as this allele is absent in the father. Given that the unborn child (II-5) is homozygous for the 6 kb allele, the 6 kb allele must be the second allele present in the mother. Since children II-2, II-3, and II-4 are heterozygous and unaffected, the disease allele cannot be associated with the 1 kb band nor the 2 kb band and the disease is most likely autosomal recessive. Therefore, the most likely RFLP pattern for the affected child (II-1) is the same as the unborn child (II-5), homozygosity for the 6 kb allele. None of the other options (choices A, B, C, D, and E) correctly account for the most likely alleles in child II-1.

7. Correct answer is **D.** The polymerase chain reaction (PCR) assay is a powerful technique used to amplify DNA by several orders of magnitude, by repeated replication of a template, in a short period of time. The process utilizes sets of specific in vitro synthesized oligonucleotides that are complementary to sequences of a target gene to prime DNA synthesis. The design of the primers is dependent upon the sequences of the DNA that is desired to be analyzed and, in this case, they would need to be complimentary to sequences of the β-globin gene. None of the other options (choices A, B, C, and E) are required elements for the PCR assay.

8. Correct answer is **E.** The most likely manifesting disease in this family is Huntington disease. Huntington disease is caused by expansion of a CAG trinucleotide repeat in the first exon of the huntingtin gene (*HTT*). The CAG repeat resides 17 codons downstream of the initiator AUG codon and its expansion results in a polyglutamine stretch in the amino terminus of the huntingtin protein that is the cause of defective function of the protein. Huntington disease is inherited as an autosomal dominant disorder so only one of the two alleles of the *HTT* gene harbor the expanded CAG repeat. Therefore, there will be two bands from the PCR results for each individual in the family. All individuals whose PCR bands are less than 800 base pairs do not have the disease, whereas each individual with one band larger than 800 base pairs is manifesting the disease. This result demonstrates that the

manifestation of an autosomal dominant trinucleotide repeat disorder, such as Huntington disease, requires a threshold number of repeats for manifestation of disease. None of the other options (choices A, B, C, and D) would be reflected in the PCR results obtained from this family.

9. Correct answer is **C.** Individuals inherit one allele of a gene from each of their parents, therefore there will be two detectable copies of a gene of interest in an assay involving DNA. There is no indication that any of the individuals, from whom the results of this PCR-based RFLP analysis are obtained, are related and therefore there is no means to determine any relationship solely from the results of this assay. However, since all individuals harbor two alleles of a given gene, the results of a PCR-based RFLP assay can easily demonstrate homozygosity versus heterozygosity by the intensity of the products of the PCR. Since the bands in lane 3 are all approximately half the intensity of the bands in all the other lanes it is most likely that this individual is heterozygous where two bands are derived from one of the two alleles and the other band is derived from the other allele. All of the other lanes (choices A, B, D, and E) represent results that would most likely be associated with homozygous individuals where the intensity of each band represents two copies of the PCR-based RFLP products.

10. Correct answer is **D.** The patient is most likely suffering from Huntington disease. Huntington disease is inherited as an autosomal dominant disorder characterized by slowly progressive neurodegeneration associated with choreic movements (abnormal involuntary movements) and dementia. Huntington disease is caused by expansion of a CAG trinucleotide repeat in the first exon of the huntingtin gene (*HTT*). The CAG repeat resides 17 codons downstream of the initiator AUG codon and its expansion results in a polyglutamine stretch in the amino terminus of the huntingtin protein that is the cause of defective function of the protein. Since this is an abnormal protein, it is an amenable target for RNA interference (RNAi) mediated therapeutic intervention. The technique of RNAi involves a mechanism of RNA-directed regulation of gene expression principally at the level of the mRNA product of the targeted gene. Interference can involve mRNA degradation and a block to translation or both. The key to the utility of RNAi is the ability to reduce or remove an abnormal protein as opposed to gene replacement therapy (choice B) which is designed to introduce a normal copy of a mutant gene. The CRISPR-Cas9 gene editing technique (choice A) is a method for editing genomes that was adapted from a naturally occurring microbial adaptive immune system that utilizes RNA-guided nucleases. The use of the CRISPR technique is not restricted to mutagenesis alone, targeted site cleavage can be exploited to promote sequence insertion or replacement by recombination. However, the CRISPR technique is not currently approved for therapeutic use in humans in the United States. Restriction fragment length polymorphism (choice C) is a diagnostic technique not a therapeutic technique. Transgenesis (choice E) refers to the replacement or addition of DNA within the germline of an organism. This process can be utilized to correct gene defects but is not currently approved for use in humans.

11. Correct answer is **D.** The RNA interference (RNAi) pathway in mammals involves the enzymatic processing of double-stranded RNA into small interfering RNAs (siRNAs) of approximately 22–25 nucleotides that may have evolved as a means to degrade the RNA genomes of RNA viruses such as retroviruses. Since RNAi reduces the level of the target mRNA, the level of the encoded protein is consequently reduced. Therefore, the RNAi technique can prove useful in treating diseases where expression of a mutant or aberrant protein is the cause of the symptoms such as the VEGFR in the progression of age-related macular degeneration. None of the other options (choices A, B, C, and E) correctly define the mechanism by which RNAi can be useful in the treatment of disease.

12. Correct answer is **C.** Genomic DNA can be isolated from any cell (excluding mature red blood cells) or tissue for cloning. Following purification of the DNA, it is digested with restriction endonucleases to generate fragments in the size range that are optimal for the vector being utilized for cloning. None of the other options (choices A, B, D, and E) correctly define the source or type of DNA used to clone genomic DNA from the human genome.

13. Correct answer is **A.** The six-nucleotide deletion identified in the patient's glucose-6-phosphate dehydrogenase gene would be consistent with removing two codons from the mRNA. The deletion of two amino acids from the glucose-6-phosphate dehydrogenase protein is likely the cause of the deficiency identified in this patient. Exon skipping (choice B) would have removed a much larger section of the mRNA. A frameshift mutation (choice C) would have resulted if the number of base pairs deleted had not been a multiple of 3. A missense mutation (choice D) would not have affected the length, only the sequence. A trinucleotide expansion (choice E) would have introduced nucleotides into the patient's mRNA.

14. Correct answer is **B.** In a Northern blot, all the mRNA from cells or tissues, isolated by the presence of the poly(A) tail at the 3'-end of almost all mRNAs, is separated by size using electrophoresis in a gel. The separated mRNAs in the gel are then transferred to a suitable membrane such as a nitrocellulose filter or a positively charged nylon filter. The filter is then incubated with the probe which will hybridize to complementary mRNAs. Following hybridization, the excess probe is washed off and the location of the hybridized probe is detected by one of a variety of different methods. The mRNA that is detected by the probe represents the expression of that particular gene in that cell or tissue. DNA sequencing (choice A) and Southern blotting (choice D) are both incorrect, since they examine the DNA of the cell, and the DNA of all the cells is identical. Polymerase chain reaction (choice C) is used to amplify DNA and could not alone determine which tissue culture expressed the gene being studied. PCR can be used to amplify the DNA probe necessary for Northern blotting. Note that in this case, however, the DNA probe was supplied in adequate amounts, making PCR unnecessary. A Western blot (choice E) is used to characterize the level of expression, and to determine the size, of a particular protein or to assay the serum for antibodies against a specific protein. Total protein is extracted and then electrophoresed on a gel and then transferred to a nitrocellulose filter. The nitrocellulose filter is incubated with a patient's serum to identify the presence of antibodies that can bind to the protein. Western blotting can also be accomplished with the use of PVDF (polyvinylidene difluoride) membranes but these do not bind low quantities of smaller proteins with the same efficacy as nitrocellulose.

15. Correct answer is **D.** The technique being employed is microarray analysis, often termed gene chip analysis. Microarray analysis allows for the determination of the level of expression of a large set of genes at the same time in a single experiment. Although there are numerous uses for gene chips, the most common experiment involves a comparison of the expression of the genes on the chip between two samples, for example, cancer cells and normal cells. The assay is carried out by preparing RNA from each sample and converting the RNA to cDNA in the presence of fluorescent nucleotides. These "tagged" cDNA preparations are called "targets" and equal amounts of each target preparation are mixed together and then hybridized to the gene chip. After washing off the unhybridized targets and image processing of the chip it is possible to see spots that are only green, only red, or a color in between that represents a mix of some red and some green. Thus, some spots will be yellow, some will be orange or degrees of these intermediate combination colors. Spots that are only red indicate that the gene was expressed only in the source of the red labeled targets and vice versa for green spots. Intermediate colors indicate different levels of expression of a gene in both samples. The CRISPR-Cas9 (choice A) system is a technique to edit the nucleotide composition of a gene. The CRISPR-Cas system involves a vector designed to encode a single-guide RNA (sgRNA) that targets a specific DNA sequence. When the sgRNA is combined with a nuclease protein (such as Cas9), efficient and flexible gene editing is possible. Fluorescence *in situ* hybridization (choice B), commonly abbreviated FISH, is a technique designed to detect specific DNA sequences within the chromosome of a cell for the purpose of identifying various genetic abnormalities like duplications, deletions, inversions, translocations, and abnormal chromosome numbers, as well as specific gene amplifications or rearrangements. Karyotype analysis (choice C) is another technique used to examine chromosomes, primarily to detect chromosomal abnormalities such as trisomy 21. Southern blotting (choice E) is a technique that is primarily used to identify specific gene fragments following their separation by size using gel electrophoresis.

16. Correct answer is **E.** The boy is most likely manifesting the symptoms of cystic fibrosis. Whereas one of the most common molecular tests for cystic fibrosis is to sequence the *CFTR* gene, it is possible to identify abnormalities in the gene using the process of Southern blotting since many of the mutations will lead to restriction fragment polymorphisms that are detectable by this technique. The CRISPR-Cas9 (choice A) system is a technique to edit the nucleotide composition of a gene. The CRISPR-Cas system involves a vector designed to encode a single-guide RNA (sgRNA) that targets a specific DNA sequence. When the sgRNA is combined with a nuclease protein (such as Cas9), efficient and flexible gene editing is possible. Karyotype analysis (choice B) is a technique used to examine chromosomes, primarily to detect chromosomal abnormalities such as trisomy 21. Microarray analysis (choice C) is a technique that is used to determine the level of expression of a large set of genes at the same time in a single experiment. Northern blotting (choice D) is a technique designed to determine the size of a particular RNA as well as whether or not the gene encoding a particular mRNA is active. Although it is possible that there are some mutations in the *CFTR* gene that result in an altered size to the encoded mRNA, a result that finds an unchanged RNA size would not benefit a diagnosis in this patient.

17. Correct answer is **B.** The infant is most likely exhibiting the signs of Down syndrome which is caused by the presence of three copies of the acrocentric chromosome 23, referred to as trisomy 23. The risk for Down syndrome increases as the age of the mother increases, and this infant was born prematurely to a 43-year-old mother. The most useful method for the postnatal determination of whether the infant has Down syndrome is to perform a karyotype analysis. Karyotyping allows for the visualization of large-scale chromosomal structural abnormalities, particularly chromosomal aneuploidies such as trisomy 21. CRISPR-Cas9 (choice A) system is a technique to edit the nucleotide composition of a gene and is therefore of no utility in making a diagnosis in this infant. Microarray analysis (choice C) is a technique that is used to determine the level of expression of a large set of genes at the same time in a single experiment and is therefore, of little diagnostic value in this infant. Northern blotting (choice D) is a technique designed to determine the size of a particular RNA and since Down syndrome is due to trisomy of chromosome 21 this technique would not be able to aid in a diagnosis. Southern blotting (choice E) is a technique that is primarily used to identify specific gene fragments following their separation by size using gel electrophoresis.

18. Correct answer is **D.** Of the techniques listed, the use of Northern blotting would be most likely to obtain the desired results. Northern blotting is a technique designed to determine the size of a particular RNA as well as whether or not the gene encoding a particular mRNA is active. Although Northern blotting could be used to determine gene expression differences, in actuality the technique of microarray analysis would be the technique of choice for this type of experiment. The enzyme-linked immunosorbent assay, ELISA (choice A) technique is designed for detecting and quantifying soluble substances such as peptides and proteins. It can detect differences in protein amount from two different samples, but these differences may not be solely due to expression difference between tumor cells and normal cells. Fluorescence *in situ* hybridization (choice B), commonly abbreviated FISH, is a technique designed to detect specific DNA sequences within the chromosome of a cell for the purpose of identifying various genetic abnormalities like duplications, deletions, inversions, translocations, and abnormal chromosome numbers, as well as specific gene amplifications or rearrangements. Karyotype analysis (choice C) is a technique used to examine chromosomes, primarily to detect chromosomal abnormalities such as trisomy 21. Southern blotting (choice E) is a technique that is primarily used to identify specific genes fragments following their separation by size using gel electrophoresis, it does not allow for determination of whether a gene is transcriptionally active or not.

19. Correct answer is **D.** The technique utilized in the clinical trials is most likely RNA interference, RNAi. The RNAi pathway involves the enzymatic processing of double-stranded RNA into small interfering RNAs, siRNAs (also referred to as microRNAs, miRNAs) of approximately 22–25 nucleotides. Processed miRNA stem-loop structures are transported from the nucleus to the cytosol where they are engaged by the RNA-induced silencing complex (RISC) which separates the two RNA strands. The active strand of the miRNA is antisense to a region of the target mRNA. The RISC then initiates degradation of the target mRNA while also interfering with translation. The end results is reduction in protein synthesis from the targeted mRNA which is, in effect, a form of post-transcriptional regulation of gene expression. The RNAi technique does not activate histone deacetylation

(choice A) or enhance proteasomal degradation of proteins (choice B) nor does it lead to interference in pre-mRNA splicing (choice C) nor to repression of transcription (choice E).

20. Correct answer is **E.** The infant is most likely showing the signs and symptoms of Tay-Sachs disease. The most common form of Tay-Sachs disease in individuals of Ashkenazi Jewish ethnicity is the result of a four nucleotide (TATC) insertion in the gene (*HEXA*) encoding the α-subunit of the lysosomal hydrolase, β-hexosaminidase A (HexA). This mutation results in the synthesis of a truncated protein whose size change would be detectable with the use of the Western blotting technique. None of the other techniques (choices A, B, C, and D) would be useful for detecting the altered HexA protein that is the underlying cause of the signs and symptoms in this infant.

PART IV INTEGRATIVE BIOCHEMISTRY

CHAPTER 28

Digestive Processes

High-Yield Terms

Mucus	A viscous mixture covering mucus membranes, produced and secreted by cells of mucus membranes, consists of glycoproteins termed mucins, water, and several other proteins such as antiseptic enzymes and immunoglobulins
Enterocytes	Columnar epithelial cells of the intestines responsible for nutrient uptake
Chief cell	Gastric chief cells are those cells in the stomach that secrete the zymogen, pepsinogen; the parathyroid gland also contains chief cells
Parietal cell	Stomach glandular epithelial cells that secrete gastric acid in response to histamine, acetylcholine, and gastrin stimulation
Oxyntic cell	Another name for parietal cells
Duct cell	Specialized cells lining the pancreatic ducts that secrete bicarbonate
Acinar cell	A cell of an acinus which is any cluster of cells that resembles a many-lobed berry-like structure that is the terminus of an exocrine gland; acinar cells of pancreas are the duct cells that secrete bicarbonate and digestive enzymes
Enteroendocrine cell	Specialized endocrine cells found in the intestines and pancreas that produce various gastrointestinal hormones and bioactive peptides
Enterochromaffin-like cell (ECL)	Neuroendocrine cells that secrete histamine and found in gastric glands of the gastric mucosa
Gut microbiota	Refers to the complex mixture of microorganisms (bacteria, fungi, viruses) that reside within the gastrointestinal tract
Prebiotic	Refers to any nondigestible substance in food that stimulates the growth and/or activity of intestinal system bacteria
Probiotic	Refers to live bacteria that can be consumed in order to confer a health benefit

TABLE 28–1 Major anatomical locations in the overall digestive process.

Location	Major Function(s)
Oral cavity	Generation of saliva to lubricate masticated food; secretion of salivary enzymes; carbohydrate digestion only
Stomach	Production of HCl; secretion of digestive enzymes; protein and lipid digestion only; secretion of gastric hormone ghrelin
Pancreas	Secretion of lipid and protein digestive enzymes; secretion of bicarbonate to neutralize gastric acid
Liver	Production and secretion of bile acids required for lipid digestion in small intestine
Gallbladder	Storage and concentration of bile
Small intestine	Production of disaccharidases required for carbohydrate digestion; terminal digestion of carbohydrates, proteins, and lipids; absorption of nutrients and electrolytes
Large intestine (colon)	Storage of digestive waste; absorption of water and electrolytes

OVERVIEW OF DIGESTIVE SYSTEM

The gastrointestinal (GI) system, with respect to the processes of food digestion, comprises the hollow organs that include the oral cavity, the esophagus, the stomach, and the small and large intestines, each of which contribute specialized functions to the processes of digestion (Table 28–1). At the gross level, the GI system can be divided into the upper GI and the lower GI. The upper GI includes the mouth, esophagus, and the stomach (Figure 28–1). The lower GI includes the small and large intestines and the rectum. In addition to these hollow organs, digestion of food requires several accessory glands and other organs that add secretions to the hollow organs of the GI. The primary accessory organs necessary for digestion are the salivary glands present within the oral cavity, the pancreas, and the liver.

The GI organs are separated from each other at key locations by specialized structures termed sphincters. Entry of food from the oral cavity to the esophagus requires passage through the upper esophageal sphincter. The bolus of food then enters the stomach by passage through the lower esophageal sphincter. When food is propelled from the stomach into the duodenum of the small intestine it passes through the pyloric sphincter. On leaving the small intestines at the level of the ileum, digested food passes through the ileocecal valve into the large intestine, also referred to as the colon. Within the colon, waste is stored until it reaches the rectum which triggers nerve impulses to initiate defecation.

OVERVIEW OF FOOD ENERGY

The conventional assessment of energy value of a food takes into account the factors such as loss during digestion and absorption and thus, indicates the value of the food to the body as a fuel. The energy content of various food components is reported on product labels as either kilojoules/gram (kJ/g) or kilocalories/gram (kcal/g) (Table 28–2). Fat is the most energy-dense macronutrient, followed by alcohol, and then protein and carbohydrate. Amino acids from proteins, and the monosaccharides derived from dietary carbohydrates, contain more oxygen, relative to carbon and hydrogen,

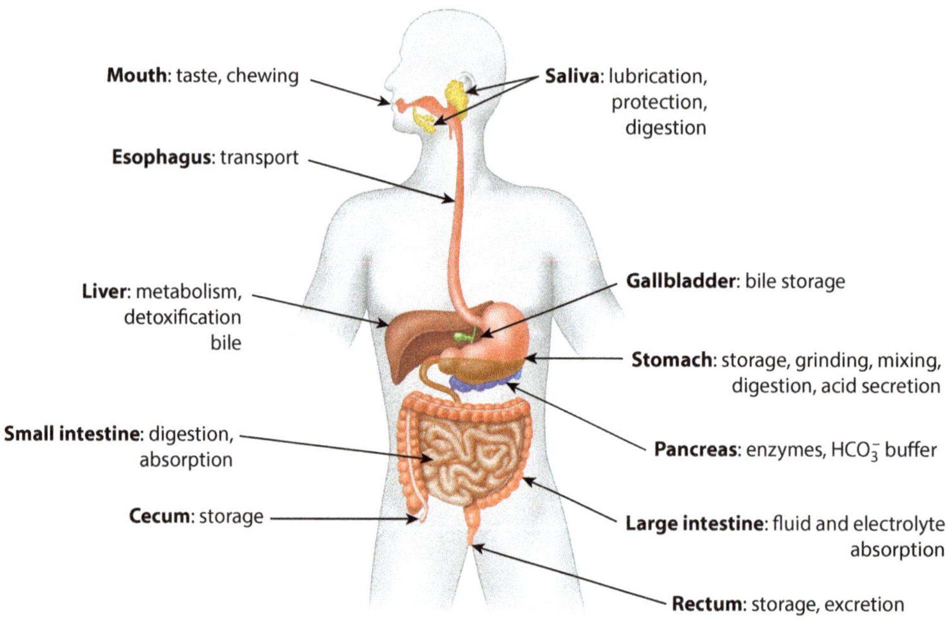

FIGURE 28–1 Overview of the major organs of digestion. Anatomical representation of the locations of the various organs of digestion from the mouth to the rectum. Each major area of digestion, along with the primary processes being carried out at those locations, are indicated. (Reproduced with permission from themedicalbiochemistrypage, LLC.)

TABLE 28–2 Standard energy composition of various food components.

Component	Energy (kJ/g)	Energy (kcal/gm)
Fat	37	9
Alcohol (specifically ethanol)	29	7
Protein	17	4
Carbohydrate	17	4
Organic acids	13	3
Sugar alcohols (sweeteners)	10	2.4
Fiber	8	2

such that they are already partially oxidized and, therefore, yield less energy than fatty acids which are in a more reduced state prior to their oxidation in the body.

Dietary fiber is not digested in the small intestines and therefore imparts limited to no caloric content to the human diet. Dietary fiber is also called roughage and consists of both soluble and insoluble components. Soluble fibers are so-called because they dissolve in water. These are easily fermented by intestinal bacteria and are referred to as prebiotics. The term probiotic refers to food or supplements that contain live bacteria intended to maintain or improve the normal microflora of the intestinal system. The advantage of insoluble fiber is that it absorbs water (particularly bulking fiber) as it transits the intestines softening the stool and thus, easing defecation. The fermentation of fiber by intestinal bacteria is known to be of physiological benefit since some of the products are absorbed and utilized for metabolic purposes such as the short-chain fatty acids (SCFA), acetate, propionate, and butyrate.

FUNCTIONS OF ORAL CAVITY

Visual and olfactory senses trigger the release of salivary fluids in preparation for mixing with the food. The primary contents of saliva include water, enzymes, and electrolytes (Table 28–3). Saliva is secreted from the parotid, submandibular, and sublingual glands within the oral cavity.

Chewing food is designed to chop, mash, and mix the contents of the mouth. The mixing of food and saliva represents the initial process of digestion. The action of α-amylase, on starch, releases glucose into the mouth. Glucose is sweet tasting which enhances the flavor of the food making it much more palatable and rewarding. When we swallow, the food is passed through the pharynx past the upper esophageal sphincter into the esophagus. Muscles in the esophagus then propel the food past the lower esophageal sphincter and into the stomach.

TABLE 28–3 Contents of saliva.

Component(s)	Functions/Comments
Water	Major component comprising almost 99% of the volume
Electrolytes	Sodium, potassium, phosphate, chloride, bicarbonate, calcium, magnesium
Mucus	A mixture of mucopolysaccharides and glycoproteins high in sialic acid and sulfated sugars, mixes with water to form a lubricant for ease of swallowing
α-Amylase	Secreted by acinar cells of the parotid and submandibular glands; initiates starch digestion into free-glucose monomers
Lingual lipase	Same enzyme as gastric lipase except within the oral cavity it is secreted by acinar cells of von Ebner glands; remains inactive until entering the acidic environment of the stomach where it functions along with gastric lipase (secreted by gastric Chief cells) to hydrolyze dietary triglycerides; functions only at acidic pH; active in the absence of bile acid emulsification as is required for pancreatic lipases
Lysozyme	Antibacterial enzyme that hydrolyzes β-1,4-glycosidic linkages between *N*-acetylmuramic acid and *N*-acetyl-D-glucosamine in cell wall peptidoglycans
Kallikrein	Secreted by acinar cells of all three major salivary glands, cleaves high molecular weight kininogen (HMWK) releasing the vasodilator, bradykinin
Antimicrobial components	Immunoglobulin, lactoperoxidase, lactoferrin, H_2O_2, thiocyanate
Opiorphin	Originally isolated from human saliva; encoded by the *PROL1* (proline-rich, lacrimal 1) gene; the five amino acid functional peptide (QRFSR) is released from the N-terminus of the preproprotein encoded by *PROL1*; functions to reduce sensations of pain via its ability to inhibit the enkephalin-inactivating peptidases neprilysin and ecto-aminopeptidase N
Transcobalamin I	Commonly called haptocorrin; encoded by the *TCN1* gene; binds vitamin B_{12} (cobalamin) to protect it from degradation in the acidic environment of the stomach; releases cobalamin in duodenum allowing it to be bound by intrinsic factor

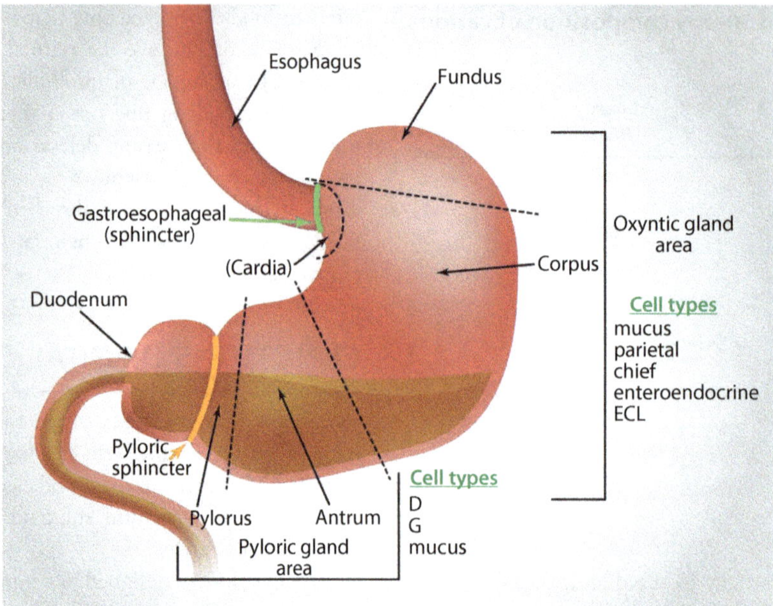

FIGURE 28–2 Organization of the major stomach segments. The three major structural areas of the stomach are denoted by the dashed lines. The cardia is indicated in parentheses due to the fact that there is controversy as to whether or not this constitutes a normal functional region of the stomach. The two major functional areas, the oxyntic gland area and the pyloric gland area, are denoted in the large brackets. The major cell types in these two functional domains are also indicated. Parietal cells secrete H^+ and Cl^- producing gastric acid and intrinsic factor which protects cobalamin (vitamin B_{12}) as it transits the small intestine to the distal ileum. Chief cells of the stomach secrete the zymogen protease, pepsinogen. ECL: enterochromaffin-like cells that secrete histamine. D: D cells that secrete somatostatin. G: G cells that secrete gastrin. The three primary enteroendocrine cells in the stomach includes ECL cells and G cells and also A (X-like) cells which release the appetite-stimulating hormone, ghrelin. (Reproduced with permission from themedicalbiochemistrypage, LLC.)

STOMACH

The role of the stomach in overall digestive processes is complex and unique. The unique digestive functions of the stomach are related to its structure and to the types of secretory products produced by various specialized exocrine cells (Figure 28–2). The stomach is tasked with storing ingested food, mixing ingested material with digestive juices and gastric acid, and then slowly emptying its contents past the pyloric sphincter into the duodenum. In addition to being responsible for digesting food, the stomach also absorbs water-soluble and lipid-soluble substances.

HIGH-YIELD CONCEPT

In addition to digestion, the stomach also plays a critical role in the sensations of appetite and satiety. These latter functions are related to the hormone ghrelin as well as to vagal nerve responses to the stomach stretching in response to uptake of the bolus of food from the esophagus.

The stomach is anatomically divided into three major segments termed the fundus (upper region of stomach), the corpus (body), and the antrum (see Figure 28–2). In addition, the stomach comprises two functional areas, the oxyntic gland and the pyloric gland areas. The oxyntic gland area comprises 80% of the stomach and encompassing both the fundus and the corpus. The pyloric gland area encompasses the antrum.

The mucosal lining of the corpus of the stomach contains two major types of specialized glands, the pyloric and oxyntic glands. The oxyntic glands are composed of parietal cells that secrete gastric acid, exocrine cells (chief cells) that secrete pepsinogen, and mucus-secreting cells. The acid secreting parietal cells are also called oxyntic cells. In addition, parietal cells of the fundus and corpus secrete intrinsic factor (see Chapter 3). The pyloric glands are located in the antrum segment of the stomach and contain cells that are responsible for secretion of gastrin (G cells), somatostatin (D cells), and mucus. Gastrin stimulates parietal cell acid secretion, and somatostatin inhibits gastric acid secretion.

There are five or six distinct types of enteroendocrine cells in the mucosal layer of the stomach which includes the G cells that secrete gastrin and the D cells that secrete somatostatin as well as the enterochromaffin-like cells (ECL) that secrete histamine, and A (X-like) cells that release the appetite-stimulating hormone, ghrelin.

Gastric Acid Production

Gastric acid production and secretion is the major exocrine function of parietal cells of the stomach. The production and secretion of gastric acid (HCl) is controlled by both hormonal- and nerve-mediated processes. The nervous system components that impact the GI tract are complex and consist of autonomic, parasympathetic (vagus), sympathetic (prevertebral ganglia), and

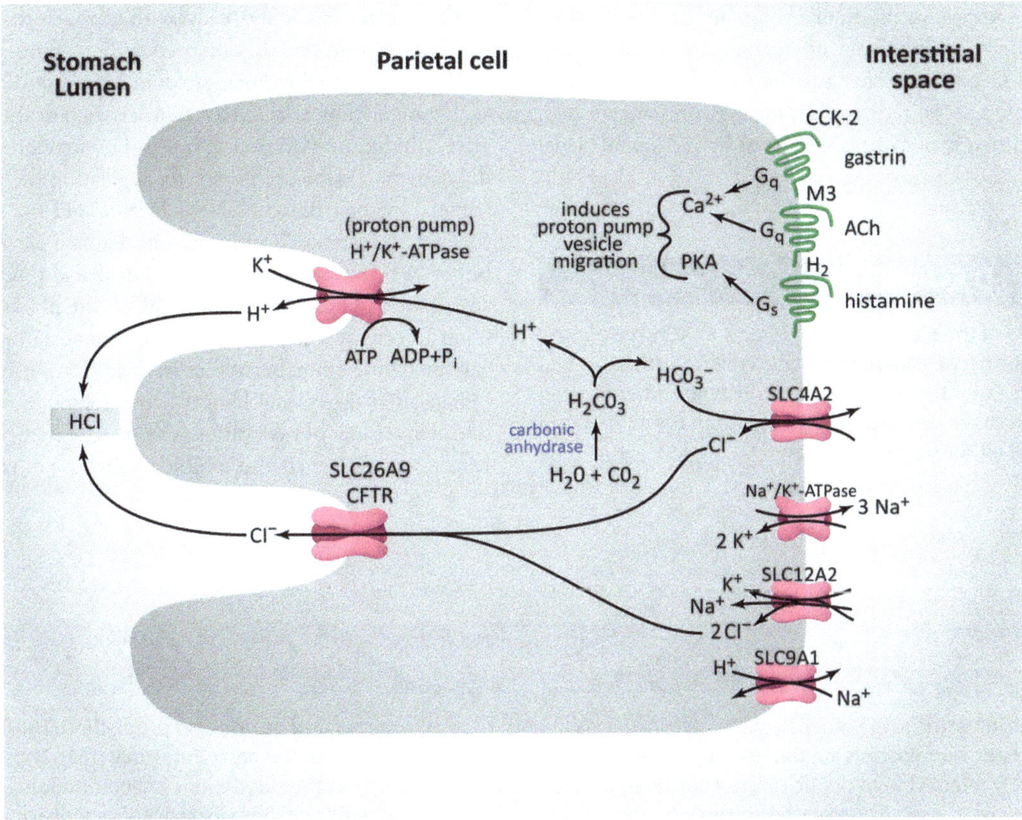

FIGURE 28–3 Biochemical and physiologic processes of gastric parietal cells. Gastric acid production by the stomach is triggered in response to the neurotransmitter acetylcholine (ACh), the gut peptide hormone gastrin, and by the neurotransmitter histamine. Stimulation of parietal cells by acetylcholine or gastrin binding to their respective G_q-coupled receptors ultimately triggers the release of intracellular calcium, Ca^{2+}. The gastric ACh receptor is the M3 receptor of the muscarinic acetylcholine receptor family. The gastrin receptor is the cholecystokinin 2 receptor, CCK-2. The released Ca^{2+} triggers the fusion of tubulovesicles containing the H^+/K^+-ATPase (proton pump) with the parietal cell apical membrane allowing transport of protons (H^+) into the canaliculus of the cell and out into the lumen of the stomach in exchange for K^+ uptake. Histamine binding to the G_s-coupled histamine H2 (H_2R) receptor on the basolateral membrane of parietal cells results in the activation of adenylate cyclase resulting in increased cAMP and activation of PKA which, via phosphorylation, triggers tubulovesicle fusion to the parietal cell apical membrane. Chloride ion loading in parietal cells, across the basolateral membrane, has been shown to be the function the Cl^-/HCO_3^- exchanger is encoded by the *SLC4A2* gene. This exchanger is commonly called anion exchanger 2 (AE2). Additional chloride transport into parietal cells occurs through the action of the $Na^+/K^+/2$ Cl cotransporter type 1 (NKCC1) encoded by the *SLC12A2* gene. Parietal cell basolateral Na^+ and K^+ exchange is carried out by the ubiquitous $\alpha1/\beta1$ Na^+/K^+-ATPase. Parietal cell basolateral membrane Na^+ and H^+ exchange is the function of one of the Na^+/H^+ exchangers (NHE) such as NHE1 encoded by the SLC9A1 gene. (Reproduced with permission from themedicalbiochemistrypage, LLC.)

enteric nerve fibers possessing both efferent (motor) and afferent (sensory) neurons. The enteric nervous system functions autonomously all along the GI tract as well as interacting with the CNS via vagal and prevertebral ganglia.

The principal stimulants for acid secretion are histamine, gastrin, and acetylcholine (ACh), the latter being released from postganglionic enteric neurons. Histamine is released from ECL cells in response to gastrin binding to these cells in fundal glands. The released histamine then binds to H_2 receptors on parietal cells. The H_2 receptor is a G_s-type GPCR (see Chapter 26) that activates adenylate cyclase, leading to elevation of intracellular cAMP concentrations and activation of PKA. With respect to gastric acid production, PKA activation leads to phosphorylation of cytoskeletal proteins involved in transport of the H^+/K^+-ATPase (proton pump) from the cytoplasm to the apical plasma membrane of the parietal cell. The H^+/K^+-ATPase transports one hydrogen ion (H^+) out of the cytoplasm of the parietal cell in exchange for one potassium ion (K^+) obtained from the lumen of the gastric gland (Figure 28–3).

The hydrogen ions are generated within the parietal cell from the ionization of carbonic acid that is generated from H_2O and CO_2 via the action of carbonic anhydrase. Carbonic acid rapidly ionizes to H^+ and bicarbonate ion. This bicarbonate is then transported to the blood, across the parietal cell basolateral membrane, in exchange for chloride ion. The chloride ions are transported into the lumen of the gastric glands via the action of anion exchangers of the solute carrier family that includes the *SLC26A9*-encoded transporter and the *CFTR*- (cystic fibrosis transmembrane conductance regulator) encoded transporter.

Vagal nerve endings on the stomach contain gastrin-releasing peptide (also known as bombesin or neuromedin B) that when released triggers G cells to secrete gastrin. Gastrin then binds to receptors on histamine-secreting cells and also on parietal cells. Gastrin exists in two major forms: little gastrin (17 amino acids) and big gastrin (34 amino acids) both of which result from a single precursor protein of 101 amino acids. Both forms of gastrin function by binding to the cholecystokinin 2 receptor (CCK2 or CCK_B).

HIGH-YIELD CONCEPT

The response of the stomach to the effects of ACh, gastrin, and histamine occur via a phenomenon referred to as potentiation. Potentiation is the effect observed where the response to two stimulants is greater than the sum of the effects of either stimulant alone.

Dysregulation of acid secretion is a significant cause of ulcerative conditions (Clinical Box 28–1), therefore, the body has developed an elaborate system for regulating the amount of acid secreted by the stomach. Gastric luminal pH is a sensitive regulator of acid secretion and protein in digested food is an excellent buffer. When the stomach is empty, or if acid production is excessive, gastric pH can fall below 3. When the pH falls, enteroendocrine D cells of the antrum secrete somatostatin which inhibits gastrin release from oxyntic cells. Acidification of the duodenal lumen also triggers mechanisms to inhibit gastric acid production. Under low pH conditions duodenal enteroendocrine S cells release secretin which also inhibits the release of gastrin.

CLINICAL BOX 28–1 DISTURBANCES IN GASTRIC ACID HOMEOSTASIS

Disturbances in gastric acid homeostasis involve increases in both basal and stimulated gastric acid production. These disturbances to gastric homeostasis are the leading causes of ulcers in the mucosal lining of the gastrointestinal tract. These ulcers are collectively referred to as peptic ulcers. Four times as many peptic ulcers arise in the duodenum (called duodenal ulcers) versus the stomach itself (called gastric ulcers). The major cause of disrupted gastric acid homeostasis (accounting for as much as 70–90% of such ulcers) is infection with *Helicobacter pylori* (*H. pylori*), a helical-shaped bacterium that lives in the acidic environment of the stomach. Around 4% of all gastric ulcers are caused by malignant tumors called gastrinomas. Stress ulcers are most often found in the proximal stomach and result from mucosal ischemia and altered mucosal defense. Although duodenal ulcers are the result of increased acid secretion, gastric ulcers are more often associated with normal or decreased basal and stimulated acid production. Gastric ulcers are, therefore, most often caused by altered gastric mucosal defense which explains the propensity for NSAID-induced ulcers to occur in the stomach. Gastric ulcers are classified into four groups according to their location and concomitant association with duodenal ulcer. Type I ulcers are found in the corpus and are generally characterized by low acid secretion, particularly at night. Type II ulcers occur in the antrum and are characterized by low, normal, or high acid secretion. Type III ulcers occur in close proximity to the pylorus and are associated with high acid output and duodenal ulcers. Type IV ulcers occur in the cardia and are characterized by low acid secretion. Treatment for gastric ulcers involves removing the injurious agent (eg, NSAID or *H. pylori*) and inhibiting acid secretion. Antacids were the first therapeutic approach for ulcers. Unfortunately, in order to neutralize luminal acid adequately they need to be taken frequently which results in noncompliance and adverse effects. Although antacids with high neutralizing capacity, given after meals and at bedtime, can accelerate ulcer healing, pain is not significantly reduced. The histamine H2 receptor antagonist (H_2RA), cimetidine, was the first of a new class of peptic ulcer treatments. H_2RA blocks both histamine-stimulated acid secretion and that induced by gastrin, which functions via stimulation of histamine release from ECL cells. The development of H^+/K^+-ATPase inhibitors (proton pump inhibitors, PPI), such as omeprazole, revolutionized the therapeutic management of gastric acid production. PPI directly inhibit the proton pump and therefore, they are capable of reducing both basal and stimulated gastric acid secretion independent of stimulus. PPI are much more effective than H_2RA at reducing gastric acid production as well as being more effective in aiding the healing of duodenal ulcers and preventing their recurrence. In addition to these more common conditions that cause abnormal gastric acid production resulting in ulcers, there are several uncommon conditions. The best characterized of the uncommon conditions is Zollinger-Ellison syndrome, ZES. ZES results from gastrin-producing tumors (gastrinomas) that result in hypersecretion of gastric acid. In any patient manifesting with refractory erosive esophagitis, multiple peptic ulcers, ulcers in the distal duodenum or jejunum, and recurrent ulcers after acid-reducing surgery, the possibility of ZES should be highly suspected. Patients with a family history of multiple endocrine neoplasia type 1 (MEN-1), or any of the endocrinopathies associated with MEN-1, that are presenting with multiple peptic ulcers should also be suspected of having ZES since approximately 25% of patients with ZES have MEN-1. MEN-1 is an autosomal dominant disorder characterized by pancreatic endocrine tumors, pituitary adenomas, and hyperparathyroidism. The PPI are used as the therapies of choice in the treatment of ZES, although very high doses are sometimes required to reduce the acid hypersecretion sufficiently. Recently, gastroesophageal reflux disease (GERD) has become the most important acid-related clinical disorder. The pathogenesis of GERD involve acid in the wrong anatomical location, not excess acid production. Numerous treatments for GERD have been attempted, but surgery is the most effective. Aside from surgery, the use of PPI are the most used drugs for treatment of GERD.

PANCREAS

The pancreas is a highly specialized organ found behind the stomach, and it is surrounded by the small intestine, liver, and spleen. The pancreas is composed primarily of two distinct types of secretory cells, endocrine and exocrine. The endocrine cells secrete a variety of hormones such as glucagon and insulin. The exocrine pancreas is involved in the secretion of numerous enzymes, electrolytes, and other substances involved in digestion (Table 28–4).

In addition to enzymes described in Table 28–4, the pancreas also secretes various cations, anions, water, and bicarbonate ion into the small intestine. Together with the pancreatic enzymes, the secretions constitute what is referred to as pancreatic juice. Pancreatic bicarbonate is critical to neutralizing the gastric acid entering the small intestine from the stomach. Like parietal cell bicarbonate production, pancreatic bicarbonate is dependent on the enzyme carbonic anhydrase. The content of bicarbonate in pancreatic juice (around 115 mEq/L) is approximately five times higher than what is normally present in plasma. This high concentration of bicarbonate makes the pH of pancreatic juice around 8.0.

Control of the secretory function of the acinar and duct cells of the pancreas is exerted via nervous and humoral mechanisms. The primary neural stimulus for pancreatic cell secretion of enzymes and bicarbonate is ACh released from postganglionic parasympathetic nerve endings. The primary hormonal triggers for acinar cell secretion are gastrin, cholecystokinin (CCK), and secretin.

SMALL INTESTINE

The intestines are divided into three major anatomical and functional segments termed the small intestine, the large intestine, and the rectum. The small intestine is further divided into three functionally distinct segments. These segments, from the stomach to the large intestines, are the duodenum, jejunum, and ileum.

The primary function of the intestines is the digestion of food and the absorption of nutrients (Table 28–5). The primary function of the large intestines is the resorption of water from food wastes thus creating fecal matter (the stool). The stool is then stored in the large intestines until it reaches the rectum where nerve impulses then stimulate the urge to defecate. In addition to water, the large intestines resorb sodium and any nutrients that may have escaped primary digestion in the ileum. The large intestine is also the site where gut bacteria (microbiota) are found. The importance of gut bacteria to human physiology is significant given that these microorganisms produce some vitamins and

TABLE 28–4 Pancreatic digestive enzymes.

Enzyme	Activator	Comments
α-Amylase	Chloride ion	Activity is the same as salivary α-amylase
Carboxyl ester lipase, CEL		Hydrolyzes cholesterol esters
Chymotrypsinogen	Trypsin	Cleaves proteins and peptides on the C-terminal side of aromatic amino acids, primarily Tyr, Pro, Trp
Colipase	Trypsin	Required at lipid-water interface for pancreatic lipase to function; the hormone enterostatin (which regulates fat intake) is derived from N-terminal end of pancreatic colipase; pentapeptide human enterostatin contains the sequence, APGPR
Deoxyribonuclease		Hydrolyzes DNA to free nucleotides
Pancreatic lipase		Hydrolyzes triglycerides to fatty acids and mono- and diacylglycerides; requires bile salt emulsified lipid droplets
Procarboxypeptidase A (A1 and A2)	Trypsin	Cleaves proteins and peptides on the C-terminal side of aromatic and aliphatic amino acids
Procarboxypeptidase B	Trypsin	Cleaves proteins and peptides on the C-terminal side of aliphatic amino acids
Proelastase	Trypsin	Cleaves proteins and peptides on the C-terminal side of basic amino acids
Ribonuclease		Hydrolyzes RNAs to free nucleotides
Secreted phospholipase A_2 ($sPLA_2$)	Trypsin	Hydrolyzes the *sn*2 position in phospholipids such as PE, PC, PI, PS releasing lysophospholipid (LPL) and a free fatty acid; at least 11 $sPLA_2$ genes; pancreatic enzyme is encoded by the *PLA2G1B* gene; lysophosphatidylcholine (LPC, lyso-PC) is a bioactive proinflammatory lipid generated by the action of $sPLA_2$
Trypsinogen	Enteropeptidase (also called enterokinase); embedded in duodenal mucosa	Cleaves proteins and peptides on the C-terminal side of Arg and Lys residues

TABLE 28–5 Nutrient absorption from various intestinal segments.

Intestinal Segment	Nutrients Absorbed
Duodenum	Calcium; magnesium; sodium; chloride; ferrous iron (Fe^{2+}), fat-soluble vitamins; glucose, galactose, and fructose
Jejunum	Heme iron; fats; fat-soluble vitamins; sucrose; lactose; proteins; amino acids; glucose; water-soluble vitamins
Ileum	Proteins; amino acids; cobalamin (vitamin B_{12}), folate, and other water-soluble vitamins; fat-soluble vitamins
Colon	H_2O; potassium; sodium; chloride; proton (H^+); bicarbonate; short-chain fatty acids (SCFA) derived from colonic microbiota metabolism of nondigestible fiber

important nutrients, and they digest molecules that cannot be degraded by human enzymes.

Within the small intestine, like the stomach, the epithelium possesses a specialized subset of cells termed enteroendocrine cells, EEC (Table 28–6).

GALLBLADDER

The gallbladder is a small organ lying just beneath the liver between the costal margin and the lateral margin of the rectus abdominis muscle. The gallbladder is the storage site for bile acids that were produced from cholesterol by the liver. The consumption of food, particularly lipid- and protein-rich foods, stimulates the release of CCK from duodenal enteroendocrine I cells which then enters the circulation and binds to receptors on the gallbladder. The binding of CCK to gallbladder cells induces pulsatile secretion of bile into the common bile duct which then meets with the pancreatic duct at the ampulla of Vater where they are secreted into the duodenum. Bile salts are involved in the emulsification of lipids in the intestines aiding their digestion by the various

TABLE 28–6 Enteroendocrine cells of the intestines.

Cell Type	Secreted Factor(s)	Major Functions
Enterochromaffin (EC) cells	Serotonin (5-HT)	Considered pan-GI cell types; found in stomach, small intestine, and large intestine; acting primarily through 5-HT_4 class receptors serotonin stimulates gastrointestinal motility and secretory processes
I cells	Cholecystokinin (CCK); serotonin (5-HT)	Predominantly found in the proximal small intestine; CCK stimulates gallbladder contractions and bile flow; increases secretion of digestive enzymes from pancreas; vagal nerves in the gut express CCK1 (CCK_A) receptors
K cells	GIP; 5-HT	Glucose-dependent insulinotropic peptide; predominantly found in the proximal small intestine; inhibits secretion of gastric acid; enhances insulin secretion; also referred to as gastric inhibitory peptide
L cells	GLP-1; PYY; OXM; GLP-2; 5-HT	Primarily located in ileum (distal small intestine) and colon; small numbers have been found in duodenum and jejunum **GLP-1:** glucagon-like peptide 1; potentiates glucose-dependent insulin secretion; inhibits glucagon secretion; inhibits gastric emptying **PYY:** protein tyrosine tyrosine; reduces gut motility; delays gastric emptying, inhibition of gallbladder contraction; exerts effects on satiety via actions in the hypothalamus **OXM:** contains all of the amino acids of glucagon; inhibits meal-stimulated gastric acid secretion similar to GLP-1 and GLP-2 action; induces satiety, decreases weight gain, and increases energy consumption; has weak affinity for GLP-1 receptor as well as the glucagon receptor, may mimic glucagon actions in liver and pancreas **GLP-2:** glucagon-like peptide 2; enhances digestion and food absorption; inhibits gastric secretions; promotes intestinal mucosal growth
M (Mo) cells	Motilin	Located in small intestine; distinct from the M cells of GI that are found in the lymph follicles termed Peyer's patches; motilin initiates inter-digestive intestinal motility; stimulates release of pancreatic polypeptide (PP); stimulates gallbladder contractions
N cells	Neurotensin	Located in jejunum; neurotensin is a 13-amino-acid peptide derived from a precursor that also produces neuromedin; involved in satiety responses and slows gastric emptying; also involved in nociception (sensation of pain)
S cells	Secretin	Located in the duodenum and jejunum; secretin induces pancreatic bicarbonate secretion; inhibits gastric secretions; stimulates PP secretion

pancreatic and duodenal lipases. Unused bile salts are returned to the gallbladder through the distal ileum and the portal circulation.

CARBOHYDRATE DIGESTION AND ABSORPTION

Dietary carbohydrates enter the body in complex forms, such as mono-, di-, and polysaccharides with the primary polysaccharides being plant starch (amylose and amylopectin) and animal glycogen. The carbohydrate polymer, cellulose, is also consumed but not digested.

The first step in the metabolism of digestible carbohydrate is the conversion of the higher polymers to simpler, soluble forms that can be transported across the intestinal wall and delivered to the tissues (Table 28–7). The breakdown of polymeric sugars begins in the mouth with salivary α-amylase. The action of salivary amylase is limited to the area of the mouth and the esophagus as it is virtually inactivated by the much stronger acid pH of the stomach. The main polymeric carbohydrate digesting enzyme of the small intestine is pancreatic α-amylase. The resulting di- and trisaccharides are hydrolyzed to monosaccharides by intestinal disaccharidases, maltase, sucrase-isomaltase, lactase (β-galactosidase), and trehalase (Table 28–7).

Glucose, fructose, and galactose represent the major monosaccharides absorbed by intestinal enterocytes. Intestinal absorption of carbohydrates occurs via passive diffusion, facilitated diffusion, and active transport (Figure 28–4). Glucose uptake involves the Na^+/glucose-dependent transporter 1 (SGLT1) and the Na^+-independent glucose transporter, GLUT2. Galactose is also absorbed from the gut via the action of SGLT1. Fructose is absorbed from the intestine via GLUT5 uptake. Transport of all three monosaccharides across the enterocyte basolateral membrane into the blood involves the action of GLUT2.

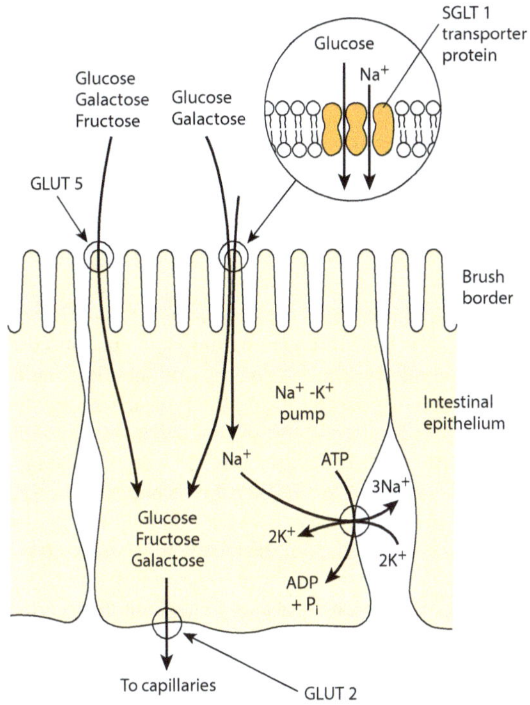

FIGURE 28–4 Transport of glucose, fructose, and galactose across the intestinal epithelium. The SGLT1 transporter is coupled to the Na^+-K^+ pump, allowing glucose and galactose to be transported against their concentration gradients. The GLUT5 Na^+-independent facilitative transporter allows fructose, as well as glucose and galactose, to be transported down their concentration gradients. Exit from the cell for all sugars is via the GLUT2 facilitative transporter. (Reproduced with permission from Rodwell VW, Bender DA, Botham KM, et al: *Harper's Illustrated Biochemistry*, 31st ed. New York, NY: McGraw Hill; 2018.)

TABLE 28–7 Carbohydrate digestive enzymes.

Enzyme	Substrate(s)	Products
Salivary and pancreatic α-amylases	α(1→4) glycosidic linkages in polysaccharides	Di- and trisaccharides and shortened polysaccharides
Maltase	Maltose: glucose disaccharide in α(1→4) glycosidic linkage	Glucose
Sucrase-isomaltase	Sucrose and isomaltose	Glucose and fructose
β-Galactosidase complex (lactase + glucosylceramidase)	Lactose, ceramides	Glucose and galactose
Trehalase	Trehalose: glucose disaccharide in α(1→1) glycosidic linkage	Glucose

Reproduced with permission from King MW: *Integrative Medical Biochemistry Examination and Board Review*. New York, NY: McGraw Hill; 2014.

PROTEIN DIGESTION AND PEPTIDE AND AMINO ACID ABSORPTION

The biological value of dietary proteins is related to the extent to which they provide all the necessary amino acids. Proteins of animal origin generally have a high biological value; plant proteins have a wide range of values from almost none to quite high. In general, plant proteins are deficient in lysine, methionine, and tryptophan, and are much less concentrated and less digestible than animal proteins. The absence of lysine in low-grade cereal proteins, used as a dietary mainstay in many underdeveloped countries, leads to an inability to synthesize protein (because of missing essential amino acids) and ultimately to a syndrome known as kwashiorkor, common among children in these countries (Clinical Box 28–2).

The digestion of dietary protein begins in the stomach and continues within the lumen of the duodenum. The initial enzyme involved in protein digestion is gastric pepsin. The zymogen, pepsinogen, is secreted from chief cells in the stomach in response

CLINICAL BOX 28–2 NUTRITION DEFICIENCY SYNDROMES

Marasmus and kwashiorkor represent two extremes of nutritional deficit in humans. Marasmus (derived from the Greek word for decay) is a form of severe malnutrition characterized by overall energy deficiency. Kwashiorkor is a form of malnutrition due to a deficiency in protein but with sufficient caloric intake. Marasmus can occur in both children and adults, whereas Kwashiorkor is only seen in children. Marasmus results from a severe deficiency of nearly all nutrients, especially protein and carbohydrates. A typical child with marasmus looks emaciated and has a body weight less than 60% of that expected for the age. Marasmus is commonly seen in children living in poverty primarily in tropical and subtropical parts of the world, particularly in countries where the diet consists mainly of corn, rice, and beans. Treatment of marasmus is normally divided into two phases. The initial acute phase of treatment involves restoring electrolyte balance, treating infections, and reversing the hypoglycemia and hypothermia. This is followed by re-feeding and ensuring that sufficient caloric and nutrient intake is maintained to enable catch-up growth in order to restore a healthy normal body mass. Kwashiorkor is an acute form of childhood protein-energy malnutrition characterized by edema causing the typical bulging stomach seen in affected children. Kwashiorkor also results in, irritability, anorexia, skin ulcers, and hepatomegaly due to fatty infiltration. The hepatomegaly also contributes to the protuberant abdomen in these children. Kwashiorkor is common in areas of famine or poor food supply. Kwashiorkor usually occurs when a baby is weaned from protein-rich breast milk and switched to protein-poor foods. This weaning usually occurs due to the birth of another child. Treatment of Kwashiorkor involves careful administration of protein with the use of carbohydrate and fat for the majority of caloric needs of the child. This is due to the fact that the administration of too much protein will lead to increased hepatic urea cycle activity. Since the liver is already compromised due to the fatty infiltration, the metabolism of protein can exacerbate the damage and lead to liver failure and death.

to the action of gastrin and to vagal nerve release of ACh. Within the small intestines there are two principal pancreatic enzymes involved in protein digestion; these are trypsin and chymotrypsin. Several additional pancreatic peptidases play a lesser role in peptide digestion (see Table 28–4).

Following digestion, free amino acids as well as peptides (2–3 amino acids in length) are absorbed by enterocytes of the proximal jejunum. Some absorption also occurs in the duodenum and a minor amount in the ileum. Endogenous proteins, such as intestinal hormones and peptides, are absorbed intact, occurring primarily within the large intestines.

The absorption of amino acids requires an active transport process that is dependent on either Na^+ or H^+ cotransport. There are several amino acid transporters encompassing seven distinct transport systems which are further grouped into three broad categories. These three categories are the neutral amino acid (monoamino monocarboxylic) transporters, the dibasic (and cysteine) amino acid transporters, and the acidic (dicarboxylic) amino acid transporters. All of the amino acid transporters are members of the solute carrier (SLC) family of transporters.

Intestinal uptake of peptides involves H^+ cotransporters which are also members of the SLC family. The most abundant peptide transporter is PepT1 (SLC15A1) but there are three additional peptide transporters within the SLC15 subfamily. Within intestinal enterocytes the absorbed peptides are hydrolyzed to free amino acids via cytoplasmic peptidases. The free amino acids are then transported across the apical membranes of enterocytes and enter the portal circulation. Patients with Hartnup disorder, due to defective neutral amino acid transport (see Clinical Box 18–1), can remain asymptomatic on a high-protein diet due to peptide absorption via PepT1.

LIPID DIGESTION AND ABSORPTION

The predominant form of dietary lipid in the human diet is triglyceride (TG or TAG). GI lipid digestion consists of several sequential steps that include physicochemical and enzymatic events. The physicochemical processes of lipid digestion involve the formation of large micelle aggregates or emulsion particles that consist of water and water-insoluble substrates. Bile acids, secreted into the duodenum, are important for lipid emulsification. Lipolysis occurs at the lipid-water interface of the micelle aggregates.

The enzymes involved in intestinal lipid digestion include gastric lipase and the pancreatic enzymes including pancreatic lipase, $sPLA_2$, carboxyl ester lipase (CEL), as well as other acylglycerol hydrolases and phospholipases (Figure 28–5).

Gastric lipase hydrolyzes primarily short- and medium-chain fatty acid linkages on the *sn*3 position of triglycerides. The liberated medium-chain fatty acids can be absorbed directly in the stomach. Secretion of gastric lipase is stimulated by both hormonal and cholinergic mechanisms that involve gastrin, CCK, and ACh. Lingual lipase and gastric lipase are not dependent on bile acids or colipase for maximal hydrolytic activity.

After passing from the stomach the digestion of triglycerides continues in the duodenum with colipase-dependent pancreatic lipase and the other pancreas-derived lipid hydrolyzing enzymes. Colipase is secreted by the pancreas in an inactive form and then activated in the intestinal lumen by trypsin. Cholesterol esters are hydrolyzed to free cholesterol and a free fatty acid via the action of CEL. Phospholipids are hydrolyzed to lysophospholipids and a free fatty acid via the action of pancreatic $sPLA_2$.

Absorption of digested lipids, free fatty acids, monoglycerides, lysophospholipids, free cholesterol, fat-soluble vitamins,

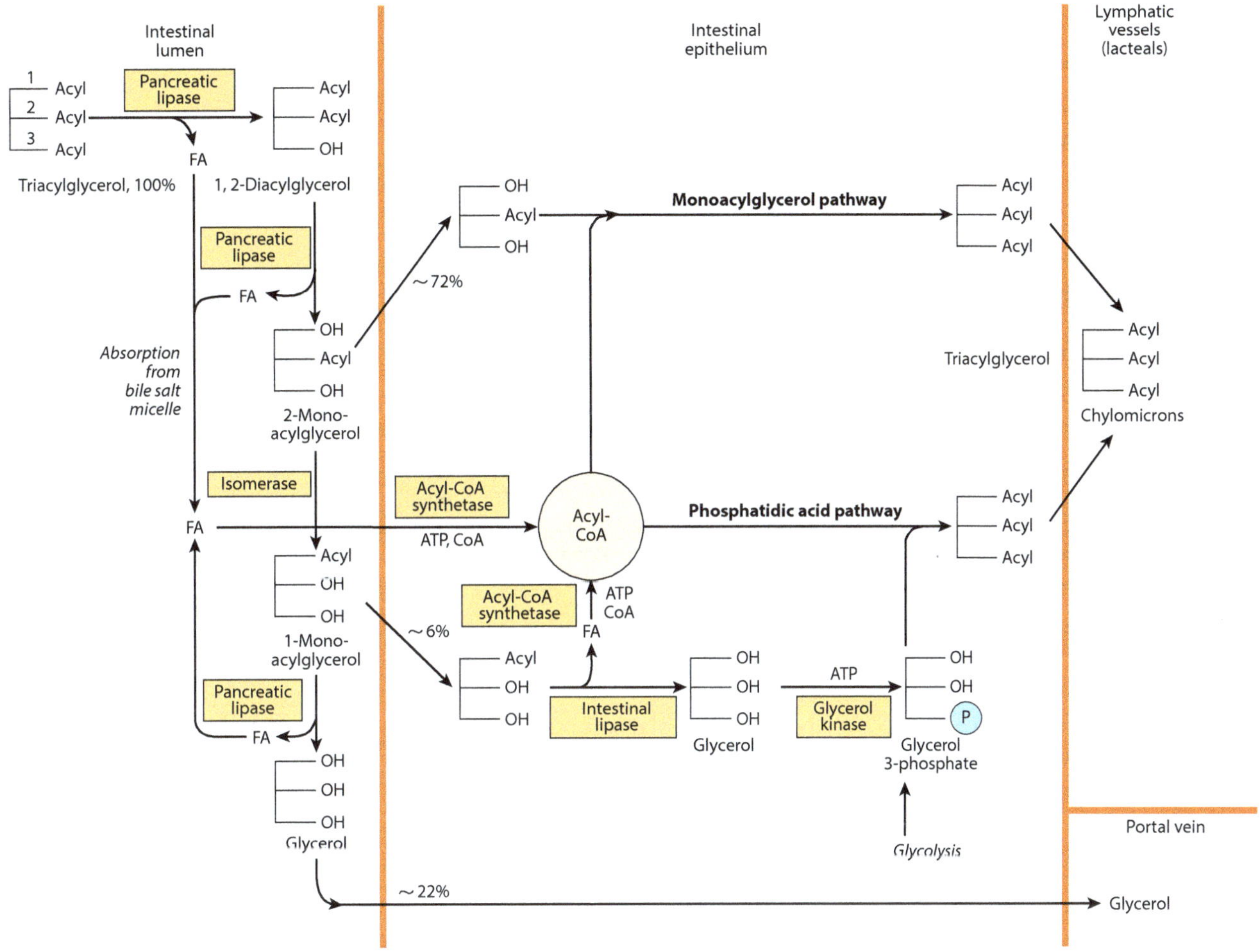

FIGURE 28–5 Digestion and absorption of triacylglycerols. The values given for percentage uptake may vary widely but indicate the relative importance of three routes shown. (Reproduced with permission from Rodwell VW, Bender DA, Botham KM, et al: *Harper's Illustrated Biochemistry*, 31st ed. New York, NY: McGraw Hill; 2018.)

occurs when mixed micelles containing these lipids interact with enterocyte brush-border membranes. Fatty acid uptake by intestinal enterocytes occurs via protein-independent diffusion and by protein-dependent transport. The fatty acid transport protein, FAT/CD36, plays a key role in the intestinal uptake of fatty acids. Another transport protein involved in facilitated fatty acid uptake is fatty acid transport protein 4, FATP4. Intestinal cholesterol uptake involves the transporter encoded by the *NPC1L1* (Niemann-Pick C1-like protein 1) gene. The cholesterol absorption inhibitor, ezetimibe, exerts its effect by inhibition of the NPC1L1 transporter.

HIGH-YIELD CONCEPT

Most monogenic forms of diabetes, termed maturity onset type diabetes of the young (MODY), are due to mutations in genes involved in pancreatic cell function (see Chapter 30). However, a rare form of MODY (termed MODY8) that is characterized by dominantly inherited childhood-onset pancreatic exocrine dysfunction and diabetes has been shown to be due to mutations in the *CEL* gene. Notably, this gene is not transcribed in pancreatic β-cells but is only expressed in the acinar cells of the pancreas and in lactating mammary gland cells. The cause of the pancreatic dysfunction in MODY8 is due to aggregation of the mutant CEL protein and the formation of amyloidotic deposits that are toxic to the pancreas resulting in an associated loss of β-cell function.

CHECKLIST

- ☑ The digestion of food involves a complex series of events that begins with the sight and smell and even the thought of food which leads to the stimulation of the salivary glands in the mouth.
- ☑ Digestion begins in the mouth with chewing and mixing of the masticated food with saliva. Contained in saliva is a-amylase, as well as many other substances, which begins the process of carbohydrate digestion.
- ☑ Chewing and swallowing represent the only voluntary processes of digestion.
- ☑ All of the involuntary processes of digestion, such as stomach and intestinal peristalsis, stomach and intestinal secretion of digestive enzymes, peptides, and hormones, gallbladder secretion of bile acids, and pancreatic secretion of digestive enzymes and bicarbonate, occur via the actions of the enteric, parasympathetic, and sympathetic nervous systems.
- ☑ The enteric nervous system acts independent of, as well as in conjunction with, the parasympathetic and sympathetic nervous systems primarily via the vagal nerve.
- ☑ The swallowing of food deposits the partially digested material into the stomach where the acidic environment denatures proteins allowing them to be hydrolyzed by pepsin secreted from cells in the stomach. Lipid hydrolysis is initiated in this acidic environment by lingual lipase secreted in saliva and gastric lipase secreted in the stomach. Both of these lipases have optimum activity in acidic pH but are no longer active when the contents of the stomach enter the duodenum and encounter the alkaline pancreatic juice.
- ☑ Once the digested material, now referred to as chime, is passed from the stomach to the small intestines the full process of carbohydrate, protein, and lipid digestion is completed via the actions of the numerous pancreatic and intestinal brush-border membrane associated enzymes.
- ☑ Within the duodenum and proximal jejunum, absorption of monosaccharides, amino acids, small peptides, monoacylglycerides, fatty acids, cholesterol, lysophospholipids, and glycerol takes place via both passive and active transport into intestinal enterocytes.

REVIEW QUESTIONS

1. A patient is being examined by his physician with complaints of cramping in the lower belly, bloating, gas, and diarrhea. These symptoms appear within 30 minutes to 2 hours after the ingestion of dairy products. On the advice of his physician, the patient agrees to cease the ingestion of foods that contain which of the following?

(A) Fructose
(B) Galactose
(C) Glucose
(D) Lactose
(E) Sucrose

2. A 29-year-old female patient has come to her physician with the primary complaint that she can no longer taste sweetness in food, particularly fruits. Suspecting that she may be suffering from glossitis her physician examines her tongue for signs consistent with this diagnosis but notes no obvious anomalies. Ultrasonic examination shows the presence of stone-like abnormalities in her salivary ducts. Given these findings, the loss of sweet taste sensation is most likely due to a defect in the secretion of which of the following?

(A) α-Amylase
(B) Haptocorrin
(C) Lingual lipase
(D) Lysozyme
(E) Mucin

3. A 19-year-old woman is being examined by her physician with complaints of fatigue, muscle cramping, intestinal pain and bloating, diarrhea, and weight loss. History reveals that these symptoms began in the past 6 months and are worse following the consumption of bread. Physical examination shows pallor. Given the signs and symptoms in this patient, which of the following is most likely to be an additional complication?

(A) Hepatomegaly
(B) Megaloblastic anemia
(C) Menorrhagia
(D) Microcytic anemia
(E) Renal lithiasis

4. A physician on a mission to treat patients in a refugee camp in Ethiopia encounters numerous children with a common cluster of signs and symptoms. The symptoms observed in these children include chronic diarrhea, dizziness, fatigue, delayed wound healing, and muscle wasting. These children have had very little food to eat, consisting of a meager daily serving of powdered milk and rice. Which of the following most likely contributed to the symptoms in these patients?

(A) Adequate daily calories that are lacking in an essential fatty acid
(B) Adequate dietary carbohydrate and fat but inadequate protein
(C) Adequate daily protein but inadequate amounts of carbohydrate and fat
(D) Too much protein precipitating renal insufficiency
(E) Total daily caloric intake that is below the level required for adequate growth

5. A 57-year-old man is being examined by his physician due to complaints of frequent gnawing and burning pain in the middle and upper stomach occurring between meals and most acutely at night. Additional symptoms reported by the patient include heartburn and blackish stools. The patients' physician suspects that he is suffering from a peptic ulcer. A defect in which of the following cells in the gastrointestinal tract would most likely be expected given this diagnosis?
(A) Chief cells
(B) Enterochromaffin-like (ECL) cells
(C) Enteroendocrine L cells
(D) Gastric mucus cells
(E) Parietal cells

6. Experiments are being carried out to test the efficacy of several novel compounds in the treatment of gastroesophageal reflux disease (GERD). Initial studies are being done with the use of cultures of gastric parietal cells. Results from the use of one compound show an inhibition of proton (H^+) secretion from the cells when they are treated with acetylcholine. This compound is most likely inhibiting the activity of which of the following?
(A) Adenylate cyclase
(B) Carbonic anhydrase
(C) Na^+/K^+-ATPase
(D) Phospholipase Cβ
(E) Protein kinase A

7. A 37-year-old woman has been taking omeprazole every day for the past 4 years as a means to control her painful acid reflux and heartburn. Which of the following represents the most likely consequence of her chronic use of this drug?
(A) Hypocalcemia
(B) Hypokalemia
(C) Iron-deficiency anemia
(D) Megaloblastic anemia
(E) Microcytic anemia
(F) Pellagra

8. A 41-year-old man has come to his physician with complaints of near constant burning pain in his upper stomach which gets worse when he lies down at night. He informs his doctor that his stools are black and that he frequently vomits up blood. A preliminary diagnosis of Zollinger-Ellison syndrome is made; however, a gastric biopsy shows no apparent gastrinoma. Abnormal activity in the secretory function of which of the following cell types would most likely be associated with the symptoms in this patient?
(A) Chief cells
(B) D cells
(C) Enterochromaffin-like (ECL) cells
(D) Enteroendocrine cells
(E) Mucus cells

9. A 63-year-old man is being seen by his physician as a follow-up to gastric surgery for the treatment of a severe duodenal ulcers. This patient has the ulcers removed by surgical resection of the proximal portion of the duodenum to the distal end of the antrum of the stomach. The patient has been prescribed a proton (H^+) pump inhibitor (PPI) because the surgery required removal of the region of the stomach that contains cells involved in the negative regulation of acid secretion. Which of the following represents the most likely cells lost in the surgery?
(A) Chief cells
(B) D cells
(C) Enterochromaffin-like (ECL) cells
(D) G cells
(E) Parietal cells

10. A 33-year-old woman has recently undergone abdominal surgery to remove a significant portion of her ileum due to damage caused by Crohn disease. Which of the following would be most likely in this patient as a consequence of her surgery?
(A) Hypocalcemia
(B) Hypokalemia
(C) Iron-deficiency anemia
(D) Megaloblastic anemia
(E) Microcytic anemia
(F) Pellagra

11. A 45-year-old woman has come to her physician with complaints of insatiable hunger that began within the past 4 months. CT scan finds a mass in the corpus of her stomach. Analysis of a biopsy sample of the mass shows significant levels of hormone secretion. Over secretion of which of the following would most likely explain the patient's primary symptom?
(A) Gastrin
(B) Ghrelin
(C) Glucagon-like peptide 1 (GLP-1)
(D) Histamine
(E) Somatostatin

12. A 43-year-old man has come to his physician with a complaint that his stools have recently acquired a foul smell and have an oily consistency. Ultrasonic examination reveals no apparent abnormalities in the gallbladder or pancreas. Biopsy of the main pancreatic duct also shows no overt pathology. Analysis of pancreatic secretions isolated during the biopsy would most likely show a reduction or loss in the presence of which of the following activities?
(A) α-Amylase
(B) Carboxyl ester lipase
(C) Pancreatic lipase
(D) Phospholipase A_2 (PLA_2)
(E) Trypsinogen

13. A physician on a mission to treat patients in a refugee camp in Ethiopia encounters numerous children with a common cluster of signs and symptoms. These include protuberant abdomens, generalized edema, loss of muscle mass, lethargy, irritability, and fatigue. Given the constellation of symptoms in these patients, treatment would most likely include which of the following?
(A) High concentration of total protein and/or essential amino acids
(B) Increased total caloric intake with a balance of protein, carbohydrate, and fat
(C) Initially begin with minimal protein
(D) Solely carbohydrate-rich foods
(E) Solely essential fatty acids

14. A 47-year-old man has come to his physician with complaints of near constant burning pain in his upper stomach which gets worse when he lies down at night. Suspecting the patient may have gastroesophageal reflux disease (GERD), his physician orders a series of tests to be performed on biopsy tissue

taken from the corpus of the stomach. Biochemical studies discover that cAMP-dependent protein kinase (PKA) is constitutively active in these cells. Molecular studies identify an activating mutation in one of the receptors that participates in gastric acid production. Which of the following most likely represents this mutant receptor?
(A) Acetylcholine M3 receptor
(B) α_1-Adrenegic receptor
(C) α_2-Adrenergic receptor
(D) Cholecystokinin 2 receptor
(E) Histamine H2 receptor

15. A 33-year-old woman has recently undergone abdominal surgery to remove a significant portion of her ileum as a result of damage done by Crohn disease. As a result of this surgery, which of the following is most likely to be elevated in the blood of this patient?
(A) Alloisoleucine
(B) Lactic acid
(C) Methylmalonic acid
(D) Phenyllactate
(E) Phytanic acid

16. A 59-year-old man is admitted to the emergency department with an 8-hour history of severe epigastric pain. History finds that the patient is a chronic alcohol consumer. The patient indicates that the pain radiates to his back and is more intense when he lies down. Physical examination reveals tachycardia, hypotension, and low-grade fever consistent with the early stage of shock. Which of the following serum measurements would be most useful in providing a diagnosis of his condition?
(A) Amylase
(B) Aspartate transaminase, AST
(C) Carbonic anhydrase
(D) Ferritin
(E) Lactate dehydrogenase
(F) Unconjugated bilirubin

17. A 32-year-old man is being examined by his physician with concerns over his recent weight loss. He reports that he cannot eat as much food as he previously could due to near constant sensations of being full. Postprandial testing finds that the rate of gastric emptying is significantly delayed. Examination by CT scan shows no abnormalities in the stomach, the pyloric sphincter, nor the small intestines. Excessive activity of which of the following would most likely account for the symptoms in this patient?
(A) Acetylcholine
(B) Cholecystokinin, CCK
(C) Gastrin
(D) Histamine
(E) Motilin
(F) Pancreatic polypeptide, PP

18. A 6-year-old girl is being examined by her pediatrician due to concerns of her parents about her abdominal pain and watery stools. History reveals that the child has had frequent colds over the past 18 months and that her symptoms appear the most severe when she drinks milk or eats ice-cream. Given the most likely diagnosis in this patient which of the following is most likely to be deficient?
(A) Calcium
(B) Cobalamin
(C) Iron
(D) Niacin
(E) Thiamine

19. A 47-year-old man has come to his physician with complaints of near constant burning pain in his upper stomach which gets worse when he lies down at night. Suspecting the patient may have gastroesophageal reflux disease (GERD), his physician prescribes an appropriate pharmacologic treatment. Which of the following is the most likely target of this therapy?
(A) Chief cells
(B) D cells
(C) Enterochromaffin-like (ECL) cells
(D) G cells
(E) Parietal cells

20. A 59-year-old man is admitted to the emergency department with an 8-hour history of severe abdominal pain. History finds that the patient is a chronic alcohol consumer. Physical examination finds a palpable mass in his left upper quadrant and CT scans confirm the presence of a tumor. Surgery is scheduled to remove the tumor and the surrounding pylorus and antrum regions of the stomach. As a result of this surgery, secretion of which of the following is most likely to be diminished in this patient?
(A) Histamine
(B) Hydrogen ion
(C) Intrinsic factor
(D) Pepsinogen
(E) Somatostatin

ANSWERS

1. Correct answer is **D.** The patient is most likely deficient in intestinal lactase and is thus, lactose intolerant. The signs and symptoms of lactose intolerance usually begin 30 minutes to 2 hours after eating or drinking foods that contain lactose. The typical symptoms of lactose intolerance include nausea, vomiting, diarrhea, bloating, gas, and painful abdominal cramping. The bloating and gas results from the bacterial fermentation of the lactose in the colon. The diarrhea is the result of the osmotic nature of lactose that interferes with intestinal water reabsorption. Ingestion of none of the other carbohydrates (choices A, B, C, and E) would result in the symptoms manifesting in this patient.

2. Correct answer is **A.** The patient is most likely experiencing the consequences of the lack of components normally found in saliva. The primary contents of saliva include water, enzymes, and electrolytes. Saliva is secreted from the parotid, submandibular, and sublingual glands within the oral cavity. The mixing of food and saliva represents the initial process of digestion. The action of α-amylase on starch releases glucose into the mouth. Glucose is sweet tasting which enhances the flavor of the food making it much more palatable and rewarding. Haptocorrin (choice B), also known as transcobalamin I, is present in saliva to protect cobalamin in the diet while it is in the acidic environment of the stomach. Lingual lipase (choice C) is an acidic lipase that functions solely in the stomach where it is involved in the initial stages of dietary lipid digestion. Salivary lysozyme (choice D) functions as an antimicrobial in the mouth. Mucin (choice E) is a mixture of mucopolysaccharides and glycoproteins high in sialic acid and sulfated sugars and it mixes with water to form a lubricant for ease of swallowing.

3. Correct answer is **D.** The patient is most likely experiencing the symptoms associated with celiac disease. In patients with celiac disease the protein, gluten, which is found in bread, oats, and many other foods containing wheat, barley, or rye, triggers an autoimmune response that causes damage to the small intestine leading to widespread manifestations of malabsorption. Iron-deficiency anemia is a common pathology in celiac disease. The typical symptoms of iron-deficiency anemia are extreme fatigue, pale skin (pallor), dizziness, headaches, and cold hands and feet. Deficiency of iron prevents the synthesis of heme in bone marrow erythroid progenitor cells. The lack of heme results in suppression of protein synthesis such that these bone marrow blast cells remain small resulting in microcytic anemia. Calcium deficiency is also a common pathology in celiac disease because it is difficult to absorb. The symptoms of hypocalcemia include muscle cramping, tetanic contractions, numbness, and tingling sensations. For sensory and motor nerves, calcium is a critical second messenger involved in normal cell function, neural transmission, and cell membrane stability. The nerves respond to a lack of calcium with hyperexcitability. None of the other symptoms (choices A, B, C, and E) are commonly associated with celiac disease.

4. Correct answer is **E.** The children being treated are most likely suffering from the nutritional disorder known as marasmus. Marasmus is a form of severe malnutrition caused by a deficiency of nearly all nutrients, especially protein and carbohydrates. A typical child with marasmus looks emaciated and has a body weight less than 60% of that expected for the age. Treatment of marasmus is normally divided into two phases. The initial acute phase of treatment involves restoring electrolyte balance, treating infections, and reversing the hypoglycemia and hypothermia. This is followed by re-feeding and ensuring that sufficient caloric and nutrient intake is maintained to enable an adequate growth rate in order to restore a healthy normal body mass. Another malnutrition disorder often encountered in children house in refugee camps is referred to as kwashiorkor. Kwashiorkor is the result of inadequate protein intake in the presence of adequate carbohydrate and fat (choice B). None of the other options (choices A, C, and D) correctly reflect the cause of the symptoms in these children.

5. Correct answer is **E.** Peptic ulcers are painful sores occurring in the lining of the stomach or in the proximal duodenum. One of the most common causes of peptic ulcers is excessive gastric acid secretion from the parietal (oxyntic) cells of the stomach. On rare occasions, this excess acid production is due to gastrinomas (Zollinger-Ellison syndrome) in the antrum of the stomach. Chief cells of the stomach (choice A) secrete the zymogen protease, pepsinogen. Enterochromaffin-like cells (choice B) secrete histamine. Overactivity of histamine release from ECL cells could result in abnormal gastric acid production given that histamine is a major stimulator of parietal cell function. However, it is more likely that a defect in these cells would lead to loss of histamine production. Enteroendocrine L cells (choice C) are present in the small intestines and do not contribute to gastric acid production. Gastric mucous cells (choice D) synthesize and secrete a mixture of mucopolysaccharides and glycoproteins high in sialic acid and sulfated sugars that form a protective lubricant within the lumen of the stomach.

6. Correct answer is **D.** Acetylcholine is one of three factors responsible for the simulation of gastric parietal cells releasing proton (H^+) into the lumen of the stomach in the process of gastric acid production. Acetylcholine activates two different classes of receptor, the muscarinic acetylcholine receptors and the nicotinic acetylcholine receptors. The muscarinic acetylcholine receptors are members of the large family of G-protein–coupled receptors, GPCR. The acetylcholine receptor on parietal cells is the M3 muscarinic acetylcholine receptor. The M3 receptor is coupled to a G_q-type G-protein that activates phospholipase Cβ (PLCβ). Activated PLCβ hydrolyzes membrane localized phosphatidylinositol-4,5-bisphosphate (PIP_2) releasing inositol-1,4,5-trisphosphate (IP_3). IP_3 binds to receptors on the endoplasmic reticulum that are calcium ion channels, the activation of which leads to calcium release to the cytosol. The increase in cytosolic calcium results in mobilization of vesicles containing the gastric proton pump (H^+/K^+-ATPase) to the apical membrane of parietal cells which allows for increased proton transport to the lumen of the stomach. None of the other proteins (choices A, B, C, and E) are directly involved in the action of acetylcholine on parietal cells.

7. Correct answer is **D.** The most likely complication resulting from chronic consumption of proton (H^+) pump inhibitors, such as omeprazole, is the consequence of a vitamin B_{12} deficiency. Vitamin B_{12} (as the hydroxocobalamin form) is synthesized exclusively by microorganisms and is primarily found in the liver of animals bound to protein as methylcobalamin or 5′-deoxyadenosylcobalamin. The vitamin must be released from these binding proteins in order to be active and this release occurs in the stomach by the gastric protease, pepsin. Pepsin is generated by autocatalytic cleavage of pepsinogen which is stimulated by gastric acid. After being released, cobalamin is bound to the salivary protein called haptocorrin (transcobalamin I) and is caried to the duodenum where it then interacts with intrinsic factor. Prolonged inhibition of the parietal H^+/K^+-ATPase (proton pump) by omeprazole will lead to increased pH of the stomach and reduced activation of pepsinogen. This will result in reduced release of cobalamin from the binding proteins leading to impaired uptake from the distal ileum. Vitamin B_{12}, specifically methylcobalamin, is a critical cofactor in the methionine synthase reaction, an enzyme that also requires folate as N^5-methyl tetrahydrofolate (methyl-THF). Inhibition of methionine synthase, as a consequence of vitamin B_{12} deficiency, results in all the folate being trapped as methyl-THF. The trapping of folate by methionine synthase due to vitamin B_{12} deficiency prevents the use of folate in the synthesis of purine nucleotides and thymidine nucleotides. The lack of adequate purine nucleotide and thymidine, in particular, prevents DNA synthesis. Erythroid progenitor cells in the bone marrow become larger during the G_1 phase of the cell cycle because the lack of thymidine prevents DNA synthesis, and these enlarged megaloblastic cells are released from bone marrow and can be visualized in a blood smear. None of the other options (choices A, B, C, E, and F) represent likely complications of chronic consumption of proton pump inhibitors.

8. Correct answer is **C.** The principal stimulants for gastric acid production are histamine, gastrin, and acetylcholine (ACh).

Gastrin is released from G cells of the stomach and acetylcholine is released from postganglionic enteric neurons. Histamine is thought to be the primary stimulus. Histamine is released from enterochromaffin-like (ECL) cells in response to gastrin binding to these cells in fundal glands of the upper stomach. The released histamine then binds to histamine H_2 receptors on parietal cells inducing a signaling cascade that results in the transport of the H^+/K^+-ATPase (proton pump) from the cytoplasm to the apical plasma membrane of the parietal cell. Increased release of histamine, resulting from excessive activity of ECL cells would, therefore, result in excessive secretion of gastric acid leading to ulceration of the mucosal lining of the stomach. Chief cells of the stomach (choice A) secrete the zymogen protease, pepsinogen. D cells (choice B) secrete somatostatin whose function is to inhibit gastrin release from G cells and histamine release from ECL cells. Enteroendocrine cells (choice D) of the stomach collectively refers to ECL cells, G cells, and A (X-like) cells which release the appetite-stimulating hormone, ghrelin. Gastric mucous cells (choice E) synthesize and secrete a mixture of mucopolysaccharides and glycoproteins high in sialic acid and sulfated sugars that form a protective lubricant within the lumen of the stomach.

9. Correct answer is **B.** The antrum of the stomach is also referred to as the pyloric gland area. The pyloric glands contain cells that secrete gastrin and somatostain. Somatostatin is secreted by D cells and exerts a tonic paracrine inhibition of gastrin secretion from G cells, thereby, controlling overall gastric acid secretion by parietal cells of the fundus and corpus of the stomach. Somatostatin can also interfere with gastric acid secretion exerted by the action of histamine. Somatostatin blocks histamine release from enterochromaffin-like cells (choice C) in the gastric mucosa. Chief cells of the stomach (choice A) are found in the corpus of the stomach, and they secrete the zymogen protease, pepsinogen. Enteroendocrine cells (choice D) of the stomach collectively refers to ECL cells, G cells, and A (X-like) cells, the latter release the appetite-stimulating hormone, ghrelin. Parietal cells (choice E) are found in the corpus of the stomach, and they secrete proton (H^+) and chloride ion (Cl^-) to generate gastric acid and also secrete intrinsic factor which binds and protects cobalamin (vitamin B_{12}) in the small intestine.

10. Correct answer is **D.** The ileum is responsible for the absorption of proteins, amino acids, cobalamin (vitamin B_{12}), folate, and several additional water-soluble vitamins, and the fat-soluble vitamins. The uptake of vitamin B_{12} occurs exclusively in the distal ileum and loss of this region of the small intestine would significantly impact levels of the vitamin. Vitamin B_{12}, specifically methylcobalamin, is a critical cofactor in the methionine synthase reaction, an enzyme that also requires folate as N^5-methyl tetrahydrofolate (methyl-THF). Inhibition of methionine synthase, as a consequence of vitamin B_{12} deficiency, results in all the folate being trapped as methyl-THF. The trapping of folate by methionine synthase due to vitamin B_{12} deficiency prevents the use of folate in the synthesis of purine nucleotides and thymidine nucleotides. The lack of adequate purine nucleotide and thymidine, in particular, prevents DNA synthesis. Erythroid progenitor cells in the bone marrow become larger during the G_1 phase of the cell cycle because the lack of thymidine prevents DNA synthesis, and these enlarged megaloblastic cells are released from bone marrow and can be visualized in a blood smear. The majority of dietary calcium is absorbed from the duodenum and thus, hypocalcemia (choice A) is unlikely. The majority of potassium is absorbed from the colon and thus, hypokalemia (choice B) is unlikely. Because iron is also absorbed from the duodenum and the jejunum, the loss of iron absorption from the ileum is not significant enough to result in the development of an iron-deficiency anemia (choice C) nor a microcytic anemia (choice E). Most water-soluble vitamins are also absorbed from the jejunum and therefore deficiency of niacin, which would result in pellagra (choice F), is not likely.

11. Correct answer is **B.** The patient is most likely experiencing the symptoms that would be associated with excessive secretion of ghrelin by the stomach. Ghrelin is produced and secreted by the A (X-like) enteroendocrine cells of the stomach oxyntic (acid secreting) glands. Because the A (X-like) cells express ghrelin they are also sometimes referred to as ghrelin cells or Gr cells. A (X-like) cells express the receptor for gastrin (gut hormone that stimulates gastric acid secretion by the stomach) and, therefore, it is believed that gastrin may directly stimulate ghrelin release. Ghrelin is the only gut hormone to induce hunger (orexigenic) sensations. The major effect of ghrelin released to the blood is exerted within the central nervous system at the level of the arcuate nucleus of the hypothalamus where it stimulates the synthesis and release of the orexigenic neuropeptides, neuropeptide Y (NPY), and agouti-related protein (AgRP). None of the other hormones (choices A, C, D, and E) elicit an orexigenic response. Indeed, GLP-1 exerts effects within the gastrointestinal system to slow gastric emptying which results in increased sensations of satiety.

12. Correct answer is **C.** The pancreas is composed primarily of two distinct types of secretory cells, endocrine and exocrine. The exocrine pancreas has ducts that are arranged in clusters called acini (singular acinus). Pancreatic digestive secretions are expelled into the lumen of the acinus and then accumulate in intralobular ducts that drain into the main pancreatic duct. The main pancreatic duct (pancreatic duct of Wirsung) joins the common bile duct coming from the gallbladder forming the ampulla of Vater. The ampulla is connected to the duodenal papilla through which the pancreatic juice, also containing bile, enters the small intestine. The pancreas secretes enzymes responsible for carbohydrate, protein, and lipid digestion. In addition to enzymes, the pancreas also secretes various cations, anions, water, and bicarbonate ion into the small intestine. Together with the pancreatic enzymes, the secretions constitute what is referred to as pancreatic juice. Pancreatic bicarbonate is critical to neutralizing the gastric acid entering the small intestine from the stomach. Pancreatic lipase is the primary lipase that hydrolyzes dietary triglycerides in the small intestines. The action of alkaline pancreatic juice results in inhibition of the activity of the acid lipases (lingual and gastric) that begin the process of triglyceride hydrolysis in the stomach. Loss of pancreatic lipase secretion would, therefore, result in incomplete digestion of dietary fats preventing their absorption and leading to increased fat content of the stools (steatorrhea). Pancreatic α-amylase (choice A) releases glucose from starch in the diet. Carboxyl ester lipase (choice B) hydrolyzes the fatty acid esterified to the hydroxyl on carbon 3 of cholesterol. Pancreatic phospholipase A_2 (choice D) hydrolyzes the fatty acid esterified to the *sn2* position of dietary phospholipids. Trypsinogen (choice E) is the precursor form of the protease, trypsin.

13. Correct answer is **C.** The children are most likely suffering from the malnutrition disorder known as kwashiorkor. Kwashiorkor is a form of malnutrition due to a deficiency in protein but with sufficient caloric intake. Kwashiorkor is an acute form of childhood protein-energy malnutrition characterized by edema causing the typical bulging stomach seen in affected children. Kwashiorkor also results in irritability, anorexia, skin ulcers, and hepatomegaly due to fatty infiltration. The hepatomegaly also contributes to the protuberant abdomen in these children. Treatment of Kwashiorkor involves careful administration of protein with the use of carbohydrate and fat for the majority of caloric needs of the child. This is due to the fact that the administration of too much protein will lead to increased hepatic urea cycle activity. Since the liver is already compromised, due to the fatty infiltration, the metabolism of protein can exacerbate the damage and lead to liver failure and death. None of the other options (choices A, B, D, and E) correctly define the most effective treatment of children with kwashiorkor.

14. Correct answer is **E.** The principal stimulants for gastric acid production are histamine, gastrin, and acetylcholine (ACh). Gastrin is released from G cells of the stomach and acetylcholine is released from postganglionic enteric neurons. Histamine is thought to be the primary stimulus. Histamine is released from enterochromaffin-like (ECL) cells in response to gastrin binding to these cells in fundal glands of the upper stomach. The released histamine then binds to histamine H_2 receptors on parietal cells inducing a signaling cascade that results in the transport of the H^+/K^+-ATPase (proton pump) from the cytoplasm to the apical plasma membrane of the parietal cell. The histamine H_2 receptor is a G_s-type G-protein–coupled receptor the activation of which results in activation of adenylate cyclase and enhanced production of cAMP. Acetylcholine binds to the M3 receptor (choice A) which is a G_q-type G-protein–coupled receptor. The adrenergic receptors (choices B and C) do not contribute to gastric acid production in parietal cells of the stomach. Gastrin binds to the cholecystokinin 2 receptor (choice D) which is a G_q-type G-protein–coupled receptor.

15. Correct answer is **C.** The ileum is responsible for the absorption of proteins, amino acids, cobalamin (vitamin B_{12}), folate, and several additional water-soluble vitamins and the fat-soluble vitamins. The uptake of vitamin B_{12} occurs exclusively in the distal ileum and loss of this region of the small intestine would significantly impact levels of the vitamin. Vitamin B_{12}, specifically methylcobalamin, is a critical cofactor for methionine synthase, and 5′-deoxyadenosyl-cobalamin is a critical cofactor for methylmalonyl-CoA mutase. The loss of adequate vitamin B_{12} would result in the accumulation of methylmalonic acid in the blood and urine as a consequence of impaired methylmalonyl-CoA mutase activity. Accumulation of alloisoleucine (choice A) is found in infants suffering from maple syrup urine disease. Numerous conditions, unrelated to gastrointestinal surgery, can lead to lactic acidemia (choice B). Accumulation of phenyllactate (choice D) results in infants suffering from phenylketonuria. Phytanic acid (choice E) would accumulate in patients with Refsum disease.

16. Correct answer is **A.** The patient is most likely experiencing the symptoms of acute pancreatitis. The hallmark of acute pancreatitis is abdominal pain that is initially localized to the epigastrium and later becomes diffuse. It typically radiates to the back and is frequently more intense in the supine position. Other common symptoms include nausea, vomiting, and tachycardia. If the pancreatitis is severe, hypotension can occur due to extravasation of blood and fluids into peritoneal spaces and shock may ensue. Measurement of both pancreatic amylase and lipase enzyme levels are useful in the diagnosis of acute pancreatitis. Amylase levels rise early in the course of the disease, while elevation of lipase levels may not occur until 24 hours after onset of illness. Although false positives and false negatives do occur, an elevated amylase level in conjunction with a consistent pattern of acute epigastric/abdominal pain is considered evidence of acute pancreatitis if other acute surgical conditions have been ruled out. Aspartate transaminase (choice B) is elevated in the blood in conditions of liver dysfunction. Humans express 15 isoforms of carbonic anhydrase (choice C) with 12 of these isoforms exhibiting functional enzymatic activity. Increased levels of serum carbonic anhydrase III are associated with myocardial infarction. Ferritin (choice D) would be elevated in the blood under conditions of iron overload, such as hemochromatosis. The measurement of lactate dehydrogenase (choice E) is especially diagnostic for myocardial infarction. Following a myocardial infarct, the serum levels of LDH rise within 24–48 hours reaching a peak by 2–3 days and return to normal in 5–10 days. Unconjugated bilirubin (choice F) in the blood is a strong indicator of hepatic dysfunction.

17. Correct answer is **B.** The major control mechanism for gastric emptying involves duodenal gastric feedback that consists of both hormonal and neural inputs. The major hormone involved in the inhibition of gastric emptying is cholecystokinin (CCK). CCK is secreted from intestinal enteroendocrine I cells predominantly in the duodenum and jejunum. The level of CCK in the blood rises within 15 minutes of food ingestion and reaches a peak by 25 minutes. The elevation in plasma CCK levels remains for approximately 3 hours following a meal. The most potent substances initiating a release of CCK from the I cells are fats and proteins. Conversely duodenal bile acids are potent suppressors of the secretion of CCK. CCK exerts its biological actions by binding to specific G-protein–coupled receptors. On binding its receptors in the gut CCK induces contractions of the gallbladder and release of pancreatic enzymes, and also inhibits gastric emptying. Within the brain (specifically the median eminence and ventromedial nucleus of the hypothalamus), CCK actions elicit behavioral responses and satiation. A reduction in gastric emptying would result from increased or excessive CCK activity resulting in rapid onset of satiety due to a feeling of fullness and the effects of CCK in the hypothalamus. Within the stomach acetylcholine (choice A), gastrin (choice C), and histamine (choice D) trigger the production of gastric acid which aids in the digestive process and would, therefore, result in increased gastric emptying. Motilin (choice E) initiates inter-digestive intestinal motility, stimulates the release of pancreatic polypeptide, and stimulates gallbladder contractions, all of which would enhance gastric emptying. Pancreatic polypeptide (choice F) is secreted from the pancreas and is synergistic with motilin in the gastrointestinal system.

18. Correct answer is **A.** The patient is most likely exhibiting the symptoms of lactose intolerance. The signs and symptoms of lactose intolerance usually begin 30 minutes to 2 hours after eating or drinking foods that contain lactose. The typical symptoms of lactose intolerance include nausea, vomiting, diarrhea, bloating, gas, and painful abdominal cramping.

The bloating and gas result from the bacterial fermentation of the lactose in the colon. The diarrhea is the result of the osmotic nature of lactose that interferes with intestinal water reabsorption. One of the richest sources of calcium is animal milk. However, lactose intolerant individuals drink less milk, so they are at increased risk for calcium deficiency. Lactose intolerant individuals are not likely to be deficient in any of the other nutrients (choices B, C, D, and E).

19. Correct answer is **E.** The principal stimulants for gastric acid production are histamine, gastrin, and acetylcholine (ACh). Histamine is thought to be the primary stimulus. All three of these stimulators of gastric acid production bind to receptors on parietal cells of the stomach. The most common treatments for gastroesophageal reflux disease are drugs that inhibit the parietal cell proton pump or the histamine receptor on parietal cells that trigger gastric acid production in response to binding histamine. Chief cells of the stomach (choice A) are found in the corpus of the stomach, and they secrete the zymogen protease, pepsinogen. D cells (choice B) secrete somatostatin whose function is to inhibit gastrin release from G cells (choice D) and histamine release from enterochromaffin-like (ECL) cells (choice C).

20. Correct answer is **E.** The antrum and pyloric region of the stomach contain primarily three types of secretory cells identified as D cells, G cells, and mucus cells. The D cells secrete somatostatin whose function is to inhibit gastrin release from G cells. Mucous cells synthesize and secrete a mixture of mucopolysaccharides and glycoproteins high in sialic acid and sulfated sugars that form a protective lubricant within the lumen of the stomach. Histamine (choice A) is released from enterochromaffin-like (ECL) cells in the corpus region of the stomach. Hydrogen ions (choice B) and intrinsic factor (choice C) are secreted from parietal cells in the corpus region of the stomach. Pepsinogen (choice D) is secreted from chief cells in the corpus region of the stomach.

CHAPTER

29

Insulin Function

High-Yield Terms

Incretin	Any gut hormone associated with food intake-stimulation of insulin secretion from the pancreas
Glucose-stimulated insulin secretion, GSIS	Process of glucose uptake and metabolism by β-cells leading to increased ATP production which inhibits a potassium-dependent ATP (KATP) channel resulting in depolarization of the membrane triggering calcium influx and insulin secretory vesicle fusion with plasma membrane
ABCC8/KCNJ11	ATP-binding cassette, sub-family C, member 8 (ABCC8-encoded protein is also known as the sulfonylurea receptor, SUR) and potassium inwardly-rectifying channel, subfamily J, member 11, protein components of the KATP channel of β-cells that regulates insulin secretion
TCF7L2	Transcription factor 7-like 2, T-cell specific HMG-box, involved in Wnt signal transduction, polymorphisms in this gene are the most highly correlated with potential for development of T2D
Insulin resistance, IR	A phenomenon whereby binding of insulin to its receptor results in impaired or failed propagation of normal signal transduction events

Insulin is a major metabolism-regulating hormone secreted by β-cells of the islets of Langerhans of the pancreas (Figure 29–1). The major function of insulin is to counter the concerted actions of a number of hormones whose effects include increased blood glucose. Thus, one major metabolic effect of insulin is to maintain low blood glucose levels. Insulin exerts this effect by stimulating glucose uptake and storage, primarily into skeletal muscle and adipose tissue, and to stimulate the storage of glucose as glycogen and glucose carbon atoms as fatty acids in triglycerides. In addition to its role in regulating glucose metabolism, insulin stimulates lipogenesis, diminishes lipolysis, and increases amino acid transport into cells.

Insulin also exerts activities typically associated with growth factors (see Figure 29–5). Insulin is a member of a family of structurally and functionally similar molecules that includes the insulin-like growth factors, IGF-1 and IGF-2. Insulin modulates transcription and stimulates protein translocation, cell growth, DNA synthesis, and cell replication, effects that it holds in common with numerous other growth factors.

Loss of insulin is incompatible with life as in the case of type 1 diabetes (T1D), whereas dysregulation in insulin function generally leads to severe hyperglycemia and shortened life span as is typically seen in poorly controlled type 2 diabetes (T2D) (see Chapter 30).

FUNCTIONAL INSULIN SYNTHESIS

Insulin is synthesized, from the *INS* gene, as a preprohormone in the β-cells of the islets of Langerhans (Figure 29–2). The signal peptide of preproinsulin is removed in the cisternae of the endoplasmic reticulum (ER) as is typical for all proteins synthesized associated with the ER. The insulin proprotein is packaged into secretory vesicles in the Golgi, folded into its native structure, and locked in this conformation by the formation of two disulfide bonds. Specific protease activity cleaves the center third of the molecule, which dissociates as C peptide, leaving the amino terminal B peptide disulfide bonded to the carboxy terminal A peptide.

GLUCOSE-STIMULATED INSULIN SECRETION (GSIS)

Insulin secretion from β-cells is principally regulated by plasma glucose levels (Figure 29–3). Increased uptake of glucose by pancreatic β-cells leads to a concomitant increase in metabolism. The increase in metabolism leads to an elevation in the ATP/ADP ratio. This in turn leads to the inhibition of an ATP-sensitive potassium channel (KATP channel). The net result is

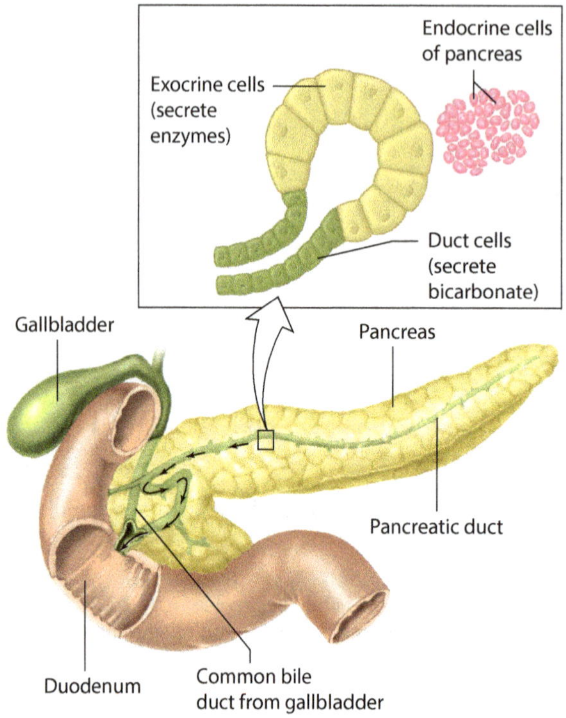

FIGURE 29–1 Structure of the pancreas. (Reproduced with permission from Widmaier EP, Raff H, Strang KT. *Vander's Human Physiology: The Mechanisms of Body Function*, 11th ed. New York, NY: McGraw Hill; 2008.)

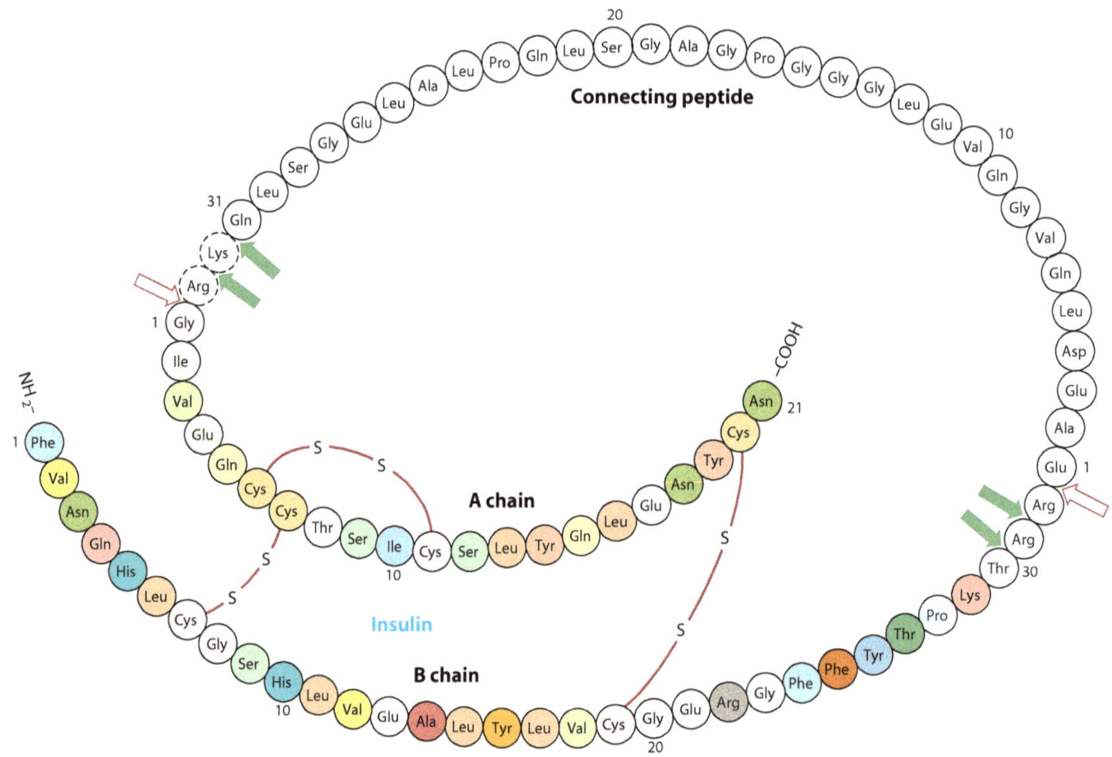

FIGURE 29–2 Structure of human proinsulin. Insulin and C-peptide molecules are connected at two sites by dipeptide links. An initial cleavage by a trypsin-like enzyme (open arrows) followed by several cleavages by a carboxypeptidaselike enzyme (solid arrows) results in the production of the heterodimeric (AB) insulin molecule (colored) and the C-peptide (white). (Reproduced with permission from Rodwell VW, Bender DA, Botham KM, et al: *Harper's Illustrated Biochemistry*, 31st ed. New York, NY: McGraw Hill; 2018.)

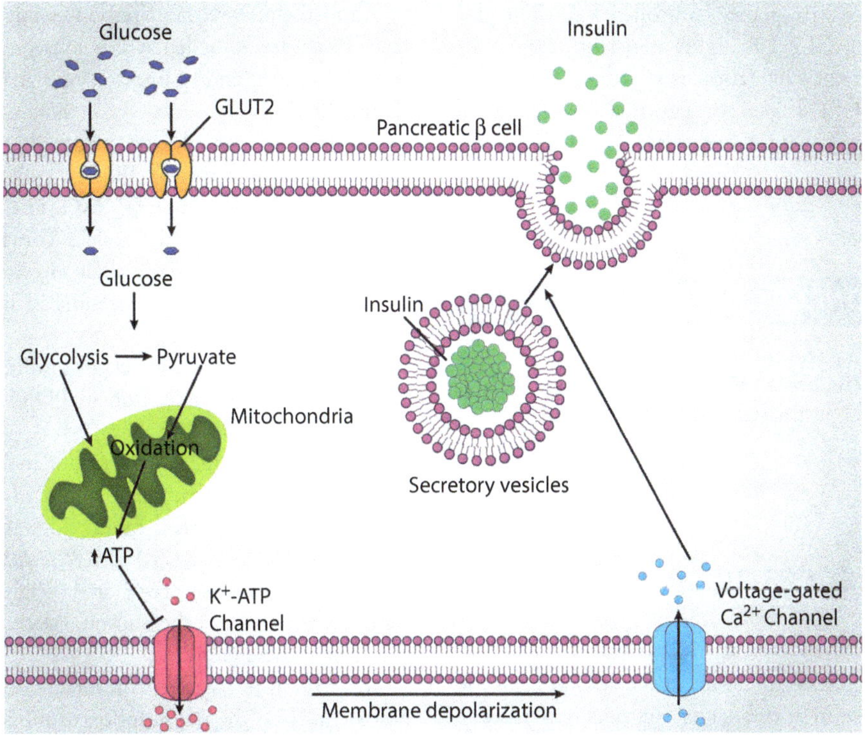

FIGURE 29–3 Glucose-stimulated insulin secretion (GSIS). Glucose, following uptake into the β-cell, is oxidized which generates ATP via mitochondrial oxidative phosphorylation. The increased ATP levels inhibit the KATP channel which leads to membrane depolarization and the opening of calcium channels. The influx of calcium triggers the fusion of insulin-containing secretory vesicles with the plasma membrane and the release of insulin to the circulation. (Reproduced with permission from themedicalbiochemistrypage, LLC.)

a depolarization of the cell leading to Ca^{2+} influx and insulin secretion.

The KATP channel is a complex of eight polypeptides comprising four copies of the protein encoded by the *ABCC8* (ATP-binding cassette, sub-family C, member 8) gene and four copies of the protein encoded by the *KCNJ11* (potassium inwardly rectifying channel, subfamily J, member 11; also known as $K_{ir}6.2$) gene. The *ABCC8*-encoded protein is also known as the sulfonylurea receptor (SUR). The *KCNJ11*-encoded protein forms the core of the KATP channel. As might be expected, the role of KATP channels in insulin secretion presents a viable therapeutic target for treating hyperglycemia due to insulin insufficiency as is typical in T2D (see Chapter 30).

As opposed to the positive role of pancreatic glucose metabolism on insulin secretion, pancreatic fatty acid uptake inhibits GSIS. Increased intracellular fatty acids interfere with the nuclear localization of two transcription factors, FOXA2 and HNF1α, that are involved in the transcription of the gene encoding the plasma membrane glucose transporter, GLUT2, as well as genes responsible for correct membrane localization of this transporter. Of significance to diabetes is the fact that defects in the *HNF1A* gene are associated with the monogenic form of diabetes, MODY3 (see Table 30–2).

NUTRIENT INTAKE AND HORMONAL CONTROL OF INSULIN RELEASE

Of the many gastrointestinal hormones (see Chapters 28 and 31), two have significant effects on insulin secretion and glucose regulation. These hormones are GLP-1 and GIP. These two hormones constitute the class of molecules referred to as the **incretins**.

HIGH-YIELD CONCEPT

Incretins are gut hormones associated with food intake-stimulation of insulin secretion from the pancreas.

On nutrient ingestion, GLP-1 is secreted from intestinal enteroendocrine L-cells that are found predominantly in the ileum. The action of GLP-1, at the level of insulin and glucagon secretion, results in significant reduction in circulating levels of glucose following nutrient intake. This activity has obvious significance in the context of diabetes, in particular the hyperglycemia associated with poorly controlled T2D. The glucose lowering activity of GLP-1 is highly transient as the half-life of this hormone in the circulation is less than 2 minutes. Removal of bioactive GLP-1 is a consequence of N-terminal proteolysis catalyzed by dipeptidylpeptidase IV (DPP IV or DPP4).

HIGH-YIELD CONCEPT

The primary physiologic responses to GLP-1 are GSIS, enhanced insulin secretion, inhibition of glucagon secretion, and inhibition of gastric acid secretion and gastric emptying.

THE INSULIN RECEPTOR SIGNALING PATHWAYS

All of the effects of insulin are the result of the activation of the insulin receptor and the resultant signal transduction cascade initiated by the activated receptor. The insulin receptor belongs to the class of cell surface receptors that exhibit intrinsic tyrosine kinase activity (see Chapter 26). The insulin receptor is a heterotetramer of two extracellular α-subunits disulfide bonded to two transmembrane β-subunits (Figure 29–4).

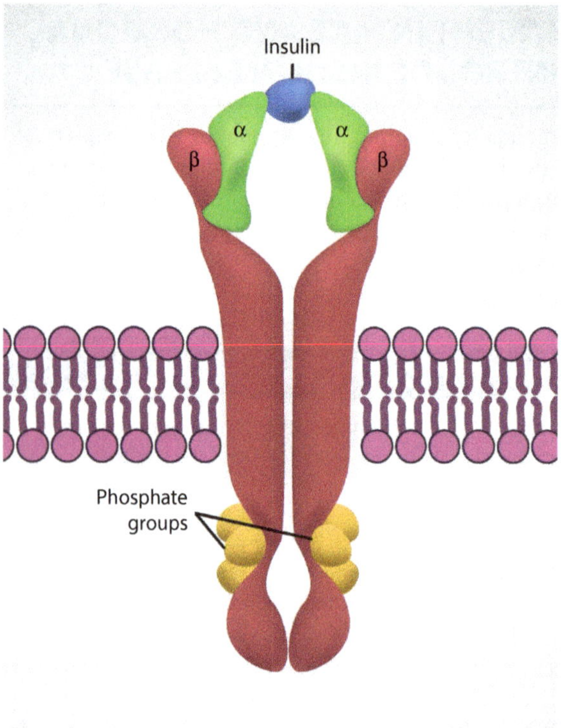

FIGURE 29–4 Structure of the insulin receptor. (Reproduced with permission from themedicalbiochemistrypage, LLC.)

All of the post-receptor responses initiated by insulin binding to its receptor are mediated as a consequence of the activation of several divergent and/or intersecting signal transduction pathways (Figure 29–5).

Insulin-mediated glucose uptake in adipocytes and skeletal muscle involves activated PDK1, which phosphorylates some isoforms of protein kinase C, PKC. The PKC isoform, PKCλ/ζ, phosphorylates intracellular vesicles containing the glucose transporter, GLUT4, resulting in their migration to, and fusion with, the plasma membrane. This results in increased glucose uptake and metabolism.

The broad metabolic effects of insulin are also exerted following insulin receptor activation of PDK1. PDK1 phosphorylates and activates the kinase identified as AKT2/PKBβ. PKB/AKT was originally identified as the tumor-inducing gene in the AKT8 retrovirus found in the AKR strain of mice. Humans express three genes in the AKT family identified as AKT1 (PKBα), AKT2 (PKBβ), and AKT3 (PKBγ). Activation of AKT2 leads to increased glycogen, fatty acid, triglyceride, and cholesterol synthesis as a result of the phosphorylation of the major regulated enzymes in these pathways.

In addition to its effects on metabolic enzyme activity, insulin exerts effects on the transcription of numerous genes. These transcriptional effects include (but are not limited to) increases in expression of the genes encoding glucokinase, liver pyruvate kinase (L-PK), lipoprotein lipase (LPL), fatty acid synthase (FAS), and acetyl-CoA carboxylase (ACC) and decreases in expression of the genes encoding glucose-6-phosphatase, fructose-1,6-bisphosphatase, and phosphoenolpyruvate carboxykinase (PEPCK).

The growth factor effects of insulin involve the activation of GRB2 resulting in signal transduction via the monomeric G-protein, RAS. Activation of RAS ultimately leads to changes in the expression of numerous growth and proliferation genes via activation of members of the MAP kinase (MAPK) and extracellular signal-regulated kinase (ERK) families.

INTESTINAL Wnt SIGNALING AND INSULIN SECRETION

The action of the Wnt protein has been shown to interact with the metabolic control exerted by insulin via its actions in both the gut and pancreas. In intestinal enteroendocrine L cells, Wnt signaling leads to enhanced expression of the *GCG* gene. In these cells, expression of the *GCG* gene results in the production of GLP-1. In the pancreas, GLP-1 induces β-cell proliferation and inhibition of β-cell apoptosis.

HIGH-YIELD CONCEPT

The GCG promoter region contains an enhancer that harbors a canonical Wnt response element that binds the TCF transcription factor, TCF7L2. Genome wide screens for polymorphisms associated with T2D have shown that two single nucleotide polymorphisms (SNPs) in the *TCF7L2* gene are the most frequently occurring SNPs associated with this disease.

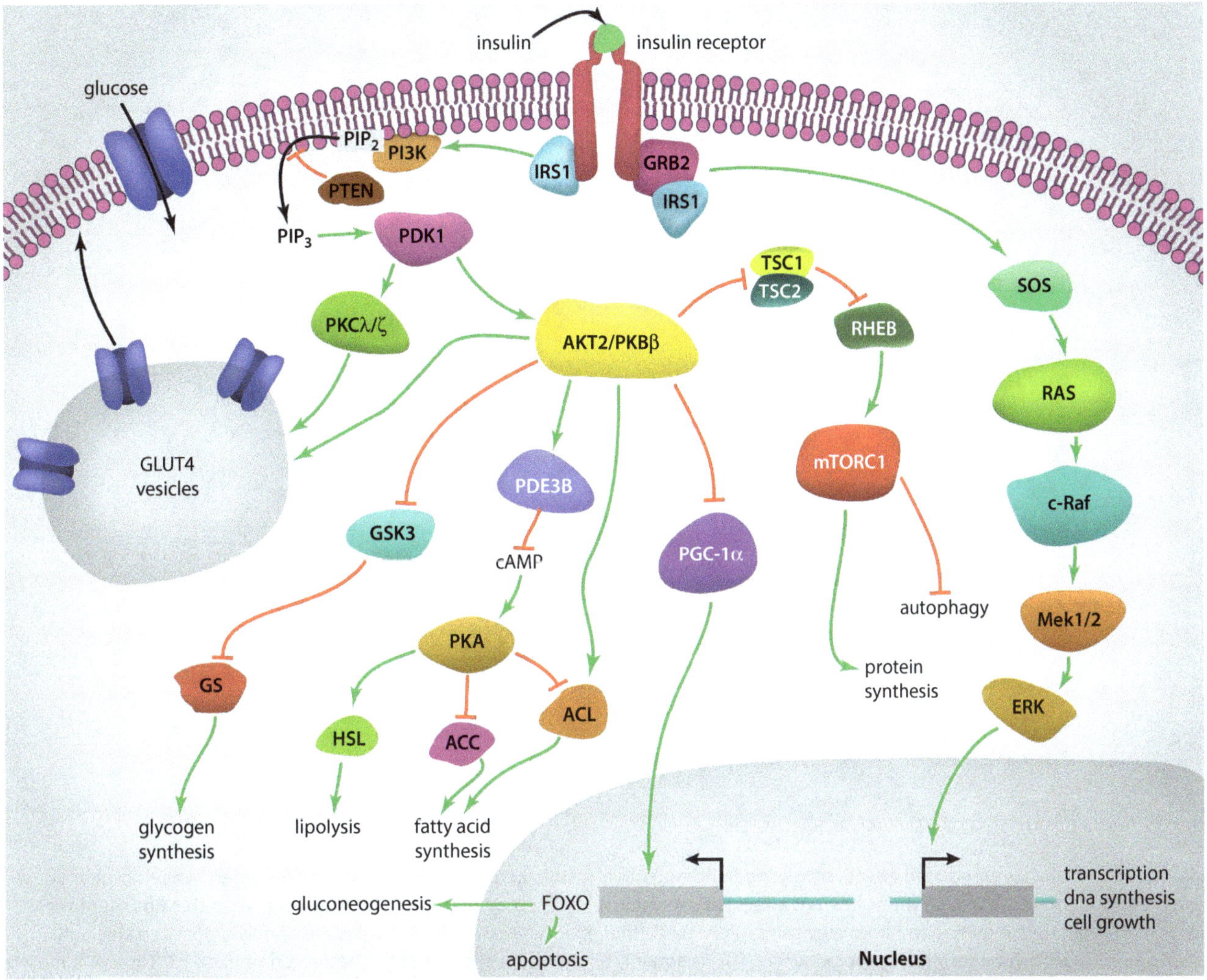

FIGURE 29–5 Multiple signal transduction pathways initiated by insulin. The indicated insulin-mediated signal transduction pathways are intended to be representative only. When insulin binds to its receptor it triggers receptor autophosphorylation that generates docking sites for insulin receptor substrate proteins (IRS, IRS2, and IRS4). IRS proteins in turn trigger the activation of a wide array of signal transducing proteins (highly simplified in this figure). The end results of insulin receptor activation are varied and in many cases cell-type specific but includes alterations in metabolism, ion fluxes, protein translocation, transcription rates, and growth properties of responsive cells. Green arrows represent positive, activating functions. Red T-lines represent inhibitory functions. PI3K: phosphatidylinositol-3-kinase. PDK1: PIP_3-dependent protein kinase 1. PTEN: phosphatase and tensin homolog. PDE3B: phosphodiesterase 3B (also called adipocyte cAMP phosphodiesterase). GS: glycogen synthase. HSL: hormone sensitive lipase. ACC: acetyl-CoA carboxylase. ACL: ATP-citrate lyase. TSC1/2: tuberous sclerosis 1 and 2. GRB2: growth factor receptor binding protein 2. SOS: son of sevenless. PGC-1α: PPARγ co-activator 1α. RHEB: Ras homolog expressed in brain. mTORC1: mechanistic target of rapamycin complex 1. (Reproduced with permission from themedicalbiochemistrypage, LLC.)

INSULIN REGULATION OF CARBOHYDRATE HOMEOSTASIS

One of the major whole-body responses to the release of insulin is the modulation of glucose homeostasis. This includes stimulated uptake of glucose from the blood, primarily by adipose tissue and skeletal muscle, followed by either storage of the glucose as glycogen or the conversion of glucose carbons into fatty acids for storage in triglycerides.

HIGH-YIELD CONCEPT

In the liver, glucose uptake is dramatically increased due to insulin-mediated increases in the activity of the enzymes glucokinase, phosphofructokinase-1 (PFK-1), and pyruvate kinase (L-PK), the key regulatory enzymes of glycolysis. These effects are induced by insulin-dependent activation of phosphodiesterase (PDE3B) which leads to decreases in cAMP levels with consequent decreases in PKA activity (see Figure 29–5).

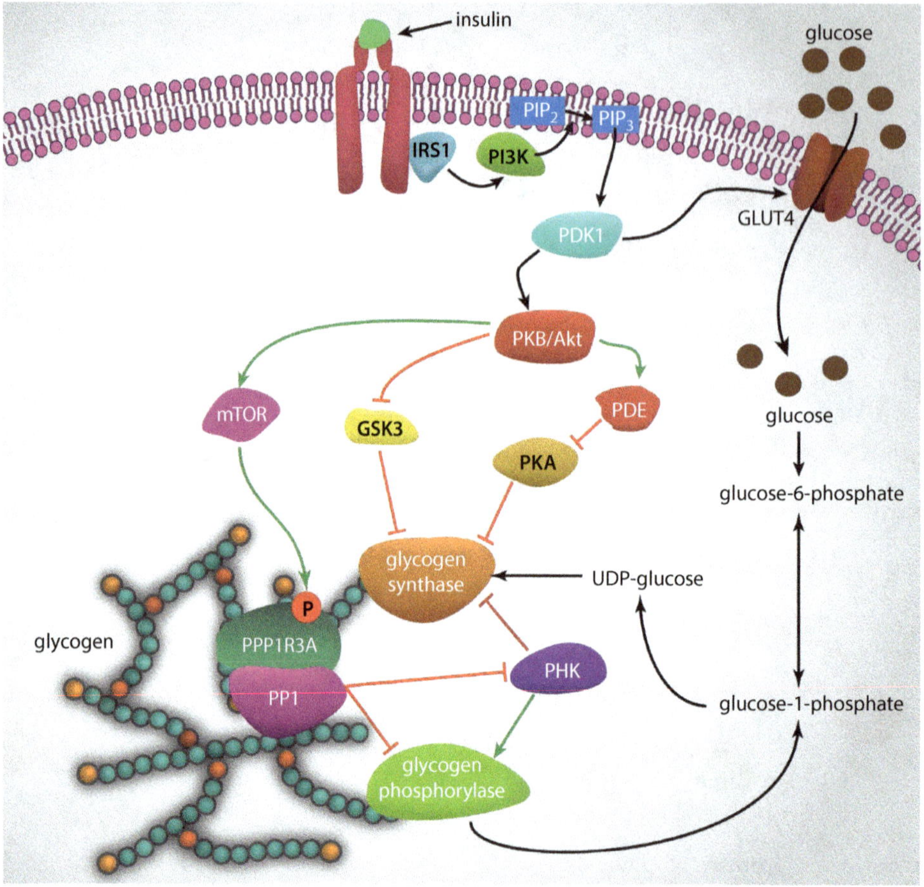

FIGURE 29–6 Insulin-mediated effects on glycogen homeostasis. Insulin activates the synthesis of glycogen, while simultaneously inhibiting glycogenolysis, through the concerted effects of several insulin receptor-activated pathways. Shown in this figure are the major insulin-regulated activities and how they can rapidly exert their effects since all the activities are closely associated through interactions with protein targeting to glycogen (PTG). PTG is actually a regulatory subunit of the heterotetrameric PP1. There is a muscle-specific PTG (PPP1R3A) and a liver-specific PTG (PPP1R3B). Also diagrammed is the response to insulin at the level of glucose transport into adipose tissue and skeletal muscle cells via GLUT4 translocation to the plasma membrane. PDK1: PIP_3-dependent protein kinase 1. GS/GP kinase: glycogen synthase: glycogen phosphorylase kinase (PHK). PP1: protein phosphatase-1. PDE: phosphodiesterase. Green arrows denote either direction of flow or positive effects. Red T lines represent inhibitory effects. (Reproduced with permission from themedicalbiochemistrypage, LLC.)

The effects of insulin on carbohydrate homeostasis result from two primary mechanisms: (1) decreased levels of cAMP via activation of phosphodiesterase and the resultant decreased level of PKA activity and (2) increased activity of protein phosphatase 1 (PP1). These effects are demonstrated for glycogen homeostasis in Figure 29–6.

INSULIN REGULATION OF LIPID HOMEOSTASIS

The net effect of insulin on global metabolism is increased storage of carbon for future use as an energy source. This includes the diversion of glucose into glycogen as well as glucose carbons into fatty acid and triglyceride synthesis. The major effects of insulin, at the level of lipid homeostasis, are activation of lipogenesis and inhibition of lipolysis, effects mediated by changes in cAMP and protein phosphorylation as in the situation for insulin-mediated changes in carbohydrate homeostasis.

INSULIN FUNCTION AS A GROWTH FACTOR

As a growth factor, insulin modulates the transcription of numerous genes involved in cell growth and differentiation. Insulin also stimulates DNA synthesis, RNA synthesis, and protein synthesis (Figure 29–7), which are required for cell proliferation. Several of

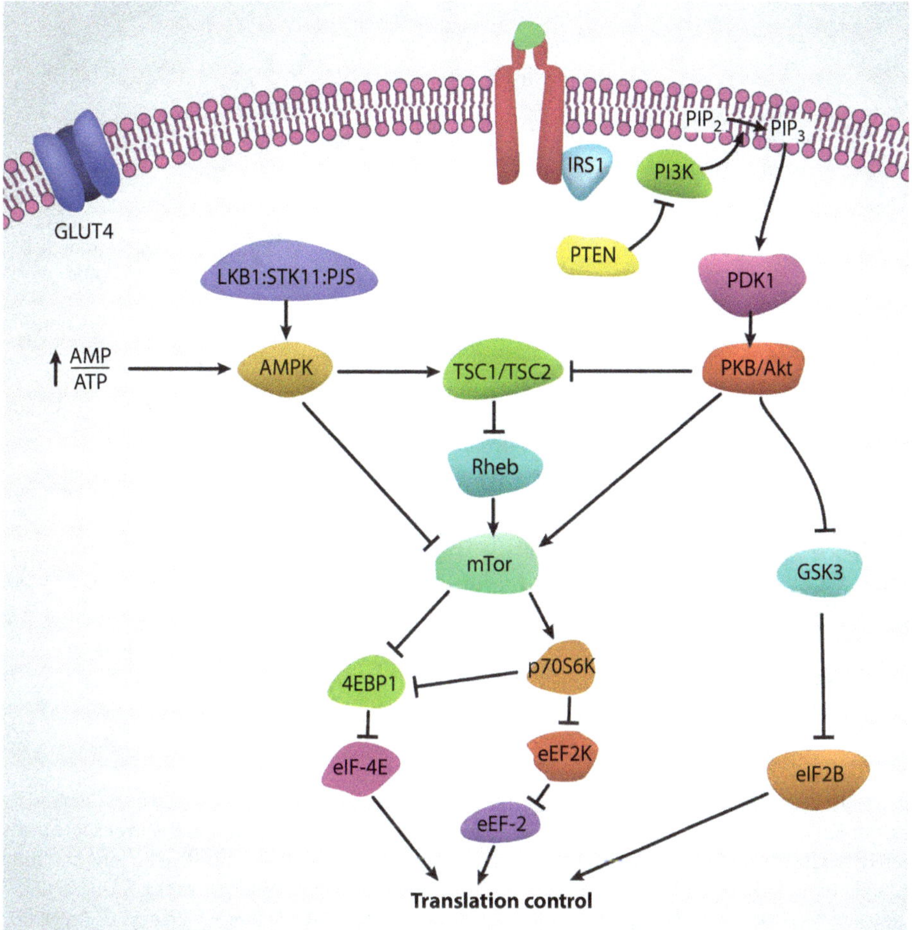

FIGURE 29–7 Insulin-mediated cascade leading to enhanced translation (not intended to be a complete description of all the targets of insulin action that affect translation rates). Also shown is the effect of an increase in the AMP to ATP ratio which activates AMP-activated kinase, AMPK. STK11-LKB1-PJS: serine-threonine kinase 11, Peutz-Jeghers syndrome gene. IRS1: insulin receptor substrate 1; PI3K: phosphatidylinositol-3 kinase; PIP_2: phosphatidylinositol 4,5-bisphosphate; PTEN: phosphatase and tensin homolog deleted on chromosome 10; PDK1: PIP_3-dependent protein kinase; TSC1 and TSC2: tuberous sclerosis tumor suppressors 1 (hamartin) and 2 (tuberin); Rheb: Ras homolog enriched in brain; mTOR: mammalian target of rapamycin. PKB/Akt: protein kinase B, GSK3: glycogen synthase kinase 3; 4EBP1: eIF-4E binding protein; p70S6K: 70kDa ribosomal protein S6 kinase, also called S6K. (Reproduced with permission from themedicalbiochemistrypage, LLC.)

the insulin-stimulated genes are involved in restricting the activation and propagation of apoptotic signals allowing for increased cell survival. The regulation of translation by initiation and elongation factors (eIF-2B, eIF-4E, and eEF-2, specifically) is reviewed in Chapter 24.

INSULIN RESISTANCE

Obesity is of epidemic proportions in the United States and one of the most serious consequences of this disorder is the development of T2D. Associated with obesity and contributing to worsening of T2D is insulin resistance (IR). Indeed, IR is a characteristic feature found associated with most cases of T2D and it is the hallmark feature of the metabolic syndrome (MetS).

HIGH-YIELD CONCEPT

Insulin resistance (IR) refers to the situation whereby insulin interaction with its receptor fails to elicit downstream signaling events (see Figure 29–8). Metabolically and clinically the most detrimental effects of IR are due to disruption in insulin-mediated control of glucose and lipid homeostasis in the primary insulin-responsive tissues: liver, skeletal muscle, and adipose tissue.

IR can occur for a number of reasons; however, the most prevalent cause is the hyperlipidemic and proinflammatory states associated with obesity. Excess free fatty acids (FFA), prevalent in obesity, exert negative effects on the insulin receptor-mediated signaling pathways in adipose tissue, liver, and skeletal muscle (Figure 29–8).

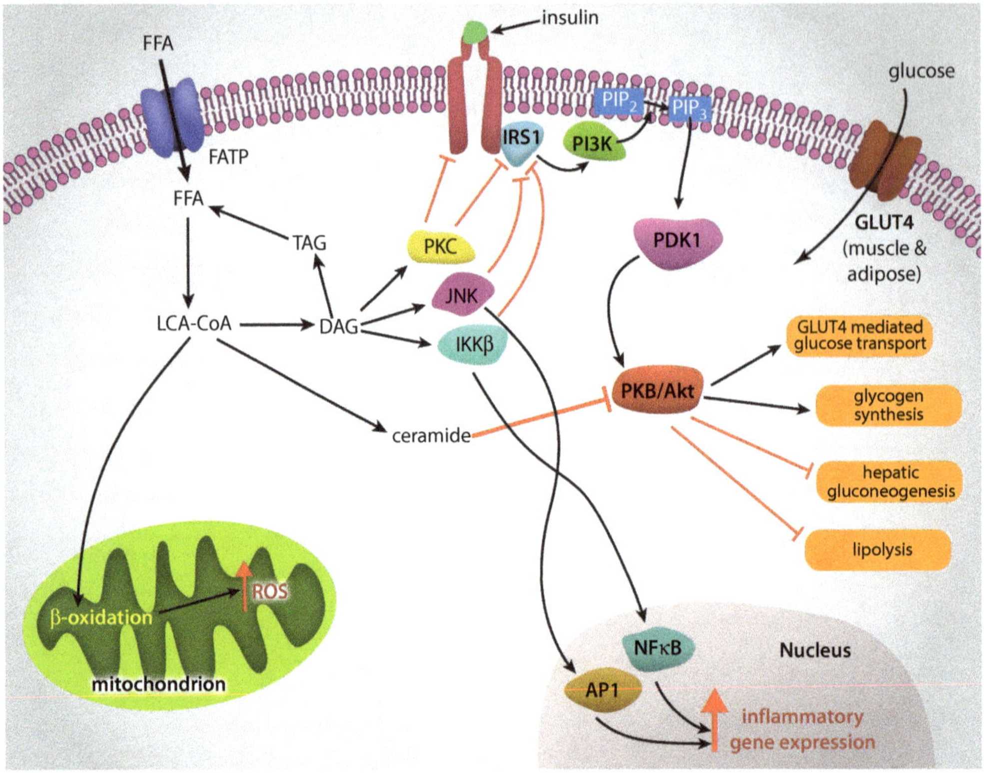

FIGURE 29–8 Insulin resistance induced by fatty acids. Model for how excess free fatty acids (FFA) lead to insulin resistance and enhanced inflammatory responses, predominantly in cells such as skeletal muscle and adipose tissue but also in the liver. Only the major pathways regulated by insulin relative to glucose and lipid homeostasis are shown. Black arrows represent positive actions and red T-lines represent inhibitory actions. JNK: Jun N-terminal kinase. PKC: protein kinase C. IKKβ: inhibitor of nuclear factor kappa B kinase beta. ROS: reactive oxygen species. PI3K: phosphatidylinositol-3 kinase. DAG: diacylglycerol. TAG: triglycerides. LCA-CoA: long-chain acyl-CoAs. NFκB: nuclear factor kappa B. (Reproduced with permission from themedicalbiochemistrypage, LLC.)

CHECKLIST

- ☑ Insulin is the most significant hypoglycemia-inducing hormone in the body.
- ☑ Insulin is produced in the β-cells of the islets of Langerhans in the pancreas. Bioactive insulin is processed from a pre-pro-protein by proteolytic digestion into a function peptide composed of an A peptide and a B peptide held together by disulfide bonds. The central portion of the proinsulin protein is called the C peptide and is not part of the functional hormone, but is released from secretory vesicles along with functional insulin.
- ☑ Secretion of insulin is stimulated primarily in response to increases in plasma glucose levels due, in part, to increased glucose oxidation within pancreatic β-cells, a process that results in increased ATP leading to inhibition of a potassium channel causing depolarization of the cell, an associated influx of calcium and insulin vesicle fusion with the plasma membrane. This is referred to as glucose-stimulated insulin secretion, GSIS.
- ☑ Gut hormones, called incretins, released in response to food intake, influence the glucose-mediated secretion of insulin.
- ☑ Increased intake of fatty acids impairs pancreatic GSIS and contributes to the etiology of obesity-induced diabetes.
- ☑ Insulin exerts activities associated with typical hormones as well as those exerted by typical growth factors. All of these dual activities are activated in response to insulin binding to its cell surface receptor. Cell-type specific responses to insulin are the result of the differential expression of signaling proteins downstream of the insulin receptor.
- ☑ The insulin receptor is a member of the class of receptors with intrinsic enzymatic activity, specifically the receptor tyrosine kinases (RTK). The insulin receptor is unique in this class in that it is a heterotetrameric receptor composed of two membrane-spanning β-subunits and two extracellular α-subunits disulfide bonded to the β-subunits.

- ☑ As a hormone, insulin stimulates glucose uptake and storage as glycogen or oxidation to acetyl-CoA for conversion to fatty acids for storage in the form of triglyceride. Insulin actions also inhibit lipolysis and stimulate lipogenesis.
- ☑ As a growth factor insulin stimulates protein synthesis, transcription profiles of numerous genes, DNA synthesis, and the inhibition of apoptosis.
- ☑ Defects in insulin-mediated signal transduction events are the basis for insulin resistance, IR. Excess free fatty acids and their metabolic intermediates are the primary culprits in the development of IR.
- ☑ IR is the precipitating event in the development of type 2 diabetes, T2D.

REVIEW QUESTIONS

1. A 54-year-old man with a past medical history of hypertension is undergoing a routine examination. He has no complaints other than some dyspnea on exertion, which has been longstanding. Current medications include a thiazide diuretic and aspirin. He does not get much physical activity during the day. Physical examination indicates he is 5 feet 11 inches tall, weighs 210 lb, has a waist circumference of 40.5 inches, and a calculated BMI of 29 kg/m^2. His blood pressure is 145/95. The rest of his physical examination is unremarkable. Blood work indicates total cholesterol of 230 mg/dL (N = <200 mg/dL), HDL 38 mg/dL (N = 40–50 mg/dL), LDL 152 mg/dL (N = <100 mg/dL), triglycerides 200 mg/dL (N = <150 mg/dL), and fasting plasma glucose 160 mg/dL (N = <100 mg/dL). Based on these observations and test results, this patient is at the greatest risk for which of the following?

(A) Elevated cortisol production
(B) Gallstones
(C) Gout
(D) Insulin resistance
(E) Liver failure
(F) Renal failure

2. A 23-year-old man is brought to the emergency department after being found unconscious and unresponsive in a parking garage. Physical examination finds no obvious signs of trauma or head injury. Blood work finds a glucose concentration of 47 mg/dL (N = 60–110 mg/dL). Following intravenous administration of glucose, the patient regains consciousness. History indicates the patient is not diabetic and does not take insulin shots. Analysis of the patient's blood for which of the following would most likely indicate the patient has developed a disorder that is contributing to his symptoms?

(A) Cortisol
(B) C peptide
(C) Epinephrine
(D) Glucagon
(E) Somatostatin

3. Clinical trials are being conducted with a novel compound designed to treat the hyperglycemia associated with type 2 diabetes. When this compound is orally administered to test subjects there is a demonstrable increase in insulin secretion. This compound is most likely exerting effects that lead to release of which of the following substances in the gut?

(A) Cholecystokinin
(B) Gastrin
(C) Glucagon-like peptide 1
(D) Pancreatic polypeptide
(E) Somatostatin

4. Experiments are being conducted on a compound designed to interfere with insulin receptor signaling. When the compound is added to cultures of adipocytes, simultaneous with insulin, there is loss of glucose uptake. In the presence of the compound, the binding of insulin to its receptor and the dissociation kinetics are identical to those determined in the absence of the compound. Which of the following most closely resembles the novel compound in its actions with respect to the insulin receptor?

(A) Acetyl-CoA
(B) Galactose
(C) Glucosamine
(D) N-acetylgalactosamine
(E) Stearic acid

5. A 15-year-old girl, with type 1 diabetes, is participating in a clinical trial of a novel compound designed to reduce circulating levels of glucose. Prior to infusion of the compound, the test patient has a postprandial serum glucose concentration of 340 mg/dL (2-h postprandial normal <150 mg/dL). Within 2 hours of infusion of the compound, her serum glucose concentration decreases to 200 mg/dL. Which of the following mechanisms best explains the effect of this novel compound?

(A) It activates GLUT4 by a cAMP-independent mechanism
(B) It increases GLUT4 mRNA
(C) It increases the K_m of GLUT4 for glucose
(D) It induces a conformational change in GLUT4
(E) It promotes GLUT4 mobilization to the plasma membrane

6. Experiments are being conducted on pancreatic β-cells derived from induced pluripotent stem cells. One compound tested in this study has been shown to cause a significant increase in insulin secretion when added to the cultures. Which of the following would most likely exert a similar effect to the compound being tested?

(A) Dapagliflozin
(B) Glyburide
(C) Metformin
(D) Pioglitazone
(E) Sitagliptin

7. Administration of insulin to an individual with type 1 diabetes results in an increase in fatty acid synthesis in the liver. Insulin-mediated inhibition of which of the following is most likely to contribute to this metabolic change?

(A) Glucokinase
(B) Glucose-6-phosphate dehydrogenase

(C) Phosphoenolpyruvate carboxykinase (PEPCK)
(D) Pyruvate dehydrogenase kinase
(E) Pyruvate kinase

8. Experiments are being carried out on a novel compound designed to mimic the metabolic effects of insulin. In testing this compound it is added to cultures of normal human hepatocytes. Measurement for a decrease in the activity of which of the following would most likely be evidence of the expected function of the compound?
(A) Acetyl-CoA carboxylase
(B) Glucokinase
(C) Lipoprotein lipase
(D) Phosphoenolpyruvate carboxykinase (PEPCK)
(E) Pyruvate kinase

9. Functional studies are being conducted using adipocytes isolated via biopsy from a 12-year-old boy who exhibits chronic hyperglycemia but with normal circulating levels of insulin. Results from these studies demonstrate that the density of insulin receptors on the patient's adipocytes is very nearly identical to adipocytes from control subjects. The insulin-binding kinetics are also identical, and the receptors become tyrosine phosphorylated in response to insulin binding. Given these observations, it is most likely that there is a defect in which of the following insulin signal transduction proteins?
(A) Cyclic nucleotide phosphodiesterase
(B) Glycogen synthase kinase 3
(C) Mechanistic target of rapamycin (mTOR)
(D) Protein kinase B (PKB/AKT)
(E) Protein kinase C (PKC)

10. The action of insulin is being examined in cells isolated from a quadriceps femoris sarcoma. When insulin is added to these cells the expected increase in glucose uptake is not observed. Failure of insulin to activate which of the following is most likely to account for the observations?
(A) Mechanistic target of rapamycin (mTOR)
(B) Phosphodiesterase
(C) Phospholipase Cβ (PLCβ)
(D) Phosphatidylinositol-3-kinase (PI3K)
(E) RAS

11. Studies are being carried out to examine the responses of myocytes in culture to the addition of insulin. Normally in myocytes when insulin binds its receptor, several proteins are phosphorylated by different kinases. One result of these studies demonstrated that several target proteins are not appropriately modified in the cultured cells. Which of the following is most likely not occurring in these cultured cells following addition of insulin?
(A) Action of a G protein in the plasma membrane
(B) Release of Ca^{2+} from the endoplasmic reticulum
(C) Release of diacylglycerol from phosphatidylinositol-4,5-bisphosphate
(D) Translocation of the glucose transporter (GLUT4) to the plasma membrane
(E) Tyrosine kinase activity of the insulin receptor

12. Experiments are being carried out in laboratory animals to identify a novel synthetic form of insulin. These experiments are carried out following the administration of a neutralizing antibody against endogenous insulin. Several hours after the administration of the anti-insulin antibodies the synthetic molecule is administered to half of the experimental animals. When comparing the metabolic profiles of the mice given the synthetic insulin, to those that did not receive the molecule, which of the following metabolic changes would most likely indicate that the synthetic insulin was functioning as expected?
(A) Decreased glycogenolysis
(B) Decreased protein synthesis
(C) Decreased triglyceride synthesis
(D) Increased gluconeogenesis
(E) Increased glucose transport into the brain
(F) Increased ketone production

13. Studies are being carried out to determine the cause of the persistent hyperglycemia in a 5-year-old girl. When blood levels of various hormones are analyzed, it is found that glucagon, epinephrine, and cortisol are all normal and changes in their levels occur as expected in response to feeding. However, there was no detectable C-peptide at any point during feeding and fasting. These results are most likely due to a defect in insulin processing in which of the following cellular locations?
(A) Cytosol
(B) Golgi apparatus
(C) Lysosomes
(D) Mitochondria
(E) Peroxisomes
(F) Rough endoplasmic reticulum

14. A 53-year-old man is being examined by his physician with the primary complaints that he has a persistent tingling in his feet and that he feels the need to urinate frequently. Physical examination finds the patient is 5 feet 9 inches tall and has a blood pressure of 147/118, a temperature of 36.3°C (97.3°F), and a BMI of 28 kg/m^2. Blood works finds that his serum glucose is 165 g/dL. Given the patient's physical signs and symptoms, which of the following is most likely inhibited in his adipose tissue?
(A) AKT2/PKBβ
(B) Glycogen phosphorylase
(C) Phosphatidylinositol-3-kinase (PI3K)
(D) Protein kinase C (PKC)
(E) Pyruvate kinase

15. Functional studies are being conducted using adipocytes isolated via biopsy from a 12-year-old boy who exhibits chronic hyperglycemia. Molecular analysis finds that the gene (*SLC2A4*) encoding GLUT4 is functional and that the protein is present in the patient's adipocytes. However, plasma membrane labeling finds less than 2% of the expected level of GLUT4. Given these experimental results, the receptor for which of the following is most likely defective in adipocytes from this patient?
(A) Amylin
(B) Epinephrine
(C) Glucagon
(D) Insulin
(E) Somatostatin

ANSWERS

1. Correct answer is **D.** The patient is most likely exhibiting the signs of type 2 diabetes as evidenced by his BMI indicating mild obesity and his elevated fasting plasma glucose level. A primary contributor to type 2 diabetes is the resistance to insulin in the periphery. Insulin resistance refers to the situation whereby insulin interaction with its receptor fails to elicit downstream signaling events. Insulin resistance is a characteristic feature found associated with obesity resulting in type 2 diabetes. In addition, insulin resistance is the hallmark feature of the metabolic syndrome (MetS). Insulin resistance can occur for a number of reasons; however, the most prevalent cause is the hyperlipidemic and pro-inflammatory states associated with overweight and obese states. Although the liver failure (choice E) and, in particular, renal failure (choice F) can result from the consequences of the chronic hyperglycemia and hyperlipidemia associated with type 2 diabetes, these pathologies are more related to the long-term risks this patient faces. None of the other pathologies (choices A, B, and C) are directly correlated with type 2 diabetes.

2. Correct answer is **B.** The patient is most likely experiencing the consequences of abnormal insulin secretion. Insulin is synthesized as a preproprotein. During its synthesis the signal peptide that directs the protein to the endoplasmic reticulum (ER) is removed in the cisternae of the ER and the proprotein is packaged into secretory vesicles in the Golgi. Within the secretory vesicles the protein is folded to its native structure which is stabilized by the formation of two disulfide bonds. Specific protease activity cleaves the center third of the molecule, which dissociates as C peptide, leaving the amino terminal B peptide disulfide bonded to the carboxy terminal A peptide. The C peptide in released, along with functional insulin, when β-cells of the pancreas are induced to secrete the hormone. In a patient in an insulin-induced coma due to injected synthetic insulin there would not be any C peptide in their blood. The presence of elevated levels of plasma C peptide in an unconscious patient could indicate an insulinoma resulting in inappropriate release of insulin leading to unexpected hypoglycemia and the resultant unconsciousness. Cortisol (choice A), epinephrine (choice C), and glucagon (choice D) would each lead to hyperglycemia, not hypoglycemia, if they were abnormally expressed. Although somatostatin (choice E) is thought to down-regulate glucagon secretion, this only occurs during periods of hyperglycemia, thus the secretion of somatostatin would not significantly induce hypoglycemia.

3. Correct answer is **C.** The glucagon-like peptides (principally glucagon-like peptide-1 [GLP-1] and glucose-dependent insulinotropic peptide, [GIP]) are gut hormones that constitute the class of molecules referred to as the incretins. Incretins are molecules associated with food intake-stimulation of insulin secretion from the pancreas. Upon nutrient ingestion GLP-1 is secreted into the blood from intestinal enteroendocrine L-cells that are found predominantly in the distal ileum and proximal colon with some production from these cell types in the duodenum and jejunum. The primary physiologic responses to GLP-1 are glucose-dependent insulin secretion, inhibition of glucagon secretion, and inhibition of gastric acid secretion and gastric emptying. The latter effect will lead to increased satiety with reduced food intake along with a reduced desire to ingest food. Within the pancreas, GLP-1 receptor activation also results in β-cell proliferation and expansion concomitant with a reduction of β-cell apoptosis. In addition, GLP-1 activity in the pancreas results in increased expression of the glucose transporter-2 (GLUT-2) and glucokinase genes. Cholecystokinin (choice A) is released from enteroendocrine I cells, predominantly in the duodenum and jejunum following the consumption of fats and proteins. A major response to cholecystokinin is secretion from the gallbladder. Gastrin (choice B) is released from enteroendocrine G cells of the antrum of the stomach. The primary function of gastrin is to stimulate parietal cells of the stomach to secrete proton (H^+) into the lumen of the stomach for the production of gastric acid. Pancreatic polypeptide, PP (choice D) is produced and secreted by type F cells within the periphery of pancreatic islets. The stimulus for the release of PP is the ingestion of food and the level of release is proportional to the caloric intake. The actions of PP include delaying gastric emptying, inhibition of gallbladder contraction, and attenuation of pancreatic exocrine secretions. Somatostatin (choice E) is produced and secreted by enteroendocrine D cells of the stomach and duodenum and δ-cells of the pancreas. Somatostatin reduces glucagon secretion in response to elevated blood glucose levels and it also inhibits gastric acid production by stomach parietal cells.

4. Correct answer is **C.** The hexosamine biosynthesis pathway (HBP), which synthesizes uridine diphospho-*N*-acetylglucosamine (UDP-GlcNAc), plays a critical role in the development of insulin resistance. Impairment in insulin-stimulated glucose uptake, under hyperglycemic and hyperinsulinemic conditions involves the HBP. Synthesis of UDP-GlcNAc initiates from glucose. Upon entering cells, glucose is converted to glucose-6-phosphate (G6P) via the action of glucokinase/hexokinase. Most of the G6P formed is oxidized in the process of glycolysis. During the process of glycolysis, phosphohexose isomerase converts G6P into fructose-6-phosphate (F6P). Whereas the majority of F6P enters glycolysis, 2–5% enters the hexosamine biosynthesis pathway (HBP) to generate UDP-GlcNAc. The first and rate-limiting enzyme in the HBP is glutamine:fructose-6-phosphate aminotransferase 1, GFAT. GFAT utilizes glutamine and F6P for the formation of glucosamine-6-phosphate (GlcN6P) and glutamate. It is possible for glucosamine to enter the HBP directly by conversion to GlcN6P via the action of hexokinase, thus bypassing the rate-limiting step of the pathway. Acetyl-CoA (choice A) is involved in the synthesis of one of the intermediates of the HBP but alone cannot contribute to elevated UDP-GlcNAc production such as is the case for glucosamine. None of the other compounds (choices B, D, and E) contribute to resistance of adipocytes to insulin signaling.

5. Correct answer is **E.** Insulin-mediated glucose uptake in adipocytes and skeletal muscle involves activation of the kinase, phosphatidylinositol-3,4,5-trisphosphate (PIP_3)-dependent kinase 1 (PDK1). Activated PDK1 phosphorylates and activates isoforms of protein kinase C (PKC) in these cells, specifically the PKCλ/ζ, isoform. Activated PKCλ/ζ, phosphorylates intracellular vesicles containing the glucose transporter, GLUT4, resulting in their migration to, and fusion with, the plasma membrane. This results in increased glucose uptake by adipocytes and skeletal muscle in response to the actions of insulin. None of the other effects (choices A, B, C, and D) correctly correspond to the mechanism by which GLUT4 is mobilized and contributes to glucose uptake.

6. Correct answer is **B.** Compounds that can induce β-cells of the pancreas to increase insulin secretion are referred to as insulin secretagogues. There are two classes of insulin secretagogues, the sulfonylureas and the meglitinides. Drugs of the sulfonylurea class include glyburide. None of the other drugs induce insulin secretion from the pancreas. Dapagliflozin

(choice A) inhibits the proximal tubule glucose reabsorption transporter, SGLT2. Metformin (choice C) is a member of the biguanide family of drugs that function to lower serum glucose levels by enhancing insulin-mediated suppression of hepatic glucose production and enhancing insulin-stimulated glucose uptake by skeletal muscle. Metformin administration does not lead to increased insulin release from the pancreas and as such the risk of hypoglycemia is minimal. Pioglitazone (choice D) is a member of the thiazolidinediones family of drugs that function by activating the transcription factor, peroxisomal proliferator activated receptor gamma, PPARγ. Sitagliptin (choice E) is a member of the dipeptidyl peptidase 4 (DPP4) inhibitors. DPP4 inhibitors reduce the proteolysis of GLP-1 allowing for prolonged activity of this gut-derived hormone. Although one of the effects of GLP-1 on the pancreas is enhanced insulin secretion, it does not result in significant increases in insulin release such as is the case for the sulfonylureas and the meglitinides.

7. Correct answer is **D.** Increased fatty acid synthesis requires sufficient levels of acetyl-CoA which is the precursor for this pathway. Within the liver, a significant contribution to the pool of acetyl-CoA comes from the oxidation of the pyruvate derived from glycolysis. Pyruvate oxidation in the mitochondria is the function of the pyruvate dehydrogenase complex, PDHc. Regulation of the PDHc involves both allosteric effectors and posttranslational modifications. The pyruvate dehydrogenase kinases (PDK1-PDK4) regulate the activity of the PDHc by phosphorylating the complex. Phosphorylation of the PDHc by PDK4 results in a lower rate of pyruvate oxidation. Reduced pyruvate oxidation lowers the pool of acetyl-CoA which is required as the substrate for fatty acid and cholesterol synthesis. One of the effects of insulin in the liver is reduced expression of the gene encoding PDK4. Since insulin action reduces the expression of PDK4, there will be less inhibition of the PDHc and thus, more acetyl-CoA for fatty acid synthesis. Insulin enhances, not inhibits, glucokinase activity (choice A) and pyruvate kinase activity (choice E) the result of which is increased oxidation of glucose to pyruvate. Glucose-6-phosphate dehydrogenase (choice B) activity is induced, not inhibited by insulin. The increased glucose-6-phosphate dehydrogenase activity is required to generate the NADPH necessary for fatty acid synthesis. The expression of phosphoenolpyruvate carboxykinase, PEPCK (choice C) is inhibited by insulin, but this is a gluconeogenic enzyme and thus, its inhibition would not be directly correlated to an increase in fatty acid synthesis.

8. Correct answer is **D.** Insulin-induced effects in hepatocytes lead to the regulated expression of a number of genes encoding metabolic enzymes. Some of these regulatory events are positive and some negative on gene expression. The expression of the genes (*PCK1, FBP1*, and *G6PC*) encoding the cytosolic isoform of phosphoenolpyruvate carboxykinase (PEPCK), fructose 1,6-bisphosphatase, and glucose 6-phosphatase, respectively, are reduced as a result of insulin action. The effect of insulin on these gluconeogenic genes ensures that glycolysis is the predominant pathway in hepatocytes. Insulin induction of hepatic glycolysis allows the excess carbons of glucose to be diverted into acetyl-CoA for input into fatty acid biosynthesis. Conversely, insulin action leads increased expression of the genes encoding acetyl CoA carboxylase (choice A), hepatic glucokinase (choice B), lipoprotein lipase (choice C), and pyruvate kinase (choice E).

9. Correct answer is **E.** One of the major functions of insulin is to stimulate the uptake of glucose from the blood. This is accomplished primarily by the responses of adipose tissue and skeletal muscle to insulin binding its receptor. The response, at the level of glucose uptake, is the stimulation of the mobilization to the plasma membrane of GLUT4-containing vesicles. The hyperglycemia observed in this patient, given normal upstream insulin responses, could most likely be explained by a reduction in GLUT4 transfer to the plasma membrane of cells of these two major insulin-responsive tissues. The migration of GLUT4 vesicles is triggered by the phosphorylation of vesicle proteins by activated PKCλ/ζ. Upon insulin binding its receptor, the receptor undergoes autophosphorylation on tyrosine residues. The presence of the phosphotyrosines promotes interaction with insulin receptor substrate 1 (IRS-1) activating this protein. Active IRS-1 in turn activates the membrane associated kinase, phosphatidylinositol-3-kinase (PI3K) which phosphorylates phosphatidylinositol-4,5-bisphosphate (PIP_2) generating phosphatidylinositol-3,4,5-trisphosphate (PIP_3). PIP_3 will then activate the kinase PIP_3-dependent kinase 1 (PDK1). Finally, PDK1 will phosphorylated and activate PKCλ/ζ. A defect in none of the other proteins (choices A, B, C, and D) would effectively explain the observations in this patient.

10. Correct answer is **D.** One of the major functions of insulin is to stimulate the uptake of glucose from the blood. This is accomplished primarily by the responses of skeletal muscle and adipose tissue to insulin binding its receptor. The response, at the level of glucose uptake, is the stimulation of the mobilization to the plasma membrane of GLUT4-containing vesicles. The hyperglycemia observed in this patient, given normal upstream insulin responses, could most likely be explained by a reduction in GLUT4 transfer to the plasma membrane of cells of these two major insulin-responsive tissues. The migration of GLUT4 vesicles is triggered by the phosphorylation of vesicle proteins by activated PKCλ/ζ. Upon insulin binding its receptor, the receptor undergoes autophosphorylation on tyrosine residues. The presence of the phosphotyrosines promotes interaction with insulin receptor substrate 1 (IRS-1) activating this protein. Active IRS-1 in turn activates the membrane associated kinase, phosphatidylinositol-3-kinase (PI3K) which phosphorylates phosphatidylinositol-4,5-bisphosphate (PIP_2) generating phosphatidylinositol-3,4,5-trisphosphate (PIP_3). PIP_3 will then activate the kinase PIP_3-dependent kinase 1 (PDK1). Finally, PDK1 will phosphorylate and activate PKCλ/ζ. Insulin normally activates mTOR (choice A) but a failure to activate this complex would result in reduced protein synthesis, not glucose transport in skeletal muscle. Insulin activates one of the phosphodiesterase (choice B) family enzymes, but this results in inhibition of glucagon and epinephrine mediated activation of PKA which is not directly involved in glucose transport in skeletal muscle. Insulin receptor signaling does not involve PLCβ (choice C). Insulin normally activates the monomeric G-protein, RAS (choice E) but a failure to activate this protein would result in impaired insulin-mediated transcriptional activation, not glucose transport in skeletal muscle.

11. Correct answer is **E.** All of the post-receptor responses initiated by insulin binding to its receptor are mediated as a consequence of the activation of several signal transduction pathways. These signal transduction cascades involve the activation of several different kinases that phosphorylate their substrates in response to activation from upstream factors

in the insulin signaling cascade. In order for these events to occur, the intrinsic tyrosine kinase activity of the insulin receptor must be activated which results in autophosphorylation of the receptor on tyrosine residues. Lack of receptor phosphorylation will prevent signaling proteins from binding to the receptor and, therefore they cannot be activated. The loss of interaction of signaling proteins with the insulin receptor will lead to loss of activation of each of the downstream kinases. Although the loss of insulin receptor autophosphorylation would ultimately decrease glucose transporter (GLUT4) translocation to the plasma membrane (choice D) the defect is more likely to be at the level of the insulin receptor. None of the other processes (choices A, B, and C) are directly associated with insulin signal transduction pathways.

12. Correct answer is **A.** The major metabolic functions of insulin are to increase carbon storage which it accomplishes primarily within the liver, skeletal muscle, and adipose tissue. Insulin accomplishes this by activating metabolic pathways that promote carbon storage. This includes activation of glycogen synthesis and activation of fatty acid synthesis, while inhibiting glycogen breakdown, lipolysis, and glucose synthesis (gluconeogenesis), the latter specifically within the liver. Activation of fatty acid synthesis occurs primarily in the liver through the actions of insulin that promote glucose oxidation to acetyl-CoA and the diversion of the acetyl-CoA into *de novo* fatty acid synthesis. These metabolic effects of insulin are the consequence of the activation of a phosphodiesterase that hydrolyzes cAMP to AMP resulting in deactivation of PKA and, consequently, reduced levels of phosphorylated metabolic enzymes. Insulin signaling also results in activation of a phosphatase that removes phosphate from numerous metabolic enzymes. At the level of glycogen synthesis and breakdown, the removal of phosphate from glycogen synthase leads to its activation, while removal of phosphate from glycogen phosphorylase leads to its deactivation. The net effect is increased storage of glucose in glycogen. All of the metabolic and growth factor mediating effects of insulin result in increased, not decreased, protein synthesis (choice B) and triglyceride synthesis (choice C). Gluconeogenesis is inhibited, not increased (choice D) and lipolysis is inhibited leading to decreased, not increased, ketone body production (choice F). Since insulin stimulates glucose uptake into adipose tissue and skeletal muscle there will be a slight, but not significant decrease in glucose uptake by the brain (choice E). Since the major glucose transporters in the brain, GLUT1 and GLUT3, are not responsive to the actions of insulin there is no significant increase in glucose transport into the brain as a result of the actions of insulin.

13. Correct answer is **B.** Like almost all secreted proteins, insulin is synthesized while being transferred into the lumen of the rough endoplasmic reticulum (RER). Following attachment to, and extrusion into, the lumen of the ER the signal sequence of the preproinsulin protein is removed. The proinsulin protein is packaged into secretory vesicles in the Golgi. Within the Golgi the proinsulin protein is folded into its native structure which is stabilized by intrachain disulfide bonds. The protease that processes proinsulin is proprotein convertase subtilisin/kexin type 1 (PCSK1). PCSK1 is also referred to as prohormone convertase 1/3 (PC1/3). PCSK1 cleaves proinsulin to remove its connecting C-peptide which liberates the disulfide bonded A and B peptides that constitutes functional insulin. The disulfide bonded A and B peptides fold into the native structure of functional insulin. Although the signal sequence of preproinsulin is removed by signal peptidase in the lumen of the ER (choice F), the remainder of the required processing occurs within vesicles of the Golgi apparatus. Synthesis and processing of insulin does not take place in any other cellular compartment (choices A, C, D, and E).

14. Correct answer is **A.** Given the patient's BMI, he is obese and is, therefore, most likely experiencing the early signs of type 2 diabetes, T2D. One hallmark consequence of T2D is peripheral insulin resistance. The hyperlipidemia that is characteristic in overweight and obese individuals results in the interference (resistance) of insulin signaling, principally within the liver, skeletal muscle, and adipose tissue. Increased uptake of free fatty acid (FFA) leads to accumulation of the metabolites of the FFA re-esterification process, including long-chain acyl-CoAs, diacylglycerol (DAG), and ceramides (see Figure 29–8). Excess FFA also participate in the relocation of several protein kinase C (PKC) isoforms, from the cytosol to the membrane compartment. DAG is a potent activator of these PKC isoforms and the membrane-associated PKCs will phosphorylate the intracellular portion of the insulin receptor on serine residues which results in impairment of insulin receptor interaction with downstream signaling proteins including insulin receptor substrate 1 (IRS1) and IRS2. Loss of IRS1 and IRS2 interaction with the receptor prevents interaction with phosphatidylinositol 3-kinase (PI3K) and its subsequent activation. When activated, PI3K phosphorylates PIP_2-generating PIP_3 which in turn activates PIP_3-dependent protein kinase 1 (PDPK1). PDPK1 phosphorylates and activates AKT2/PKBβ. The increased levels of ceramides that result from hyperlipidemic states result in direct inhibition of AKT2. The actions of AKT2, in adipose tissue, normally lead to increased GLUT4-mediated glucose uptake and inhibition of lipolysis. In the absence of normal insulin-mediated signaling, glycogen phosphorylase will remain active, not inhibited (choice B). Although the activity of PI3K (choice C) will be reduced as a result of impaired signaling from IRS1 and IRS2, its activity is not inhibited. PKC activity (choice D) is also not inhibited as a result of obesity-induced insulin resistance. Indeed, several PKC isoforms remain active, but toward membrane-associated targets as opposed to their normal cytosolic targets. Pyruvate kinase (choice E) activity will also be reduced as a result of insulin resistance in adipose tissue but it is not inhibited.

15. Correct answer is **D.** The absence of GLUT4 glucose transporters from the plasma membrane of adipocytes isolated from this patient most likely indicates that functional insulin receptors are not present in these cells. Insulin signaling in adipose tissue, and skeletal muscle, leads to activation of AKT2/PKBβ and specific isoforms of PKC. These enzymes phosphorylate proteins associated with GLUT4-containing vesicles, the consequences of which are migration to, and fusion with, the plasma membrane leading to increased glucose transport into these cells. None of the other hormones (choices A, B, C, and E) activate signaling processes that lead to increased mobilization of GLUT4 to the plasma membrane of adipocytes or skeletal muscle myocytes.

CHAPTER

30

Diabetes Mellitus

High-Yield Terms

Polyuria	Excessive urine output as is typical in most forms of diabetes
Polyphagia	Excessive hunger typically associated with type 1 diabetes
Polydipsia	Excessive thirst as is often associated with diabetes
Oral glucose tolerance test, OGTT	A test to measure the plasma responses to intake of a bolus of glucose; used to determine insulin function and the potential for diabetes
Type 1 diabetes, T1D	Insulin-dependent diabetes mellitus (IDDM), insulin-deficient form of diabetes most often manifesting in children as a result of autoimmune destruction of the β-cells of the pancreas
Diabetic ketoacidosis, DKA	A potentially life-threatening condition of excess ketone production by the liver in response to uncontrolled fatty acid release from adipose tissue resulting from excess glucagon secretion
Type 2 diabetes, T2D	Noninsulin-dependent diabetes mellitus (NIDDM), a form of the disease associates with peripheral insulin resistance progressing to loss of insulin production
Gestational diabetes mellitus, GDM	A specific form of diabetes mellitus characterized by glucose intolerance first appearing during pregnancy
Maturity-onset type diabetes of the young, MODY	A class of T2D caused by inherited or somatic mutations in any of several genes involved in pancreatic function
Neonatal diabetes	Hyperglycemia resulting from dysfunction in insulin action within the first 6 months of life and thus, not type 1 diabetes
HbA_{1c}	Designates the glycosylated form of adult hemoglobin; is a measure of the level of glucose in the plasma

DIABETES DEFINED

Diabetes is any disorder characterized by excessive urine excretion. The most common form of diabetes is diabetes mellitus, a metabolic disorder in which there is an inability to maintain carbohydrate and lipid homeostasis due to disturbances in insulin function, resulting in hyperglycemia and excess urinary excretion of glucose as well as hyperlipidemia. Diabetes mellitus is characterized by chronic hyperglycemia and the potential for episodic ketoacidosis. Additional symptoms of diabetes mellitus include excessive thirst, (polydipsia) glucosuria, polyuria, lipemia, and excessive hunger (polyphagia). There are two primary forms of diabetes mellitus, type 1 and type 2. Type 1 diabetes (T1D) is defined by the loss of insulin production by the pancreas and type 2 diabetes (T2D) is defined by loss of peripheral responses to insulin. If left untreated T1D can lead to fatal ketoacidosis. Of the two major forms of diabetes mellitus, T2D represents the prevalent form of the disease.

Two primary criteria are used to clinically establish an individual as suffering from diabetes mellitus, particularly T2D. One is a fasting plasma glucose (FPG) level in excess of 126 mg/dL (7 mmol/L), where normal levels should be less than 100 mg/dL (5.6 mmol/L). The second is defined by the results of an oral glucose tolerance test (OGTT) where having plasma glucose levels in excess of 200 mg/dL (11 mmol/L) at two times points, one of which must be within 2 hours of ingestion of glucose (Figure 30–1). Different clinical labs may use different units for the measurement of serum glucose concentrations, either in mmol/L or mg/dL. One can easily interconvert these values using the following formulas where mg/dL × 0.0555 = mmol/L or simply divide mg/dL by 18 to get the approximate mmol/L value.

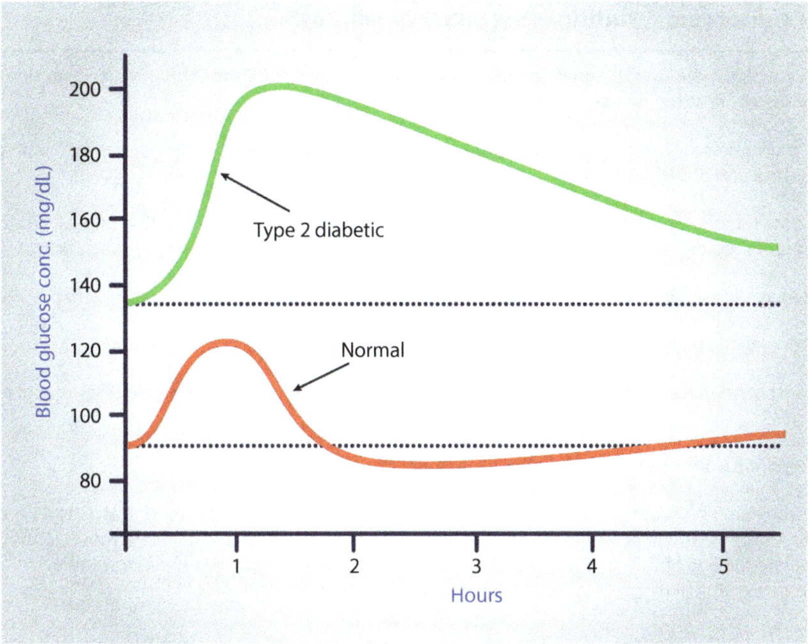

FIGURE 30–1 Glucose tolerance curve for a normal person and one with noninsulin-dependent diabetes mellitus (NIDDM, type 2 diabetes). The dotted lines indicate the boundaries for the range of glucose concentration expected in a normal individual. (Reproduced with permission from themedicalbiochemistrypage, LLC.)

TYPES OF DIABETES MELLITUS

Diabetes mellitus is a heterogeneous clinical disorder with numerous causes. Two main classifications of diabetes mellitus exist, **idiopathic** and **secondary**.

Idiopathic diabetes is divided into two main types: insulin-dependent and noninsulin-dependent diabetes mellitus. Insulin-dependent diabetes mellitus, IDDM (more commonly referred to as T1D) is defined by the development of ketoacidosis in the absence of insulin therapy. T1D most often manifests in childhood (hence, also called juvenile-onset diabetes) and is the result of an autoimmune destruction of the β-cells of the pancreas. Non-insulin-dependent diabetes mellitus, NIDDM (more commonly referred to as T2D) is characterized by persistent hyperglycemia but rarely leads to ketoacidosis. T2D generally manifests after age 40 and therefore has the obsolete name of adult onset-type diabetes. However, due to the rising rates of adolescent obesity in industrialized countries there is an increasing incidence of T2D in pre- and postpubescent children. T2D can also result from genetic defects that cause both insulin resistance and insulin deficiency.

Secondary causes of diabetes mellitus are numerous and can be associated with the pharmacology of certain drugs and as a consequence of unrelated diseases and disorders (Table 30–1). Many other genetic syndromes have either diabetes or impaired glucose tolerance associated with them such as Down syndrome, Huntington disease, and Turner syndrome.

MATURITY-ONSET TYPE DIABETES IN THE YOUNG: MODY

Maturity-onset type diabetes of the young (MODY) is a form of diabetes characterized by onset prior to age 25 but not associated with autoimmune loss of pancreatic β-cells. MODY was previously considered to be a third form of type 2 diabetes; however, with the discovery that specific gene mutations are the causes of the various forms of MODY, they are now classified as monogenic forms of diabetes mellitus.

All cases of MODY are associated with some level of impaired β-cell function characterized by defective GSIS (see Chapter 29). Patients may also exhibit insulin resistance and late β-cell failure. Evidence indicates that mutations in at least 14 different genes have been correlated with the development of MODY with 11 reviewed in Table 30–2. All cases of MODY are rare or very rare except for MODY2.

ADDITIONAL TYPES OF DIABETES

Other forms of diabetes include gestational diabetes, diabetes insipidus, brittle diabetes, and bronze diabetes. Diabetes insipidus is characterized by the excess output (3–20 L per day; normal is less than 3 L per day) of dilute urine. There are four major classifications of diabetes insipidus, each of which is related to the primary site/cause of the excess urine output.

TABLE 30–1 Diseases/disorders resulting in secondary diabetes.

Gestational diabetes	Form of diabetes mellitus that appears during pregnancy, generally in third trimester; women experiencing this form of diabetes are at higher risk for future development of T2D
Pancreatic disease	Pancreatectomy leads to the clearest example of secondary diabetes; cystic fibrosis and pancreatitis can also lead to destruction of the pancreas
Endocrine disease	Some tumors can produce counter-regulatory hormones that oppose the action of insulin or inhibit insulin secretion; counter-regulatory hormones include glucagon, epinephrine, growth hormone, and cortisol
Glucagonomas	Pancreatic cancers that secrete glucagon
Pheochromocytomas	Adrenal medullary tumors that secrete excess epinephrine
Cushing syndrome (see Clinical Box 31–2)	Most often due to excess ACTH secretion from a pituitary adenoma, results in excess cortisol secretion from adrenal glands
Acromegaly	Resulting from excess growth hormone production
Mutations in insulin receptor gene (INSR)	Two related syndromes, Donohue and Rabson-Mendenhall; three common clinical features are insulin resistance, acanthosis nigricans, and hyperandrogenism (the latter being observed only in females); most Donohue syndrome children die before the age of 2; most Rabson-Mendenhall patients die in their teens or early twenties

TABLE 30–2 Forms of MODY.

Type	Gene	Encoded Protein	Comments
MODY1	*HNF4A*	Hepatocyte nuclear factor-4α, HNF-4α	Gene is also known as transcription factor-14 (TCF14); HNF-4α is a member of the nuclear receptor family of transcription factors, specifically identified as NR2A1; expression of HNF-4α is associated with the growth and normal functioning of the pancreas; many genes are known to be regulated by HNF-4α including those encoding HNF-1α, PPARα, insulin, glucose-6-phosphatase, GLUT2, the liver pyruvate kinase isoform (L-PK) which is also expressed in the pancreas, glyceraldehyde-3-phosphate dehydrogenase (GAPDH), aldolase B, and uncoupling protein 2, UCP2.
MODY2	*GCK*	Glucokinase	Because the enzyme is responsive to glucose uptake, it is often referred to as the pancreatic glucose sensor.
MODY3	*HNF1A*	Hepatocyte nuclear factor-1α, HNF-1α	Also called transcription factor-1 (TCF1); is involved in a regulatory loop with HNF-4α controlling many genes involved in pancreatic and liver function such as the gene encoding *GLUT2* and *L-PK*. The designations of *GLUT2* and *L-PK* are not the gene identities but the protein identities.
MODY4	*PDX1*	Pancreas duodenum homeobox-1	A homeodomain-containing transcription factor; also called insulin promoter factor-1 (IPF-1); involved in pancreatic precursor determination in cells of the developing gut; major activator of insulin gene transcription in mature pancreas.
MODY5	*HNF1B*	Hepatocyte nuclear factor-1β, HNF-1β	Also called transcription factor-2 (TCF2); is a critical regulator of a transcriptional network that controls the specification, growth, and differentiation of the embryonic pancreas; mutations in *HNF1B* are associated with pancreatic hypoplasia, defective kidney development, and genital malformations.
MODY6	*NEUROD1*	Neurogenic differentiation 1, NeuroD1	A basic helix-loop-helix (bHLH) type transcription factor first identified as a neural fate-inducing gene; regulates insulin gene transcription.
MODY7	*KLF11*	Krüpple-like factor 11, KLF11	A zinc-finger transcription factor involved in activation at the insulin promoter; is a TGF-β-inducible transcription factor.
MODY8	*CEL*	Carboxyl-ester lipase, CEL	Involved in dietary lipid metabolism (see Chapter 13); frameshift deletions in the variable number tandem repeats (VNTR) of the *CEL* gene are associated with pancreatic exocrine and β-cell dysfunction.
MODY9	*PAX4*	Paired box 4, PAX4	A paired box domain-containing transcription factor; involved in the differentiation of endoderm-derived endocrine pancreas.
MODY10	*INS*	Insulin	This form of MODY is associated with heterozygosity for missense mutations in the *INS* gene.
MODY11	*BLK*	B-lymphocyte specific tyrosine kinase, Blk	Polymorphisms in *BLK* are associated with a higher prevalence of obesity and diabetes than with other MODY loci.

TABLE 30–3 Most common autoantibodies detected in type 1 diabetics.

Autoantibodies	Comments
Islet cell cytoplasmic antibodies, ICCA	These are the primary antibodies found in 90% of T1D patients; presence of ICCA is a highly accurate predictor of future development of T1D; ICCA are not specific for β-cells antigens, but the autoimmune attack appears to selectively destroy β-cells; whether a direct cause or an effect of islet cell destruction, the titer of the ICCA tends to decline over time
Islet cell surface antibodies, ICSA	Found in up to 80% of T1D patients; titer of ICSA declines over time; some patients with T2D have been identified that are ICSA positive
Glutamic acid decarboxylase, GAD	Found in up to 80% of T1D patients; titer of anti-GAD declines over time; two GAD genes, *GAD1* and *GAD2*; *GAD1* encodes GAD67, *GAD2* encodes GAD65 (reflects protein MW); *GAD1* and *GAD2* genes expressed in the brain, *GAD2* expression also in pancreas; presence of anti-GAD antibodies (both anti-GAD65 and anti-GAD67) is a strong predictor of the future development of T1D
Anti-insulin antibodies, IAA	Detectable in around 40% of children with T1D

These forms are referred to as central, nephrogenic, dipsogenic, and gestational.

Another form of diabetes is diabetes insipidus which is the result of a deficiency of antidiuretic hormone (ADH, also referred to as vasopressin or arginine vasopressin, AVP). The major symptom of diabetes insipidus (excessive output of dilute urine) results from an inability of the kidneys to resorb water.

TYPE 1 DIABETES (T1D), INSULIN-DEPENDENT DIABETES MELLITUS (IDDM)

Type 1 diabetes has been shown to be the result of an autoimmune reaction to antigens of the islet cells of the pancreas (Table 30–3). There is a strong association between T1D and other endocrine autoimmune disorders (eg, Addison disease). Additionally, there is an increased prevalence of autoimmune disease in family members of T1D patients.

Pathophysiology of Type 1 Diabetes

The autoimmune destruction of pancreatic β-cells in T1D leads to a deficiency of insulin secretion. In addition to loss of insulin production there is abnormal glucagon secretion. The loss of insulin secretion, coupled with glucagon dysregulation, results in the metabolic derangements associated with T1D. The major metabolic derangements which result from insulin deficiency in T1D are impaired glucose, lipid, and protein metabolism (Figure 30–2).

HIGH-YIELD CONCEPT

In addition to the loss of insulin secretion, the function of pancreatic α-cells is also abnormal resulting in dysregulation in secretion of glucagon in T1D patients. Normally, hyperglycemia leads to reduced glucagon secretion. However, in patients with T1D, glucagon secretion is not suppressed by hyperglycemia.

The most pronounced example of this metabolic disruption is that patients with T1D rapidly develop diabetic ketoacidosis (DKA) in the absence of insulin administration. Particularly problematic for long-term T1D patients is an impaired ability to secrete glucagon in response to hypoglycemia. This leads to potentially fatal hypoglycemia in response to insulin treatment in these patients.

A. Glucose Metabolism in T1D

Insulin normally stimulates hepatic and skeletal muscle glycogen synthesis while repressing hepatic gluconeogenesis. The activity of hepatic glucokinase is also regulated by insulin. Taken together the hepatic consequences, at the level of glucose homeostasis, of T1D are excessive glucose output resulting in hyperglycemia. The insulin deficiency simultaneously impairs nonhepatic tissue utilization of glucose, primarily adipose tissue and skeletal muscle, due to loss of GLUT4 mobilization to the plasma membrane. This ultimately exacerbates the hyperglycemia.

When the capacity of the kidneys to absorb glucose is surpassed, **glucosuria** ensues. Glucose is an osmotic diuretic and an increase in renal glucose excretion is accompanied by loss of water and electrolytes, termed **polyuria**. The result of the loss of water (and overall volume) leads to the hyperactivation of the thirst mechanism (**polydipsia**). The negative caloric balance which results from the glucosuria and tissue catabolism leads to an increase in appetite and food intake (**polyphagia**).

B. Lipid Metabolism in T1D

Insulin normally represses adipose tissue triglyceride breakdown while stimulating glucose uptake to promote triglyceride synthesis. Conversely, glucagon stimulates adipose tissue triglyceride breakdown. The consequences in T1D is excess free fatty acids (FFA) in the circulation: lipemia.

Normally, hepatic oxidation of fatty acids is repressed in the presence of insulin due to activation of acetyl-CoA carboxylase (ACC) and the resultant levels of malonyl-CoA that inhibit carnitine palmitoyltransferase 1 (CPT1). Thus, in the absence of insulin, malonyl-CoA levels fall and fatty acid oxidation is elevated.

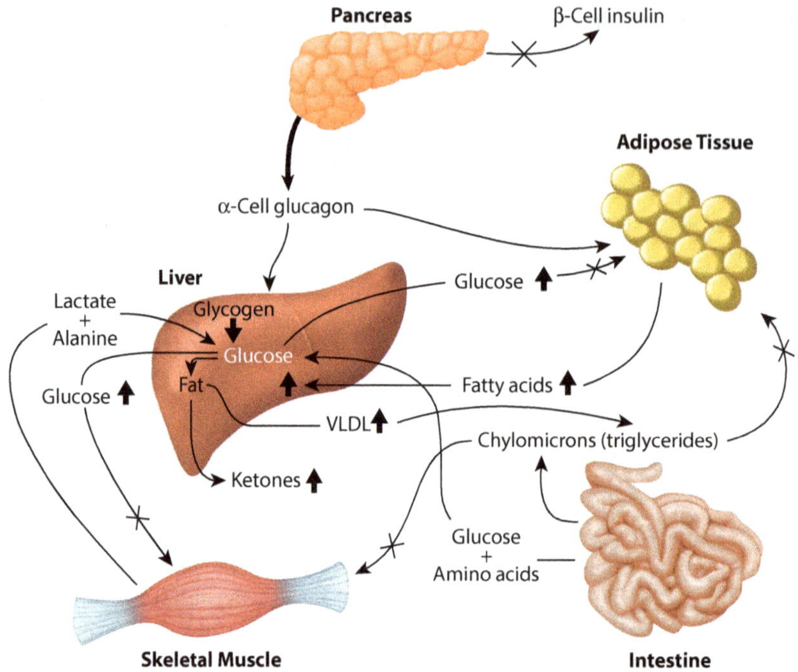

FIGURE 30–2 Metabolic disruptions occurring in T1D. The major metabolic disturbances associated with T1D are the result of the loss of insulin and uncontrolled increases in glucagon secretion from the pancreas. Glucagon stimulates triglyceride hydrolysis in adipose tissue and increases glycogen breakdown and gluconeogenesis in the liver. The glucose released from the liver is not taken up by adipose tissue or muscle due to loss of insulin-mediated GLUT4 migration to the plasma membrane. Lipid homeostasis in the liver is shifted to oxidation resulting in elevated ketone production. Whatever triglyceride that is incorporated into very-low-density lipoprotein (VLDL) in the liver and in chylomicrons from the gut cannot be taken up by adipose tissue due to the enhanced lipolysis occurring in this tissue. Skeletal muscle alanine and lactate contribute to glucose production by the liver exacerbating the hyperglycemia resulting from impaired insulin responses. (Reproduced with permission from themedicalbiochemistrypage, LLC.)

The increased fat oxidation leads to increased mitochondrial acetyl-CoA which the liver diverts into ketone body synthesis (see Chapter 10).

HIGH-YIELD CONCEPT

Production of ketone bodies, in excess of the ability to utilize them leads to ketoacidosis which is called diabetic ketoacidosis (DKA, Clinical Box 30–1) in T1D. If the DKA is not treated, it can lead to fatal consequences in T1D patients. Ketoacidosis can be easily diagnosed by smelling the breath since acetone, a spontaneous breakdown product of acetoacetate, is volatilized by the lungs producing a distinctive odor.

Fatty acid removal from plasma triglycerides is catalyzed by adipose tissue, skeletal muscle, and cardiac muscle lipoprotein lipase (LPL). The level and activity of LPL are induced by insulin; therefore, in the absence of insulin in T1D the result of loss of LPL activity is hypertriglyceridemia.

C. Protein Metabolism in T1D

Insulin regulates the synthesis of many genes, either positively or negatively that then affect overall metabolism. Insulin has a global effect on protein metabolism, increasing the rate of protein synthesis and decreasing the rate of protein degradation. Insulin deficiency in T1D leads to increased catabolism of protein which in turn increases plasma amino acids, particularly alanine and glutamine. These two amino acids serve as precursors for hepatic, intestinal, and renal gluconeogenesis. In liver, the increased gluconeogenesis further contributes to the hyperglycemia of T1D.

TYPE 2 DIABETES (T2D), NONINSULIN-DEPENDENT DIABETES MELLITUS (NIDDM)

Type 2 diabetes refers to the common form of idiopathic diabetes mellitus. Type 2 diabetes is generally characterized by late-onset (hence the archaic term of adult-onset diabetes) and a reduced likelihood for ketoacidosis. Development of T2D is the result of multifactorial influences that include lifestyle, environment, and genetics. The primary cause of T2D is resistance to the peripheral tissue effects of insulin.

The major clinical complications of T2D are the result of persistent hyperglycemia which leads to numerous pathophysiologic consequences (Figure 30–3). Hyperglycemia increases blood viscosity reducing microvascular circulation. The reduced circulation results in diabetic retinopathy (referred to as diabetic blindness), peripheral neuropathy (resulting in numbness in the extremities

CLINICAL BOX 30–1 DIABETIC KETOACIDOSIS

The most severe and life-threatening complication of poorly controlled type 1 diabetes is diabetic ketoacidosis (DKA). DKA is characterized by metabolic acidosis, hyperglycemia, and hyperketonemia. Diagnosis of DKA is accomplished by detection of hyperketonemia and metabolic acidosis (as measured by the anion gap) in the presence of hyperglycemia. The anion gap refers to the difference between the concentration of cations other than sodium and the concentration of anions other than chloride and bicarbonate. The anion gap, therefore, represents an artificial assessment of the unmeasured ions in plasma. Calculation of the anion gap involves sodium (Na^+), potassium (K^+), chloride (Cl^-), and bicarbonate (HCO_3^-) measurements, and it is defined as $[(Na^+ + K^+) - (Cl^- + HCO_3^-)]$ where the ion concentrations are measured as mEq/L or in mmol/L. Using this calculation, the normal anion gap is around 10–20 mEq/L. Normal plasma concentrations of potassium are quite low, so the normal practice is to ignore this ion in the anion gap calculation such that the equation becomes: $[Na^+ - (Cl^- + HCO_3^-)]$. Using this formula, the normal anion gap is 5–15 mEq/L. The anion gap will increase when the concentration of plasma K^+, Ca^{2+}, or Mg^{2+} is decreased, when organic ions such as lactate are increased (or foreign anions accumulate), or when the concentration or charge of plasma proteins increases. A higher than normal anion gap is diagnostic of metabolic acidosis. Rapid and aggressive treatment is necessary as the metabolic acidosis can result in cerebral edema and coma, eventually leading to death. The hyperketonemia in DKA is the result of insulin deficiency and unregulated glucagon secretion from α-cells of the pancreas. Circulating glucagon stimulates the adipose tissue to release fatty acids stored in triglycerides. The free fatty acids enter the circulation and are taken up primarily by the liver where they undergo fatty acid β-oxidation to acetyl-CoA. Normally, acetyl-CoA is completely oxidized to CO_2 and water in the TCA cycle. However, the level of fatty acid β-oxidation is in excess of the ability of the liver to fully oxidize the excess acetyl-CoA and, thus, the compound is diverted into the ketogenesis pathway. The ketones (ketone bodies) are β-hydroxybutyrate and acetoacetate with β-hydroxybutyrate being the most abundant. Acetoacetate will spontaneously (nonenzymatic) decarboxylate to acetone. Acetone is volatile and is released from the lungs giving the characteristic sweet smell to the breath of someone with hyperketonemia. The ketones are released into the circulation and because they are acidic lower the pH of the blood resulting in metabolic acidosis. Insulin deficiency also causes increased triglyceride and protein metabolism in skeletal muscle. This leads to increased release of glycerol (from triglyceride metabolism) and alanine (from protein metabolism) to the circulation. These substances then enter the liver where they are used as substrates for gluconeogenesis which is enhanced in the absence of insulin and the elevated glucagon and the increased acetyl-CoA which activates pyruvate carboxylase. The increased rate of glucose production in the liver, coupled with the glucagon-mediated inhibition of glucose storage into glycogen results in the increased glucose release from the liver and consequent hyperglycemia. The resultant hyperglycemia produces an osmotic diuresis that leads to loss of water and electrolytes in the urine. The ketones are also excreted in the urine, and this results in an obligatory loss of Na^+ and K^+. The loss in K^+ is large, sometimes exceeding 300 mEq/L/24 h. Initial serum K^+ is typically normal or elevated because of the extracellular migration of K^+ in response to the metabolic acidosis. The level of K^+ will fall further during treatment as insulin therapy drives K^+ into cells. If serum K^+ is not monitored and replaced as needed life-threatening hypokalemia may develop. Hypokalemia results in slowed cardiac conductance, delated ventricular repolarization, a shorter refractory period, and an increase in automaticity. Using ECG to monitor DKA patients will show ventricular dysrhythmia, prolonged QT intervals, and mild ST wave depression. Each case of DKA must be treated on an individual basis. Table 30–4 shows a general scheme for diagnosis and treatment of DKA.

HIGH-YIELD CONCEPT

Unlike patients with T1D, those with T2D have detectable levels of circulating insulin. On the basis of oral glucose tolerance testing the essential elements of T2D can be divided into four distinct groups; those with normal glucose tolerance, chemical diabetes (called impaired glucose tolerance), diabetes with minimal fasting hyperglycemia (FPG <140 mg/dL), and diabetes in association with overt fasting hyperglycemia (FPG >140 mg/dL). Most patients with T2D will first exhibit normal to high insulin secretion but have impaired peripheral tissue responses, primarily reduced adipose tissue, and skeletal muscle glucose disposal.

HIGH-YIELD CONCEPT

Assessment of therapeutic efficacy in the treatment of the hyperglycemia in T2D is accomplished by routine measurement of the circulating levels of glycated hemoglobin, designated as the level of HbA_{1c}, often designated as just A1C (Clinical Box 30–2). HbA_1 is the major form of adult hemoglobin in the blood and the "c" refers to the glycated form of the protein.

and tingling in fingers and toes), poor wound healing, renal failure, and erectile dysfunction. Similar to the situation in T1D, the hyperglycemia in T2D results in osmotic diuresis (polyuria) and the water loss results in excessive thirst (polydipsia).

Glycation of hemoglobin (as well as numerous other proteins and macromolecules) occurs as a result of nonenzymatic covalent sugar attachment to the protein subunits of hemoglobin. These glycated macromolecules are referred to as advanced glycation end-products (AGE). Glycation can involve fructose or glucose but in the context of hemoglobin glycation it is almost exclusively glucose that is attached to the hemoglobin proteins. Glycation of hemoglobin is sometimes referred to as glycosylation but it is a nonenzymatic attachment of the sugar, so the use of the term glycosylated hemoglobin is incorrect as it infers an enzyme catalyzed reaction.

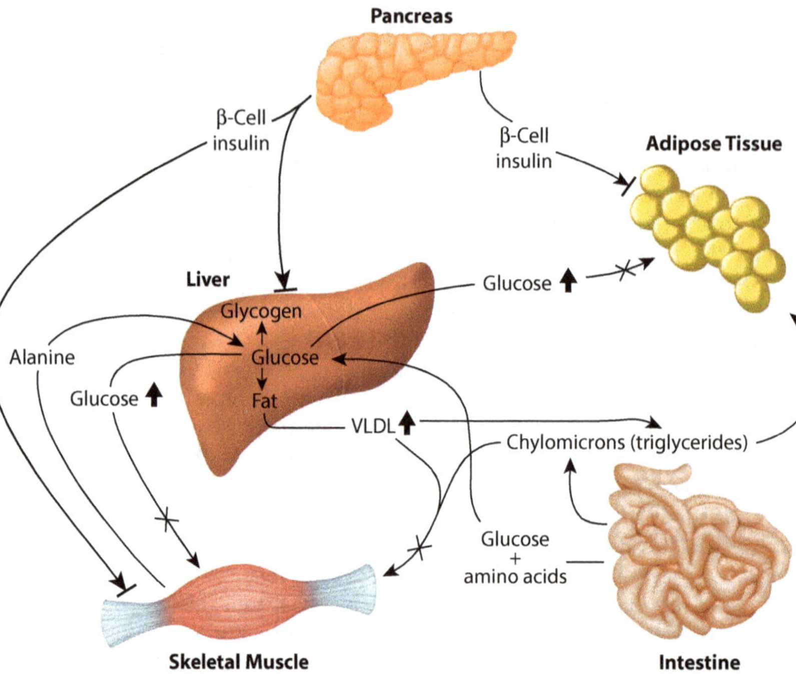

FIGURE 30–3 Metabolic disruptions occurring in T2D. The major metabolic disturbances associated with T2D are the result of impaired peripheral tissue responses to insulin, primarily the liver, skeletal muscle, and adipose tissue. The bars at the ends of the insulin arrows denote the failure of the hormone to activate normal signaling in these tissues. The insulin resistance results in elevated glucose and VLDL output by the liver; this coupled to impaired glucose uptake by skeletal muscle and adipose tissue results in hyperglycemia and hyperlipidemia. (Reproduced with permission from themedicalbiochemistrypage, LLC.)

TABLE 30–4 Assessment and treatment of diabetic ketoacidosis.

Initial Assessment of DKA	Blood glucose >250 mg/dL
	Arterial pH <7.3
	Serum bicarbonate <15 mEq/L
	Urinary ketones ≥3+ and/or serum ketones are positive
Monitoring	Vital signs every hour
	Serum glucose every hour and as needed
	Blood gas pH every 2 h (use arterial for first measurement then can use venous)
	Electrolytes every 1–2 h
	Urine ketones on each void
	Fluid input and output continuously
	Magnesium and phosphorous immediately and then every 1–2 h
Fluid management	Start normal saline at 1 L/h or 15–20 mL/kg/h initially
	Determine hydration status, goal being to replace 50% of estimated volume loss in the first 4 h then remainder over next 8–12 h
	Infuse normal saline 125–500 mL/h, rate dependent on hydration status
	Once serum Na^+ is corrected infuse ½ normal saline at 4–14 mL/kg/h
	When serum glucose reaches 250 mg/dL change fluid to D5W ½ normal saline at same rate

(Continued)

TABLE 30–4 Assessment and treatment of diabetic ketoacidosis. (*Continued*)

Insulin management	Discontinue all oral diabetic medications and previous insulin orders Give regular insulin IV bolus of 10 units Start insulin infusion usually at a rate of 0.15 unit/kg Insulin administration goal is to reduce serum glucose 50–70 mg/dL/h When serum glucose is ≤150 mg/dL then can switch to adult sq insulin with basal insulin
Potassium management	If serum K^+ is <3.3, give 40 mEq/h until it is >3.3 If serum K^+ is >3.3 but <5.0, give 20–30 mEq/L of IV fluids to keep serum K^+ between 4–5 mEq/L If serum K^+ is ≥5.0, do not give K^+ but check serum levels every 2 h when replacing K^+, both potassium chloride and potassium phosphate can be used Hold K^+ replacement if patient urine output is <30 mL/h
Bicarbonate management	Assess need for bicarbonate by arterial pH measurement If pH <6.9, give 100 mEq sodium bicarbonate in 1 L D5W and infuse at 200 mL/h If pH is 6.9–7.0, give 50 mEq sodium bicarbonate in 1 L D5W and infuse at 200 mL/h If pH >7.0, do not give bicarbonate Continue sodium bicarbonate administration until pH is >7.0 Monitor serum K^+

The presence of AGE within the plasma leads to severe pathological consequences which include enhanced oxidative stress, oxidation of LDL (oxLDL), induced secretion of various proinflammatory cytokines, inhibition of the dilating effects of nitric oxide (NO), increased vascular permeability, and arterial stiffening.

CLINICAL BOX 30–2 MEASUREMENT OF HbA_{1c} LEVELS

Typical values for HbA_{1c} measurement (using the previous standard Diabetes Control and Complications Trial, DCCT units of %) are shown in Table 30–5, where values above 6% represent prolonged hyperglycemia. Beginning in 2011, a new international standard (International Federation of Clinical Chemistry, IFCC units) for the measurement of HbA_{1c} levels was developed. This new standard equates the mmol of HbA_{1c} per mole of total measured hemoglobin, Hb (mmol/mol). The method for calculating the relationship between these two measurement values is to use the following formula:

$$\text{IFCC-HbA}_{1c}\ (\text{mmol/mol}) = [\text{DCCT-HbA}_{1c}\ (\%) - 2.15] \times 10.929.$$

To calculate the estimated average glucose (eAG) level in the blood using the DCCT (%) values, one would use the following formula:

$$\text{eAG(mg/dL)} = 28.7 \times \text{A1C} - 46.7 \text{ (for glucose level in mM use: eAG(mM)} = 1.59 \times \text{A1C} - 2.59$$

With new IFCC standard, the target range of HbA_{1c} for healthy levels is 48–59 mmol/mol.

THERAPEUTIC INTERVENTION FOR HYPERGLYCEMIA

Many, if not all, of the vascular consequences of insulin resistance are due to the persistent hyperglycemia seen in T2D. For this reason, a major goal of therapeutic intervention in T2D is to reduce circulating glucose levels. There are many pharmacologic strategies to accomplish these goals (Table 30–6).

TABLE 30–5 Comparison of various HbA_{1c} measurements.

HbA_{1c}	HbA_{1c}/Hb mmol/mol	eAG (mg/dL)	eAG (mM)
4%	20	68	3.8
5%	31	97	5.4
6%	42	125	7
7%	53	154	8.5
8%	64	183	10
9%	75	212	11.7
10%	86	240	13.3
11%	97	270	15
12%	108	298	16.5
13%	119	326	18

TABLE 30–6 Hypoglycemia inducing drugs used in the treatment of T2D.

Drug Class	Primary Target	Comments
SGLT2 antagonists	Na^+-glucose cotransporter 2 (SGLT2)	SGLT2 is expressed nearly exclusively in the apical membranes of epithelial cells of the proximal tubule of the kidney; responsible for approximately 90% of renal glucose reabsorption; all drugs in this class contain the suffix "-gliflozin"
Thiazolidinediones, TZD	PPARγ	Includes rosiglitazone and pioglitazone; agonists of PPARγ; net effect of TZD is a potentiation of the actions of insulin in liver, adipose tissue, and skeletal muscle, increased peripheral glucose disposal and a decrease in glucose output by the liver; TZD stimulate expression and release of adiponectin (see Chapter 31); adiponectin stimulates glucose uptake and fatty acid oxidation in skeletal muscle; mutations in PPARγ correlate to familial insulin resistance
Mimetics, inhibitors	GLP-1 or DPP4	GLP-1 inhibits pancreatic glucagon secretion and enhances GSIS; GLP-1 is rapidly degraded by dipeptidylpeptidase IV (DPP4); GLP-1 mimetics (GLP-1 receptor agonists, GLPRA) and DPP4 inhibitors induce dramatic reductions in plasma glucose concentrations; currently there are seven GLP-1 receptor agonist drugs that have been approved for use in the treatment of T2D in the United States; dual-acting drugs have been developed that function as GLP1RA and glucose-dependent insulinotropic peptide (GIP) receptor agonists (GIPRA); due to the appetite suppressing effects of the GLP1RA and GIPRA, these drugs are now also being used for the treatment of obesity; the GLP1RA and GIPRA all contain the suffix "-tide"; DDP4 inhibitors all contain the suffix "-gliptin"
Biguanides		Enhance insulin-mediated suppression of hepatic glucose production and insulin-stimulated glucose uptake by skeletal muscle; metformin is the most widely prescribed insulin-sensitizing drug in current clinical use; because the major site of action for metformin is the liver its use can be contraindicated in patients with liver dysfunction; improves insulin sensitivity by increasing insulin receptor tyrosine kinase activity, enhancing glycogen synthesis and increasing recruitment and transport of GLUT4 transporters to the plasma membrane; metformin also has a mild inhibitory effect on complex I of oxidative phosphorylation, has antioxidant properties, and activates both glucose-6-phosphate dehydrogenase and AMPK; in adipose tissue, metformin inhibits lipolysis while enhancing re-esterification of fatty acids; metformin is highly recommended to reduce the incidence as well as the potential for polycystic ovarian syndrome, PCOS
Sulfonylureas	SUR protein (encoded by ABCC8 gene), component of pancreatic KATP	Referred to as endogenous insulin secretagogues because they induce the pancreatic release of endogenous insulin; have been in use for over 50 years; tolbutamide, acetohexamide, chlorpropamide, and tolazamide were first generation in the class but are no longer routinely used; glipizide, glimepiride, and glyburide are second-generation drugs in class; all function by binding to and inhibiting the pancreatic KATP channel involved in GSIS
Meglitinides	SUR protein (encoded by *ABCC8* gene), component of pancreatic KATP, different binding site than sulfonylureas	Non-sulfonylurea insulin secretagogues; includes repaglinide and nateglinide; function by binding to site on KATP distinct from the sulfonylureas
Glucosidase inhibitors	α-Glucosidase	Function by interfering with the action of the α-glucosidases present in small intestinal brush-border cell membranes thereby reducing intestinal uptake of glucose; includes acarbose and miglitol; function locally in the intestine and have no major systemic action; common adverse side effects of these inhibitors are abdominal bloating and discomfort, diarrhea, and flatulence.

CHECKLIST

- ☑ Diabetes mellitus is a metabolic disorder primarily associated with deregulated glucose homeostasis.
- ☑ There are two major types of diabetes: type 1 and type 2. Type 1 diabetes is associated with loss of the insulin-producing cells of the pancreas and usually manifests in childhood. Type 2 diabetes is associated with a progression from peripheral tissue resistance to normal levels of insulin to eventual loss of insulin production and usually manifest later in life.
- ☑ Type 1 diabetes is characterized by frequent episodes of potentially life-threatening ketoacidosis due, in part, to abnormal regulation of pancreatic glucagon secretion.
- ☑ Due to abnormal glucagon secretion and lack of insulin secretion in type 1 diabetes, the primary metabolic disruption are in carbohydrate, lipid, and protein homeostasis.

- ☑ Type 2 diabetes is most frequently associated with obesity and it is the hyperlipidemia typically seen in obesity that plays a major role in peripheral resistance to the actions of insulin. Due to rising juvenile diabetes rates, type 2 diabetes is appearing now with much higher frequency in children and young adult.
- ☑ Several related forms of diabetes are the result of defects in genes responsible for normal pancreatic function and these disorders are referred to as the maturity-onset type diabetes of the young, MODY.
- ☑ Several diseases are associated with disruptions in insulin secretion, and or, action resulting is what are referred to as secondary diabetes.
- ☑ Gestational diabetes mellitus (GDM) is a special situation whereby glucose intolerance is first apparent during pregnancy. Women who experience GDM are likely to develop type 2 diabetes later in life.
- ☑ Neonatal diabetes refers to a circumstance in which hyperglycemia results from dysfunction in insulin action within the first 6 months of life and presents a potentially life-threatening condition.
- ☑ Type 1 diabetes is highly associated with polymorphisms in genes of the major histocompatibility cluster (MHC).
- ☑ The hyperglycemia associated with diabetes can be assessed by the measurement of glycosylated hemoglobin, identified as HbA_{1c} (A1c). The efficacy of type 2 diabetes drugs is reflected, in part, by the degree to which they can lower and control A1c levels.
- ☑ Numerous classes of drug have been developed to exert hypoglycemia-inducing effects as a means to treat the hyperglycemia associated with type 2 diabetes.

REVIEW QUESTIONS

1. A 48-year-old woman is being seen for a routine physical examination as a new patient in a general medicine clinic. Her present medical history is significant for BMI of 27 kg/m^2 and an 8-year history of noninsulin-dependent diabetes. The patient reports that her diabetes had been fairly well controlled with metformin and a strict diet regimen. However, she is now anxious about her condition and admits to recently developing poor and irregular eating habits, and frequently forgetting to take her medication. Laboratory studies find her non-fasting plasma glucose is 280 mg/dL (N = <100 mg/dL) and her HbA_{1c} value is 7.3% (N = 4–5.6%). Given the signs and symptoms in this patient, which of the following would most likely be decreased with respect to her cardiovascular system?

(A) Blood flow
(B) Cardiac output
(C) Systolic blood pressure
(D) Total peripheral resistance

2. A 31-year-old woman is being examined by her physician with complaints of sweating and heart palpitations in the mornings. The patient states that these symptoms started approximately 5 months ago but that she wasn't initially concerned because they resolved following eating her breakfast. Physical examination finds no obvious abnormalities. Fasting plasma studies find a glucose concentration of 47 mg/dL (N = 60–110 mg/dL). Additional fasting plasma findings include elevated levels of insulin and C-peptide. Based on the findings in this patient, which of the following is the most likely cause of her symptoms?

(A) Administration of exogenous insulin
(B) Autoantibodies activating the insulin receptor
(C) Increased somatostatin production
(D) Loss of pancreatic α-cells
(E) Pancreatic β-cell tumor

3. Experiments are being conducted on a novel compound designed to treat the hyperglycemia associated with type 2 diabetes. The compound has been designed to act as a competetive inhibitor of the liver isoform of glycogen phosphorylase. Which of the following best explains why inhibition of this enzyme would result in reduced concentrations of serum glucose?

(A) Hepatic fatty acid β-oxidation will decrease leading to reduced energy production needed for gluconeogenesis
(B) Hepatocytes will have a reduced capacity to store glucose following meals
(C) Liver glucose output will be reduced early during fasting
(D) The resultant increase in glycogen storage will inhibit glucose uptake by the liver leading to increased utilization in skeletal muscle
(E) There will be an increase in hepatic gluconeogenesis

4. Combinatorial chemistry is being exploited to identify novel orally acting drugs that can be used to treat the hyperlipidemia associated with type 1 diabetes. A drug that is identified as being able to enhance the activity of which of the following would be most useful?

(A) Acyl-CoA dehydrogenase
(B) Carnitine palmitoyltransferase 1
(C) Glucose-6-phosphatase
(D) Hepatic lipase
(E) Lipoprotein lipase

5. Experiments are being conducted on a novel compound designed to treat the hyperglycemia associated with type 2 diabetes. The compound is structurally similar to glipizide. This novel compound is most likely to exert it's effects by which of the following mechanisms?

(A) Activating PPARγ leading to increased hepatic glucose metabolism
(B) Inhibiting pancreatic ATP-dependent potassium channels inducing insulin secretion

(C) Interfering with carbohydrate digestion, thus reducing glucose intake
(D) Restricting hepatic glucose output, thereby reducing serum glucose concentration
(E) Stimulating pancreatic glucose metabolism leading to increased insulin secretion

6. Combinatorial chemistry is being exploited to identify novel orally acting drugs that can be used to treat the hyperlipidemia associated with type 2 diabetes. Using preliminary assays on cultured hepatocytes, one compound has been identified as being associated with increased phosphorylation of acetyl-CoA carboxylase 1 (ACC1). Given this result, it is most likely that this novel compound is related to which of the following?
(A) Dapagliflozin
(B) Glipizide
(C) Liraglutide
(D) Metformin
(E) Pioglitazone

7. A 42-year-old man with chronic, poorly controlled type 2 diabetes is undergoing an examination following a suspected heart attack. Analysis of serum finds highly elevated levels of advanced glycation end products (AGE). Which of the following is the most likely reason this finding can be correlated to the patient's cardiovascular disease?
(A) Decreased production of immune cell-derived IL-2
(B) Enhanced turnover of erythrocytes
(C) Enhanced oxidation of LDL
(D) Inhibition of lysyl oxidase
(E) Inhibition of vascular endothelial cell nitric oxide production

8. Experiments are being conducted on a novel compound designed to treat the hyperglycemia associated with type 2 diabetes. The compound has been shown to inhibit the activity of the protease, dipeptidyl peptidase 4 (DPP4). Which of the following is most likely to exhibit enhanced activity as a result of administration of this novel compound?
(A) Cholecystokinin
(B) Glucagon
(C) Glucagon-like peptide-1 (GLP-1)
(D) Insulin
(E) Somatostatin

9. Clinical trials are being carried out to test the efficacy of a novel drug designed to reduce the likelihood of ketoacidosis in type 1 diabetics. Observation of which of the following would most likely indicate the drug was exerting the expected effect?
(A) A decrease in adipocyte cAMP levels leading to accelerated fatty acid release
(B) A substantial decrease in the rate of hepatocyte fatty acid β-oxidation
(C) An increase in hepatic glucose conversion to acetyl-CoA
(D) An increase in the rate of the TCA cycle
(E) Elevation of acetyl-CoA levels in skeletal muscle driving ketone body utilization

10. A 31-year-old woman is being examined by her physician with complaints of sweating and heart palpitations in the mornings. The patient states that these symptoms started approximately 5 months ago but that she wasn't initially concerned because they resolved following eating her breakfast. Physical examination finds no obvious abnormalities. Fasting plasma studies find a glucose concentration of 47 mg/dL (N = 60–110 mg/dL). The hormone inducing her hypoglycemia exerts its effects by binding a cell surface receptor, an event that most likely activates which of the following?
(A) cAMP-dependent protein kinase A (PKA)
(B) Mitogen activated protein kinase (MAPK)
(C) Phospholipase Cβ (PLCβ)
(D) Phosphorylation of serine residues in the receptor
(E) Phosphorylation of tyrosine residues in the receptor
(F) Transcription factor binding to DNA

11. A 42-year-old man with chronic, poorly controlled type 2 diabetes is undergoing an examination following a suspected heart attack. Analysis of serum finds highly elevated levels of advanced glycation end products (AGE). Which of the following is the most likely protein contributing to this finding?
(A) Albumin
(B) Ceruloplasmin
(C) Hemoglobin
(D) Lysyl oxidase
(E) Transferrin

12. Combinatorial chemistry is being exploited to identify novel orally acting drugs that can be used to treat the hyperglycemia associated with type 2 diabetes. Using preliminary assays on cultured hepatocytes, one compound has been identified as being associated with increased activation of AMPK. Given this result, which of the following processes is most likely inhibited by this compound, thereby contributing to the expected beneficial effects?
(A) Fatty acid β-oxidation
(B) Gluconeogenesis
(C) Glycogen synthesis
(D) Glycolysis
(E) Ketogenesis

13. A 17-year-old boy with type 1 diabetes is undergoing a routine physical examination. History reveals that the patient does not routinely control his serum glucose levels with self-injection of insulin. Serum studies find fasting glucose concentration of 430 mg/dL (N = 60–110 mg/dL) and triglyceride concentration of 490 mg/dL (N <150 mg/dL). Which of the following represents the most likely cause of the hypertriglyceridemia in this patient?
(A) Deficiency in LDL receptors
(B) Deficiency of hormone-sensitive lipase
(C) Deficiency of lipoprotein lipase activity
(D) Increased hepatic cholesterol synthesis
(E) Increased hepatic glycogen metabolism
(F) Increased hepatic triglyceride synthesis

14. A 48-year-old woman moved to a new area and is being seen for a routine physical examination as a new patient in a general medicine clinic. Her present medical history is significant for a 30-lb weight excess and an 8-year history of type 2 diabetes, which she reports has been fairly well controlled with oral agents and a strict diet regimen. However, she is now anxious about her condition and admits to recently developing poor and irregular eating habits, and occasionally missing a medication dosage due to the high stress level surrounding her recent move. The most accurate estimation of this patient's recent glucose control would best be accomplished by measuring for the level of which of the following?
(A) Fasting insulin and C peptide levels
(B) Glucose tolerance test

(C) Level of glycated hemoglobin
(D) Random serum glucose
(E) Urine ketone body level

15. A 15-year-old girl is being examined by her pediatrician with complaints of frequent urination, excessive thirst, and unexplained weight loss. Post-prandial blood work demonstrates that her glucose levels are well above normal. In addition, she has above normal levels of urinary ketones. Which of the following would most likely be an additional finding in this patient?
(A) Decreased concentration of fructose 2,6-bisphosphate in the hepatocytes
(B) Decreased rate of gluconeogenesis from alanine
(C) Decreased renal threshold for glucose reabsorption
(D) Increased cholesterol synthesis
(E) Increased expression of GLUT4 transporters in skeletal muscle
(F) Increased renal gluconeogenesis from glutamine

16. A 16-year-old boy, who has type 1 diabetes, measures his blood glucose level after his most recent meal which shows it to be 290 mg/dL. He self-injects his normal dose of insulin. As a result of his actions, which of the following is most likely to be increased in his hepatocytes?
(A) cAMP-dependent protein kinase (PKA) activity
(B) cAMP levels
(C) Glucose-6-phosphatase activity
(D) Level of pyruvate kinase phosphorylation
(E) Phosphofructokinase-1 (PFK1) activity

17. A 24-year-old woman is being examined in the emergency department with complaints of nausea, vomiting, and difficulty breathing for the past 5 hours. History reveals that the patient is a type 1 diabetic but that she has been too distressed to inject her insulin for at least the last 24 hours. Physical examination indicates lethargy, dehydration, and deep respirations. Serum studies find a glucose concentration of 270 mg/dL (random normal = <140 mg/dL), pH 7.24 (N = 7.35–7.45), and an anion gap 13.3 (N = 8–12 mEq/L). Given the observations in this patient, which of the following best describes the current activity of the metabolic pathways in her liver?

	Gluconeogenesis	Glycogen Synthesis	Fatty Acid Oxidation	Glycolysis
A.	↑	↑	↑	↓
B.	↑	↑	↓	↓
C.	↑	↓	↑	↓
D.	↓	↑	↑	↑
E.	↓	↓	↓	↓

18. Experiments are being conducted on the metabolic profiles in two different groups of individuals. One group of individuals are fasting, and the other are type 1 diabetics who have not properly controlled their insulin levels. Although these two groups represent distinct populations, measurement of urine ketone levels finds that they elevated in all test subjects. Which of the following would best explain these findings?
(A) Increased fatty acid β-oxidation
(B) Increased gluconeogenesis
(C) Increased glycogenolysis
(D) Inhibition of fatty acid β-oxidation
(E) Inhibition of gluconeogenesis
(F) Inhibition of glycogenolysis

19. A 15-year-old girl who is type 1 diabetic is undergoing a routine examination by her endocrinologist. History reveals that the patient does not routinely control her insulin injections. Blood work finds serum glucose of 275 mg/dL (normal random <140 mg/dL) and A1c of 7.5% (N = 4–5.6%). Which of the following best explains the A1c finding in this patient?
(A) Glucose competes with other sugars for glycation of hemoglobin
(B) Hemoglobin is glycated in erythrocyte Golgi complexes
(C) Hemoglobin is glycated when serum glucose concentrations are increased
(D) Hyperglycemia inhibits erythrocyte degradation by spleen cells
(E) Hyperglycemia inhibits lysosomal degradation of hemoglobin

20. Patients who have undergone total pancreatectomy due to pancreatic cancer will require insulin injections. Individuals who are type 1 diabetic also require insulin injections. Which of the following best explains why the type 1 diabetic patients will require more insulin?
(A) Hyperglucagonemia in addition to insulin deficiency
(B) Insulin receptor defects
(C) Post-receptor resistance to insulin
(D) Production of insulin with abnormal structure
(E) Receptor-mediated increases in glucagon release

21. A 47-year-old man is being examined by his physician with complaints of muscle weakness. History indicates the patient is diabetic and hypertensive. The patient takes both insulin and metoprolol. Serum studies show potassium of 6.0 mM (N = 3.6–5.2 mM) and BUN of 24 mg/dL (N = 7–20 mg/dL). Two weeks after adjusting the patient insulin level and eliminating the metoprolol the patient reports no more muscle weakness. Which of the following most likely contributed to the muscle symptoms in this patient?
(A) High potassium-mediated block of acetylcholine receptors
(B) High potassium-mediated block of skeletal muscle calcium channels
(C) Hyperpolarization of neuromuscular junctions
(D) Skeletal muscle depolarization with resultant sodium channel inactivation
(E) Skeletal muscle hyperpolarization with resultant sodium channel blockade

22. Common symptoms in both type 1 and type 2 diabetes include polyuria and polydipsia. The polyuria is the consequence of hyperglycemia resulting in osmotic diuresis. Which of the following represents the primary region of the nephron where this pathology is exerted?
(A) Ascending limb of the loop of Henle
(B) Bowman's capsule
(C) Collecting duct
(D) Descending limb of the loop of Henle
(E) Distal convoluted tubule
(F) Glomerulus
(G) Juxtaglomerular apparatus
(H) Proximal tubule

23. A 57-year-old woman was taken to the Emergency Department after being found unconscious in a parking lot. With a distinct odor of alcohol, the attending physician orders a blood alcohol test which shows it to be 0.22%. Now conscious, the patient states that she was drinking with friends that evening but does not recall how she got to the parking lot, nor does she recall losing consciousness. History reveals that the patient has early-onset alcohol-related liver dysfunction, hypertension, hyperlipidemia, and recently diagnosed type 2 diabetes. Additional laboratory studies done on the patient's blood find glucose is 185 mg/dL (normal nonfasting is <125 mg/dL), bicarbonate is 17.5 mEq/L (N = 22–29 mEq/L), lactate is 5.7 mmol/L (N = 0.5–2.2 mmol/L), BUN is 27 mg/dL (N = 6–21 mg/dL), ALT is 195 U/L(N = 7–45 U/L), and AST is 415 U/L (N = 8–33 U/L). The patient reports that she has been taking an oral medication that her family doctor prescribed for her diabetes 5 months ago. She indicates that she does not recall the name but that she takes the medication once a day with her dinner. Which of the following is the most likely mechanism of action of the drug that this patient has most likely been prescribed?

(A) Activation of peroxisome proliferator-activated receptor γ (PPARγ)
(B) Inhibition of dipeptidyl peptidase-4 (DPP4)
(C) Inhibition of hepatic gluconeogenesis
(D) Interference with renal proximal tubule glucose reabsorption
(E) Stabilization of glucagon-like peptide-1 (GLP-1)

24. A 14-year-old boy is being examined in the Emergency Department, having been brought there by his concerned mother. The mother states that her son, who is a type 1 diabetic, has been experiencing confusion, weakness, and nausea all day. When questioned, the mother states that her son takes his insulin as instructed by his endocrinologist. Physical examination finds the patient is quite lethargic and his mucous membranes are dry. The attending physician orders blood tests, but the results are still pending. Given the signs and symptoms in this patient, which of the following sets of lab results is most likely to be associated with the laboratory studies?

	Anion Gap	Arterial pH	Glucose	Bicarbonate
A.	9 mEq/L	7.52	15 mg/dL	18 mEq/L
B.	10 mEq/L	7.55	235 mg/dL	25 mEq/L
C.	12 mEq/L	7.25	190 mg/dL	12 mEq/L
D.	16 mEq/L	7.20	265 mg/dL	11 mEq/L
E.	20 mEq/L	7.15	35 mg/dL	13 mEq/L

25. A 57-year-old woman, who is overweight, is hypertensive, and has type 2 diabetes is being assessed by her physician during a routine physical examination. When queried, the patient indicates that she has been adherent to her prescribed medications that include lisinopril and metformin. In the course of the examination, the physician orders routine blood tests, the results of which show that the patient's glucose level is 157 mg/dL and her HbA_{1c} level is 8.2%. The physician explains that to further reduce the patient's glucose and HbA_{1c} levels, he is going to prescribe an additional medication. He states that the most commonly observed side effect of this new medication is an increased risk for urinary tract infections. Which of the following is the most likely target of the medication that the patient's physician is prescribing?

(A) Dipeptidyl peptidase-4 (DPP4)
(B) Glucagon-like peptide-1 (GLP-1)
(C) Glucagon-like peptide-1 receptor (GLP-1R)
(D) Pancreatic β-cell KATP
(E) Peroxisome proliferator activated receptor γ (PPARγ)
(F) Sodium-glucose co-transporter 2 (SGLT2)

ANSWERS

1. Correct answer is **A.** Blood flow refers to the movement of blood through a vessel, tissue, or organ, and is usually expressed in terms of volume of blood per unit of time. As the viscosity of blood increases there is increased resistance to blood flow. Viscosity is an intrinsic property of a fluid that is related to the internal friction of adjacent fluid layers sliding past one another. This internal friction contributes to the resistance to flow as described by Poiseuille's equation. Blood is a non-Newtonian fluid because its viscosity increases at low flow velocities. The low flow velocities of blood allow for increased interactions to occur between cells and plasma proteins. This interaction can result in erythrocytes sticking together within the microcirculation leading to increased viscosity. Indeed, as hematocrit increases so too does viscosity. Another contributor to increased blood viscosity is the level of glucose in the blood. As blood viscosity increases cardiac output increases, not decreases (choice B), total peripheral resistance (TPR) increases, not decreases (choice D), and systolic blood pressure increases, not decreases (choice C). With increasing TPR (also known as systemic vascular resistance, SVR), there is a concomitant decrease in blood flow.

2. Correct answer is **E.** The patient is most likely experiencing the initial symptoms associated with a pancreatic β-cell cancer, an insulinoma. Typical symptoms associated with β-cell tumors are dizziness, weakness, sweating, confusion, anxiety, tremors, and hunger. These symptoms are the result of the tumor continuously secreting insulin even when blood glucose levels are low and can, in fact, result in precipitously low fasting plasma glucose as seen in this patient. Although dangerously low fasting plasma glucose levels can result from injection of insulin (choice A) this patients' symptoms have been chronic and there is no indicated history that she is a diabetic requiring insulin. Autoantibodies to the insulin receptor (choice B) have been demonstrated to antagonize the physiologic actions of insulin and the most common result is hyperglycemia unresponsive to massive doses of insulin. This condition represents a very rare cause of insulin resistant diabetes. Increased pancreatic δ-cell somatostatin production (choice C) and loss of pancreatic α-cell production of glucagon (choice D) would not lead to the severe fasting hypoglycemia and attendant symptoms present in this patient.

3. Correct answer is **C.** During early fasting, as the level of glucose in the blood falls, the pancreas releases glucagon, and the adrenal glands release epinephrine, into the circulation to stimulate hepatic gluconeogenesis. The glucagon receptor is coupled to a G_s-type G-protein which activates adenylate cyclase to produce cAMP which in turn activates PKA. Epinephrine binds both the α_1-adrenergic and β_2-adrenergic receptors present on hepatocytes. The response to activated β-adrenergic receptors is identical to that initiated by the glucagon receptor. PKA phosphorylates and activates phosphorylase kinase. The α_1-adrenergic receptor is coupled to a G_q-type G-protein, the consequences of which are increased free intracellular calcium. The calcium binds to the calmodulin subunit of phosphorylase kinase resulting in its activation. Active phosphorylase kinase phosphorylates both glycogen synthase and glycogen phosphorylase resulting in reduced glycogen synthesis and enhanced glucose release from glycogen, respectively. The combined effects of glucagon and epinephrine, acting on the liver in periods of low blood glucose, are increased glucose output from glycogen. Thus, an inhibition of glycogen phosphorylase would limit the ability of the liver to provide glucose to the blood. Negatively affecting the activity of glycogen phosphorylase would not significantly affect the rate of hepatic fatty acid β-oxidation (choice A). Glycogen synthesis is the function of glycogen synthase whose activity would not be affected by an inhibitor of glycogen phosphorylase, therefore there would be no inhibition to glucose storage post feeding (choice B). Inhibition of glycogen phosphorylase would not affect skeletal muscle glucose usage (choice D) nor lead to an increase in hepatic gluconeogenesis (choice E).

4. Correct answer is **E.** One of the normal effects of insulin is to increase the level of lipoprotein lipase (LPL) on the surface of endothelial cells of the vasculature in adipose tissue, skeletal muscle, and cardiac muscle. The lack of normal levels of circulating insulin in type 1 diabetics, even in response to injected insulin, results in impaired regulation of LPL levels. The reduced levels of LPL in type 1 diabetics contributes to the hyperlipidemia associated with this disorder. Therefore, a drug designed to enhance either residual LPL activity or the amount of LPL, or both, would be beneficial at lowering blood lipid levels in type 1 diabetics. Activation of acyl-CoA dehydrogenases (choice A) and carnitine palmitoyltransferase 1 (choice B) would lead to increased fatty acid β-oxidation which could, in theory, reduce overall blood lipid. However, due to the reduced levels of LPL activity in type 1 diabetes the fatty acid substrates for these enzymes would not be efficiently released from circulating triglycerides. Enhanced activity of glucose-6-phosphatase (choice C) would exacerbate the hyperglycemia of type 1 diabetes and have no effect on the level of blood lipids in this disorder. Hepatic lipase (choice E) only removes fatty acids from triglycerides in HDL and, therefore, activation of this enzyme would have limited capacity to lower total blood lipids.

5. Correct answer is **B.** Glipizide is a member of the sulfonylurea family of hypoglycemia-inducing drugs. The sulfonylurea drugs function by binding to and inhibiting the pancreatic ATP-dependent K^+ channel (KATP) that is responsible for glucose-mediated insulin secretion. The normal pancreatic response to increased blood glucose is an increased uptake by β-cells with concomitant oxidation. The increase in glucose oxidation leads to an elevation in the ATP/ADP ratio. The increased level of ATP results in an inhibition of the KATP channel. Inhibition of the pancreatic β-cell KATP channel results in depolarization of the β-cell. The depolarization results in the activation of plasma membrane-associated L-type calcium channels leading to increased influx of calcium into the β-cell. This influx of calcium results in mobilization of secretory vesicles containing insulin to the plasma membrane and the secretion of insulin into the blood. The thiazolidinedione class of hypoglycemia inducing drugs activate PPARγ (choice A). The α-glucosidase inhibitors function by interfering with the action of the α-glucosidases present in the small intestinal brush border. The consequence of this inhibition is a reduction in digestion and the consequent absorption of glucose into the systemic circulation (choice C). The biguanide, metformin, exerts its effects, in part, by inhibiting hepatic gluconeogenesis and, therefore, hepatic glucose output (choice D). There are currently no hypoglycemia-inducing drugs that function by stimulating pancreatic glucose metabolism to activate insulin secretion (choice E).

6. Correct answer is **D.** The biguanide, metformin, exerts numerous effects that contribute to reductions in blood glucose. It improves insulin sensitivity by increasing insulin receptor tyrosine kinase activity, it enhances glycogen synthesis in hepatocytes, and it increases recruitment and transport of GLUT4 transporters to the plasma membrane in adipose tissue. Metformin also has a mild inhibitory effect on complex I of oxidative phosphorylation. The reduced activity of complex I of mitochondrial oxidative phosphorylation results in reduced ATP synthesis with a concomitant rise in AMP. The increasing levels of AMP are while result in the metformin-mediated activation of AMPK. The importance of AMPK in the actions of metformin stems from the role of AMPK in the regulation of both lipid and carbohydrate metabolism. AMPK is a master metabolic regulatory kinase whose role is to shift cells from ATP consumption to ATP production. One of the targets of AMPK is acetyl-CoA carboxylase 1, the rate limiting enzyme of *de novo* fatty acid biosynthesis. A reduction in hepatic fatty acid biosynthesis would lead to reduced VLDL production and release, thereby contributing to reductions in overall circulating lipids. Dapagliflozin (choice A) exerts its hypoglycemia-inducing effects by inhibiting the renal glucose transporter, SGLT2, which is responsible for glucose reabsorption from the blood. Glipizide (choice B) exerts its hypoglycemia-inducing effects by stimulating insulin secretion from the pancreas. Liraglutide (choice C) exerts its hypoglycemia-inducing effects by functioning as a GLP-1 receptor agonist. Activation of the GLP-1 receptor on pancreatic β-cells results in increased insulin synthesis and release. Pioglitazone (choice E) is a member of the thiazolidinediones family of hypoglycemia-inducing drugs that function through the activation of PPARγ.

7. Correct answer is **C.** Chronic hyperglycemia, such as in type 2 diabetes, promotes a proinflammatory state that contributes to the glycation of proteins and lipids. These glycated macromolecules are referred to as advanced glycation end-products (AGE). One of the most significant glycated proteins in diabetes is hemoglobin. Glycated hemoglobin is identified as HbA_{1c}. Numerous pathologic consequences result from the presence of AGE and include enhanced oxidative stress, oxidation of LDL (oxLDL), induced secretion of various proinflammatory cytokines, inhibition of the dilating effects of nitric oxide (NO), increased vascular permeability, and arterial stiffening. A receptor that binds AGE is present in the plasma membrane of numerous cell types including immune cells, vascular endothelial cells, and smooth muscle cells. This receptor was originally identified as Receptor for Advanced Glycation End-products (RAGE). RAGE is a member of the human class J scavenger receptor family (specifically SCARJ1). This receptor is encoded by the *AGER* (advanced glycosylation end-product specific receptor) gene. None of the other

options (choices A, B, D, and E) correlate with the pathology from advanced glycation end products.

8. Correct answer is **C.** Dipeptidyl peptidase 4 (DPP4) is a serine exopeptidase that catalyzes the release of an N-terminal dipeptide provided that the next to last residue is proline, hydroxyproline, dehydroproline, or alanine. DPP4 substrates include neuropeptides, chemokines, and the incretin hormones, glucagon-like peptide-1 (GLP-1) and glucose-dependent insulinotropic peptide (GIP, formerly known as gastric inhibitory peptide). GLP-1 stimulates postprandial insulin secretion and has also been shown to stimulate proliferation and inhibit apoptosis of pancreatic β-cells. GLP-1 also inhibits glucagon release from pancreatic α-cells, inhibits gastric emptying, and reduces the desire for food intake. The utility of DPP4 inhibitors is that they act to prevent inactivation of GLP-1 and, therefore, prolong the duration of action of GLP-1. The efficacy and safety of second-generation selective DPP4 inhibitors in the treatment of type 2 diabetes has been well established and have been shown to reduce HbA_{1c} by about 0.6–0.7%. None of the other proteins (choices A, B, D, and E) are targets for the proteolytic activity of DPP4 and therefore would not exhibit enhanced activity in the presence of a DPP4 inhibitor.

9. Correct answer is **B.** The most frequent consequence of poorly controlled type 1 diabetes is ketoacidosis, referred to as diabetic ketoacidosis, DKA. The hyperketonemia in DKA is the result of insulin deficiency and unregulated glucagon secretion from α-cells of the pancreas. Circulating glucagon stimulates adipose tissue to release fatty acids which are taken up, and oxidized, primarily by the liver. Under these conditions, the level of fatty acid β-oxidation is in excess of the livers' ability to fully oxidize the excess acetyl-CoA and, thus, the compound is diverted into ketone synthesis. The ketones are released into the circulation and because they are acidic lower the pH of the blood resulting in metabolic acidosis. A drug designed to decrease hepatic fatty acid β-oxidation would, therefore, result in reduced ketogenesis and reduced incidence of DKA. None of the other processes (choices A, C, D, and E) would contribute to a reduction in the potential for diabetic ketoacidosis in type 1 diabetes.

10. Correct answer is **E.** The patient is most likely experiencing the initial symptoms associated with a pancreatic β-cell cancer, an insulinoma. Typical symptoms associated with β-cell tumors are dizziness, weakness, sweating, confusion, anxiety, tremors, and hunger. These symptoms are the result of the tumor continuously secreting insulin even when blood glucose levels are low and can, in fact, result in precipitously low fasting plasma glucose as seen in this patient. Insulin exerts its effects by binding to its receptor on target cells such as adipocytes skeletal muscle cells, and hepatocytes. The insulin receptor possesses intrinsic tyrosine kinase activity and upon binding of insulin the kinase function is activated. The initial substrate for insulin receptor-mediated phosphorylation is the receptor itself. Downstream of the activated insulin receptor is the activation of members of the MAP kinase family (choice B) and enhnaced transcription factor binding to DNA (choice F). However, neither of these events constitute the immediate response to insulin binding to its receptor. None of the other activities (choices A, C, and D) directly correspond to the binding of insulin to its receptor.

11. Correct answer is **C.** Chronic hyperglycemia, such as in type 2 diabetes, promotes a proinflammatory state that contributes to the glycation of proteins and lipids. These glycated macromolecules are referred to as advanced glycation end-products (AGE). One of the most significant glycated proteins in diabetes is hemoglobin. Numerous pathologic consequences result from the presence of AGE and include enhanced oxidative stress, oxidation of LDL (oxLDL), induced secretion of various pro-inflammatory cytokines, inhibition of the dilating effects of nitric oxide (NO), increased vascular permeability, and arterial stiffening. Glycated hemoglobin is identified as HbA_{1c}, often designated as just A1C. Since hemoglobin is present in erythrocytes and these cells have a limited life span of around 120 days in the circulation, measurement of HbA_{1c} levels is a relatively accurate measure of the amount of glucose in the blood and the length of time the level has been elevated. None of the other proteins (choices A, B, D, and E) represent significant contributors to the generation of advanced glycation end products.

12. Correct answer is **B.** The novel compound is most likely mimicking the effects of the biguanide, metformin. Metformin exerts numerous effects that contribute to reductions in blood glucose. It improves insulin sensitivity by increasing insulin receptor tyrosine kinase activity, it enhances, not inhibits (choice C) glycogen synthesis in hepatocytes, and it increases recruitment and transport of GLUT4 transporters to the plasma membrane in adipose tissue. Metformin also has a mild inhibitory effect on complex I of oxidative phosphorylation. The reduced activity of complex I of mitochondrial oxidative phosphorylation results in reduced ATP synthesis with a concomitant rise in AMP. The increasing levels of AMP are what result in the metformin-mediated activation of AMPK. AMPK is a master metabolic regulatory kinase whose role is to shift cells from ATP consumption to ATP production. One of the targets of AMPK is the transcription factor that activates expression of the genes encoding the hepatic gluconeogenic enzymes, phosphoenolpyruvate carboxykinase (PEPCK) and glucose-6-phosphatase. Phosphorylation of this transcription factor by AMPK renders it incapable of activating its target genes. The net effect is reduced glucose output from the liver through inhibition of gluconeogenesis. All the other processes (choices A, C, D, and E) would be enhanced as a result of activated AMPK as each of these provides for the production of energy either within the hepatocyte or in peripheral tissues (choice E).

13. Correct answer is **C.** The triglyceride components of VLDL and chylomicron are hydrolyzed to free fatty acids and glycerol in the vasculature of adipose tissue, skeletal muscle, cardiac muscle by the actions of lipoprotein lipase, LPL. Insulin exerts numerous effects on overall metabolic homeostasis where one of its effects directly relates to the symptoms in this patient. The level of LPL on the surface of endothelial cells of the vasculature is regulated via the actions of insulin. Since type 1 diabetics do not synthesize insulin, they do not properly regulate the level of LPL which contributes to hypertriglyceridemia in these individuals. None of the other processes (choices A, B, D, E, and F) directly correlate with the cause of the hypertriglyceridemia evident in this patient.

14. Correct answer is **C.** When present in high concentration, glucose can react nonenzymatically with protein amino groups to form an unstable intermediate, or Schiff base, which subsequently undergoes an internal rearrangement to form a stable glycated protein. The glycation of the amino acids valine and lysine on the β-globin proteins of hemoglobin results in the

formation of glycated hemoglobin identified as HbA_{1c}, or simply as A1C. Because erythrocytes circulate for an average of 90–120 days, assaying HbA_{1c} provides an index of a diabetic patient's glucose control over the preceding 3–4 months. Although normal values vary between laboratories, on average nondiabetic subjects have HbA_{1c} levels roughly between 4% and 5.6%, whereas in type 2 diabetics, especially when poorly controlled, the HbA_{1c} level can be higher than 8%. None of the other measurements (choices A, B, D, and E) would be useful in determining this patient's recent glucose control.

15. Correct answer is **A.** The patient most likely has type 1 diabetes. Associated with insulin deficiency in type 1 diabetes is unregulated glucagon secretion. In the absence of injected insulin these patients will experience exacerbated responses to the increased glucagon. Glucagon action in the liver includes activation of PKA. One of the targets of PKA is PFK2. When PFK2 is phosphorylated, it hydrolyzes the potent PFK1 activator, fructose-2,6-bisphosphate (F2,6BP) resulting in reduced levels of F2,6BP and reduced activity of PFK1. Given that hyperglycemia is associated with type 1 diabetes the threshold of glucose reabsorption in the kidney would be increased, not decreased (choice C). As a result of the elevated glucagon release in type 1 diabetics there would be increased gluconeogenesis, not decreased (choice B) and decreased cholesterol synthesis, not increased (choice D). The lack of insulin production in type 1 diabetes would result in decreased, not increased (choice E) expression of GLUT4 transporters in skeletal muscle. Renal gluconeogenesis is not likely to be affected (choice F) in type 1 diabetics.

16. Correct answer is **E.** The ability of insulin to modify the metabolic processes in cells, such as hepatocytes, is through the induction of a phosphodiesterase and a phosphatase. Activation of a phosphodiesterase results in the hydrolysis of cAMP which will lead to reduced, not increased levels of cAMP (choice B) and reduced, not increased (choice A) activation of PKA. One of the targets of PKA is the bifunctional enzyme, phosphofructokinase-2 (PFK2). When PFK2 is phosphorylated, it functions as a phosphatase and it hydrolyzes the potent PFK1 activator, fructose-2,6-bisphosphate (F2,6BP) resulting in reduced activity of PFK1. However, in the presence of insulin the reduced level of active PKA prevents PFK2 from being phosphorylated. In addition, the insulin-mediated activation of phosphatase enhances phosphate removal from PFK2. When PFK2 is dephosphorylated, it functions as a kinase and synthesizes F2,6BP from the glycolytic intermediate, fructose-6-phosphate. The F2,6BP then potently activates PFK1. The level of glucose-6-phosphatase activity (choice C) is not affected by the actions of insulin. Another target of hepatic PKA is pyruvate kinase. Since PKA activity is significantly reduced by insulin, the level of pyruvate kinase phosphorylation would be decreased, not increased (choice D).

17. Correct answer is **C.** Associated with insulin deficiency in type 1 diabetes is uncontrolled glucagon secretion. In the absence of injected insulin in this patient, she will have exacerbated responses to the increased glucagon. Within the liver, glucagon exerts its effects by binding to is G_s-type G-protein–coupled receptor. The activation of this G-protein results in activation of adenylate cyclase resulting in increased production of cAMP. The increased cAMP results in activation of PKA. All of the hepatic responses to glucagon are mediated by PKA phosphorylating numerous substrates. One of the targets of PKA is the bifunctional enzyme, phosphofructokinase-2 (PFK2). When PFK2 is phosphorylated, it functions as a phosphatase and it hydrolyzes the potent PFK1 activator, fructose-2,6-bisphosphate (F2,6BP) resulting in reduced activity of PFK1. F2,6BP is also an allosteric inhibitor of the gluconeogenic enzyme, fructose-1,6-bisphosphatase. The net effect of phosphorylated PFK2 is decreased glycolysis and increased gluconeogenesis. Another target of PKA is phosphorylase kinase which is activated by being phosphorylated. Active phosphorylase kinase phosphorylates glycogen synthase, reducing its activity, and glycogen phosphorylase, increasing its activity. The net effect of activated phosphorylase kinase is inhibition of glycogen synthesis and activation of glycogen breakdown. Another target of PKA is the rate limiting enzyme of *de novo* fatty acid biosynthesis, acetyl-CoA carboxylase 1 (ACC1). Phosphorylation of ACC1 reduces its activity, therefore decreasing fatty acid biosynthesis. The reduced synthesis of malonyl-CoA, the product of ACC1, results in less inhibition of carnitine palmitoyltransferase 1 and a resultant increase in fatty acid β-oxidation. None of the other options (choices A, B, D, and E) correctly correspond to the overall changes in carbohydrate and lipid homeostasis that result in type 1 diabetics from the dysregulation of glucagon release.

18. Correct answer is **A.** Type 1 diabetes is not only associated with loss of insulin secretion but also abnormal secretion of glucagon. An individual on a fast would have reduced levels of blood glucose and the compensation for this would be increased secretion of pancreatic glucagon and adrenal epinephrine to stimulate gluconeogenesis in the liver. Glucagon and epinephrine also stimulate adipose tissue lipolysis. The released fatty acids are taken up by tissues, primarily by the liver, where they are oxidized. In the liver the oxidation of fatty acids exceeds the capacity of the TCA cycle to fully oxidize the acetyl-CoA resulting in increased synthesis of the ketones, acetoacetate, and β-hydroxybutyrate. Because both the fasting subjects and the type 1 diabetics have elevated glucagon there will be increased ketogenesis in both populations. Although glucagon enhances gluconeogenesis (choice B) and glycogenolysis (choice C) in the liver, these processes do not contribute to ketogenesis. Fatty acid β-oxidation, gluconeogenesis, and glycogenolysis are each increased, not inhibited (choices D, E, and F) as a result of the actions of glucagon.

19. Correct answer is **C.** When present in high concentration, glucose can react nonenzymatically with protein amino groups to form an unstable intermediate, or Schiff base, which subsequently undergoes an internal rearrangement to form a stable glycated protein. The glycation of the amino acids valine and lysine on the β-globin proteins of hemoglobin results in the formation of glycated hemoglobin identified as HbA_{1c}, or simply as A1C. Because erythrocytes circulate for an average of 90–120 days, assaying HbA_{1c} provides an index of a diabetic patient's glucose control over the preceding 3–4 months. None of the other options (choices A, B, D, and E) correctly define the process of hemoglobin glycation generating A1C.

20. Correct answer is **A.** In addition to the loss of insulin production and secretion typical of type 1 diabetes, there is abnormal regulation of pancreatic α-cells. Normally, hyperglycemia leads to reduced glucagon secretion from pancreatic α-cells. However, in patients with type 1 diabetes, glucagon secretion is not suppressed by hyperglycemia. The resultant inappropriately elevated glucagon levels exacerbate the metabolic defects due to insulin deficiency. The dysregulation of glucagon secretion in type 1 diabetics is the basis for the requirement for more insulin, relative to a patient who has undergone total pancreatectomy. None of the other options (choices B, C, D, and E) correctly explains why type 1 diabetics require insulin at higher levels than patients who have undergone total pancreatectomy.

21. Correct answer is **D.** Elevated serum potassium levels cause membrane depolarization with a resulting sodium channel inactivation. Under these conditions, muscle fibers are less able to initiate and propagate action potentials, leading to impaired excitation contraction coupling, with an associated muscle weakness. The hyperkalemia in this patient is probably due to multiple factors. Insulin normally promotes potassium uptake into cells via stimulation of Na^+/K^+-ATPase activity, therefore if the dose of insulin this patient administers is lower than optimal it could contribute to hyperkalemia. Metoprolol is a member of the β-blocker class of antihypertensive drugs. The β-blockers partially inhibit Na^+/K^+-ATPase activity, thereby contributing to hyperkalemia. Finally, the elevated BUN indicates some level of renal dysfunction. Failing kidneys cannot efficiently excrete potassium into the urine, further contributing to hyperkalemia. None of the other options (choices A, B, C, and E) correctly explain the muscle symptoms in this patient.

22. Correct answer is **H.** The proximal tubule reabsorbs the majority (about two-thirds) of sodium and water present in the glomerular filtrate. Both the luminal sodium concentration and the luminal osmolality remain constant (and equal to plasma values) along the entire length of the proximal tubule. Water and sodium are reabsorbed proportionally because the water is dependent on, and coupled with, the active reabsorption of Na^+. The water permeability of the proximal tubule is high, and therefore a significant transepithelial osmotic gradient is not possible. Sodium is actively reabsorbed from the lumen of the proximal tubule via the action of the Na^+/H^+ antiporter 3 (NHE3) encoded by the *SLC9A3* gene. Increased glucose reabsorption by the Na^+-dependent glucose transporter, SGLT2, in diabetes will osmotically prevent water reabsorption resulting in diuresis. Although water reabsorption does occur in the collecting duct (choice C) in response to vasopressin activation of aquaporin 2, this activity does not contribute to osmotic diuresis. None of the other sections of the nephron (choices A, B, D, E, F, and G) represent regions of significant reabsorption of sodium or water.

23. Correct answer is **C.** The patient has most likely been prescribed metformin, an oral medication, to control her blood glucose levels due to her type 2 diabetes. Metformin is most often the first drug prescribed to treat a patient's hyperglycemia resulting from their type 2 diabetes. Typically, metformin is initially prescribed to be taken as a single dose, usually 500 mg once per day and to be taken with the evening meal. The patient's blood analysis shows clear signs of metabolic acidosis due, in large part, to the excessive level of lactate in her blood. The consumption of ethanol impairs lactate dehydrogenase conversion of lactate to pyruvate and promotes the conversion of pyruvate to lactate which leads to lactic acidemia and consequent metabolic acidosis. The elevated AST and ALT levels, and the ratio of AST/ALT being greater than 2 is confirmation of the alcohol-induced cirrhosis in this patient. Metformin has a mild inhibitory effect on complex I of oxidative phosphorylation, has antioxidant properties, and activates both glucose-6-phosphate dehydrogenase (G6PD; also identified as G6PDH) and AMP-activated protein kinase (AMPK). Within hepatocytes, the metformin-mediated activation of AMPK results in suppression of both glycogenolysis and gluconeogenesis, effects that limit glucose output by the liver. Whereas all of the other mechanisms (choices A, B, D, and E) represent effects of type 2 diabetes treatments, only metformin, which inhibits hepatic gluconeogenesis, is considered as a first choice due to its effectiveness at lowering blood glucose levels and it is well-tolerated by most patients. The thiazolidinedione drugs that inhibit PPARγ (choice A) have the potential for serious side effects and are either no longer used or only used in conjunction with other drugs, particularly metformin. The DPP4 inhibitor drugs (choice B), which lead to stabilization of GLP-1 (choice E) are most often prescribed in combination with metformin. The SGLT2 inhibitors, which block renal glucose reabsorption (choice D), are usually only prescribed to diabetes patients who have not achieved adequate blood glucose reduction with other medications.

24. Correct answer is **D.** The patient is most likely experiencing the symptoms of diabetic ketoacidosis, DKA. DKA is characterized by metabolic acidosis (low pH of the blood), hyperglycemia, and hyperketonemia (elevated ketones in the blood). Diagnosis of DKA is accomplished by detection of hyperketonemia and metabolic acidosis (as measured by the anion gap) in the presence of hyperglycemia. In the context of DKA, the anion gap will be elevated. In addition to lactic acidosis, DKA is one of the most common causes of an elevated anion gap. An initial assessment of DKA is made in type 1 diabetes patients whose blood glucose is >250 mg/dL, with arterial pH <7.3, serum bicarbonate <15 mEq/L, and an anion gap >15 mEq/L. None of the other laboratory results (choices A, B, C, and E) present the overall conditions of DKA.

25. Correct answer is **F.** The most likely diabetes medications that are associated with a risk for urinary tract infections, particularly in female patients, are the SGLT2 inhibitors. SGLT2 is expressed nearly exclusively in the apical membranes of epithelial cells of the proximal tubule of the kidney and has been shown to be responsible for approximately 90% of the renal glucose reabsorption. Therefore, the inhibition of the renal SGLT2 activity results in greatly enhanced glucose release in the urine. Several drugs, all of which carry the suffix "-gliflozin," that inhibit SGLT2 have been developed. The use of the SGLT2 inhibitor drugs can increase the risk of urinary tract infections (UTIs) in some patients due to the increased glucose in the urine (glycosuria), which can promote bacterial growth. However, the overall risk of UTI with SGLT2 inhibitors is generally considered low. The use of none of the other diabetes medications (choices A, B, C, D, and E) is associated with a risk for UTI.

CHAPTER 31

Peptide and Amino Acid–Derived Hormones

High-Yield Terms

Endocrine glands	Secrete chemicals or hormones into the circulation
Exocrine glands	Excrete chemicals or hormones via ducts
Paracrine	Refers to any substance secreted by one cell which acts on cells next to or in close proximity to the source
Autocrine	Refers to any substance secreted by one cell which acts on the secreting cell itself
Thyrotoxicosis	The condition resulting from hyperthyroidism leading to excess production and release of thyroid hormones

PEPTIDE HORMONE STRUCTURE AND FUNCTION

The endocrine system represents different tissues that secrete hormones into the circulatory system for dissemination throughout the body, thereby, regulating the function of distant tissues and maintaining homeostasis. Classically, endocrine hormones are considered to be derived from amino acids, proteins/peptides (examples in Table 31–1), or sterols (see Chapter 32). The site of action of hormones can be distant from the site of synthesis (endocrine hormones), close to the cells that secrete them (paracrine hormones), or directly on the cell that secreted them (autocrine hormones).

Once a hormone is secreted by an endocrine tissue, it generally binds to a specific plasma protein carrier, with the complex being disseminated to distant tissues. Carrier proteins for peptide hormones prevent hormone destruction by plasma proteases. Carriers for steroid and thyroid hormones allow these very hydrophobic substances to be present in the plasma at concentrations several 100-fold greater than their solubility in water would permit. Carriers for small, hydrophilic amino acid–derived hormones prevent their filtration through the renal glomerulus, greatly prolonging their circulating half-life.

RECEPTORS FOR PEPTIDE AND AMINO ACID–DERIVED HORMONES

With the exception of the thyroid hormone receptors, the receptors for amino acid–derived and peptide hormones are located in the plasma membrane. Receptor structure for amino acid and peptide hormones is varied and includes single transmembrane-spanning receptors, multisubunit membrane-spanning receptors, and multipass membrane receptors of the G-protein–coupled receptor (GPCR) family. Single-pass and multipass receptors can possess intrinsic enzymatic activity. For example, the insulin receptor is a heterotetrameric receptor that possesses intrinsic tyrosine kinase activity. The receptor for the natriuretic factor peptides (ANP and BNP) possesses intrinsic guanylate cyclase activity. As reviewed in Chapter 26, GPCR family receptors couple to three major classes of G-protein: G_s, G_i, and G_q.

On hormone binding to receptor, signals are transduced to the interior of the cell, where second messengers and phosphorylated proteins generate appropriate metabolic responses. The main second messengers are cAMP, Ca^{2+}, inositol-1,4,5-trisphosphate (IP_3), diacylglycerol (DAG), and cGMP.

GPCR that couple to G_s-type G-proteins activate adenylate cyclase resulting in conversion of ATP to cAMP. The cAMP in turn activates the kinase, PKA. GPCR that couple to G_i-type G-proteins primarily lead to inhibition of adenylate cyclase resulting in reduced cAMP production and thus, reduced levels of active PKA. GPCR that couple G_q-type G-proteins activate phospholipase C-β (PLCβ) which then hydrolyzes membrane phosphatidylinositol 4,5-bisphosphate (PIP_2) to produce two messengers: IP_3, which is soluble in the cytosol, and DAG, which remains in the membrane phase. Cytosolic IP_3 binds to receptors on the ER that are ligand-activated Ca^{2+} channels allowing stored Ca^{2+} to flood the cytosol. There it activates numerous enzymes, many by activating their calmodulin or calmodulin-like subunits. Along with Ca^{2+}, DAG activates kinases of the PKC family. Intracellular cGMP activates kinases of the protein kinase G (PKG) family. The enzymes of the PKA, PKC, and PKG families are all serine/threonine kinases whose activities propagate the biological effects of most peptide and amino acid–derived hormones.

TABLE 31–1 Major peptide and amino acid–derived hormones.*

Hormone	Structure	Functions
Skeletal Muscle Hormones/Myokines		
Irisin	22 kDa proteolytic fragment of the transmembrane protein FNDC5 (fibronectin type III domain-containing protein 5)	Expression induced, in skeletal muscle, by PGC1-α in response to exercise, induces a conversion of white adipose tissue (WAT) into a more brown fat (BAT) type, generally referred to as beige or brite fat cells
Pituitary Hormones		
Adrenocorticotropic hormone (ACTH); also called corticotropin	Anterior pituitary peptide derived from POMC; polypeptide; ACTH is 39 amino acids	Stimulates cells of adrenal gland to increase steroid synthesis and secretion
Follicle-stimulating hormone (FSH)	Anterior pituitary peptides; two proteins: ± peptide is 96 amino acids;^{2} peptide is 120 amino acids	Ovarian follicle development and ovulation, increases estrogen production; acts on Sertoli cells of seminiferous tubule to increase spermatogenesis
Growth hormone (GH, or somatotropin)	Anterior pituitary peptide; protein of 191 amino acids	General anabolic stimulant, increases release of insulin-like growth factor-I (IGF-I), cell growth, and bone sulfation
Lipotropin (LPH)	Anterior pituitary peptides derived from POMC; β polypeptide is 93 amino acids, γ polypeptide is 60 amino acids	Increases fatty acid release from adipocytes
Luteinizing hormone (LH); human chorionic gonadotropin (hCG) is similar and produced in placenta	Anterior pituitary peptides; two peptides: α peptide is 96 amino acids; β peptide is 121 amino acids	Increases ovarian progesterone synthesis, luteinization; acts on Leydig cells of testes to increase testosterone synthesis and release and increase interstitial cell development
Melanocyte-stimulating hormones (MSH)	Anterior pituitary peptides derived from POMC; α polypeptide is 13 amino acids, β polypeptide is 18 amino acids, γ polypeptide is 12 amino acids	α-MSH most significant, involved in control of appetite and feeding behaviors via melanocortin receptor (MC4R)-expressing neurons in hypothalamus, immunomodulation via MC1R-expressing monocytes, macrophages, and dendritic cells (DC), downregulates the production of proinflammatory and immunomodulating cytokines (IL-1, IL-6, TNF-α, IL-2, IFN-γ, IL-4, IL-13) as well as the expression of costimulatory molecules (CD86, CD40, ICAM-1) on antigen-presenting DCs
Oxytocin	Posterior pituitary peptide; polypeptide of nine amino acids CYIQNCPLG (C residues are disulfide bonded)	Uterine contraction, causes milk ejection in lactating females (the "let-down" response), responds to suckling reflex and estradiol, lowers steroid synthesis in testes
Prolactin (PRL)	Anterior pituitary peptide; protein of 197 amino acids	Stimulates differentiation of secretory cells of mammary gland and stimulates milk synthesis
Thyroid-stimulating hormone, TSH (thyrotropin)	Anterior pituitary peptides; two peptides: α peptide is 96 amino acids; β peptide is 112 amino acids	Acts on thyroid follicle cells to stimulate thyroid hormone synthesis
Vasopressin (antidiuretic hormone, ADH)	Posterior pituitary peptide; polypeptide of nine amino acids CYFQNCPRG (C residues are disulfide bonded)	Responds to osmoreceptor which senses extracellular [Na^+], blood pressure regulation, increases H_2O reabsorption from distal tubules in kidney, loss results in dilute urine and polydipsia (constant thirst) condition termed diabetes insipidus
Hypothalamic Hormones and Peptides		
Corticotropin-releasing factor (CRF or CRH)	Protein of 41 amino acids	Acts on corticotrope to release ACTH and β-endorphin (lipotropin)
Gonadotropin-releasing factor (GnRF or GnRH)	Polypeptide of 10 amino acids	Acts on gonadotrope to release LH and FSH
Growth hormone-releasing factor (GRF or GRH)	Protein of 40 and 44 amino acids	Stimulates GH secretion
Melanin-concentrating hormone, MCH	19 Amino acid cyclic peptide	Important orexigenic (appetite stimulating) hormone
Neuropeptide Y, NPY	36 Amino acids, five receptors termed Y receptors	Effects on hypothalamic function in appetite, controls feeding behavior and energy homeostasis, levels increase during starvation to induce food intake

TABLE 31–1 Major peptide and amino acid–derived hormones.* (*Continued*)

Hormone	Structure	Functions
Orexins	Two peptides from single preproprotein; orexin A is 33 amino acids, orexin B is 28 amino acids	Important roles in the emotional and motivational aspects of feeding behavior, increases food consumption (orexigenic) hence derivation of peptide name; increases wakefulness and suppresses REM sleep
Prolactin-release inhibiting factor (PIF or PIH)	Is the neurotransmitter dopamine that is derived from the amino acid tyrosine	Acts on lactotrope to inhibit prolactin release
Somatostatin (SIF, also called growth hormone-release inhibiting factor, GIF)	Polypeptide of 14 and 28 amino acids	Inhibits GH and TSH secretion
Thyrotropin-releasing factor (TRF; also called thyrotropin-releasing hormone: TRH)	Peptide of 3 amino acids derived from a 242 amino acid precursor; when fully processed the C-terminal Gln residue is converted to pyroglutamate which is a cyclic amino acid; active peptide is NH_2-Pro-His-Glu(pyro)	Stimulates TSH and prolactin secretion
Thyroid Hormones		
Thyroxine and triiodothyronine	Iodinated dityrosine derivatives; released from the thyroid protein, thyroglobulin	Responds to TSH and stimulates oxidations in many cells
Calcitonin	Protein of 32 amino acids	Produced in parafollicular C cells of the thyroid, its role in the regulation of Ca^{2+} homeostasis is insignificant in humans
Calcitonin gene-related peptide (CGRP)	Hormone is termed αCGRP; protein of 37 amino acids; product of the calcitonin gene (*CALCA*) as a result of alternative splicing of the precursor mRNA in the brain; a related protein (βCGRP) is derived from the *CALCB* gene	Functions in nociception (sensation of pain) and in homeostasis of the cardiovascular system through functioning as a potent vasodilator
Parathyroid Hormone		
Parathyroid hormone (PTH)	Protein of 84 amino acids	Regulation of Ca^{2+} and P_i homeostasis, stimulates renal reabsorption of Ca^{2+} and bone Ca^{2+} release thus increasing serum Ca^{2+}, also stimulates renal phosphate (PO_4^{3-}) efflux
Adipose Tissue Hormones/Adipokines		
Adiponectin	244 Amino acid protein with four distinct functional domains	Major biological actions are increases in insulin sensitivity and fatty acid oxidation
Adipsin (also called complement factor D)		Produced by adipocytes, liver, monocytes, and macrophages; rate-limiting enzyme in complement activation
C-reactive protein (CRP)		Produced by adipocytes and hepatocytes; is a member of the pentraxin family of calcium-dependent ligand binding proteins; assists complement interaction with foreign and damaged cells; enhances phagocytosis by macrophages; levels of expression regulated by circulating IL-6; modulates endothelial cell functions by inducing expression of various cell adhesion molecules, eg, ICAM-1, VCAM-1, and selectins; induces MCP-1 expression in endothelium; attenuates NO production by downregulating NOS expression; increase expression and activity of PAI-1
Leptin	167 Amino acid precursor processed to 146 amino acids	Regulation of overall body weight by limiting food intake and increasing energy expenditure, regulation of the neuroendocrine axis, inflammatory responses, blood pressure, and bone mass
Resistin	108 Amino acid preprotein in humans	Produced by adipocytes, spleen, monocytes, macrophages, lung, kidney, bone marrow, and placenta; induces insulin resistance; levels of protein increase in obesity; modulates endothelial cell function by enhancing expression of the cell adhesion molecule VCAM-1 and the chemoattractant MCP-1

(*Continued*)

TABLE 31–1 Major peptide and amino acid–derived hormones.* (*Continued*)

Hormone	Structure	Functions
Gut Hormones		
Cholecystokinin, CCK	Predominant form is 33 amino acids	Produced by enteroendocrine I cells predominantly in the duodenum, jejunum; stimulates gallbladder contraction and bile flow, increases secretion of digestive enzymes from pancreas
Enterostatin	Derived from N-terminal end of pancreatic colipase; pentapeptide existing in three forms in mammals: APGPR (human), VPDPR, and VPGPR	Regulates fat intake, peripheral or central administration inhibits its consumption of a high-fat diet but not a low-fat diet
Fibroblast growth factor 19, FGF19	216 Amino acids; member of the large FGF family of growth factors	Produced in ileum, expression of *FGF19* gene activated by transcription factor FXR; FXR is activated when ileal enterocytes absorb bile acids, when released to the portal circulation FGF19 stimulates hepatic glycogen and protein synthesis while inhibiting glucose production; reduces the expression and activity of CYP7A1 which is the rate-limiting enzyme in bile acid synthesis; acts in the gallbladder to induce relaxation and refilling with bile acids
Gastrin	17 Amino acids (little gastrin) and 34 amino acids (big gastrin)	Produced by stomach antrum, stimulates acid and pepsin secretion, also stimulates pancreatic secretions
Gastrin-releasing peptide (GRP); a bombesin-like peptide family member	27 Amino acids	Stimulates release of gastrin from G cells of the stomach and CCK from small intestinal enteroendocrine I cells
Ghrelin	28 Amino acids derived from preproghrelin protein; acylated on Ser3 with *n*-octanoic acid, non-acylated forms found in circulation also but not bioactive	Primary site of production is A (X-like) enteroendocrine cells of the stomach oxyntic (acid secreting) glands, minor synthesis in intestine, pancreas and hypothalamus; appetite stimulation, stimulates NPY release, regulation of energy homeostasis, glucose metabolism, gastric secretion and emptying, insulin secretion
Glucagon-like peptide 1 (GLP-1) formerly called enteroglucagon	Two forms: 31 amino acids, GLP-1(7-37) and 30 amino acids, GLP-1(7-36)amide	Produced by enteroendocrine L cells predominantly in the ileum and colon; potentiates glucose-dependent insulin secretion, inhibits glucagon secretion, inhibits gastric emptying
Glucose-dependent insulinotropic polypeptide (GIP) originally called gastric inhibitory polypeptide	42 Amino acids	Produced by enteroendocrine K cells of the duodenum and proximal jejunum; inhibits secretion of gastric acid, enhances insulin secretion
Motilin	22 Amino acids	Controls gastrointestinal muscles, stimulates release of PP, stimulates gallbladder contractions
Neuromedin B; a bombesin-like peptide family member	10 Amino acids (amidated)	Secretion of gastrin, CCK, GIP, insulin; smooth muscle contraction; enhances food intake
Obestatin	23 Amino acids derived from preproghrelin protein	Primary site of synthesis is stomach, minor synthesis in intestine; acts in opposition to ghrelin action on appetite
Oxyntomodulin	37 Amino acids, the first 29 are identical to glucagon	Produced by enteroendocrine L cells predominantly in the ileum and colon; contains all of the amino acids of glucagon; inhibits meal-stimulated gastric acid secretion similar to GLP-1 and GLP-2 action; induces satiety, decreases weight gain, and increases energy consumption; has weak affinity for GLP-1 receptor as well as glucagon receptor, may mimic glucagon actions in liver and pancreas
Peptide tyrosine tyrosine: PYY	36 Amino acids	Produced by enteroendocrine L cells predominantly in the ileum and colon; reduces gut motility, delays gastric emptying, inhibition of gallbladder contraction, induces satiety via actions in the arcuate nucleus (ARC) of the hypothalamus
Secretin	27 Amino acids	Secreted from duodenum at pH values below 4.5, stimulates pancreatic acinar cells to release bicarbonate and H_2O

TABLE 31–1 Major peptide and amino acid–derived hormones.* (*Continued*)

Hormone	Structure	Functions
Somatostatin	14 Amino acid version	Inhibits release and action of numerous gut peptides such as CCK, OXM, PP, gastrin, secretin, motilin, GIP; also inhibits insulin and glucagon secretion from pancreas
Substance P, a member of the tachykinin family that includes neurokinin A (NKA) and neurokinin B (NKB)	11 Amino acids	CNS function in pain (nociception), involved in vomit reflex, stimulates salivary secretions, induces vasodilation; antagonists have antidepressant properties
Pancreatic Polypeptide (polypeptide fold) Family		
Amphiregulin	Two peptides: 78 amino acid truncated form and 84 amino acid form with six additional N-terminal amino acids	Homology to epidermal growth factor (EGF) and binds to the EGF receptor (EGFR)
Pancreatic Polypeptide, PP	36 Amino acids	Suppresses glucose-induced insulin secretion, inhibits bicarbonate and protein secretion from pancreas
Peptide Tyrosine Tyrosine, PYY	see Hypothalamic Hormones and Peptides above	see Hypothalamic Hormones and Peptides above
Neuropeptide Y, NPY	36 Amino acids, five receptors termed Y receptors	see Hypothalamic Hormones and Peptides above
Pancreatic Hormones		
Amylin	37 Amino acids, intrachain disulfide bonded	Also called islet amyloid polypeptide (IAPP), produced by β-cells of the pancreas, co-secreted with insulin; reduces the rate of gastric emptying, suppresses food intake, and suppresses post-meal glucagon secretion
Glucagon	Polypeptide of 29 amino acids	see text
Insulin	Disulfide-bonded dipeptide of 21 and 30 amino acids	Produced by β-cells of the pancreas, increases glucose uptake and utilization, increases lipogenesis, general anabolic effects; reviewed in Chapter 29
Pancreatic polypeptide, PP	see Pancreatic Polypeptide Family above	see Pancreatic Polypeptide Family above
Somatostatin	see Gut Hormones above	see Gut Hormones above
Placental Hormones		
Chorionic gonadotropin	Two proteins: α is 96 amino acids; β is 147	Activity similar to LH
Chorionic somatomammotropin, also called placental lactogen	Protein of 191 amino acids	Acts like prolactin and GH
Relaxin	2 Proteins of 22 and 32 amino acids	Produced in ovarian corpus luteum, inhibits myometrial contractions, secretion increases during gestation
Gonadal Hormones		
Inhibins A and B	The inhibin alpha (α) peptide is 134 amino acids and is encoded by the *INHA* gene; the α-peptide forms disulfide bonds with either the inhibin beta A (115 amino acids encoded by the *INHBA* gene) peptide forming inhibin A or with the inhibin beta B (116 amino acid encoded by the *INHBB* gene) peptide forming inhibin B	Inhibition of FSH secretion

(Continued)

TABLE 31–1 Major peptide and amino acid–derived hormones.* (*Continued*)

Hormone	Structure	Functions
Adrenal Medullary Hormones		
Epinephrine (adrenalin)	Derived from tyrosine	Classic "fight-or-flight" response, increases glycogenolysis, lipid mobilization, smooth muscle contraction, cardiac function, binds to all classes of catecholamine receptors (α- and β-adrenergic)
Norepinephrine (noradrenalin)	Derived from tyrosine	Classic "fight-or-flight" response, lipid mobilization, arteriole contraction, also acts as neurotransmitter in the CNS, released from noradrenergic neurons, binds all catecholamine receptors except β_2-adrenergic
Liver Hormones/Hepatokines		
Angiotensin II	Polypeptide of 8 amino acids derived from angiotensinogen (present in the α_2-globulin fraction of plasma) which is cleaved by the kidney enzyme renin to give the decapeptide, angiotensin I, the C-terminal 2 amino acids are then released (by action of angiotensin-converting enzyme, ACE) to yield angiotensin II	Responsible for essential hypertension through stimulated synthesis and release of aldosterone from adrenal cells
Cardiac and Vascular Hormones		
Atrial natriuretic peptide (ANP)	28-Amino acid peptide containing a 17-amino acid ring formed by intrachain disulfide bonding	Released from heart right atrium in response to hypervolemia; actions include natriuresis, diuresis, vasorelaxation, inhibition of renin and aldosterone secretion, also plays a key role in cardiovascular homeostasis
Endothelins	Three family members: ET-1, ET-2, ET-3; all are 21-amino-acid peptides with two Cys-Cys disulfide bonds	Released from endothelial cells; interact with G-protein–coupled receptors (GPCR) identified as ETA, ETB; endothelins primarily mediate smooth muscle contraction on binding to endothelin receptors on these cells; can elicit smooth muscle relaxation through interactions with endothelin receptors on endothelial cells which results in increased nitric oxide (NO) production; the ETB receptor had been suggested to exist in two forms, ETB1 and ETB2, but there is no pharmacologic evidence to support the existence of two forms in humans; an additional endothelin receptor identified as ETC was proposed but no gene in the human genome has been identified
Natriuretic peptide B (BNP)	Precursor BNP is cleaved intracellularly and then also when released to the blood	Released from heart ventricles in response to hypervolemia; original mammalian BNP was isolated from brain but the human brain natriuretic factor is CNP; BNP and ANP act by binding to the same receptor; actions include natriuresis, diuresis, vasorelaxation, inhibition of renin and aldosterone secretion, also plays a key role in cardiovascular homeostasis
Kidney Hormones		
Erythropoietin, EPO	Derived from 193 amino acid precursor protein	Highly glycosylated hormone (40% of total mass) that is also considered a growth factor; is required for erythropoiesis in the bone marrow; exerts its effects by binding the EPO receptor, EPOR
Pineal Hormones		
Melatonin	Derived from tryptophan; structure is *N*-acetyl-5-methoxytryptamine	Regulation of circadian rhythms

*Not intended to represent a complete listing of all hormones.

THE HYPOTHALAMIC-PITUITARY AXIS

The hypothalamus is located below the thalamus and just above the brain stem and is composed of several domains (nuclei) that perform a variety of functions. The hypothalamus is involved in the control of certain metabolic processes as well as other functions of the autonomic nervous system. The hypothalamus synthesizes and secretes a variety of neurohormones, referred to as hypothalamic-releasing hormones (or factors), that act on the pituitary to direct the release of the various pituitary hormones.

The pituitary gland has two lobes called the posterior and anterior lobes (Figure 31–1). Each lobe secretes peptide hormones that exert numerous effects on the body. The posterior pituitary excretes the two hormones, oxytocin and vasopressin. The anterior pituitary secretes six hormones: adrenocorticotropic hormone (ACTH, also called corticotropin), thyroid-stimulating hormone (TSH), follicle-stimulating hormone (FSH), luteinizing hormone (LH), growth hormone (GH), and prolactin (PRL). ACTH is derived from a large precursor protein identified as pro-opiomelanocortin (POMC). The posterior pituitary secretes oxytocin and vasopressin.

The secretion of the anterior pituitary hormones is under control of the hypothalamus, hence the description of the system as the hypothalamic-pituitary axis. The secretion of the hormones ACTH, TSH, FSH, LH, and GH are stimulated by signals from

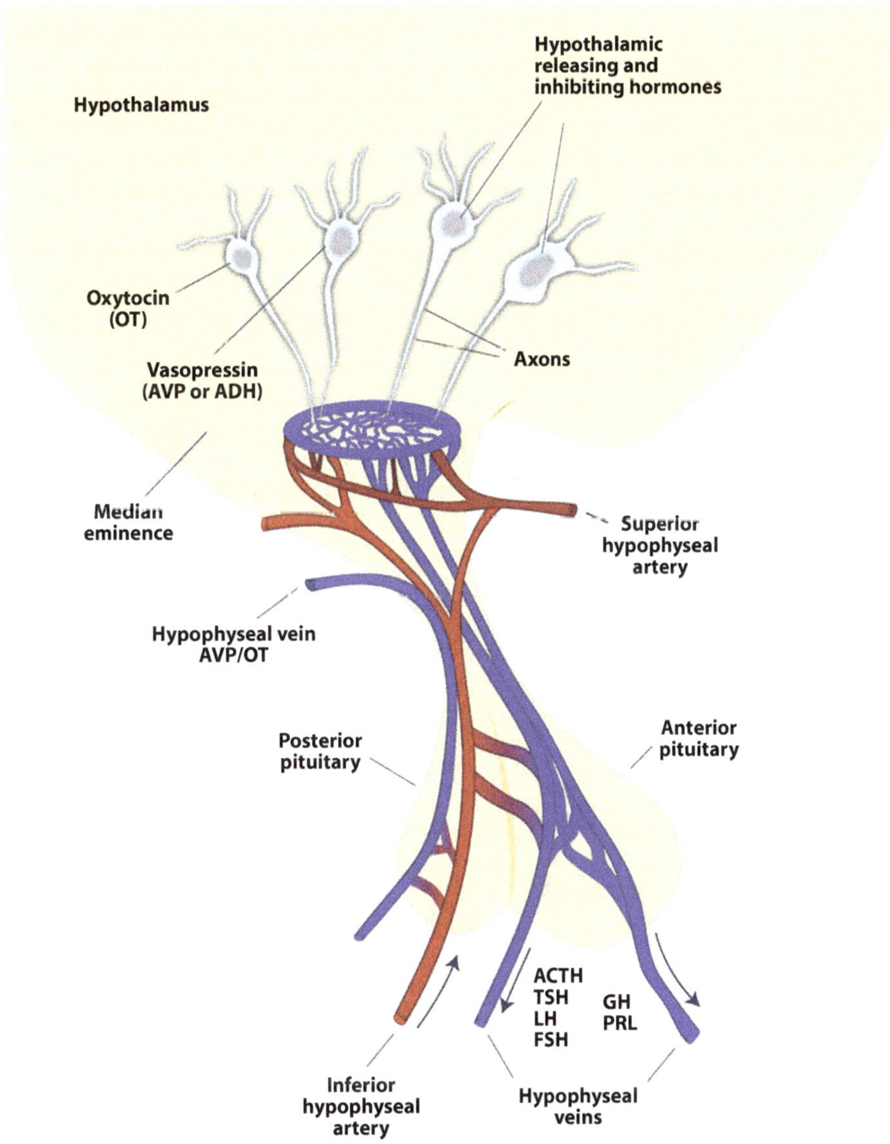

FIGURE 31–1 Diagrammatic representation of the interactions between the hypothalamus and the pituitary. The hypothalamic releasing and inhibiting hormones exert their effects on the release of anterior pituitary hormones. Oxytocin and vasopressin (antidiuretic hormone) are released directly from hypothalamic axons that terminate in the posterior pituitary, and the hormones are secreted from there directly into the systemic circulation. (Reproduced with permission from themedicalbiochemistrypage, LLC.)

the hypothalamus, whereas, PRL secretion is inhibited by hypothalamic signals.

HIGH-YIELD CONCEPT

The cell types that synthesize and secrete the various anterior pituitary hormones are specialized secretory cells. The cells that secrete ACTH are called corticotropes (or corticotrophs). The cells that secrete thyroid-stimulating hormone are called thyrotropes (or thyrotrophs). The cells that secrete follicle-stimulating hormone and luteinizing hormone are called gonadotropes (or gonadotrophs). The cells that secrete prolactin are called lactotropes (or lactotrophs). The cells that secrete growth hormone are called somatotropes (or somatotrophs).

The synthesis and secretion of anterior pituitary hormones occurs in response to hypothalamic releasing or inhibiting hormones. There are six hypothalamic releasing and inhibiting hormones: corticotropin-releasing hormone (CRH), thyrotropin-releasing hormone (TRH), gonadotropin-releasing hormone (GnRH), luteinizing hormone-releasing hormone (LHRH), growth hormone-releasing hormone (GHRH), growth hormone release-inhibiting hormone (GHIH, more commonly called somatostatin), and prolactin release-inhibiting hormone (which is dopamine). GnRH has been shown to stimulate the release of both FSH and LH and as such the term GnRH is more appropriately used than LHRH.

ANTERIOR PITUITARY HORMONES AND THEIR FUNCTIONS

ACTH

Adrenocorticotropic hormone (ACTH) is a member of the POMC-derived family of factors (Figure 31–2). The primary protein product of the *POMC* gene is a 285 amino acid precursor that can undergo differential processing to yield at least eight peptides, dependent on the location of synthesis and the stimulus leading to their production.

The processing of POMC involves glycosylations, acetylations, and extensive proteolytic cleavage at sites shown to contain regions of basic protein sequence (see Figure 31–2). The proteases that recognize these cleavage sites are tissue-specific so, for example, the physiologically active product of the anterior pituitary is ACTH.

ACTH is the main physiologically active product of the actions of the hypothalamic-releasing hormone, CRH, on the anterior pituitary. Although CRH is the primary stimulus for ACTH release, other hormones also exert effects on ACTH release. CRH stimulates a pulsatile secretion of ACTH with peak levels seen before waking and declining as the day progresses. Negative

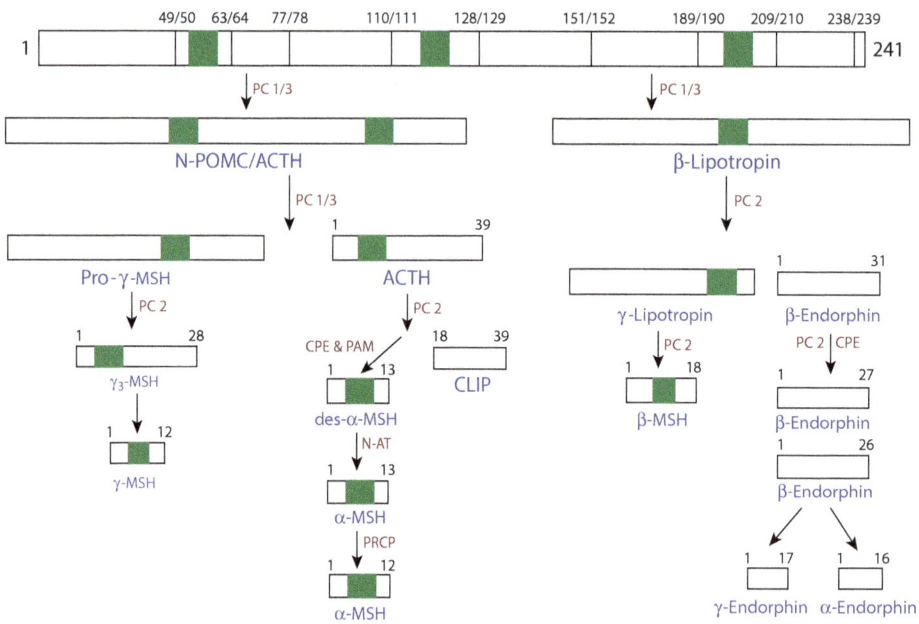

FIGURE 31–2 Processing of the POMC precursor protein. Cleavage sites consist of the sequences, Arg-Lys, Lys-Arg, or Lys-Lys. Enzymes responsible for processing of POMC peptides include prohormone convertase 1/3 (PC1/3), prohormone convertase 2 (PC2), carboxypeptidase E (CPE), peptidyl α-amidating monooxygenase (PAM), *N*-acetyltransferase (N-AT), and prolylcarboxypeptidase (PRCP). Adrenocorticotropic hormone (ACTH) and β-lipotropin are products generated in the corticotrophic cells of the anterior pituitary under the control of corticotrophin-releasing hormone (CRH). Alpha-melanocyte– stimulating hormone (α-MSH), corticotropin-like intermediate lobe peptide (CLIP), γ-lipotropin, and β-endorphin are products generated in the intermediate lobe of the pituitary under the control of dopamine. α-, β-, and γ-MSH are collectively referred to as melanotropin or intermedin. The blue-shaded boxes represent the heptapeptide sequence that constitutes the MSH core. (Reproduced with permission from themedicalbiochemistrypage, LLC.)

feedback on ACTH secretion is exerted by cortisol at both the hypothalamic and anterior pituitary levels. Additional factors (stressors) influence ACTH secretion primarily as a result of the actions of vasopressin and CRH.

The biological role of ACTH is to stimulate the production of adrenal cortex steroids, principally the glucocorticoids, cortisol, and corticosterone. ACTH also stimulates the adrenal cortex to produce the mineralocorticoid, aldosterone as well as the androgen, androstenedione. ACTH exerts its effects on the adrenal cortex by binding to a specific receptor that is a member of the melanocortin receptor family, melanocortin-2 receptor (MC2R). The main cortical cell response to ACTH is increased activity of CYP11A1 which converts cholesterol to pregnenolone during steroid hormone synthesis (see Chapter 32).

Primary adrenal insufficiency (adrenal hypoplasia) is characteristic of Addison disease (see Clinical Box 32–1). Secondary adrenal insufficiency occurs in patients with deficiencies in pituitary ACTH production or secretion. Secondary adrenal insufficiency is characterized by weakness, fatigue, nausea, vomiting, and anorexia. On the opposite side of the abnormal ACTH spectrum are the adrenal hyperplasias. These include the congenital adrenal hyperplasias (CAH; see Chapter 32) and Cushing syndrome (see Clinical Box 32–2).

Growth Hormone

Growth hormone (GH) is synthesized in acidophilic pituitary somatotropes as a single polypeptide chain that exists in functional form as a disulfide-bonded hormone. Expression of GH occurs only in the pituitary. The growth-promoting effects of GH are due to induced secretion of insulin-like growth factor 1 (IGF-1). The metabolic effects of GH include the promotion of gluconeogenesis and amino acid uptake by cells, and it induces the breakdown of tissue lipids which provides the energy needed to support the stimulated protein synthesis.

Growth hormone elicits its effects by binding to a plasma membrane localized receptor (GHR) that is a member of the class I cytokine receptor family. The activated GHR interacts with intracellular members of the Janus kinase (JAK) family of kinases. Activation of the JAK family kinases leads to docking of proteins of the STAT (signal transducer and activator of transcription) family to the GHR and subsequent activation of the RAS/ERK (extracellular signal-regulated kinase) and PI3K (phosphatidylinositol-3-kinase)/AKT signal transduction pathways.

There are a number of genetic deficiencies associated with GH. GH-deficient dwarfs lack the ability to synthesize or secrete GH, and these short-statured individuals respond well to GH therapy. Pygmies lack the IGF-1 response to GH but not its metabolic effects. Laron dwarfs have normal or excess plasma GH but lack liver GH receptors and have low levels of circulating IGF-1. The production of excessive amounts of GH before epiphyseal closure of the long bones leads to gigantism, and when GH becomes excessive after epiphyseal closure, acral bone growth leads to the characteristic features of acromegaly.

Prolactin

Prolactin is produced by acidophilic pituitary lactotropes. Prolactin is known to bind zinc (Zn^{2+}) and the binding of this metal stabilizes prolactin in the secretory pathway. Prolactin is the lone tropic hormone of the pituitary that is routinely under negative control by dopamine. Decreased hypophyseal dopamine production, or damage to the hypophyseal stalk, leads to rapid upregulation of PRL secretion. Prolactin does not appear to play a role in normal gonadal function yet hyperprolactinemia in humans results in hypogonadism.

Prolactin secretion increases during pregnancy and promotes breast development in preparation for the production of milk and lactation. During pregnancy the increased production of estrogen enhances breast development but it also suppresses the effects of prolactin on lactation. Following parturition estrogen (as well as progesterone) levels fall allowing lactation to occur. This is to ensure that lactation is not induced until the baby is born.

Prolactin elicits its effects by binding to a plasma membrane localized receptor (PRLR) that is a member of the class I cytokine receptor family. The activated PRLR interacts with intracellular members of the Janus kinase (JAK) family of kinases. Activation of the JAK family kinases leads to docking of proteins of the STAT (signal transducer and activator of transcription) family to the PRLR and subsequent activation of the RAS/ERK (extracellular signal-regulated kinase) and PI3K (phosphatidylinositol-3-kinase)/AKT signal transduction pathways.

Thyroid-Stimulating Hormone

TSH is a member of the glycoprotein hormone family that includes the gonadotropins, FSH, LH, and hCG. All members of the family are highly glycosylated. Each of the glycoprotein hormones is an (α:β) heterodimer, with the β-subunit being identical in all members of the family. The biological activity of the hormone is determined by the β-subunit, which is not active in the absence of the β subunit. The β-subunit gene is identified as chorionic gonadotropin, alpha: CGA.

The synthesis and release of TSH is controlled by two principal pathways. The first is exerted by the level of triiodothyronine (T_3, or T3; see Chapter 32) within thyrotropic cells which regulates TSH expression, translation, and release. The second mode of regulation is exerted by hypothalamic TRH (Figure 31–3). TRH binding to its receptor on thyrotropes leads to TSH secretion as well as increased TSH transcription and posttranslational glycosylation. The TRH-mediated release of TSH is pulsatile with peak secretion being exerted between midnight and 4 am.

TSH binds to receptors on the basal membrane of thyroid follicles triggering increased secretion of the thyroid hormones, T3 and thyroxine (T_4 or T4). TSH-binding to its receptor also results in increased TSH synthesis and thyroid cell growth. TSH causes an increase in the synthesis of a major thyroid hormone precursor, thyroglobulin. Thyroglobulin is a glycosylated protein whose tyrosine residues are sites for iodination and are used to synthesize T3 and T4 (see Chapter 32). Lysosomal proteases degrade thyroglobulin-releasing amino acids and T3 and T4, which are secreted into the circulation.

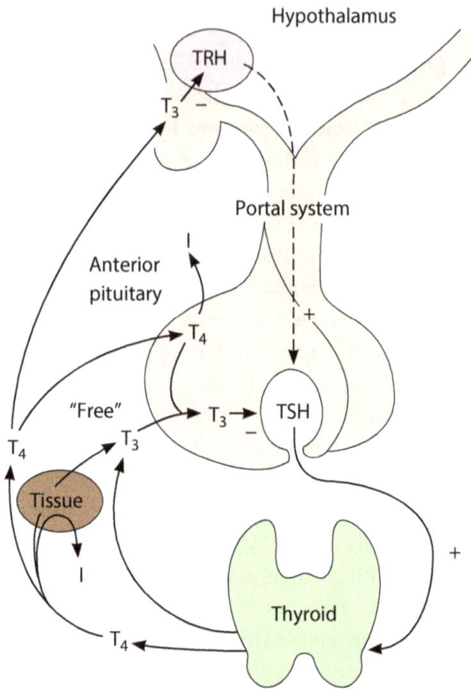

FIGURE 31–3 The hypothalamic-hypophysial-thyroidal axis. TRH produced in the hypothalamus reaches the thyrotrophs in the anterior pituitary by the hypothalamohypophysial portal system and stimulates the synthesis and release of TSH. In both the hypothalamus and the pituitary, it is primarily T3 that inhibits TRH and TSH secretion, respectively. T4 undergoes monodeiodination to T3 in neural and pituitary as well as in peripheral tissues. (Reproduced with permission from Gardner DG, Shoback D. *Greenspan's Basic and Clinical Endocrinology*, 10th ed. New York, NY: McGraw Hill; 2018.)

Numerous congenital and acquired forms of hypothyroidism and hyperthyroidism are the result of alterations in the expression, processing, and function of the TSH receptor (TSHR). The most common TSHR disorder resulting in hyperthyroidism (thyrotoxicosis) is Graves disease (Clinical Box 31–1).

Follicle-Stimulating Hormone and Luteinizing Hormone

The synthesis and release of FSH and LH is controlled by the action of the hypothalamic releasing factor GnRH. The function of GnRH is to induce an episodic release of both FSH and LH that determines the onset of puberty and ovulation in females. In females, FSH stimulates follicular development and estrogen synthesis by granulosa cells of the ovary. In males, FSH promotes testicular growth and within the Sertoli cells of the seminiferous tubules of the testis FSH enhances the synthesis of androgen-binding proteins, ABP. The function of ABP is to bind testosterone (T) and dihydrotestosterone (DHT), as well as 17α-estradiol, resulting in the concentration of the male sex hormones within these cells.

The FSH receptor (FSHR) and the LH-choriogonadotropin receptor (LHCGR) are both members of the large GPCR family and both are coupled to G_s-type G-proteins. Binding of FSH and LH to their respective receptors results in activation of adenylate cyclase leading to increased PKA activity. The LHCGR is expressed in the ovary, thecal cells, stromal cells, luteinizing granulosa, and luteal cells of the ovary and in Leydig cells of the testes.

CLINICAL BOX 31–1 GRAVES DISEASE

Graves disease is a disorder that was originally described by the Irish physician, Robert James Graves in 1835. His original description referred to the disease as "exophthalmic goiter." Graves disease is now known to be a syndrome that manifests as hyperthyroidism with a diffuse goiter. Specifically, Graves disease is associated with thyrotoxicosis which is defined as a state of thyroid hormone excess but is not synonymous with hyperthyroidism (result of excessive thyroid function). The major causes of thyrotoxicosis are the hyperthyroidism of Graves disease, toxic adenomas, and toxic multinodular goiter. In addition to hyperthyroidism and goiter, Graves disease is associated with eye disease characterized by inflammation and involvement of intra-orbital structures, dermopathy referred to as pretibial myxoedema, and rare involvement of the nails, fingers, and long bones known as acropachy. Graves disease is an autoimmune disease caused by autoantibodies to the thyroid-stimulating hormone (TSH) receptor, TSH-R. These antibodies (identified as TSI: TSH-R-stimulating immunoglobulins) bind to the TSH-R on thyroid follicular cells and mimic the receptor activation actions of TSH. The consequences of this hyperactivation of the thyroid are stimulated follicular cell growth, resulting in diffuse thyroid enlargement and increased production of thyroid hormones. With respect to the thyroid hormones, the fraction of triiodothyronine (T3) production relative to thyroxine (T4) is increased. Graves disease is the most common autoimmune disease in the United States affecting 0.5% of the population. Graves disease accounts for 60–80% of all forms of thyrotoxicosis with the prevalence being higher among women than men. Smokers and those individuals with other autoimmune disorders or with a family history of thyroid autoimmunity are more likely to develop the disease than the general population. The disease rarely begins prior to adolescence and typically manifests between 20 and 50 years of age. Across different populations, the rate of the disease can vary dependent on the intake of iodine with increased prevalence of Graves disease associated with higher iodine intake. The onset of Graves disease is usually acute, reflecting the sudden production of TSI. Most patients will report the classical symptoms of hyperthyroidism that include weight loss despite increased appetite, heat intolerance, irritability, insomnia, sweatiness, diarrhea, palpitations, muscular weakness, and menstrual irregularity. On physical examination, the classic clinical signs of Graves disease will be diffuse goiter, eye disease, warm smooth skin, hyperreflexia, fine resting tremor, and tachycardia. All of these symptoms of Graves disease are related to the effects of thyroid overstimulation of metabolism and exacerbation of sympathetic nervous system responses. The sympathomimetic effects include the aforementioned

CLINICAL BOX 31–1 (CONTINUED)

tachycardia as well as hand tremors, anxiety, and gastrointestinal hypermotility. Less common findings include atrial fibrillation and a thyroid bruit reflecting the marked increase in thyroid vascularity. Older presenting patients are more likely to present with depression, weight loss, atrial fibrillation, and congestive heart failure then will be present in younger patients. Although less likely, some Graves disease patients will present with proximal myopathy, cardiomyopathy, malabsorption, hypercalcemia, hepatitis, gynecomastia, and loss of glycemic control in patients with diabetes. Eye disease affects up to 50% of patients with Graves disease. The pathophysiology of the ocular issues associated with Graves disease is distinct from the sympathomimetic ocular effects of thyroid hormone excess which are identified as thyroid stare, known as the Dalrymple sign (wide open eyes and eyelid spasm). The cardinal features of thyroid eye disease include exophthalmos (abnormal eyeball protrusion), chemosis (conjunctive edema) and when severe, impaired extra-ocular muscle movement. The impaired eye movement is most easily seen during a vertical and lateral gaze test. The consequences of chemosis include infections leading to swollen, congested, watery or gritty eyes. Vision changes also result resulting in loss of visual fields or acuity and diplopia (double vision). In any patient suspected of hyperthyroidism it is extremely important to perform a comprehensive clinical assessment of disturbances in biochemical processes. To this end, serum TSH is a sensitive index for primary thyroid disease and therefore, the most important initial screening test. Patients who are identified with reduced levels of TSH are likely to have suppression of the hypothalamic-pituitary axis. In these patients it is necessary to subsequently measure for the level of free T3 and T4. In Graves disease associated hyperthyroidism both of these hormones will be elevated in the serum. Care must be taken in interpreting free thyroid hormone levels as artifacts in their measurements are associated with critical illness, disturbances in binding proteins due to drugs or pregnancy, and to the use of heparin as an anticoagulant. The measurement of serum TSH-receptor antibodies is highly correlated to the confirmation of a diagnosis of Graves disease. In 90% of patients with presumed Graves disease, TSI and TSH-receptor binding immunoglobulins (TBII) are found and are directly related to the disruption in thyroid function. However, routine measurement of TSI or TBII is unnecessary in patients in whom the diagnosis of Graves disease is confirmed due to thyrotoxicosis with eye changes suggestive of thyroid eye disease. The measurement of TSI and TBII are also useful for assessing the risk of relapse after a course of drug treatment for Graves disease. These drugs include the thionamides, methimazole (MMI), carbimazole, and propylthiouracil (PTU). Measurement of the autoantibodies is also highly useful when assessing the risk of neonatal Graves disease in pregnant women with Graves disease. Other antibodies, including thyroid peroxidase (TPO) and thyroglobulin (Tg) antibodies, may be significantly elevated in Graves disease but they are not specific to a diagnosis of the disease. These latter autoantibodies may also be detected in Hashimoto disease (chronic lymphocytic thyroiditis resulting in hypothyroidism). Hashimoto disease is the most common form of hypothyroidism in the United States.

POSTERIOR PITUITARY HORMONES AND THEIR FUNCTIONS

Vasopressin

Vasopressin is also known as antidiuretic hormone (ADH), because it is the main regulator of body fluid osmolarity through induced renal reabsorption of water. Vasopressin increases the reabsorption rate of water in principal cells of the collecting ducts of the kidney tubule, causing the excretion of urine that is concentrated in Na^+ and, thus, yielding a net drop in osmolarity of body fluids.

Vasopressin exerts its effects in the tubule by binding to receptors of the GPCR family. There are three kinds of vasopressin receptors designated V_1A (V1A or just V1), V_1B (V1B: also known as the V_3 receptor), and V_2 (V2). Although there are three vasopressin receptors, the major actions of vasopressin are elicited through activation of the V_1A and V2 receptors. The V_1A and V_1B receptors are GPCR that activate G_q-type G-proteins leading to the activation of PLCβ and the subsequent hydrolysis of PIP_2 which results in increased intracellular Ca^{2+} concentration and the activation of PKC. The V_2 receptor is a GPCR that activates a G_s-type G-protein leading to the activation of adenylate cyclase resulting in increased cAMP levels and activation of PKA.

The V_1A (V1) receptors are found in vascular smooth muscle cells and vasopressin binding to these receptors triggers vascular contraction resulting in increased blood pressure. The V_1A receptor is also expressed in smooth muscle cells of the uterus (myometrium), in hepatocytes, and in platelets. The V_1B (V3) receptor is expressed in the anterior pituitary.

HIGH-YIELD CONCEPT

Vasopressin deficiency leads to production of large volumes of watery urine and polydipsia. These symptoms are diagnostic of a condition known as diabetes insipidus. Diabetes insipidus has numerous causes that include effects on the hypothalamic-pituitary-axis and the kidneys. Mutations in the gene encoding the V_2 receptor are responsible for X-linked nephrogenic diabetes insipidus.

Oxytocin

Oxytocin is produced in the magnocellular neurosecretory cells of the hypothalamus and is then stored in axon terminals of the anterior pituitary. Secretion of oxytocin is stimulated by electrical activity of the oxytocin cells of the hypothalamus.

The actions of oxytocin are elicited via the interaction of the hormone with the oxytocin receptor. The oxytocin receptor is a GPCR that is coupled to a G_q type G-protein leading to activation of PLCβ and thus, the hydrolysis of PIP_2 resulting in increased intracellular Ca^{2+} concentration and the activation of PKC.

Oxytocin secretion in nursing women is stimulated by direct neural feedback obtained by stimulation of the nipple during suckling. This response to oxytocin is referred to as the "let-down response." Its physiologic effects include the contraction of mammary gland myoepithelial cells, which induces the ejection of milk from mammary glands. The other primary action of oxytocin is the stimulation of uterine smooth muscle contraction leading to childbirth. The uterine effect of oxytocin is due, in part, to increased production and release of the prostaglandin $PGF_2\alpha$ from the myometrium and to a lesser extent from the decidua. In males, the circulating levels of oxytocin increase at the time of ejaculation. It is believed that the increase in oxytocin levels causes increased contraction of the smooth muscle cells of the vas deferens thereby propelling the sperm toward the urethra.

NATRIURETIC HORMONES

Natriuresis refers to enhanced urinary excretion of sodium. Three natriuretic hormones have been identified and are referred to as ANP, BNP, and CNP. Atrial natriuretic peptide (ANP: also called atrial natriuretic factor, ANF) is secreted by atrial cardiac myocytes in the wall of the right atrium. BNP was originally identified as brain natriuretic peptide since it was first isolated from porcine brain. In humans BNP is secreted by cardiac ventricular myocytes. ANP and BNP both exert the same effects as a consequence of binding to the same receptor. In humans, a third natriuretic peptide (CNP) is present in the brain but not in the heart.

Active ANP is a 28-amino acid peptide containing a 17-amino acid ring formed by intrachain disulfide bonding. Active BNP is a 32-amino acid peptide that also contains a 17-amino acid ring. ANP and BNP are released in response to increased venous volume returning to the heart. ANP and BNP exert their systemic effects in the vasculature by binding to specific receptors.

Three different natriuretic peptide receptors have been identified. These receptors are ANPR-A, ANPR-B, and ANPR-C. The natriuretic peptide receptors are members of the larger family of single transmembrane spanning guanylate cyclase enzymes. Expression of the ANPR-A is highest in adipocytes but is also high in kidney, adrenal glands, vascular endothelium, and heart. Expression of the ANPR-B is highest in smooth muscle with the next highest levels of expression being found in the brain, and endometrial tissue. ANP and BNP are the natural ligands for the ANPR-A receptor and bind with relatively equivalent affinity and elicit the same responses. CNP is the ligand for the ANPR-B receptor. The function of the ANPR-C protein is to serve as a clearance receptor removing natriuretic peptides from the blood via receptor-mediated endocytosis.

When ANP or BNP bind to receptor, an increase in the intrinsic guanylate cyclase activity results leading to production of cGMP. Within vascular smooth muscle cells, the increased cGMP exerts numerous effects resulting in smooth muscle relaxation and vasodilation. Activation of cGMP-dependent protein kinase (specifically PKGIα) leads to phosphorylation of regulatory subunits of myosin light-chain phosphatases leading to enhanced removal of phosphates from myosin light chains and reduced contractile activity. The activity of cGMP is also direct in that it inhibits smooth muscle plasma membrane L-type Ca^{2+} channels resulting in reduced intake of Ca^{2+} and, as a consequence, reduced activation of myosin light-chain kinases leading to reductions in vasoconstriction.

The actions of ANP and BNP are to cause natriuresis by increasing glomerular filtration. This effect results from relaxation of the mesangial cells of the glomeruli and thus may increase the surface area of these cells so that filtration is increased. Alternatively, ANP and BNP may act on tubule cells to increase sodium excretion. Other effects of ANP and BNP include reducing blood pressure, decreasing the responsiveness of adrenal glomerulosa cells to stimuli that result in aldosterone production and secretion, inhibition of vasopressin secretion, and decreasing vascular smooth muscle cell responses to vasoconstrictive agents. ANP and BNP also lower renin secretion by the kidneys, thus lowering circulating angiotensin II levels.

RENIN-ANGIOTENSIN SYSTEM

The renin-angiotensin system (RAS; also commonly called the renin-angiotensin-aldosterone system, RAAS) is responsible for regulation of blood pressure (Figure 31–4). Bioactive angiotensin (angiotensin II) is derived from the precursor protein, angiotensinogen, predominantly produced by the liver. Renin is a protease/hormone produced by the kidneys and is responsible for cleavage of angiotensinogen initiating the production of bioactive

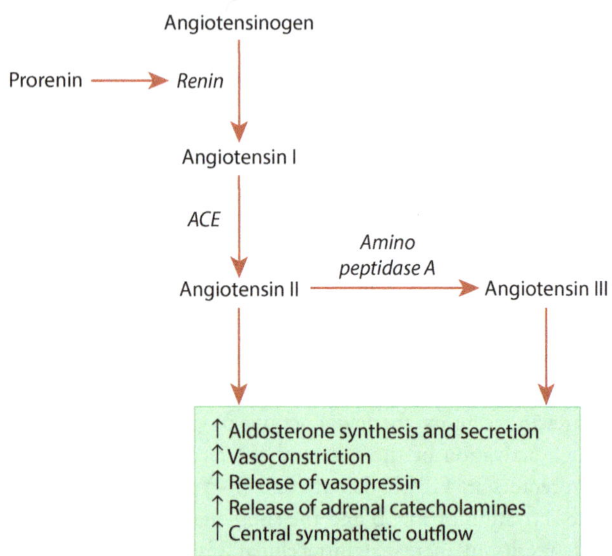

FIGURE 31–4 Steps in the production of angiotensin peptides by the renin-angiotensin system (ACE, angiotensin-converting enzyme). (Reproduced with permission from King MW: *Integrative Medical Biochemistry Examination and Board Review*. New York, NY: McGraw Hill; 2014.)

angiotensin II. The only enzymatic function for renin is to cleave a 10-amino acid peptide from the N-terminal end of angiotensinogen. This cleaved decapeptide is called angiotensin I. Angiotensin I is then cleaved by the action of angiotensin-converting enzyme (ACE) generating the bioactive octapeptide hormone, angiotensin II. Unlike renin which has a single substrate, ACE exhibits activity to a wide range of substrates ranging in size from tripeptides to proteins of 42 amino acids. The major substrates for ACE are angiotensin I and bradykinin, both of which are involved in the regulation of blood pressure.

The intra-renal baroreceptor system is a key mechanism for regulating renin secretion. A drop in blood pressure results in the release of renin from juxtaglomerular cells (JG cells; also called granular cells) which are specialized smooth muscle cells in the wall of the afferent arterioles at the base of the glomerulus in the juxtaglomerular apparatus. These are the only cells in the human body that synthesize and secrete renin. Renin secretion is also regulated by the rate of Na^+ and Cl^- transport across the apical (tubular lumen side) membrane of epithelial cells of the macula densa which resides just distal to the loop of Henle.

Angiotensin II is one of the most potent naturally occurring vasoconstrictors (see Clinical Box 31–2). In addition to its effects on the vasculature, angiotensin II (and its derivative angiotensin III) acts on the kidneys to increase renal tubular Na^+ and Cl^- reabsorption, water retention, and K^+ excretion, on the posterior pituitary to induce the release of vasopressin, stimulates the zona glomerulosa cells of the adrenal cortex to secrete aldosterone, and exerts effects in the central nervous system resulting in increased sympathetic outflow from the rostral ventrolateral medulla of the brain stem.

Two distinct types of angiotensin II receptors have been identified, AT1R and AT2R. The AT1R is a GPCR coupled to both G_q-type and G_i-type G-proteins. AT1R is expressed in the heart, blood vessels, kidney, adrenal cortex, lung, and brain. AT2R is also a GPCR and is coupled to activation of a G_i-type G-protein. Expression of the AT2R is limited, in the adult, to the brain (predominantly the cerebellum), adrenal gland, and myometrium. Within the brain, the primary AT2R ligand is angiotensin III.

CLINICAL BOX 31–2 PHARMACOLOGY OF ANGIOTENSIN II

The vasoconstrictive action of angiotensin II is primarily exerted on the arterioles and leads to a rise in both systolic and diastolic blood pressure. It is this action of angiotensin II on blood pressure that led to the development of a class of drugs called the ACE inhibitors for use as antihypertensive drugs. As the name implies, ACE inhibitors prevent ACE from converting angiotensin I to angiotensin II. All of the drugs that inhibit the activity of ACE contain the suffix "–pril" (eg, captopril). One side-effect of the use of ACE inhibitors is a persistent dry cough leading to lack of compliance with the drugs in a number of patients. The cause of the dry cough is due to reduced degradation of bradykinin, a known substrate for ACE. Although bradykinin is primarily involved in the contractile activity of vascular smooth muscle, it also induces constriction of the bronchioles in the lungs and it is this latter activity that contributes to the dry cough with the use of ACE inhibitors. Due primarily to the development of a dry hacking cough with the use of ACE inhibitors, drugs that block the activity of the AT1R were developed for the treatment of hypertension. This class of drug is called the angiotensin receptor blocker (ARB) class. All of the ARB drugs are AT1R antagonists and thus, exert their antihypertensive effects at the level of the receptor itself. All drugs in the ARB class contain the suffix "–sartan" (eg, losartan). In addition to their use in the treatment of hypertension the ARBs are used to treat diabetic nephropathy and congestive heart failure.

PARATHYROID HORMONE

Parathyroid hormone (PTH) is synthesized and secreted by chief cells of the parathyroid glands. Secretion of PTH from the parathyroid gland is controlled via the activity of the Ca^{2+}-sensing receptor (CaSR). The CaSR is expressed in the parathyroid glands, renal tubule cells, bone marrow, thyroid gland C-cells, gastrin-secreting cells in the stomach, several areas of the brain, and in several other tissues. The CaSR is a GPCR whose ligand is Ca^{2+}. The CaSR is coupled to the activation of G_i, G_q, and G_{12}-type G-proteins resulting in decreased production of cAMP and increased production of DAG and IP_3. Calcium activation of the CaSR results in proteolysis of PTH within chief cells of the parathyroid glands.

The role of PTH is to regulate Ca^{2+} concentration in extracellular fluids which it accomplishes in concert with calcitriol (see Chapter 3). PTH acts by binding to GPCR family receptors that are coupled to G_s- and G_q-type G-proteins. There are two receptors that recognize PTH identified as the PTH-1 and PTH-2 receptors (PTH1R and PTH2R). The PTH-1 receptor is found predominantly in bone and kidney. The body response to PTH is complex but is aimed in all tissues at increasing Ca^{2+} levels in extracellular fluids. PTH induces the demineralization of bone by indirectly stimulating osteoclast activity (through initial activation of osteoblasts which express the PTH-1 receptor), which leads to elevated plasma Ca^{2+} and phosphate. In the kidney, PTH reduces renal Ca^{2+} clearance by stimulating its reabsorption. At the same time, PTH reduces the reabsorption of phosphate and thereby increases its clearance. Finally, PTH acts on the liver, kidney, and intestine to stimulate the production of calcitriol which is responsible for enhancing Ca^{2+} absorption in the intestine.

PANCREATIC HORMONES

The pancreas is composed of both endocrine and exocrine glands. The exocrine glands are composed of the digestive enzyme secreting cells (see Chapter 28). The endocrine glands are called islets of Langerhans and these glands are composed of at least five cell

TABLE 31–2 Secretory products of Islets of Langerhans cells in the pancreas.

Cell Type	Substances Secreted
α-cell	Proglucagon, glucagon, ghrelin
β-cell	Insulin, amylin, proinsulin, C peptide, GABA
δ-cell	Somatostain-14
ε-cell	Ghrelin
PP cell (F cell)	Pancreatic polypeptide

Reproduced with permission from King MW: *Integrative Medical Biochemistry Examination and Board Review*. New York, NY: McGraw Hill; 2014.

types, each of which secrete different hormones (Table 31–2). The functions of insulin are reviewed in Chapter 29.

Glucagon

Glucagon is a 29-amino acid hormone derived by proteolytic processing from the very much larger proglucagon protein. The primary effect of glucagon is to stimulate hepatic glycogen breakdown and activation of gluconeogenesis. The net effect of glucagon is increased delivery of hepatic glucose to the blood. Glucagon exerts its effects by binding to the glucagon receptor which is a GPCR coupled to a G_s-type G-protein. The major site of expression of the glucagon receptor is the liver with the second highest level of expression seen in the kidney and to a lesser extent, in adipose tissue, heart, endocrine pancreas, adrenal glands, spleen, and cerebral cortex.

HIGH-YIELD CONCEPT

Skeletal muscle cells do not respond to glucagon due to the lack of glucagon receptors on these cells.

The binding of glucagon to its receptor in adipose tissue results in increased activation of hormone-sensitive lipase, HSL resulting in increased release of fatty acids that were stored in the triglycerides in adipose tissue. The released fatty acids are oxidized in the liver providing the necessary energy needed for gluconeogenesis which is activated in liver in response to glucagon. Within the endocrine pancreas, the glucagon receptor is found on the β-cells that secrete insulin. The effect of glucagon on these cells is to stimulate insulin release so that there results in a fine regulatory control over the overall level of circulating glucose.

In addition to direct changes in metabolic activity, exerted primarily via PKA-mediated phosphorylation, glucagon exerts effects on gene expression. Increased hepatic PKA activity results in phosphorylation of cytoplasmic cAMP response element binding protein, CREB. When phosphorylated CREB migrates to the nucleus and binds to cAMP response elements (CRE) in target genes resulting in altered transcription. An important CREB target is the gene encoding the gluconeogenic enzyme, phosphoenolpyruvate carboxykinase, PEPCK.

Somatostatin

Somatostatin is secreted by enteroendocrine D cells of the stomach and duodenum, δ-cells of the pancreas, and is also secreted by the hypothalamus. There are two forms of somatostatin identified as SS-28 and SS-14. The primary function of the somatostatin is the suppression of secretory activities of numerous cell types. Somatostatin suppresses the secretion of growth hormone, prolactin, ACTH, cholecystokinin (CCK), gastrin, secretin, glucose-dependent insulinotropic peptide (GIP), vasoactive intestinal peptide (VIP), glucagon, insulin, renin, and aldosterone. Within the CNS, somatostatin functions as a neurotransmitter and neuromodulator.

Somatostatin exerts these effects by binding to receptors of the GPCR family called the somatostatin receptors of which there are five identified as SSTR1-SSTR5. All five receptors are coupled to a G_i-type G-protein that inhibits adenylate cyclase. The somatostatin receptors form complex signaling networks as a result of homodimerization and heterodimerization. In addition to inhibition of adenylate cyclase, somatostatin receptor activation is also coupled to activation of MAPK and protein tyrosine phosphatases, activation of PLCβ and PLA_2, the regulation of inwardly rectifying K^+ channel function, and the inhibition of voltage-dependent Ca^{2+} channel activity.

Amylin

Amylin is a 37 amino acid peptide that is secreted from β-cells of the pancreas simultaneously with insulin. Amylin has also been called islet amyloid polypeptide (IAPP). The primary actions attributable to amylin secretion are reduction in the rate of gastric emptying, suppression of food intake, and suppression of post-meal glucagon secretion. Collectively these three actions compliment the plasma glucose regulating actions of insulin.

HIGH-YIELD CONCEPT

A stable analog of amylin called pramlintide (Symlin) is used as an adjunct to insulin treatment for T1D and T2D. Patients who use pramlintide show a modest degree of weight loss. Current trials are being undertaken to establish the efficacy of pramlintide in the treatment of obesity in patients without diabetes.

Amylin exerts its effect via interaction with three distinct GPCR complexes. These complexes all contain the calcitonin receptor (CTR) as a core protein and either one of three receptor activity-modifying proteins (RAMP), RAMP1, RAMP2 or RAMP3. The specific amylin receptors result from the dimerization of various splice variants of the calcitonin receptor (CTRa or CTRb) with either RAMP1, RAMP2, and RAMP3. These receptors are commonly referred to as AMY_1, AMY_2, and AMY_3 with either an a or b in the subscript designating which CTR splice variant of the calcitonin receptor is in the complex. Amylin receptors are expressed in the nucleus accumbens, the dorsal raphe, and the area postrema in the hind brain. The satiety-inducing effects of amylin are primarily the result of activation of its receptors in the area postrema.

CHECKLIST

- ☑ The endocrine system is composed of a number of tissues that secrete their products, endocrine hormones, into the circulatory system; from there they are disseminated throughout the body, regulating the function of distant tissues and maintaining homeostasis.
- ☑ Peptide hormones constitute the largest class of endocrine system molecules.
- ☑ Peptide hormones of the endocrine system can function in the classical sense which involves secretion from one cell type followed by dissemination via the blood to distance responsive cells. Peptide hormones can also exert highly local effects termed paracrine hormones, or they can even act on the secreting cell itself, termed autocrine hormones.
- ☑ Peptide hormones can be quite small encompassing only a few amino acids to several hundred.
- ☑ All peptide hormones exert their biological effects by binding to cell surface plasma membrane receptors. The peptide hormone receptors are most often members of the GPCR family, but also include members of the single transmembrane family of receptors.
- ☑ Some of the most important whole body homeostatic regulating peptide hormones are produced and secreted by the hypothalamic-pituitary axis.
- ☑ Most peptide hormones are produced from a single gene. A critically relevant exception to this is the pro-opiomelanocortin (*POMC*) gene which produces a pro-peptide of 241 amino acids that, depending on the source of synthesis, can be processed into several different peptides, each with distinct biological functions.

REVIEW QUESTIONS

1. A 32-year-old woman is being examined by her physician with complaints of fatigue, muscle weakness, weight gain, and constipation. A decrease in which of the following would allow her physician to differentiate a diagnosis of primary from secondary hypothyroidism?

(A) Reverse triiodothyronine (rT3)
(B) Thyroglobulin
(C) Thyroid-stimulating hormone
(D) Thyroxine (T4)
(E) Triiodothyronine (T3)

2. A 51-year-old woman comes to the physician because of losing weight despite being continuously hungry and eating more than usual. She also reports that she is experiencing irritability, insomnia, diarrhea, muscle weakness, heart palpitations, and intolerance to heat. Which of the following receptor types is most likely to be stimulated in this patient?

(A) G-protein coupled
(B) Guanylate cyclase
(C) Protein phosphatase
(D) Serine/threonine kinase
(E) Tyrosine kinase

3. A 59-year-old postmenopausal woman is being examined by her physician with the primary complaint that she no longer has the ability to stand erect without pain. History reveals that she recently suffered a minor fracture of her ulna by bumping into the door frame entering her bathroom. An X-ray of her spine demonstrates vertebral thinning. Which of the following hormones would be the most useful in attempting to treat this patient's condition?

(A) Adrenocorticotropic hormone (ACTH)
(B) Calcitriol
(C) Growth hormone
(D) Parathyroid hormone
(E) Thyroid hormone

4. A 31-year-old man is being examined to ascertain the sudden onset of his severe hypertension. The patient reports that he has not consumed any alcohol, nor does he uses any medications or illegal drugs. Analysis of serum electrolytes indicates a reduced level of potassium and elevated levels of sodium and chloride. The patient's physician suspects that he is experiencing a disruption in the normal physiological responses to vascular volume. If this diagnosis is correct, which of the following could most likely be the cause of the patients' condition?

(A) Cushing syndrome
(B) Graves' disease
(C) Hyperparathyroidism
(D) Posterior pituitary adenoma
(E) Renal glomerular carcinoma

5. Experiments are being conducted on renal function in laboratory animals with the use of synthetic peptides. When one of the peptides is administered to the animals the level of urine sodium increases significantly. The effects of this peptide most closely mimics which of the following?

(A) Angiotensin II
(B) Atrial natriuretic peptide
(C) Oxytocin

(D) Prolactin
(E) Renin

6. A 59-year-old postmenopausal woman is being examined by her physician with the primary complaint that she no longer has the ability to stand erect without pain. History reveals that she recently suffered a minor fracture of her ulna by bumping into the door frame entering her bathroom. An X-ray of her spine demonstrates vertebral thinning. Aside from pharmacologic parathyroid hormone therapy, which of the following would be most useful in treating this woman's condition?
(A) Adrenocorticotropic hormone (ACTH)
(B) Calcitonin
(C) Corticotropic-releasing hormone
(D) Growth hormone
(E) Thyroid-stimulating hormone

7. A 29-year-old woman is being examined by her physician during a routine annual physical examination. History includes no personal or family history of disease. The patient does not take any prescription medications. Physical examination shows her blood pressure to be 164/112. Blood chemistry shows potassium of 2.4 mM (N = 3.6–5.2 mM) and bicarbonate of 31 mM (N = 19–25 mM). Additional laboratory studies find the level of epinephrine is normal whereas renin and aldosterone levels are above normal. Which of the following would most likely explain the observations in this patient?
(A) Activated epithelial Na^+ channels in the kidney
(B) Adrenocorticotropic hormone-secreting neoplasm
(C) Aldosterone-secreting adenoma
(D) 21-Hydroxylase deficiency
(E) Renin-secreting neoplasm

8. A 23-year-old woman is being examined in a fertility clinic to try to ascertain if she is the reason she and her husband have been unable to conceive a child. Ultrasonic examination of her abdomen finds her ovaries are smaller than normal and they contain poorly developed follicles. A deficiency in which of the following would most likely explain these findings?
(A) Corticotropin-releasing hormone
(B) Follicle-stimulating hormone
(C) Gonadotropin-releasing hormone
(D) Growth hormone
(E) Luteinizing hormone-releasing hormone

9. A 42-year-old woman is being examined by her physician with complaints of extreme thirst. She gets the greatest relief from consuming large quantities of ice water or by sucking on ice cubes. She reports that she also must frequently urinate. Suspecting her patient has developed diabetes mellitus, a urine glucose test is performed but this finds no abnormal level of the sugar. However, it is found that the patient has significantly dilute urine. Which of the following is most likely to be observed in this patient given these findings?
(A) Adrenocorticotropic hormone (ACTH) excess
(B) Cortisol deficiency
(C) Oxytocin excess
(D) Renin deficiency
(E) Thyroid-stimulating hormone excess
(F) Vasopressin deficiency

10. Clinical trials are being performed to ascertain the efficacy of a novel compound in the suppression of appetite. If these trials are successful, it is most likely that the compound is inhibiting the activity of which of the following?
(A) Adiponectin
(B) Cholecystokinin
(C) Ghrelin
(D) Glucagon-like peptide 1 (GLP-1)
(E) Peptide tyrosine tyrosine (PYY)

11. A 44-year-old man is being examined by his physician as he is concerned about the yellowish color of his eyes. Physical examination shows his blood pressure to be 90/58 and the presence of icteric sclera. Blood tests shout elevations in both AST and ALT. Given the signs in this patient, an imbalance in the levels of which of the following is most likely to be found?
(A) Adrenocorticotropic hormone (ACTH)
(B) Aldosterone
(C) Angiotensin II
(D) Corticotropin releasing hormone (CRH)
(E) Cortisol

12. Experiments are being conducted on several novel compounds to determine their effects on the cardiovascular system. One of the compounds is structurally related to enalapril. If this compound is administered to humans, the levels of which of the following would most likely be affected?
(A) Adrenocorticotropic hormone (ACTH)
(B) Aldosterone
(C) Corticotrophin-releasing hormone (CRH)
(D) Follicle-stimulating hormone (FSH)
(E) Renin

13. Laser ablation experiments are being carried out in laboratory animals to ascertain the effects, on feeding behaviors, of damage to certain regions of the hypothalamus. In one series of experiments, it is found that loss of the targeted region causes the animals to eat nearly continuously, no matter the time of day, nor the composition of the chow. Ablation of which of the following structures is most likely to have occurred?
(A) Lateral hypothalamic area
(B) Paraventricular nucleus
(C) Posterior nucleus
(D) Suprachiasmatic nucleus
(E) Ventromedial nucleus

14. Experiments are being conducted on the effects of synthetic peptides on the feeding behaviors of laboratory mice. Following the administration of one of the peptides it is observed that the mice eat continuously regardless of the light-dark cycle. This synthetic peptide is most likely mimicking the effects of which of the following?
(A) Cholecystokinin
(B) Ghrelin
(C) α-Melanocyte stimulating hormone, α-MSH
(D) Peptide tyrosine tyrosine, PYY
(E) Thyroid-stimulating hormone

15. A 34-year-old man is being examined by his physician with the chief complaint being frequent nausea and indigestion. In addition, the patient reports that he has a constant sensation of fullness and bloating, and a sour taste in his mouth. The patient's physician suspects he is experiencing functional dyspepsia and orders tests to confirm his preliminary diagnosis. Which of the following is most likely contributing to this patient's symptoms?
(A) Cholecystokinin
(B) Gastrin
(C) Glucagon-like peptide 1

(D) Secretin
(E) Vasoactive intestinal polypeptide

16. A 63-year-old man is being examined in the emergency department following a 24-hour bout of severe diarrhea. Physical examination shows respirations of 30 per minute, heart rate of 120 beats per minute, and a temperature of 39°C. Cultures of blood, cerebrospinal fluid, urine, and stool are all negative for pathogens. Analysis of the patients' blood finds levels of vasoactive intestinal peptide that are three times higher than normal. Which of the following would be most useful to intervene in the consequences of the patient's hormonal imbalance?
(A) Cholecystokinin
(B) Histamine
(C) Glucagon-like peptide 1
(D) Pancreatic polypeptide
(E) Somatostatin

17. A 19-year-old man is being examined by his physician due to concerns about his inability to obtain an erection and by the increased fatty infiltration of his chest giving him the appearance of having breasts. Overproduction of which of the following is most likely responsible for this patient's symptoms?
(A) Corticotropin-releasing hormone
(B) Follicle-stimulating hormone
(C) Gonadotropin-releasing hormone
(D) Growth hormone
(E) Melanocyte-stimulating hormone
(F) Prolactin

18. A 29-year-old man has experienced a gradual change in his physical appearance that includes enlargement of his tongue, protrusion of his jaw, enlargement of his hands and feet, and a bulging of his chest. These physical changes are most likely the result of the excessive production of which of the following?
(A) Adrenocorticotropic hormone (ACTH)
(B) Corticotropin-releasing hormone
(C) Follicle-stimulating hormone
(D) Gonadotropin-releasing hormone
(E) Growth hormone
(F) Triiodothyronine (T3)

19. A 41-year-old man is being examined by his physician with complaints of chronic headaches, fatigue, tingling in his fingers and toes, and heart palpitations. Blood chemistry shows potassium of 2.4 mM (N = 3.6–5.2 mM) and bicarbonate of 31 mM (N = 19–25 mM). X-rays discover a mass on his right adrenal gland. Which of the following is most likely decreased in this patient?
(A) Aldosterone
(B) Angiotensinogen
(C) Calcitriol
(D) Cortisol
(E) Renin

20. A 47-year-old man is being examined in the emergency department for extreme abdominal pain. Ultrasonic examination finds that his pancreas is enlarged and there are numerous clearly visible lobular structures. Biopsy of the tissue finds that the tumors are derived from α-cell islets. Given these findings, which of the following would most likely be expected in this patient?
(A) Decreased (<6%) hemoglobin A_{1c}
(B) Decreased insulin production
(C) Hyperglycemia
(D) Hypoglycemia
(E) Increased serum amylin
(F) Increased serum somatostatin

21. A 29-year-old man has experienced a gradual change in his physical appearance that includes enlargement of his tongue, protrusion of his jaw, enlargement of his hands and feet, and a bulging of his chest. Given the symptoms in this patient, which of the following would provide the greatest therapeutic benefit?
(A) Follicle-stimulating hormone
(B) Growth hormone-releasing hormone
(C) Insulin
(D) Somatostatin
(E) Triiodothyronine (T3)

22. Experiments are being carried out with a novel compound to test its efficacy in the treatment of obesity. When this compound is administered to laboratory animals, it is discovered that the level of glucose metabolism in the hypothalamus is dramatically reduced. Based upon this observation, hypothalamic release of which of the following is most likely to be elevated?
(A) Agouti-related peptide, AgRP
(B) Cocaine- and amphetamine-regulated transcript, CART
(C) Galanin
(D) Melanin concentrating hormone, MCH
(E) Neuropeptide Y, NPY

23. A 48-year-old woman is being examined by her physician with the primary complaint of thinning hair and unexplained weight loss. She states that the weight loss has occurred even though she has not significantly changed her dietary habits. When questioned, she indicates that she frequently feels overly warm and sweaty and that she has trouble sleeping. Physical examination shows an otherwise healthy female with warm smooth skin and a mild resting tremor in both hands. Her physician orders blood tests to be performed. Given the signs and symptoms in this patient, which of the following would most likely be detected in the blood tests?
(A) Autoantibodies to thyroid-stimulating hormone (TSH)
(B) Autoantibodies to thyroid peroxidase
(C) Elevated thyroid-stimulating hormone (TSH) level
(D) Significantly reduced levels of thyroxine
(E) Thyroid-stimulating hormone (TSH) receptor stimulating immunoglobulins

24. A 46-year-old man is brought to the Emergency Department by his wife because of the onset of swelling in his tongue, lips, and face that began within the past 2 hours. The patient states that he does not have chest pain or heart palpitations, does not have any abdominal pain, and is not experiencing nausea or vomiting. He does indicate that he has had a dry, unproductive cough for the past week. History reveals that the patient has been treated for hypertension and type 2 diabetes for the past year. He states that he cannot recall the names of his medications, but he does recall that his physician changed his blood pressure medication 2 weeks ago. The attending physician suspects that the patient is experiencing adverse side effects to one of his medications. Which of the following is the most likely type of medication responsible for the patient's symptoms?
(A) Angiotensin converting enzyme (ACE) inhibitor
(B) Angiotensin II receptor blocker

(C) Beta blocker
(D) Calcium channel blocker
(E) Diuretic

25. A 42-year-old man is being examined by his physician because he is concerned about his weight loss, fatigue, and agitation that has begun to manifest over the past 6 months. Physical examination finds cutaneous and mucosal hyperpigmentation. His blood pressure is 92/60 mm Hg, pulse is 80 beats per minute, and respirations are 14 per minute. The physician suspects his patient is suffering the consequences of a specific disorder and orders a series of tests to confirm her diagnosis. Which of the following is most likely to be found as a result of the tests that were ordered?
(A) Low ACTH, high cortisol, high potassium, high sodium
(B) Low ACTH, high cortisol, high potassium, low sodium
(C) Low ACTH, low cortisol, low potassium, high sodium
(D) High ACTH, high cortisol, high potassium, high sodium
(E) High ACTH, low cortisol, high potassium, low sodium
(F) High ACTH, low cortisol, low potassium, low sodium

ANSWERS

1. Correct answer is **C.** Primary hypothyroidism refers to the loss of thyroid hormone production resulting from defects or disease of the thyroid gland itself. Secondary hypothyroidism refers to the loss of thyroid hormone production resulting from an insufficient stimulation of the thyroid gland, most commonly due to lack of thyroid-stimulating hormone (TSH) production from the anterior pituitary gland. Carrying out an assay for the level of plasma TSH is, therefore the preferred means to assess whether a patient is experiencing the symptoms of a primary or secondary hypothyroidism where a high level of TSH is indicative of primary hypothyroidism and normal or low level of TSH would be indicative of secondary hypothyroidism. Reverse triiodothyronine (choice A) is a metabolite of thyroxine (T4) and, therefore it would be low in both primary and secondary hypothyroidism. Measurement for levels of thyroglobulin (choice B) can be inconclusive if the thyroid pathology causing hypothyroidism is also associated with autoantibodies to thyroglobulin. The levels of thyroxine, T4 (choice D) and triiodothyronine, T3 (choice E) would be low in both primary and secondary hypothyroidism.

2. Correct answer is **A.** The patient is most likely experiencing the symptoms of Graves disease. Graves disease is a form of hyperthyroidism with a diffuse goiter. Specifically, Graves disease is associated with thyrotoxicosis which is defined as a state of thyroid hormone excess but is not synonymous with hyperthyroidism (result of excessive thyroid function). Graves disease is an autoimmune disease caused by autoantibodies to the thyroid-stimulating hormone (TSH) receptor, TSHR. These antibodies (identified as TSI:TSHR-stimulating immunoglobulins) bind to the TSHR on thyroid follicular cells and mimic the receptor activation actions of thyroid-stimulating hormone, TSH. The consequences of this hyperactivation of the thyroid are stimulated follicular cell growth resulting in diffuse thyroid enlargement and increased production of thyroid hormones. The TSHR is a member of the G-protein–coupled receptor (GPCR) family of receptors. Graves disease is the most common autoimmune disease, affecting 0.5% of the population in the United States, and represents 50–80% of cases of hyperthyroidism. The disorder occurs more commonly in women, smokers, and patients with other autoimmune diseases. None of the other receptor types (choices B, C, D, and E) represent the TSH receptor.

3. Correct answer is **D.** Parathyroid hormone (PTH) exerts both catabolic and anabolic effects in bone which are dependent upon the type of bone and the specific cell types responding to PTH binding its receptor. PTH stimulates osteoclast formation by binding to its receptor on stromal/osteoblastic cells and stimulating the production of Receptor Activator of NFKappaB Ligand (RANKL) and inhibiting the expression of RANKL decoy receptor, osteoprotegerin (OPG). PTH binds to PTH1R on cells of the osteoblastic lineage including osteoprogenitor cells, lining cells, immature osteoblasts, mature osteoblasts, and osteocytes. The binding of PTH stimulates a variety of factors resulting in increased proliferation of mesenchymal stem cells, such that these cells are committed into the osteoblast lineage. In addition, the actions of PTH result in enhanced osteoblast differentiation leading to new bone matrix production and ultimately mineralization of bone tissue. Osteoblastic cells also produce RANKL whose function is to stimulate osteoclast production and function. Osteoblasts also produce the soluble RANKL decoy receptor, osteoprotegerin (OPG). PTH enhances production of RANKL and inhibits production of OPG leading to increased osteoclastic bone resorption. Bone resorption leads to the release of Ca^{2+} and P_i as a result of the degradation of hydroxyapatite, the major mineral component of bone. The actions of PTH can result in the stimulation of bone turnover leading to either a net increase in bone formation or a net increase in bone resorption. The primary function of PTH is to respond to reduced circulating Ca^{2+} levels and to stimulate resorption of bone Ca^{2+}. However, recombinant PTH (rPTH) has proven to be of significant benefit in the treatment of osteoporosis. Although PTH increases bone resorption it also increases the formation of new bone which is the more pronounced response to rPTH. Intermittent infusion of rPTH results in new bone formation and has shown efficacy in the treatment of the bone loss associated with osteoporosis. This PTH-induced phenomenon occurs as a result of the laying down of protein matrix and mineralization that occurs not only in the previous existing matrix, but in the new matrix that is formed. Patients receiving rPTH show an increase in bone density as well as a decrease in fractures when compared to other forms of treatment. Whereas continuous elevation of PTH levels, as occurs in humans due to abnormal secretion from the parathyroid glands, results in loss of bone mass leading to osteoporosis, intermittent elevation of PTH that occurs with the daily injections of rPTH has the opposite effect of building bone. Administration of none of the other hormones (choices A, B, C, and E) will provide significant utility in the treatment of osteoporosis.

4. Correct answer is **E.** The patient is most likely experiencing the symptoms caused by cancer of the kidney which is affecting the intra-renal baroreceptor system. This system is a key mechanism for regulating renin secretion. A drop in blood pressure results in the release of renin from juxtaglomerular cells (JG cells; also called granular cells) which are specialized smooth muscle cells in the wall of the afferent arterioles at the base of the glomerulus in the juxtaglomerular apparatus. These are the only cells in the human body that synthesize and secrete renin. The renin-angiotensin system (RAS; also commonly called the renin-angiotensin-aldosterone system, RAAS) is responsible for regulation of blood pressure. Bioactive angiotensin (angiotensin II) is derived from the precursor protein, angiotensinogen, predominantly produced by the liver. Renin is a protease/hormone produced by the kidneys whose sole enzymatic function is to cleave a 10-amino acid peptide from the N-terminal end of angiotensinogen generating angiotensin I. Angiotensin I is then cleaved by the action of angiotensin-converting enzyme (ACE) generating the bioactive octapeptide hormone, angiotensin II. Angiotensin II is one of the most potent naturally occurring vasoconstrictors. In addition to its effects on the vasculature, angiotensin II acts on the kidneys to increase renal tubular Na^+ and Cl^- reabsorption, water retention, and K^+ excretion, on the posterior pituitary to induce the release of vasopressin, stimulates the zona glomerulosa cells of the adrenal cortex to secrete aldosterone, and exerts effects in the central nervous system resulting in increased sympathetic outflow from the rostral ventrolateral medulla of the brain stem. The consequences of a renal glomerular carcinoma are elevated and unregulated release of renin resulting in the sudden onset of severe hypertension evident in this patient. None of the other disorders (choices A, B, C, and D) would be associated with sudden onset of severe hypertension.

5. Correct answer is **B.** Natriuresis refers to enhanced urinary excretion of sodium. This can occur in response to specific hormonal signals, in certain disease states, and through the action of diuretic drugs. At least three peptides of the natriuretic hormone family have been identified. Atrial natriuretic peptide (ANP: also called atrial natriuretic factor, ANF) was the first cardiac natriuretic hormone identified. This hormone is secreted by cardiac myocytes when sodium chloride intake is increased and when the volume of the extracellular fluid expands. Specifically, ANP is released from cardiomyocytes in the wall of the right atrium of the heart in response to increased venous volume returning to the heart via the inferior and superior vena cava. The action of ANP is to cause natriuresis via several distinct mechanisms. ANP induces relaxation of the mesangial cells of the glomeruli increasing the surface area of these cells so that filtration is increased. ANP also acts on renal tubule cells to increase sodium excretion. The increased sodium excretion mediated by ANP results from its inhibition of the basolateral membrane localized Na^+/K^+-ATPase throughout the nephron, reduced activity of the apical membrane localized Na^+/H^+ antiporter 3 (NHE3; encoded by the *SLC9A3* gene) in the proximal tubule, and decreasing Na^+-K^+-$2Cl^-$ cotransporter 1 (NKCC1; encoded by the *SLC12A2* gene) activity and renal concentration efficiency in the thick ascending limb (TAL) of the loop of Henle. In the medullary collecting duct, ANP reduces sodium reabsorption by inhibiting the epithelial sodium channel (ENaC) and vasopressin-induced water reabsorption. None of the other hormones (choices A, C, D, and E) directly interfere with sodium reabsorption in the kidney.

6. Correct answer is **B.** Calcitonin is a 32-amino acid peptide secreted by C cells of the thyroid gland. Calcitonin is a hypocalcemia-inducing peptide that exerts its effects in numerous species by antagonizing the effects of PTH and strongly inhibiting osteoclast function. In humans, however, the role of calcitonin in calcium homeostasis is of limited physiologic significance. In humans the major benefits of calcitonin are the use of salmon calcitonin in the treatment of osteoporosis and to suppress bone resorption in Paget disease. None of the other hormones (choices A, C, D, and E) would provide significant benefit treatment of osteoporosis.

7. Correct answer is **E.** The patient's hypertension is most likely the result of excessive renin secretion from the kidneys. The renin-angiotensin system (RAS; also commonly called the renin-angiotensin-aldosterone system, RAAS) is responsible for regulation of blood pressure. Bioactive angiotensin (angiotensin II) is derived from the precursor protein, angiotensinogen, predominantly produced by the liver. Renin is a protease/hormone produced by the kidneys whose sole enzymatic function is to cleave a 10-amino acid peptide from the N-terminal end of angiotensinogen generating angiotensin I. Angiotensin I is then cleaved by the action of angiotensin-converting enzyme (ACE) generating the bioactive octapeptide hormone, angiotensin II. Angiotensin II is one of the most potent naturally occurring vasoconstrictors. In addition to its effects on the vasculature, angiotensin II acts on the kidneys to increase renal tubular Na^+ and Cl^- reabsorption, water retention, and K^+ excretion, on the posterior pituitary to induce the release of vasopressin, stimulates the zona glomerulosa cells of the adrenal cortex to secrete aldosterone, and exerts effects in the central nervous system resulting in increased sympathetic outflow from the rostral ventrolateral medulla of the brain stem. The consequences of a renin-secreting neoplasm would be elevated blood pressure and hypokalemia as is evident in this patient. None of the other options (choices A, B, C, and D) would correctly count for the signs and symptoms in this patient.

8. Correct answer is **B.** The patient is most likely experiencing the consequences of deficient follicle-stimulating hormone (FSH) synthesis and release. The anterior pituitary gonadotropins, luteinizing hormone (LH), and FSH are responsible for the development and maturation of ovaries and sperm. In females, FSH stimulates follicular development and estrogen synthesis by granulosa cells of the ovary, whereas LH (choice E) induces thecal cells of the ovary to synthesize estrogens and progesterone and promotes estradiol secretion. The surge in LH release that occurs in mid-menstrual cycle is the responsible signal for ovulation. A deficiency in FSH production would result in poor development and maturation of the ovaries as is evident in this patient. Deficiency in none of the other hormones (choices A, C, and D) would account for the reduced ovarian development and maturation seen in this patient.

9. Correct answer is **F.** The patient is most likely manifesting the signs and symptoms of diabetes insipidus. Diabetes insipidus is a disorder characterized by the production of excessive and dilute urine. There are several causes of diabetes insipidus including disorders affecting hypothalamic vasopressin production (central diabetes insipidus), disturbances in thirst control exerted by the hypothalamus (dipsogenic diabetes insipidus), loss of the effects of vasopressin in the kidney (nephrogenic diabetes insipidus), or gestational diabetes insipidus. The secretion of vasopressin is regulated in the hypothalamus by osmoreceptors which sense water and Na^+ concentration and stimulate increased vasopressin secretion when plasma osmolarity increases. The secreted vasopressin increases the reabsorption rate of water in kidney tubule cells, causing the excretion of urine that is concentrated in Na^+ and thus yielding a net drop in osmolarity of body fluids. Vasopressin deficiency leads to production of large volumes of watery urine and to polydipsia. These symptoms are

diagnostic of diabetes insipidus. Deficiency or excess in none of the other hormones (choices A, B, C, D, and E) would result in diabetes insipidus.

10. Correct Answer is **C.** Numerous factors produced in the gut and in the brain regulate feeding behavior either by increasing the desire to consume food (orexigenic) or by suppressing this desire (anorexigenic). Ghrelin is the only hormone produced in the gastrointestinal system, specifically the stomach, that exerts an orexigenic response in the brain. Ghrelin is produced and secreted by the A (X-like) enteroendocrine cells of the stomach oxyntic (acid secreting) glands. Because the A (X-like) cells express ghrelin they are also sometimes referred to as ghrelin cells or Gr cells. A (X-like) cells express the receptor for gastrin (gut hormone that stimulates gastric acid secretion by the stomach) and, therefore, it is believed that gastrin may directly stimulate ghrelin release. Smaller amounts of ghrelin are released from the small intestine and even less from the colon. The major effect of ghrelin released to the blood is exerted within the central nervous system at the level of the arcuate nucleus (ARC) of the hypothalamus where it stimulates the synthesis and release of the orexigenic neuropeptides, neuropeptide Y (NPY) and agouti-related protein (AgRP). The appetite-inducing effects of ghrelin are, therefore, the result of its stimulation of hypothalamic release of these orexigenic neuropeptides. Adiponectin (choice A) is a hormone secreted by adipose tissue. The major biological actions of adiponectin are increases in insulin sensitivity and fatty acid oxidation, but it does not contribute to changes in feeding behavior. Cholecystokinin, CCK (choice B) is secreted from intestinal enteroendocrine I cells predominantly in the duodenum and jejunum. Within the brain (specifically the median eminence and ventromedial nucleus of the hypothalamus) CCK actions elicit behavioral responses and satiation. Glucagon-like peptide 1, GLP-1 (choice D) is secreted into the blood from intestinal enteroendocrine L-cells that are found predominantly in the distal ileum and proximal colon with some production from these cell types in the duodenum and jejunum. The primary physiologic responses to GLP-1 are glucose-dependent insulin secretion, inhibition of glucagon secretion, and inhibition of gastric acid secretion and gastric emptying. The latter effect will lead to increased satiety with reduced food intake along with a reduced desire to ingest food. Peptide tyrosine tyrosine, PYY (choice E) is produced by, and secreted from, intestinal enteroendocrine L-cells of the ileum and colon. Both CCK and gastrin are involved in the rapid release of PYY in response to eating. The amount of PYY released in response to the ingestion of food is proportional to the caloric intake. The release of PYY results in reduced gut motility and a delay in gastric emptying, both of which contribute to satiety. Within the CNS, PYY exerts its effects on satiety via actions in the hypothalamus, specifically the ARC of the hypothalamus.

11. Correct answer is **C.** The patient is most likely exhibiting the signs and symptoms of liver disease or dysfunction as evidenced by the hyperbilirubinemia-induced jaundice and elevated serum levels of AST and ALT, the so-called liver function enzymes. The liver is a critical organ for synthesis of proteins involved in numerous processes throughout the body. One important protein made by the liver that is involved in the regulation of blood pressure is angiotensinogen, the precursor to angiotensin II. The renin-angiotensin system is responsible for regulation of blood pressure. The intrarenal baroreceptor system is a key mechanism for regulating renin secretion. A drop in pressure results in the release of renin from the juxtaglomerular cells of the kidneys. The only function for renin is to cleave a 10-amino acid peptide from the N-terminal end of angiotensinogen generating angiotensin I. Angiotensin I is then cleaved by angiotensin-converting enzyme yielding angiotensin II. Angiotensinogen is produced by and secreted from hepatocytes. In individuals that have liver disease the pressive actions of angiotensin II are greatly reduced, which would account for the low blood pressure observed in this patient. None of the other hormones (choices A, B, D, and E) are produced by the liver and therefore would not be affected in an individual with liver disease or dysfunction.

12. Correct answer is **B.** Enalapril is an angiotensin converting enzyme (ACE) inhibitor. ACE is responsible for the cleavage of two amino acids from angiotensin I, generating angiotensin II. Angiotensin II is a peptide hormone of the rennin-angiotensin system responsible for regulation of blood pressure. The intra-renal baroreceptor system is a key mechanism for regulating renin secretion. A drop in pressure results in the release of renin from the juxtaglomerular cells of the kidneys. Renin secretion is also regulated by the rate of Na^+ and Cl^- transport across the macula densa. The higher the rate of transport of these ions the lower is the rate of renin secretion. The only function for renin is to cleave a 10-amino acid peptide from the N-terminal end of angiotensinogen yielding angiotensin I. ACE action then generates angiotensin II, one of the most potent naturally occurring vasoconstrictors. In addition to its effects in the vascular, other physiologic responses to angiotensin II include induction of adrenal cortex synthesis and secretion of aldosterone. Release of aldosterone leads to further Na^+ retention by the kidneys with the consequences being an additional pressive effect on the vasculature. Thus, the use of ACE inhibitors would not only reduce the production of angiotensin II but also aldosterone. None of the other hormones (choices A, C, D, and E) would be directly affected in patients taking ACE inhibitors such as enalapril.

13. Correct answer is **E.** The hypothalamus is located below the thalamus and just above the brain stem and is composed of several domains (nuclei) that perform a variety of functions. The primary nuclei of the hypothalamus that are involved in feeding behaviors and satiety (the sensation of being full) include the arcuate nucleus of the hypothalamus (ARC, also abbreviated ARH), the dorsomedial hypothalamic nucleus (DMH or DMN), and the ventromedial hypothalamic nucleus (VMH or VMN). All three of these nuclei are located in the tuberal medial area of the hypothalamus. The ARC is involved in the control of feeding behavior as well as in the secretion of various pituitary-releasing hormones. The DMH is involved in stimulating gastrointestinal activity. The VMH is involved in neural signals that elicit the sensations of satiety. Lesions in the VMH and the DMH of the hypothalamus result in hyperphagia (excessive hunger) and obesity. The lateral hypothalamic area (choice A) is responsible for transmitting orexigenic signals (desire for food intake) and lesions in this region results in starvation. The paraventricular nucleus (choice B) plays essential roles in regulation of neuroendocrine and autonomic functions but is not directly involved in the regulation of feeding behaviors. The posterior nucleus (choice C) functions in the regulation of blood pressure, pupillary dilation, and thermoregulation. Lesions in this region result in hypothermia. The suprachiasmatic nucleus (choice D) is responsible for the regulation of circadian rhythms.

14. Correct answer is **B.** Continued feeding in laboratory animals regardless of light and dark cycles is most likely exerted via the effects of ghrelin. Ghrelin is produced and secreted by the A (X-like) enteroendocrine cells of the stomach oxyntic (acid secreting) glands. Because the A (X-like) cells express ghrelin they are also sometimes referred to as ghrelin cells or Gr cells. A (X-like) cells express the receptor for gastrin (gut hormone that stimulates gastric acid secretion by the stomach) and, therefore, it is believed that gastrin may directly stimulate ghrelin release. Smaller amounts of ghrelin are released from the small intestine and even less from the colon. The major effect of ghrelin released to the blood is exerted within the central nervous system at the level of the arcuate nucleus (ARC) of the hypothalamus where it stimulates the synthesis and release of the orexigenic neuropeptides, neuropeptide Y (NPY) and agouti-related protein (AgRP). The appetite-inducing effects of ghrelin are, therefore, the result of its stimulation of hypothalamic release of these orexigenic neuropeptides. Administration of ghrelin will overcome the normal light-dark cycle-mediated regulation of feeding behavior. Cholecystokinin (choice A), α-melanocyte-stimulating hormone (choice C), and peptide tyrosine tyrosine (choice D) are all appetite-suppressing hormones. Thyroid-stimulating hormone, TSH (choice E) regulates metabolic rate by inducing the thyroid gland to secrete the thyroid hormones, thyroxine (T4) and triiodothyronine (T3). Increased TSH results in decreased food intake.

15. Correct answer is **B.** Functional dyspepsia is a term for recurring signs and symptoms of indigestion that have no obvious cause. Functional dyspepsia is associated with recurrent stomach and epigastric pain and burning sensation, uncomfortable postprandial fullness, and satiety upon consumption of small amounts of food. A potential cause of functional dyspepsia can be abnormal stimulation of gastric acid production of no apparent etiology. Gastrin is produced by enteroendocrine G cells of the gastric antrum and duodenum. Gastrin stimulates the production of gastric acid by binding to the cholecystokinin receptor 2 (CCK2; also called CCKB) on parietal cells. Cholecystokinin (choice A) is released from enteroendocrine I cells predominantly of the duodenum and jejunum in response to fat and protein intake. Cholecystokinin stimulates gallbladder contraction and bile flow and increases secretion of digestive enzymes from the pancreas. Glucagon-like peptide 1, GLP-1 (choice C) is secreted into the blood from intestinal enteroendocrine L-cells that are found predominantly in the distal ileum and proximal colon. The primary physiologic responses to GLP-1 are glucose-dependent insulin secretion, inhibition of glucagon secretion, and inhibition of gastric acid secretion and gastric emptying. The latter effect will lead to increased satiety with reduced food intake along with a reduced desire to ingest food. Secretin (choice D) is released from enteroendocrine S cells of the duodenum and to a lesser extent the jejunum. Secretin stimulates pancreatic bicarbonate secretion and inhibits gastric secretions. Vasoactive intestinal polypeptide (choice E) does stimulate intestinal and pancreatic secretions, but it acts as neurotransmitter in the enteric nervous system and is mainly released by mechanical and neuronal stimulation.

16. Correct answer is **E.** Vasoactive intestinal polypeptide (VIP) is a neurotransmitter expressed in both the peripheral and central nervous systems. In the brain and in the parasympathetic nerves of the digestive tract it also acts as a hormone. VIP has a secretin-like effect on the pancreas. It increases the volume of water and bicarbonate output and affects gastrointestinal blood flow through its vasodilatory effects. All these responses to VIP contribute to severe secretory diarrhea in the case of VIP overproduction. Somatostatin administration would be the most useful in a patient with excessive VIP because it has a broad range of inhibitory effects including inhibition of gastrointestinal secretions, slowing gastrointestinal motility, and reducing splanchnic blood flow. Administration of none of the other hormones (choices A, B, C, and D) would be as effective as somatostatin at countering the consequences of excessive VIP production.

17. Correct answer is **F.** The patient is most likely experiencing the consequences of inappropriate production of prolactin. Prolactin is produced by acidophilic pituitary lactotrophs. Prolactin is the lone trophic hormone of the pituitary that is routinely under negative control by prolactin release-inhibiting hormone (PIH or PIF), which is, in fact, the catecholamine neurotransmitter, dopamine. Decreased hypophyseal dopamine production, or damage to the hypophyseal stalk, leads to rapid up-regulation of PRL secretion. Prolactin secretion increases in females during pregnancy and promotes breast development in preparation for the production of milk and lactation. Endocrine dysfunction leading to excessive prolactin production is associated with breast enlargement and impotence in males. None of the other hormones (choices A, B, C, D, and E), if over produced, would result in fatty infiltration of the chest in males.

18. Correct answer is **E.** The patient is most likely exhibiting the signs and symptoms of acromegaly. Acromegaly is a disorder manifesting in adults as a consequence of the overproduction of growth hormone by the pituitary. Specifically, acromegaly results when there is an excess production of growth hormone after epiphysial closure and cessation of long bone growth. The typical symptoms of acromegaly include enlargement of the face, hands, and feet. Excessive production of none of the other hormones (choices A, B, C, D, and F) would result in the manifestation of the acromegaly apparent in this patient.

19. Correct answer is **E.** The patient is most likely manifesting the symptoms associated with primary aldosteronism. The presence of primary aldosterone excess, as opposed to insufficiency (choice A) is associated with a triad of symptoms that includes hypertension, unexplained hypokalemia, and metabolic alkalosis. The most common cause of primary aldosteronism is an adrenal adenoma. The increased plasma aldosterone concentration leads to increased renal Na^+ reabsorption, which results in plasma volume expansion. The increase in plasma volume suppresses renin release from the juxtaglomerular apparatus and these patients usually have low plasma renin levels. None of the other hormones (choices B, C, and D) would be decreased in a patient with primary aldosteronism.

20. Correct answer is **C.** Tumors of pancreatic α-cell islets are termed glucagonomas. A glucagonoma results in enhanced secretion of glucagon. The metabolic effects of the hyperglucagonemia would be increased hepatic gluconeogenesis and glycogen breakdown and enhanced fatty acid release from adipose tissue. The glucose released from glycogen and the glucose generated by gluconeogenesis would then be transported to the blood resulting in hyperglycemia, not hypoglycemia (choice D). The oxidation of this glucose within the hepatocyte's would be restricted due to glucagon-mediated inhibition of the glycolytic enzyme, phosphofructokinase 1 (PFK1).

The hyperglycemia would result in an increase, not a decrease (choice A) in the level of hemoglobin A_{1c}. Unless the tumor infiltrated and affected pancreatic β-cells and pancreatic δ-cells there would be no change in the production and release of insulin (choice B), amylin (choice E), or somatostatin (choice F).

21. Correct answer is **D.** The patient is most likely exhibiting the signs and symptoms of acromegaly. Acromegaly is a disorder manifesting in adults as a consequence of the overproduction of growth hormone by the pituitary. Specifically, acromegaly results when there is an excess production of growth hormone after epiphysial closure and cessation of long bone growth. The typical symptoms of acromegaly include enlargement of the face, hands, and feet. One treatment option for acromegaly is medication with somatostatin. Somatostatin suppresses the secretion of growth hormone, prolactin, ACTH, cholecystokinin (CCK), gastrin, secretin, glucose-dependent insulinotropic peptide (GIP: also known as gastric inhibitory peptide), vasoactive intestinal peptide (VIP), glucagon, insulin, renin, and aldosterone. Synthetic forms of somatostatin are the drugs of choice in the treatment of acromegaly since they have longer half-lives than the natural somatostatin. Administration of none of the other hormones (choices A, B, C, and E) would result in inhibition of growth hormone secretion and therefore would provide no benefit in the treatment of acromegaly.

22. Correct answer is **E.** Oxidation of different fuel sources within the hypothalamus exerts effects on the synthesis and release of some of the neuropeptides generated in this structure. The activation of neuropeptide Y (NPY) producing neurons in the hypothalamus exhibits fuel source specificity in that oxidation of glucose and fatty acids exert differing effects. Glucose oxidation signals ample energy supply and thus results in reduced NPY expression. On the other hand, fatty acid oxidation has limited, if any, effect on NPY release. Inhibition of glucose oxidation results in dramatically increased NPY release even in the presence of fatty acid metabolism. Thus, a compound that blocks glucose oxidation in the hypothalamus would be expected to result in a significant increase in the level of NPY expression. Decreases in hypothalamic glucose metabolism do not result in increased release of any of the other neuropeptides (choices A, B, C, and D).

23. Correct answer is **E.** The patient is most likely exhibiting the signs and symptoms associated with Graves disease. Graves disease is a form of hyperthyroidism with a diffuse goiter. Specifically, Graves disease is associated with thyrotoxicosis which is defined as a state of thyroid hormone excess but is not synonymous with hyperthyroidism (result of excessive thyroid function). Graves disease is an autoimmune disease caused by autoantibodies to the thyroid-stimulating hormone (TSH) receptor, TSHR. These antibodies (identified as TSHR-stimulating immunoglobulins, TSI) bind to the TSHR on thyroid follicular cells and mimic the receptor activation actions of thyroid-stimulating hormone, TSH. The consequences of this hyperactivation of the thyroid are stimulated follicular cell growth resulting in diffuse thyroid enlargement and increased, not decreased (choice D) production of thyroid hormones, triiodothyronine (T3) and thyroxine (T4). Graves disease is the most common autoimmune disease, affecting 0.5% of the population in the United States, and represents 50–80% of cases of hyperthyroidism. The disorder occurs more commonly in women, smokers, and patients with other autoimmune diseases. Autoantibodies to TSH (choice A) have not been described in humans, but they would lead to hypothyroidism, not hyperthyroidism, such as in Graves disease. Autoantibodies to thyroid peroxidase (choice B), designated TSOAb, are more commonly associated with the autoimmune form of hypothyroidism termed Hashimoto thyroiditis. Although some of the symptoms of Graves disease and Hashimoto thyroiditis are similar, Hashimoto patients gain weight, not lose weight, despite no change in diet or level of exercise and they are intolerant to cold, not heat, as in Graves disease. The excessive thyroid hormone production in Graves disease results from autoantibodies to the TSHR, not to overproduction of thyroid-stimulating hormone, TSH (choice C).

24. Correct answer is **A.** The patient is most likey experiencing the adverse effects of an antihypertensive drug of the angiotensin converting enzyme (ACE) inhibitor family. ACE inhibitors prevent ACE from converting angiotensin I to angiotensin II. All of the drugs that inhibit the activity of ACE contain the suffix "–pril," for example, captopril. One side-effect of the use of ACE inhibitors is a persistent dry cough leading to lack of compliance with the drug in a number of patients. The cause of the dry cough is due to reduced degradation of bradykinin, a known substrate for ACE. Although bradykinin is primarily involved in the contractile activity of vascular smooth muscle, it also induces constriction of the bronchioles in the lungs, and it is this latter activity that contributes to the dry cough with the use of ACE inhibitors. Another consequence of ACE inhibitors leading to increased levels of bradykinin is angioedema that most often affects the face and lips. Bradykinin causes angioedema because it acts as a vasodilator by stimulating nitric oxide production within vascular endothelial cells, subsequently leading to smooth muscle cell relaxation. It is possible for drugs of the angiotensin II receptor blocker (ARB) class (coice B) to cause angioedema but this is much more rare than ACE inhibitor-induced angioedema. None of the other antihypertensive drug classes (choices C, D, and E) are associated with the negative side effect of angioedema.

25. Correct answer is **E.** The patient is most likely manifesting the signs and symptoms of Addison disease, a disease of adrenal insufficiency. Addison disease results from the inability of the adrenal cortex to synthesize and secrete glucocorticoid (primarily cortisol) and mineralocorticoid (primarily aldosterone) hormones resulting in excessive production of the anterior pituitary peptide hormone, ACTH. The hallmark features of Addison disease are asthenia (fatigability and weakness), weight loss, and hyperpigmentation (particularly on sun-exposed skin). Addison disease is also associated with a characteristic sequela of biochemical presentations. These include hyponatremia, hypoglycemia, hyperkalemia, unexplained eosinophilia, and mild prerenal azotemia (accumulation of urea and creatinine in the body). The consequence of adrenal cortical hormone synthesis failure, principally cortisol, is increased secretion of ACTH, not decreased (choices A, B, and C). The high ACTH associated with Addison disease is the result of reduced, not increased (choice E), cortisol production and release. Due to the high ACTH, there is an associated increase, not a decrease (choice F), in serum potassium and a decrease in serum sodium, not an increase (choice D). These changes in serum electrolyte levels are the result of insufficient mineralocorticoid (aldosterone) synthesis.

C H A P T E R

32

Steroid and Thyroid Hormones

High-Yield Terms

Androstanes	Any 19-carbon steroid hormone, such as testosterone or androsterone, that controls the development and maintenance of male secondary sex characteristics
Estranes	Any 18-carbon steroid hormone, such as estradiol and estrone, produced chiefly by the ovaries and responsible for promoting estrus and the development and maintenance of female secondary sex characteristics
Pregnanes	Any 21-carbon steroid hormone, such as progesterone, responsible for changes associated with luteal phase of the menstrual cycle; differentiation factor for mammary glands
Cytochrome P450, CYP	Any of a large number of enzymes produced from the cytochrome P450 genes; are involved in the synthesis and metabolism of various molecules and chemicals
Glucocorticoids	Any of the group of corticosteroids predominantly involved in carbohydrate metabolism
Mineralocorticoids	Steroid hormones characterized by their influence on salt and water balance
Hormone response elements, HREs	Specific nucleotide sequences, residing upstream of steroid target genes, that are bound by steroid hormone receptors

INTRODUCTION TO THE STEROID HORMONES

The steroid hormones are all derived from cholesterol. The conversion of cholesterol to the 18-, 19-, and 21-carbon steroid hormones involves the rate-limiting, irreversible cleavage of a six-carbon residue from cholesterol, producing pregnenolone (C21).

Steroids with 21 carbon atoms are known systematically as pregnanes, whereas those containing 19 and 18 carbon atoms are known as androstanes and estranes, respectively. The high-yield human steroid hormones are listed in Table 32–1 along with the structure of the precursor, pregnenolone.

All the steroid hormones and thyroid hormones exert their actions by binding to intracellular receptors, termed nuclear receptors. Ligand-bound receptors bind to specific nucleotide sequences in the DNA of responsive genes termed hormone response elements, HRE. The interaction of steroid-receptor complexes with the HRE leads to altered rates of transcription of the associated genes.

INTRODUCTION TO THE THYROID HORMONES

The thyroid hormones (called thyronines) are all derived from the amino acid tyrosine within specific follicle cells of the thyroid gland. The primary hormone secreted from the thyroid gland is thyroxine (T4: 3,5,3′5′-tetraiodothyronine). Another hormone secreted from the thyroid, but at much lower levels, is triiodothyronine (T3).

T3 is the most biologically active form of thyroid hormone and exerts its effects by binding to the thyroid hormone receptor (TR). TR is a member of the steroid hormone/thyroid hormone superfamily of nuclear receptors and binds to specific HRE in thyroid hormone target genes.

STEROID HORMONE BIOSYNTHESIS

Many of the enzymes of steroid hormone biosynthesis are members of the cytochrome P450 family of enzymes and they have common, preferred, and official nomenclatures. These enzymes are most correctly identified by the CYP acronym and include the family number, subfamily letter, and polypeptide number. Many of these enzymes are still identified by their historically common names or by the P450 nomenclature which includes a number designating the site of action of the particular enzyme (Table 32–2).

REGULATION OF CYP11A1 ACTIVITIES

The principal rate-limiting step of steroid hormone synthesis is catalyzed by the CYP11A1 enzyme which is also known as desmolase or P450 side-chain cleavage enzyme (P450scc).

TABLE 32–1 Structures of the mammalian steroid hormones.

Structure	Description
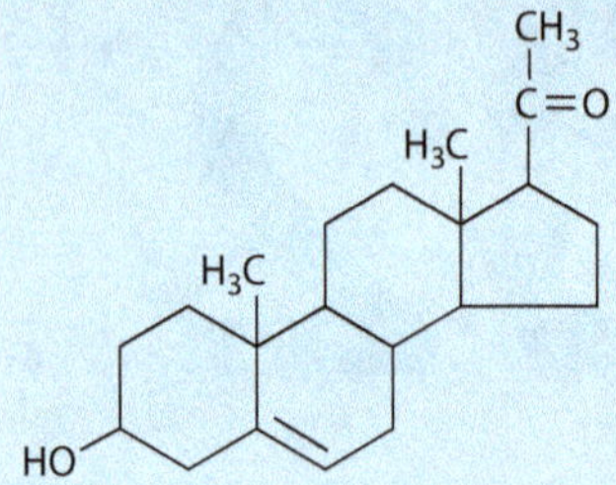	**Pregnenolone:** produced directly from cholesterol, the precursor molecule for all C_{18}, C_{19}, and C_{21}, steroids
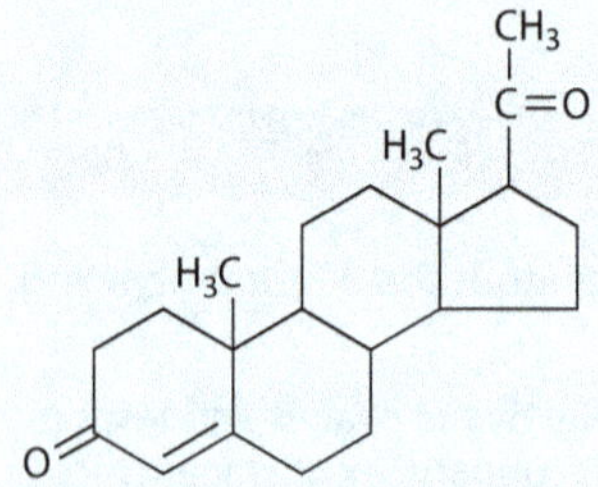	**Progesterone:** a progestogen, produced directly from pregnenolone and secreted from the *corpus luteum*, responsible for changes associated with luteal phase of the menstrual cycle, differentiation factor for mammary glands
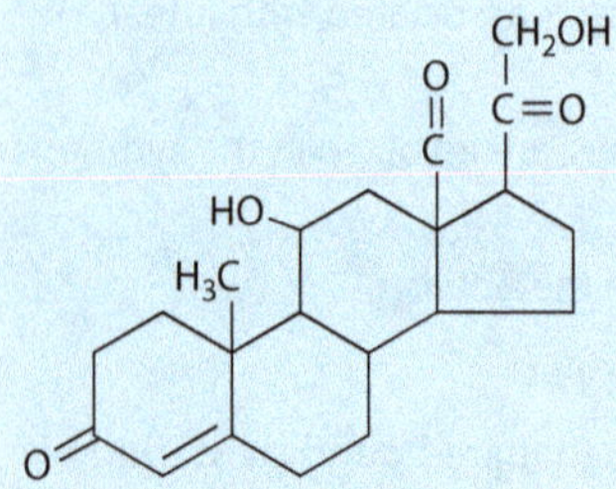	**Aldosterone:** the principal mineralocorticoid, produced from progesterone in the *zona glomerulosa* of adrenal cortex, raises blood pressure and fluid volume, increases Na^+ uptake
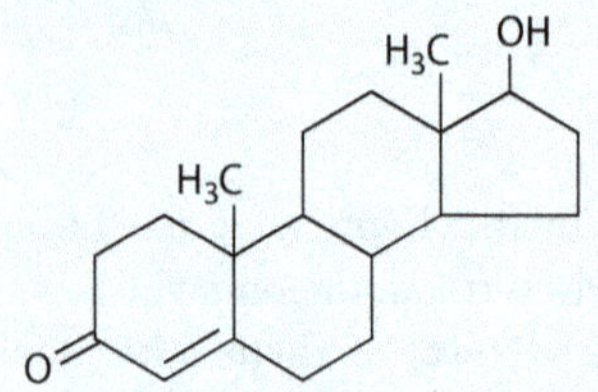	**Testosterone:** an androgen, male sex hormone synthesized in the testes, responsible for secondary male sex characteristics, produced from progesterone
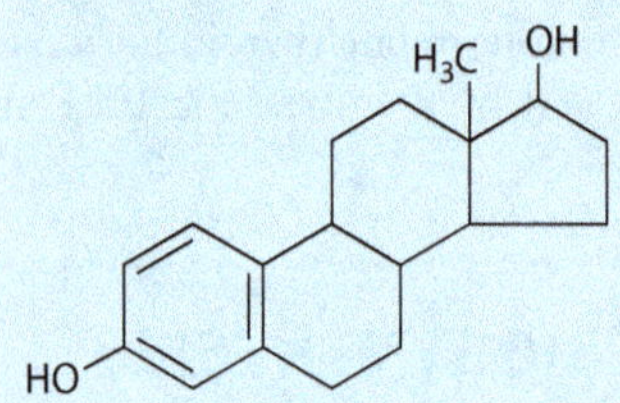	**Estradiol:** an estrogen, principal female sex hormone, produced in the ovary, responsible for secondary female sex characteristics
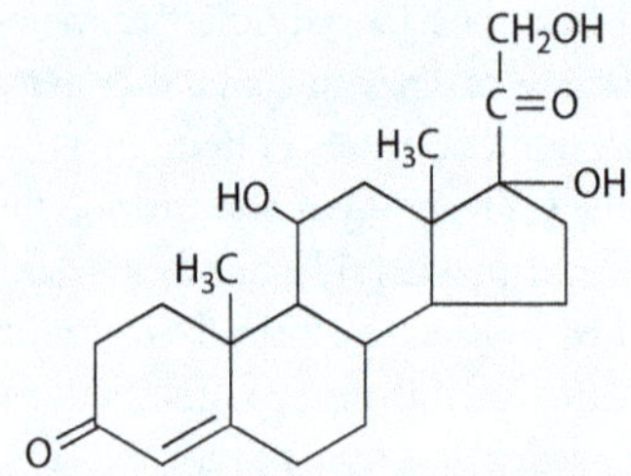	**Cortisol:** dominant glucocorticoid in humans, synthesized from progesterone in the *zona fasciculata* of the adrenal cortex, involved in stress adaptation, increases gluconeogenesis in liver, elevates blood pressure, increases Na^+ uptake by the kidney, numerous effects on the immune system

Reproduced with permission from King MW: *Integrative Medical Biochemistry Examination and Board Review*. New York, NY: McGraw Hill; 2014.

TABLE 32–2 Primary activities required for steroid hormone synthesis.

Common Name(s)	Gene	Activities	Primary Site of Expression
Steroidogenic acute regulatory protein (StAR)	*STAR*	Mediates transport of cholesterol from outer mitochondrial membrane to the inner membrane; transport process represents the rate-limiting step in steroidogenesis	All steroidogenic tissues except placenta and brain
Desmolase, P450ssc	*CYP11A1*	Cholesterol-20,23-desmolase; functions in complex consisting of CYP11A1, ferredoxin reductase (also known as adrenodoxin reductase) and ferredoxin 1 (also known as adrenodoxin); catalyzes the committed and regulated step in steroid biosynthesis	Steroidogenic tissues
3β-Hydroxysteroid dehydrogenase type 1	*HSD3B1*	3β-Hydroxysteroid dehydrogenase	Placental for progesterone synthesis; dual-function enzyme; approved name is hydroxy-delta-5-steroid dehydrogenase, 3 beta- and steroid delta-isomerase 1
3β-Hydroxysteroid dehydrogenase type 2	*HSD3B2*	3β-Hydroxysteroid dehydrogenase; dual-function enzyme; approved name is hydroxy-delta-5-steroid dehydrogenase, 3 beta- and steroid delta-isomerase 2	Steroidogenic tissues
P450c11	*CYP11B1*	11β-Hydroxylase	Only in zona fasciculata and zona reticularis of adrenal cortex
P450c17	*CYP17A1*	Two activities: 17α-hydroxylase and 17,20-lyase	Steroidogenic tissues
P450c21	*CYP21A2*	21-Hydroxylase	Not expressed in the zona reticularis of adrenal cortex
Aldosterone synthase	*CYP11B2*	18α-Hydroxylase	Exclusive to zona glomerulosa of adrenal cortex
Estrogen synthetase	*CYP19A1*	Aromatase	Gonads, brain, adrenals, adipose tissue, bone
17β-Hydroxysteroid dehydrogenase type 3	*HSD17B3*	17-ketoreductase; humans express 18 enzymes of the 17β-hydroxysteroid dehydrogenase type, all of which are members of the short-chain dehydrogenase/reductase (SDR) superfamily; this family of enzymes is involved in several reactions of steroid hormone synthesis including adrenal steroids, and male and female sex hormones	Steroidogenic tissues
Sulfotransferase	*SULT2A1*	Sulfotransferase	Liver, adrenals
5α-Reductase type 3	*SRD5A3*	5α-Reductase; primary enzyme carrying out the testosterone to DHT conversion	Steroidogenic tissues

CYP11A1-mediated cholesterol side-chain cleavage occurs through a series of three interconnected reactions each of which is regulated by cAMP- and PKA-dependent processes. In response to the actions of ACTH in adrenal cortical cells, the level of cAMP rises resulting in stimulated activity of PKA. PKA phosphorylates StAR (Table 32–2) and hormone-sensitive lipase, HSL. The activation of HSL results in the removal of the fatty acid esterification at the C-3 position of cholesterol, thereby increasing the concentrations of free cholesterol. Free cholesterol is the substrate for CYP11A1.

Long-term regulation of steroid synthesis is also controlled via regulated expression of the *CYP11A1* gene. This gene contains a cAMP response element (CRE) that binds the transcription factor identified as cAMP-response element-binding protein (CREB), specifically CREB1. CREB1 is phosphorylated by PKA in the nucleus which allows interaction with the coactivator, CREB-binding protein (CBP), and binding to CRE in target genes such as *CYP11A1*.

STEROIDS OF THE ADRENAL CORTEX

The adrenal cortex is responsible for production of three major classes of steroid hormones (Figure 32–1): glucocorticoids, which regulate carbohydrate metabolism; mineralocorticoids, which regulate the body levels of sodium and potassium; and androgens, whose actions are similar to those of steroids produced by the male gonads (Figure 32–2).

The adrenal cortex is composed of three main tissue regions: zona glomerulosa, zona fasciculata, and zona reticularis. Although the pathway to pregnenolone synthesis is the same in all zones of the cortex, the zones are histologically and enzymatically distinct, with the exact steroid hormone product being dependent on the enzymes present in the cells of each zone.

The primary steroid hormones produced by adrenal cortical zona fasciculata cells are the glucocorticoids, cortisol, and corticosterone.

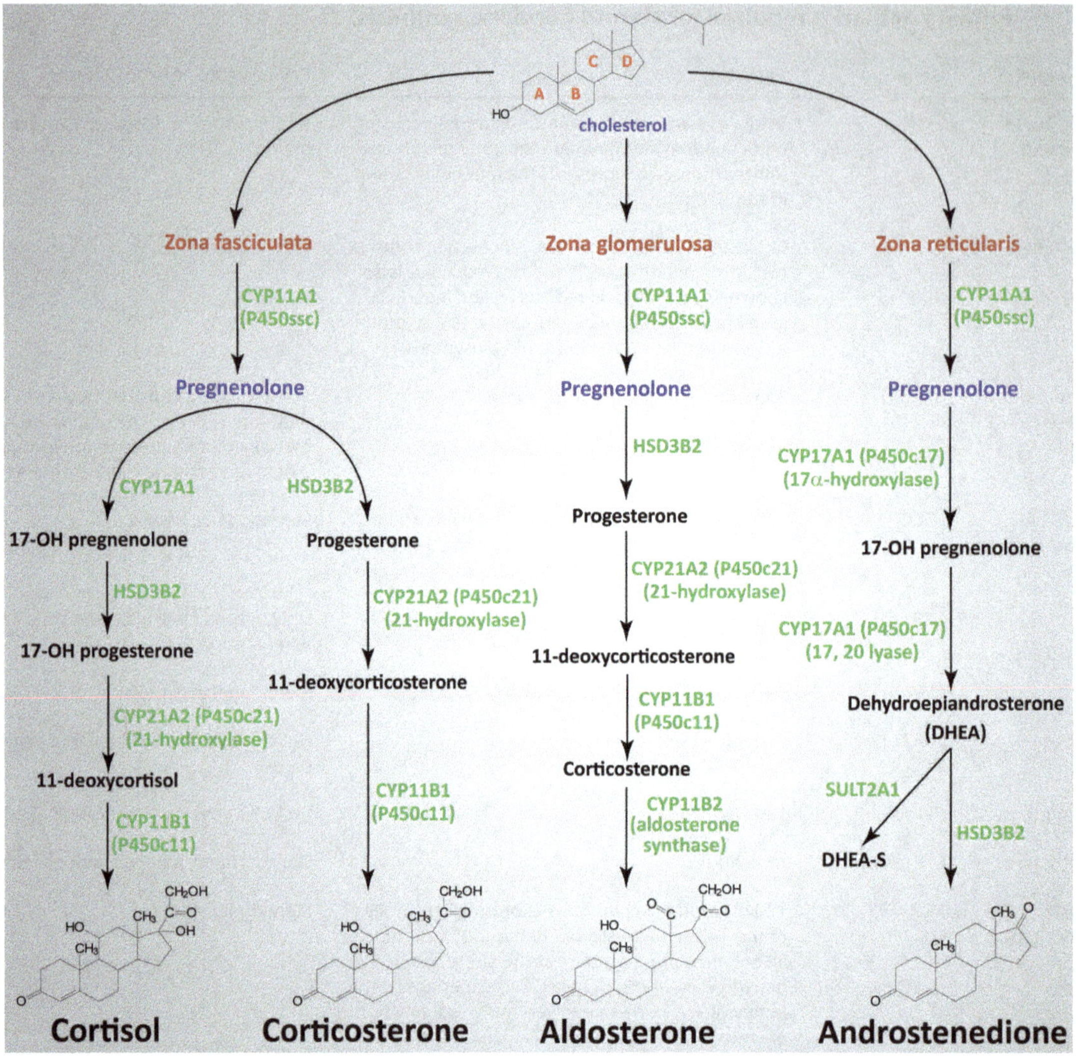

FIGURE 32–1 Synthesis of the various adrenal steroid hormones from cholesterol. Only the terminal hormone structures are included. HSD3B2 is 3β-hydroxysteroid dehydrogenase type 2. The activities of the HSD3B2-encoded enzyme are 3β-dehydrogenase and Δ4,5-isomerase. CYP11B1 is 11β-hydroxylase (also known as P450c11). CYP17A1 (also known as P450c17) is a single microsomal enzyme that has two steroid biosynthetic activities: 17α-hydroxylase which converts pregnenolone to 17-hydroxypregnenolone (17-OH pregnenolone) and 17,20-lyase which converts 17-OH pregnenolone to DHEA (dehydroepiandrosterone). CYP21A2 (also known as P450c21) is 21-hydroxylase. CYP21A2 is sometimes identified as CYP21 or CYP21B. CYP11B2 is aldosterone synthase which is also known as 18α-hydroxylase. SULT2A1 is sulfotransferase. (Reproduced with permission from themedicalbiochemistrypage, LLC.)

The primary steroid hormone produced by adrenal cortical zona glomerulosa cells is the mineralocorticoid, aldosterone. The primary steroid hormones produced by adrenal cortical zona reticularis cells are the androgens, androstenedione, and dehydroepiandrosterone (DHEA). A portion of DHEA is sulfated to DHEA-S via the sulfotransferase encoded by the *SULT2A1* gene.

REGULATION OF ADRENAL STEROID SYNTHESIS

Adrenocorticotropic hormone (ACTH) regulates steroid hormone production in the adrenal cortex, primarily within cells of the zona fasciculata and zona reticularis. ACTH exerts its effects by binding the ACTH receptor which is identified as MC2R for melanocortin-2 receptor. The ACTH receptor is a G_s-type G-protein–coupled GPCR, and ACTH binding triggers activation of adenylate cyclase, elevation of cAMP, and increased PKA. Activation of

HIGH-YIELD CONCEPT

The effect of ACTH on the production of cortisol is particularly important, with the result that a classic feedback loop results in cortisol inhibiting ACTH release from the pituitary. The ACTH-cortisol regulatory loop is required to the regulation of the circulating levels of corticotropin-releasing hormone (CRH), ACTH, and cortisol.

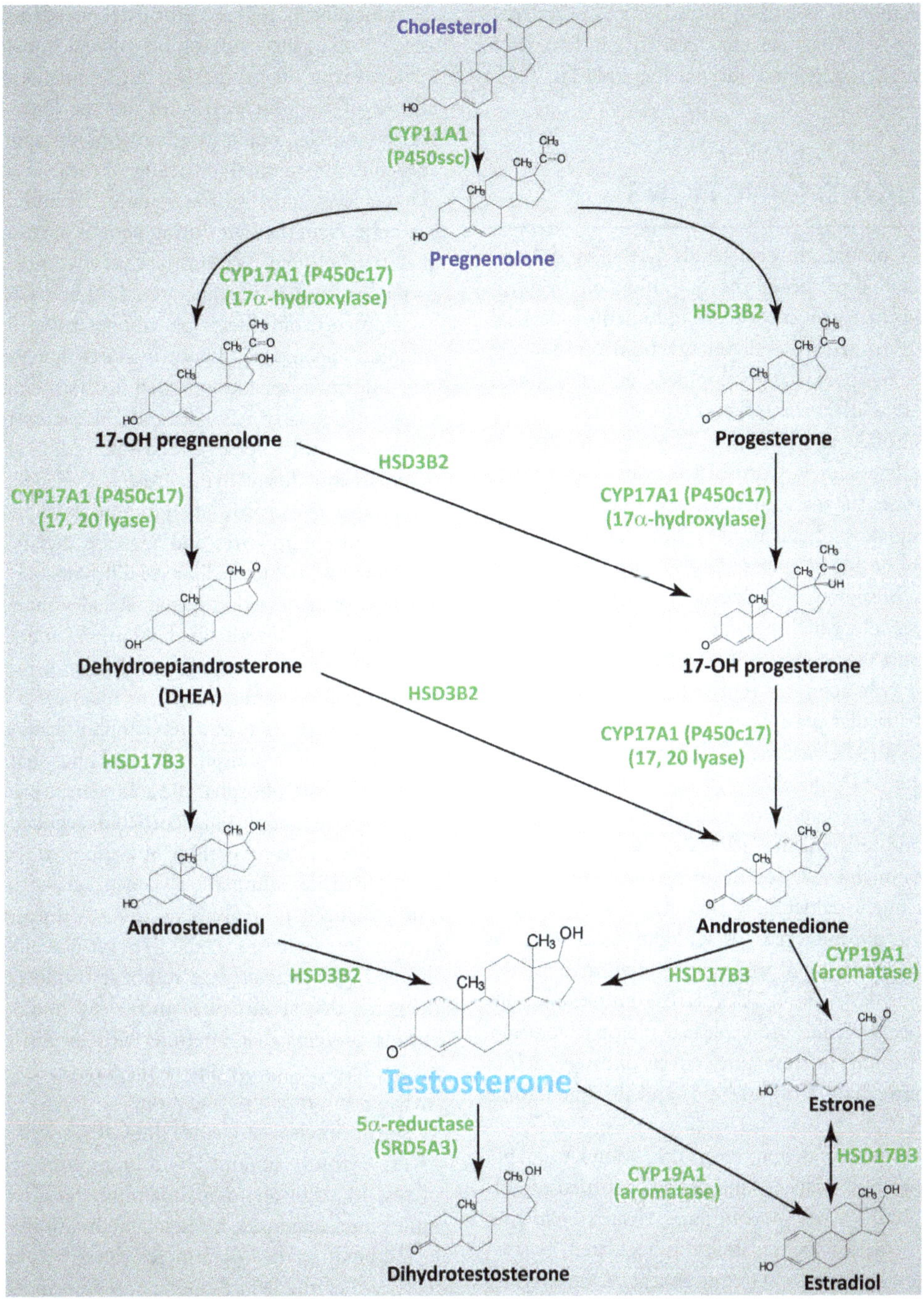

FIGURE 32–2 Synthesis of the male sex hormones in Leydig cells of the testis. CYP11A1, HSD3B2, and CYP17A1 are the same enzymes as those needed for adrenal steroid hormone synthesis (Figure 32–1). CYP19A1 is also referred to as aromatase or estrogen synthetase. HSD17B3 is 17β-hydroxysteroid dehydrogenase type 3 (also called 17-ketoreductase). SRD5A3 is 5α-reductase type 3 (referred to simply as 5α-reductase). (Reproduced with permission from themedicalbiochemistrypage, LLC.)

PKA leads to phosphorylation and activation of hormone-sensitive lipase (HSL) leading to increased concentrations of free cholesterol, the substrate for steroid hormone synthesis.

Aldosterone secretion from the zona glomerulosa is stimulated by angiotensin II, and to a lesser extent angiotensin III (see Chapter 31). The interplay between renin from the kidney and plasma angiotensinogen is important in regulating plasma aldosterone levels, sodium and potassium levels, and ultimately blood pressure. This hormonal regulatory process is referred to as the renin-angiotensin-aldosterone system, RAAS (see Chapter 31).

Although fasciculata and reticularis cells each have the capability of synthesizing androgens and glucocorticoids, the main pathway normally followed is that leading to glucocorticoid production. However, when genetic defects occur in the three enzyme complexes leading to glucocorticoid production, large amounts of the most important androgen, dehydroepiandrosterone (DHEA), are produced. These mutations lead to hirsutism and other masculinizing changes in secondary sex characteristics in females as is seen in several of the congenital adrenal hyperplasias, CAH (see Clinical Box 32–3).

GLUCOCORTICOID FUNCTIONS

The major function of the glucocorticoids is the modulation of carbohydrate metabolism, hence the derivation of the term, glucocorticoid. The primary glucocorticoid in humans is cortisol. Glucocorticoids also regulate overall energy homeostasis, they modulate embryonic and postnatal development, and they modulate stress responses that affect survival and reproduction.

Cortisol inhibits uptake and utilization of glucose resulting in elevations in blood glucose levels. Cortisol acts as an insulin antagonist and also suppresses the release of insulin, both effects leading to reduced glucose uptake and enhanced hepatic gluconeogenesis. The effect of cortisol on blood glucose levels is further enhanced through stimulated breakdown of skeletal muscle protein and adipose tissue triglycerides which provides substrates and energy, respectively, for gluconeogenesis. Cortisol's effects on hepatic gluconeogenesis involve enhancing the transcription of several genes in the pathway in particular phosphoenolpyruvate carboxykinase (PEPCK, encoded by the *PCK1* gene) and glucose-6-phosphatase (G6P, encoded by the *G6PC* gene).

Glucocorticoids also exert inhibitory effects on the inflammatory processes. The anti-inflammatory activity of the glucocorticoids is exerted, in part, through inhibition of phospholipase A_2 (PLA_2) activity with a consequent reduction in the release of arachidonic acid from membrane phospholipids. Arachidonic acid serves as the precursor for the synthesis of various proinflammatory bioactive lipids such as leukotriene B_4 (LTB_4). The immune modulating effects of glucocorticoids are exploited pharmacologically and is the basis for the anti-inflammatory effects of drugs such as prednisone (an intermediate-acting steroid) and dexamethasone (a long-acting steroid).

When released to the circulation, cortisol is bound to a specific glycosylated α-globulin called transcortin (or corticosteroid-binding globulin, CBG) for transport to target tissues. Following uptake into tissues cortisol bioavailability is regulated by two enzymes that function in opposition to one another. One enzyme, 11β-hydroxysteroid dehydrogenase 2 (encoded by the *HSD11B2* gene) oxidizes cortisol to its inactive metabolite, cortisone. The other enzyme, 11β-hydroxysteroid dehydrogenase 1 (encoded by the *HSD11B1* gene) reduces the 11-oxo group (11-oxoreductase activity) in cortisone and 11-dehydrocorticosterone generating the active glucocorticoids, cortisol, and corticosterone.

Once inside the cell, glucocorticoids exert their effects by binding to the glucocorticoid receptor (GR) which is a member of the large nuclear receptor family. The GR-encoding gene (*NR3C1*) is constitutively expressed in virtually every cell type, but tissue-specific expression patterns of the alternative GR isoforms result in tissue-specific transcriptional outcomes. The predominant GR species are identified as GRα (777 amino acids) and GRβ (742 amino acids). It is also important to note that most glucocorticoids bind to the mineralocorticoid receptor (MR encoded by the *NR3C2* gene) as well, and as such, can exhibit mineralocorticoid-like activities.

The major organs that are targets for the metabolic regulatory actions of the glucocorticoids are the liver, adipose tissue, and skeletal muscle. Similar to the role of glucagon in the liver, glucocorticoids are essential to the role of the liver in maintaining blood glucose levels during fasted states. In addition, glucocorticoids exert effects on the liver during periods of stress to ensure adequate glucose is released. Within the liver, two primary target genes for cortisol, as outlined earlier, are *PCK1* and *G6PC*.

Glucocorticoid effects on adipose tissue lipid homeostasis are complex, encompassing both increased lipogenesis through adipocyte differentiation and increased lipolysis. Glucocorticoids increase adipose tissue fatty acid release by increasing the expression of the hormone-sensitive lipase gene (symbol: *LIPE*) and the gene encoding monoglyceride lipase (symbol: *MGLL*). Under normal physiologic conditions, glucocorticoids promote preadipocyte differentiation into mature adipocytes and increase dietary fat intake. During glucocorticoid-induced adipocyte differentiation, a lipolytic transcriptional program is activated and includes numerous genes involved in triglyceride synthesis, lipid transport, and lipid storage. Triglyceride synthesis genes turned on by cortisol include several AGPAT (acylglycerol-3-phosphate acyltransferase) genes that encode enzymes that incorporate a fatty acid into lysophosphatidic acid and the *LPIN1* gene that encodes phosphatidic acid phosphatase that removes the phosphate from phosphatidic acid generating a diglyceride.

In skeletal muscle, glucocorticoids regulate protein and glucose metabolism. During periods of fasting, stress, or during exercise, glucocorticoids stimulate glycogen breakdown and proteolysis. The enhanced proteolysis occurs as a means to provide amino acid carbon skeletons to the liver for gluconeogenesis, a pathway that is highly activated in response to glucocorticoids. Many of the genes that are activated in skeletal muscle by glucocorticoids encode proteins that interfere with insulin signaling in skeletal muscle resulting in the observed decreases in protein synthesis and increases in protein degradation.

In the absence of ligand, the GR (as well as the MR) remains in the cytosol contained within multiprotein chaperone complexes. In addition to maintaining the GR in the cytosol, the multiprotein complex facilitates high-affinity ligand binding. On ligand binding, the GR complex changes its conformation leading to release of the ligand-bound receptor and exposure of the two nuclear localization signals in the GR allowing for rapid transport into the nucleus. Within the nucleus, the ligand-bound GR interacts with HRE in target genes.

MINERALOCORTICOID FUNCTIONS

Mineralocorticoids control the excretion of electrolytes (minerals). The major circulating mineralocorticoid is aldosterone. Aldosterone exerts its primary effects through actions on the kidneys but also functions in the colon and sweat glands. The principal effect of aldosterone is to enhance sodium (Na^+) reabsorption in the connecting tubule (CNT) and cortical collecting duct of the nephrons in the kidneys (see Clinical Box 32–1). Secondary to

CLINICAL BOX 32–1 ADRENAL INSUFFICIENCY AND ADDISON DISEASE

Adrenal insufficiency describes a related group of disorders that are generally divided into two broad categories. Disorders that are due to a primary inability of the adrenal glands to synthesize and secrete hormone constitute the primary adrenal insufficiency syndromes. Disorders of adrenal function that result from inadequate adrenocorticotropic hormone (ACTH) synthesis or release from the anterior pituitary constitute the secondary adrenal insufficiency syndromes. The major primary adrenal insufficiency syndrome is Addison disease. Addison disease was first described by Thomas Addison in 1855. It is now known that Addison disease results from the inability of the adrenal cortex to synthesize and secrete glucocorticoid (primarily cortisol) and mineralocorticoid (primarily aldosterone) hormones. Although most of the early cases were the result of infection with *Mycobacterium tuberculosis*, today the most frequent cause of Addison disease is idiopathic atrophy, most often the result of autoimmune destruction of the cortical tissue of the adrenal glands. Rare instances of Addison disease are associated with adrenoleukodystrophy, tumor metastases, HIV infection, cytomegalovirus (CMV) infection, bilateral hemorrhage, amyloidosis, and sarcoidosis. The consequence of adrenal cortical hormone synthesis failure is increased secretion of ACTH, from anterior pituitary corticotropes, in an effort to stimulate the adrenal glands. In addition, the loss of adrenal cortisol production results in loss of the normal feedback inhibitory loop that cortisol exerts on ACTH secretion. Primary and secondary adrenal insufficiency share many clinical features yet have easily distinguishable differences. The associated increase in ACTH secretion in Addison disease contrasts with secondary adrenal insufficiency which is due to ACTH deficiency. In addition, Addison disease is associated with hyperpigmentation. The hyperpigmentation in Addison disease is related to melanocyte stimulation by ACTH and α-melanocyte-stimulating hormone (α-MSH), where ACTH is the more potent stimulator of melanogenesis. In secondary adrenal insufficiency syndromes, mineralocorticoid synthesis is essentially normal, whereas glucocorticoid synthesis is insufficient. The normal mineralocorticoid synthesis in secondary adrenal insufficiency is due to the fact that it is primarily regulated by salt and water metabolism rather than by ACTH. Without treatment, adrenal insufficiency can be fatal, hence, early recognition is extremely important. The characteristic clinical presentation of acute primary adrenal insufficiency includes an insidious onset of asthenia (fatigability and weakness), cutaneous and mucosal pigmentation, agitation, nausea, vomiting, anorexia, weight loss, orthostatic (postural) hypotension (drop in blood pressure on standing), confusion, circulatory collapse, abdominal pain, and fever. Indeed, one can consider the hallmark features of Addison disease to be asthenia, weight loss, and pigmentation (particularly on sun-exposed skin), as these three symptoms are present in more than 97% of patients. Addison disease is also associated with a characteristic sequelae of biochemical presentations. These include hyponatremia, hypoglycemia, hyperkalemia, unexplained eosinophilia, and mild prerenal azotemia (accumulation of urea and creatinine in the body). The typical history and clinical findings of chronic primary adrenal insufficiency include a protracted history of malaise, fatigue, anorexia, weight loss, joint and back pain, and darkening of the skin. In addition, patients may crave salt and may develop preferences for salty foods and fluids. The hyperpigmentation associated with Addison disease may be homogeneous or blotchy and occurs in all racial and ethnic groups. In addition, isolated darker areas occur at the palmar creases, flexural areas, sites of friction, recent scars, vermilion border of the lips, and genital skin. Mucosal membranes, in particular the buccal, periodontal, and vaginal mucosa may also show patchy macular areas of increased pigmentation. The cutaneous and mucosal pigmentation increases with age and advancement of the symptoms of Addison disease. Autoimmune destruction is the most common cause of primary adrenal insufficiency in industrialized countries and may be the sole cause or, in rare instances, be associated with inherited autoimmune polyglandular syndromes. These latter syndromes tend to present either in childhood (type 1), in association with hypoparathyroidism and mucocutaneous candidiasis, or in adulthood (type 2), in association with insulin-dependent diabetes mellitus, autoimmune thyroid disease, and vitiligo (autoimmune destruction of melanocytes). Suspicion of Addison disease should be high in individuals with AIDS as well as other viral disorders such as CMV necrotizing adrenalitis. On suspicion of Addison disease, biochemical testing is needed to confirm the diagnosis of adrenal insufficiency. As the disease advances, serum sodium, chloride, and bicarbonate levels will be reduced while serum potassium levels will be elevated all of which results from insufficient levels of aldosterone. Aldosterone exerts its primary effects through actions on the kidneys but also functions in the colon and sweat glands. The principal effect of aldosterone is to enhance sodium (Na^+) reabsorption in the connecting tubule (CNT) and cortical collecting duct of the nephrons in the kidneys. Within these regions of the nephron aldosterone induces the expression of the Na^+,K^+-ATPase subunit genes (*ATP1A1* and *ATP1B1*), the genes encoding the subunits (*SCNN1A, SCNN1B,* and *SCNN1C*) of the epithelial sodium channel (ENaC), and the *SLC12A3* gene (encoding the Na^+-Cl^- cotransporter, NCC). The net effect of the induction of these transporter genes, by aldosterone, is enhanced Na^+ reabsorption as a function of the apical membrane localized ENaC and NCC transporters and delivery to the blood via the action of the basolateral membrane localized Na^+,K^+-ATPase. Secondary to the Na^+ uptake is efflux of potassium (K^+) to the tubular lumen. In addition to K^+ excretion, aldosterone enhances the excretion of hydrogen (H^+) ions from the collecting duct. Therefore, the hyponatremia of Addison disease results from both the loss of sodium to the urine and to the movement of sodium into the intracellular compartment. As sodium moves into the cell, fluid depletion in the vasculature ensues which exacerbates the hypotension of Addison disease. The hyperkalemia, primarily due to loss of aldosterone, is also a result of acidosis and impaired glomerular filtration. Plasma levels of cortisol and aldosterone are reduced below normal levels. In addition, neither hormone levels rise in response to administration of ACTH as would be expected in a normal individual. Normal cortisol levels in the hypotensive state, due to the absence of adrenal insufficiency, are expected to be in the range of 18 μg/dL (495 nmol/L) following administration of cosyntropin (250 μg administered IM or IV). In individuals in whom the cosyntropin administration test results in cortisol values greater than 19 μg/dL (524 nmol/L), Addison disease can be excluded as the cause of

CLINICAL BOX 32–1 (CONTINUED)

associated symptomology. Alternatively, if the cortisol level is less than 3 μg/dL (83 nmol/L) it is virtually assured that the patient's symptoms are due to Addison disease. Measurement of free cortisol in the urine is not at all useful in the correct diagnosis of Addison disease. Measurement of plasma ACTH helps to determine if the observed symptoms and biochemical results are due to primary or secondary adrenal insufficiency. With primary insufficiency the values of plasma ACTH will be above the normal range, whereas, in secondary insufficiency the plasma levels will be lower than normal. Identification of hypokalemia in the presence of elevated plasma renin levels signifies a mineralocorticoid deficiency and, therefore, allows for discrimination of primary adrenal insufficiency. All patients with primary adrenal insufficiency should be treated via physiologic replacement of the deficient glucocorticoid and mineralocorticoid hormones. Patients with acute adrenal insufficiency should also receive fluid resuscitation. Administration of hydrocortisone (cortisol) IV (100 mg every 8 h) is the standard treatment protocol for acute treatment of Addison disease. For chronic therapy, oral hydrocortisone (12–15 mg/day) provides adequate glucocorticoid replacement. Administration can be in divided doses during the day to grossly recapitulate the normal diurnal pattern of cortisol secretion. In obese individuals or in patients being treated with anticonvulsants, the dosage of hydrocortisone needs to be increased. Conversely, in patients with type 2 diabetes or who are hypertensive, the hydrocortisone dosage needs to be reduced. Administration of hydrocortisone does not replace the mineralocorticoid component missing in Addison disease. For this deficiency patients take oral fludrocortisone (0.05–0.1 mg/day). In order to prevent excessive sodium loss during this therapy, patients need to take 3–4 g/day of sodium. Also, when patients are experiencing an additional illness, especially accompanied with fever, the dose of hydrocortisone should be doubled. Due to the increased risk for excessive sodium loss, patients are advised to take this increased dosage with a salty broth such as beef or chicken bouillon. Due to the fact that there is no simple way to assess whether the replacement dose of glucocorticoid is correct, clinical evaluation is necessary to identify signs and symptoms of over- or under-replacement. A recurrence of symptoms of adrenal insufficiency clearly suggest that the dose of hydrocortisone is insufficient. These symptoms may be vague, such as malaise, and may be difficult to ascribe solely to glucocorticoid deficiency. Development of Cushing syndrome-like features such as weight gain, hyperglycemia, hypertension, or osteopenia, is indicative of excessive hydrocortisone administration. The dosage of fludrocortisone should be adjusted so that plasma renin activity is normal. Measurement of plasma renin levels should be considered first in patients with continued salt craving or hypotension. If abnormal then adjustment of fludrocortisone dosage, and addition of salt should be considered before the glucocorticoid dose is increased in order to avoid excessive glucocorticoid treatment.

the Na^+ uptake is efflux of potassium (K^+) to the tubular lumen. In addition to K^+ excretion, aldosterone enhances the excretion of hydrogen (H^+) ions from the collecting duct which is a compensating action to counter the accumulation of the positive charge imparted by increased Na^+ reabsorption.

Aldosterone, like all steroid hormones, functions as a ligand activating the transcriptional activity of the mineralocorticoid receptor, MR. The MR is a member of the nuclear receptor superfamily and is encoded by the *NR3C2* gene. In addition to aldosterone, the glucocorticoids, cortisol and corticosterone, bind to and activate the MR. In aldosterone target tissues the expression of the 11β-hydroxysteroid dehydrogenase 2 (*HSD11B2*) gene ensures that cortisol is deactivated by conversion to cortisone and corticosterone is deactivated by conversion to 11-dehydrocorticosterone. Deoxycorticosterone (DOC; 11-deoxycorticosterone) exhibits some mineralocorticoid action but only about 3% of that of aldosterone.

In the absence of ligand, the MR remains in the cytosol contained within multiprotein chaperone complexes. The cytosolic MR-containing complex is highly similar to that of the cytosolic GR complex. On ligand binding, the MR complex changes its conformation leading to release of the ligand-bound receptor and exposure of the two nuclear localization signals in the MR allowing for rapid transport into the nucleus. Within the nucleus, the ligand-bound MR binds to the same type of HRE to which the GR binds.

DEFECTS IN ADRENAL STEROIDOGENESIS

Defective synthesis of the steroid hormones produced by the adrenal cortex can have profound effects on human development and homeostasis. Addison disease (Clinical Box 32–1) represents a disorder characterized by adrenal insufficiency that was first identified in a patient who presented with chronic adrenal insufficiency resulting from progressive lesions of the adrenal glands caused by tuberculosis. In addition to diseases that result from the total absence of adrenocortical function, there are syndromes that result from hypersecretion of adrenocortical hormones. Disorders that manifest with adrenocortical hyperplasia are referred to as Cushing syndrome (Clinical Box 32–2).

The congenital adrenal hyperplasias (CAH) are a group of inherited disorders that result from loss-of-function mutations in one of several genes involved in adrenal steroid hormone synthesis. In the virilizing forms of CAH the mutations result in impairment of cortisol production and the consequent accumulation of steroid intermediates proximal to the defective enzyme. The majority of CAH cases (90–95%) are the result of defects in *CYP21A2* with a frequency of between 1 in 5,000 and 1 in 15,000 (Clinical Box 32–3).

CLINICAL BOX 32–2 CUSHING DISEASE

Hypercortisolemia is the hallmark symptom in both Cushing disease and Cushing syndrome. Cushing syndrome is the disorder first described by Harvey Cushing in 1932 in several patients with adrenocortical hyperplasia that was the result of basophilic adenomas of the anterior pituitary. Cushing described this syndrome as patients with truncal (central) adiposity, hypertension, weakness, fatigability, purplish abdominal striae ("stretch" marks), amenorrhea, edema, glucosuria, osteoporosis, and hirsutism. Some confusion can result given that the current distinction between Cushing syndrome and Cushing disease is that the former is associated with adrenal dysfunction (most usually due to tumors) resulting in excess cortisol production and secretion, whereas the latter results from anterior pituitary dysfunction (mostly due to tumors) resulting in excess ACTH secretion. The excess ACTH overstimulates the adrenal glands resulting, secondarily, in excess cortisol secretion. Sometimes Cushing disease is referred to as ACTH-dependent Cushing syndrome. Considering all cases of hypercortisolemia, 80–85% are caused by pituitary corticotrope adenomas resulting in excess ACTH secretion. The other 10–15% of cases result from unilateral benign and malignant adrenal tumors resulting directly in excessive cortisol secretion. Central obesity was and continues to be the most common finding in Cushing syndrome. This feature is apparent in approximately 95% of adult patients and in 100% of pediatric patients. In addition to truncal adiposity, Cushing syndrome patients exhibit unique fat accumulations over the face and neck giving the classical "moon" facies and "buffalo hump." In addition to the unique patterns of fat deposition, Cushing syndrome patients have thin extremities (spider appearance) that are due to the effects of cortisol on protein disposition in skeletal muscle. Hypertension is observed in at least 80% of Cushing syndrome patients. This associated hypertension is a major contributing factor to cardiovascular morbidity in this disease. The hypertension in Cushing syndrome results from the effects of glucocorticoids on plasma volume, peripheral vascular resistance, and cardiac output. These latter effects of glucocorticoids are due, in part, to the fact that glucocorticoids also bind and activate the mineralocorticoid receptor in addition to the glucocorticoid receptor. Although the hypertension usually improves with surgical removal of the precipitating tumor, patients may still require some form of pharmacologic antihypertensive intervention. This therapy may be required only preoperatively but is required postoperatively as well in some patients. The thiazides and furosemide can worsen the hypokalemia caused by the excess cortisol and, therefore, should be avoided. The renin-angiotensin system is augmented in Cushing syndrome due to the hypercortisolemia and, therefore, ARB (angiotensin II receptor blockers) and ACE (angiotensin-converting-enzyme) inhibitors are the recommended drugs of choice to treat hypertension in these patients. Cushing syndrome patients can manifest with virilization due to the excess cortisol and adrenal androgens. Therefore, women often present with amenorrhea combined with hirsutism, acne, signs of virilization (clitoral enlargement, deepening of the voice, male pattern baldness). Male patients frequently present with diminished libido or impotence associated with subnormal testosterone production. The most common, and recommended, initial tests for Cushing syndrome are urinary free cortisol (UFC) at least two times, late night salivary cortisol, at least two measurements, a 1 mg overnight dexamethasone suppression test (DST), or longer low-dose DST (2 mg/day for 48 h). Sometimes patients will show normal test results but present with distinctive clinical features highly suggestive of Cushing syndrome. In these individuals it is recommended to periodically repeat the tests. The gold standard screening test for determination of Cushing syndrome is to assay for ACTH and cortisol levels following a dose of dexamethasone. In this test, a failure to see ACTH and cortisol secretion be suppressed is highly indicative of Cushing syndrome. The 1 mg dexamethasone test is usually given between 11 pm and midnight (12 am) with cortisol levels being measured between 8 am and 9 am the following morning. Positive cortisol suppression, in this test, is evident if the serum level is less than 1.8 mg/dL in patients with pituitary causes of Cushing syndrome. In patients with adrenal causes of Cushing syndrome, a positive result is evident with cortisol suppression to 5 mg/dL. In patients with underlying psychiatric disorders (depression, anxiety, obsessive-compulsive disorder) and in patients with morbid obesity or in alcoholics, the recommended test is the 2 days, 2 mg/day DST assay. Once hypercortisolemia is diagnosed, its cause needs to be identified. An ACTH level is the next step to further investigate the source of Cushing syndrome. ACTH levels below 5 pg/mL at two separate occasions support the diagnosis of ACTH-independent Cushing disease. If serum ACTH is more than 15 pg/mL the disease is most likely to be ACTH-dependent Cushing syndrome. Surgery is the preferred treatment for both ACTH-dependent and -independent Cushing syndrome. In patients with Cushing disease, the initial treatment is selective pituitary adenomectomy. Postoperative hypocortisolemia is the measure for surgical success and this varies between 70% and 90%. In patients with persistent or recurrent disease it is necessary to carry out transsphenoidal surgery and add radiation therapy. In addition, it is often recommended to include bilateral adrenalectomy as a definitive treatment option that provides immediate control of hypercortisolemia. Although recommended in many cases, this latter surgical approach is not without potential for serious complications in addition to the problem of patient compliance with lifelong glucocorticoid and mineralocorticoid replacement therapy. Patients who undergo bilateral adrenalectomy are at risk for Nelson syndrome. Nelson syndrome is growth of a pituitary corticotrope adenoma which can cause neurologic symptoms due to compression from the mass and can also lead to increased ACTH secretion. Following surgical intervention, Cushing syndrome patients require pharmacologic management that is usually directed at decreasing adrenal steroid secretion. Steroidogenesis inhibitors like metyrapone, ketoconazole aminoglutethimide, and etomidate have been successfully used to lower cortisol level. Metyrapone is effective in controlling in 80% of patients with Cushing disease and adrenal tumor. Adrenal insufficiency is the major unwanted effect. In addition, hirsutism and acne may worsen in patients due to the accumulation of androgenic precursors from metyrapone blockade of cortisol synthesis. Ketaconazole is an oral antimycotic that when taken in larger doses inhibits cortisol synthesis. An advantage to ketaconazole is that adrenal androgen concentrations and serum cholesterol concentrations fall, whereas they rise with metyrapone treatment.

CLINICAL BOX 32-2 (CONTINUED)

Aminoglutethimide blocks adrenal synthesis of cortisol, aldosterone, and androgens, as well as the production of estrogens in extra-glandular tissues. Etomidate, normally used as an anesthetic, is a potent inhibitor of cortisol secretion when administered parenterally at low doses. Mifepristone is a synthetic steroid with high affinity for both the glucocorticoid and the progesterone receptors. Administration of mifepristone leads to inhibition of glucocorticoid receptor activation and, as a result, inhibition of transcriptional activation of cortisol target genes.

CLINICAL BOX 32-3 CONGENITAL ADRENAL HYPERPLASIAS

The congenital adrenal hyperplasias (CAH) are a group of inherited disorders that result from loss-of-function mutations in one of several genes involved in adrenal steroid hormone synthesis. In the virilizing forms of CAH the mutations result in impairment of cortisol production and the consequent accumulation of steroid intermediates proximal to the defective enzyme. In the virilizing forms of CAH there is increased ACTH secretion which leads to elevated synthesis of adrenal androgens. In addition, there is adrenal cortical hyperplasia, the symptom that imparts the name to these disorders. All forms of CAH are inherited in an autosomal recessive manner. There are two common and at least three rare forms of virilizing CAH. The common forms are caused by mutations in either *CYP21A2* (21-hydroxylase, also identified as just CYP21 or CYP21B) or *CYP11B1* (11β-hydroxylase). The majority of CAH cases (90–95%) are the result of defects in *CYP21A2* with a frequency of between 1 in 5,000 and 1 in 10,000. Three rare forms of virilizing CAH result from defects in either 3β-hydroxysteroid dehydrogenase (*HSD3B2*), placental aromatase (*CYP19A1*), or P450-oxidoreductase (POR). The typical signs of virilizing CAH are reflective of the androgen excess as well as the mineralocorticoid and glucocorticoid deficiencies. In general, the degree to which a given mutation results in reduction of enzyme activity is correlated to the level of glucocorticoid and mineralocorticoid deficiency. An additional CAH is caused by mutations that affect either the 17β-hydroxylase, 17,20-lyase or both activities encoded in the *CYP17A1* gene. Unlike the virilizing forms of CAH, in individuals harboring *CYP17A1* mutations that result in severe loss of enzyme activity there is absent sex steroid hormone production accompanied by hypertension resulting from mineralocorticoid excess. The reactions catalyzed by the 21-hydroxylase enzyme, encoded by the *CYP21A2* gene, include the conversion of 17α-hydroxyprogesterone to 11-deoxycortisol and the conversion of progesterone to 11-deoxycorticosterone. The synthesis of 11-deoxycortisol occurs within adrenal cortical cells of the zona fasciculata while synthesis of 11-deoxycorticosterone occurs in adrenal cortical cells of the zona glomerulosa. CAH resulting from deficiencies in the *CYP21A2* gene represent the most commonly occurring forms (>95%) of the disease. The majority of the mutations in *CYP21A2* that result in CAH have been identified and the severity of the disorder can be correlated to specific mutations and the consequent effect of the mutation on enzyme activity. Deficiencies in CYP21A2 result in decreased secretion and plasma concentration of cortisol. The reduced levels of cortisol result in a reduction in the negative feedback exerted by this hormone on the hypothalamic-pituitary axis. The reduced negative feedback leads to increased secretion of corticotropin-releasing hormone (CRH) and ACTH. The resultant high plasma concentrations of ACTH are responsible for the adrenocortical hyperplasia characteristic of this disorder. CAH resulting from CYP21A2 deficiencies is divided into three distinct clinical forms. The most severe enzyme impairment mutations result in the salt-losing form. Females with this form of the disease present at birth due to ambiguity in the external genitalia. Males with the salt-losing form present with acute adrenal crisis shortly after birth or in early infancy. Females who present with no acute adrenal crisis and only mild masculinization of the external genitalia and males who present with virilism early in life are considered to be suffering from the simple virilizing form of CAH. The final clinical form of CAH manifests only in females at puberty or shortly thereafter with symptoms of mild excess androgen development resulting in hirsutism, amenorrhea, and infertility. This form of the disorder is referred to as the attenuated form or the late onset or non-classic form. The 21-hydroxylase gene (*CYP21A2, CYP21, CYP21B*) is located within the class III region of the major histocompatibility complex (MHC) on chromosome 6. There are in fact, two *CYP21* genes within this MHC locus but one of the two is a pseudogene and is identified as CYP21P. Older nomenclature identifies the *CYP21P* gene as the 21-hydroxylase A gene (or *CYP21A1*) and *CYP21A2* as the 21-hydroxylase B gene. All 21-hydroxylase activity is synthesized from the mRNA encoded by the *CYP21A2* gene.

Salt-losing CYP21A2 deficiency: In the salt-losing form of this disorder, the degree of loss of enzyme activity is severe to complete. As a result of the level of enzyme deficiency, the synthesis of cortisol is negligible. Because CYP21A2 is also needed for the synthesis of aldosterone, which is a major hormone involved in Na^+ retention by the kidney, there is excessive salt loss leading to hyponatremic dehydration which can be fatal if not treated. Although there is some aldosterone made, the level of salt loss exceeds the ability of the adrenal cortex to make sufficient aldosterone to compensate. The net result is an acute adrenal crisis. The near complete, or complete, loss in cortisol production results in loss of the normal cortisol-mediated feedback inhibition of the hypothalamic-pituitary (CRH-ACTH) axis. The excess ACTH release from the pituitary leads to maximal adrenal androgen secretion with the result being masculinization of the female genitalia. The first sign of CAH due to CYP21A2 deficiency is, in fact, the ambiguous female genitalia in neonates. The masculinization can be so extreme as to result in the fusion of the labia and the formation of a penile urethra. Diagnosis of the salt-losing form of this disorder is made in females born with masculinized genitalia, who are of normal 46,XX karyotype, with marked elevation in plasma 17α-hydroxyprogesterone and androstenedione, as well as serum chemistry showing hyponatremia, hypochloremia, and hyperkalemic acidosis.

CLINICAL BOX 32–3 (CONTINUED)

Simple virilizing CYP21A2 deficiency: In the simple virilizing form of the disorder, the deficiency in CYP21A2 is not complete or as severe as in the salt-losing form. As a result, the adrenal cortex can compensate for salt loss with increased aldosterone synthesis and release. In addition, although there is increased ACTH release there is near normal plasma cortisol levels and thus, there is no glucocorticoid deficit. However, as in the salt-losing form the CRH-ACTH axis is hyperactive leading to excessive adrenal androgen synthesis with consequent masculinization of the female genitalia.

Attenuated CYP21A2 deficiency: As the name of this form of disease implies, patients with the attenuated form exhibit only mild reductions in CYP21A2 activity. Symptoms associated with this form of the disorder manifest in females at puberty. There are no signs of masculinization of the genitalia in females with this form of the disease. Although females have relatively normal breast development, the androgen excess results in excessive body hair (hirsutism), amenorrhea, and the development of small ovarian cysts.

MALE SEX HORMONES

Synthesis of testosterone and estradiol is under tight biosynthetic control, with short and long negative feedback loops that regulate the secretion of follicle-stimulating hormone (FSH) and luteinizing hormone (LH) by the pituitary and gonadotropin-releasing hormone (GnRH) by the hypothalamus (see Chapter 31). FSH and LH stimulate CYP11A1 activity resulting in sex hormone production.

In males, LH binds to Leydig cells, stimulating production of testosterone (Figure 32–2). Testosterone is secreted to the blood and is also carried to Sertoli cells where the double bond of testosterone is reduced, by the action of steroid 5α-reductase, producing dihydrotestosterone (DHT). Testosterone is also produced by Sertoli cells but in these cells its synthesis is regulated by FSH. Testosterone and DHT are carried in the blood and delivered to target tissues, by a specific gonadal-steroid binding globulin (GBG). Dihydrotestosterone is the most potent of the male steroid hormones, with an activity that is 10 times that of testosterone.

Humans express three different steroid 5α-reductase genes, *SRD5A1*, *SRD5A2*, and *SRD5A3*, where *SRD5A3* is the primary enzyme carrying out the testosterone to DHT conversion. Mutations in the *SRD5A2* gene are the cause of a form of male pseudohermaphroditism. In addition to DHT formation, the *SRD5A3*-encoded enzyme (also called polyprenol reductase) is required for the conversion of polyprenol to dolichol which is necessary for the synthesis of *N*-linked glycoproteins (see Chapter 24). Mutations in the *SRD5A3* gene are associated with the development of a particular form of congenital disorder of glycosylation (CDG) identified as CDG-Iq (see Clinical Box 24–5).

FSH stimulates Sertoli cells to secrete androgen-binding protein (ABP), which transports testosterone and DHT from Leydig cells to sites of spermatogenesis. There, testosterone acts to stimulate protein synthesis and sperm development.

FEMALE SEX HORMONES

In females, LH binds to thecal cells of the ovary, where it stimulates the synthesis of androstenedione and testosterone (Figure 32–3). CYP19A1 (aromatase, also called estrogen synthetase) is responsible for the final conversion of the latter two molecules into the estrogens.

CYP19A1 activity is also found in granulosa cells, but in these cells the activity is stimulated by FSH. Normally, thecal cell androgens produced in response to LH diffuse to granulosa cells, where granulosa cell CYP19A1 converts these androgens to estrogens. Granulosa cell estrogens are largely, if not all, secreted into follicular fluid. Thecal cell estrogens are secreted largely into the circulation, where they are delivered to target tissues by the same globulin (GBG) used to transport testosterone.

THYROID HORMONES

The thyroid hormones, referred to as the thyronines, are synthesized from the amino acid tyrosine within specialized cells of the thyroid gland. The two major thyroid hormones are triiodothyronine (T3 or T_3) and thyroxine (T4 or T_4) (Figure 32–4). Within the periphery the major actions of thyroid hormone are exerted via T3. Synthesis of the thyroid hormones is controlled via the action of the anterior pituitary hormone, thyroid-stimulating hormone, TSH (see Chapter 31). In addition to pituitary control, synthesis of the thyroid hormones requires iodine uptake into the thyroid gland and incorporation into tyrosine residues in the major thyroid protein, thyroglobulin.

The primary functions for the thyroid hormones are fetal and postnatal development, development of the CNS, modulation of cardiac function through regulation of myocardial contraction and relaxation, renal water clearance, gastrointestinal motility, thermal regulation, energy expenditure, and regulation of lipid metabolism.

Iodine is a critical micronutrient due to its role in the generation of functional thyroid hormones. The basolateral membrane of thyroid gland cells (thyrocytes) transports iodide into the cell from the circulation (Figure 32–5). The transporter is called the Na^+/I^- symporter (NIS), which is encoded by the *SLC5A5* gene. The NIS transporter moves two moles of Na^+ and one mole of I^- into the thyrocyte. The expression of the thyrocyte *SLC5A5* gene is controlled via the actions of TSH. In addition to regulated expression, TSH controls the migration of NIS into and out of the

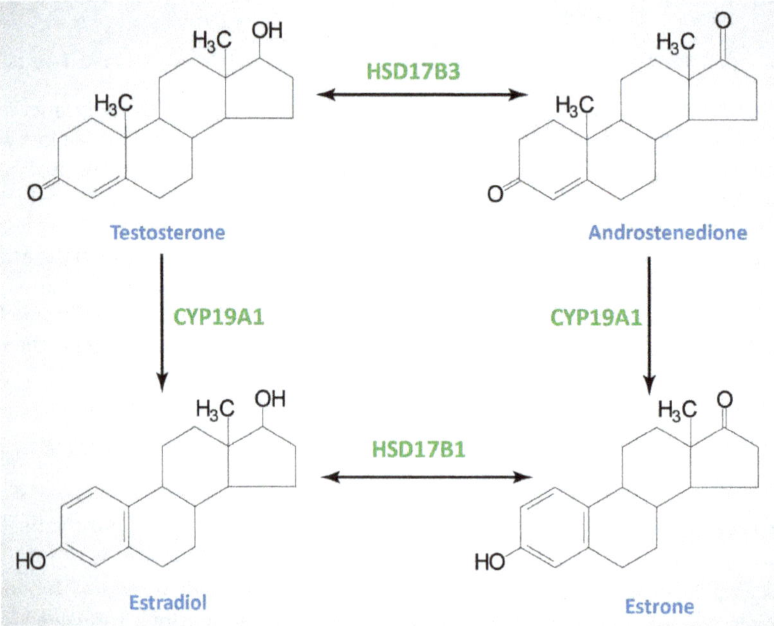

FIGURE 32–3 Synthesis of the major female sex hormones in the ovary. Synthesis of testosterone and androstenedione in the ovary occurs by the same pathways as indicated for synthesis of the male sex hormones (Figure 32–2). CYP19A1 is aromatase (also called estrogen synthetase). HSD17B1 and HSD17B3 are 17β-hydroxysteroid dehydrogenase type 1 and 17β-hydroxysteroid dehydrogenase type 3, respectively. (Reproduced with permission from themedicalbiochemistrypage, LLC.)

basolateral membranes of the thyrocyte. Mutations in the *SLC5A5* gene result in thyroid dyshormonogenesis type 1 (TDH1).

Within the colloid, iodide (I^-) is oxidized to I^+ by thyroid peroxidase (TPO; also called thyroperoxidase) found only in thyroid tissue. Mutations in the *TPO* gene are associated with several disorders of thyroid hormone biogenesis which includes congenital hypothyroidism, thyroid hormone organification defect IIA, and congenital goiter. The oxidation reaction catalyzed by TPO requires hydrogen peroxide (H_2O_2) which is produced by an NADPH oxidase complex often referred to as thyroid oxidase. The NADPH oxidase is composed of multiple subunits including dual oxidase 1 (DUOX1) and dual oxidase 2 (DUOX2). Another gene required for the function of the NADPH oxidase complex is *DUOXA2* (dual oxidase maturation factor 2) which is involved in the maturation and membrane localization of DUOX2. The activity of the NADPH oxidase is also regulated via the actions of TSH.

The incorporation of iodine into tyrosine residues in thyroglobulin occurs in the lumen of thyroid follicles (the colloid) and it is transported across the thyrocyte apical membrane via the action of a $Cl^-/I^-/HCO_3^-$ exchanger identified as pendrin (*SLC26A4*). Mutations in the *SLC26A4* gene are the cause of

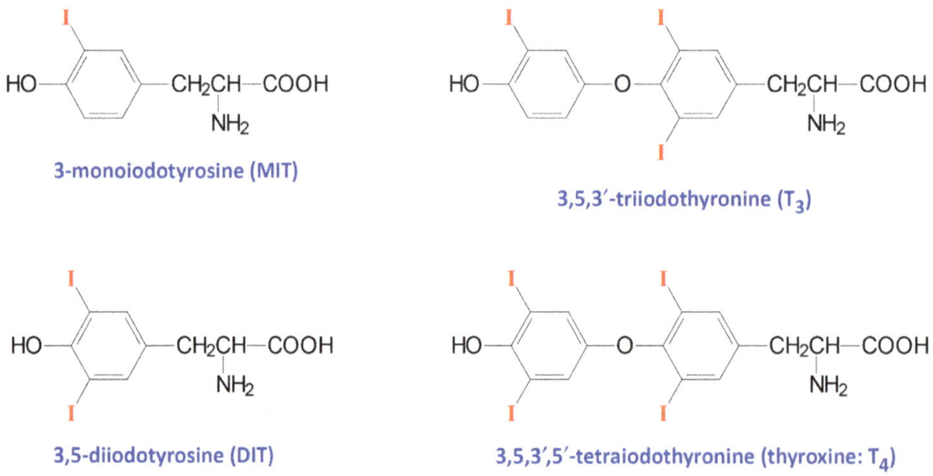

FIGURE 32–4 Structures of primary thyroid hormones. (Reproduced with permission from themedicalbiochemistrypage, LLC.)

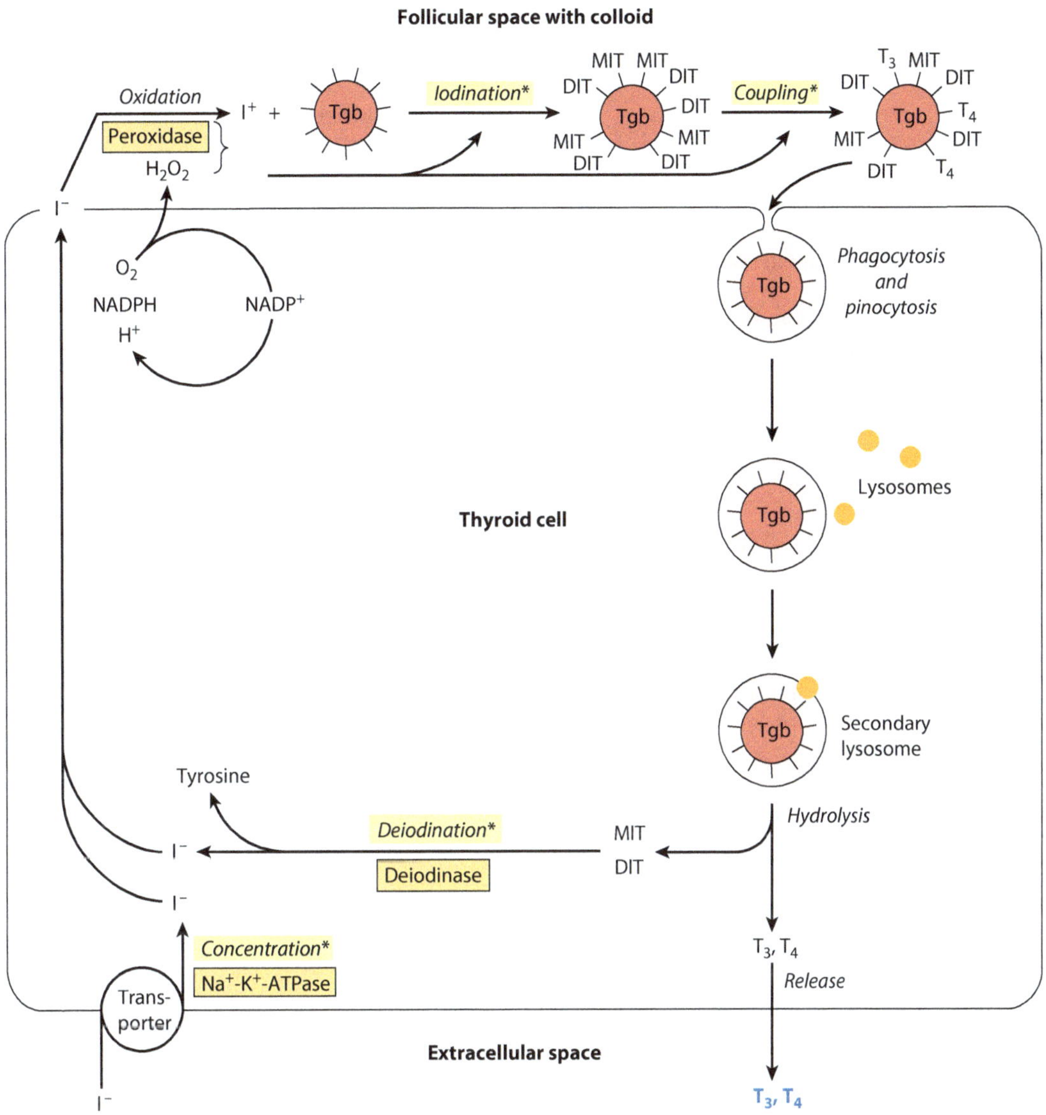

FIGURE 32–5 Model of iodide metabolism in the thyroid follicle. A follicular cell is shown facing the follicular lumen (top) and the extracellular space (bottom). Iodide enters the thyroid primarily through a transporter (bottom left). Thyroid hormone synthesis occurs in the follicular space through a series of reactions, many of which are peroxidase-mediated. Thyroid hormones, stored in the colloid in the follicular space, are released from thyroglobulin by hydrolysis inside the thyroid cell. (DIT, diiodotyrosine; MIT, monoiodotyrosine; Tgb, thyroglobulin; T3, triiodothyronine; T4, tetraiodothyronine.) Asterisks indicate steps or processes where inherited enzyme deficiencies cause congenital goiter and often result in hypothyroidism. (Reproduced with permission from Rodwell VW, Bender DA, Botham KM, et al: *Harper's Illustrated Biochemistry*, 31st ed. New York, NY: McGraw Hill; 2018.)

Pendred syndrome (PDS), also known as thyroid dyshormonogenesis type 2B (TDH2B). Mature, iodinated thyroglobulin is taken up in vesicles by thyrocytes and fuses with lysosomes. Lysosomal proteases degrade thyroglobulin releasing amino acids and T_3 and T_4, which are secreted into the circulation.

The addition of I^+ to tyrosine residues of thyroglobulin is catalyzed by TPO at the thyrocyte apical membrane-colloid interface. The products of this reaction are thyroglobulin complexes containing monoiodotyrosyl (MIT) and diiodotyrosyl (DIT) residues (see Figure 32–4). Two molecules of DIT condense to form T4 while a molecule of MIT and one of DIT condense to form T3. Mutations in the *TPO* gene are associated with thyroid dyshormonogenesis type 2A (THD2A).

T3 is the more biologically active thyroid hormone and T4 is converted to T3 within peripheral tissues via the actions of a 5′-deiodinase (thyroxine deiodinase type 1; encoded by the *DIO1* gene). This deiodinase is also present in the thyroid gland and plays a critical role in overall regulation of iodide homeostasis in this tissue. Deiodination of MIT and DIT also takes place within the thyroid gland. These reactions are catalyzed by an

TABLE 32–3 Etiology of hypothyroidism.

Primary: 1. Hashimoto thyroiditis: • With goiter • "Idiopathic" thyroid atrophy, presumably end-stage autoimmune thyroid disease, following either Hashimoto thyroiditis or Graves disease • Neonatal hypothyroidism due to placental transmission of TSH-R blocking antibodies 2. Radioactive iodine therapy for Graves, disease 3. Subtotal thyroidectomy for Graves, disease, nodular goiter, or thyroid cancer 4. Excessive iodide intake (kelp, radiocontrast dyes) 5. Subacute thyroiditis (usually transient) 6. Iodide deficiency (rare in North America) 7. Inborn errors of thyroid hormone synthesis 8. Drugs • Lithium • Interferon-alfa • Amiodarone
Secondary: Hypopituitarism due to pituitary adenoma, pituitary ablative therapy, or pituitary destruction
Tertiary: Hypothalamic dysfunction (rare)
Peripheral resistance to the action of thyroid hormon

Reproduced with permission from Gardner DG, Shoback D. *Greenspan's Basic and Clinical Endocrinology*, 10th ed. New York, NY: McGraw Hill; 2018.

NADPH-dependent flavoprotein (iodotyrosine deiodinase; IYD), which recognizes MIT and DIT but not T3 nor T4. The iodine released from MIT and DIT is reused for hormone biogenesis.

Thyroid hormones exert their effects by binding to cytosolic receptors of the steroid-thyroid hormone receptor superfamily (nuclear receptors) identified as thyroid hormone receptors (TR). There are two TR receptors designated TRα and TRβ encoded by the THRA and THRB genes, respectively.

HYPO- AND HYPERTHYROIDISM

Numerous congenital and acquired forms of hypothyroidism and hyperthyroidism are the result of alterations in the expression, processing, and function of the TSHR. The most common TSHR disorder resulting in hyperthyroidism (thyrotoxicosis) is Graves disease (see Clinical Box 31–1). At the other end of the spectrum are disorders that lead to hypothyroidism (Table 32–3). Deficiency in iodine is the most common cause of hypothyroidism worldwide. Indeed, the practice of producing iodized table salt was to stem the occurrence of hypothyroidism. When hypothyroidism is evident in conjunction with sufficient iodine intake it is either autoimmune disease (Hashimoto thyroiditis) or the consequences of treatments for hyperthyroidism that are the causes. In the embryo, thyroid hormone is necessary for normal development and hypothyroidism in the embryo is responsible for cretinism, which is characterized by multiple congenital defects and intellectual impairment.

HIGH-YIELD CONCEPT

Hypothyroidism refers to the clinical syndrome resulting from deficiency in the thyroid hormones. The general manifestation of hypothyroidism is a reduced level of metabolic processes. Hyperthyroidism, commonly called thyrotoxicosis, refers to the clinical syndrome resulting when tissues are exposed to high levels of the thyroid hormones.

STEROID AND THYROID HORMONE RECEPTORS

Steroid and thyroid hormone receptors are ligand-activated proteins that directly regulate transcription of target genes. Unlike peptide hormone receptors, steroid hormone receptors are found in the cytosol and the nucleus. The steroid and thyroid hormone receptor super-family of proteins is known as the nuclear receptors (reviewed in Chapter 26).

CHECKLIST

- ☑ All steroid hormones are derived from cholesterol and contain either 18-, 19-, or 21-carbon atoms.
- ☑ The thyroid hormones are iodinated derivatives of the amino acid tyrosine.
- ☑ The steroid hormones can be grouped into the adrenal cortical steroids and the gonadal steroids.
- ☑ The major adrenal cortical steroids are the glucocorticoids, the mineralocorticoids, and the androgens. Each of these hormones is synthesized in one of three specialized zones of the adrenal cortex called the zona glomerulosa, zona reticularis, and zona fasciculata.
- ☑ Synthesis of the adrenal steroids is under the control of the hypothalamic-pituitary axis with specific anterior pituitary hormones exerting influence on adrenal steroidogenesis, primarily controlled by ACTH.
- ☑ Glucocorticoids, primarily cortisol, exert a feedback regulation on the rate and level of their synthesis by inhibiting ACTH release from the pituitary.

- ☑ Synthesis of the mineralocorticoids is also influenced by the renin-angiotensin system of the kidneys and liver.
- ☑ Defects in several of the adrenal steroid biosynthesizing enzymes as well as defects in hypothalamic-pituitary function results in potential severe and life-threatening disorders.
- ☑ The synthesis of gonadal steroid hormones is also controlled by the hypothalamic-pituitary axis, primarily involving pituitary follicle-stimulating hormone and luteinizing hormone.
- ☑ Thyroid hormones are the dityrosine derivatives, triiodothyronine (T3), and thyroxine (T4). Synthesis of the thyroid hormones is regulated by the anterior pituitary hormone, TSH. Thyroid hormone synthesis is dependent on iodine.
- ☑ The steroid and thyroid superfamily of hormones, which also includes vitamin D and retinoic acid, all bind to intracellular receptors referred to as nuclear receptors.

REVIEW QUESTIONS

1. A neonate is being examined following birth because of partial fusion of the labia and an enlarged clitoris. Serum studies show potassium concentration of 8.2 mEq/L (N = 3.5–5.0 mEq/L) and a sodium concentration of 112 mEq/L (N = 136–145 mEq/L). Given the findings in this neonate, which of the following serum steroids is most likely to be found at elevated levels?

(A) Aldosterone
(B) Corticosterone
(C) Cortisol
(D) 11-Deoxycortisol
(E) 17α-Hydroxyprogesterone

2. A 37-year-old man is being examined by his physician with complaints of fatigue, unexplained weight gain, constipation, and dry itchy skin. Physical examination finds a heart rate of 52 beats per minute and a temperature of 35.9°C. Serum studies find normal levels of thyroid-stimulating hormone (TSH), and only slightly elevate levels of thyroxine (T4), and triiodothyronine (T3). Which of the following would best explain the signs and symptoms in this patient?

(A) Autoantibodies to TSH receptors
(B) Decreased production of T4-binding globulin
(C) Impaired intracellular signaling by the TSH receptor
(D) Impaired nuclear receptors for T4 and T3
(E) Increased secretion of thyrotropin-releasing hormone (TRH)

3. A 49-year-old woman comes to the emergency department with excruciating pain in her wrist after a low impact fall. X-ray results show the patient has sustained a Colles fracture. The patient says that she has been seen by her primary care physician on a regular basis for management of her 5-year history of type 2 diabetes, refractory hypertension, and subsequent chronic kidney disease. Her diabetes required early insulin treatment. She reports that, of late, she has had weight gain, easy bruising, flushing, and low mood. The emergency department physician attributes these latter symptoms to obesity and menopause. When asked, she indicates that she has not taken any glucocorticoids. Which of the following laboratory findings would most likely be seen in this patient?

(A) Decreased free plasma testosterone
(B) Decreased plasma levels of thyroid-stimulating hormone
(C) Decreased urinary cortisol output
(D) Increased levels of plasma adrenocorticotropic hormone (ACTH)
(E) Increased levels of plasma vasopressin
(F) Increased urinary triiodothyronine (T3) output

4. A 32-year-old woman comes to the physician because of continuous nausea and frequent bouts of vomiting over the past week. She says that she has had to stop her involvement in ballet lessons due to loss of energy and poor concentration over the past 6 months. In addition to her nausea, she says that she has had a poor appetite for months and that she has lost 10 lb over the past 3 months. Physical examination shows dryness and darkening of the skin in several areas. When asked by her physician, she denies any abnormal diet or food restricting behaviors. She says that she has not experienced abdominal pain, diarrhea, fever, dysuria, or headache. Which of the following laboratory findings are most likely in this patient?

(A) Decreased plasma adrenocorticotropic hormone (ACTH)
(B) Decreased plasma estrogen
(C) Decreased urinary cortisol output
(D) Increased plasma aldosterone
(E) Increased plasma cortisol
(F) Increased urinary triiodothyronine (T3) output

5. A 43-year-old woman is being examined by her physician with complaints of dizziness, extreme fatigue, nausea, and weight loss during the prior 8-month period. Additional symptoms include dizziness, easy fatigability, nausea with occasional vomiting, and progressive weight loss over the prior 8 months. Physical examination shows areas of skin hyperpigmentation, heart rate of 106 beats per minute, and supine blood pressure of 120/75. The patient has trouble standing due to severe postural dizziness. Abdominal ultrasound shows normal liver, spleen, pancreas, and pelvic organs. A CT scan of the abdomen showed a nonenhancing oval-shaped left suprarenal mass with calcification. The signs and symptom in this patient are most likely the result of which of the following?

(A) Addison disease
(B) Cushing syndrome
(C) Graves disease
(D) Hyperthyroidism
(E) Pituitary adenoma

6. A 5-month-old infant is undergoing an examination to determine the cause of her lack of weight gain, poor feeding, vomiting, and diarrhea. Physical examination finds that the infant has an enlarged clitoris and partially fused labia. Genetic testing reveals her karyotype is 46,XX. Blood work finds serum

glucose of 38 mg/dL (N = 45–126 mg/dL) and sodium of 115 mEq/L (N = 136–145 mEq/L). Which of the following would most likely explain the hyponatremia in this infant?
(A) Cortisol production is negligible resulting in increased ACTH release from the pituitary
(B) Cortisol production is negligible due to loss of ACTH control of hypothalamic responses
(C) The adrenal cortex is producing excess aldosterone
(D) The adrenal cortex is producing no androstenedione
(E) There is dysregulation of androgen synthesis which normally controls aldosterone synthesis

7. A 61-year-old man is being examined by his physician with complaints of fatigue and feeling cold all the time. History reveals that the patient is being treated with amiodarone for persistent ventricular fibrillation. Physical examination finds dry flaky skin, brittle fingernails, and blood pressure of 107/84. His temperature is 36.1°C, heart rate is 68 beats per minute, and respirations are 12 per minute. Examination of the thyroid gland shows no obvious abnormalities. Which of the following metabolic changes are most likely to be associated with the signs and symptoms in this patient?

	Thyroxine (T4) synthesis	Thyroid-stimulating hormone synthesis	Triiodothyronine (T3) synthesis
A.	↑	↑	↑
B.	↑	↑	↓
C.	↑	↓	↑
D.	↑	↓	↓
E.	↓	↑	↑
F.	↓	↑	↓

8. A neonate is being examined following birth because of partial fusion of the labia and an enlarged clitoris. Serum studies show potassium concentration of 8.2 mEq/L (N = 3.5–5.0) and a sodium concentration of 112 mEq/L (N = 136–145 mEq/L). Given the findings in this neonate, which of the following serum steroids is most likely to be found at significantly reduced levels?
(A) Androstenedione
(B) Corticosterone
(C) Dehydroepiandrosterone (DHEA)
(D) 17α-Hydroxypregnenolone
(E) 17α-Hydroxyprogesterone

9. A 45-year-old woman is being examined by her physician because she is concerned about her weight gain, fatigue, muscle weakness, and thinning hair. Physical examination shows facial hirsutism and red striae in abdominal and underarm areas. She indicates that she is not on any medication and there is no significant family history of disease. Laboratory studies show a fasting plasma glucose of 198 mg/dL (N = 75–115 mg/dL) and a 24-hour urinary free cortisol of 375 μg (N = 50–100 μg/24 h). These signs and symptoms are most likely the result of which of the following?
(A) Addison disease
(B) Cushing syndrome
(C) Graves disease
(D) Hyperthyroidism
(E) Hypothyroidism

10. A 32-year-old woman is diagnosed with hypertension, hypernatremia, and hypokalemia. Measurements of plasma glucocorticoid levels show them to be within the normal range; however, renin and angiotensin II levels are elevated. Ultrasound examination finds the presence of a mass in the left kidney. Which of the following is most likely produced in excess in this woman?
(A) Aldosterone
(B) Androstenedione
(C) Dehydroepiandrosterone (DHEA)
(D) Estradiol
(E) Testosterone

11. A 63-year-old woman is being examined by her physician with complaints of dizziness, extreme fatigue, nausea, and weight loss during the prior 8-month period. Physical examination shows areas of darkening skin. Her heart rate is 106 beats per minute. Blood pressure lying down is 100/60 and she has trouble standing due to severe postural dizziness. Abdominal ultrasound shows normal liver, spleen, pancreas, and pelvic organs. A CT scan of the abdomen showed a nonenhancing oval-shaped left suprarenal mass with calcification. The signs and symptoms in this patient are most likely the result of a deficiency in which of the following?
(A) Adrenocorticotropic hormone (ACTH)
(B) Corticotropin-releasing hormone
(C) Cortisol
(D) Parathyroid hormone
(E) Renin

12. A baby girl is born with ambiguous genitalia and diagnosed with severe classical congenital deficiency of adrenal 21-hydroxylase enzyme. Without any treatment, which of the following would most likely be evident in analysis of the infants' blood?
(A) Hypercalcemia
(B) Hyperchloremia
(C) Hyperphosphatemia
(D) Hypocalcemia
(E) Hypokalemia
(F) Hyponatremia

13. A routine examination of a neonate finds serum potassium concentration of 8.2 mEq/L (N = 3.5–5.0) and a serum sodium concentration of 112 mEq/L (N = 136–145 mEq/L). Loss of function of which of the following steroids is most likely to account for the findings in this infant?
(A) Aldosterone
(B) Androstenedione
(C) Cortisol
(D) 11-Deoxycorticosterone
(E) 11-Deoxycortisol

14. A 45-year-old woman is being examined by her physician because she is concerned about her weight gain, fatigue, muscle weakness, and thinning hair. Physical examination shows facial hirsutism and red striae in abdominal and underarm areas. She indicates that she is not on any medication and there is no significant family history of disease. Laboratory studies show a fasting plasma glucose of 198 mg/dL (N = 75–115 mg/dL) and a 24-hour urinary free cortisol of 375 μg (N = 50–100 μg/24 h). Which of the following is

most likely to be found at elevated levels in the blood of this patient?
(A) Adrenocorticotropic hormone (ACTH)
(B) Aldosterone
(C) Angiotensinogen
(D) 11-Deoxycorticosterone
(E) Thyrotropin releasing hormone

15. A 57-year-old woman was diagnosed with rheumatoid arthritis 1 year ago. Her therapeutic intervention has been the daily administration of prednisone since her diagnosis. Which of the following is the most likely complication of her therapy?
(A) Acromegaly
(B) Adrenal insufficiency
(C) Hypokalemia
(D) Hypernatremia
(E) Hyperthyroidism

16. A 4-year-old boy is being examined by his pediatrician due to parental concerns about his apparent signs of precocious puberty. Genetic testing reveals his karyotype is 46,XY. Serum studies find elevated levels of adrenocorticotropic hormone (ACTH). Given the findings in this child, which of the following is most likely?
(A) Adrenal cortical atrophy
(B) Adrenal medullary hypertrophy
(C) Excessive production of cortisol
(D) Serum cholesterol will decline
(E) Serum levels of 17α-hydroxypregnenolone will be elevated

17. A 29-year-old body builder has been using testosterone patches in an attempt to augment his accumulation of muscle mass. He and his wife have been trying to conceive for the past 6 months with no success. Testing in a fertility clinic finds that he has an extremely low sperm count. Which of the following effect of testosterone is most likely contributing to his infertility?
(A) Activation of inhibin
(B) Feedback activation of follicle-stimulating hormone
(C) Feedback inhibition of gonadotropin-releasing hormone
(D) Inhibition of follicle-stimulating hormone
(E) Inhibition of the mineralocorticoid receptor

18. A 37-year-old woman is being examined by her physician with complaints of chronic fatigue, nausea, unexplained weight loss, and abdominal pain. A basic metabolic panel finds sodium of 111 mEq/L (N = 136–145 mEq/L), potassium 5.7 mEq/L (N = 3.5–5.0 mEq/L), chloride 78 mEq/L (N = 98–106 mEq/L), and bicarbonate 23 mM (N = 19–25 mM). Serum hormone analysis finds ACTH is 540 pg/mL (N = 9–52 pg/mL) and cortisol is 0.2 mg/dL (N = 5–25 mg/dL). Given the signs and symptoms in this patient, which of the following is most likely?
(A) Adrenal adenoma
(B) Adrenal insufficiency
(C) Hyperthyroidism
(D) Hypothyroidism
(E) Pheochromocytoma

19. A 44-year-old woman is being examined by her physician with complaints of chronic fatigue, aching muscles, and general weakness. Physical examination shows dry flaky skin and slow reflexes. Laboratory studies find thyroid stimulating hormone (TSH) is 12 mU/mL (N = 0.4–5 mU/mL) and free T4 is 4 mg/dL (N = 5–12 mg/dL). With of the following is the most likely explanation of the signs and symptoms in this patient?
(A) Hyperthyroidism due to autoimmune thyroid disease
(B) Hyperthyroidism due to iodine excess
(C) Hyperthyroidism secondary to a hypothalamic-pituitary defect
(D) Hypothyroidism due to autoimmune thyroid disease
(E) Hypothyroidism secondary to a hypothalamic-pituitary defect
(F) Hypothyroidism due to adrenal insufficiency

20. A 3-month-old girl is being examined by her pediatrician because her parents are concerned about her excessive sleeping and lack of activity when she is awake. History revels the infant has had persistent hyperbilirubinemia. Physical examination reveals abnormal deep tendon reflexes, hypothermia, and muscular hypotonia. Given the signs and symptoms in this infant, which of the following would be the best therapeutic intervention?
(A) Cortisol
(B) Growth hormone
(C) Thiamine
(D) Thyroxine
(E) Vitamin D

21. A 27-year-old woman and her 29-year-old husband are being evaluated for infertility. They have been unable to conceive a child despite regular intercourse for the past 12 months. The infertility clinic performs an ovulation test on the woman and obtains a negative result. Given this result, which of the following is most likely deficient in this woman?
(A) Estradiol
(B) Follicle-stimulating hormone (FSH)
(C) Luteinizing hormone (LH)
(D) Progesterone
(E) Testosterone

22. A 35-year-old woman is being examined by her physician with complaints of chronic fatigue, unexplained weight gain, constipation, and irregular menstrual cycles. Physical examination finds the presence of a goiter. Serum studies show slight elevation in TSH but normal levels of thyroxine (T4) and triiodothyronine (T3). No antibodies to the TSH receptor can be detected in serum. Given the symptoms and findings in this patient, which of the following is most likely?
(A) Graves disease
(B) Hashimoto disease
(C) Iodine intoxication
(D) Subacute thyroiditis
(E) Thyroid dyshormonogenesis type 1

23. Clinical trials are being carried out on the efficacy of an orally administered analog of cortisol. Following the administration of the analog, assays are carried out to determine the transcription profile in adrenal tissue. The gene encoding which of the following enzymes is most likely to be seen expressed at higher levels when compared to control tissue?
(A) Acetyl-CoA carboxylase
(B) Homocysteine methyltransferase
(C) Methionine adenosyltransferase
(D) Methylmalonyl-CoA racemase
(E) Phenylethanolamine *N*-methyltransferase

24. Patients with osteoarthritis are often given injections of dexamethasone to repress inflammation. Following injection, the dexamethasone is cleared from the body with a half-life of around 4 hours. After the drug has been eliminated which of the following is most likely to be observed?
    (A) Induced proteins are specifically targeted for degradation
    (B) Induced proteins remain functional after the drug is eliminated
    (C) Target genes are silenced by incorporation into heterochromatin
    (D) Target genes remain transcriptionally active
    (E) Unoccupied receptors remain associated with target DNA sequence

25. A 2-month-old newborn is being examined for failure to thrive. Physical examination finds the infant has ambiguous genitalia. Serum analysis finds the infant's sodium concentration is 115 mEq/L (N: 135–145 mEq/L) and potassium concentration is 6 mEq/L (N: 3.5–5.5 mEq/L). Karyotype analysis finds the infant to be genetically female with 46,XX genotype. This infant most likely has a defect in the synthesis of which of the following hormones?
    (A) Cortisol
    (B) Dehydroepiandrosterone (DHEA)
    (C) Estradiol
    (D) Progesterone
    (E) Testosterone

ANSWERS

1. Correct answer is **E.** The infant is most likely manifesting the signs and symptoms of a congenital adrenal hyperplasia (CAH). CAH are a group of inherited disorders that result from loss-of-function mutations in one of several genes involved in adrenal steroid hormone synthesis. The most common forms of CAH are caused by defects in either *CYP21A2* (21-hydroxylase, also identified as just CYP21 or CYP21B) or *CYP11B1* (11β-hydroxylase). The majority of CAH cases (90–95%) are the result of defects in *CYP21A2*. In the virilizing forms of CAH the mutations in *CYP21A2* result in impairment of cortisol and corticosterone production in the *zona fasciculata* and aldosterone production in the *zona glomerulosa*, and the consequent accumulation of steroid intermediates proximal to the defective enzyme. In the virilizing forms of CAH there is increased ACTH secretion which leads to elevated synthesis of adrenal androgens. In addition, there is adrenal cortical hyperplasia. The 21-hydroxylase enzyme possesses two different substrate binding sites, one for 17α-hydroxyprogesterone and one for progesterone. The reactions catalyzed by the 21-hydroxylase enzyme include the conversion of 17α-hydroxyprogesterone to 11-deoxycortisol and the conversion of progesterone to 11-deoxycorticosterone. The 21-hydroxylase functions in both the *zona fasciculata* and the *zona glomerulosa* of the cortex of the adrenal glands. Loss of 21-hydroxylase function results in the accumulation of the two substrates for this enzyme, progesterone and 17α-hydroxyprogesterone. Within the *zona glomerulosa*, loss of 21-hydroxylase activity will result in reduced, not increased, synthesis of aldosterone (choice A). Within the *zona fasciculata*, the loss of 21-hydroxylase activity will result in reduced, not increased, levels of corticosterone (choice B), cortisol (choice C), and 11-deoxycortisol (choice D).

2. Correct answer is **D.** The patient is most likely exhibiting the typical signs and symptoms of hypothyroidism. Deficiency in iodine is the most common cause of hypothyroidism worldwide. Indeed, the practice of producing iodized table salt was to stem the occurrence of hypothyroidism. When hypothyroidism is evident in conjunction with sufficient iodine intake it is most likely autoimmune disease (Hashimoto thyroiditis) or the consequences of treatments for hyperthyroidism that are the cause. However, in this patient there is no evidence of loss of thyroid function given that the serum levels of thyroxine (T4) and triiodothyronine (T3) are detectable indicating a normal response of the thyroid gland to thyroid-stimulating hormone, TSH. The presence of T4 and T3 clearly indicates that the TSH receptor is functional (choice C) in the thyroid gland. Therefore, the most likely cause of the symptoms of hypothyroidism in this patient would be a defect in the function of the thyroid hormone receptors, TR. The presence of autoantibodies to the TSH receptor (choice A) results in overstimulation of the receptor and a consequent hyperthyroidism. This is the situation in patients with Graves disease. Given that the serum level of T4 was slightly elevated it is indicative that thyroid hormone-binding globulin, which protects the thyroid hormones in the circulation, was present, not decreased (choice B). Increased secretion of thyrotropin releasing hormone (choice E) from the hypothalamus would result in increased TSH synthesis and release from the anterior pituitary. However, results from this patient showed normal levels of TSH.

3. Correct answer is **D.** The patient most likely suffering from Cushing syndrome, a form of hypercortisolemia. Indeed, hypercortisolemia is the hallmark symptom in both Cushing disease and Cushing syndrome. Cushing syndrome is the disorder first described by Harvey Cushing in 1932 in several patients with adrenocortical hyperplasia that were the result of basophilic adenomas of the anterior pituitary. Some confusion can result given that the current distinction between Cushing syndrome and Cushing disease is that the former is associated with adrenal dysfunction (most usually due to tumors) resulting in excess cortisol production and secretion, whereas the latter results from anterior pituitary dysfunction (most usually due to tumors) resulting in excess ACTH secretion. The excess ACTH overstimulates the adrenal glands resulting, secondarily, in excess, not decreased (choice C) cortisol secretion. Sometimes Cushing disease is referred to as ACTH-dependent Cushing syndrome. Considering all cases of hypercortisolemia, 80–85% are caused by pituitary corticotrope adenomas resulting in excess ACTH secretion. The other 10–15% of cases result from unilateral benign and malignant adrenal tumors resulting directly in excessive cortisol secretion. None of the other laboratory findings (choices A, B, E, and F) would correspond to the signs and symptoms presenting in a patient with hypercortisolemia.

4. Correct answer is **C.** The patient is most likely experiencing the symptoms of the adrenal insufficiency associated with Addison disease. Adrenal insufficiency describes a related group of disorders that are generally divided into two broad categories. Disorders that are due to a primary inability of the adrenal glands to synthesize and secrete hormone, such as cortisol, constitute the primary adrenal insufficiency syndromes. Disorders of adrenal function that result from inadequate adrenocorticotropic hormone (ACTH) synthesis or release from the anterior pituitary constitute the secondary adrenal

insufficiency syndromes. The major primary adrenal insufficiency syndrome is Addison disease whose frequency is higher in females than in males. The reduced adrenal cortical synthesis of cortisol in Addison disease results in the loss of the feedback control that cortisol normally exerts on the pituitary leading to increased, not decreased (choice A), ACTH output. The characteristic clinical presentation of acute primary adrenal insufficiency includes an insidious onset of asthenia (fatigability and weakness), cutaneous and mucosal pigmentation, agitation, nausea, vomiting, anorexia, weight loss, orthostatic (postural) hypotension (drop in blood pressure upon standing), confusion, circulatory collapse, abdominal pain, and fever. Indeed, one can consider the hallmark features of Addison disease to be asthenia, weight loss, and pigmentation (particularly on sun-exposed skin), as these three symptoms are present in more than 97% of patients. The typical history and clinical findings of Addison disease include a protracted history of malaise, fatigue, anorexia, weight loss, joint and back pain, and darkening of the skin. In addition, patients may crave salt and may develop preferences for salty foods and fluids. None of the other findings (choices B, D, E, and F) would be parent in a patient with Addison disease.

5. Correct answer is **A.** The patient is most likely experiencing the symptoms of the adrenal insufficiency associated with Addison disease. The reduced adrenal cortical synthesis of cortisol in Addison disease results in the loss of the feedback control that cortisol normally exerts on the pituitary leading to increased adrenocorticotropic hormone (ACTH) output. The characteristic clinical presentation of acute primary adrenal insufficiency includes an insidious onset of asthenia (fatigability and weakness), cutaneous and mucosal pigmentation, agitation, nausea, vomiting, anorexia, weight loss, orthostatic (postural) hypotension (drop in blood pressure upon standing), confusion, circulatory collapse, abdominal pain, and fever. Indeed, one can consider the hallmark features of Addison disease to be asthenia, weight loss, and pigmentation (particularly on sun-exposed skin), as these three symptoms are present in more than 97% of patients. The typical history and clinical findings of Addison disease include a protracted history of malaise, fatigue, anorexia, weight loss, joint and back pain, and darkening of the skin. Cushing syndrome (choice B) is characterized by hypercortisolemia which is the precise opposite of the lack of cortisol production characteristic of Addison disease. Cushing syndrome is characterized by truncal (central) adiposity, hypertension, weakness, fatigability, purplish abdominal striae (stretch marks), amenorrhea, edema, glucosuria, osteoporosis, and hirsutism. Cushing syndrome and Cushing disease refer to related pathologies resulting from different primary causes. Cushing syndrome is associated with adrenal dysfunction (most usually due to tumors) resulting in excess cortisol production and secretion, whereas Cushing disease results from anterior pituitary dysfunction, most usually due to tumors (choice E), resulting in excess ACTH secretion. Graves disease (choice C) is associated with thyrotoxicosis which is defined as a state of thyroid hormone excess but is not synonymous with hyperthyroidism (choice D) which is the result of excessive thyroid function. The major causes of thyrotoxicosis are the hyperthyroidism of Graves disease, toxic adenomas, and toxic multinodular goiter. In addition to hyperthyroidism and goiter, Graves disease is associated with eye disease characterized by inflammation and involvement of intra-orbital structures, dermopathy referred to as pretibial myxedema, and rare involvement of the nails, fingers, and long bones known as acropachy.

6. Corect Choice **A**. The infant is most likely manifesting the signs and symptoms of a congenital adrenal hyperplasia, CAH. CAH are a group of inherited disorders that result from loss-of-function mutations in one of several genes involved in adrenal steroid hormone synthesis. The most common forms of CAH are caused by defects in either CYP21A2 (21-hydroxylase, also identified as just CYP21 or CYP21B) or CYP11B1 (11β-hydroxylase). The majority of CAH cases (90–95%) are the result of defects in *CYP21A2*. In the virilizing forms of CAH the mutations in *CYP21A2* result in impairment of cortisol and corticosterone production in the *zona fasciculata* and aldosterone production in the *zona glomerulosa*. Aldosterone exerts its primary effects through actions on the kidneys but also functions in the colon and sweat glands. The principal effect of aldosterone is to enhance sodium (Na^+) reabsorption in the connecting tubule (CNT) and cortical collecting duct of the nephrons in the kidneys. Within these regions of the nephron, aldosterone induces the expression of the Na^+/K^+-ATPase subunit genes (*ATP1A1* and *ATP1B1*), the genes encoding the subunits (*SCNN1A, SCNN1B,* and *SCNN1C*) of the epithelial sodium channel (ENaC), and the *SLC12A3* gene (encoding the Na^+-Cl^- cotransporter, NCC). The net effect of the induction of these transporter genes, by aldosterone, is enhanced Na^+ reabsorption as a function of the apical membrane localized ENaC and NCC transporters and delivery to the blood via the action of the basolateral membrane localized Na^+/K^+-ATPase. Therefore, loss of aldosterone production due to 21-hydroxylase deficiency results in excessive sodium loss accounting for the hyponatremia in this patient. None of the other options (choices B, C, D, and E) correctly account for the cause of the hyponatremia in patients with 21-hydroxylase deficient CAH.

7. Correct answer is **F.** The patient is most likely exhibiting the typical signs and symptoms of hypothyroidism that are exacerbated by the patient's use of the antiarrhythmic, amiodarone. The signs and symptoms of hypothyroidism are the result of the generalized decrease in metabolic processes. Deficiency in iodine is the most common cause of hypothyroidism worldwide. Indeed, the practice of producing iodized table salt was to stem the occurrence of hypothyroidism. When hypothyroidism is evident in conjunction with sufficient iodine intake it is most likely the result of autoimmune disease (Hashimoto thyroiditis) or the consequences of treatments for hyperthyroidism. Amiodarone is a class III antiarrhythmic drug, and its use is associated with a number of side effects, including thyroid dysfunction (both hypo- and hyperthyroidism). The thyroid dysfunction associated with amiodarone use is a result of the high iodine content of the drug and its direct toxic effect on the thyroid gland. As a result of the reduction in thyroid hormone production and output by the thyroid gland there is increased hypothalamic release of thyrotropin-releasing hormone (TRH) which then enhances the release of thyroid-stimulating hormone (TSH) from the pituitary in an attempt to increase thyroid production of the thyroid hormones. The typical findings in patients with Hashimoto thyroiditis are increased plasma TSH and reduced plasma thyroxine (T4) and triiodothyronine (T3). None of the other changes in hormone levels (choices A, B, C, D, and E) would be associated with hypothyroidism.

8. Correct answer is **B.** The infant is most likely manifesting the signs and symptoms of a congenital adrenal hyperplasia, CAH. CAH are a group of inherited disorders that result from loss-of-function mutations in one of several genes involved in adrenal steroid hormone synthesis. The most common forms of CAH are caused by defects in either *CYP21A2* (21-hydroxylase, also identified as just CYP21 or CYP21B) or *CYP11B1* (11β-hydroxylase). The majority of CAH cases (90–95%) are the result of defects in *CYP21A2.* In the virilizing forms of CAH the mutations in *CYP21A2* result in impairment of cortisol and corticosterone production in the *zona fasciculata* and aldosterone production in the *zona glomerulosa*, and the consequent accumulation of steroid intermediates proximal to the defective enzyme. In the virilizing forms of CAH there is increased ACTH secretion which leads to elevated, not reduced, synthesis of the adrenal androgens, androstenedione (choice A) and dehydroepiandrosterone (choice C), in the *zona reticularis.* Intermediates in adrenal cortical steroid hormone synthesis are elevated, not reduced, as a result of 21-hydroxylase deficiency and include 17α-hydroxypregnenolone (choices D) and 17α-hydroxyprogesterone (choice E).

9. Correct answer is **B.** The patient most likely suffers from Cushing syndrome, a form of hypercortisolemia. Indeed, hypercortisolemia is the hallmark symptom in both Cushing disease and Cushing syndrome. Cushing syndrome is the disorder first described by Harvey Cushing in 1932 in several patients with adrenocortical hyperplasia that were the result of basophilic adenomas of the anterior pituitary. Some confusion can result given that the current distinction between Cushing syndrome and Cushing disease is that the former is associated with adrenal dysfunction (most usually due to tumors) resulting in excess cortisol production and secretion, whereas the latter results from anterior pituitary dysfunction (most usually due to tumors) resulting in excess ACTH secretion. Cushing syndrome may mimic common conditions such as obesity, poorly controlled diabetes, and hypertension, which progress over time and often coexist in patients with the metabolic syndrome. The characteristic features of Cushing syndrome are psychiatric disturbances (depression, mania, and psychoses), central obesity, hypertension, diabetes, moon-shaped face, thin fragile skin, easy bruising, and purple striae (stretch marks). In addition, Cushing syndrome patients manifest with gonadal dysfunction that is characteristic of hyperandrogenism with excess body and facial hair (hirsutism) and acne. The most common symptoms that lead to a diagnosis of Cushing syndrome are weight gain, depression, subjective muscle weakness, and headache. Addison disease (choice A) results from adrenal insufficiency. The characteristic clinical presentation of Addison disease is asthenia, weight loss, and skin pigmentation. Graves disease (choice C) is associated with thyrotoxicosis which is defined as a state of thyroid hormone excess but is not synonymous with hyperthyroidism (choice D) which is the result of excessive thyroid function. In addition to hyperthyroidism and goiter, Graves disease is associated with eye disease characterized by inflammation and involvement of intra-orbital structures and dermopathy referred to as pretibial myxedema. Hypothyroidism (choice E) is characterized by a general reduction in metabolic processes resulting in fatigue, slow movement and slow speech, cold intolerance, constipation, and weight gain.

10. Correct answer is **A.** The presence of the mass in the left kidney in this patient is suggestive of cancer and the patient's symptoms are indicative of the excessive renin production by the kidney. The intra-renal baroreceptor system is a key mechanism for regulating renin secretion. A drop in blood pressure results in the release of renin from juxtaglomerular cells (JG cells; also called granular cells) which are specialized smooth muscle cells in the wall of the afferent arterioles at the base of the glomerulus in the juxtaglomerular apparatus. These are the only cells in the human body that synthesize and secrete renin. The only enzymatic function for renin (an aspartyl protease) is to cleave a 10-amino acid peptide from the N-terminal end of angiotensinogen. This cleaved decapeptide is called angiotensin I. Angiotensin I is then cleaved by the action of angiotensin-converting enzyme (ACE) generating the bioactive octapeptide hormone, angiotensin II. Angiotensin II is one of the most potent naturally occurring vasoconstrictors. In addition to its effects on the vasculature, angiotensin II acts on the kidneys to increase renal tubular Na^+ and Cl^- reabsorption, water retention, and K^+ excretion, on the posterior pituitary to induce the release of vasopressin (antidiuretic hormone, ADH), and stimulates the *zona glomerulosa* cells of the adrenal cortex to secrete aldosterone. Aldosterone exerts its primary effects through actions on the kidneys but also functions in the colon and sweat glands. The principal effect of aldosterone is to enhance sodium (Na^+) reabsorption in the connecting tubule (CNT) and cortical collecting duct of the nephrons in the kidneys. Within these regions of the nephron, aldosterone induces the expression of the Na^+/K^+-ATPase subunit genes (*ATP1A1* and *ATP1B1*), the genes encoding the subunits (*SCNN1A, SCNN1B,* and *SCNN1C*) of the epithelial sodium channel (ENaC), and the *SLC12A3* gene (encoding the Na^+-Cl^- cotransporter, NCC). The net effect of the induction of these transporter genes, by aldosterone, is enhanced Na^+ reabsorption as a function of the apical membrane localized ENaC and NCC transporters and delivery to the blood via the action of the basolateral membrane localized Na^+/K^+-ATPase. The combined effects of excess renin and aldosterone secretion are the hypertension, hypernatremia, and hypokalemia present in this patient. Excessive the production of none of the other hormones (choices B, C, D, and E) would manifest with the symptoms present in this patient.

11. Correct answer is **C.** The patient is most likely experiencing the symptoms the adrenal insufficiency associated with Addison disease. The reduced adrenal cortical synthesis of cortisol in Addison disease results in the loss of the feedback control that cortisol normally exerts on the pituitary leading to increased, not decreased (choice A), adrenocorticotropic hormone (ACTH) output. The characteristic clinical presentation of acute primary adrenal insufficiency includes an insidious onset of asthenia (fatigability and weakness), cutaneous and mucosal pigmentation, agitation, nausea, vomiting, anorexia, weight loss, orthostatic (postural) hypotension (drop in blood pressure upon standing), confusion, circulatory collapse, abdominal pain, and fever. Indeed, one can consider the hallmark features of Addison disease to be asthenia, weight loss, and pigmentation (particularly on sun-exposed skin), as these three symptoms are present in more than 97% of patients. The typical history and clinical findings of Addison disease include a protracted history of malaise, fatigue, anorexia, weight loss, joint and back pain, and darkening of the skin. One of the most common causes of Addison disease is an adrenocortical adenoma which in this patient is evident from the CT scan showing a suprarenal mass. Deficiency in none of the other hormones (choices B, D, and E) would manifest with the signs and symptoms presenting in this patient.

12. Correct answer is **F.** The infant is most likely manifesting the signs and symptoms of a congenital adrenal hyperplasia, CAH. CAH are a group of inherited disorders that result from loss-of-function mutations in one of several genes involved in adrenal steroid hormone synthesis. The most common forms of CAH are caused by defects in either *CYP21A2* (21-hydroxylase, also identified as just CYP21 or CYP21B) or *CYP11B1* (11β-hydroxylase). The majority of CAH cases (90–95%) are the result of defects in CYP21A2. In the virilizing forms of CAH the mutations in *CYP21A2* result in impairment of cortisol and corticosterone production in the *zona fasciculata* and aldosterone production in the *zona glomerulosa*, and the consequent accumulation of steroid intermediates proximal to the defective enzyme. The principal effect of aldosterone is to enhance sodium (Na^+) reabsorption in the connecting tubule (CNT) and cortical collecting duct of the nephrons in the kidneys. Within these regions of the nephron, aldosterone induces the expression of the Na^+/K^+-ATPase subunit genes (*ATP1A1* and *ATP1B1*), the genes encoding the subunits (*SCNN1A, SCNN1B,* and *SCNN1C*) of the epithelial sodium channel (ENaC), and the *SLC12A3* gene (encoding the Na^+-Cl^- cotransporter, NCC). The net effect of the induction of these transporter genes, by aldosterone, is enhanced Na^+ reabsorption as a function of the apical membrane localized ENaC and NCC transporters and delivery to the blood via the action of the basolateral membrane localized Na^+/K^+-ATPase. The loss of aldosterone production in 21-hydroxylase deficient CAH patients is, therefore, associated with hyponatremia and hyperkalemia, not hypokalemia (choice E). None of the other options (choices A, B, C, and D) would be evident in a patient with 21-hydroxylase deficiency.

13. Correct answer is **A.** The electrolyte values identified in this infant are most likely the result of a loss of the adrenal cortical steroid, aldosterone. The principal effect of aldosterone is to enhance sodium (Na^+) reabsorption in the connecting tubule (CNT) and cortical collecting duct of the nephrons in the kidneys. Within these regions of the nephron, aldosterone induces the expression of the Na^+/K^+-ATPase subunit genes (*ATP1A1* and *ATP1B1*), the genes encoding the subunits (*SCNN1A, SCNN1B,* and *SCNN1C*) of the epithelial sodium channel (ENaC), and the *SLC12A3* gene (encoding the Na^+-Cl^- cotransporter, NCC). The net effect of the induction of these transporter genes, by aldosterone, is enhanced Na^+ reabsorption as a function of the apical membrane localized ENaC and NCC transporters and delivery to the blood via the action of the basolateral membrane localized Na^+/K^+-ATPase. The loss of aldosterone production, such as in the case of 21-hydroxylase deficient CAH patients is, therefore, associated with the hyponatremia and hyperkalemia found in this patient. Loss of function of none of the other steroid (choices B, C, D, and E) would result in hyponatremia and hyperkalemia.

14. Correct answer is **A.** The patient most likely suffers from Cushing syndrome, a form of hypercortisolemia. Indeed, hypercortisolemia is the hallmark symptom in both Cushing disease and Cushing syndrome. Cushing syndrome is the disorder first described by Harvey Cushing in 1932 in several patients with adrenocortical hyperplasia that were the result of basophilic adenomas of the anterior pituitary. Some confusion can result given that the current distinction between Cushing syndrome and Cushing disease is that the former is associated with adrenal dysfunction (most usually due to tumors) resulting in excess cortisol production and secretion, whereas the latter results from anterior pituitary dysfunction (most usually due to tumors) resulting in excess ACTH secretion. The excess ACTH over stimulates the adrenal glands resulting in excess cortisol secretion. Sometimes Cushing disease is referred to as ACTH-dependent Cushing syndrome. Considering all cases of hypercortisolemia, 80–85% are caused by pituitary corticotrope adenomas resulting in excess ACTH secretion. The other 10–15% of cases result from unilateral benign and malignant adrenal tumors resulting directly in excessive cortisol secretion. Elevated levels of none of the other hormones (choices B, C, D, and E) would result in the signs and symptoms manifesting in this patient.

15. Correct answer is **B.** Chronic exogenous glucocorticoid (prednisone) administration suppresses the hypothalamic-pituitary-adrenal axis. Specifically, glucocorticoids feedback and inhibit pituitary adrenocorticotropic hormone (ACTH) secretion. The biological role of ACTH is to stimulate the production of adrenal cortical steroids, principally the glucocorticoids, cortisol, and corticosterone. ACTH also stimulates the adrenal cortex to produce the mineralocorticoid, aldosterone as well as the androgens, dehydroepiandrosterone androstenedione. The principal effect of aldosterone is to enhance sodium (Na^+) reabsorption in the connecting tubule (CNT) and cortical collecting duct of the nephrons in the kidneys. Patients chronically treated with glucocorticoids will eventually suffer from secondary adrenal insufficiency. As a result of the secondary adrenal insufficiency, resulting from chronic glucocorticoid therapy, the loss of sufficient aldosterone production leads to hyponatremia, not hypernatremia (choice C) and hyperkalemia, not hypokalemia (choice E). Neither of the other options (choices A and D) would result from chronic prednisone therapy.

16. Correct answer is **E.** The patient is most likely exhibiting the signs of the congenital adrenal hyperplasia (CAH) resulting from mutations in the gene, *CYP21A2*, encoding 21-hydroxylase. Deficiency in 21-hydroxylase results in the failure of adrenal *zona fasciculata* and *zona glomerulosa* cells to make the glucocorticoids, cortisol and corticosterone, and the mineralocorticoid, aldosterone, respectively. The lack of cortisol production results in an inability to provide negative feedback suppression of ACTH production. As a result, the adrenal glands are under constant stimulation to maximize steroidogenesis. Adrenal cortical steroid hormone intermediates above the 21-hydroxylase reaction, such as 17α-hydroxypregnenolone, accumulate and contribute to increased synthesis of the androgens, dehydroepiandrosterone and androstenedione, within adrenal *zona reticularis* cells. The increased androgen synthesis in this patient is the cause of his precocious puberty. None of the other options (choices A, B, C, and D) would be apparent in a patient with a 21-hydroxylase deficiency.

17. Correct answer is **C.** Testosterone directly inhibits the secretion of gonadotropin-releasing hormone (GnRH) from the hypothalamus. The gonadotropins, luteinizing hormone (LH) and follicle-stimulating hormone (FSH), are anterior pituitary hormones whose synthesis and release is controlled by hypothalamic GnRH. In males, FSH promotes testicular growth and within the Sertoli cells of the seminiferous tubules of the testis. FSH enhances the synthesis of androgen-binding proteins (ABP) whose function is to bind testosterone (T) and dihydrotestosterone (DHT), as well as 17β-estradiol, resulting in the concentration of the male sex hormones within these cells. The concentration of T and DHT leads to the enhancement of spermatogenesis. Therefore, testosterone-mediated inhibition of GnRH release results in reductions in circulating levels of the gonadotropins where the net effect in males would be a decrease in sperm count. None of the other options (choices A, B, D, and E) correctly explain the effects that testosterone exerts on spermatogenesis leading to infertility.

18. Correct answer is **B.** The patient is most likely experiencing the symptoms the adrenal insufficiency associated with Addison disease. The reduced adrenal cortical synthesis of cortisol in Addison disease results in the loss of the feed-back control that cortisol normally exerts on the pituitary. The loss of this feed-back control process results in increased adrenocorticotropic hormone (ACTH) output by the pituitary. The loss of adrenal cortical aldosterone synthesis results in disturbed electrolyte homeostasis. The principal effect of aldosterone is to enhance sodium (Na^+) reabsorption in the connecting tubule (CNT) and cortical collecting duct of the nephrons in the kidneys. Within these regions of the nephron, aldosterone induces the expression of the Na^+/K^+-ATPase subunit genes (*ATP1A1* and *ATP1B1*), the genes encoding the subunits (*SCNN1A, SCNN1B,* and *SCNN1C*) of the epithelial sodium channel (ENaC), and the *SLC12A3* gene (encoding the Na^+-Cl^- cotransporter, NCC). The net effect of the induction of these transporter genes, by aldosterone, is enhanced Na^+ reabsorption as a function of the apical membrane localized ENaC and NCC transporters and delivery to the blood via the action of the basolateral membrane localized Na^+/K^+-ATPase. The loss of aldosterone production is, therefore, associated with the hyponatremia and hyperkalemia found in this patient. Adrenal adenomas (choice A) that result in active secretion of adrenocortical hormones results in hypercortisolemia as is typical in Cushing syndrome. Hyperthyroidism (choice C), such as in Graves disease, is associated with thyrotoxicosis, goiter (enlarged thyroid gland), an ophthalmopathy in the form of exophthalmos (eyes bulge out), and dermopathy in the form of pretibial myxedema. Hypothyroidism (choice D) can have a primary or secondary causes. Primary hypothyroidism directly impacts the thyroid gland resulting in reduced synthesis and release of the thyroid hormones. Typical symptoms of hypothyroidism can include chronic fatigue, unexplained weight gain, cold intolerance, dry flaky skin, and constipation. Pheochromocytoma (choice E) is a neuroendocrine tumor of adrenal medullary chromaffin cells. Adrenal medullary chromaffin cells synthesize and secrete the catecholamines, epinephrine and norepinephrine. Typical symptoms associated with pheochromocytoma are hypertension, headaches, tachycardia, and diaphoresis.

19. Correct answer is **D.** The patient is most likely experiencing the signs and symptoms of hypothyroidism. A primary thyroid gland deficiency leads to low thyroxine (T4) levels and high TSH levels. The most common cause of thyroid gland failure is called autoimmune thyroiditis or Hashimoto thyroiditis. It develops slowly due to persistent inflammation of the thyroid. Hashimoto thyroiditis is most often observed in middle-aged women. The measurement of elevated TSH levels in the blood is of high diagnostic value since it helps determine even minor degrees of hypothyroidism. Correct diagnosis is critical because treatment usually continues for life. Hyperthyroidism (choices A, B, and C) is also known as thyrotoxicosis. The most common hyperthyroidism is Graves disease. Graves disease is associated with goiter, eye disease characterized by inflammation and involvement of intra-orbital structures, and dermopathy referred to as pretibial myxedema. Central hypothyroidism is the term describing hypothyroidism resulting from a defect in the hypothalamic pituitary axis (choice E) where the most common causes are pituitary lesions. However, central hypothyroidism does not represent a significant cause of this condition. Adrenal insufficiency does not result in hypothyroidism (choice F).

20. Correct answer is **D.** The infant is most likely manifesting the signs of cretinism. In the embryo, thyroid hormone is necessary for normal development and hypothyroidism in the embryo is responsible for cretinism, which is characterized by multiple congenital defects and intellectual impairment. Because the neurological consequences of congenital hypothyroidism are severe, neonatal screening for thyroid hormone levels at birth is routine. Most infants born with congenital hypothyroidism appear normal at birth. However, if left untreated the symptoms will include a thick protruding tongue, poor feeding, prolonged jaundice (which exacerbates the neurological impairment), hypotonia (recognized as "floppy baby syndrome"), episodes of choking, and delayed bone maturation resulting in short stature. The most common therapeutic intervention for cretinism is administration of thyroxine (10 to 15 μg/kg of body weight per day). Therapeutic intervention with none of the other substances (choices A, B, C, and E) would provide benefit to this patient.

21. Correct answer is **C.** The most likely cause of the negative ovulation test in this patient is a lack of functional anterior pituitary gonadotropins, luteinizing hormone (LH) or follicle-stimulating hormone (FSH). In females FSH stimulates follicular development and estrogen synthesis by granulosa cells of the ovary. In females, LH induces thecal cells of the ovary to synthesize estrogens and progesterone and promotes estradiol secretion. The surge in LH release that occurs in mid-menstrual cycle is the responsible signal for ovulation. Therefore, the lack of ovulation in this patient is most likely the result of deficiency in LH. Deficiency in none of the other hormones (choices A, B, D, and E) would significantly contribute to the negative ovulation test in this patient.

22. Correct answer is **B.** The patient is most likely experiencing the symptoms of Hashimoto disease. Patients with chronic autoimmune thyroiditis or Hashimoto disease may demonstrate several different serum thyroid autoantibodies, but these vary from patient to patient. Thyroid peroxidase antibodies are found in roughly 85% of patients with Hashimoto disease, about 40% of patients with Graves disease, and in less than 15% of patients with other thyroid disorders. Typical symptoms of Hashimoto disease are extreme fatigue, weight gain, hair loss, depression, and chronic low-level pain. In the early stages of Hashimoto disease, the thyroid enlarges explaining the goiter in this patient. The absence of TSH receptor antibodies rules out Graves disease (choice A). Iodine intoxication (choice C) is extremely rare and is associated with nausea, vomiting, delirium, and shock. Subacute thyroiditis (choice D) is an acute inflammatory disease of the thyroid gland most often the result of a viral infection. The symptoms of subacute thyroiditis are not chronic as they are in this patient. Thyroid dyshormonogenesis type 1, TDH1 (choice E) results from mutations in the gene (*SLC5A5*) that encodes the iodine transporter present in the basolateral membranes of thyroid gland cells (thyrocytes). The transporter is called the Na^+/I^- symporter (NIS) and it functions to transport iodide into thyrocytes from the circulation.

23. Correct answer is **E.** Cortisol is a steroid hormone that exerts its effects by binding to its intracellular receptor, the glucocorticoid receptor. The glucocorticoid receptor is a member of the large family of nuclear receptors that are ligand-activated transcription factors. The major organs that are targets for the transcriptional regulatory actions of the glucocorticoids are the liver, adipose tissue, and skeletal muscle. Numerous additional tissues, including the adrenal glands are targets for the actions of the glucocorticoids. Phenylethanolamine *N*-methyltransferase (PNMT) is an adrenal medullary enzyme whose activity is induced by cortisol. PNMT catalyzes the conversion of norepinephrine to epinephrine. The cortisol-mediated increase in the synthesis and release of epinephrine will trigger fatty acid release from adipose tissue and gluconeogenesis and glycogen breakdown in the liver. These latter effects on hepatic glucose homeostasis define the original identification of the adrenal cortical hormones, cortisol and corticosterone, as glucocorticoids. Genes encoding none of the other enzymes (choices A, B, C, and D) are directly regulated by glucocorticoids.

24. Correct answer is **B.** The glucocorticoids, cortisol and corticosterone, and the synthetic mimetics such as dexamethasone, exert their effects by binding to an intracellular receptor called the glucocorticoid receptor, GR. The GR is a member of the large family of nuclear receptors that are ligand activated transcription factors. Numerous tissues are targets for the actions of the glucocorticoids and the resultant activation of target genes in these tissues results in increased levels of the encoded proteins. Many of the induced proteins may have a prolonged half-life such that several hours after the removal of the dexamethasone from the body the proteins may likely still be present in the target cells. None of the other options (choices A, C, D, and E) correctly define the long-term effects of dexamethasone.

25. Correct answer is **A.** The infant is manifesting the signs and symptoms of a congenital adrenal hyperplasia, CAH. CAH are a group of inherited disorders that result from loss-of-function mutations in one of several genes involved in adrenal steroid hormone synthesis. The most common forms of CAH are caused by defects in either *CYP21A2* (21-hydroxylase, also identified as just CYP21 or CYP21B) or *CYP11B1* (11β-hydroxylase). The majority of CAH cases (90–95%) are the result of defects in *CYP21A2*. In the virilizing forms of CAH the mutations in *CYP21A2* result in impairment of cortisol and corticosterone production in the *zona fasciculata* and aldosterone production in the *zona glomerulosa*, and the consequent accumulation of steroid intermediates proximal to the defective enzyme. In the virilizing forms of CAH there is increased ACTH secretion due to loss of cortisol-mediated feedback inhibition of its release from the pituitary. The excess ACTH stimulates adrenal cortical hormone synthesis where the androgens, dehydroepiandrosterone (choice B) and androstenedione, synthesized by *zona reticularis* cells, are the only ones possible due to 21-hydroxylase deficiency. Defects in the synthesis of none of the other hormones (choices C, D, and E) occur in congenital adrenal hyperplasia.

CHAPTER

33

Blood Coagulation

High-Yield Terms

Hemostasis	Refers to the process of blood clotting and then the subsequent dissolution of the clot following repair of the injured tissue
Intrinsic pathway	Pathway of coagulation initiated in response to contact of blood with a negatively charged surface, primarily represents a pathophysiologic reaction
Extrinsic pathway	Pathway of coagulation initiated in response to release of tissue factor in response to vascular injury; represents the normal physiologic pathway of coagulation
Platelets	Also called thrombocytes, are small, disk-shaped non-nucleated fragments released from megakaryocytes involved in initiating hemostasis
Platelet glycoproteins	Refers to several types of platelet surface receptors (eg, GPIIb-GPIIIa) involved in the processes of platelet activation and aggregation
Kallikrein	Any of several serine proteases that cleave kininogens to form kinins; includes plasma and tissue kallikreins
Kinin	Any of a group of vasoactive polypeptides (eg, bradykinin) formed by kallikrein-catalyzed cleavage of kininogens causing vasodilation and altering vascular permeability
Tenase complex	The complex of calcium ions and factors VIIIa, IXa, and X on the surface of activated platelets
Prothrombinase complex	A complex composed of platelet phospholipids, calcium ions, factors Va and Xa, and prothrombin
Thrombus	Refers to the blood clot which is the final product of the blood coagulation
von Willebrand factor, vWF	A complex multimeric glycoprotein that is produced by and stored in the α-granules of platelets and found associated with subendothelial connective tissue
Factor V Leiden	An inherited disorder of blood clotting resulting from a variant factor V that causes a hypercoagulability disorder
Partial thromboplastin time (PTT)	Assay for defects in activities of the intrinsic pathway of coagulation
Prothrombin time (PT)	Assay for defects in activities of the extrinsic pathway of coagulation

EVENTS OF BLOOD COAGULATION

The process of blood clotting and then the subsequent dissolution of the clot following repair of the injured tissue is termed hemostasis. Hemostasis proceeds through a series of four coordinated events required to respond to the loss of vascular integrity.

1. The initial phase of the process is vascular constriction. This limits the flow of blood to the area of injury.
2. Activation of platelets is absolutely required for hemostasis to proceed. Platelets become activated by thrombin and aggregate at the site of injury, forming a temporary, loose platelet plug. Platelets clump by binding to collagen that becomes exposed following rupture of the endothelial lining of vessels. On activation, platelets release contents of their granules that are critical for the coagulation cascade. In addition to induced secretion, activated platelets change their shape to accommodate the formation of the plug.
3. To ensure stability of the initially loose platelet plug, a fibrin mesh (also called the clot) forms and entraps the plug. If the plug contains only platelets and fibrin, it is termed a **white thrombus**; if red blood cells are present, it is called a **red thrombus.**

4. Finally, the clot must be dissolved in order for normal blood flow to resume following tissue repair. The dissolution of the clot occurs through the action of plasmin.

PLATELET ACTIVATION AND von WILLEBRAND FACTOR (vWF)

The initial activation of platelets is induced by thrombin binding to specific receptors on the surface of platelets, thereby initiating a signal transduction cascade (Figure 33–1). The thrombin receptors are protease-activated receptors (PAR) that are members of the large GPCR family. There are three PAR to which thrombin binds identified as PAR-1 (PAR1), PAR-3 (PAR3), and PAR-4 (PAR4).

In order for platelets to fully participate in blood coagulation, they must adhere to the collagen of the subendothelial ECM that is exposed on vascular injury. On adhering, platelets release the contents of their granules and aggregate.

The adhesion of platelets to the collagen exposed on endothelial cell surfaces is mediated by vWF. Inherited deficiencies of vWF are the causes of von Willebrand disease, (vWD) (Clinical Box 33–1). The function of vWF is to act as a bridge between a specific glycoprotein complex on the surface of

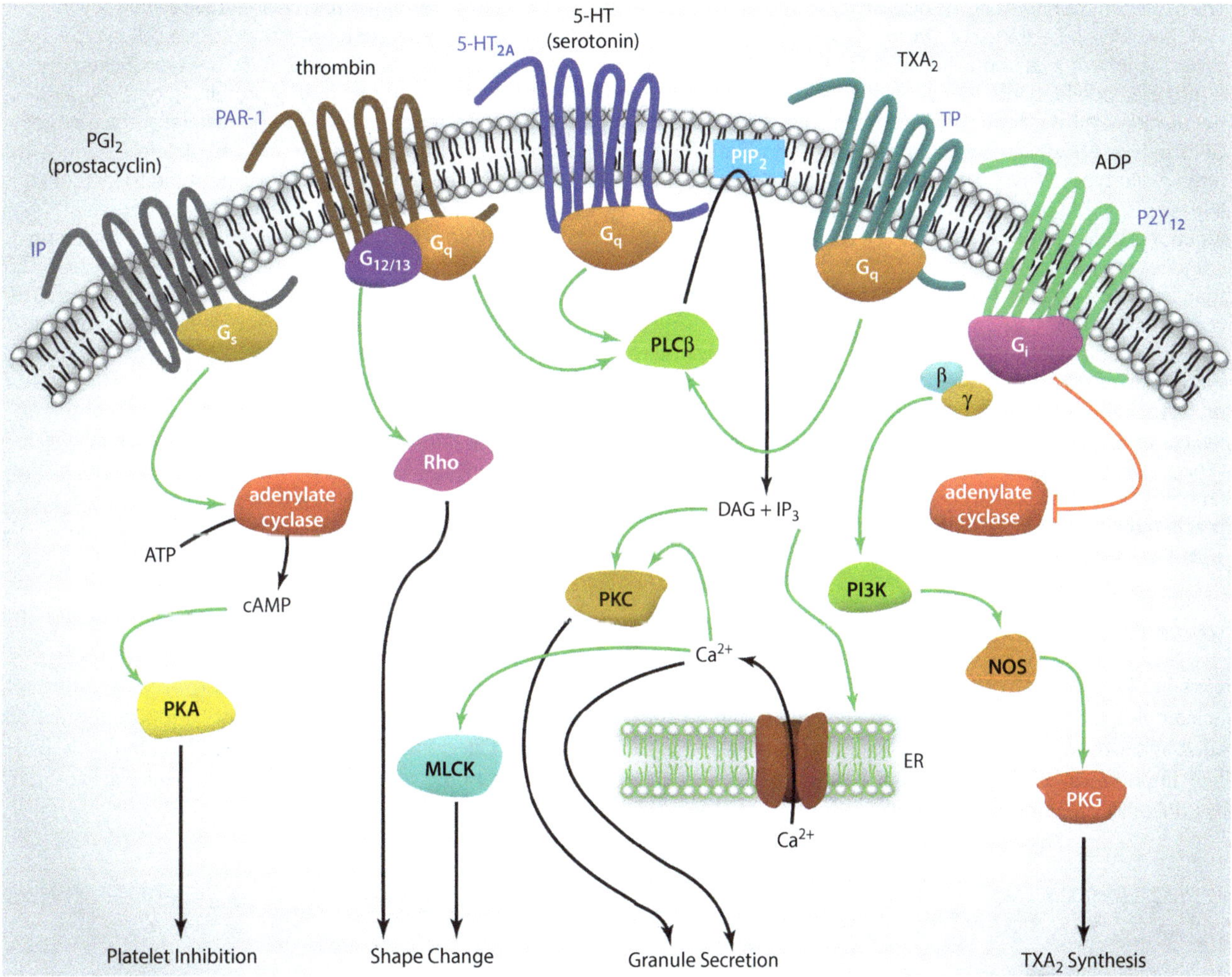

FIGURE 33–1 Signaling pathways involved in the regulation of platelet activation. Regulation of platelet activation occurs via the interaction of numerous effector molecules with receptors present in the plasma membranes of platelets. Two important receptors are the glycoproteins GPIb-GPIX-GPV and GPIIb-GPIIIa. Numerous G-protein–coupled receptors (GPCR) are also involved in platelet functions. Five different GPCR, their respective ligands, and brief representations of their signal transduction pathways are shown. The prostacyclin receptor is IP. The represented thrombin receptor is protease-activated receptor-1 (PAR-1). PAR-1 is known to activate both G_q– and G_{12}-type G-proteins. The platelet serotonin receptor is $5HT_{2A}$. The thromboxane (TXA_2) receptor is TP. The platelet ADP receptor is $P2Y_{12}$. Although complex, the complete signaling pathways are not shown for simplicity. Rho represents a typical member of the Rho family of monomeric G-proteins. The β and γ subunits of the G_i-type G-protein associated with the ADP receptor can activate the kinase, PI3K while the α subunit simultaneously inhibits the activation of adenylate cyclase. NOS is nitric oxide synthase. MLCK: myosin light-chain kinase. (Reproduced with permission from themedicalbiochemistrypage, LLC.)

CLINICAL BOX 33-1 von WILLEBRAND DISEASE

von Willebrand disease (vWD) is caused by deficiencies in the protein von Willebrand factor (vWF). vWF is a multi-subunit glycoprotein that is found in subendothelial connective tissue, the blood, and in the α granules of platelets. vWD and vWF get their name from Erik von Willebrand who first described a bleeding disorder whose mode of inheritance was autosomal rather than X-linked (as in hemophilia A and hemophilia B). In addition, the disease resulted in bleeding from mucocutaneous sites (typical skin and mucous membranes) rather than from deep tissues and joints. vWD is the most commonly occurring bleeding disorder with clinically significant forms affecting approximately 1 in 1000 individuals. However, abnormalities in vWF have been estimated to occur with a frequency of 1 in 100 persons, thus a relatively small fraction of persons harboring mutations in vWF actually experience symptoms. vWF is involved in two important reactions of hemostasis (blood coagulation). The first is the interaction of vWF with specific receptors on the surface of platelets and the subendothelial connective tissue. This interaction allows platelets to adhere to areas of vascular injury. The second role of vWF is to bind to and stabilize factor VIII allowing factor VIII to survive in the blood. As a consequence of these roles for vWF, deficiencies result in defective platelet adhesion and to secondary deficiencies in factor VIII. Since factor VIII deficiency results in hemophilia A, it is not surprising that vWF deficiencies can manifest with clinical symptoms that appear to be hemophilia A. There are both dominant and recessive forms of vWD. The most common form of the disease (type 1) is an autosomal dominant disorder resulting from quantitative deficiency in vWF. Recessive inheritance of a virtual lack of vWF protein characterizes the clinically severe form of the disease called type 3 vWD. The inheritance of qualitative defects in vWF (dysfunctional protein) is characteristic of type 2 vWD. The type 2 category is further subdivided into four variants that are based on the functional characteristics of the mutant protein. In type 2A vWD the residual vWF has reduced function. In type 2B vWD the mutant vWF has an increased affinity for the platelet surface protein GPIb. In type 2M vWD there is the presence of normal vWF multimeric complexes, but they exhibit reduced platelet-dependent function. In type 2N vWD there are factor VIII deficiencies that are the result of mutations in vWF that do not bind to factor VIII. In patients with type 1 and type 3 vWD (the quantitative deficiencies) the severity of the disease is related to the degree of functional deficiency in vWF. Clinically, type 1 and 3 vWD patients can manifest from insignificant problems to life-threatening complications. Patients with type 2 vWD (the qualitative deficiencies) may exhibit symptoms whose severity may be greater than would be expected based on a knowledge of the functional defect. Symptoms of vWD often present shortly after birth. The common symptoms are easy bruising, bleeding from the gums, cutaneous hematomas, and prolonged bleeding from cuts and abrasions. Individuals with severe forms of vWD can have bleeding complications because they either lack sufficient vWF to promote platelet adhesion at the site of vascular injury or they are factor VIII deficient due to the lack of the stabilizing action of vWF on factor VIII. The therapeutic response to vWD requires an understanding of the distinct functions of vWF. Mucocutaneous and postsurgical bleeding can be treated by raising the level of factor VIII. In order to address the platelet adhesion deficit in vWD it is necessary to increase the level of functional vWF. THIS can be accomplished using fresh frozen plasma or cryoprecipitates. The limitation to these approaches is that a large volume of frozen plasma is needed to deliver sufficient amount of vWF and cryoprecipitates are known to be associated with possible disease transmission. Platelet transfusions can be helpful in some patients with vWD, especially those who are refractory to factor VIII-vWF concentrates.

platelets (GPIb-GPIX-GPV) and collagen fibrils. The GPIb part of the complex is composed of two proteins, GPIbα and GPIbβ encoded by separate genes.

The importance of the interaction between vWF and the GPIb-GPIX-GPV complex of platelets is demonstrated by the inheritance of bleeding disorders caused by defects in three of the four proteins of the complex. The most common disorder resulting from defects in the GPIb-GPIX-GPV complex is Bernard-Soulier syndrome which is also known as giant platelet syndrome (Clinical Box 33–2).

CLINICAL BOX 33-2 BERNARD-SOULIER SYNDROME

Bernard-Soulier syndrome (BSS) is a bleeding disorder that was first described in 1948 by Jean Bernard and Jean Pierre Soulier. Although the frequency of BSS is approximately 1 in 1,000,000 it is still the second most common inherited bleeding disorder that results as a consequence of defects in platelet function. BSS is characterized by, among other symptoms, the presence of giant platelets. Hence the disorder is also known as Giant Platelet syndrome. In addition to the presence of giant platelets, patients experience a prolonged bleeding time. Although platelets from these individuals will aggregate in response to the presence of epinephrine, collagen, and/or ADP they will not aggregate in the presence of ristocetin. Ristocetin is an antibiotic isolated from *Amycolatopsis lurida* that was once used to treat staphylococcal infections. Ristocetin induces binding of von Willebrand factor to platelet glycoprotein Ib (GPIb) and, as a consequence of this activity, the compound is used in a diagnostic assay for von Willebrand disease. Bernard-Soulier syndrome is an autosomal recessive disorder in which most patients have either a decrease or absence of all four proteins of the platelet surface glycoprotein complex identified as the GPIb complex. This platelet glycoprotein complex

CLINICAL BOX 33–2 (CONTINUED)

serves as a binding site for von Willebrand factor (vWF) which then acts as a bridge between subendothelial extracellular matrix collagen fibrils exposed at the site of injury and platelets. This interaction between the platelet GPIb complex, vWF, and collagen is absolutely required for platelet adhesion and subsequent aggregation at the site of injury. The absence of platelet aggregation results in failure of the blood coagulation cascade. At least 18 different molecular defects have been identified resulting in Bernard-Soulier syndrome. The GPIb complex is composed of four different proteins encoded by four distinct genes. The proteins are identified as GPIbα, GPIbβ, GPIX, and GPV. The GPIbα and GPIbβ subunits form a disulfide-bonded heterodimer. The association of GPV and GPIX proteins into the complex is noncovalent. Mutations in GPIbα result in type A BSS, mutations in GPIbβ result in type B BSS, and mutations in GPIX result in type C BSS. The first identified mutation in BSS was found in the *GP1BA* gene and there are now at least 11 known alleles of this gene comprising nonsense and missense mutations. The clinical manifestations of Bernard-Soulier syndrome are similar to those in patients with dysfunctional platelets. These symptoms include mucocutaneous bleeding (bleeding from mucous membranes and skin), gastrointestinal hemorrhage, and purpuric skin bleeding (bleeding from purplish patches on the skin). In female patients there is the additional complication of menorrhagia. Evaluation of Bernard-Soulier patients is done by analysis of platelet number and size. All patients will have some level of thrombocytopenia (decreased platelet number) and platelets that are from 3 to 20 times normal size. Bleeding times are increased in Bernard-Soulier syndrome, but the distinguishing abnormality is the failure of platelet aggregation (agglutination) in the presence of ristocetin. This aggregation defect cannot be corrected by the addition of normal plasma. Treatment of bleeding in Bernard-Soulier patients is accomplished by local application of pressure, topical thrombin, and platelet transfusion. In female patients, hormonal management of menses is important.

In addition to its role as a bridge between platelets and exposed collagen on endothelial surfaces, vWF binds to and stabilizes coagulation factor VIII. Binding of factor VIII by vWF is required for normal survival of factor VIII in the circulation.

Once adherent to the endothelium, further activation of platelets involves binding of thrombin as well as several factors released from platelet granules such as ADP and TXA_2 (see Figure 33–1). Platelets contain three types of granules termed dense, alpha, and lysosomal. Dense granules contain serotonin, calcium ions, and ADP. Alpha granules contain fibronectin, vWF, fibrinogen, factor V, factor IX, protein S, high-molecular-weight kininogen (HMWK), platelet factor-4 (PF-4), thrombospondin-1, and plasminogen activator inhibitor-1 (PAI-1). Lysosomal granules contain acid hydrolases, β-galactosidase, and β-glucuronidase.

ADP signaling occurs by binding to a GPCR of the P2Y family ($P2Y_{12}$). Activation of this receptor on platelets results in exposure of the platelet glycoprotein receptor complex: GPIIb-GPIIIa. The important role of ADP in platelet activation can be appreciated from the use of the ADP receptor antagonist, clopidogrel, in the control of blood coagulation.

The importance of the GPIIb-GPIIIa complex in platelet activation and coagulation is demonstrated by the fact that bleeding disorders result from inherited defects in this glycoprotein complex. The most common inherited platelet dysfunction is Glanzmann thrombasthenia (Clinical Box 33–3) which results from defects in the GPIIb protein. In addition, the importance of this complex in overall hemostasis is demonstrated by the use of complex antagonists as anticoagulants (eg, abciximab).

CLINICAL BOX 33–3 GLANZMANN THROMBASTHENIA

Glanzmann thrombasthenia (weak platelets) is an autosomal recessive disorder affecting the processes of blood coagulation that was originally described in 1918 by the Swiss pediatrician W.E. Glanzmann as a heterogenous group of bleeding disorders. The hallmark of the disease is the failure of platelets to bind fibrinogen and aggregate in the presence of a variety of physiological agonist such as ADP, thrombin, epinephrine, or collagen. Glanzmann thrombasthenia is a bleeding disorder in which the underlying defect in all patients is an abnormality in the gene encoding either the GPIIb (integrin α2b) or GPIIIa (integrin β3) protein of the GPIIb-GPIIIa complex. The GPIIb-GPIIIa complex is a member of integrin family of cell surface receptors and is also called integrin α2bβ3 (also written as αIIbβ3). The platelet GPIIb-GPIIIa complex is the most abundant platelet receptor representing approximately 15% of the total protein on the surface of platelets. Although Glanzmann thrombasthenia is a rare disorder it is the most recognized inherited disorder of platelet function. Over 200 individuals have been described as having Glanzmann thrombasthenia and in more than 60 cases the molecular defect has been identified. The molecular abnormalities causing Glanzmann thrombasthenia range from major gene deletions and inversions to single-point mutations. These mutations have been grouped according to the biochemical consequences and include transcriptional and protein functional defects. Among the functional defects there are protein stability mutants, glycoprotein complex maturation mutants, and ligand-binding mutants. The clinical manifestations of Glanzmann thrombasthenia are significant mucocutaneous bleeding that is evidenced at an early age. Lifelong repeated bleeding at sites of minor trauma such as the gums (gingival) and the nose (epistaxis). In females heavy bleeding during menstruation may require therapeutic intervention. Severe intracranial or gastrointestinal hemorrhage can occur spontaneously (ie, unprovoked by injury) and is a significant cause of mortality in 5–10% of Glanzmann thrombasthenia patients. Treatment of the disorder is limited to local measures such as the application of pressure. Platelet transfusion may be useful but only on a limited basis as resistance will develop to the infused platelets.

THE CLOTTING CASCADES

Activation of platelets is required for their consequent aggregation with fibrin to form a platelet plug. Two pathways lead to the formation of a fibrin clot: the intrinsic and extrinsic pathways (Figure 33–2). Fibrin clot formation in response to tissue injury is the most clinically relevant event of hemostasis under normal physiological conditions. This process is the result of the activation of the extrinsic pathway. The intrinsic pathway has low significance under normal physiologic conditions.

Although both the extrinsic and intrinsic coagulation pathways are initiated by distinct mechanisms, the two converge on a common pathway that leads to clot formation. Both pathways are complex and involve numerous different proteins termed clotting factors (Table 33–1).

HIGH YIELD CONCEPT

Many of the clotting factors are modified post-translationally by the addition of a second carboxylic acid group to glutamate (Glu) residues in the proteins. These modified Glu are referred to as "gla" residues. The gla residues are added via the actions of a vitamin K-dependent enzyme, gamma-glutamyl carboxylase (GGCX). The presence of a gla residue allows for the chelation of calcium ions, a key regulatory process for activation of these coagulation factors. The gla residue containing clotting factors are prothrombin (factor II), factors VII, IX, and X, and protein C and protein S. Calcium ions (Ca^{2+}) were, at one time, considered factor IV of the coagulation cascades.

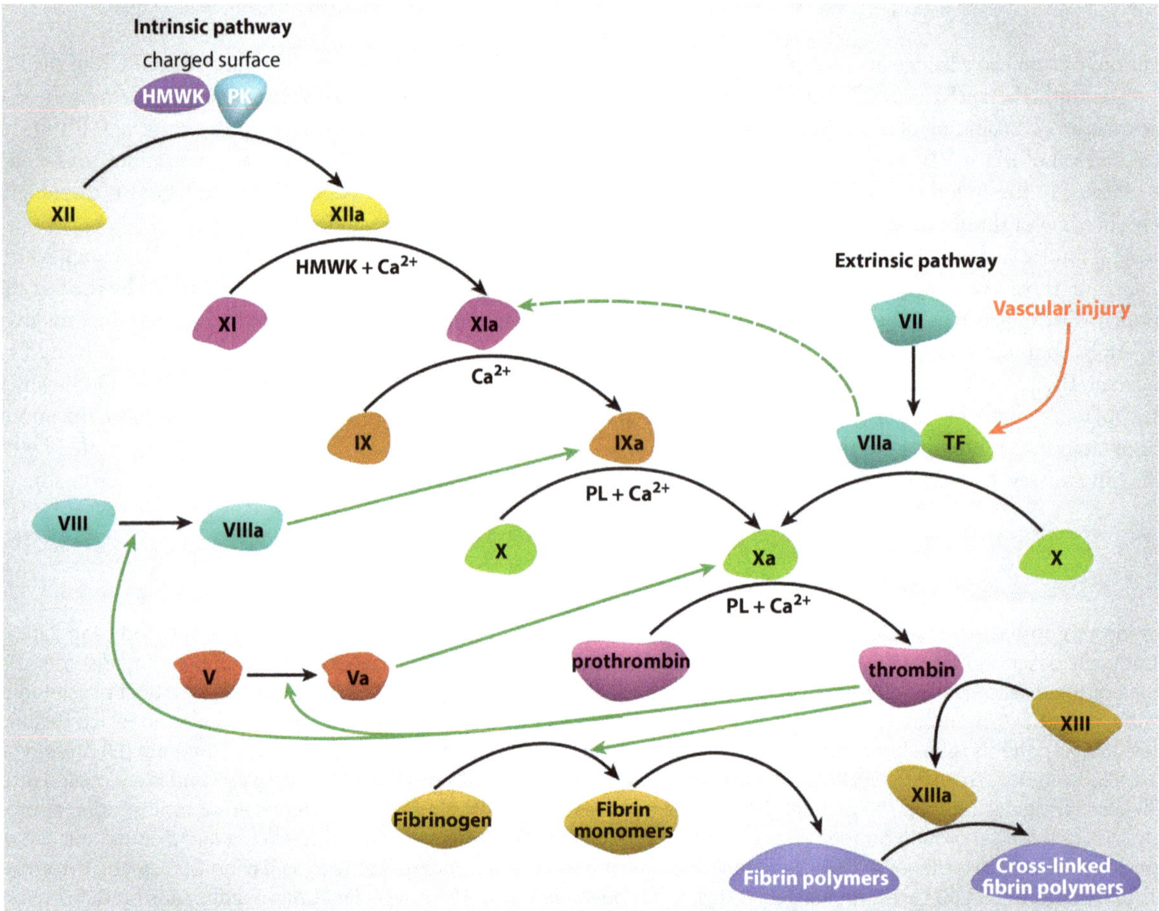

FIGURE 33–2 The clotting cascades. The intrinsic cascade (which has less in vivo significance in normal physiologic circumstances than the extrinsic cascade) is initiated when contact is made between blood and exposed negatively charged surfaces. The extrinsic pathway is initiated on vascular injury which leads to exposure of tissue factor, TF (also identified as factor III), a subendothelial cell-surface glycoprotein that binds phospholipid. The green dotted arrow represents a point of crossover between the extrinsic and intrinsic pathways. The two pathways converge at the activation of factors X to Xa. Factor Xa has a role in the further activation of factors VII to VIIa as depicted by the green arrow. Active factor Xa hydrolyzes and activates prothrombin to thrombin. Thrombin can then activate factors XI, VIII, and V, furthering the cascade. Ultimately the role of thrombin is to convert fribrinogen to fibrin and to activate factors XIII to XIIIa. Factor XIIIa (also termed transglutaminase) cross-links fibrin polymers solidifying the clot. HMWK: high-molecular-weight kininogen. PK: prekallikrein. PL: phospholipid. (Reproduced with permission from themedicalbiochemistrypage, LLC.)

TABLE 33–1 Proteins involved in blood coagulation.

Factor	Trivial Name(s)	Pathway	Characteristic/Activities
Prekallikrein (PK)	Fletcher factor	Intrinsic	Functions with HMWK and factor XII
High-molecular-weight kininogen (HMWK)	Contact activation cofactor; Fitzgerald, Flaujeac Williams factor	Intrinsic	Cofactor in kallikrein and factor XII activation, necessary in factor XIIa activation of XI, precursor for bradykinin (a potent vasodilator and inducer of smooth muscle contraction)
Fibrinogen	Factor I	Both	Cleaved by thrombin into fibrin monomers allowing for self-assembly into a regular array that forms a weak fibrin clot
Prothrombin	Factor II	Both	Contains N-term. *gla* segment; while on the surface of activated platelets the prothrombinase complex (platelet phospholipids, Ca^{2+}, factors Va and Xa, and prothrombin) hydrolyzes prothrombin-releasing active thrombin
Tissue factor	Factor III	Extrinsic	A subendothelial cell-surface glycoprotein that acts as a cofactor for factor VII
V	Proaccelerin, labile factor, accelerator (Ac-) globulin	Both	Activated by minute amounts of thrombin; factor Va is a primary cofactor of the prothrombinase complex that utilizes factor Xa proteolysis of prothrombin to active thrombin
VII	Proconvertin, serum prothrombin conversion accelerator (SPCA), cothromboplastin	Extrinsic	Activated by thrombin in presence of Ca^{2+}; factor VIIa functions with tissue factor in the activation of factor X
VIII	Antihemophiliac factor A, antihemophilic globulin (AHG)	Intrinsic	Activated by thrombin; factor VIIIa is a component of the tenase complex that includes factors VIIIa, IXa, and X, as well as Ca^{2+}; functions as the scaffold for the formation of the tenase complex
IX	Christmas factor, antihemophilic factor B, plasma thromboplastin component (PTC)	Intrinsic	Activated by factor XIa in presence of Ca^{2+}; factor IXa is a component of the tenase complex (factors VIIIa, IXa, X, and Ca^{2+})
X	Stuart-Prower Factor	Both	Activated on surface of activated platelets by tenase complex and by factor VIIa in presence of tissue factor and Ca^{2+}
XI	Plasma thromboplastin antecedent (PTA)	Intrinsic	Component of the contact phase complex; is activated by factor XIIa; factor XIa activates factor IX to IXa
XII	Hageman factor	Intrinsic	Binds to exposed collagen at site of vessel wall injury which autoactivates the enzyme; factor XIIa activates prekallikrein to kallikrein and kallikrein cleaves HMWK-releasing bradykinin; reciprocal activation of factor XII by kallikrein resulting in amplification of the system
XIII	Protransglutaminase, fibrin-stabilizing factor (FSF), fibrinoligase	Both	Activated by thrombin in presence of Ca^{2+}; stabilizes fibrin clot by covalent cross-linking of fibrin monomers
von Willebrand factor		Intrinsic	Associated with subendothelial connective tissue; serves as a bridge between platelet glycoprotein GPIb/IX and collagen
Protein C		Both	Activated to protein Ca by thrombin bound to thrombomodulin; then degrades factors VIIIa and Va
Protein S		Both	Acts as a cofactor of protein C; both proteins contain *gla* residues
Thrombomodulin		Both	Protein on the surface of endothelial cells; binds thrombin, which then activates protein C
Serpin family A member 10 (SERPINA10)	Protein Z-dependent protease inhibitor (PZI)	Both	Degrades activated factor X (Xa) and activated factor XI (XIa) in complex with protein Z, Ca^{2+}, and phospholipids
Protein Z		Both	Required cofactor for the activation of PZI; deficiency is associated with a procoagulant state caused by excessive Xa and thrombin production, dysfunction is linked with several thrombotic disorders, including arterial vascular and venous thromboembolic diseases

INTRINSIC PATHWAY AND THE ROLE OF THE KALLIKREIN-KININ SYSTEM

Activation of the intrinsic pathway of coagulation, in part, involves the contribution of the kallikrein-kinin system. This system comprises a complex of proteins that when activated leads to the release of vasoactive kinins. The kinins are released from both high-molecular-weight kininogen (HMWK) and low molecular weight kininogen (LMWK) via activation of either plasma kallikrein or tissue kallikrein, respectively.

The kinins are involved in many physiologic and pathologic processes including regulation of blood pressure and flow (via modulation of the renin-angiotensin pathway), blood coagulation, cellular proliferation and growth, angiogenesis, apoptosis, and inflammation. Kinin action on endothelial cells leads to vasodilation, increased vascular permeability, release of tissue plasminogen activator (tPA), production of nitric oxide (NO), and the mobilization of arachidonic acid, primarily resulting in prostacyclin (PGI_2) production by endothelial cells. With respect to hemostasis the most important kinin is bradykinin which is released from HMWK. Bradykinin is a 9-amino acid vasoactive peptide that induces vasodilation and increases vascular permeability.

The plasma kinin forming system is composed of factor XII, factor XI, prekallikrein, and HMWK. Factor XII, prekallikrein, and HMWK reversibly bind to endothelial cells, platelets, and granulocytes. Interaction with a charged surface (referred to as contact activation) results in autoactivation of factor XII to factor XIIa. Factor XIIa then activates prekallikrein to kallikrein and kallikrein cleaves HMWK-releasing bradykinin.

Several physiological substances serve as the charged surface to which the contact system binds. These substances include phospholipids, oxidized LDL (oxLDL), hematin (hydroxide of heme), fatty acids, sodium urate crystals, protoporphyrin, sulfatides, heparins, chondroitin sulfates, articular cartilage, endotoxin, homocysteine, and amyloid β-protein.

EXTRINSIC CLOTTING CASCADE

The extrinsic pathway is initiated at the site of injury in response to the release of tissue factor and thus, is also known as the tissue factor pathway. Tissue factor is a cofactor in the factor VIIa-catalyzed activation of factor X. Factor VIIa cleaves factor X to factor Xa in a manner identical to that of factor IXa of the intrinsic pathway. Indeed, activated factor Xa is the site at which the intrinsic and extrinsic coagulation cascades converge. The activation of factor VII occurs through the action of thrombin or factor Xa. The ability of factor Xa to activate factor VII creates a link between the intrinsic and extrinsic pathways. An additional link between the two pathways exists through the ability of tissue factor and factor VIIa to activate factor IX.

HIGH-YIELD CONCEPT

The formation of a complex between factor VIIa and tissue factor is believed to be a principal step in the overall clotting cascade. Evidence for this stems from the fact that persons with hereditary deficiencies in the components of the contact phase of the intrinsic pathway do not exhibit clotting problems.

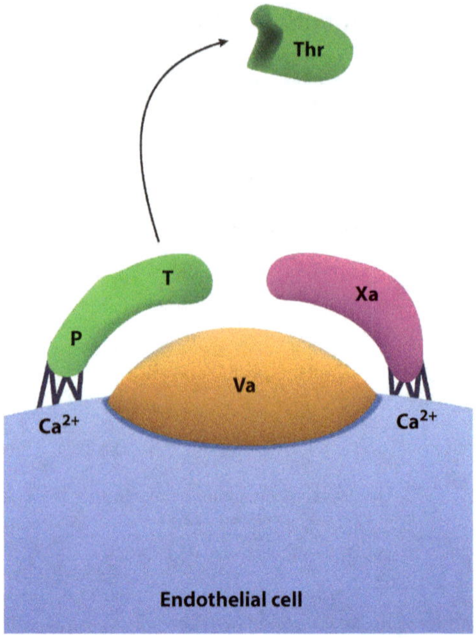

FIGURE 33–3 Formation of the prothrombinase complex and release of active thrombin. Prothrombin (PT) binds to the complex of calcium ion, active factor V (Va), and active factor X (Xa) which then leads to the catalytic release of active thrombin. (Reproduced with permission from themedicalbiochemistrypage, LLC.)

ACTIVATION OF PROTHROMBIN TO THROMBIN

Prothrombin conversion to active thrombin is the function of activated factor X (Xa) in the complex referred to as the prothrombinase complex (Figure 33–3). Activated factor V (Va) serves as the primary cofactor in the formation of the prothrombinase complex, similar to the role of factor VIIIa in the tenase complex formation. Active thrombin, in turn, converts fibrinogen to fibrin.

THROMBIN ACTIVATION OF FIBRIN CLOT FORMATION

A major role of thrombin in blood coagulation is the catalytic digestion of fibrinogen to release fibrin monomers termed fibrinopeptides (Figure 33–4). Fibrinogen consists of three pairs of polypeptides designated: $([A\alpha][B\beta][\gamma])_2$. The A and B portions of the Aα and Bβ chains comprise the **fibrinopeptides**, A and B, respectively. The released of the fibrin monomers associate into a subunit structure designated $(\alpha\beta\gamma)_2$. These fibrin structures spontaneously aggregate in a regular array, forming a somewhat weak fibrin clot.

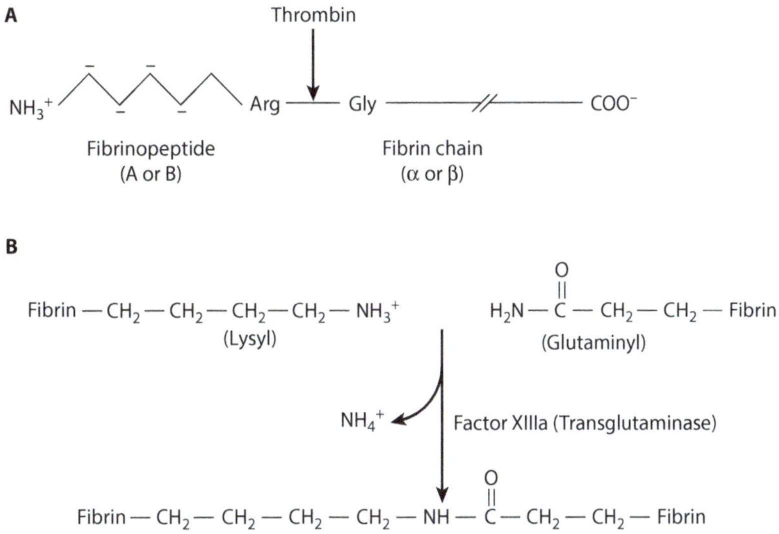

FIGURE 33–4 Formation of a fibrin clot. **(A)** Thrombin-induced cleavage of Arg-Gly bonds of the Aα and Bβ chains of fibrinogen to produce fibrinopeptides (left-hand side) and the α and β chains of fibrin monomer (right-hand side). **(B)** Cross-linking of fibrin molecules by activated factor XIII (factor XIIIa). (Reproduced with permission from Murray RK, Bender DA, Botham KM, et al: *Harper's Illustrated Biochemistry*, 29th ed. New York, NY: McGraw Hill; 2012.)

In addition to fibrin activation, thrombin converts factor XIII to factor XIIIa, a highly specific transglutaminase that introduces cross-links between the fibrin monomers generating an insoluble fibrin clot (Figure 33–4).

CONTROL OF THROMBIN LEVELS

There are two principal mechanisms by which thrombin activity is regulated. The predominant mechanism is the regulated conversion of prothrombin to thrombin via the prothrombinase complex. The level of active thrombin is also regulated by specific thrombin inhibitors. Antithrombin III is the most important since it can also inhibit the activities of factors IXa, Xa, XIa and XIIa, plasmin, and kallikrein.

The activity of antithrombin III is potentiated in the presence of heparan and heparan sulfate on the surface of vessel endothelial cells or by heparin released from basophils and mast cells. Heparin binds to a specific site on antithrombin III inducing a new conformation that has a higher affinity for thrombin as well as its other substrates. This effect of heparin is the basis for its clinical use as an anticoagulant.

PROTEIN C: CONTROL OF COAGULATION AND INTRAVASCULAR INFLAMMATION

Protein C (PC) is a trypsin-like serine protease that serves as a major regulator of the coagulation process. Protein S (PS) serves as a cofactor for the functions of activated protein C (abbreviated aPC). Protein C is activated by thrombin. The activation of PC by thrombin occurs on the surface of the endothelium when thrombin binds to thrombomodulin and "captures" circulating PC (Figure 33–5). Following activation, aPC interacts with PS and cleaves VIIIa and Va, thereby inactivating both of these factors.

The importance of aPC in controlling factor Va activity is evident from the hypercoagulopathy (thrombophilia) referred to as factor V Leiden (Clinical Box 33–4). This thrombophilia is caused by mutations in the factor V gene resulting in a protein that is not effectively degraded by aPC.

CLINICAL BOX 33–4 FACTOR V LEIDEN

The importance of aPC in controlling Va activity can be seen in the hypercoagulopathy (thrombophilia) referred to as factor V Leiden. This thrombophilia is caused by mutations in the factor V gene resulting in a protein that is not effectively degraded by activated protein C (aPC). Factor V Leiden is an autosomal recessive disorder that represents the most common inherited thrombophilia in Caucasian populations of European descent. Overall, 5% of the world population harbors the factor V Leiden mutation. The symptoms of factor V Leiden are deep vein thrombosis (DVT) and pulmonary embolism, both of which can be fatal. In fact, it is estimated that in as many as 30% of patients who experience DVT and/or pulmonary embolisms are carriers of the factor V Leiden mutation. Anyone below the age of 45 experiencing a thromboembolic event, or anyone with a family history of venous thrombosis, may likely be a factor V Leiden individual. Loss of protein C results in massive and usually lethal thrombotic complications in infants with homozygous PC deficiency. In individuals who are heterozygous for PC deficiencies there is an increased risk for venous thrombosis.

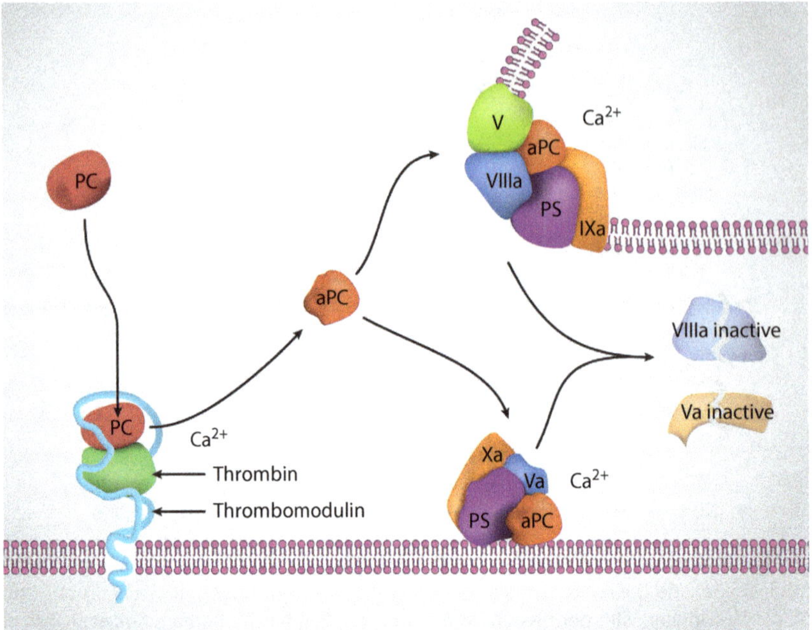

FIGURE 33–5 Role of thrombomodulin in thrombin activation of protein C (PC). Thrombomodulin is an endothelial cell surface glycoprotein that binds thrombin and protein C. The "capture" of thrombin and protein C allows thrombin to activate protein C. Active protein C (APC) then interacts with its cofactor protein S (PS) and cleaves active factors VIII (VIIIa) and V (Va) into inactive forms, thereby terminating their role in coagulation. (Reproduced with permission from themedicalbiochemistrypage, LLC.)

Activated PC is not only functional as an anticoagulation but also serves anti-inflammatory and cytoprotective functions at the level of the endothelial cells of the vasculature and monocytes. Activated PC binds to the endothelial protein C receptor (EPCR) resulting in activation of PAR-1 which elicits cytoprotective and anti-inflammatory responses within endothelial cells. The cytoprotective effects elicited via aPC activation of PAR-1 include protection of the endothelial cell barrier and induction of anti-apoptotic signaling pathways as well as expression of eNOS. Additional endothelial responses to aPC activation of PAR-1 occur via inhibition of the expression and actions of the potent pro-inflammatory transcription factor, NFκB. The suppression of NFκB action results in downregulation of the synthesis of endothelial pro-inflammatory cytokines such as IL-6 and IL-8.

DISSOLUTION OF FIBRIN CLOTS

Degradation of fibrin clots is the function of plasmin, a serine protease that circulates as the inactive pro-enzyme, plasminogen. Plasminogen binds to both fibrinogen and fibrin allowing it to be incorporated into a clot as it is formed. Tissue plasminogen activator (tPA) and, to a lesser degree, urokinase are serine proteases which convert plasminogen to plasmin. Inactive tPA is released from vascular endothelial cells, following injury, and binds to fibrin where it is consequently activated. Active tPA cleaves plasminogen to plasmin which then digests the fibrin (Figure 33–6). The level of active tPA is controlled by binding to specific inhibitory proteins with plasminogen activator-inhibitor type 1 (PAI-1) and PAI-2 being of the greatest physiologic significance. Soluble plasminogen and plasmin are rapidly inactivated primarily by α_2-antiplasmin.

COAGULATION DISORDERS

Disorders in coagulation can result from defects in any of the processes of platelet adherence and activation or with any of the proteins required for coagulation. Assays for coagulation factor function (Clinical Box 33–5) aid in the correct diagnosis of disorders of coagulation.

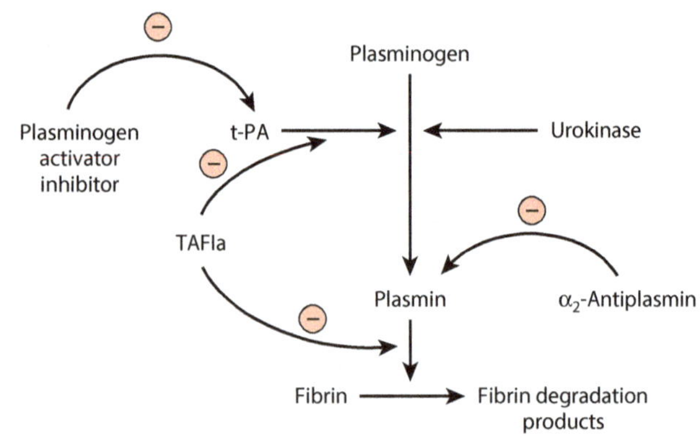

FIGURE 33–6 Initiation of fibrinolysis by the activation of plasmin. Scheme of sites of action of tissue plasminogen activator (t-PA), urokinase, plasminogen activator inhibitor, α2-antiplasmin, and thrombin-activatable fibrinolysis inhibitor (TAFIa) (the last three proteins exert inhibitory actions). (Reproduced with permission from Rodwell VW, Bender DA, Botham KM, et al: *Harper's Illustrated Biochemistry*, 31st ed. New York, NY: McGraw Hill; 2018.)

CLINICAL BOX 33–5 BLOOD COAGULATION TESTS AND INTERPRETATIONS

The primary tests for determination of coagulation activity are bleeding time, prothrombin time (PT), partial thromboplastin time (PTT), and activated partial thromboplastin time (aPTT).

Bleeding time assays are used to evaluate the vascular and platelet responses that are associated with hemostasis. The bleeding time is a frequent assay performed on preoperative patients to ensure there is an adequate response to vessel injury prior to surgery. As indicated earlier, the rapid responses to vascular injury (occurring within seconds) are vessel constriction and platelet adhesion to the vessel wall. The Ivy method for determining the bleeding time involves the use of a blood pressure cuff (sphygmomanometer) which is placed on the forearm and inflated to 40 mm Hg. A superficial incision is then made on the forearm and the time it takes for bleeding to stop is recorded. With the Ivy method bleeding should stop within 1–9 minutes. Any bleeding time greater than 15 minutes would be indicative of a defect in the initial responses of vessels and platelets to vascular injury. A less invasive bleeding time assay involves the use of a lancet or special needle and a 3–4-mm deep prick is made on the fingertip or earlobe. This bleeding time assay is referred to as the Duke method and in this assay bleeding should cease within 1–3 minutes. The bleeding time is affected (prolonged) by any defect in platelet function, by vascular disorders, and in von Willebrand disease but is not affected by other coagulation factors. Disorders that are commonly associated with an increased bleeding time include thrombocytopenia, disseminated intravascular coagulation (DIC), Bernard-Soulier syndrome, and Glanzmann thrombasthenia. Abnormal bleeding times are also found in patients with Cushing syndrome, severe liver disease, leukemia, and bone marrow failure.

The **prothrombin time (PT)** is an assay designed to screen for defects in fibrinogen, prothrombin, and factors V, VII, and X and thus measures activities of the extrinsic pathway of coagulation. When any of these factors is deficient then the PT is prolonged. A normal PT is 11.0–12.5 seconds. A PT greater than 20 seconds is indicative of coagulation deficit. The PT is measured using plasma after the blood cells are removed. A blood sample is collected in a tube containing citrate or EDTA to chelate any calcium and thus inhibit coagulation and then the cells are removed by centrifugation. After the cells are removed, excess calcium is added to the plasma to initiate coagulation. The most common measure of PT is to divide the time of coagulation of a patients' blood by that of a known standard and this value is referred to as the international normalized ratio (INR). Normal INR values range from 0.8–1.2. PT is used to determine the correct dosage of the warfarin class of anticoagulation drugs (eg, Coumadin), for the presence of liver disease or damage, and to evaluate vitamin K status.

The **partial thromboplastin time (PTT)** is used to assay for defects in the intrinsic pathway of coagulation. The PTT assay has been modified by the addition of activators that shorten the normal clotting time, and this form of the assay is referred to as the activated partial thromboplastin time (aPTT). The PTT is normally prescribed for patients with unexplained bleeding or clotting. The assay will evaluate the function of fibrinogen, prothrombin, and factors V, VIII, IX, X, XI, and XII. A defect in any of these factors will result in a prolonged PTT (or aPTT). A normal PTT is 60–70 seconds, whereas for the aPTT the normal range is 30–40 seconds. The PTT is a standard assay used to assess the efficacy of heparin anticoagulant therapy. Prolonged PTTs are associated with acquired or congenital bleeding disorders resulting from coagulation factor deficiency, vitamin K deficiency, liver disease, DIC, von Willebrand disease, leukemia, hemophilia, and during heparin administration.

Coagulation disorders can result in hypercoagulation (referred to as the coagulopathies) or in an inability to coagulate. The most common coagulopathy is Factor V Leiden (see Clinical Box 33–4). Hemophilia A (Clinical Box 33–6) and hemophilia B (Clinical Box 33–7) are probably the most well-known of the coagulation disorders. However, the most common cause of defective coagulation is von Willebrand disease, vWD (see Clinical Box 33–1).

CLINICAL BOX 33–6 HEMOPHILIA A

Hemophilia A is referred to as classic hemophilia and was first recognized in the second century AD. The disease is an X-linked recessive bleeding disorder caused by defects in the clotting cascade enzyme factor VIII. Factor VIII serves as a cofactor in the activation of factor X to Xa in a reaction referred to as the "tenase" complex. The actual enzyme responsible for activating factor X to Xa is activated factor IX (factor IXa). A total of 2537 mutations have been identified in the *F8* gene leading to hemophilia A. These mutations include frameshift mutations, missense mutations, nonsense mutations, gene inversions, large deletions, and splicing errors. Patients with hemophilia A suffer from joint (hemarthrosis) and muscle hemorrhage, easy bruising, and prolonged bleeding time from wounds. Almost all patients with hemophilia A have normal platelet function so the bleeding from minor cuts or abrasions is generally not severe. Hemophilia A can be divided into severe or moderate disease. Approximately 50–60% of hemophilia A patients suffer from the severe form of the disease and have less than 1% normal factor VIII activity. Patients with moderate hemophilia A have from 1 to 20% of normal factor VIII. Because hemophilia A is an X-linked disease almost all patients are male, and the occurrence worldwide is 1 in 5000 male births. It is possible that an affected female can result from the mating of an affected male with a carrier female but the Mendelian frequency for such a situation is approximately

CLINICAL BOX 33-6 (CONTINUED)

1 in 50 million female births. Nonetheless, there have been cases described of female hemophilia A patients. A more common mechanism for presentation of hemophilia A in females is the process of X chromosome inactivation which could lead to inactivation of the X chromosome that harbors the wild-type factor VIII gene. Other rare possibilities also exist for the generation of female hemophilia A but are not discussed here. The frequency and severity of the bleeding in hemophilia A patients is inversely correlated to the level of residual factor VIII protein circulating in the blood. The weight bearing joints are the ones most affected in the disease and include the hips, knees, ankles, and elbows. If the bleeding in the joints is left untreated it will lead to severe swelling and pain, joint stiffness, and inflammation. Blood in the synovial fluid of the joints is highly irritating causing synovial overgrowth and a tendency to cause additional bleeding from the vascular tissues of the joint. The bleeding results in the deposition of iron in chondrocytes with the consequences being the development of degenerative arthritis. Muscle bleeding, like joint bleeding, is most prevalent in large load-bearing muscle groups such as in the thigh, calf, buttocks, and posterior abdominal wall. Since all of these untoward clinical symptoms are the result of a lack of factor VIII in the blood, replacement of factor VIII by intravenous infusion completely normalizes the hemophiliac's blood coagulation (hemostasis) processes.

CLINICAL BOX 33-7 HEMOPHILIA B

Hemophilia B, also known as factor IX deficiency or Christmas disease, is an X-linked recessive bleeding disorder caused by defects in the vitamin K-dependent enzyme, factor IX, of the clotting cascade. Factor IX is also known as the Christmas factor, hence the association of hemophilia B with the term Christmas disease. Activated Factor IX (factor IXa) is the enzyme responsible for the activation of factor X to Xa in a reaction referred to as the "tenase" complex. A cofactor in this reaction is activated factor VIII (factor VIIIa), deficiencies in which result in hemophilia A. Hemophilia B results in a bleeding disorder that is clinically indistinguishable from the more common hemophilia A. Hemophilia B occurs in approximately 1 in 30,000 male births. At least 1094 mutations have been identified in the *F9* gene leading to hemophilia B. The major symptom of hemophilia B is spontaneous bleeding into the joints and the soft tissues of the body. The disease exhibits three levels of manifestation. The severe disease results in patients with less than 1% of normal factor IX protein in the circulation, moderate disease results from 1–5% of normal factor IX protein and mild disease is found when patients have 6–30% of normal factor IX. The most common clinical symptoms of hemophilia B that requires therapeutic intervention are soft tissue hemorrhage and hemarthroses (bleeding in the joints). The leading cause of morbidity and mortality in hemophilia B patients is intracranial hemorrhage. Severely affected patients are usually diagnosed before age 1. The most effective treatment for hemophilia B patients is the administration of highly purified factor IX concentrates or, as is the more common therapeutic practice, the injection of recombinant factor IX protein.

PHARMACOLOGIC INTERVENTION IN BLEEDING

Inhibitors of Vitamin K-Dependent *gla* Residue Formation

The coumarin drugs, such as warfarin inhibit coagulation by inhibiting the vitamin K-dependent γ-carboxylation reactions necessary to the function of functional thrombin, factors VII, IX, and X, as well as proteins C and S, and protein Z. The coumarin drugs take several days for their maximum anticoagulant effects to be realized. For this reason, heparin is normally administered first followed by warfarin or warfarin-related drugs. Protein C is the least stable of the *gla* residue factors and so its anticoagulant function will be lost earliest in coumarin therapies. The early loss of protein C necessitates the need to coadminister heparin in the early stage of coumarin therapies to prevent a hypercoagulopathy.

Activation of Antithrombin III

Heparin functions as an anticoagulant because it binds to, and activates, antithrombin III which then inhibits the serine proteases of the coagulation cascade.

Plasminogen Activators

Recombinant tPA is highly effective for prevention of thrombotic episodes following cardiac ischemia. This is particular true in the short period following myocardial infarct. Streptokinase is another plasminogen activator useful from a therapeutic standpoint.

Inhibition of Eicosanoid Synthesis

Nonsteroidal anti-inflammatories (NSAIDs), such as aspirin function as anticoagulants via inhibition of platelet activation. By virtue of inhibiting the activity of cyclooxygenase (COX), NSAIDs reduce the production of TXA_2 by platelets as well as reducing endothelial cell production of prostacyclin (PGI_2), an inhibitor of platelet aggregation and a vasodilator. Localized to the site of coagulation is a balance between the levels of platelet-derived TXA_2 and endothelial cell-derived PGI_2. This allows for platelet aggregation and clot formation but also prevents excessive accumulation of the clot, thus maintaining blood flow around the site of the clot. Since endothelial cells replenish COX, and thus prostacyclin, the net effect of NSAIDs is inhibition of platelet activation.

Inhibition of Platelet Activation/Function

Several anticoagulation drugs, in addition to NSAIDs, function by inhibiting the activation of platelets and their subsequent aggregation. Clopidogrel is an irreversible inhibitor of the ADP receptors on platelet membranes preventing platelet-derived ADP from participating in further platelet activation. The GPIIb-GPIIIa antagonists more completely inhibit platelet aggregation than do NSAIDs or clopidogrel. The current family of these drugs includes abciximab (a monoclonal antibody), eptifibatide (a cyclic hexapeptide), and tirofiban (a synthetic organic non-peptide molecule).

Inhibition of Thrombin

The direct reversible inhibitor of thrombin, dabigatran, is prescribed to patients suffering from atrial fibrillation (AF) to prevent the occurrence of stroke in these patients. The primary use of dabigatran is in patients being switched from warfarin.

Inhibition of Factor Xa

Inhibition of factor Xa is also useful in patients with atrial fibrillation. The drugs rivaroxaban and apixaban are direct inhibitors of factor Xa either free or within the prothrombinase complex. In addition to prevention of stroke risk in AF patients, rivaroxaban is useful in the prevention of venous thromboembolism.

CHECKLIST

- ☑ Hemostasis is the process of blood clotting and then the subsequent dissolution of the clot following repair of the injured tissue. This involves platelets, interaction of blood with vessel walls, and numerous coagulation factors, many of which are synthesized as pro-enzymes (serine protease zymogens) in the liver.
- ☑ Blood coagulation requires a coordinated series of four events that begins with vasoconstriction to slow the loss of blood, then platelets adhere to the collage exposed at the site of injury leading to activation and aggregation, coagulation factor cascade is initiated terminating with the formation of a cross-linked fibrin clot; when the damage is repaired the clot must be dissolved returning the vessel to normal function.
- ☑ Effective and efficient hemostasis requires that platelets adhere to the exposed ECM at the site of vessel injury. The adherence of platelets results in their activation leading to the release of platelet granule contents and platelet aggregation.
- ☑ Platelet adhesion requires exposed collagen as well as the subendothelial glycoprotein, von Willebrand factor.
- ☑ There are two primary coagulation cascades that are initiated under distinctly different circumstance but that converge by activation of factor X. The intrinsic pathway of coagulation is initiated in response to contact of blood with a negatively charged surface and primarily represents a pathophysiologic reaction. The extrinsic pathway is initiated in response to release of tissue factor in response to vascular injury and represents the normal physiologic pathway of coagulation.
- ☑ For clotting to come to completion, the clotting cascades converge on the activation of factor X which then activates thrombin. Thrombin hydrolyzes fibrinogen and the resulting fibrinopeptides aggregate. Thrombin also activates factor XIII which catalyzes cross-linking of the fibrin monomers.
- ☑ Regulation of the clotting cascades is also initiated by thrombin such that thrombin serves not only to ensure a clot forms but also ensures that the clotting process does not become excessive. Thrombin regulates the extent of coagulation by activating protein C which then hydrolyzes and inhibits the activities of factor VIII and factor V.
- ☑ Clot dissolution following tissue repair is catalyzed by plasmin. Plasmin is released from plasminogen via the action of tissue plasminogen activator (tPA) or urokinase.
- ☑ Numerous bleeding disorders and hypercoagulation disorders result from defects in the processes of hemostasis including platelet function and clotting cascade factors. Deficiencies in von Willebrand factor are the leading cause of bleeding disorders. Hemophilia A and B are the most widely recognized bleeding disorders.
- ☑ Numerous pharmacologic agents are used to control the rate of coagulation including those that interfere with platelet function and those that interfere with clotting factor processing or function.

REVIEW QUESTIONS

1. A 38-year-old woman is being treated for a venous thromboembolism (VTE) that resulted in partial blockage of the hepatic portal vein. The patient's history indicates that she has smoked for 20 years and had experienced two first trimester miscarriages. Which of the following hemostasis disorders is most likely associated with the cause of this patient's miscarriages and VTE?
   (A) Antithrombin III deficiency
   (B) Bernard-Soulier syndrome
   (C) Factor V Leiden
   (D) Glanzmann thrombasthenia
   (E) Hemophilia A
   (F) Hemophilia B
   (G) von Willebrand disease

2. A 7-year-old boy is being examined by a physician because his parents are concerned about his unexplained problems with bleeding. History reveals that the boy has had frequent issues with prolonged bleeding since shortly after birth. The parents report that he experiences easy bruising, bleeding from the gums, and frequent epistaxis. The patient's parents are first cousins, but they themselves showed no issues with bleeding. Hemostatic analysis of the patient's blood showed dramatically prolonged plasma prothrombin clotting time (PT). Given the frequency and type of bleeding evident in this patient and the results of the PT, which of the following is most likely deficient in this patient?
   (A) Factor VIII
   (B) Factor XI
   (C) Factor XIII
   (D) Fibrinogen
   (E) High-molecular-weight kininogen, HMWK
   (F) Platelets

3. A 5-year-old boy is being treated for a suspected case of congenital deficiency in coagulation. He had bled from the umbilical and circumcision sites during his first week of life. He experiences frequent ecchymoses and hematomas within 12–24 hours each time he falls or bumps his legs against a hard surface. His parents are first cousins but there is no family history of bleeding disorders. A bleeding disorder workup is initiated, and the results indicate that PT, PTT, fibrinogen, platelet aggregation studies, and von Willebrand factor are normal. The patient's plasma was incubated with thrombin and Ca^{2+} and the resultant clot dissolved in the presence of urea. Which of the following is most likely defective or deficient in this patient?
   (A) Factor V
   (B) Factor VII
   (C) Factor VIII
   (D) Factor XIII
   (E) Prothrombin

4. A 66-year-old man is admitted to the hospital for a grade III draining ulceration and underlying osteomyelitis of the left fifth metatarsal head. Medical history is significant for type 1 diabetes. Surgical history is significant for a resection of an infected tibial sesamoid of the right foot. Prior to treatment of the ulceration, routine clotting tests were performed and showed an aPTT time of 69.5 seconds (N = 30–40 seconds) while PT was normal. Which of the following factors of coagulation is most likely defective in this patient?
   (A) Factor VII
   (B) Factor XI
   (C) Prekallikrein
   (D) Tissue factor
   (E) Tissue factor pathway inhibitor, TFPI

5. Experiments are being carried out to test the efficacy of several compounds at modifying the process of blood coagulation. Assay of these compounds involves determination of fibrin clot formation. Addition of one compound to whole blood is associated with the formation of a fibrin clot within 3 seconds. Control assays in the absence of the compound generate a fibrin clot in 12 seconds. Given the observed results, which of the following proteins is most likely targeted for inhibition by the test compound?
   (A) Factor V
   (B) Factor XIII
   (C) Fibrinogen
   (D) Protein C
   (E) Thrombin

6. A 3-year-old boy is brought to the emergency department because of persistent blood in his mouth, which is the result of a fall nearly 6 hours ago. His mother says that the child tends to bleed for prolonged periods from his immunization sites, but there is no history of bruising or hematomas. There is no family history of bleeding disorders. Physical examination shows no petechia, no bruising, and no joint swelling. Laboratory studies show a PT of 11.3 seconds (N = 11–12.5 seconds) and an aPTT of 59.7 seconds (N = 30–40 seconds). Which of the following is the most likely diagnosis?
   (A) Afibrinogenemia
   (B) Antithrombin III deficiency
   (C) Factor XI deficiency
   (D) Hemophilia A
   (E) von Willebrand disease

7. A 39-year-old man is being examined to determine the cause of his frequent deep vein thrombotic (DVT) episodes. Analysis of his blood coagulation process indicates a clear hypercoagulopathy. Which of the following is the most likely cause of this patient's pathology?
   (A) Afibrinogenemia
   (B) Bernard-Soulier syndrome
   (C) Factor V Leiden
   (D) Hemophilia A
   (E) von Willebrand disease

8. A 4-year-old boy is brought to his physician because of repeated episodes of easy bruising and epistaxis. Laboratory studies show a bleeding time (utilizing the Duke method) of 1.5 minutes (N = 1–3 minutes), a PTT of 135 seconds (N = 60–90 seconds), and PT of 11.8 seconds (N = 11–12.5 seconds). Platelet count is 285,000 (N = 150,000–450,000). Based on these laboratory findings, which of the following is most likely defective in this patient?
   (A) Factor X
   (B) Platelet adhesion
   (C) Protein C
   (D) Tissue factor
   (E) Vitamin K-dependent carboxylation
   (F) von Willebrand factor

9. A 12-year-old boy is being examined by his pediatrician due to concerns his parents have about his frequent bruising. The

pediatrician performs a coagulation test and determines that the patient's aPTT time is 60 seconds (N = 30–40 seconds). A deficiency in which of the following would most likely explain the findings in this patient?
(A) Factor VII
(B) Factor XIII
(C) Factor IX
(D) Protein C
(E) Tissue factor pathway inhibitor, TFPI

10. Clinical trials are being carried out on a novel regulator of coagulation for use in the therapeutic intervention in patients undergoing percutaneous coronary intervention (PCI) as well as patients with Glanzmann thrombasthenia. This novel compound is most likely targeting which of the following?
(A) GPIa-GPIIa
(B) GPIb-GPIX-GPV
(C) GPIIb-GPIIIa
(D) Prothrombinase complex
(E) Tenase complex

11. A 2-year-old boy is being examined by his pediatrician to determine the cause of his severe and frequent bruising, particularly in his joints. Clotting tests are performed and the patient's aPTT was 65 seconds (N = 30–40 seconds), the PT was 12 seconds (N = 11–12.5 seconds), and platelet count was 230,000 (N = 150,000–450,000). Which of the following is most likely deficient in this patient?
(A) Factor V
(B) Factor IX
(C) GPIIb-GPIIIa
(D) Protein C
(E) Thrombin

12. A 47-year-old fireman is admitted to the emergency room for extensive burns received while battling a fire. He develops pregangrenous changes in multiple digits of both hands, his left foot, and his nose. A short time later, he experiences bleeding from his mucous membranes and IV site, as well as the development of multiple petechiae. Which of the following is the most likely initiating mechanism of this clinical scenario?
(A) Antithrombin III deficiency
(B) Failure of platelet aggregation
(C) Gram-negative bacterial infection
(D) Tissue hypoxemia
(E) Tissue thromboplastin

13. An 8-year-old child has a long history of bleeding dysfunction characterized by spontaneous nontraumatic hemorrhages into joint spaces, skeletal muscle, and mucous membranes. Laboratory studies reveal a normal prothrombin time (PT), elevated partial thromboplastin time (PTT), normal levels of factor X, and normal platelet aggregation studies with ristocetin. Which of the following is the most likely diagnosis?
(A) Bernard-Soulier syndrome
(B) Factor XI deficiency
(C) Glanzmann thrombasthenia
(D) Hemophilia A
(E) von Willebrand disease

14. A 4-year-old girl is being examined to ascertain the cause of her tendency to bleed profusely. History reveals the patient bruises easily and has bleeding from her gums. Analysis of coagulation factors in her blood shows normal levels of factor V but low levels of factor VIII. A platelet aggregation test finds that combination of the patient's serum with normal platelets results in only 20% of the platelet aggregation seen with both samples from a normal individual. Based on these findings this patient is most likely to be deficient in which of the following?
(A) Factor IX
(B) Factor X
(C) Fibrinogen
(D) GPIIb-GPIIIa
(E) von Willebrand factor

15. A 7-year-old boy is being examined by his pediatrician to determine the reason for his bleeding dysfunction. Molecular studies have identified a deletion of exon 2 in the gene encoding prothrombin. Given this mutation, which of the following processes is most likely to be directly affected in this patient?
(A) Activation of high-molecular-weight kininogen
(B) Activation of protein S
(C) Activation of von Willebrand factor
(D) Cleavage of factor IX to IXa
(E) Cleavage of factor X to Xa
(F) Cleavage of factor XIII to XIIIa

16. Clinical trials are being carried out on a novel compound structurally related to acetylsalicylate. When this compound is administered to trial participants, the average platelet aggregation time increases by 70%. The effects of this compound are most likely exerted at the level of which of the following platelet activities or functions?
(A) ADP receptor
(B) Cyclooxygenase
(C) GPIIb-GPIIIa
(D) Phospholipase A_2
(E) von Willebrand factor

17. A 36-year-old man is being examined to determine the cause of his frequent deep vein thrombotic (DVT) episodes. Analysis of his blood coagulation process indicates a definitive hypercoagulopathy. Further studies find that the normal regulation of the extrinsic pathway is defective in this patient. Given these findings, which of the following is most likely to be deficient in this patient?
(A) Antithrombin III
(B) High-molecular-weight kininogen (HMWK)
(C) Lipoprotein-associated coagulation factor (LACI)
(D) Protein C
(E) von Willebrand factor

18. A 12-year-old girl is being attended to in the emergency department due to the fact that she has been bleeding from her nose over the past 60 minutes. History reveals that she has had numerous episodes of epistaxis and gingival bleeding. Analysis of her platelet function finds that binding of von Willebrand factor is greatly reduced most likely due to defective platelet glycoprotein receptor complexes. Given these findings, which of the following is most likely impaired in this patient?
(A) Activation of protein kinase C (PKC), thus, preventing changes to platelet morphology
(B) Adhesion of platelets to vascular endothelial cells
(C) Cleavage and activation of high-molecular-weight kininogen
(D) Induction of platelet crosslinking
(E) Release of prothrombin from platelet granules

19. A 15-year-old boy has frequent episodes of prolonged mucocutaneous bleeding. Coagulation studies determine that his coagulation time, clot retraction, and platelet counts are all within the normal range for his age. Assay for the levels of prothrombin, fibrinogen, factor IX, and factor X finds that all are within the normal range. The level of factor VIII was found to be significantly below normal. Given the symptoms and findings in this individual, which of the following would most likely be defective?
(A) Factor V
(B) GPIIb-GPIIIa
(C) High-molecular-weight kininogen
(D) Tissue factor
(E) von Willebrand factor

20. A 7-year-old girl is being examined by her pediatrician to determine the reason for her bleeding dysfunction. Molecular studies have identified a deletion of exon 2 in the gene (*F2*) encoding prothrombin. Given this mutation, activation of which of the following is most likely to be directly affected in this patient?
(A) Factor V
(B) Factor VII
(C) Factor IX
(D) Factor XI
(E) Factor XIII

21. A 2-year-old boy is being examined by his pediatrician to determine the cause of his severe and frequent bruising, particularly in his knees and elbows. Clotting tests are performed and the patient's aPTT was 75 seconds (N = 30–40 seconds), whereas the PT and platelet counts were within the normal ranges. Which of the following is most likely deficient in this patient?
(A) Factor VIII
(B) Fibrinogen
(C) GPIIb-GPIIIa
(D) Thrombin
(E) von Willebrand factor

22. Experiments are being conducted on a novel monoclonal antibody that was designed to interfere with the coagulation process. The results of these experiments show that the antibody functions very similarly to a previously approved monoclonal antibody, abciximab. Given this finding, which of the following is the most likely target of this new antibody?
(A) Factor Xa
(B) Fibrinogen
(C) GPIIb-GPIIIa
(D) Receptor $P2Y_{12}$
(E) Thrombin

23. A 3-year-old boy is being examined in the Emergency Department for a possible fracture after having fallen off a chair at home. Physical examination shows the patient to be in significant distress with painful erythematous edema on the left knee and multiple bruises on his left thigh and buttocks. An x-ray does not find any evidence of a fracture in the leg or hips. The patient's parents report that their son had significant bleeding when he was circumcised. Blood is taken for analysis and finds that the patient's hemoglobin, hematocrit, and platelet levels are all within the expected normal ranges. Bleeding function tests find bleeding time is 8 minutes (N = 2–7 minutes), prothrombin time, PT, is 11.3 seconds (N = 11–12.5 seconds), and activated partial thromboplastin time, aPTT, is 47 seconds (N = 30 – 40 seconds). Which of the following is the most likely cause of symptoms in this patient?
(A) Defect of platelet activation
(B) Deficiency of vitamin K
(C) Impaired inactivation of factor V
(D) Inactivating mutation in the gene encoding GPIIb
(E) Insufficient thrombin activation

24. A 35-year-old woman is brought to the Emergency Department due to an acute onset of chest pain and shortness of breath. The patient indicates that the pain is stabbing and that it gets worse when she inhales. History reveals that the patient has had recurrent episodes of deep vein thrombosis (DVT) and that her mother succumbed as a result of a pulmonary embolism. The patient states that she does not smoke or utilize oral contraceptives. Physical examination shows an otherwise healthy-looking female with the exception of a swollen lower left leg that is tender to the touch. Duplex ultrasound shows the presence of an occlusive thrombus in the left femoral vein. The attending physician orders blood test that included blood coagulation studies. The results of these tests show that the patient has a normal level of hemoglobin and platelets, and that her hematocrit is also within normal limits. The prothrombin time, PT, is 14 seconds (N = 11–12.5 seconds) and partial thromboplastin time, PTT, is 74 seconds (N = 60–70 seconds). She is a nonsmoker, does not take oral contraceptive pills, and takes aspirin daily. Her temperature is 37.0°C (98.6°F), pulse is 112/min, respirations are 27/min, blood pressure is 134/93 mm Hg, and oxygen saturation is 88% on room air. Breath sounds are clear bilaterally. There are no murmurs. Her right lower extremity is swollen and tender. Given the signs and symptoms in the patient, which of the following is the most likely contributing factor?
(A) Deficiency in vitamin K
(B) Factor V Leiden mutation
(C) Inactivating mutation in the gene encoding factor VIII
(D) Inactivating mutation in the gene encoding GPIIb
(E) Inappropriate protein C activation

25. A 12-year-old boy has been brought to the Emergency Department by his mother for treatment of a nosebleed that began in the absence of any trauma and has been bleeding for the past 2 hours. Physical examination confirms that there is no obvious trauma to the external nose or the nasal cavities, and there are no petechia or purpura on the patient's skin. Close examination of the nasal mucosa does not reveal any dilated or abnormal vessels. The mother reports that her son's gums bleed for several minutes to an hour after every routine dental examination and cleaning. History reveals that the patient's older sister and maternal aunt each have a history of heavy menstruation and prolonged bleeding from their gums following routine dental examinations and cleanings. Given the most likely diagnosis in this patient, which of the following represents the most likely results from bleeding function tests?

Prothrombin Time	Activated Partial	Thromboplastin Time	Bleeding Time
(A)	Normal	Increased	Normal
(B)	Normal	Increased	Increased
(C)	Normal	Normal	Increased
(D)	Increased	Increased	Increased
(E)	Increased	Normal	Increased
(F)	Increased	Normal	Normal

(A)
(B)
(C)
(D)
(E)
(F)

26. A 67-year-old man is undergoing a routine follow-up examination with his cardiologist following coronary bypass surgery that included angioplasty and the placement of a stent. This surgical intervention occurred following the patient's admittance to the Emergency Department as the result of an acute myocardial infarction. The patient's history is significant for hypercholesterolemia, hypertension, and type 2 diabetes for which he takes atorvastatin, lisinopril, and metformin. Following the placement of the stent, the patient was prescribed medication to reduce his risk of experiencing another myocardial infarction or a stroke. Given the most likely prescribed medication, which of the following bleeding time results would be most likely to be found in this patient?

Prothrombin Time	Activated Partial	Thromboplastin Time	Bleeding Time
(A)	Increased	Increased	Increased
(B)	Increased	Increased	Normal
(C)	Increased	Normal	Increased
(D)	Normal	Increased	Increased
(E)	Normal	Increased	Normal
(F)	Normal	Normal	Increased

(A)
(B)
(C)
(D)
(E)
(F)

27. A 38-year-old woman is being treated in the Emergency Department due to her inability to get her nosebleed to stop. The bleeding has been occurring over the past 4 hours. History reveals that the patient suffers from inflammatory bowel disease and has been adherent to a fat-free diet for the past 10 months in an attempt to reduce her bowel discomfort. Her family physician prescribed vancomycin 8 days ago to treat an infection with *Clostridium difficile*. The attending physician orders blood tests that find that the patient's platelet count and red blood cell numbers are within the expected normal ranges. Assay for vitamin K finds that the patient's blood level is 0.08 ng/mL (N = 0.1–2.2 ng/mL). Given the findings in this patient, which of the following values for bleeding tests would be most likely to be observed?

Prothrombin Time	Activated Partial	Thromboplastin Time	Bleeding Time
(A)	Increased	Increased	Increased
(B)	Increased	Increased	Normal
(C)	Increased	Normal	Normal
(D)	Normal	Increased	Increased
(E)	Normal	Increased	Normal
(F)	Normal	Normal	Increased

(A)
(B)
(C)
(D)
(E)
(F)

28. A 17-year-old girl is being examined by her personal physician, having been brought there by her father after briefly losing consciousness. She tells her physician that she is on her period, and it has been quite heavy for the past 3 days. History reveals that her mother and maternal aunt both had frequent heavy menstruation. Her physician orders blood tests including coagulation studies with the results showing normal levels of hemoglobin and platelets. Bleeding time and activated partial thromboplastin times (aPTT) were both prolonged but the prothrombin time (PT) was normal. Given these signs and symptoms, which of the following is the most likely underlying disorder in this patient?
(A) Bernard-Soulier syndrome
(B) Glanzmann thrombasthenia
(C) Hemophilia A
(D) Thrombocytopenia
(E) von Willebrand disease

29. A 10-year-old child, with a long history of bleeding dysfunction characterized by spontaneous nontraumatic hemorrhages into joint spaces, skeletal muscle, and mucous membranes, is being treated in the Emergency Department for uncontrolled bleeding from his gums following a routine dental exam and cleaning. History reveals that the patient's maternal uncle also suffered from episodes of prolonged bleeding. Given the most likely diagnosis in this patient, which of the following is most likely to be found to be abnormal in this patient?
(A) Activated partial thromboplastin time (aPTT)
(B) Bleeding time
(C) Platelet count
(D) Prothrombin time (PT)
(E) Serum levels of vitamin K

30. A 5-year-old boy is being treated for a suspected case of congenital deficiency in coagulation. He had bled from the umbilical and circumcision sites during his first week of life. He experiences frequent ecchymoses and hematomas within 12–24 hours each time he falls or bumps his legs against a hard surface. His parents are first cousins but there is no family history of bleeding disorders. A bleeding disorder workup is initiated, and the results indicate that PT, PTT, fibrinogen, platelet aggregation studies, and von Willebrand factor are normal. The patient's plasma was incubated with thrombin and Ca^{2+} and the resultant clot dissolved in the presence of urea. Given the findings in this patient, which of the following values for bleeding tests would be most likely to be observed?

Prothrombin Time	Activated Partial	Thromboplastin Time	Bleeding Time
(A)	Increased	Increased	Increased
(B)	Increased	Increased	Normal
(C)	Increased	Normal	Normal
(D)	Normal	Increased	Increased
(E)	Normal	Normal	Normal
(F)	Normal	Normal	Increased

(A)
(B)
(C)
(D)
(E)
(F)

ANSWERS

1. Correct answer is **C.** The patient is most likely exhibiting the symptoms associated with the hyercoagulopathy known as factor V Leiden. Factor V Leiden is a hereditary thrombophilia that causes activated protein C (aPC) resistance. The molecular basis of factor V Leiden is a missense mutation in the factor V (*FV*) gene that changes a G to an A (G1691A), resulting in arginine (R) at amino acid position 506 being changed to glutamine (R506Q). Overall, 5% of the world population harbors this factor V Leiden mutation. The normal interaction between aPC and factor V involves thrombin. Thrombin cleavage of protein C (PC) removes the activation peptide generating aPC. When activated through cleavage by thrombin, aPC cleaves both activated factor V (designated Va) and activated factor VIII (designated VIIIa) into inactive enzymes. This results in the termination of the role of VIIIa as the scaffold for the formation of the tenase complex, and Va as a cofactor in the conversion of prothrombin to thrombin in the prothrombinase complex. The net effect, at the level of coagulation, of the activation of PC is termination of further increases in thrombin production and a halt to further fibrin clot formation. The factor V Leiden mutation results in a protein that is not effectively degraded by aPC such that there is limited control of thrombin activation by Va and a consequent hypercoagulopathy. The symptoms of factor V Leiden are deep vein thrombosis (DVT; also termed venous thromboembolism, VTE) and pulmonary embolism, both of which can be fatal. The presence of the factor V Leiden mutation in females is a serious risk factor for miscarriage. Antithrombin III deficiency (choice A) is the result of mutations in the gene (*SERPINC1*) encoding the serine protease inhibitor called antithrombin III. Antithrombin III deficiency can lead to deep vein thrombosis and pulmonary embolism. Arterial thrombosis is rare in antithrombin III deficiency. Thrombosis may occur spontaneously or in association with surgery, trauma, or pregnancy. However, there is no increased risk for miscarriage in women with antithrombin III deficiency. Bernard-Soulier syndrome, BSS (choice B) is the second most common inherited bleeding disorder that results as a consequence of defects in platelet function. BSS is characterized by, among other symptoms, the presence of giant platelets. Hence the disorder is also known as Giant Platelet syndrome. In addition to the presence of giant platelets, patients experience a prolonged bleeding time. Glanzmann thrombasthenia (choice D) mutation in the gene encoding the GPIIb (integrin α2b) or GPIIIa (integrin β3) protein of the platelet GPIIb-GPIIIa complex. The GPIIb-GPIIIa complex is a member of integrin family of cell surface receptors and is also called integrin α2bβ3 (also written as αIIbβ3). Glanzmann thrombasthenia is associated with significant mucocutaneous bleeding that is evidenced at an early age, and lifelong repeated bleeding at sites of minor trauma such as the gums (gingival) and the nose (epistaxis) is common. Severe intracranial or gastrointestinal hemorrhage can occur spontaneously (ie, unprovoked by injury) and is a significant cause of mortality in 5–10% of Glanzmann thrombasthenia patients. Hemophilia A (choice E) is the result of mutations in the factor VIII (*F8*) gene and hemophilia B (choice F) results from mutations in the factor IX (*F9*) gene. Both hemophilias are associated with joint and muscle hemorrhage, easy bruising, and prolonged bleeding time from wounds. von Willebrand disease (choice G) comprises a spectrum of bleeding dysfunction all of which result from mutations in the gene encoding von Willebrand factor (vWF). The common symptoms of von Willebrand disease are easy bruising, bleeding from the gums, cutaneous hematomas and prolonged bleeding from cuts and abrasions.

2. Correct answer is **D.** The patient is most likely experiencing the symptoms of a deficiency in fibrinogen. Defects associated with factors of the pathways of blood coagulation can be assessed with specific assays. The prothrombin time (PT) is an assay designed to screen for defects in fibrinogen, prothrombin, and factors V, VII, and X and thus measures activities of the extrinsic pathway of coagulation. When any of these factors is deficient then the PT is prolonged. A normal PT is 11.0–12.5 seconds. A PT greater than 20 seconds is indicative of coagulation deficit. To assess for deficiency in the function of factor VIII (choice A) or factor IX (choice B) the optimal assay is the partial thromboplastin time, PTT. The PTT will evaluate the function of fibrinogen, prothrombin, and factors V, VIII, IX, X, XI, and XII. A defect in any of these factors will result in a prolonged PTT (or activated partial thromboplastin time. aPTT). A normal PTT is 60–70 seconds, whereas for the aPTT the normal range is 30–40 seconds. Factor XIII deficiency (choice C) is a rare bleeding disorder whose symptoms are normally seen soon after birth, usually with abnormal bleeding from the umbilical cord stump. If the condition is not treated, affected individuals may have episodes of excessive and prolonged bleeding that can be life-threatening. High-molecular-weight kininogen deficiency (choice E) is not associated with a tendency to bleeding dysfunction but affected individuals will exhibit abnormal surface-mediated activation of fibrinolysis. Numerous bleeding disorders are associated with platelet deficiencies (choice F) such as Bernard-Soulier

syndrome and Glanzmann thrombasthenia, but they are not associated with prolonged PT.

3. Correct answer is **D.** The patient is most likely experiencing the symptoms of a deficiency in factor XIII. Factor XIII is converted to its active form (XIIIa) by thrombin in the presence of Ca^{2+}. Deficiency in factor XIII is characterized by delayed bleeding even though primary hemostasis is normal. Typical symptoms include neonatal bleeding from the umbilical cord, intracranial hemorrhage, soft tissue hematomas, and abnormal wound healing. Umbilical cord bleeding after birth occurs in over 90% of afflicted individuals. Deficiency in factor V (choice A), factor VII (choice B), factor VIII (choice C), and prothrombin (choice E) would be apparent with a prolonged PT or PTT which was not the case in this patient.

4. Correct answer is **B.** The patient is most likely experiencing the symptoms of a deficiency in factor XI. When factor XI is activated to XIa by activated factor XII (XIIa) its function is to activate factor IX to IXa. The most common feature of factor XI deficiency is prolonged bleeding after trauma or surgery. The partial thromboplastin time (PTT) is used to assay for defects in the intrinsic pathway of coagulation. The PTT assay has been modified by the addition of activators that shorten the normal clotting time and this form of the assay is referred to as the activated partial thromboplastin time (aPTT). The PTT is normally prescribed in patients with unexplained bleeding or clotting. The assay will evaluate the function of fibrinogen, prothrombin, and factors V, VIII, IX, X, XI, and XII. A defect in any of these factors will result in a prolonged PTT (or aPTT). Deficiency in factor VII (choice A) would be detectable with the prothrombin time, PT, assay since this was normal there is not likely a deficiency in factor VII in this patient. Although prekallikrein deficiency (choice C) is associated with a prolonged aPTT and normal PT, the frequency of this disorder is extremely rare (<80 identified individuals worldwide) especially in comparison to factor XI deficiency. Tissue factor deficiency (choice D) will result in reduced levels of thrombin which would be evident by a prolonged PT, which was not apparent in this patient. Tissue factor pathway inhibitor deficiency (choice E) would result in excessive production of thrombin and as a consequence a hypercoagulopathy as opposed to prolonged bleeding.

5. Correct answer is **D.** Protein C (PC) is a trypsin-like serine protease that serves as a major regulator of the coagulation process. Thrombin cleavage of PC removes the activation peptide generating activated protein C, aPC. When activated through cleavage by thrombin, aPC cleaves both factor Va and factor VIIIa into inactive enzymes. This results in the termination of the role of VIIIa as the scaffold for the formation of the tenase complex and Va as a cofactor in the conversion of prothrombin to thrombin in the prothrombinase complex. The net effect, at the level of coagulation, of the activation of PC is termination of further increases in thrombin production and a halt to further fibrin clot formation. A lack of aPC activity would be apparent if fibrin clotting was accelerated due to lack of inhibition of factors Va and VIIIa. Inhibition of none of the other factors (choices A, B, C, and E) would result in a more rapid formation of a fibrin clot. Indeed, inhibition of these factors would result in reduced or nonexistent fibrin clot formation.

6. Correct answer is **E.** The patient is most likely experiencing the bleeding dysfunction known as von Willebrand disease. von Willebrand disease (vWD) is caused by deficiencies in the protein von Willebrand factor (vWF). vWF is a multisubunit glycoprotein that is found in subendothelial connective tissue, the blood and in the α granules of platelets. The disorder is characterized by bleeding from mucocutaneous sites (typical skin and mucous membranes) rather than from deep tissues and joints. The second role of vWF is to bind to and stabilize factor VIII allowing factor VIII to survive in the blood. As a consequence of these roles for vWF, deficiencies result in defective platelet adhesion and to secondary deficiencies in factor VIII. Afibrinogenemia (choice A) refers to a complete lack of fibrinogen. Afibrinogenemia is characterized by neonatal umbilical cord hemorrhage, ecchymoses, mucosal hemorrhage, internal hemorrhage, and recurrent spontaneous abortion. Antithrombin III deficiency (choice B) is the result of mutations in the gene (*SERPINC1*) encoding this serine protease inhibitor. Antithrombin III deficiency would result in elevated levels of active thrombin thereby resulting in significant reduction in both PT and aPTT. Factor XI deficiency (choice C) is associated with prolonged bleeding after trauma or surgery. Hemophilia A (choice D) is the result of mutations in the factor VIII (*F8*) gene and is associated with joint and muscle hemorrhage, easy bruising, and prolonged bleeding time from wounds.

7. Correct answer is **C.** The patient is most likely experiencing the symptoms of mutation in the factor V gene which is the cause of the disorder referred to as factor V Leiden. The mutation in the factor V gene results in a protein that is not effectively degraded by activated protein C, aPC. Factor V Leiden is the most common inherited thrombophilia in Caucasian populations of European descent. Overall, 5% of the world population harbors the factor V Leiden mutation. The symptoms of factor V Leiden are deep vein thrombosis (DVT) and pulmonary embolism, both of which can be fatal. In fact, it is estimated that as many as 30% of patients, who experience DVT and/or pulmonary embolisms, are carriers of the factor V Leiden mutation. Afibrinoginemia (choice A), Bernard-Soulier syndrome (choice B), hemophilia A (choice D), and von Willebrand disease (choice E) are all associated with reduced blood coagulation not hypercoagulopathy.

8. Correct answer is **F.** The patient is most likely suffering the bleeding dysfunction known as von Willebrand disease. von Willebrand disease (vWD) is caused by deficiencies in the protein von Willebrand factor (vWF). vWF is a multi-subunit glycoprotein that is found in subendothelial connective tissue, the blood and in the α granules of platelets. Individuals with von Willebrand disease show bleeding after minor trauma, with the most common sites including skin (easy bruising) and mucous membranes (epistaxis). Coagulation tests reveal a prolonged PTT, a normal PT, and a prolonged bleeding time with normal platelet count, all of which are characteristic of the test results in this patient. Deficiency in factor X (choice A) and tissue factor (choice D), as well as a deficiency in vitamin K-dependent carboxylation (choice E) of coagulation factors such as prothrombin, factor VII, factor IX, and factor X would all result in a prolonged PT as opposed to the normal PT found in this patient. A deficiency in platelet adhesion (choice B), which is associated with Bernard-Soulier syndrome and Glanzmann thrombasthenia, would not be associated with an increased PTT as evidenced in this patient. Deficiency in protein C (choice C) would result in a hypercoagulopathy due to the fact that the function of activated protein C (aPC) is to inhibit the activity of the procoagulation factors, activated factor VII (VIIa) and activated factor V (Va).

9. Correct answer is **C.** This patient is most likely deficient in factor IX as evidenced by the results of the aPTT assay. The partial thromboplastin time (PTT) is used to assay for defects in the intrinsic pathway of coagulation. The PTT assay has been modified by the addition of activators that shorten the normal clotting time and this form of the assay is referred to as the activated partial thromboplastin time (aPTT). The assay will evaluate the function of fibrinogen, prothrombin, and factors V, VIII, IX, X, XI, and XII. A defect in any of these factors will result in a prolonged PTT (or aPTT). Deficiencies in none of the other factors (choices A, B, D, and E) would correlate with the prolonged aPTT assay identified in this patient.

10. Correct answer is **C.** The novel compound is most likely targeting a protein complex associated with platelet function since this is what is the defect associated with Glanzmann thrombasthenia. Glanzmann thrombasthenia (weak platelets) is an autosomal recessive disorder affecting the processes of blood coagulation. The hallmark of the disease is the failure of platelets to bind fibrinogen and aggregate in the presence of a variety of physiological agonist such as ADP, thrombin, epinephrine, or collagen. The underlying defect in all patients with Glanzmann thrombasthenia is an abnormality in the gene encoding either the GPIIb (integrin α2b) or GPIIIa (integrin β3) protein of the GPIIb-GPIIIa complex. The GPIIb-GPIIIa complex is a member of integrin family of cell surface receptors and is also called integrin α2bβ3 (also written as αIIbβ3). The platelet GPIIb-GPIIIa complex is the most abundant platelet receptor representing approximately 15% of the total protein on the surface of platelets. GPIIb-GPIIIa antagonists represent anticoagulant drugs that inhibit platelet aggregation regardless of the agonist. Therefore, abcixamab more completely inhibits platelet aggregation than does aspirin or clopidogrel. None of the other complexes (choices A, B, D, and E) are defective in Glanzmann thrombasthenia and therefore would not represent the target for the novel regulator of coagulation.

11. Correct answer is **B.** The patient most likely has the bleeding disorder known as hemophilia B. Hemophilia is most often suspected in a patient with unexplained hemarthroses, a prolonged aPTT, a normal PT, and normal platelet count. Hemophilia B results from deficiencies in factor IX. The prevalence of hemophilia B is approximately one-tenth that of hemophilia A. All patients with hemophilia B have prolonged coagulation time and decreased factor IX clotting activity. Similar to the situation where hemophilia A, there are severe, moderate, and mild forms of hemophilia B and these forms reflect the level of factor IX activity in plasma. A deficiency of the factor V (choice A) would manifest with bleeding dysfunction similar to that observed in this patient, however the PT is prolonged with factor V deficiency. Deficiency of the platelet glycoprotein receptor complex, GPIIb GPIIIa (choice C) would result. Deficiency of protein C (choice D) would result in a hypercoagulopathy, not a reduced ability of blood to clot. Deficiency of thrombin (choice E) would be associated with a prolonged PT unlike the normal PT found in this patient.

12. Correct answer is **E.** The patient is most likely exhibiting the typical findings of disseminated intravascular coagulation, DIS. DIS is initiated by the release of tissue factor or thromboplastin (either exogenous, eg, amniotic fluid, or endogenous, eg, tissue damage as in this case) into the circulation. Thromboplastin is a complex of phospholipids and tissue factor. The excessive release of tissue factor results in activation of the extrinsic coagulation cascade, resulting in the formation of multiple thrombi that can block the microcirculation and produce ischemia and necrosis in vulnerable tissues. As thrombus formation continues, platelets and clotting factors can be exhausted, allowing hemorrhage to occur. The ischemic changes and hemorrhage characteristic of DIS are both apparent in this patient. None of the other options (choices A, B, C, and D) would correctly define the initiating mechanism of the disseminated intravascular coagulation as evidenced in this patient.

13. Correct answer is **D.** The patient most likely has the bleeding disorder known as hemophilia A. Hemophilia is most often suspected in a patient with unexplained hemarthroses, a prolonged aPTT, a normal PT, and normal platelet count. Hemophilia A results from deficiencies in factor VIII. The bleeding dysfunction associated with hemophilia A is characterized by spontaneous hemarthrosis (hemorrhaging into joints), soft tissue bleeding, and bleeding into mucosal surfaces. Blood from hemophilia A patients will show normal platelet aggregation in the presence of ristocetin. Ristocetin is an antibiotic isolated from *Amycolatopsis lurida* and it induces the binding of von Willebrand factor to the GPIb-GPIX-GPV glycoprotein complex on the surface of platelets. The ristocetin-induced platelet aggregation assay is an ex vivo assay for live platelet function. Bernard-Soulier syndrome (choice A) and Glanzmann thrombasthenia (choice C) are bleeding disorders that are both the result of abnormal platelet function which is not the case in this patient. Deficiency in factor XI (choice B) confers an injury-related bleeding tendency as opposed to the spontaneous bleeding in this patient. Since the ristocetin-induced platelet aggregation assay was normal in this patient the bleeding dysfunction cannot be von Willebrand disease (choice E).

14. Correct answer is **E.** The patient is most likely experiencing the bleeding disorder known as von Willebrand disease (vWD) which results from mutations in the gene encoding von Willebrand factor (vWF). The disorder is characterized by bleeding from mucocutaneous sites (typical skin and mucous membranes) rather than from deep tissues and joints. vWF is involved in two important reactions of blood coagulation. The first is the interaction of vWF with specific receptors on the surface of platelets and the subendothelial connective tissue. This interaction allows platelets to adhere to areas of vascular injury. The second role of vWF is to bind to and stabilize factor VIII allowing factor VIII to survive in the blood. Given the functions of vWF, deficiencies in this protein will result in defective platelet adhesion and to secondary deficiencies in factor VIII. Since factor VIII deficiency results in hemophilia A, vWF deficiencies can manifest with clinical symptoms that appear to be similar to those of hemophilia A. Deficiency in factor IX (choice A), factor X (choice B), and fibrinogen (choice C) would not be associated with reduced levels of factor VIII nor the reduced platelet aggregation capability as evidenced in this patient. Deficiency in platelet glycoprotein complex, GPIIb GPIIIa (choice D), would result in deficiency of platelet aggregation but would not lead to reduced levels of factor VIII in the blood.

15. Correct answer is **F.** Thrombin possesses numerous activities that regulate the processes of hemostasis. Thrombin cleaves fibrinogen releasing fibrinopeptides. The thrombin-mediated release of the fibrinopeptides generates fibrin monomers that spontaneously aggregate in a regular array, forming a somewhat weak fibrin clot. Thrombin activates factor XIII to factor XIIIa. Factor XIIIa is a highly specific transglutaminase that introduces cross-links composed of covalent bonds between the amide nitrogen of glutamines and ε-amino group of lysines in the fibrin monomers forming a stable clot. Thrombin also activates factor V to Va and factor VIII to VIIIa resulting in promotion of both the prothrombinase and tenase complexes, respectively. These two events lead to dramatic elevation in the rate of coagulation. However, thrombin also activates protein C (PC) to aPC which serves to limit the extent of coagulation because aPC cleaves and inactivates factors Va and VIIIa. Thrombin also activates platelets by binding to a class of G-protein-coupled receptors (GPCR) called protease activated receptors (PAR), specifically PAR-1, PAR-3, and PAR-4, leading to increased platelet activation. Thrombin is not directly involved in the proteolytic activation of any of the other proteins (choices A, B, C, D, and E).

16. Correct answer is **B.** Acetylsalicylate (aspirin) is an important inhibitor of platelet activation. By virtue of inhibiting the activity of cyclooxygenase, aspirin reduces the production of TXA_2 by platelets. Aspirin also reduces endothelial cell production of prostacyclin (PGI_2), an inhibitor of platelet aggregation and a vasodilator. Localized to the site of coagulation is a balance between the levels of platelet derived TXA_2 and endothelial cell derived PGI_2. This allows for platelet aggregation and clot formation but preventing excessive accumulation of the clot, thus maintaining blood flow around the site of the clot. Endothelial cells regenerate active cyclooxygenase faster than platelets because mature platelets cannot synthesize the enzyme, requiring new platelets to enter the circulation (platelet half-life is approximately 4 days). Therefore, the rate of PGI_2 synthesis is greater than that of TXA_2 in the presence of aspirin. The net effect of aspirin is more in favor of endothelial cell-mediated inhibition of the coagulation cascade. Acetylsalicylate does not exert its effects on platelet activity through any of the other proteins (choices A, C, D, and E).

17. Correct answer is **C.** A major mechanism for the inhibition of the extrinsic pathway occurs at the tissue factor-factor VIIa-Ca^{2+}-Xa complex. The protein, lipoprotein-associated coagulation inhibitor (LACI) specifically binds to this complex. LACI is also referred to as extrinsic pathway inhibitor (EPI) or tissue factor pathway inhibitor (TFPI) and was formerly named anticonvertin. Deficiency of antithrombin III (choice A), protein C (choice D), and von Willebrand factor (choice E) would result in hypercoagulopathy regardless of whether the intrinsic and extrinsic coagulation cascades was activated. Defective high-molecular-weight kininogen (choice B) is only involved in the activation of the intrinsic coagulation cascade and does not contribute to the regulation of the extrinsic coagulation cascade.

18. Correct answer is **D.** In order for hemostasis to occur, platelets must adhere to the subendothelial cell extracellular matrix-associated collagen. Upon binding to collagen, platelets become activated and release the contents of their granule and aggregate. Contained in the dense granules of platelets is ADP. The release of ADP further stimulates platelets thereby increasing the overall activation cascade. ADP also modifies the platelet membranes leading to exposure of the platelet glycoprotein receptor complex, GPIIb-GPIIIa. GPIIb-GPIIIa constitutes a receptor for von Willebrand factor (vWF) and fibrinogen. Upon binding to GPIIb-GPIIIa, vWF acts as a bridge between another specific glycoprotein complex on the surface of platelets (GPIb-GPIX-GPV) and the exposed collagen at the site of vessel injury. The net effect is that these platelet glycoprotein complexes contribute to fibrinogen-induced platelet crosslinking and resultant increased aggregation and activation. None of the other options (choices A, B, C, and E) correctly reflect the consequences of defective platelet glycoprotein receptor complexes.

19. Correct answer is **E.** The patient is most likely exhibiting the bleeding dysfunction known as von Willebrand disease, vWD. This disorder results from defects in von Willebrand factor (vWF). von Willebrand disease is characterized by bleeding from mucocutaneous sites (typically skin and mucous membranes) rather than from deep tissues and joints. vWF is involved in two important reactions of blood coagulation one of which is to bind to and stabilize factor VIII allowing factor VIII to survive in the blood. Deficiencies in vWF can, therefore, result in deficiencies in factor VIII. None of the other proteins (choices A, B, C, and D) contribute to the stability of factor VIII in the blood.

20. Correct answer is **E.** A deletion of exon 2 in the *F2* gene would result in the loss of production of prothrombin. Prothrombin, when activated to thrombin, possesses numerous activities that regulate the processes of hemostasis. Thrombin cleaves fibrinogen releasing fibrinopeptides. The thrombin-mediated release of the fibrinopeptides generates fibrin monomers that spontaneously aggregate in a regular array, forming a somewhat weak fibrin clot. Thrombin activates factor XIII to factor XIIIa. Factor XIIIa is a highly specific transglutaminase that introduces cross-links composed of covalent bonds between the amide nitrogen of glutamines and ε-amino group of lysines in the fibrin monomers forming a stable clot. Thrombin also activates factor V to Va and factor VIII to VIIIa resulting in promotion of both the prothrombinase and tenase complexes, respectively. These two events lead to dramatic elevation in the rate of coagulation. However, thrombin also activates protein C (PC) to aPC which serves to limit the extent of coagulation because aPC cleaves and inactivates factors Va and VIIIa. Thrombin is not directly involved in the proteolytic activation of any of the other proteins (choices A, B, C, and D).

21. Correct answer is **A.** The patient most likely has the bleeding disorder known as hemophilia A. Hemophilia is most often suspected in a patient with unexplained hemarthroses, a prolonged aPTT, a normal PT, and normal platelet count. Hemophilia A results from deficiencies in factor VIII. The bleeding dysfunction associated with hemophilia A is characterized by spontaneous hemarthrosis (hemorrhaging into joints), soft tissue bleeding, and bleeding into mucosal surfaces. Deficiency in fibrinogen (choice B) and thrombin (choice D) would both result in increased PT. Deficiency in GPIIb-GPIIIa (choice C) would result in abnormal platelet counts. Although von Willebrand disease (vWD), which results from deficiency in von Willebrand factor, vWF (choice E) results in an elongated aPTT, a normal PT, and normal platelet counts, as seen in this patient, the sites of bleeding are distinct from hemophilia A. The locations of frequent bleeding in vWD are most often the skin and mucous membranes whereas in hemophilia A the sites of bleeding are deep tissue such as in the joints.

22. Correct answer is **C.** The novel monoclonal antibody is most likely targeting the platelet glycoprotein complex, GPIIb GPIIIa, which is the same target for the drug, abciximab. The utility of GPIIb-GPIIIa antagonists is that they more completely inhibit platelet aggregation than do drugs such as aspirin or the platelet receptor, $P2Y_{12}$ (choice D), antagonists such as clopidogrel. Drugs that inhibit factor Xa, either free or within the prothrombinase complex, such as is the case for the drug rivaroxaban, are useful in the prevention of venous thromboembolism. The coumadin-based drugs, such as warfarin, that interfere with the function of the vitamin K-dependent carboxylation of factor X (choice A) and prothrombin (choice E), do not target the same coagulation factors as abciximab. Currently there are no anticoagulants that are designed to target the functions of fibrinogen (choice B).

23. Correct answer is **E.** The patient is most likely exhibiting the typical bleeding consequences of hemophilia, most likely hemophilia A since this is the most common form of hemophilia. Hemophilia is most often suspected in a patient with unexplained hemarthroses, a prolonged aPTT, a normal PT, and normal platelet count. Hemophilia A results from deficiencies in factor VIII. Patients with hemophilia A suffer from joint and muscle hemorrhage, easy bruising, and prolonged bleeding time from wounds. Almost all patients with hemophilia A have normal platelet function so the bleeding from minor cuts or abrasions is generally not severe. Hemophilia A can be divided into severe or moderate disease. Approximately 50%–60% of hemophilia A patients suffer from the severe form of the disease and have <1% normal factor VIII activity. Although the patient has normal levels of platelets, defective activation of the platelets (choice A) could lead to prolonged bleeding. However, the characteristic bleeding seen in patients with platelet dysfunction, such as in Glanzmann thrombasthenia or Bernard-Soulier syndrome, is typically cutaneous and mucosal as opposed to the deep tissue (hemarthrosis) bleeding seen in this patient. Vitamin K (choice B) is required for the functional modification of prothrombin, factors VII, IX, and X, as well as protein C and protein S. Thus, a deficiency in the vitamin would be associated with a prolonged PT which was not found in this patient. Inactivation of factor V (choice C), specifically the activated form (Va), is carried out by activated protein C (aPC). Factor V, when activated (Va), is a cofactor in the tenase complex which is required for the activation of factor X to Xa. Factor Xa is responsible for the activation of prothrombin to thrombin. Therefore, inactivation of factor V is required to prevent excessive coagulation, and the consequences of impaired inactivation would be hypercoagulation, not excessive bleeding. GPIIb (choice D) is a glycoprotein present in the platelet receptor complex, GPIIb-GPIIIa, which is a receptor for vWF and fibrinogen, responsible for fibrinogen-induced platelet aggregation. Defective GPIIb is one cause of Glanzmann thrombasthenia, which is characterized by frequent and significant cutaneous and mucosal bleeding, as opposed to the deep tissue bleeding evident in this patient.

24. Correct answer is **B.** The patient is most likely exhibiting the signs and symptoms associated with the hypercoagulopathy identified as factor V Leiden. Factor V Leiden is a hereditary thrombophilia that causes activated protein C (aPC) resistance. The molecular basis of factor V Leiden is a missense mutation in the factor V (*FV*) gene that changes a G to an A (G1691A), resulting in arginine (R) at amino acid position 506 being changed to glutamine (R506Q). Overall, 5% of the world population harbors this factor V Leiden mutation. The normal interaction between aPC and factor V involves thrombin. Thrombin cleavage of protein C (PC) removes the activation peptide generating aPC. When activated through cleavage by thrombin, aPC cleaves both activated factor V (designated Va) and activated factor VIII (designated VIIIa) into inactive enzymes. This results in the termination of the role of VIIIa as the scaffold for the formation of the tenase complex, and Va as a cofactor in the conversion of prothrombin to thrombin in the prothrombinase complex. The net effect, at the level of coagulation, of the activation of PC is termination of further increases in thrombin production and a halt to further fibrin clot formation. The factor V Leiden mutation results in a protein that is not effectively degraded by aPC such that there is limited control of thrombin activation by Va and consequent hypercoagulopathy. The symptoms of factor V Leiden are deep vein thrombosis (DVT; also termed venous thromboembolism, VTE) and pulmonary embolism, both of which can be fatal. Vitamin K (choice A) is required for the functional modification of prothrombin, factors VII, IX, and X, as well as protein C and protein S. Thus, a deficiency in the vitamin would be associated with a significantly prolonged PT and PTT which was not found in this patient. Inactivating mutations in factor VIII (choice C) are associated with hemophilia A. The *F8* gene is located on the X chromosome so the disorder is almost never observed in females. GPIIb (choice D) is a glycoprotein present in the platelet receptor complex, GPIIb-GPIIIa, which is a receptor for vWF and fibrinogen, responsible for fibrinogen-induced platelet aggregation. Defective GPIIb is one cause of Glanzmann thrombasthenia, which is characterized by frequent and significant cutaneous and mucosal bleeding, as opposed to the deep vein thrombosis evident in this patient. Inappropriate activation of protein C (choice E) would lead to an increase in the inactivation of factors V and VIII resulting in a reduced capacity for coagulation not a hypercoagulopathy as is typically the cause of deep vein thromboses.

25. Correct answer is **B.** The patient is most likely experiencing the bleeding dysfunction known as von Willebrand disease, vWD. vWD is the most commonly occurring bleeding disorder with clinically significant forms affecting approximately 1 in 1000 individuals. However, abnormalities in vWF have been estimated to occur with a frequency of 1 in 100 people. vWD is caused by deficiencies in the protein von Willebrand factor (vWF). There are both dominant and recessive forms of vWD with the most common form of the disease (type 1) being the autosomal dominant form. vWF is a multi-subunit glycoprotein that is found in subendothelial connective tissue, the blood, and in the α granules of platelets. The disorder is characterized by bleeding from mucocutaneous sites (typical skin and mucous membranes) rather than from deep tissues and joints. The second role of vWF is to bind to and stabilize factor VIII allowing factor VIII to survive in the blood. As a consequence of these roles for vWF, deficiencies in the protein result in defective platelet adhesion and secondary deficiencies in factor VIII. As a result of the defect in platelet adhesion in vWD, bleeding time will be prolonged, thus eliminating choices A and F. The PT test is used to assess the extrinsic pathway of coagulation by assaying for the activities of fibrinogen, prothrombin, V, VII, and X. These factors are not directly impacted by deficiencies in vWF so the PT is almost always normal in patients with vWD, thus eliminating choices D, E, and F. The aPTT measures the intrinsic pathway of coagulation, which includes factors VIII and IX. Since the stability of factor VIII depends upon vWF, deficiencies in vWF will lead to reduced levels of factor VIII leading to increases in the aPTT which eliminates choices C, E, and F.

26. Correct answer is **F.** The patient was most likely prescribed clopidogrel as this anti-coagulant drug is the drug of choice for the prevention of myocardial infarction and stroke in patients following balloon angioplasty and stent placement during coronary bypass surgery. Clopidogrel is an irreversible inhibitor of the ADP receptors on platelet membranes. The primary platelet ADP receptor is a member of the G-protein coupled (GPCR) purinergic receptor family identified as the P2Y12 receptor. When ADP binds to the P2Y12 receptor on platelets they are activated and aggregate leading to amplification of the coagulation response, thus clopidogrel interferes with this process. Since clopidogrel interferes with platelet activation, bleeding time is prolonged, which eliminates choices B and E. However, there is no direct effect on either the intrinsic or extrinsic pathways of coagulation so an individual's aPTT (measures intrinsic) and PT (measures extrinsic) will be within normal limits, thus eliminating all choices except F.

27. Correct answer is **B.** Vitamin K is required for the functional modification of prothrombin, factors VII, IX, and X, as well as protein C and protein S. Thus, a deficiency in the vitamin would be associated with a prolonged PT (measures extrinsic pathway function) and a prolonged aPTT (measures intrinsic pathway function). Therefore, choices C, D, E, and F can be eliminated. However, platelet function would not be directly affected by a deficiency in vitamin K, thus bleeding time would be normal which eliminates choices A, D, and F.

28. Correct answer is **E.** The patient is most likely manifesting the symptoms of von Willebrand disease (vWD) which is the most common bleeding disorder. There are both dominant and recessive forms of vWD and, given this patient's family history, she most likely has the dominant form. Indeed, the most common form of the disease (type 1) is an autosomal dominant disorder resulting from quantitative deficiency in von Willebrand factor, vWF. vWF is a multi-subunit glycoprotein that is found in subendothelial connective tissue, the blood, and in the α granules of platelets. The disorder is characterized by bleeding from mucocutaneous sites (typical skin and mucous membranes) rather than from deep tissues and joints. The second role of vWF is to bind to and stabilize factor VIII allowing factor VIII to survive in the blood. As a consequence of these roles for vWF, deficiencies result in defective platelet adhesion and secondary deficiencies in factor VIII. As a consequence of these roles for vWF, deficiencies in the protein result in defective platelet adhesion and secondary deficiencies in factor VIII. As a result of the defect in platelet adhesion in vWD, bleeding time will be prolonged. The PT test is used to assess the extrinsic pathway of coagulation by assaying for the activities of fibrinogen, prothrombin, V, VII, and X. These factors are not directly impacted by deficiencies in vWF so the PT is almost always normal in patients with vWD. The aPTT measures the intrinsic pathway of coagulation, which includes factors VIII and IX. Since the stability of factor VIII depends on vWF, deficiencies in vWF will lead to reduced levels of factor VIII leading to increases in the aPTT. Bernard-Soulier syndrome (choice A) and Glanzmann thrombasthenia (choice B) are both due to disorders in platelet function so they would also be associated with an increase in the measured bleeding time. However, since there is no direct effect on the intrinsic or extrinsic pathways the PT and aPTT results would be within normal ranges in patients with either of these disorders. Hemophilia A (choice C) is caused by deficiency in factor VIII, the gene for which is located on the X chromosome. Although bleeding time and aPTT would be increased, and PT would be normal, in a patient with hemophilia A, the frequency of females with this disorder is extremely rare. Thrombocytopenia (choice D) is a disorder of platelet production resulting in low platelet counts. A reduction in platelets would result in a prolonged bleeding time but would not be associated with a significant change in PT or aPTT.

29. Correct answer is **A.** The patient most likely has the bleeding disorder known as hemophilia A. Hemophilia is most often suspected in a patient with unexplained hemarthroses, a prolonged aPTT, a normal PT (choice D), and normal platelet count (choice C). Hemophilia A results from deficiencies in factor VIII. The bleeding dysfunction associated with hemophilia A is characterized by spontaneous hemarthrosis (hemorrhaging into joints), soft tissue bleeding, and bleeding into mucosal surfaces. Bleeding time (choice B) can be somewhat abnormal in patients with hemophilia A, but it is most often found to be within the expected normal range. Hemophilia A is always associated with a prolonged aPTT as seen in this patient. Vitamin K (choice E) is required for the functional modification of prothrombin, factors VII, IX, and X, as well as protein C and protein S. Thus, abnormal levels of the vitamin would be associated with a prolonged PT which is not observed in this patient.

30. Correct answer is **E.** The patient is most likely experiencing the symptoms of a deficiency in factor XIII. Factor XIII is converted to its active form (XIIIa) by thrombin in the presence of Ca^{2+}. Deficiency in factor XIII is characterized by delayed bleeding even though primary hemostasis is normal. Typical symptoms include neonatal bleeding from the umbilical cord, intracranial hemorrhage, soft tissue hematomas, and abnormal wound healing. Umbilical cord bleeding after birth occurs in over 90% of afflicted individuals. Patients with deficiency in factor XIII will exhibit normal bleeding time, normal prothrombin time (PT), and normal activated partial thromboplastin time (aPTT). The bleeding in factor XIII deficiency occurs due to impairment in the stability of a fibrin clot. Factor XIII is also referred to as fibrin stabilizing factor (FSF) and as fibrinoligase, the latter due to the role of factor XIII in inducing cross-links between fibrin monomers, thereby stabilizing fibrin clots. None of the other blood test values (choices A, B, C, D, and F) are reflective of normal results for all three tests.

CHAPTER

34

Cancer Biology

High-Yield Terms

Warburg effect	Refers to the observation made by Otto Warburg in 1924 of the altered metabolic profile of cancer cells, specifically that they "fermented" glucose to lactate at higher rates than would be expected
PKM2	Isoform of pyruvate kinase that is expressed in all cancers and most proliferating cells and contributes to altered metabolism in these cells
Neoplasm	Any abnormal mass of tissue, medically synonymous with the term tumor
Malignancy	Medically describes any condition that becomes progressively more severe; with respect to cancers the term characterizes invasiveness and the tendency to metastasize
Metastasis	Refers to the spread of cancer from a site of origin to a new organ or another part of the body
Apoptosis	Highly regulated and coordinated process of programmed cell death, PCD
Proto-oncogene	Any normal gene that can become an oncogene due to gene mutation or abnormal expression
Oncogene	Any gene that has the potential to cause cancer; in tumor cells, these gene are often mutated or expressed at high levels
Tumor suppressor	Any gene that prevents the unregulated growth of cells, loss of function of this class of gene can result in cancer, also called antioncogene

CANCER DEFINED

Cancer, in the broadest terms, is a term that refers to a wide array of disorders typified by unregulated cell growth. The medical and biological term is **neoplasm** and defines an abnormal tissue that grows more rapidly than normal and continues to grow and proliferate in the absence of the originating growth signal.

Neoplasms are transformed cells that can also harbor the characteristics of immortality. Transformation is a multistep process which results in the generation of the neoplastic cells. Immortalization refers to cells with unlimited life span but is not directly associated with aberrant growth or malignancy. Neoplasms can be benign or malignant. In the strictest sense, malignancy is defined as the ability to generate invasive tumors when cells are transplanted *in vivo*. However, medically this is not a useful definition due to the time required for the assessment of this capability. Therefore, it is more appropriate to define a malignant tumor, or a mass, by its potential to worsen, to invade the surrounding tissues, and to exhibit the potential for metastases.

Metastasis is the ability of cells from a tumor to break away from the original mass and spread to another location in the body. Although these terms broadly define all cancers, different types of cancers from different tissues exhibit a wide range of altered characteristics (Figure 34–1).

GENETIC ALTERATIONS AND CANCER

All cancer cells contain some form of genetic damage that appears to be the responsible event leading to **tumorigenesis** (the generation of cancer). The genetic damage present in a parental tumorigenic cell is maintained (ie, not correctable) such that it is a heritable trait of all daughter cells of subsequent generations of the parental cancer cell. This is referred to as clonal expansion such that all subsequent cells of a tumor contain the same genetic alteration that was present in the originating cell.

The genetic damage present in a cancer cell can arise either spontaneously or the mutation can be inherited. Familial cancers are those that arise from the inheritance of a mutated gene or chromosomal abnormality that predisposes an individual to cancer. This of course does not always mean that an individual acquiring an inherited mutation will develop cancer just that the individual has an increased likelihood relative to an individual who does not possess the mutant gene.

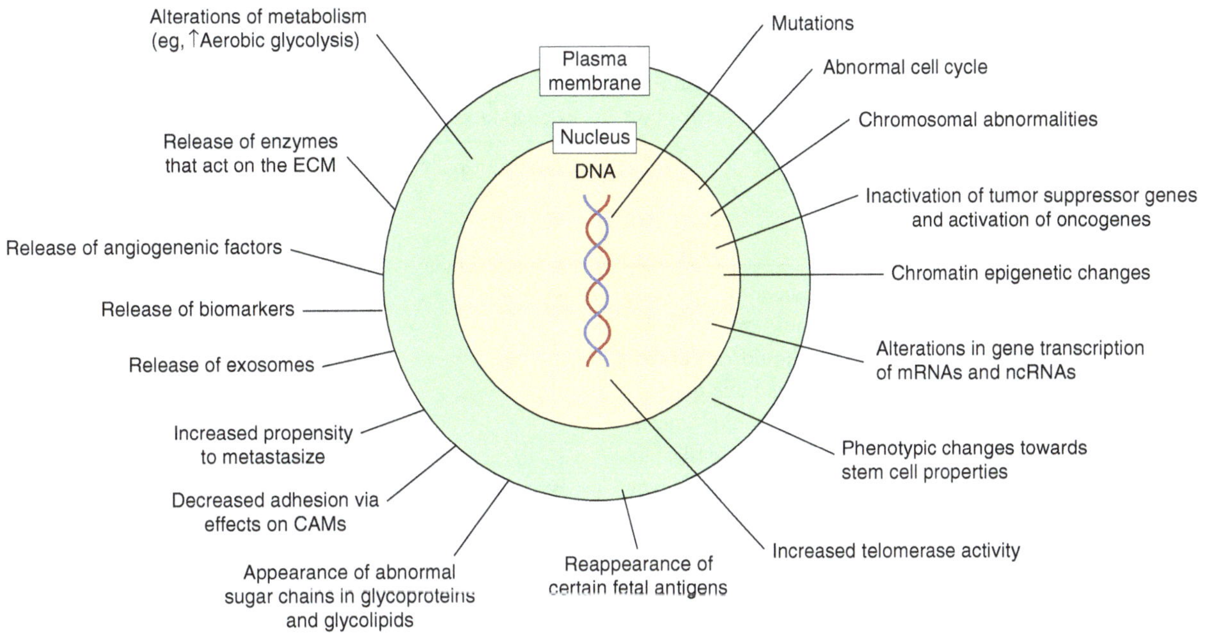

FIGURE 34–1 Some biochemical and genetic changes that occur in human cancer cells. Many changes can be observed in cancer cells; only some of these are shown here. The roles of mutations in activating oncogenes and inactivating tumor-suppressor genes are discussed in the text. Abnormalities of cell cycle progression and of chromosome and chromatin structure, including aneuploidy, are common. Alterations of expression of specific mRNAs and regulatory ncRNAs have been reported, and the relationship of stem cells to cancer cells is a very active area of research. Telomerase activity is often detectable in cancer cells. Tumors sometimes synthesize certain fetal antigens, which may be measurable in the blood. Changes in plasma membrane constituents (eg, alteration of the sugar chains of various glycoproteins—some of which are cell adhesion molecules—and glycolipids) have been detected in many studies, and may be of importance in relation to decreased cell adhesion and metastasis. Various molecules are released from cancer cells, in either soluble or membrane-bound vesicular forms (exosomes), and can be detected in the blood or extracellular fluid; these include metabolites, lipids, carbohydrates, proteins, and nucleic acids. Angiogenic factors and various proteinases are also released by some tumors. Many changes in metabolism have been observed; for example, cancer cells often exhibit a high rate of aerobic glycolysis. (CAM, cell adhesion molecule; ECM, extracellular matrix.) (Reproduced with permission from Rodwell VW, Bender DA, Botham KM, et al: *Harper's Illustrated Biochemistry*, 31st ed. New York, NY: McGraw Hill; 2018.)

Spontaneous mutations resulting in cancer are most often the result of exposure to some form of carcinogen. Carcinogens can be chemicals, radiant energies (such as UV or gamma irradiation), or oncogenic viruses. Chemical carcinogens and radiant energies generally lead to DNA damage that exceeds the capability of a cell to repair and thus, the damage is propagated in the resultant daughter cells. Often, individuals who harbor existing mutations in genes whose encoded proteins are involved in the processes of DNA repair are highly susceptible to cancers caused by these types of exposures.

The genetic damage found in cancer cells is of two types referred to as dominant or recessive. Dominant mutations are associated with genes defined as **proto-oncogenes** (Table 34–1). The distinction between the terms proto-oncogene and oncogene relates to the activity of the protein product of the gene. A proto-oncogene is a gene whose protein product has the capacity to induce cellular transformation provided it sustains some genetic insult. An oncogene is a gene that has sustained some genetic damage and, therefore, produces a protein capable of cellular transformation. The process of activation of proto-oncogenes to oncogenes can include retroviral transduction or retroviral integration, point mutations, insertion mutations, gene amplification, chromosomal translocation, and/or protein-protein interactions.

TABLE 34–1 Differences between oncogenes and tumor suppressor genes.

Oncogenes	Tumor Suppressor Genes
Mutation in one of the two alleles is sufficient to produce oncogenic effects.	Mutations in both alleles are required to produce oncogenic effects.
Oncogenic effect is due to gain-of-function of a protein that stimulates cell growth and proliferation	Oncogenic effect is due to loss-of-function of a protein that inhibits cell growth and proliferation.
Mutations in oncogenes arise in somatic cells, and hence are not inherited.	Mutations in tumor suppressor genes may be present in somatic or germ cells (and hence, may be inherited)
Usually do not show tissue preference with respect to the type of cancers in which they are found	Often demonstrate strong tissue preference with respect to the type of cancers in which they are found (eg, mutations in the *RB* gene result in retinoblastoma)

Data from Levine AJ. The p53 tumor-suppressor gene. N Engl J Med. 1992;326(20): 1350–1352.

Recessive mutations are associated with genes referred to as **tumor suppressors**, growth suppressors, recessive oncogenes or anti-oncogenes. The loss-of-function, as opposed to gain-of-function, of the gene products of tumor suppressors predisposes an individual to the development of certain cancers.

TYPES OF CANCER

Human cancers can be divided into two broad categories with one representing solid tumors and the second the liquid cancers. Solid cancers are the sarcomas and carcinomas. The liquid cancers are the cancers that originate in cells derived from the bone marrow. In broad terms there are three defined types of liquid cancers; leukemias, multiple myelomas, and lymphomas. Leukemias are blood cancers that originate in the bone marrow from a single type of progenitor cell. Multiple myelomas are bone marrow-derived cancers that are derived from the antibody producing cells. Lymphomas are cancers of the lymphatic system and are associated with lymphocyte lineage cells. Although there are many types of lymphoma they are broadly categorized as Hodgkin or non-Hodgkin lymphoma.

Sarcomas are cancers derived from transformed cells with a mesenchymal origin. These cancers include those affecting bone, muscle, connective tissue, fat, and the vasculature. Although hematopoietic cells (the cells of blood) are derived from mesenchymal stem cells and thus, hematopoietic cancers (leukemias and lymphomas) are strictly defined as sarcomas, they are more commonly separated into the separate category of liquid cancers.

Carcinomas are cancers derived from transformed epithelial cells that originate from the endoderm or ectoderm layer of the developing embryo. These cells are found in the lining of the mouth, throat, stomach, and intestines, the mammary ducts, the pancreas, the prostate gland, and the lungs. Carcinomas represent the most common types of cancers in humans and can be divided into several distinct variants defined by histology (Table 34–2).

TABLE 34–2 Histologically defined types of carcinomas.

Carcinoma	Characteristics
Adenocarcinoma	Originates in glandular tissues; the cancerous cells do not need to be part of a gland, but they exhibit secretory properties
Adenosquamous carcinoma	Mixed tumor containing both adenocarcinoma and squamous cell carcinoma cell types
Anaplastic carcinoma	A heterogeneous group of high-grade carcinomas whose cells lack distinct histological or cytological evidence of the more specifically differentiated neoplasms
Large cell carcinoma	Large rounded or overtly polygonal-shaped cells with abundant cytoplasm; most commonly found in lung cancers
Small cell carcinoma	Small, round, primitive-appearing cells with little evident cytoplasm; commonly found in lung cancers, also called oat-cell carcinomas
Squamous cell carcinoma	Derived from the most superficial epithelial layers, consist of flat, scale-like cells called squamous epithelial cells

METABOLIC ALTERATIONS ASSOCIATED WITH CANCER

All cancers exhibit altered metabolic processes that allow the cells to grow by having enhanced access to nutrients in the blood and diverting the carbon atoms of nutrients into the biomass required for their altered growth properties. One of the earliest observations of altered metabolism in cancer cells was made by Otto Warburg in 1924 for which he won the Nobel Prize in Medicine in 1931. His observations of cancer metabolism became known as the Warburg hypothesis or the Warburg effect.

GLUCOSE METABOLISM AND THE WARBURG EFFECT

In his studies on cancer cell metabolism, Otto Warburg discovered that, unlike most normal tissues, cancer cells tended to "ferment" glucose into lactate even in the presence of sufficient oxygen to support mitochondrial oxidative phosphorylation. He originally postulated this represented mitochondrial dysfunction in cancer cells; however, it was subsequently shown that this was not the mitigating reason for the increased production of lactate in cancer cells.

It might seem counterintuitive that highly proliferative cells, such as is characteristic of cancers, would bypass oxidation of pyruvate (from glucose) in mitochondria since this is the organelle where the vast majority of the ATP from glycolysis is generated. However, it has been shown that oncogenic mutations can result in the uptake of nutrients, particularly glucose and glutamine, that meet or exceed the bioenergetic demands of cell growth and proliferation. Proliferating cells, including cancer cells, require altered metabolism to efficiently incorporate the carbons from glucose and the carbons and nitrogen from glutamine into biomass. The ultimate fate of glucose depends not only on the proliferative state of the cell but also on the activities of the specific glycolytic enzymes that are expressed. This is particularly true for pyruvate kinase, the terminal enzyme in glycolysis.

PYRUVATE KINASE ISOFORMS AND CANCER

Humans express various forms of pyruvate kinase from two distinct genes identified as *PKLR* and *PKM* (see Chapter 5). Expression of PKM1 predominates in cardiac muscle, skeletal muscle, smooth muscle, brain, adrenal medulla, and mature sperm. Expression of PKM2 occurs in most proliferating cells, including in all cancer cell lines and tumors tested to date (Figure 34–2; see also Clinical Box 5–2), embryonic tissues, epithelial cells of the distal tubule of the kidney, spleen, ovaries, testes, intestine, leukocytes, thymus, and adrenal cortex.

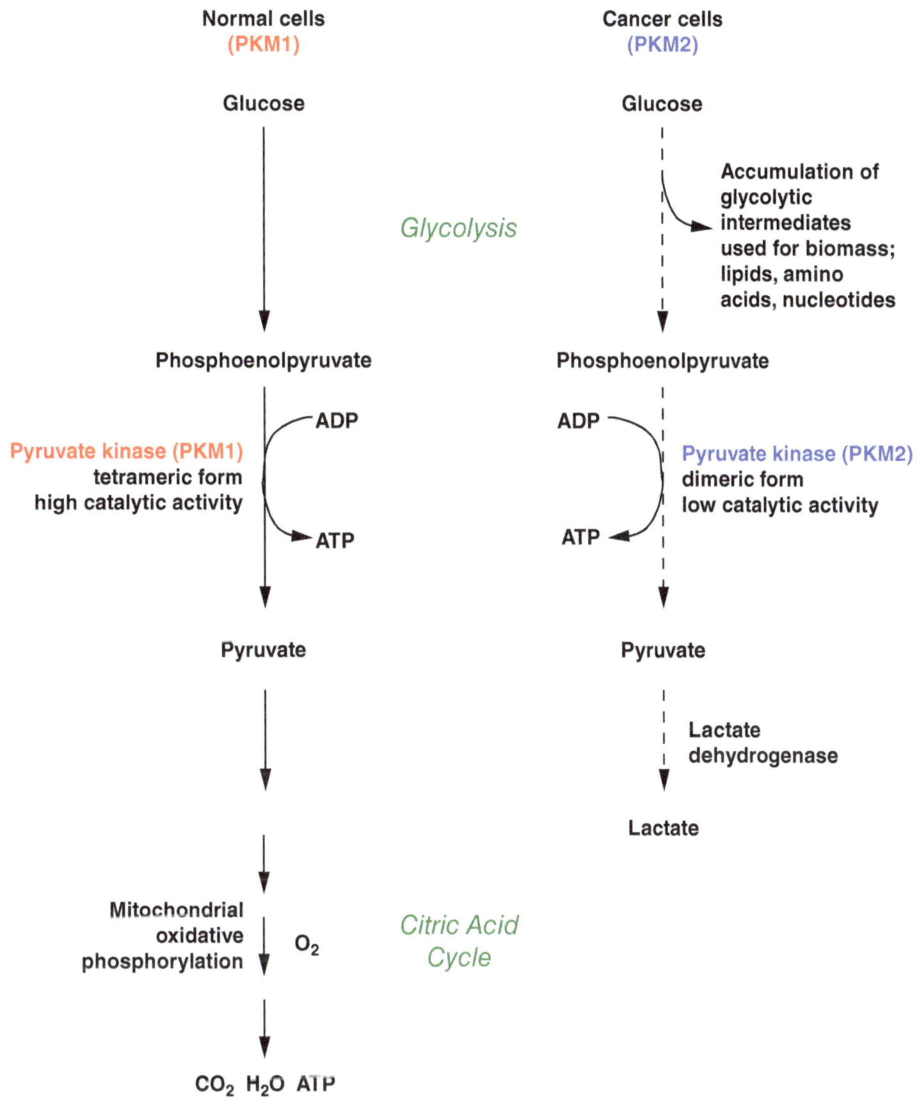

FIGURE 34–2 Pyruvate kinase isozymes and glycolysis in normal and in cancer cells. In normal cells, the major source of ATP is oxidative phosphorylation. Some ATP is obtained from glycolysis. The major pyruvate kinase (PK) isozyme in normal cells is PKM1. In cancer cells, aerobic glycolysis is prominent, lactic acid is produced via the action of lactate dehydrogenase (LDH) and production of ATP from oxidative phosphorylation is diminished (not shown in the figure). In cancer cells, PKM2 is the major PK isozyme. For complex reasons not as yet fully understood, this change of isozyme profile in cancer cells is associated with decreased net production of ATP from glycolysis, but increased use of metabolites to build up biomass. (Reproduced with permission from Rodwell VW, Bender DA, Botham KM, et al: *Harper's Illustrated Biochemistry*, 31st ed. New York, NY: McGraw Hill; 2018.)

PKM2 STRUCTURE-FUNCTION RELATIONSHIPS

PKM2 can exist as a homodimeric or as a homotetrameric enzyme. The tetrameric form of PKM2 exhibits high catalytic activity in the conversion of phosphoenolpyruvate (PEP) to pyruvate and this is associated with ATP synthesis and catabolic metabolism of glucose. In contrast, the dimeric form of PKM2 has low catalytic activity and this low activity, in part, facilitates the diversion of glycolytic intermediates into glucose metabolic branch pathways that including glycerol synthesis and the pentose phosphate pathway. Of significance to proliferating cells, as well as cancer, is that the NADPH produced by the pentose phosphate pathway is used to reduce the level of reactive oxygen species (ROS) and is used in numerous reductive biosynthetic pathways. In addition, the ribose-5-phosphate is used for nucleotide synthesis.

The regulation of the dimeric versus tetrameric forms of PKM2 is under complex control that includes allosteric effectors and posttranslational modifications. The various posttranslational modifications include phosphorylation, acetylation, and oxidation. The upstream glycolytic metabolite (see Chapter 5), fructose-1,6-bisphosphate (FBP), promotes the formation of the tetrameric form of the enzyme. The amino acid serine, which can be derived from the glycolytic intermediate, 3-phosphoglycerate, is also an allosteric activator promoting the tetrameric form of PKM2. Another allosteric stimulator of the tetrameric form of PKM2 is 5-aminoimidazole-4-carboxyribonucleotide (SAICAR) which is an intermediate in purine nucleotide biosynthesis.

PKM2 AS A TRANSCRIPTIONAL CO-ACTIVATOR

When PKM2 is phosphorylated on a particular serine residue (Ser 37) it migrates into the nucleus where it functions as a transcriptional coactivator of β-catenin in the activation of the *MYC* gene. MYC is a potent transcription factor and elevated expression of MYC contributes to the transformed state of cancer cells. Phosphorylation of another serine (Ser 202) also results in migration of PKM2 to the nucleus and this modification allows PKM2 to serve as a transcriptional coactivator of the transcription factor, identified as signal transducer and activator of transcription 5A (STAT5A), resulting in enhanced transcription of a member of the cyclin family (cyclin D1) of cyclin-dependent kinase (CDK) regulators leading to enhanced cell cycle progression.

GLUTAMINE METABOLISM IN CANCER

Glutamine represents the most abundant amino acid in the blood with levels that are in the range of 500 μM. This level of glutamine accounts for over 20% of the total pool of free amino acids in the blood. Although the diet serves as a principal source of glutamine from digested proteins that is then absorbed through the small intestine, another major source of blood glutamine is the ammonia scavenging reactions that take place in skeletal muscle and liver as well as many other tissues.

By circulating in the plasma glutamine represents a major contributor to the energy needs of cells, as a major molecule for movement of ammonia in a nontoxic form, as a carbon source for the synthesis of glucose via gluconeogenesis in the kidney and small intestine, and as a critical substrate for the hexosamine biosynthesis pathway which synthesizes UDP-GlcNAc.

UDP-GlcNAc is added to numerous cytoplasmic and nuclear proteins (referred to as *O*-GlcNAcylation) altering their activities. *O*-GlcNAcylation also represents a mode of epigenetic modification of histone proteins. The need for UDP-GlcNAc for glycoprotein synthesis also demonstrates the role of glutamine in endoplasmic reticulum (ER) homeostasis preventing the activation of ER stress pathways. Glutamine carbons and nitrogen atoms also serve as substrates for the synthesis of other amino acids, nucleotides, and the antioxidant, glutathione. All of these roles of glutamine metabolism, referred to as glutaminolysis, in the generation of biomass contribute to the growth of cancer cells (Figure 34–3).

Glutamine is transported into cells through the actions or various transporters such as the one encoded by the *SLC1A5* gene (also known as ASCT2: Alanine Serine Cysteine Transporter 2). Within the cytosol glutamine and aspartate combine through the action of asparagine synthase to form asparagine and glutamate. Cytosolic glutamine is also a required substrate for the synthesis of UDP-GlcNAc in the hexosamine biosynthesis pathway.

In the mitochondria glutamine is deaminated by the glutaminase encoded by the *GLS2* gene (one of the two glutaminase genes in humans) forming glutamate. Within the mitochondria the glutamate can be converted to 2-oxoglutarate (α-ketoglutarate) via transamination reactions or through the action of glutamate dehydrogenase (encoded by the *GLUD1* gene).

In numerous cancer cells the GLS-encoded enzyme (often referred to as KGA for kidney-type glutaminase) is found in the cytosol allowing for high levels of glutamate to be formed in this location. The glutamate can be used in a series of transamination reactions ultimately contributing to the synthesis of proline, alanine, and aspartate. Glutamate is also used to make glutathione which serves a potent antioxidant function in proliferating and cancer cells. Within the cytosol the glutamate is also converted to 2-oxoglutarate via transamination reactions.

In cancer cells the cytosolic IDH1-encoded enzyme can convert 2-oxoglutarate to isocitrate which then contributes to the cytoplasmic pool of citrate. In the mitochondria, the 2-oxoglutarate can enter the TCA cycle where it can be oxidized to malate and oxaloacetic acid (OAA). The malate can be transported to the cytosol and converted to pyruvate through the action of malic enzyme (encoded by the *ME1* gene). This latter reaction has the benefit of contributing to the NADPH pool which cancer cells can use for reductive biosynthetic reactions such as fatty acid, cholesterol, and nucleotide biosynthesis. The OAA generated from glutamine can be transaminated to aspartate and transported to the cytosol where it can be used in the process of nucleotide biosynthesis.

In many cancer cells expression of the *IDH2* gene is enhanced and, like the cytosolic IDH1-encoded enzyme, can carry out the reverse TCA cycle reaction, converting 2-oxoglutarate to isocitrate. It should be pointed out that in this context these are normal activities of the wild-type IDH1- and IDH2-encoded enzymes. Mutant forms of IDH1 and IDH2 are also found in cancer cells but catalyze distinct reactions as a result of mutations.

Many cancer cells also activate a reductive oxidation process that allows isocitrate to be converted to citrate. The citrate can be transported into the cytosol and hydrolyzed to acetyl-CoA and OAA. The acetyl-CoA can serve as a precursor for the synthesis of fatty acids and cholesterol promoting the ability of cancer cells to generate membranes for rapid cell division.

The glutamine and the aspartate that result from the transamination of OAA, as well as by the routes utilizing glutamate, both serve in the processes of nucleotide biosynthesis. In addition to the carbons of glutamine, the nitrogen is critical to the formation of carbamoyl phosphate which is the first step in pyrimidine nucleotide biosynthesis.

Glutamine can also be transported out of cells, through the action of the LAT1 antiporter, in exchange for leucine. The increased intracellular levels of leucine can activate the mTOR complex 1 (mTORC1) which prevents apoptosis. Export of glutamine can also occur through the action of the xCT antiporter allowing cystine uptake. The cystine is reduced to cysteine which contributes to glutathione synthesis as well as overall protein synthesis.

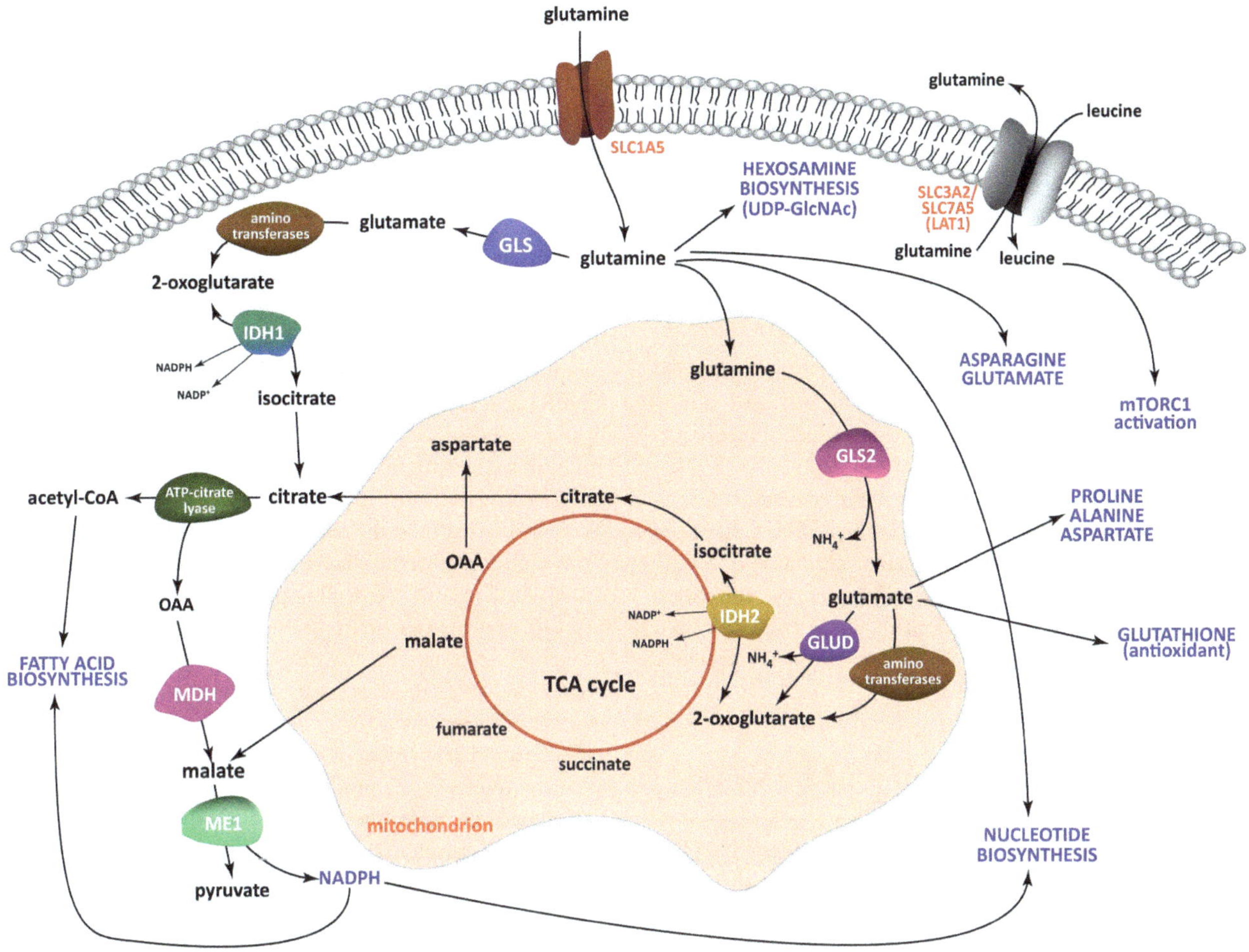

FIGURE 34–3 Metabolic pathways that utilize glutamine in proliferating and cancer cells. Glutamine is the most abundant amino acid in the blood, and it is transported into cells through the actions or various transporters (see text). Within the cytosol the carbons and nitrogens from glutamine serve as substrates for the synthesis of numerous other amino acids, the synthesis of the nucleotides, the synthesis of the antioxidant glutathione, as well as serving to generate the reduced electron carrier, NADPH, which is required for many of the biosynthetic processes taking place at accelerated levels in cancer cells. Mitochondrial glutamine carbons are shuttled into the TCA cycle keeping it operating at maximal rates allowing for the electrons from NADH and $FADH_2$ to drive the synthesis of ATP. (Reproduced with permission from themedicalbiochemistrypage, LLC.)

LACTATE METABOLISM AND CANCER

The altered metabolism of glucose in cancer cells, leading to increased lactate production, results in enhanced level of lactate transport out of the cells via transporters of the monocarboxylate transporter (MCT) family which are encoded by genes of the SLC16 family. Contributing to enhanced lactate production is induction of the hypoxia-induced factor 1 (HIF-1) transcription factor pathway, one target of which is the *LDHA* gene. The increased production of lactate, by cancer cells, contributes to the acidification of the tumor microenvironment which, in turn, promotes further activation of the HIF-1 pathway.

Lactate accumulation also results in pyruvate accumulation in cancer cells. Pyruvate is a known inhibitor of the prolyl hydroxylases that hydroxylate the HIF1α subunit protein of the HIF-1 complex. Loss of HIF1α proline hydroxylation results in increased HIF1α stability and, therefore, increased HIF-1 transcriptional activity. Thus, accumulation of lactate and pyruvate, which occurs as a result of both altered *PKM2* gene expression and activation of the HIF-1 pathway, further promotes activation of the HIF-1 pathway leading to a controlled and enhanced metabolic profile within cancer cells.

6-PHOSPHOGLUCONATE DEHYDROGENASE AND CANCER

The third enzyme of the pentose phosphate pathway, 6-phosphogluconate dehydrogenase (6PGD), is encoded by the phosphogluconate dehydrogenase (*PGD*) gene. Enhanced expression of the *PGD* gene has been reported in numerous different human cancers such as colorectal carcinomas, breast and ovarian cancers, cervical cancers, hepatocellular carcinomas, thyroid cancer, lung cancers, and leukemias.

Altered expression of the *PGD* gene and activity of the encoded 6PGD enzyme is mediated via both posttranscriptional and posttranslational mechanisms. In addition, 6PGD activity is modified by direct protein-protein interactions with malic enzyme 1 (ME1).

Overexpression of the epidermal growth factor receptor (*EGFR*) gene has been identified in up to 50% of human cancers. Recent evidence has shown that the activation of the EGFR signal transduction cascade leads to tyrosine phosphorylation of 6PGD. Tyrosine phosphorylation of 6PGD results in upregulated binding of $NADP^+$ and a consequent increase in the production of NADPH and ribose-5-phosphate. NADPH is critical for biomass production in cancer cells as well as being important in the detoxification of reactive oxygen species, ROS. The increased ribose-5-phosphate enhances nucleotide biosynthesis which subsequently enhances DNA synthesis.

Acetylation of lysine residues in metabolic enzymes is associated with altered catalytic activity. Acetylation of 6PGD has been identified in numerous human cancer cells. Acetylation of 6PGD promotes the formation of active dimers of the enzyme. Inhibition of the deacetylation of 6PGD has been shown to enhance tumor progression most likely as a result of the enhanced metabolic advantage of increased 6PGD activity.

MALIC ENZYME AND 6PGD IN CANCER

The malic enzyme encoded by the *ME1* gene is an $NADP^+$-dependent enzyme that functions as a major contributor to the transfer of acetyl-CoA from the mitochondria to the cytosol where it can serve as a substrate for fatty acid and cholesterol biosynthesis as well as cytosolic protein acetylation. Increased expression of the *ME1* gene, in several cancers, has been shown to be associated with increased activity of 6PGD and overall elevated activity of the pentose phosphate pathway. Increased levels of ME1 activity are associated with hetero-oligomerization with 6PGD which enhances the activity of 6PGD. ME1-mediated activation of 6PGD results in enhanced $NADP^+$ binding and NADPH production. Like the consequences for tumor promotion from 6PGD acetylation, interaction of 6PGD with ME1 leads to enhanced production of NADPH and ribose-5-phosphate, in turn resulting in enhanced biomass production and DNA synthesis in cancer cells.

CANCER CELL EVASION OF APOPTOSIS

Apoptosis refers to the highly regulated and coordinated processes of programmed cell death (PCD) (Figure 34–4). The control of apoptosis represents a balance between the activity of proapoptotic genes and prosurvival (antiapoptotic) genes, processes that many cancers evade allowing them to continue to proliferate. Within cancer cells, mutations associated with the loss of function of proapoptotic genes (eg, *TP53* which encodes p53, see Clinical Box 34–2) and/or overexpression of antiapoptotic genes contribute to the transformed nature of cancer cells.

In general, cell survival pathways predominate, provided cells have adequate access to the appropriate growth (trophic) promoting signals. Under certain conditions some cells will actually release specific hormones that triggers the apoptotic program of adjacent or nearby cells. Two primary pathways exist for the initiation of the apoptotic process in a wide variety of different cell types. These two pathways are termed the intrinsic and extrinsic pathways of apoptosis.

The intrinsic apoptotic pathway is predominantly centered around, and/or regulated by, the mitochondria. An additional intrinsic pathway involves the activation of apoptosis in response to endoplasmic reticulum (ER) stress. The major extrinsic pathway is mediated by receptors that represent a subfamily of the tumor necrosis factor receptor (TNFR) superfamily that includes TNFR1 and FAS. These receptors are activated by an appropriate ligand, such as TNFα and the FAS ligand (FASL), respectively, and initiate a specific apoptotic program. Since these ligands and receptors activate a pathway of PCD these pathways are collectively referred to as the death receptor pathways of apoptosis.

Within the context of the various apoptotic programs, there are similar features and overlapping protein functions. One family of proteins, the caspases, are central to both the intrinsic and extrinsic apoptotic programs. Caspases are so-called because they are **c**ysteine **asp**artate prote**ases**. Caspases are synthesized as precursor inactive proteins (zymogens) that are proteolytically processed, often by another member of the caspase family. The proteolysis of a caspase results in the production of a large and a small subunit that dimerize to form the catalytically active caspase. Within the large caspase family, several members serve as initiators of the apoptotic program and others serve as effectors of the upstream inducing signals.

Apoptosis must not only be efficiently and correctly activated in response to the appropriate signals, but the process must also be tightly controlled at the level of inhibition. Inhibition of apoptosis can occur through the action of antiapoptotic proteins, also referred to as pro-survival factors. Several pro-survival (antiapoptotic) proteins are encoded by genes of the BCL-2 superfamily of apoptosis regulators. Another class of proteins that serve to prevent apoptosis are collectively referred to as inhibitors of apoptosis (IAP).

Proteins of the BCL-2 superfamily are classified as either initiators, cell survival proteins, or effector proteins. The prosurvival proteins are commonly referred to as guardians or as antiapoptotic proteins and are exemplified by BCL-2 itself. The effector proteins are commonly referred to as proapoptotic proteins. Although there are several proapoptotic effector proteins, the BAK (BCL-2 antagonist/killer 1) and BAX (BCL-2 associated protein X) proteins are the most prevalent. BAK is localized to the outer mitochondrial membrane while BAX is localized to the cytosol but activation of apoptotic signaling induces its interaction with the mitochondria. Both BAK and BAX function in the context of mitochondrial (intrinsic pathway) apoptosis.

METASTASES

A significant factor leading to mortality associated with cancer is the spread of the cancer from the site of its origination to another, or many other, locations. The process of cancer spreading is

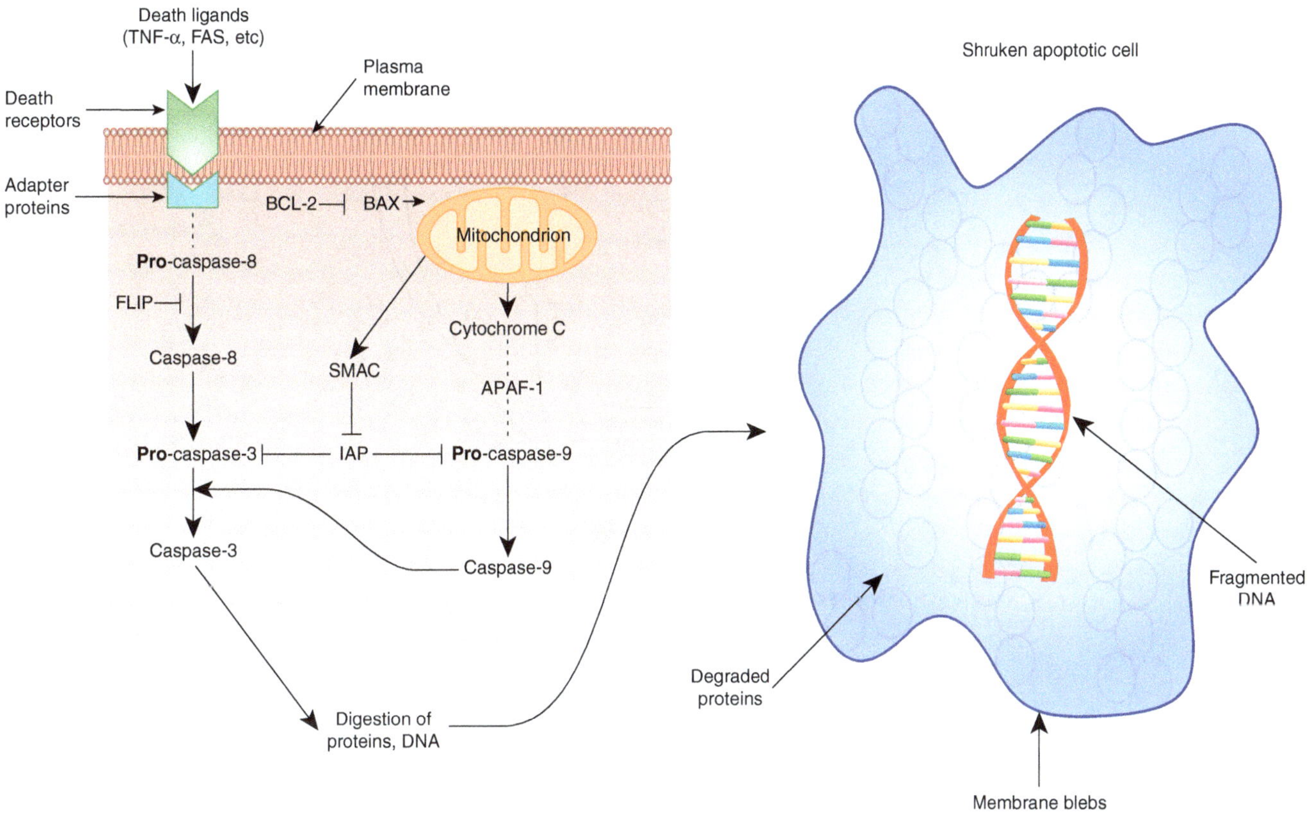

FIGURE 34–4 Simplified scheme of apoptosis. The major molecular events in the extrinsic pathway are shown on the left: Death signals includee TNF-α and FAS (present on the surface of lymphocytes and some other cells). The signals (ligands) interact with specific death receptors (there are a number of them). The activated receptor then interacts with an adapter protein (FADD is one of a number of them), and then forms a complex with procaspase-8. (The complex is indicated by the interrupted line between the adapter protein and procaspase-8 in the Figure). Through a series of further steps, active caspase-3 is formed, whichh is a major effector (executioner) of cell damage. Regulation of the extrinsic pathway can occur due to the inhibitory effect of FLIP on the conversion of procaspase-8 to caspase-8, and also the inhibitory effect of IAP on procaspase-3. On the right are the major cellular events in the intrinsic (mirochondrial) pathway. Various cell stresses affect the permeability of the mitochondrial outer membrane, resulting in efflux of cytochrome c into the cytopasm. This forms a complex with APAF-1 and procaspase-9, called an apoptosome. Through these interactions, procaspase-9 is converted to caspase-9. This, in turn, can act on procaspase-3 to convert it to its active form. Regulation of the intrinsic pathway can occur at the level of BAX, whichh facilitates increasing mitochondrial permeability permitting efflux of cytochrome c, and is thus pro-apoptotic. BCL-2 opposes this effect of BAX and is thus antiapoptotic. IAP also inhibits procaspase-9; this effect of IAP can be overcome by SMAC. (APF-1, apoptotic protease activating factor-1; BAX, BCL-2-associatred X protein; BCL-2, B-cell CLL/lymphoma 2 (CLL represents chronic lymphatic leukemia); FADD, FAS-associated death domain; FAS, FAS antigen; FLICE, FADD-like ICE; FLIP, FLICE inhibitory protein; IAP, inhibitor of apoptosis protein; ICE, interleukin-1-β convertase; SMAC, second mitochondria-derived activator of caspase; signifies opposes the action of; arrows indicate activation.

referred to clinically as metastasis (Figure 34–5). In order for a cancer cell to metastasize, it must first break away from the primary tumor and enter the blood stream. The process by which the cell enters the blood is called **intravasation**. The cell can then migrate to a new location usually where its migration is arrested in a small capillary. There the cell migrates into the local extracellular matrix (ECM) and begins to grow and divide. The process of migration into the ECM is referred to as **extravasation**.

To metastasize, a tumor cell must be released from the ECM of the primary tumor. Two mechanisms are involved in this process. One is a reduction in the expression of cell adhesion molecules, in particular members of the cadherin family. The other mechanism required for cancer cells to metastasize is that the ECM of the tumor must be locally degraded. One of the most important class of enzymes involved in ECM remodeling is the matrix metalloproteinases (MMPs). Many metastatic cancers express elevated levels of MMPs, particularly MMP-2 and MMP-9, leading to degradation of the basement membrane and ECM allowing the cells to escape to the blood.

In order for a new tumor to form, there must be an adequate blood supply to the site and this is accomplished via the secretion of angiogenic factors. Angiogenesis is the process of new vessel synthesis and this process is a target of several anticancer therapies. One of the growth factors involved in stimulating angiogenesis is vascular endothelial growth factor (VEGF). The monoclonal antibody (bevacizumab) targets VEGF and in so doing prevents the growth of new vessels in various types of cancers.

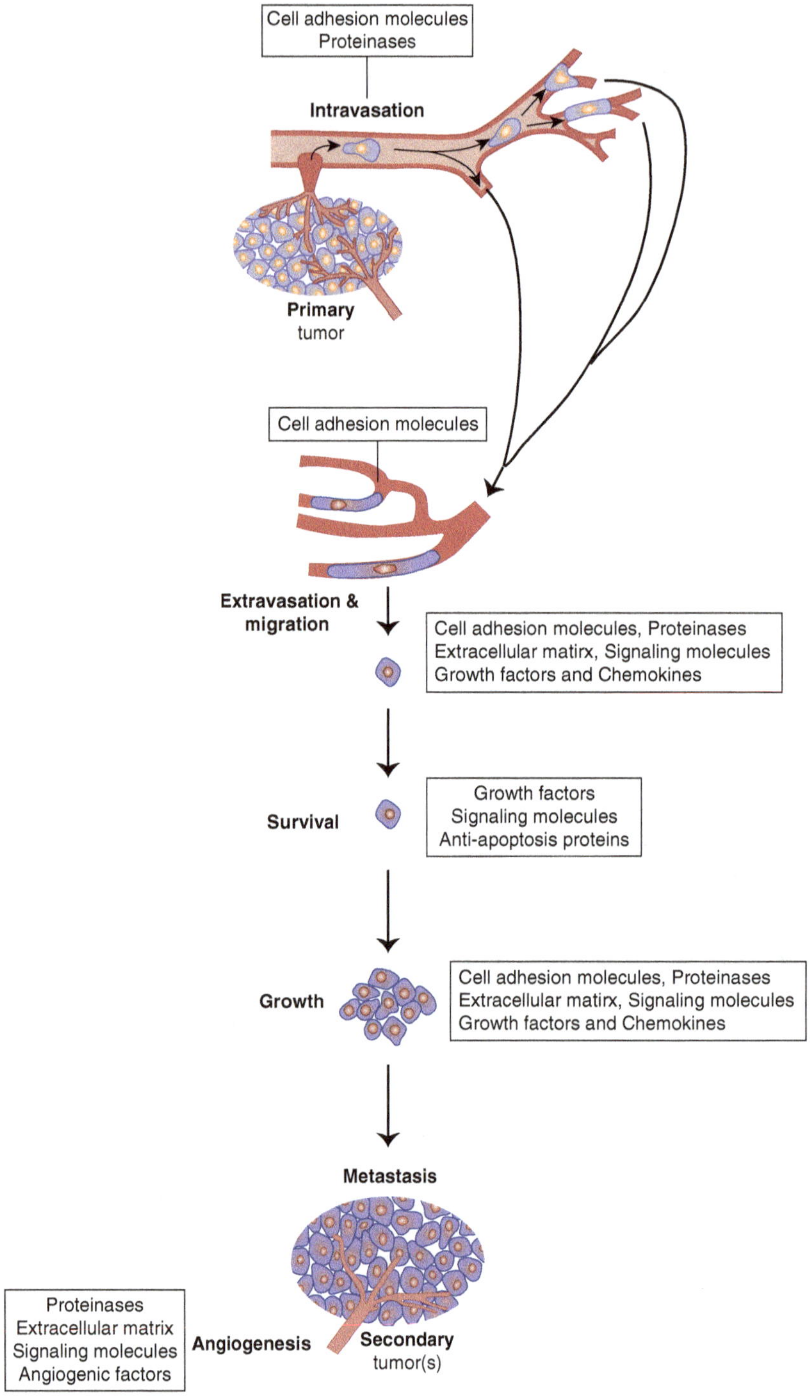

FIGURE 34–5 Simplified scheme of metastasis. Schematic representation of the sequence of steps in metastasis, indicating some of the factors believed to be involved. (Adapted with permission from Chambers AF, Groom AC, MacDonald IC. Dissemination and growth of cancer cells in metastatic sites, Nat Rev Cancer. 2002;2(8):563–572.)

VIRUSES AND CANCER

Tumor cells can arise by the carcinogenic actions of specific tumor viruses (Table 34–3). Tumor viruses are of two distinct types. There are viruses with DNA genomes (eg, papilloma and adenoviruses) and those with RNA genomes called the retroviruses. It should be noted that not all DNA or RNA viruses cause cancer in animals, for example the influenza (orthomyxoviridae family) and measles (paramyxoviridae family) viruses, which are RNA viruses, are not tumor viruses.

TABLE 34–3 Some viruses that cause or are associated with human cancers.

Virus	Genome	Cancer
Epstein-Barr virus	DNA	Burkitt lymphoma, nasopharyngeal cancer, B-cell lymphoma
Hepatitis B	DNA	Hepatocellular carcinoma
Hepatitis C	RNA	Hepatocellular carcinoma
Human herpesvirus 8 (HHV-8)	DNA	Kaposi sarcoma
Human papilloma viruses (types 16 and 18)	DNA	Cancer of the cervix
Human T-cell leukemia virus type 1	RNA	Adult T-cell leukemia

Reproduced with permission from Rodwell VW, Bender DA, Botham KM, et al: *Harper's Illustrated Biochemistry*, 31st ed. New York, NY: McGraw Hill; 2018.

Tumor-causing retroviruses are rare in humans. Nonetheless, the human T-cell leukemia viruses (HTLVs) and human immunodeficiency virus (HIV) are the most notable examples of RNA tumor viruses in humans. The HTLV belongs to the oncovirinae family of viruses and HIV belongs to the lentivirinae family. Another human RNA virus that causes cancer is the hepatitis C virus (HCV) which belongs to the flaviviridae family of viruses.

Retroviruses can induce the transformed state within the cells they infect by two mechanisms. Both of these mechanisms are related to the life cycle of these viruses. One mechanism is associated with the viral infection process. When a retrovirus infects a cell its RNA genome is converted into DNA by the viral encoded RNA-dependent DNA polymerase (reverse transcriptase). The DNA then integrates into the genome of the host cell where it can remain, being copied as the host genome is duplicated during the process of cellular division. Retroviral genomes contain sequence elements termed long terminal repeats (LTR). These LTRs possess strong transcriptional enhancer activity. If viral integration occurs near a highly regulated gene and the presence of the LTR results in dysregulation the result can lead to cellular overgrowth typical of the transformed state.

The other mechanism of retroviral induction of cancer is related to the production of new viral particles and reinfection of surrounding cells. At some frequency the integration process leads to rearrangement of the viral genome and the consequent incorporation of a portion of the host genome into the viral genome. This process is termed transduction. Occasionally this transduction process leads to the virus acquiring a gene from the host that is normally involved in cellular growth control. Because of the alteration of the host gene during the transduction process as well as the gene being transcribed at a higher rate due to its association with the retroviral LTRs the transduced gene confers a growth advantage to subsequent infected cells. The end result of this process is unrestricted cellular proliferation leading to tumorigenesis.

Cellular transformation by DNA tumor viruses, in most cases, has been shown to be the result of protein-protein interaction. Proteins encoded by the DNA tumor viruses, termed tumor antigens or T antigens, can interact with cellular proteins. This interaction effectively sequesters the cellular proteins away from their normal functional locations within the cell. The predominant types of proteins that are sequestered by viral T antigens have been shown to be of the tumor-suppressor type, such as the retinoblastoma susceptibility gene-encoded protein, pRB (see Clinical Box 34–1). It is the loss of their normal suppressor functions that results in cellular transformation.

HEREDITARY CANCER SYNDROMES

Hereditary cancer syndromes have their origin in random genetic mutations that occur in the germ cells and thus, are passed on in the germline of an individual with typical Mendelian patterns of inheritance. Specific hereditary susceptibility syndromes have been characterized that increase the risk of malignancies of the breast, ovary, colon, endometrium, and endocrine organs. The most prevalent hereditary cancer syndromes are Lynch syndrome (also known as hereditary nonpolyposis colorectal cancer, HNPCC), familial adenomatous polyposis (FAP, Clinical Box 34–3), hereditary breast and ovarian cancer (HBOC), and multiple endocrine neoplasia type 2 (MEN2).

The identification of hereditary cancer susceptibility syndromes, at the level of the gene, has significant medical implications. One major benefit of being able to test for cancer susceptibility genes is that individuals in high-risk families, who did not themselves inherit the susceptibility gene, can avoid unnecessary medical interventions.

TUMOR SUPPRESSORS

Tumor-suppressor genes are genes that regulate the growth of cells and when these genes are functioning properly, they can prevent and inhibit the growth of tumors (see Table 34–4). When a tumor-suppressor gene is altered, for example due to sustaining a mutation, the protein product of the gene may lose the ability to properly control cell growth. Under these conditions the cell can grow and proliferate in an uncontrolled way leading to development of cancer. Several familial cancers have been shown to be associated with the loss of function of a tumor-suppressor gene such as *RB1* (Clinical Box 34–1) and *TP53* (Clinical Box 34–2).

There are three main classifications of tumor-suppressor genes. These include genes that encode proteins that tell cells to stop growing and dividing. Another class encodes proteins responsible for repairing DNA damage prior to allowing cells to complete the cell cycle. The third class encodes proteins that are involved in regulating cell death processes, called apoptosis.

TABLE 34–4 Representative tumor-suppressor genes.

Familial Cancer Syndrome	Tumor Suppressor Gene	Function	Tumor Types Observed
Li-Fraumeni Syndrome	*TP53*	Cell cycle regulation, apoptosis	Brain tumors, sarcomas, leukemia, breast cancer
Familial retinoblastoma	*RB1*	Cell cycle regulation	Retinoblastoma, osteogenic sarcoma
Wilms tumor	*WT1*	Transcriptional regulation	Pediatric kidney cancer, most common form of childhood solid tumor
Neurofibromatosis type 1	*NF1*	Catalysis of RAS inactivation	Neurofibromas, sarcomas, gliomas
Familial adenomatous polyposis	*APC*	Signaling through adhesion molecules to nucleus	Colon cancer
Deleted in colorectal carcinoma	*DCC*	Transmembrane receptor involved in axonal guidance via netrins	Colorectal cancer
Familial breast cancer	*BRCA1*	Functions in transcription, DNA binding, transcription-coupled DNA repair, homologous recombination, chromosomal stability, ubiquitination of proteins, and centrosome replication	Breast and ovarian cancer
Familial breast cancer	*BRCA2*: same as the FANCD1 locus	Transcriptional regulation of genes involved in DNA repair and homologous recombination	Breast and ovarian cancer
Lynch syndrome (also known as hereditary nonpolyposis colon cancer HNPCC)	*MLH1, MSH2, MSH6, PMS2*	DNA mismatch repair	Colon cancer, endometrial cancer, ovarian cancer, pancreatic cancer, prostate cancer, brain cancer
von Hippel-Lindau Syndrome	*VHL*	Is a component of a ubiquitin ligase complex that ubiquitylates HIF-1α; also involved in inhibition of transcription elongation	Renal cancers, hemangioblastomas, pheochromocytoma, retinal angioma
Multiple endocrine neoplasia type 1	*MEN1*	Serves as a scaffold protein for processes of histone modification	Parathyroid and pituitary adenomas, islet cell tumors, carcinoid

CLINICAL BOX 34–1 TUMOR SUPRESSOR RB1 AND RETINOBLASTOMA

Retinoblastoma (RB) is a rare type of eye cancer that forms in immature cells of the retina and most often manifest in early childhood prior to the age of 5. Retinoblastoma results from loss of function of the protein encoded by the *RB1* gene. Diagnosis of retinoblastoma after the age of 6 is extremely rare due to the terminal differentiation of retinal epithelial cells. In most children with retinoblastoma, the disease affects only one eye. However, in about 30% of children with retinoblastoma the cancer develops in both eyes. The most common first sign of retinoblastoma is a visible whiteness in the pupil referred to as leukocoria. This is also called amaurotic cat's eye reflex. Additional symptoms of retinoblastoma include crossed eyes or eyes that do not point in the same direction (strabismus), persistent eye pain, redness, or irritation; and blindness or poor vision in the affected eye(s). Retinoblastoma is often curable when it is diagnosed early. If not treated promptly, the cancer can spread to other parts of the body leading to life-threatening metastasis. When retinoblastoma is associated with a gene mutation that occurs in all of the body's cells, it is known as germinal retinoblastoma. Individuals with this form of retinoblastoma also have an increased risk of developing several other cancers outside the eye. Specifically, they are more likely to develop a cancer of the pineal gland in the brain (pinealoma), a type of bone cancer known as osteosarcoma, cancers of soft tissues such as muscle, and an aggressive form of skin cancer called melanoma. In the familial form of retinoblastoma individuals inherit a mutant, loss of function allele from an affected parent. A subsequent later somatic mutational event (referred to as loss of heterozygosity, LOH) inactivates the normal allele resulting in retinoblastoma development. This leads to an apparently dominant mode of inheritance. The requirement for an additional somatic mutational event at the unaffected allele means that penetration of the defect is not always complete. Indeed, the penetration frequency for retinoblastoma is not 100% but closer to 90%, meaning not all individuals who inherit, what is supposed to be genetically a dominant disease, actually develop retinoblastoma. In addition, due to the terminal

CLINICAL BOX 34–1 (CONTINUED)

differentiation of pigmented retinal epithelial cells, if a child does not suffer a somatic mutation in the wild-type *RB* gene before the age of 6–8 they will never develop the disease. In the sporadic forms of retinoblastoma involving the RB1 gene, two somatic mutational events must occur, the second of which must occur in the descendants of the cell receiving the first mutation. This combination of mutational events is extremely rare. The pRB protein is a nuclear localized phosphoprotein. pRB is not detectable in any retinoblastoma cells. However, surprisingly detectable levels of pRB can be found in most proliferating cells even though there is a restricted number of tissues affected by mutations in the RB gene (ie, retina, bone, and connective tissue). Many different types of mutation occur to result in loss of pRB function. The largest percentage (30%) of retinoblastomas contain large scale deletions. Splicing errors, point mutations, and small deletions in the promoter region have also been observed in some retinoblastomas. The germ-line mutations in *RB1* occur predominantly during spermatogenesis as opposed to oogenesis. However, the somatic mutations occur with equal frequency at the paternal or maternal locus. In contrast, somatic mutations at RB1 in sporadic osteosarcomas occur preferentially at the paternal locus. This may be the result of genomic imprinting. The major function of pRB is in the regulation of cell cycle progression. Its ability to regulate the cell cycle correlates to the state of phosphorylation of pRB. Phosphorylation is maximal at the start of S phase and lowest after mitosis and entry into G1. Stimulation of quiescent cells with mitogen induces phosphorylation of pRB, while in contrast, differentiation induces hypophosphorylation of pRB. It is, therefore, the hypophosphorylated form of pRB that suppresses cell proliferation. One of the most significant substrates for phosphorylation by the G_1 cyclin-CDK complexes that regulate progression through the cell cycle is pRB. pRB forms a complex with proteins of the E2F family of transcription factors, a result of which renders E2F inactive (Figure 34–6). The original E2F proteins was so-called due to its binding to the adenovirus E2 promoter. When pRB is phosphorylated by G_1 cyclin-CDK complexes it is released from E2F allowing E2F to transcriptionally activate genes. In the context of the cell cycle, E2F increases the transcription of the S-phase cyclins as well as leads to increases in its' own transcription. There are six members of the E2F family identified as E2F1–E2F6. The proteins E2F1, E2F2, and E2F3 are regulated by pRB. When released from pRB, the E2F transcription factors can form homodimers and bind to target DNA sequences or they can form heterodimers to activate transcription.

CLINICAL BOX 34–2 TUMOR SUPPRESSOR P53 AND LI-FRAUMENI SYNDROME (LFS)

Li-Fraumeni syndrome (LFS) is a rare autosomal dominant disorder that greatly increases the risk of developing several types of cancer, particularly in children and young adults. The disorder is named for the two physicians who first recognized and described the syndrome: Frederick Pei Li and Joseph F. Fraumeni, Jr. The cancers most often associated with Li-Fraumeni syndrome include breast cancer, a form of bone cancer called osteosarcoma, and cancers of soft tissues (such as muscle) called soft tissue sarcomas. Other cancers commonly seen in this syndrome include brain tumors, cancers of blood-forming tissues (leukemias), and a cancer called adrenocortical carcinoma that affects the outer layer of the adrenal glands. LFS is linked to germline mutations in the tumor suppressor gene, *TP53* that encodes the protein identified as p53. The p53 protein is involved in the blocking of cell cycle progression (see Figure 34–7) while DNA repair takes place or if the DNA damage is severe enough p53 initiates a program of apoptosis. Mutant p53 involvement in neoplasia is more frequent than any other known tumor suppressor or dominant proto-oncogene. The p53 protein is a nuclear localized phosphoprotein. A domain near the N-terminus of the p53 protein is highly acidic like similar domains found in various transcription factors. p53 regulates the transcription of genes involved in suppression of cell growth. p53 binds to DNA sequences containing two copies of the motif: 5′-PuPuC(A/T)(A/T)GPyPyPy-3′ (Pu = any purine; Py = any pyrimidine). This sequence motif indicated that that p53 bound to DNA as a homotetramer. Binding as a tetrameric complex explains the fact that mutant p53 proteins act in a dominant manner to interfere with the activity of wild-type proteins present in the tetrameric complex. Like pRB, p53 forms a complex with SV40 large T antigen, as well as the E1B transforming protein of adenovirus and E6 protein of human papilloma viruses. Complexing with these tumor antigens increases the stability of the p53 protein. This increased stability of p53 is characteristic of mutant forms found in tumor lines. The complexes of T antigens and p53 renders p53 incapable of binding to DNA and inducing transcription. A cellular protein, identified as MDM2 binds to p53 resulting in loss of p53-mediated transactivation of gene expression. The MDM2 protein is a member of the large family of E3 ubiquitin ligases. When associated with p53 the MDM2 protein ubiquitylates p53. This ubiquitylation leads to proteasome-mediated degradation of p53. Several other ubiquitin ligases ensure that p53 activity is kept in check by ensuring it has a very short half-life in the cells. The transcriptional activity of p53 is regulated by various posttranslational mechanisms in addition to ubiquitylation and includes phosphorylation, acetylation, and methylation. Under normal cellular conditions the level of p53 is low following mitosis but increases during G_1. During S-phase the protein becomes phosphorylated by the M-phase cyclin-CDK complex of the cell cycle. This phosphorylation of p53 allows it to dissociate from MDM2 and migrate to the nucleus and activate the expression of target genes. Under conditions of cellular stress, or when DNA is damaged by ionizing or UV irradiation, various kinases become activated and result in the hyperphosphorylation of p53 dramatically increasing p53-mediated transcription. These stress-induced and DNA damage-induced kinases include ataxia telangiectasia mutated kinase (ATM), ataxia telangiectasia and Rad3-related protein (ATR), casein kinase I (CKI), and AMPK. One major cell-cycle regulating gene that is a target for p53 is the CDK inhibitory protein (CIP), $p21^{CIP}$. Activation of p53, particularly in response to stress or DNA-damage, results in increased expression of $p21^{CIP}$ resulting in cell cycle arrest at several points (Figure 34–7).

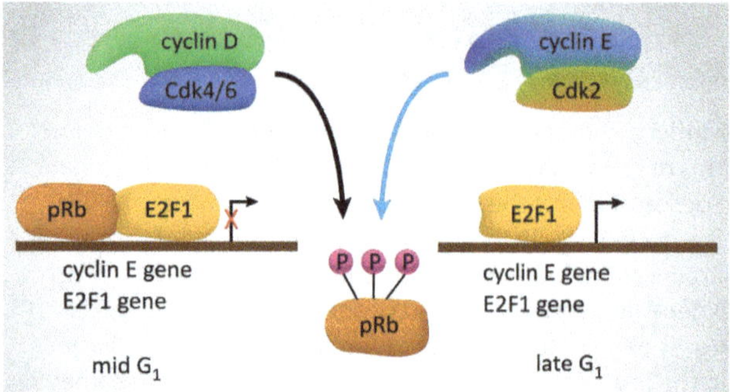

FIGURE 34–6 Regulation of E2F activity by pRB. During early G_1 the transcription factor E2F is inhibited by interaction with pRB in the cytosol. Activation of the G_1 cyclin-CDK complex (cyclin D-CDK4/6) results in the phosphorylation of pRB which then releases E2F. Free from pRB, E2F migrates to the nucleus where it activates the transcription of several genes including the cyclin E gene and the E2F gene itself. The autoregulation of E2F allows for high level activity of this critical cell cycle regulatory factor. In addition, the activation of cyclin E expression results in formation of active cyclin E-CDK2 complexes which keep pRB phosphorylated ensuring transit through to S-phase of the cell cycle. (Reproduced with permission from themedicalbiochemistrypage, LLC.)

DNA METHYLATION AND TUMOR SUPPRESSORS

The link between the epigenetic phenomenon of DNA methylation (see Chapter 22) and cancer is reflected in the fact that alterations in DNA methylation contribute to nearly half of all human cancers. In most cases the higher the level of DNA methylation the more transcriptionally repressed is the methylated gene. The best characterized epigenetic "lesions" in malignant cells are the promoter CpG island hypermethylation events that lead to transcriptional repression of tumor-suppressor genes. These changes have been observed in numerous cancers and were first fully characterized in retinoblastomas (the *RB1* gene), breast cancers (the *BRCA1* gene), renal carcinomas (the *VHL* gene), and numerous types of cancers involving hypermethylation of the cyclin-dependent kinase (CDK) inhibitory gene, p16. Hypermethylation of the gene (*CDKN2A*) encoding p16 has been observed in nearly 20% of all primary human neoplasms.

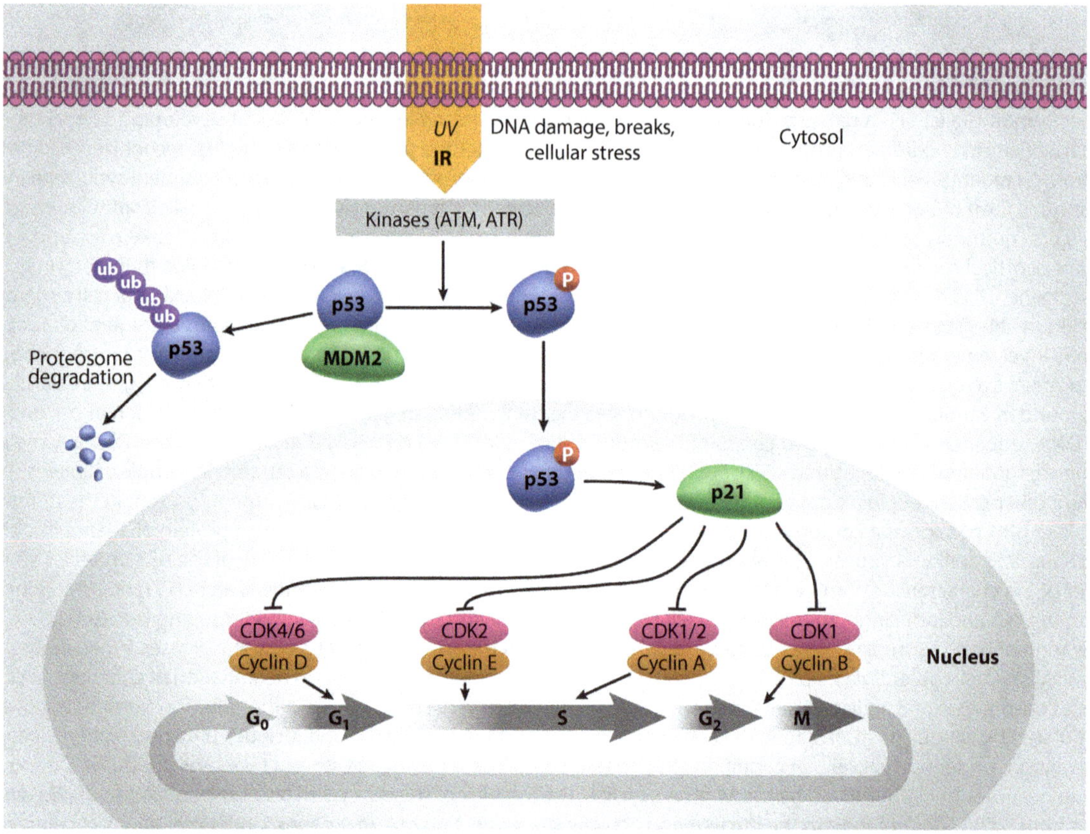

FIGURE 34–7 DNA damage induction of p53 and activation of $p21^{CIP}$. Ionizing radiation, or other causes of DNA damage, activate the ataxia-telangiectasia mutated (ATM) kinase. ATM phosphorylates p53 which stabilizes the protein and releases it from the ubiquitin ligase, MDM2. The phosphorylated p53 then migrates to the nucleus where it activates transcription of various target genes. One target of p53 is the gene encoding CDK inhibitory protein, $p21^{CIP}$. Increased expression of $p21^{CIP}$ results in inhibition of G_1-S- and S-cyclin-CDK complexes ensuring that cells do not progress through S phase of the cell cycle until DNA damage is repaired. (Reproduced with permission from themedicalbiochemistrypage, LLC.)

TABLE 34–5 Breast and ovarian cancer susceptibility genes.

Gene	Function, Role in Cancer
ATM	**a**taxia **t**elangiectasia **m**utated, first identified as causing ataxia telangiectasia, is a PI3K-type kinase activated by DNA damage
BRCA1	**br**east **ca**ncer **1**, early onset, along with BRCA2, the first genes identified as being mutated in inherited forms of breast and ovarian cancer, both are tumor suppressors involved in DNA repair and chromosomal stability
BRCA2	**br**east **ca**ncer **2**, early onset, is also known as Fanconi anemia complementation group D1 (*FANCD1*) gene, plays a major role in high-risk breast cancer predisposition
BRIP1	**BR**CA1 **i**nteracting **p**rotein C-terminal helicase 1, functions in double-strand DNA break repair in concert with BRCA1, is also known as Fanconi anemia complementation group J (FANCJ)
CHEK2	cell cycle **che**ckpoint **k**inase 2. CHEK2 is a serine threonine kinase that is activated by ATM protein in response to DNA double-strand breaks, regulates function of BRCA1 protein in DNA repair, exerts a number of critical roles in cell cycle control and apoptosis
PALB2	**pa**rtner and **l**ocalizer of **B**RCA2, binds directly to BRCA1 and serves as the molecular scaffold in the formation of the BRCA1-PALB2-BRCA2 complex, is also known as Fanconi anemia complementation group N (FANCN)
RAD51C	a member of the RAD51 family of related proteins involved in recombinational DNA repair and meiotic recombination

BREAST CANCERS

Breast cancers include any cancer originating from breast tissue but are most commonly seen in cells of the inner lining of milk ducts or the lobules that supply the ducts with milk. Cancers originating from milk ducts are known as ductal carcinomas, whereas, those originating from lobules are known as lobular carcinomas. Breast cancers account for almost 23% of all cancers in women worldwide. Most forms of breast cancer are spontaneous and not due to the inheritance of a specific mutant gene.

The primary risk factors for breast cancer include smoking, dietary life style including high-fat diets, obesity, and alcohol consumption. Although most breast (and ovarian) cancers are spontaneous, inherited mutations in several genes have been shown to be associated with an increased risk of developing these types of cancers (Table 34–5). To date seven loci have been identified that when mutated predispose an individual to breast and ovarian cancer. These loci are *BRCA1*, *BRCA2*, *ATM*, *CHEK2*, *BRIP1*, *PALB2*, and *RAD51C*. Of significance is that all of these breast cancer susceptibility genes encode proteins that function in some aspect of DNA damage repair (see Chapter 22).

GASTROINTESTINAL CANCERS

The gastrointestinal (GI) system is the site of more malignant tumors than any other organ system. The most common locations for GI cancers are the large intestine (colon) and the rectum (colorectal cancers) but cancers of the mouth, esophagus, stomach, and small intestines, are included when discussing overall GI cancer rates. Almost all colon cancers are adenocarcinomas that result from adenomatous polyps (Figure 34–7). Although most colon cancers arise from adenomatous polyps the majority of them do not give rise to cancer. Routine colonoscopy is designed to examine for the presence of these polyps and they can be removed during the procedure.

With respect to overall GI cancers, the differences in worldwide distribution rates can be explained almost entirely by environmental factors. There are, however, several well-defined inherited genetic disorders that predispose an individual to colorectal carcinomas. Cancers of the upper GI, mouth, esophagus, and stomach are almost entirely due to influences of the diet. The most prevalent dietary causes of GI cancers are high fat, high calorie, and low-fiber diets, typical of what is seen in the Western-style diet. Cancers of the lower GI, the colorectal cancers, are much more often related to genetic factors including inheritance or somatic acquisition of gene mutations predisposing one to the development of cancer.

Many colorectal cancers are initiated due to inheritance of mutated tumor suppressor genes or through somatic mutations in these same genes. One of the most frequently mutated tumor-suppressor genes responsible for initiation of colorectal cancers is the adenomatous polyposis coli gene (*APC*). Inherited mutations in *APC* are the cause of familial adenomatous polyposis, FAP (Clinical Box 34–3).

Another well-characterized inherited colorectal carcinoma syndrome is Lynch syndrome, also known as hereditary non-polyposis colorectal cancer, HNPCC. Lynch syndrome is a family of inherited cancer syndromes that results from mutations in at least four different genes involved in the repair of DNA damage. Specifically, these four genes, *MLH1*, *MSH2*, *MSH6*, and *PMS2*, are all involved in DNA mismatch repair (MMR) during DNA replication. Lynch syndrome accounts for 5% of all cases of colorectal cancer and patients who inherit a mutation in any of these genes have an 80% chance of developing colorectal cancer. Because the inheritance of a mutated DNA mismatch repair gene is present in all cell types, these individuals have increased risk of cancers in multiple other locations. In women with Lynch syndrome, uterine (endometrial) cancers are quite common.

CLINICAL BOX 34–3 TUMOR SUPPRESSOR APC AND FAMILIAL ADENOMATOUS POLYPOSIS

Familial adenomatous polyposis (FAP) is an inherited disorder characterized by a highly elevated risk of developing colorectal carcinoma. FAP is associated with germline mutations in the adenomatous polyposis coli (*APC*) gene. Somatic mutations in APC are also highly correlated to the initiation of colorectal cancer in the general population. Multiple colonic polyp development, within the first decades of life, is characteristic of FAP. These polyps become malignant carcinomas and adenomas later in life. FAP adenomas appear as a result of loss-of function mutations to the APC gene which characterizes the gene as a tumor suppressor. To date, more than 120 different germ line and somatic mutations have been identified in the *APC* gene. The vast majority of these mutations lead to C-terminal truncation of the APC protein. The protein coding region of the *APC* gene is extremely large encompassing 2844 amino acids. The APC protein is found associated with other proteins in the cytosol. One of these APC-associated proteins is β-catenin. The catenins are a family of proteins that interact with the cytoplasmic portion of the cadherins (cell-cell adhesion family of proteins), thus linking the cadherins to the actin cytoskeleton. Catenins are equally important in the signaling cascade initiated by the Wnt family of proteins that are involved in embryonic patterning and development of the nervous system. The Wnt proteins are secreted factors that interact with cell-surface receptors. Wnt-receptor interaction induces the activity of the cytoplasmic phosphoprotein dishevelled. Activated dishevelled inhibits the serine/threonine kinase glycogen synthase kinase-3β (GSK-3β). When GSK-3β is inhibited, β-catenin becomes hypophosphorylated. The hypophosphorylated form of β-catenin migrates to the nucleus and interacts with transcription factors, in particular with T-cell factor/lymphoid enhancer-binding factor-1 (TCF/LEF-1), thereby, inducing expression of various genes. The suspected role of APC in this pathway is to bind phosphorylated β-catenin. The APC-β-catenin complex stimulates the ubiquitination of β-catenin resulting in its degradation in the proteosome. Mutations which lead to a loss of APC, or to a loss of APC interaction with β-catenin, result in constitutive activation of TCF/LEF-1 and unrestricted cell growth. Within the colon this leads to development of adenomatous polyps. Subsequent mutations (see Figure 34–8) in other genes results in the eventual progression to adenocarcinoma.

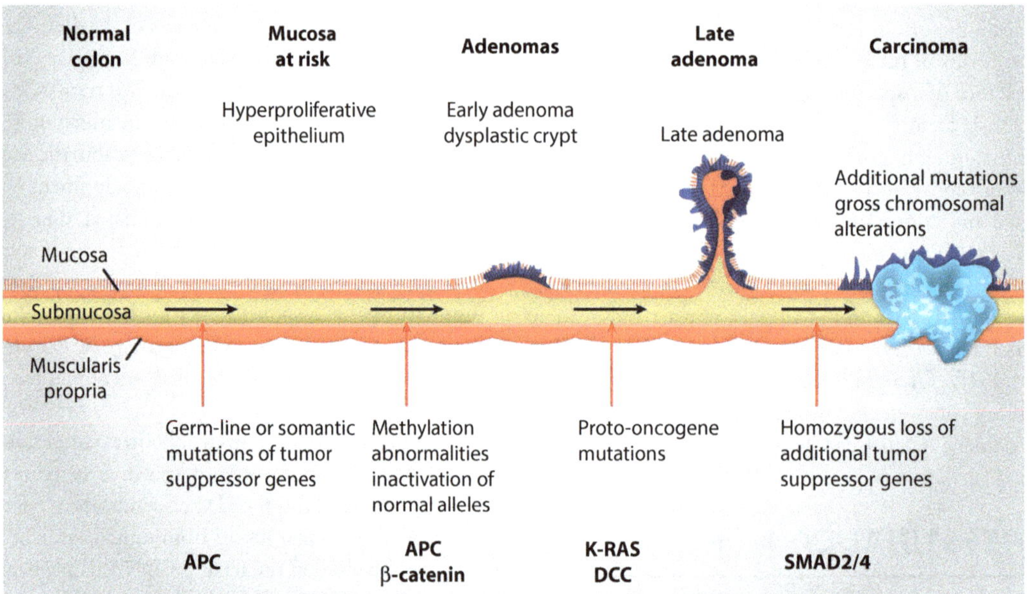

FIGURE 34–8 Progression of normal colonic mucosa to full-blown adenocarcinoma. The initial step in colorectal carcinoma is formation of an adenoma, most often associated with loss of adenomatous polyposis coli (*APC*) gene function. Larger adenomas and early carcinomas acquire progressively more and more mutations such as in the β-catenin and small GTPase (K-RAS) genes. This is followed by loss of chromosome 18q which disrupts SMAD2/4 function. Many additional mutations are known to be associated with this progressive development to a full-blown carcinoma but are not depicted here. (Reproduced with permission from themedicalbiochemistrypage, LLC.)

HEMATOPOIETIC AND LYMPHOID CANCERS

Hematological cancers represent those cancers affecting cells of the blood and bone marrow, the myeloid cancers, as well as cancers of the lymphatic system, the lymphoid cancers. Myeloid lineage cancers include the erythroid cells, granulocytes, monocytes, megakaryocytes, and mast cells. The lymphoid lineage cancers include the lymphomas, the lymphocytic leukemias, and the myelomas. There is a close association between gross chromosomal abnormalities and the development of leukemias and lymphomas. The lymphomas account for approximately 4% of all cancers in the United States. The leukemias, account for approximately 2–4% of all incidences of cancer in the United States and for 3–5% of all cancer deaths. The leukemias are particularly devastating emotionally because they are the most common cancers in children.

The most commonly occurring types of leukemias are acute lymphoblastic leukemia (ALL), acute myelogenous leukemia (AML), chronic lymphocytic leukemia (CLL), and chronic myelogenous leukemia (CML, Clinical Box 34–4). Lymphomas account for approximately 56% of all hematologic cancers and are classified as Hodgkin or non-Hodgkin lymphomas. There are four generalized categories of Hodgkin lymphoma all of which are characterized by the spread of the disease from one lymph node to another. Hodgkin lymphoma can be diagnosed by histological examination of the affected lymph cells. These cells have a characteristic multinucleated appearance and are called Reed-Sternberg cells (RS cells).

Non-Hodgkin lymphomas (NHL) represent all other lymphomas that are not distinctly Hodgkin lymphomas. There are at least 16 different types of characterized NHL. Like most hematologic cancers, 80–90% of NHL are associated with gross chromosomal abnormalities. The most common chromosomal aberrations are translocations between chromosomes 8 and 14 [identified as t(8:14)] and those between chromosomes 14 and 18 [t(14:18)].

The t(8:14) translocation was the first chromosome abnormality to be molecularly characterized. The MYC proto-oncogene on chromosome 8 becomes fused to the immunoglobulin heavy chain enhancer region on chromosome 14 causing highly unregulated expression of the *MYC* gene resulting in abnormal cell growth and proliferation. The t(14:18) translocation disrupts the *BCL2* gene on chromosome 18 resulting in loss of BCL-2-mediated regulation of apoptosis.

CLINICAL BOX 34–4 CHRONIC MYELOGENOUS LEUKEMIA

Chronic myelogenous leukemia (CML) is a cancer associated with unregulated growth of myeloid lineage cells of the bone marrow which then accumulate in the blood. The affected cells are mature granulocytes (eosinophils, basophils, and neutrophils) and granulocyte precursors. In the first stages of CML, many patients do not have any symptoms of the disease and can remain symptom-free for several years. CML is most often diagnosed between the ages of 45 and 55 with 30% of diagnosed patients being over the age of 65. CML is most often discovered through routine blood tests (a complete blood count, CBC), not due to the presentation of overt symptoms. Detection of CML through a CBC is due to the identification of increased numbers of granulocytes of all types. During the progression of CML the number of cancer cells accumulates to the point of interference with normal functions resulting in the manifestation of symptoms. These symptoms can include bleeding and bruising, anemia, fatigue, loss of weight, loss of appetite, night sweats, enlarged lymph nodes, and recurrent infections. Definitive diagnosis of CML is accomplished via the detection of a specific chromosomal translocation in metaphase cells. This translocation is referred to as the Philadelphia chromosome and its presence is denoted as Ph^+. The Philadelphia chromosome results from a translocation between chromosomes 9 and 22 [t(9:22)]. The t(9:22) translocation fuses the Ableson tyrosine kinase (ABL) on chromosome 9 with the BCR locus on chromosome 22. The *ABL* gene was first identified as an oncogene in murine leukemias. The BCR locus was originally identified as a region of frequent chromosomal breakage and thus, termed the breakpoint cluster region, BCR. The BCR-ABL fusion protein results in constitutive activation of the tyrosine kinase activity of ABL. The normal function of ABL is to regulate the activity of a number of cell cycle regulating proteins. Loss of regulated ABL activity therefore leads to unregulated cell cycle progression leading to malignancy. The drug imatinib mesylate was the first drug specifically designed to target the tyrosine kinase activity of the BCR-ABL oncoprotein and has been used with high success in the treatment of Ph^+ CML.

CHECKLIST

- ☑ Cancers are the result of some form of insult to the genetic makeup of a cell. These insults can, and do, include point mutations, insertions, deletions, gross chromosomal abnormalities (eg, translocations), and viral disruption of the genome.
- ☑ The vast majority of cancers are the result of alterations in the function of genes involved in aspects of cell signaling from growth factors, receptors, intracellular signaling molecules, and transcription factors. Additional classes of affected genes in cancer are those that regulate progression through the cell cycle.
- ☑ Cancers can continue to grow unrestricted due to induced loss of growth regulatory signals as well as the induction of unregulated nutrient intake. Solid tumors can expand because they induce the expression of factors involved in the production of new vessels (angiogenesis).
- ☑ Cancer cells acquire the ability to modify metabolic programs to maximize the diversion of carbon and nitrogen from the blood, primarily glucose and glutamine, into biomass: lipids, amino acids and proteins, nucleotides and nucleic acids.
- ☑ With respect to nutrient intake and metabolism, all cancer cells express a particular form of the glycolytic enzyme, pyruvate kinase (specifically the PKM2 isoform), that leads to most glycolysis proceeding to lactate instead of to complete oxidation in the TCA cycle. This unique glycolytic metabolism is referred to as the Warburg effect and it allows glucose carbons to be diverted into the biomass necessary for cancer cell proliferation.
- ☑ The vast majority of human cancers result from genetic alterations in somatic cells. However, there are many cancers that result from germline transmission (inheritance) of altered genes that predispose an individual to a particular form of cancer.
- ☑ Cancers are the result of changes in two distinct classes of gene: the dominant cancer causing genes are referred to as oncogenes and cancer results from any gain-of-function mutation in the original proto-oncogene; the recessive cancer-causing genes are referred to as the tumor suppressors and cancer results from and loss-of-function mutation to the gene.
- ☑ Epigenetics plays a role in cancer and is most often related to changes in DNA methylation status. Many cancers have been found to result from hypermethylation of tumor-suppressor genes resulting in their transcriptional silencing.
- ☑ Cancer metastasis is the process by which a tumor cell can break away from the originating tumor and migrate to a new location in the body forming new tumor sites. Metastasis requires several properties unique to cancer that include loss of cell adhesion, breakdown of the ECM, penetration into the vasculature, evasion of immune surveillance, and colonization of the new site.
- ☑ Overall, cancer is a multistep process that occurs in different pathways in different individuals even when considering the same type of cancer. This makes treatments difficult within the context of a given type of cancer in different individuals.

REVIEW QUESTIONS

1. A 43-year-old woman is being examined by her physician with complaints of severe fatigue, chronic headaches, and radiating pain and fullness on her left side. A routine blood test indicates the presence of increased immature white cells (blasts), reduced platelets, and reduced leukocytes. Her physician orders a karyotype analysis of cells from a bone marrow aspirate with the results showing the following: 46,XY,t(9;22)(q34.1;q11.2). This finding is most consistent with which of the following?

(A) Acute lymphocytic leukemia
(B) Chronic myelogenous leukemia
(C) Hodgkin lymphoma
(D) Multiple myeloma
(E) Non-Hodgkin lymphoma

2. A 12-year-old girl is being treated for glioblastoma. Molecular studies performed on cells isolated from biopsy tissue discover the presence of an altered arginine codon in the gene encoding isocitrate dehydrogenase 1 (IDH1). Given these findings, which of the following molecular processes is most likely to be altered?

(A) DNA replication
(B) Epigenetic regulation of gene expression
(C) Function of miRNA
(D) Homologous recombination during meiosis
(E) Splicing of mRNA

3. A 34-year-old man is being examined by his physician with complaints of abdominal distension, night sweats, and shortness of breath, all of which have developed over the last 5 weeks. Physical examination finds decreased breath sounds in the right lung base and a 2-cm lymph node appreciated on the left inguinal region. Karyotyping of cells extracted from biopsy tissue from the inguinal lymph node shows 46,XY,t(14;18)(q32;q21). Based on the signs and findings in this patient, which of the following is most likely?

(A) Acute lymphocytic leukemia
(B) Acute myelogenous leukemia
(C) Chronic myelogenous leukemia
(D) Hodgkin lymphoma
(E) Non-Hodgkin lymphoma

4. A 53-year-old woman has undergone a diagnostic test following a routine mammogram showing a potential cancerous lesion.

Biopsy tissue was taken at the time of the mammogram, and the results were positive for an invasive ductal carcinoma. Her prescribed course of treatment includes removal of the affected tissue followed by oral tamoxifen therapy. The use of tamoxifen will most likely modulate the action of estrogen in this patient via which of the following mechanisms?

(A) Activation of the MAP kinase pathway downstream of the estrogen receptor
(B) Activation of the tyrosine kinase activity of the estrogen receptor
(C) Binding to the nuclear receptor for estrogen
(D) Binding to the transcriptional coactivator of the estrogen receptor
(E) Dimerization of the estrogen receptor in the cytosol
(F) Dimerization of the estrogen receptor in the plasma membrane

5. A 57-year-old woman is being examined by her physician with complaints of chronic severe fatigue, chronic headaches, and radiating pain and fullness on her left side for the past 5 months. Due to suspicion of leukemia, her physician orders a detailed analysis of cells from a bone marrow aspirate. Results from these studies show the presence of a particular cytological defect referred to as the Philadelphia chromosome. Based on this finding, which of the following is most likely contributing to the symptoms in this patient?

(A) Defective DNA mismatch repair
(B) Loss of DNA damage-mediated cell cycle arrest
(C) Reduced activity of the RAS G-protein
(D) Unregulated serine phosphorylation
(E) Unregulated tyrosine phosphorylation

6. A 39-year-old man is being examined by his physician with complaints of chronic fatigue and unexplained weight loss. Physical examination finds massive splenomegaly. Blood work shows a leukocyte count of 125,000/μL (N = 45,000–11,000/μL). The physician suspects his patient may have a form of leukemia and orders cytogenetic analysis of cells from a bone marrow aspirate. The results of this assay find the following karyotype: 46,XY,t(9;22)(q34.1;q11.2). Which of the following is most likely associated with this karyotype?

(A) Amplification of an oncogene
(B) Creation of a frame-shift mutation in a tumor suppressor gene
(C) Deletion of genetic material
(D) Formation of a fusion gene
(E) Production of a nonsense mutation in a proto-oncogene

7. A 27-year-old man is being examined by his physician to ascertain the cause of the bumps appearing on his skull and jaw. Physical examination of the patient finds several epidermoid cysts. Family history indicates that his mother died of colorectal cancer when the patient was only 6 years old. Given the external signs apparent in this patient, the physician recommends a colonoscopy, the results of which show hundreds of polyps. Given the signs and symptoms in the patient, which of the following genes is most likely to be altered?

(A) APC
(B) NF1
(C) RB1
(D) TP53
(E) VHL

8. A 34-year-old woman has sought genetic counseling following obtaining results from an online genetic testing company. The results of this genetic test showed that she harbored a mutation in the gene (*PALB2*) encoding the protein, partner and localizer of *BRCA2*. Given this finding, which of the following is most likely?

(A) Colorectal cancer
(B) Fibrosarcoma
(C) Glioblastoma
(D) Lymphoma
(E) Ovarian cancer

9. A 12-year-old girl is being treated for glioblastoma. Molecular studies performed on cells isolated from biopsy tissue discover the presence of an altered arginine codon in the gene encoding isocitrate dehydrogenase 1 (IDH1). Given these findings, which of the following is most likely to found at elevated levels?

(A) 2-Hydroxyglutarate
(B) Isocitrate
(C) α-Ketoglutarate
(D) Oxaloacetate
(E) Succinate

10. A 5-year-old woman is in the emergency department having a fracture of her right ulna casted. The attending physician notes that the child has several large and dark café-au-lait patches on her back and upper legs. The physician relates to the child's parents that she may harbor a mutant form of the *NF1* gene. If this is indeed found to be true, which of the following is most likely to be found in this patient?

(A) Brachydactyly
(B) Breast cancer
(C) Leukemia
(D) Lisch nodules
(E) Osteoporosis

11. A 24-year-old man who was treated for exudative macular edema has been found to have retinal and central nervous system hemangioblastomas, adrenal pheochromocytoma, as well as multiple pancreatic and renal cysts. History reveals that his father, who had been treated for uncontrolled blood pressure, died from a cerebral vascular accident at the age of 54. Loss of which of the following is the most likely contributor to the signs and symptoms in this patient?

(A) Regulation of β-catenin
(B) Regulation of cell cycle progression
(C) Regulation of E2F activity
(D) Regulation of hypoxia-induced factor-1 activity
(E) Regulation of the RAS G-protein

12. A 4-year-old man is being examined by an ophthalmologist due to his failing vision. Physical examination finds that his eyes appear to look in different directions and his pupils appear white through the physician's ophthalmoscope. Which of the following is the most likely explanation for the observation in this patient?

(A) Hypophosphorylation of pRB so that it can no longer interact with E2F
(B) Increased in the expression of pRB resulting in increased binding of pRB to E2F
(C) Loss of expression of pRB rendering E2F inactive
(D) Mutation in phosphorylation site in pRB preventing its interaction with a coactivator of E2F
(E) Mutation in the domain of pRB to which E2F binds resulting in constitutive E2F activity

13. A 62-year-old woman with chronic hepatitis B infection and a 3-year history of cirrhosis presents with jaundice, increasing ascites, left upper quadrant pain, and chronic fatigue. Liver biopsy is performed after an abdominal CT scan reveals the presence of an 18-cm mass in the left lobe. Histopathology of the biopsy tissue finds abnormally thickened hepatic cords composed of moderately well-differentiated hepatocytes with an increased nuclear to cytoplasmic ratio and prominent nucleoli. Which of the following mechanisms is the most likely initiating event underlying the changes in the patient's liver?
(A) Failure of immune surveillance
(B) Hepatic conversion of procarcinogen to a carcinogenic metabolite
(C) Loss of p53 tumor-suppressor gene
(D) Spontaneous chromosomal deletion
(E) Viral DNA insertion into the host genome

14. A 43-year-old woman has just been informed that the cancer that originated in her left breast has metastasized to her liver. Loss of expression of which of the following is most likely to have contributed to this finding?
(A) E-cadherin
(B) Fibronectin
(C) Intercellular adhesion molecule-1 (ICAM-1)
(D) Laminin-211
(E) P-selectin

15. Experiments are being conducted on the functions of the tumor suppressor, p53. These experiments are being carried out using normal cells in culture and involve the effects of ionizing radiation. Following exposure of the cells to ultraviolet light, which of the following is most likely to occur?
(A) Apoptosis is inhibited
(B) Cells are prevented from entering S phase
(C) The concentration of p53 decreases
(D) Replication of DNA is enhanced
(E) Transcription of metaphase cyclins is increased

16. A 27-year-old man has undergone a routine colonoscopy because of his concern over a family history of colon cancer. There is no family history of any other types of cancer. During the colonoscopy biopsy tissue was taken from an area of abnormal growth. Molecular analysis of the cells from the biopsy found that three of five microsatellite markers showed evidence of instability. Which of the following processes is most likely to be defective in these cells?
(A) Cell adhesion regulation
(B) Control of cell cycle progression
(C) DNA mismatch repair
(D) DNA replication
(E) Regulation of apoptosis

17. A 42-year-old man is being examined by his family physician due to concerns that he has blood in his stool. He also complains of chronic fatigue over the past 2 months. His physician orders blood tests to be performed and the results indicate the patient has an iron deficiency anemia. Family history is significant for colorectal carcinoma in his father and endometrial cancer in his younger sister. Given the symptoms in the patient, and family history, his physician recommends that the patient undergo a diagnostic colonoscopy. During the colonoscopy a mass was detected in the ascending colon. A biopsy of the mass is taken and analyzed, which confirms it is an adenocarcinoma. Given these findings, autosomal dominant inheritance of a mutation in which of the following genes is most likely to be responsible for this patient's condition?
(A) *APC*
(B) *MEN1*
(C) *MSH2*
(D) *NF1*
(E) *TP53*

18. Experiments are being conducted to identify novel compounds that can block the process of apoptosis with the aim of targeting certain neurodegenerative disorders. The ideal compound is expected to be nontoxic to neural tissues and to be able to target both the intrinsic and extrinsic pathways of apoptosis. If the experiments identify the ideal molecule, which of the following is most likely to be its identified mechanism of action?
(A) Activation of pore formation in the outer mitochondrial membrane
(B) Blocking FAS ligand (FASL) binding to FAS
(C) Enhancement of BAX interaction with mitochondria
(D) Inhibition of BCL-2 activation
(E) Inhibition of initiator caspases

19. A 42-year-old man is being examined by his family physician due to concerns that he has blood in his stool. He also complains of chronic fatigue over the past 2 months. His physician orders blood tests to be performed and the results indicate the patient has an iron deficiency anemia. Family history is significant for colorectal carcinoma in his father and endometrial cancer in his younger sister. Given the symptoms in the patient, and family history, his physician recommends that the patient undergo a diagnostic colonoscopy. During the colonoscopy a mass was detected in the ascending colon. A biopsy of the mass is taken and analyzed, which confirms it is an adenocarcinoma. Which of the following is the most likely cause of the adenocarcinoma detected in this patient?
(A) Chronic hepatitis C infection
(B) Defective mismatch repair during DNA replication
(C) Defective repair of double-strand breaks in DNA
(D) Increased expression of the *MLH1* gene
(E) Spontaneous mutation in the *BRCA1* gene

20. Experiments are being conducted to identify novel compounds that can enhance tumor cell killing via activation of apoptosis. When one novel compound is added to colorectal carcinoma cells in culture it is found that there is increased activation of p53 along with increased cytosolic levels of cytochrome *c*. Given these findings, which of the following processes is most likely affected because of the actions of the novel compound?
(A) Blocking FAS ligand (FASL) binding to FAS
(B) Enhancement of BCL-2 activity
(C) Increased mitochondrial permeability
(D) Inhibition of BAX association with outer mitochondrial membrane
(E) Inhibition of the activation of initiator caspase activity

ANSWERS

1. Correct answer is **B.** The findings in this patient are most indicative of chronic myelogenous leukemia, CML. CML is a cancer associated with unregulated growth of myeloid lineage cells. The affected cells are mature granulocytes (eosinophils, basophils, and neutrophils) and granulocyte precursors. CML is most often discovered through routine blood tests (a complete blood count, CBC), not due to the presentation of overt symptoms. Detection of CML through a CBC is due to the identification of increased numbers of granulocytes of all types. Definitive diagnosis of CML can be accomplished via the detection of specific chromosomal translocations in metaphase cells. One type of translocation is referred to as the Philadelphia chromosome and its presence is denoted as Ph^+. The Philadelphia chromosome results from a translocation between chromosomes 9 and 22 [t(9;22)]. The t(9;22) translocation fuses the Ableson tyrosine kinase (ABL) on chromosome 9 with the BCR (breakpoint cluster region) locus on chromosome 22. The BCR-ABL fusion protein results in constitutive activation of the tyrosine kinase activity of ABL which prevents proper differentiation of myeloid lineage cells. Acute lymphocytic leukemia, ALL (choice A), also known as acute lymphoblastic leukemia, is characterized by clonal expansion and increased proliferation, prolonged survival, and impaired differentiation of lymphoid hematopoietic progenitors. Although the more common translocation found in patients with ALL is t(12;21)(p13;q22), some patients do harbor the Ph^+ chromosome. Hodgkin lymphoma (choice C) is not normally identifiable by a CBC with differential. The most common abnormality is a lump or mass in a lymph node. Multiple myeloma (choice D) is associated with low levels of white blood cells, red blood cells, and platelets. The chromosomal abnormalities in multiple myeloma include trisomies and translocations involving the immunoglobulin heavy chain (IgH) genes such as t(11;14), t(4;14), t(6;14), t(14;16), and t(14;20). Non-Hodgkin lymphoma (choice E), similar to Hodgkin lymphoma, is not normally identifiable by a CBC with differential. The most common abnormality is a lump or mass in a lymph node. The most common chromosomal abnormality in non-Hodgkin lymphoma is t(14;18)(q32;q21).

2. Correct answer is **B.** Clinical significance is associated with the *IDH1* gene as there has been a close association made between mutations in this gene and the development of certain forms of cancer, specifically gliomas of the brain. All of the mutations in *IDH1* that are associated with gliomagenesis are missense mutations that alter the normal Arg residue at position 132 to a histidine (R132H). Normally IDH1 converts isocitrate to 2-oxoglutarate (α-ketoglutarate) while also generating NADPH. The R132H mutation in IDH1 results in a loss of isocitrate binding while at the same time altering the catalytic activity of the enzyme such that it reduces 2-oxoglutarate to 2-hydroxyglutarate (2-HG) while simultaneously oxidizing NADPH to $NAPD^+$. Increases in 2-HG levels, coupled with decreases in 2-oxoglutarate levels, result in competitive inhibition of several important 2-oxoglutarate and Fe^{2+}-dependent dioxygenases (2OG-oxygenases) such as DNA demethylases and histone demethylases that are involved in regulating chromatin structure and the consequent epigenetic regulation of gene expression. In addition, inhibition of prolyl hydroxylase domain (PDH) containing enzymes, such as those that are involved in cellular responses to hypoxia, also results from increased 2-HG levels. None of the other processes (choices A, C, D, and E) are affected in cells harboring mutations in the *IDH1* gene.

3. Correct answer is **E.** The symptoms in this patient, coupled with the karyotype, indicate that he is most likely experiencing the symptoms of non-Hodgkin lymphoma. Non-Hodgkin lymphomas (NHLs) are a diverse group of blood cancers that include any kind of lymphoma except Hodgkin lymphomas. There are at least 16 different characterized types of NHL that vary significantly in their severity, from indolent to very aggressive. Non-Hodgkin lymphoma is not normally identifiable by a CBC with differential. The most common abnormality is a lump or mass in a lymph node. Many NHL cells contain gross chromosomal aberrations including translocations. The most common chromosomal translocation found in NHL is t(14;18)(q32;q21). Acute lymphocytic leukemia, ALL (choice A), acute myelogenous leukemia, AML (choice B), and chronic myelogenous leukemia, CML (choice C) are all associated with abnormalities detectable through a complete blood count (CBC) with differential. The most common chromosomal abnormality in ALL is t(12;21)(p13;q22). Chromosomal abnormalities in AML included structural and numerical abnormalities with common translocations being t(8;21) and t(15,17). The most common chromosomal abnormality in the CML is t(9;22)(q34.1;q11.2). Hodgkin lymphoma (choice D), like non-Hodgkin lymphoma, is most often detected by the presence of a mass or a lump in a lymph node. Chromosomal abnormalities in Hodgkin lymphoma include both numerical and structural abnormalities.

4. Correct answer is **C.** Tamoxifen is referred to as a selective estrogen receptor modulator (SERM). This designation refers to the fact that the drug acts like an anti-estrogen in breast cells, but it acts like an estrogen in other tissues. In breast tissue, tamoxifen acts as an estrogen receptor antagonist by competing with estrogen for the receptor. The result is that the transcription of estrogen-responsive genes is inhibited. However, in other tissues, such as in bone, tamoxifen acts as an agonist of the estrogen receptor. As an anticancer drug tamoxifen does not kill cancer cells but prevents them from growing, hence it is cytostatic not cytocidal. None of the other mechanisms (choices A, B, D, E, and F) correspond to the mechanism by which tamoxifen functions as an anticancer drug.

5. Correct answer is **E.** The patient most likely has chronic myelogenous leukemia, CML. CML is a cancer associated with unregulated growth of myeloid lineage cells. The affected cells are mature granulocytes (eosinophils, basophils, and neutrophils) and granulocyte precursors. CML is most often discovered through routine blood tests (a complete blood count, CBC), not due to the presentation of overt symptoms. Definitive diagnosis of CML is accomplished via the detection of a specific chromosomal translocation in metaphase cells. This translocation is referred to as the Philadelphia chromosome and its presence is denoted as Ph^+. The Philadelphia chromosome results from a translocation between chromosomes 9 and 22 [t(9;22)]. The t(9;22) translocation fuses the Ableson tyrosine kinase (ABL) on chromosome 9 with the BCR (breakpoint cluster region) locus on chromosome 22. The BCR-ABL fusion protein results in constitutive activation of the tyrosine kinase activity of ABL which prevents proper differentiation of myeloid lineage cells. None of the other mechanisms (choices A, B, C, and D) represent relevant contributing factors to the symptoms in this patient.

6. Correct answer is **D.** The patient most likely has chronic myelogenous leukemia, CML. CML is a cancer associated with unregulated growth of myeloid lineage cells. The affected cells are mature granulocytes (eosinophils, basophils, and neutrophils) and granulocyte precursors. The karyotype identified in this patient reflects the Philadelphia chromosome, denoted as Ph^+. The Philadelphia chromosome results from a translocation between chromosomes 9 and 22 [t(9;22)]. The t(9;22) translocation fuses the Ableson tyrosine kinase (ABL) on chromosome 9 with the BCR (breakpoint cluster region) locus on chromosome 22. The BCR-ABL fusion protein results in constitutive activation of the tyrosine kinase activity of ABL which prevents proper differentiation of myeloid lineage cells. None of the other options (choices A, B, C, and E) correctly represent the consequences of the translocation identified in this patient.

7. Correct answer is **A.** The patient is most likely experiencing the signs of familial adenomatous polyposis, FAP. Germ-line mutations in the adenomatous polyposis coli (*APC*) gene are responsible for FAP. Multiple colonic polyp development characterizes the disease. These polyps arise during the second and third decades of life and become malignant carcinomas and adenomas later in life. In addition to polyps in the gastrointestinal system, individuals with FAP often have other signs including lumps or bumps on the skull and jaw (osteomas), cysts on the skin (epidermoid cysts), dental changes (extra teeth), noncancerous tumors most often found in the abdomen (desmoid tumors), and freckle-like spots on the inside of the eye. Mutations in the *NF1* gene (choice B) are the cause of neurofibromatosis type 1, a disorder associated with a predisposition to the development of multiple neurofibromas, café-au-lait spots, and Lisch nodules. Loss of function of the *RB1* gene (choice C) is the cause of the childhood eye cancer, retinoblastoma. Loss of function of the *TP53* gene (choice D) is found in numerous different types of cancer. The inheritance of one mutant allele of *TP53* is known as Li-Fraumeni syndrome. Loss of function of the *VHL* gene (choice E) is the cause of von Hippel-Lindau syndrome. Individuals with von Hippel-Lindau syndrome are predisposed to a wide array of tumors that include renal cell carcinomas, retinal angiomas, cerebellar hemangioblastomas, and pheochromocytomas.

8. Correct answer is **E.** Not all breast and ovarian cancers are caused by inherited mutations in specific genes. However, several genetic loci have been shown to predispose an individual to these types of cancer. To date seven loci have been identified that when mutated predispose an individual to breast and ovarian cancer. These loci are BRCA1, BRCA2, ATM, CHEK2, BRIP1, PALB2, and RAD51C. Of significance is that all of these breast cancer susceptibility genes encode proteins that function in some aspect of DNA damage repair. The *PALB2* gene is partner and localizer of *BRCA2* and encodes a protein that interacts with BRCA2 protein in the nucleus. PALB2 binds directly to BRCA1 and serves as the molecular scaffold in the formation of the BRCA1-PALB2-BRCA2 complex. Mutations in the *PALB2* gene result in defective BRCA1-BRCA2 complexes leading to defective DNA repair and increased potential for ovarian and breast cancer. The of the other cancers (choices A, B, C, and D) are directly related to mutations in the *PALB2* gene.

9. Correct answer is **A.** Clinical significance is associated with the *IDH1* gene as there has been a close association made between mutations in this gene and the development of certain forms of cancer, specifically gliomas of the brain. All of the mutations in IDH1 that are associated with gliomagenesis are missense mutations that alter the normal Arg residue at position 132 to a histidine (R132H). Normally IDH1 converts isocitrate to 2-oxoglutarate (α-ketoglutarate) while also generating NADPH. The R132H mutation in IDH1 results in a loss of isocitrate binding while at the same time altering the catalytic activity of the enzyme such that it reduces 2-oxoglutarate to 2-hydroxyglutarate (2-HG) while simultaneously oxidizing NADPH to $NAPD^+$. Increases in 2-HG levels, coupled with decreases in 2-oxoglutarate (α-ketoglutarate) levels, result in competitive inhibition of several important 2-oxoglutarate and Fe^{2+}-dependent dioxygenases (2OG-oxygenases) such as DNA demethylases and histone demethylases that are involved in regulating chromatin structure and the consequent epigenetic regulation of gene expression. None of the other metabolites (choices B, C, D, and E) are significantly elevated as a consequence of mutations in the *IDH1* gene.

10. Correct answer is **D.** Mutations in the *NF1* gene are the cause of neurofibromatosis type 1, a disorder associated with a predisposition to the development of multiple neurofibromas, café-au-lait spots, and Lisch nodules. Some patients also develop benign pheochromocytomas and tumors in the central nervous system, CNS. A small percentage of patients develop neurofibrosarcomas which are likely to be Schwann cell derived. Development of benign neurofibromas versus malignant neurofibrosarcomas may be the difference between inactivation of one *NF1* allele versus both alleles, respectively. None of the other abnormalities (choices A, B, C, and E) are associated with mutations in the *NF1* gene.

11. Correct answer is **D.** The patient most likely is experiencing the symptoms of von Hippel-Lindau syndrome. von Hippel-Lindau syndrome (VHL) results from inheritance of a mutated copy of the *VHL* gene. As a consequence of somatic mutation or loss of the normal *VHL* gene, individuals are predisposed to a wide array of tumors that include renal cell carcinomas, retinal angiomas, cerebellar hemangioblastomas, and pheochromocytomas. One characteristic feature of tumors from VHL patients is the high degree of vascularization, primarily as a result of the constitutive expression of the vascular endothelial growth factor (*VEGF*) gene. Many of the hypoxia-inducible factor 1 (HIF-1) controlled genes are also constitutively expressed in the tumors that harbor mutations in the *VHL* gene. The correlation between VHL and HIF-1 is that VHL is a ubiquitin ligase and one of its targets is the HIF-1α protein of the HIF-1 complex. Loss of the regulation of β-catenin (choice A) is observed in patients sustaining mutations in the gene (*APC*) encoding the adenomatous polyposis coli (APC) protein. Loss of the regulation of cell cycle progression (choice B) is observed in cancers caused by loss of function of the transcription factor, p53. Loss of regulation of E2F function (choice C) is the result of loss of function of the pRB protein. Loss of regulation of the monomeric G-protein RAS (choice E) would be observed in cells having lost the function of neurofibromin which is encoded by the *NF1* gene.

12. Correct answer is **E.** The patient is most likely experiencing the symptoms of retinoblastoma. Retinoblastoma results from loss of function of the tumor suppressor, pRB, encoded by the retinoblastoma susceptibility gene, *RB1*. The major function of pRB is in the regulation of cell cycle progression. Its ability to regulate the cell cycle correlates to the state of phosphorylation of pRB. Phosphorylation is maximal at the start of S phase and lowest after mitosis and entry into G_1. Stimulation of quiescent cells with mitogen induces phosphorylation of pRB, while in contrast, differentiation induces hypophosphorylation of pRB. It is, therefore, the hypophosphorylated form of pRB that suppresses cell proliferation. One of the most significant substrates for phosphorylation by the G_1 cyclin-CDK complexes that regulate progression through the cell cycle is pRB. pRB forms a complex with proteins of the E2F family of transcription factors, a result of which renders E2F inactive. When pRB is phosphorylated by G_1 cyclin-CDK complexes it is released from E2F allowing E2F to transcriptionally activate its target genes. Any defect in the ability of pRB to bind to E2F will lead to constitutive activation of DNA synthesis leading to unrestrained proliferation. None of the other options (choices A, B, C, and D) correspond to the role of pRB in the regulation of cell cycle progression via its interactions with E2F family transcription factors.

13. Correct answer is **E.** This patient's history of chronic hepatitis B infection and cirrhosis greatly increases her risk for hepatocellular carcinoma. A diagnosis of hepatocellular carcinoma is confirmed by the microscopic description of the liver biopsy findings, which are classical for hepatocellular carcinoma. This type of carcinoma usually arises in a cirrhotic liver and hepatitis B infection is a major cause of cirrhosis worldwide. In such individuals, hepatitis virus DNA integration into host DNA can be demonstrated and is strongly suspected of having a role in the initiation of hepatocellular carcinoma. There are other factors that are also suspected of having a role but given the patient's relevant medical history and the high prevalence of hepatocellular carcinoma in hepatitis B-positive populations, viral-mediated oncogenesis is the most likely scenario. None of the other options (choices A, B, C, and D) correctly correspond to the initiating event predisposing a patient to hepatocellular carcinoma.

14. Correct answer is **A.** Metastasis is the spread of cancer cells to tissues and organs beyond where the tumor originated, and the formation of new tumors in these remote sites. The process of metastasis involves several events. The loss of cell-cell adhesion capacity allows malignant tumor cells to dissociate from the primary tumor mass. Changes in the interaction between cells and the extracellular matrix enable the tumor cells to invade the surrounding stroma in a process termed invasion. The process of invasion involves the secretion of substances to degrade the basement membrane and extracellular matrix and also the suppression of proteins involved in the control of motility and migration. One important cell adhesion molecule shown to play a critical role in tumor metastatic potential is E-cadherin. E-cadherin is an epithelial cell adhesion molecule whose expression is often downregulated during carcinoma progression and metastatic spread of tumors. Although many other cell adhesion molecules can play a role in cancer cell migration away from a primary tumor, adenocarcinomas are epithelial in origin and thus, E-cadherin is the most likely molecule whose expression is altered in this patient. Loss of none of the other extracellular matrix-associated proteins (choices B, C, D, and E) play a critical role in the ability of epithelium-derived tumor cells to metastasize.

15. Correct answer is **B.** The p53 protein functions as a transcription factor that regulates the expression of numerous genes involved in suppression of cell growth specifically by inhibiting cell cycle progression. The p53 protein is normally retained in the cytosol through its interaction with a ubiquitin ligase identified as MDM2. Under conditions of cellular stress, or when DNA is damaged by ionizing or UV irradiation, various kinases become activated and phosphorylate p53. When p53 is phosphorylated, it is released from MDM2 and migrates into the nucleus where it can activate the transcription of numerous target genes. One major cell-cycle regulating gene that is a target for p53 is the gene encoding the CDK inhibitory protein (CIP), $p21^{CIP}$. Activation of p53 results in increased expression of $p21^{CIP}$ with a resultant arrest in the G_1 phase of the cell cycle so they cannot begin DNA synthesis in S phase. If the DNA damage is severe enough, such that the cell cannot repair it, p53 is involved in activating expression of genes that will trigger apoptosis as opposed to inhibiting it (choice A). The response of cells to UV irradiation, at the level of p53, is an increase, not a decrease (choice C) in p53 concentration. DNA replication is inhibited, not enhanced (choice D), upon activation of p53. p53 does not directly enhance transcription of metaphase cyclins (choice E).

16. Correct answer is **C.** Microsatellite instability (MSI) is a characteristic feature associated with the development of colorectal carcinomas defined as Lynch syndrome (also known as hereditary non-polyposis colorectal carcinoma, HNPCC). The underlying causes of Lynch syndrome are mutations in one of four genes (*MLH1*, *MSH2*, *MSH6*, and *PMS2*) whose encoded proteins are required for the process of DNA mismatch repair. DNA mismatch repair involves a series of enzymes that recognize and repair erroneous insertions, deletions and mis-incorporation of bases that can arise during DNA replication and recombination, as well as repairing some forms of DNA damage. DNA mismatching during replication can occur with high frequency in regions of highly repetitive DNA sequences such as microsatellites. Microsatellite instability refers to a condition of genetic hypermutability that results from impaired DNA mismatch repair mechanisms. Defects in none of the other processes (choices A, B, D, and E) are correlated to microsatellite instability.

17. Correct answer is **C.** The patient is most likely manifesting the signs and symptoms of Lynch syndrome. Lynch syndrome represents a family of inherited cancers that result from mutations in genes whose encoded proteins function in the process of mismatch repair during DNA replication. Lynch syndrome is also known as hereditary nonpolyposis colorectal carcinoma, HNPCC. The cancers that are found in patients with Lynch syndrome include colorectal, endometrial, ovarian, stomach, small intestine, pancreatic, and urinary tract cancers. Currently there are five genes whose disruptions are associated with the inheritance of Lynch syndrome. These genes are *MLH1*, *MSH2*, *MSH6*, *PMS2*, and *EPCAM*. Although the *EPCAM*-encoded protein is not directly involved in DNA mismatch repair, mutations at the end of *EPCAM* gene disrupt the function of the closely associated *MSH2* gene. Inherited mutations in the *APC* gene (choice A) are the cause of familial adenomatous polyposis, a form of colorectal carcinoma that results from the formation of thousands of adenomatous polyps that eventually transform into adenocarcinomas. Inherited mutations in the *MEN1* gene (choice B) are the causes of multiple endocrine neoplasia type 1 which is associated with parathyroid and pituitary adenomas and islet cell tumors. Inherited mutations in the *NF1* gene (choice D) are the causes of neurofibromatosis type 1, NF1. NF1 is primarily associated with neurofibromas, sarcomas, and gliomas. Inherited mutations in the *TP53* gene (choice E) are the cause of Li Fraumeni syndrome, a cancer syndrome associated with brain tumors, sarcomas, leukemias, and breast cancers.

18. Correct answer is **E.** Within the context of the intrinsic and extrinsic apoptotic programs, there are similar features and overlapping protein functions. One family of proteins, the caspases, is central to both the intrinsic and extrinsic apoptotic programs. Caspases are synthesized as precursor inactive proteins (zymogens) that are proteolytically processed, often by another member of the caspase family. The proteolysis of a caspase results in the production of a large and a small subunit that dimerize to form the catalytically active caspase. Thus, to inhibit both intrinsic and extrinsic apoptosis the primary target(s) will be the caspase proteins. Activation of pore formation in the outer mitochondrial membrane (choice A) would actually lead to activation of the intrinsic pathway of apoptosis as opposed to inhibiting it. The FAS receptor, to which FASL binds, is one of the activators of the extrinsic pathway of apoptosis. Although blocking FASL binding (choice B) would interfere with the activation of the extrinsic pathway, it would not affect the intrinsic pathway. The function of BAX (choice C) is to participate in the activation of the intrinsic (mitochondrial) pathway of apoptosis so enhancing BAX interaction with the mitochondrial membrane would enhance apoptosis, not inhibit it. BCL-2 (choice D) is a prosurvival protein that is associated with the outer mitochondrial membrane where it interferes with the release of cytochrome *c* induced by activated BAK and/or BAX. BCL-2 also inhibits activation of caspase cascades thereby preventing apoptosis. Thus, the inhibition of BCL-2 activation would lead to enhanced, not inhibited, activation of the intrinsic apoptotic pathway.

19. Correct answer is **B.** The patient is most likely manifesting the signs and symptoms of Lynch syndrome. Lynch syndrome represents a family of inherited cancers that result from mutations in genes whose encoded proteins function in the process of mismatch repair during DNA replication. Lynch syndrome is also known as hereditary nonpolyposis colorectal carcinoma, HNPCC. The cancers that are found in patients with Lynch syndrome include colorectal, endometrial, ovarian, stomach, small intestine, pancreatic, and urinary tract cancers. Currently, there are five genes whose disruptions are associated with the inheritance of Lynch syndrome. These genes are *MLH1*, *MSH2*, *MSH6*, *PMS2*, and *EPCAM*. Although the *EPCAM*-encoded protein is not directly involved in DNA mismatch repair, mutations at the end of *EPCAM* gene disrupt the function of the closely associated *MSH2* gene. Chronic hepatitis C infection (choice A) is associated with hepatocellular carcinomas, not colorectal carcinomas. Defective repair of double-strand breaks (DSB) in DNA (choice C) and the development of cancer are typical of inherited mutations in the *BRCA1* and *BRCA2* genes as well as several other genes that encode proteins involved in the process of DSB repair. Whereas colorectal carcinoma can result from defective DSB repair, it is not commonly associated with the development of endometrial cancers in women. Increased expression of the *MLH1* gene (choice D) would actually result in an enhanced ability for mismatch repair to take place during DNA replication, the exact opposite of what causes Lynch syndrome, the most likely disorder manifesting in this patient. Spontaneous mutation in the *BRCA1* gene (choice E) is not likely to be associated with colorectal carcinoma and also would have no genetic bearing on the apparent dominant familial connection between the cancer in this patient, his father, and his younger sister.

20. Correct answer is **C.** The two primary pathways for the initiation of the apoptotic process are termed the intrinsic and extrinsic pathways of apoptosis. The intrinsic apoptotic pathway is predominantly centered around and/or regulated by the mitochondria. When mitochondrial permeability is enhanced, there is an associated release of cytochrome *c* which is a direct activator of the intrinsic apoptotic pathway. The FAS receptor and the FAS ligand (choice A) are activators of the extrinsic pathway of apoptosis and as such do not result in enhanced mitochondrial permeability and release of cytochrome *c*. BCL-2 is a prosurvival protein that is associated with the outer mitochondrial membrane where it interferes with the release of cytochrome *c* induced by activated BAK and/or BAX. Thus, enhancement of BCL-2 activation (choice B) would lead to enhanced, not inhibited, activation of the intrinsic apoptotic pathway. The function of BAX (choice D) is to participate in the activation of the intrinsic (mitochondrial) pathway of apoptosis so inhibiting BAX interaction with the mitochondrial membrane would decrease apoptosis, not activate it. Inhibition of initiator caspase activity (choice E) would be associated with decreased, not increased apoptosis which is the aim of this study.

PART V MEDICAL GENETICS

CHAPTER

35

Medical Genetics

High-Yield Terms

Autosome	Any one of the 22 non-sex determining chromosomes
Pedigree	An orderly diagram of a family's genetic features, relative to a particular disease in the family, extending over several generations
Punnett square	A Punnett square is a graphical representation of the possible genotypes of offspring arising from a particular mating
Polymorphism	Refers to any one of two or more variants of a particular gene or DNA sequence. The most common are single nucleotide polymorphisms, SNP ("snip")
Incomplete penetration	The lack of phenotype in an individual harboring a dominant mutant allele
Obligate carrier	Specifically refers to females carrying a mutant allele for an X-linked gene. Can often be seen used when describing the parents of a child manifesting an autosomal recessive disease
Concordance/ Discordance	Concordance refers to the probability that a pair of individuals will both have a certain characteristic such as the presence of the same trait in both members of a pair of twins. Discordance refers to the lack of the same trait in both members of a pair of twins
Karyotype	Refers to a picture of the number and types of chromosomes in an individual
Linkage disequilibrium	When an observed haplotype frequency does equal the product of the frequencies of the alleles constituting that haplotype

GENETIC BASIS OF INHERITANCE

Medical genetics can be defined as the diagnosis and management of inherited disorders. Specifically, medical genetics is the application of genetics to the practice of medical care. Genetics requires an understanding of the nature of the hereditary material (Table 35–1) and the mechanisms for how this information is transmitted from cell to cell. The hereditary material is, of course, the DNA in the nucleus that constitutes the human genome.

The human genome consists of approximately 3.2×10^9 nucleotides (bases) that are organized into chromosomes of varying sizes. The human genome consists of 22 pairs of chromosomes, termed the **autosomes**, and two different sex chromosomes. The autosomes are numbered based upon their sizes with the largest being chromosome 1 and the smallest chromosome 22 (Figure 35–1). The two sex chromosomes are identified as X and Y where males possess both an X and a Y chromosome and females possess two X chromosomes. Although females possess two copies

TABLE 35–1 Basic genetic terminologies.

Term	Description
Locus	Refers to the particular location, or position, of a segment of DNA; can refer to the position of a single gene or to the position of a segment of DNA containing many genes such as the β-globin locus on chromosome 11 which contains five functional genes and one pseudogene
Gene	The term that defines a unit of heredity; there are both coding (protein-coding genes) and noncoding genes
Allele	All humans inherit a copy of their DNA from each parent and each parental set of chromosomes contains different versions (approximately 3–5 million different bases) termed alleles; for any given gene there are two alleles: the maternal and the paternal versions; for any given gene there is a common allele referred to as the wild-type allele
Variant (Mutant)	Refers to the sequence differences in a gene relative to that of the wild-type gene due to the presence of a mutation; can refer to mutation causing disease but does not necessarily imply difference in function
Polymorphism	Denotes variant alleles of a particular DNA sequence; the most common polymorphisms are single nucleotide polymorphisms (SNP) but the term can refer to much larger sequences of DNA
Genotype	Refers to the overall genetic composition of a genome in an organism
Phenotype	Refers to the observable characteristics resulting from an organism's genotype; genotype does not always specifically control phenotype due to the processes of epigenetics (see Chapter 22)
Homozygous/ homozygote	Refers to having the same allele on both homologous chromosomes at a particular locus
Heterozygous/ heterozygote	Refers to having different alleles on both homologous chromosomes at a particular locus
Compound heterozygote	Defines the genotype in which two different mutant alleles of a gene are present as opposed to one wild-type allele and one mutant allele; an individual that inherit a sickle cell anemia allele (HbS) from one parent and a hemoglobin C allele from the other is an example of a compound heterozygote; designated HbSC
Hemizygous/ hemizygote	Refers to the situation where there is only one copy of a gene such as in males with respect to the X chromosome or likewise in Turner syndrome females resulting from loss of one of the two X chromosomes
Dominant allele	Represents a variant of a gene that will produce a phenotype even in the presence of other alleles
Recessive allele	Represents a variant of a gene that will not produce a phenotype on its own; two copies of these types of alleles are required to manifest a phenotype
Allelic heterogeneity	Represents the situation where multiple different mutations in the same gene result in the same clinical disorder, possibly with variable phenotypic expression; cystic fibrosis, of varying severity, results from over 1500 different mutations in the *CFTR* gene
Locus heterogeneity	Represents the situation where the same, or highly similar, clinical phenotype arises due to mutations in different genes; osteogenesis imperfecta is a generalized fragile bone disease that results from mutations in at least 13 different genes
Loss of heterozygosity (LOH)	Refers to the situation where a chromosome has lost an entire gene or an entire section of a chromosome; LOH is common in the development of many cancers
Pleiotropy	Refers to the circumstance when a single gene produces multiple diverse phenotypes in different organ system; Marfan syndrome results from mutations in the fibrillin gene (*FBN1*) and manifests with arachnodactyly (bone), lens dislocation (eye), and dissecting aortic aneurysms (heart)
Penetrance	Refers to the likelihood that a gene, such as a mutant gene, can manifest a phenotype; in some individuals the presence of a mutant allele that should manifest a clinical phenotype does not and this circumstance is referred to as incomplete penetrance
Expressivity	Refers to the extent or degree to which a genetic defect is expressed such as mild, severe, early, late (does not relate to penetrance)
Anticipation	Refers to the phenomenon where an inherited disease manifest at earlier ages and with increased severity in each subsequent generation; this phenomenon was originally described for type 1 myotonic dystrophy and has subsequently been shown to be associated with most trinucleotide repeat expansion disorders
Imprinting	Refers to the epigenetic phenomenon of parent-of-origin specificity in gene expression; results from differential parental chromosomal methylation status

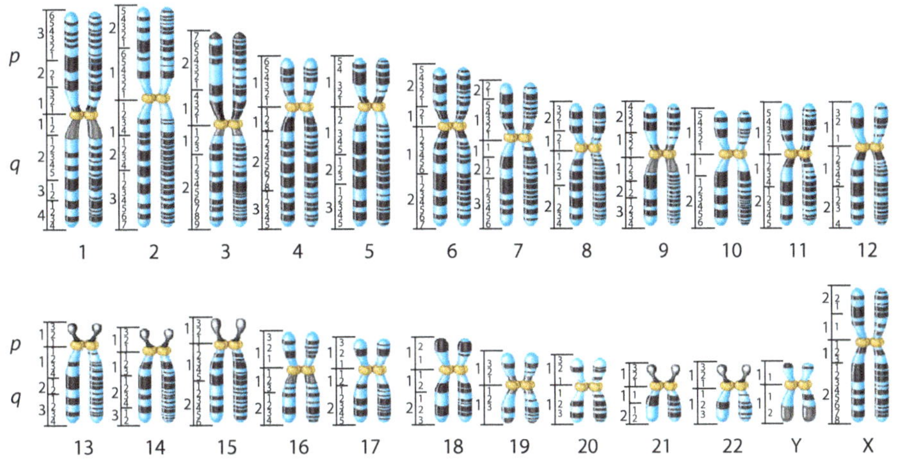

FIGURE 35–1 Conventional numbering system of G bands in human chromosomes. Karyotypes are ways of organizing and presenting the chromosomal makeup of an individual. (Reproduced with permission from Brooker RJ: *Genetics: Analysis & Principles*, 7th ed. New York, NY: McGraw Hill, 2021.)

of the X chromosome, not all genes on both chromosomes are expressed due to the process of X chromosome inactivation, XCI (see Chapter 22).

In addition to being of different sizes the chromosomes are divided into two distinct arms on either side of the centromeric domains of each chromosome. The centromere of each chromosome is a highly condensed region of exclusively repetitive DNA (termed satellite DNA) that is the site at which the microtubules of the spindle attach, via the kinetochore, during cell division (see Chapter 22). The longer of the two chromosome arms is referred to as the q arm and the shorter as the p arm.

In some chromosomes, the size of the p and q arms is very similar such that the centromere is very nearly in the middle of the chromosome. These latter chromosomes are termed **metacentric** chromosomes (1, 3, 16, 19, 20). Chromosomes with longer q arms are referred to as **submetacentric** chromosomes (2, 4-12, 17, 18, and X). A small subset of chromosomes (13, 14, 15, 21, 22, and Y) have nearly nonexistent p arms and these chromosomes are termed the **acrocentric** chromosomes.

The contribution of DNA from both the human male and female constitutes the inherited genetic material that defines the characteristics of their offspring. These characteristics are determined primarily by the composition of protein-coding genes in the inherited chromosomes. Of the vast amount of DNA in the human genome only around 1% is devoted to protein-coding genes. Indeed, the current estimate is that there are approximately 21,000 protein-coding genes in the human genome. However, due to alternative promoter usage and alternative mRNA splicing (see Chapter 23) a vastly larger total number of distinct proteins is derived from the human genome.

SINGLE-GENE GENETICS

Many diseases and disorders are the result of the inheritance of different alleles of a single gene and are, therefore, appropriately referred to as singe-gene disorders. Single-gene disorders follow classical Mendelian inheritance patterns in families and are the result of mutations in genes on the autosomes or the sex chromosomes. Inheritance of autosomal diseases can be recessive, requiring two mutant alleles, or dominant where only a single mutant allele can manifest a phenotype. Sex chromosome inheritance can be X-linked or, in males, Y-linked. The Y chromosome only contains around 200 genes and diseases are very rare and thus, they will not be reviewed. One important gene on the Y chromosome is the gene encoding testis determining factor (TDF) which is also known as sex-determining region Y (SRY) protein.

Another important mode of inheritance involves the mitochondrial genome, mtDNA (see Chapter 10). Because mitochondrial DNA is derived nearly exclusively from the maternal gametes, inheritance of mutations or deletions in the mtDNA is strictly maternal. This is not to say that all diseases of mitochondrial dysfunction are exclusively maternal in inheritance. The mtDNA only encodes 13 of the several hundred proteins required for mitochondrial function. Therefore, inheritance of mutations in any of the nuclear genes encoding functions of the mitochondrial will also result in mitochondrial dysfunction.

The inheritance patterns of single-gene disorders in families can be obtained from a family history of the patient and summarized using a pedigree (Figure 35–2). A pedigree is simply a graphical representation of a family tree using a defined set of symbols (Figure 35–3). Pedigrees are organized according to generations and individuals in that generation. The generations are designated by Roman numerals and the individuals in a generation are designated with Arabic numerals (see Figure 35–2).

PEDIGREE INTERPRETATION

Basic pedigree interpretation involves asking a series of simple questions. The first question to ask is whether the disease is transmitted in a dominant or recessive manner. This can be ascertained by determining if the disease is vertically penetrant, meaning

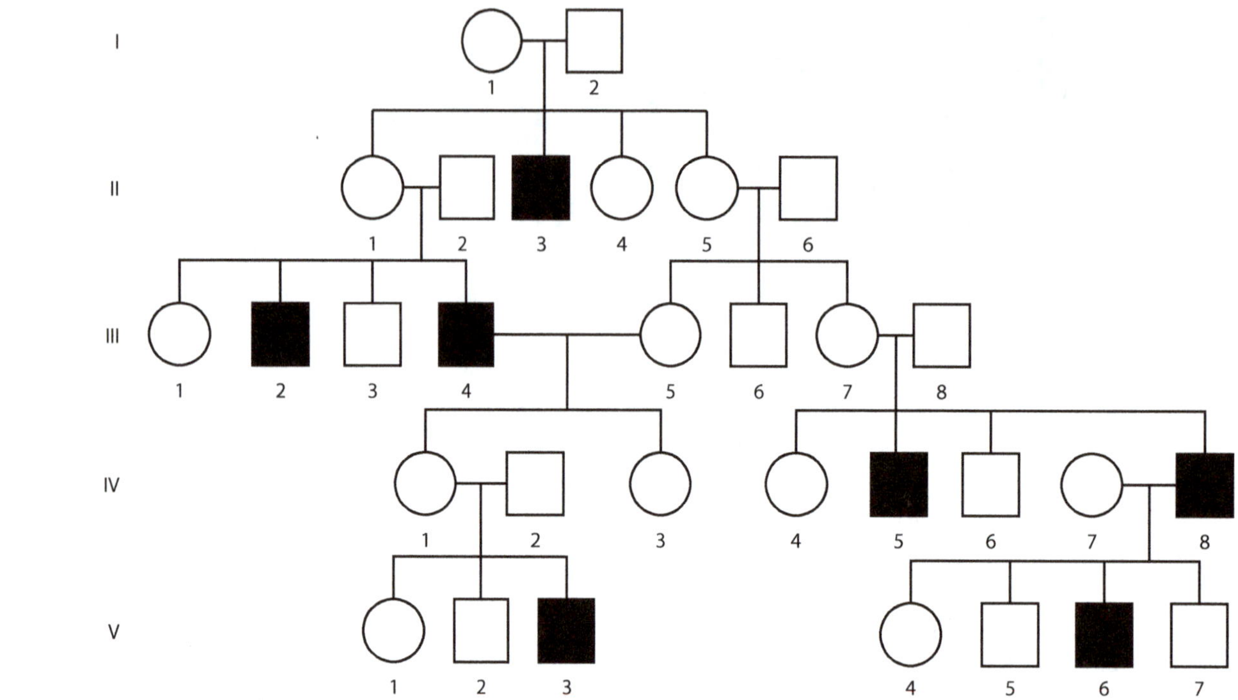

FIGURE 35–2 Pedigree of an autosomal recessive disease. (Reproduced with permission from themedicalbiochemistrypage, LLC.)

there is at least one affected individual in every generation. If vertical penetration is evident the disease is highly likely to be dominantly inherited. On the other hand, if there is one or more generation (generational skipping) with no affected individuals the disease is highly likely to be recessively inherited. The next step is to determine if the inheritance of the disease is autosomal or sex-linked. Autosomal inheritance, whether dominant or recessive, will show very nearly identical numbers of affected males and females. Sex-linked inheritance, specifically X-linked, can be determined by the absence of transmission from affected males to their male children.

Using the pedigree in Figure 35–2, it can easily be determined that the represented disease is recessive in inheritance since neither individual in generation I have the disease, that is, there is a skipped generation. The next step is to determine if the disease is sex linked or autosomal. Autosomal diseases will show relatively equal numbers of affected males and females and since in this pedigree there are only affected males one might conclude that the disease is X-linked and recessive. However, the next step in pedigree interpretation is to examine for the presence, or absence, of male-to-male transmission. Since male IV-8 has an affected son (V-6), the disease cannot be X-linked inheritance and thus, must be autosomal recessive.

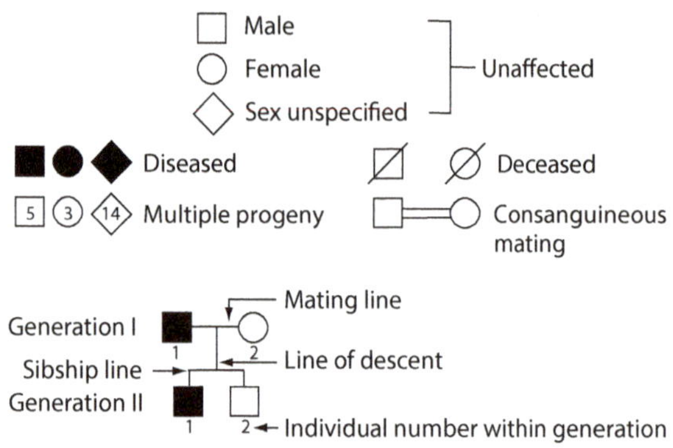

FIGURE 35–3 Symbols used in pedigree analysis. In the simple two-generation pedigree shown at the bottom the affected father in the first generation is designated I-1 and his affected son is designated II-1. (Reproduced with permission from Goldberg ML, Fischer JA, Hood L, et al: Genetics: From Genes to Genomes, 7th ed. New York, NY: McGraw Hill; 2021).

PUNNETT SQUARES

A Punnett square is a graphical representation (Figure 35–4) of the possible genotypes of offspring arising from a particular mating. These tables were developed by the geneticist, Reginald C. Punnett and thus, bear his name. Creating a Punnett square requires knowledge of the genetic composition of the parents. Punnett squares can be used for the analysis of the outcomes of the crosses between not only single genes but also two or more genes. However, in the analysis of the recurrence risk for the majority of human diseases, which are single-gene disorders, the Punnett square represents the outcomes of a single-gene (monohybrid) cross. Each box in the Punnett square represents one possible genotype for a single fertilization event.

Female gametes \ Male gametes	A	a
A	A A 1/4	A a 1/4
a	A a 1/4	a a 1/4

FIGURE 35–4 Punnett square of the two alleles of a single gene (monohybrid cross). The genotypic segregation for a monohybrid cross is shown to exhibit the pattern of 1:2:1 (1 A/A, 2 A/a, 1 a/a). For a single-gene disorder, the Punnett square demonstrates that for a recessive allele (a) there is a 25% (1/4) chance of having an affected child when both parents are carriers. If the disease is dominant (A), 75% (3/4) of the children of heterozygotes will inherit the disease allele. (Reproduced with permission from themedicalbiochemistrypage, LLC.)

AUTOSOMAL RECESSIVE DISORDERS

Single-gene autosomal recessive disorders result from the inheritance of two mutant alleles of a gene. The defining feature of these disorders is that the parents of an affected individual are both carriers such that their genotypes are designated A/a, where the lower case "a" represents the mutant allele. Pedigrees of families demonstrating an autosomal recessive disease (see Figure 35–2) exhibit horizontal transmission meaning there are generations where the disease is not apparent (skipped generations). Transmission of autosomal recessive disorders is commonly seen in consanguineous matings.

The distribution of affected individuals for autosomal recessive conditions is equal between males and females. Affected family members typically do not have affected parents. The siblings of an affected individual have a 25% likelihood of themselves being affected if the parents are the more common heterozygous genotype. This recurrence risk can be easily determined using a Punnett square. Since each parent carries the mutant allele and each has a 50% (1/2) chance of donating the mutant allele to any child the overall chance of any child being born with the a/a genotype and thus, manifesting the disease is ½ × ½ = ¼ (25%).

HIGH-YIELD CONCEPT

The incidence of carriers for an autosomal recessive allele (disease allele "*q*") will always be twice the frequency of that disease allele in the population.

In calculating the recurrence risk for any child of a sibling of an affected individual, who they themselves are not affected by the disease, it is necessary to understand that their likelihood of being a carrier is 2/3 (67%) and not ½ (50%) as would be predicted from the use of a Punnett square. Although examination of a Punnett square would find that there is a 50% chance of an individual having the A/a genotype from the mating of carrier parents, the fact that the individual is unaffected by the disorder necessarily eliminates the a/a genotype leaving only three (not four) possible genotypes for the unaffected sibling, two of which are carrier (A/a) genotypes.

AUTOSOMAL DOMINANT DISORDERS

Single-gene autosomal dominant disorders result from the inheritance of only one abnormal allele. Dominant conditions demonstrate vertical transmission, meaning at least one individual in each generation is observed to be affected (Figure 35–5). Transmission from males and females is equally likely and the distribution of affected individuals is equal between males and females. The vast majority of individuals affected by an autosomal dominant condition are heterozygotes harboring one wild-type allele and one mutant allele for the causative gene. Their genotype is designated A/a, where the capital "A" denotes the mutant allele.

As in all cases, each parent has a 50% (1/2) chance of donating one of their two alleles for any given gene to their child. In the case of autosomal dominant diseases, a child need only receive one mutant allele to manifest the disease. Therefore, any child of a parent with an autosomal dominant disease (who themselves is very likely to be heterozygous for the mutant allele) has a 50% chance of inheriting the mutant allele and being affected. In the rare circumstance where both parents are heterozygotes for an autosomal dominant disorder, each child has a 75% chance of being affected. In the even rarer circumstance where a parent is homozygous for a dominant allele there is a 100% chance of having an affected child. Using Punnett squares makes these recurrence risk assignments extremely easy.

HIGH-YIELD CONCEPT

The frequency of an autosomal dominant disease in a population will always be twice the frequency of the mutant allele ("*q*") in the population.

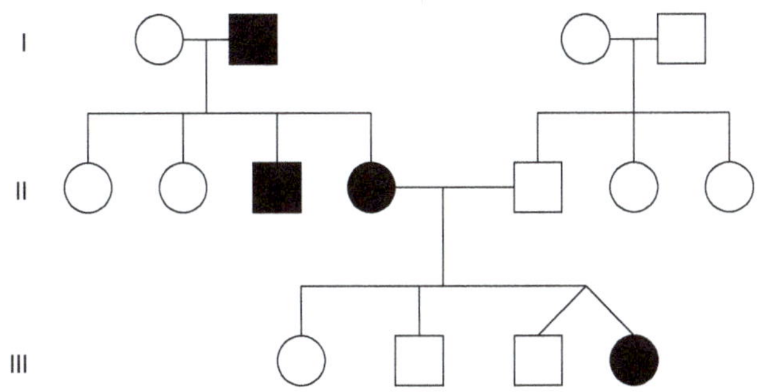

FIGURE 35–5 Sample pedigree for a simple dominant trait. (Reproduced with permission from Schaefer GB, Thompson Jr. JN: *Medical Genetics: An Integrated Approach*. New York, NY: McGraw Hill; 2014.)

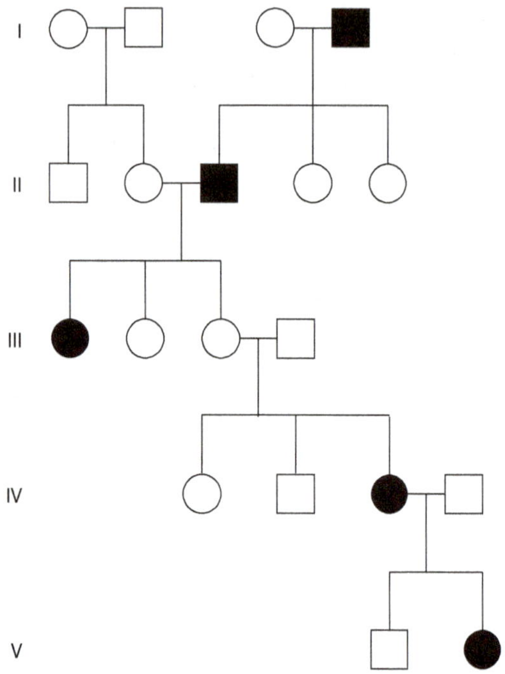

FIGURE 35–6 This pedigree is consistent with dominant inheritance, except for individual III-3, who apparently passes on the dominant trait but does not express it. This can be interpreted as an example of incomplete penetrance. (Reproduced with permission from Schaefer GB, Thompson Jr. JN: *Medical Genetics: An Integrated Approach*. New York, NY: McGraw Hill; 2014.)

Phenotypically normal members of a family generally do not transmit the dominant mutant allele. However, in rare cases an individual harboring a mutant allele may be phenotypically normal due to the process of **incomplete penetration** (Figure 35–6). It is important to be able to recognize the phenomenon of incomplete penetration from a pedigree for the purposes of calculating the penetration rate of an autosomal dominant disorder. The penetration rate is determined by dividing the total number of affected individuals in a particular pedigree by the total number of individuals who should be affected. Once the penetration rate has been calculated, this value is multiplied by the normal 50% recurrence risk for autosomal dominant diseases to obtain the actual likelihood of a child manifesting the disease.

Using Figure 35–6 as an example for calculation of penetration rate, individuals I-1, II-3, III-1, IV-3, and V-2 (a total of 5 individuals) are affected by the dominant trait. Individual III-3 most likely carriers the mutant allele but does not manifest the disorder so the total number of individuals who have/should have the disease is 6 and therefore the penetration rate is 5/6 = 83%. The normal recurrence risk for a child of parents where one manifests an autosomal dominant disorder is 50%; however, in the pedigree shown in Figure 35–6 the recurrence risk for a child of individuals III-3 and III-4, as an example, would be 50% × 83% (the penetration rate) = 42%.

In some families, an affected individual may not have an affected parent because the disease arose as the result of a **new mutation** (spontaneous mutation). In these circumstances, if the new mutation is on an autosome, any subsequent siblings of the affected individual have essentially no risk for the disorder. However, any children of the individual affected by the new mutation will have the same likelihood (50%) of manifesting the disease as for any autosomal dominant disorder. New mutations can also arise on the X chromosome such as is the case in approximately 30% of individuals suffering from Duchene muscular dystrophy.

There are varying forms of autosomal dominant conditions. True dominant conditions will demonstrate the same phenotype in heterozygous and homozygous individuals. A classic example of this type of dominant disorder is Huntington disease. In some cases, a disease is incompletely dominant where homozygous individuals demonstrate a much more severe phenotype than heterozygotes. A classic example of this type of dominant disorder is the form of familial hypercholesterolemia that results from mutations in the LDL-receptor gene.

Codominance refers to the circumstance when both alleles at a locus in a compound heterozygote are contributing to a phenotype. One clinically significant example of codominance is expression of the ABO blood group antigens (see Figure 12–9). Individuals that have type AB blood are exhibiting a phenotype due to codominant expression of both the A and B alleles.

X-LINKED DISORDERS

Although historically the X-linked disorders have been defined as recessive or dominant, the current practice is to no longer use these terms. For an X-linked disorder that is only observed in hemizygous individuals (ie, males and rarely, Turner females) and very rarely in heterozygotes (ie, females), it was classically defined as an X-linked recessive disorder. When the phenotype is always evident in heterozygotes, as well as in hemizygotes, it was classically defined as X-linked dominant. However, due to X chromosome inactivation and epigenetic regulation of X-linked gene expression it can be difficult to ascertain if the pattern is recessive or dominant and thus, the distinctions are not used by most medical geneticists. As for all X-linked disorders there is never male-to-male transmission.

Classic X-linked recessive disorders, such as glucose-6-phosphate dehydrogenase deficiency, will show a much higher incidence in males than in females (Figure 35–7). An affected male will transmit the disease allele to all of his daughters, thus all daughters of affected males are termed **obligate carriers** of the mutant X-linked allele. Likewise, all the mothers of affected sons had to be harboring the mutant X-linked allele and thus are also

HIGH-YIELD CONCEPT

Because females harbor two X chromosomes the rate of female carriers for X-linked recessive type diseases will always be twice the incidence rate of the disease in males. For example, if the frequency of an X-linked recessive type disease found in males in a population is 1 in 10,000, the frequency of obligate carrier females in that population is twice that rate or 1 in 5000.

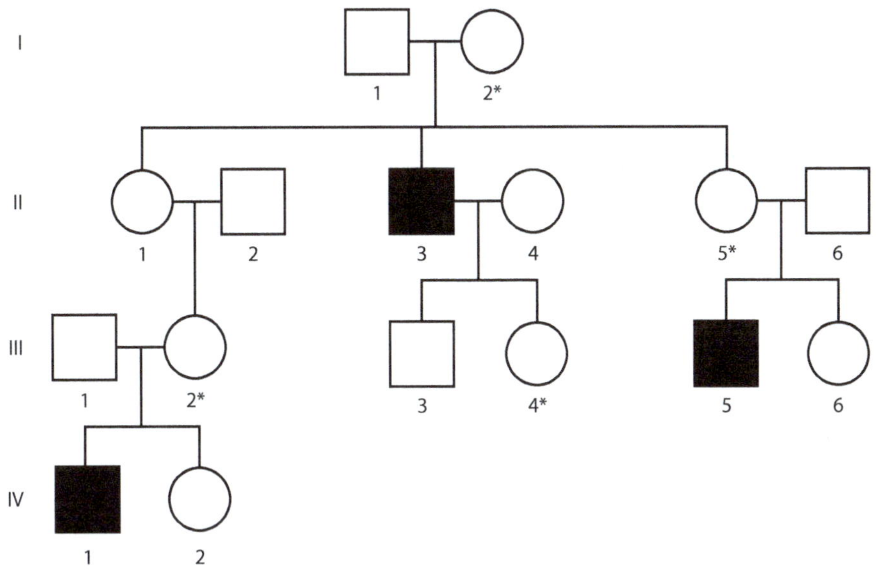

FIGURE 35–7 X-linked recessive pedigree. Typical of recessive inheritance there is at least one skipped generation (generation I). Typical of X-linked recessive inheritance there are only males in the family with the disease. Although females can manifest an X-linked recessive disease, the incidence is very rare, especially in a small population represented by a family pedigree. The asterisks point out the obligate female carriers which can easily be determined since all daughters of affected fathers and all mothers of affected sons are obligate carriers. (Reproduced with permission from themedicalbiochemistrypage, LLC.)

referred to as obligate carriers. For obligate carrier females of X-linked disorders, 50% of their sons are at risk for the disorder and 50% of their daughters are likely to be carriers of the mutant X-linked allele.

Classic X-linked dominant diseases, such as fragile X syndrome and Rett syndrome, will show an incidence rate in females that is twice that of males. This is due to the fact that females possess two X chromosomes and thus, have twice the likelihood of harboring a dominant X-linked mutant allele. Because the X-linked allele in these disorders is dominant, all daughters of affected males will themselves manifest the disease (Figure 35–8). For affected females, who are most likely to be heterozygotes (X/x), who have children with unaffected males, 50% of their children, regardless of their sex, will manifest the disease.

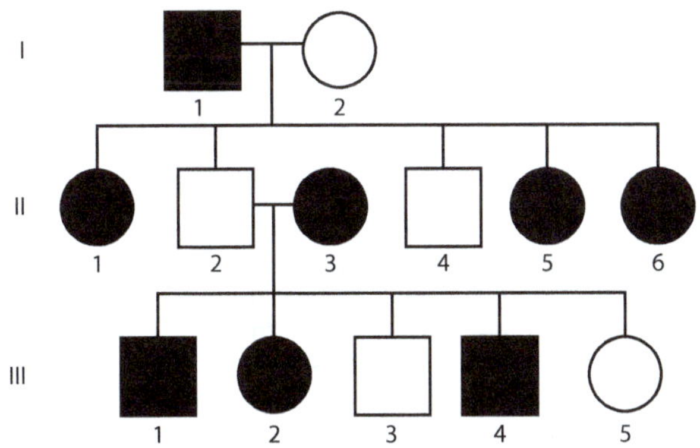

FIGURE 35–8 X-linked dominant pedigree. Typical of a dominant disease, X-linked dominance demonstrates vertical penetration in a family pedigree. Discrimination between autosomal dominance and X-linked dominance can be made by examining the pedigree for male-to-male transmission as well as by the inheritance in female children of an affected male, all of whom must have the disease to clearly define X-linked dominant inheritance. (Reproduced with permission from themedicalbiochemistrypage, LLC.)

HIGH-YIELD CONCEPT

Because females harbor two X chromosomes the frequency of X-linked dominant type diseases in females will always be twice the frequency of the disease in males.

SEX-LIMITED AND SEX-INFLUENCED DISORDERS

Sex-linked diseases are those that are primarily the result of mutations in genes on the X chromosome but generally do not reflect gender-specific differences. However, sex-limited and sex-influenced phenotypes and disorders are clearly related to gender. The idea of a sex-limited gene was first postulated by Charles Darwin in his book, *The Descent of Man and Selection in Relation to Sex*, where he referred to any gene that expresses differently between sexes as a sex-limited gene.

For example, genes that control the processes of sperm development are present in the genomes of females, but sperm production only occurs in males, hence these genes are sex-limited. Male pattern baldness is an example of a sex-influenced phenotype and is due to the differences in androgen and estrogen production in the two sexes. In males a single dominant gene is responsible for the phenotype of male pattern baldness and while the gene is expressed in females it is recessive and, therefore, does not manifest a phenotype.

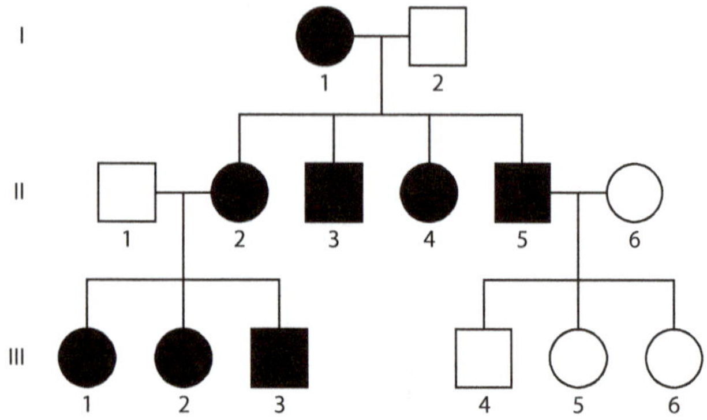

FIGURE 35–9 Mitochondrial inheritance pedigree. Pedigrees of mitochondrial inheritance demonstrate the vertical penetration feature typical of autosomal dominance. No children of an affected male (III-4, III-5, and III-6) can manifest the disease. However, all children, regardless of their sex, of an affected female will get the disease (II-2, II-3, II-4, II-5, III-1, III-2, and III-3). (Reproduced with permission from themedicalbiochemistrypage, LLC.)

MATERNAL EXCLUSIVE MITOCHONDRIAL DISORDERS

Inheritance of mutations in genes encoded by the mitochondrial genome (mtDNA) demonstrate several unique features compared to the inheritance of mutations in genes in the nuclear genome. Mutations in mtDNA genes are inherited strictly from the maternal lineage. The mitochondria of the sperm are not present in the zygote such that only maternal mtDNA is transmitted to a subsequent generation.

When analyzing a pedigree for a family in which a mtDNA mutation is transmitted it will bear the characteristic vertical penetration of an autosomal dominant disorder (Figure 35–9). However, since only mothers transmit their mtDNA to their children (except in extremely rare instances), the disease will never be transmitted from an affected father to his children, regardless of their sex. On the other hand, all the children of an affected mother, regardless of their sex, will be affected by the disease.

The manifestation of the symptoms of mtDNA-associated disorders is quite variable due to several characteristics of mitochondria. Each mitochondrion contains multiple copies of the mtDNA and at cell division the replicated copies of the mtDNA sort randomly to the newly synthesized mitochondria. In addition, the mitochondria themselves distribute randomly to the two resulting daughter cells, a process referred to as **replicative segregation**. Replicative segregation is one of the mechanisms that accounts for the significant variability in the manifestation of symptoms associated with mtDNA-associated disorders.

Given that mitochondria contain multiple copies of the mtDNA they can possess both wild-type mtDNA and mutant mtDNA. Mitochondria also undergo fission during cell division allowing for the wild-type and mutant mtDNA to be randomly distributed into daughter mitochondria. The result of this process is that there is a random assortment, and therefore proportion, of mutant and wild-type mtDNA. The daughter cells that result from cell division may, therefore, receive a mixture of mitochondria, some with mutant mtDNA and some wild-type mtDNA. This phenomenon is referred to as **mitochondrial heteroplasmy**. In some instances, a daughter cell may acquire a population of mitochondria that harbor only wild-type mtDNA or only mutant mtDNA. This latter phenomenon is referred to as **mitochondrial homoplasmy**.

Mitochondria are the major energy-producing organelles of cells, and as a result of mtDNA mutations, the ability to produce ATP can be severely compromised. The brain and skeletal muscle require large amounts of mitochondrial ATP and are, therefore, the most severely affected tissues as a result of mtDNA mutations. Because of the brain and skeletal muscle involvement, these mtDNA disorders are most often referred to as the mitochondrial encephalomyopathies (Clinical Box 35–1).

CLINICAL BOX 35–1 MITOCHONDRIAL ENCEPHALOMYOPATHIES

Mitochondrial diseases are some of the most common inherited disorders in metabolism. Because the brain and skeletal muscle are dependent on high rates of mitochondrial ATP production, these tissues tend to be the most severally affected in inherited diseases resulting from defects in mitochondrial function. Therefore, these disorders are referred to as the mitochondrial encephalomyopathies. This large class of disorders can be the result of mutations in genes of the nuclear genome as well as genes of the mitochondrial genome. A hallmark of the mitochondrial diseases is that, depending on the particular disease, symptom manifestation can occur at any age and can cause symptoms in any organ system. Most mitochondrial proteins are nuclear-encoded and so it is not surprising that the vast majority of mitochondrial diseases are the result of mutations in genes from the nuclear genome. Mutations in 228 nuclear genes and all 13 mitochondrial mRNA genes are associated with rare monogenic syndromes in which mitochondrial dysfunction is central to the resulting pathology of the disease. The most common causes of mitochondrial disorders in humans are mutations in the genes that encoded the proteins of complex I of the oxidative phosphorylation pathway. Although many mitochondrial disorders result from monogenic mutation, many reflect changes in the normal processes of mitochondrial biogenesis triggered by changes in the cellular milieu. It is also important to note that numerous conditions, that are not classically considered to involve mitochondria, such as cancers, cardiovascular diseases, and neurodegenerative diseases, are impacted by alterations in overall mitochondrial dynamics. Many of the disorders that result from defects in mitochondrial biogenesis and/or function have multiple genetic causes such that

CLINICAL BOX 35–1 (CONTINUED)

manifestation can result from maternal inheritance, X-linked inheritance, autosomal recessive inheritance, or autosomal dominant inheritance, or they can be the result of sporadic somatic mutation. Several of the more commonly occurring mitochondrial disorders result from not one single gene defect but can result from mutations or deletions in multiple different genes, each of which result in similar pathologies. Leigh syndrome represents this latter class of mitochondrial disorder given that the general pathology of Leigh syndrome has been shown to result from mutations in at least 16 different genes that include both mitochondrial DNA (mtDNA) genes and nuclear genome genes. Several defined mitochondrial disorders have been shown to result from mutations in the same gene leading to potential diagnostic complications. For example, mitochondrial encephalopathy, lactic acidosis, with stroke-like episodes (MELAS) and myoclonic epilepsy with ragged-red fibers (MERFF) are both associated with mutations in the mtDNA-encoded genes MT-TK, MT-TL1, MT-TH, MT-TS1, and MT-ND5. Mitochondrial diseases can be caused by mutations in genes required for mtDNA replication as well as genes required for mtDNA maintenance. Mitochondrial diseases can also result from mutations in genes that encode proteins of the complexes of the oxidative phosphorylation machinery or genes that encode proteins required for proper assembly of these complexes. Mutations in several of the genes required to synthesize coenzyme Q (ubiquinone) also result in mitochondrial disorders whose symptoms overlap with those of the common disorders such as Leigh syndrome. Mutations in genes encoding proteins required for mitochondrial protein synthesis also cause pathologies resulting from defects in mitochondrial function. Several of the more common mitochondrial encephalomyopathies (Table 35–2) are the result of exclusively mtDNA mutations and as a result are strictly maternal in their inheritance.

TABLE 35–2 Maternally inherited mitochondrial diseases.

Disorder	Causative Genes	Symptoms
Mitochondrial encephalopathy, lactic acidosis, stroke-like episodes: MELAS	MT-TL1, MT-TQ, MT-TH, MT-TK, MT-TC, MT-TS1, MT-ND1, MT-ND5, MT-ND6, MT-TS2	All mutations causing MELAS are in mtDNA-encoded genes; inheritance is strictly maternal; most common cause (80% of cases) of MELAS is inheritance of an A → G transition mutation in the *MT-TL1* gene which is a *mtDNA* gene that encodes a Leu (L) tRNA that recognizes the codons UUA and UUG; symptoms usually appear in early childhood following a period of normal growth; earliest symptoms include muscle weakness and pain, recurrent headaches, loss of appetite, vomiting, and seizures; common pathology is lactic acidosis resulting in vomiting, abdominal pain, extreme fatigue, muscle weakness, and difficulty breathing; most individuals with MELAS experience stroke-like episodes beginning before age 40
Myoclonic epilepsy with ragged red fibers: MERFF	MT-TK, MT-TL1, MT-TH, MT-TS1, MT-TS2, MT-TF, MT-ND5	All mutations causing MERFF are in mtDNA-encoded genes; inheritance is strictly maternal; most common cause (80% of cases) of MERFF is inheritance of mutations in the *MT-TK* gene which is a *mtDNA* gene that encodes a Lys (K) tRNA; symptoms of MERFF begin to appear in childhood or early adolescence; MERFF is characterized by myoclonus (muscle twitching), muscle weakness (myopathy), and progressive stiffness (spasticity); additional common symptoms of MERFF are seizures, ataxia, peripheral neuropathy, optic neuropathy, hearing loss, and dementia; many MERFF patients are of short stature
Leber hereditary optic neuropathy: LHON	MT-ND1, MT-ND2, MT-ND4, MT-ND4L, MT-ND5, MT-ND6, MT-CYB, MT-CO3, MT-ATP6	All mutations causing LHON are in mtDNA-encoded genes; inheritance is strictly maternal; symptoms of LHON usually present in midlife (mean age of onset 27–35 years); symptoms are predominantly restricted to the visual system; symptoms include acute or subacute central vision loss that initially manifests with blurring and clouding of vision ultimately leading to blindness; mutations in the mtDNA that cause LHON can act autonomously or in association with each other in the manifestation of the pathology of LHON; males manifest symptoms more often than females; often individuals who harbor LHON mutations never experience symptoms with more than 50% of males and 85% of females remaining symptom free
Kearns-Sayre syndrome: KSS	mtDNA deletions	The mtDNA deletions observed in KSS range from 1.3–8 kbp and can vary in position; the most common deletion (35% of patients) is a 4997 bp deletion of nucleotide 8469–13,147 (encompassing 12 genes); symptoms of KSS usually appear before age 20 and most commonly affect the eyes; characteristic symptoms include chronic progressive external ophthalmoplegia (PEO) which represents weakness or paralysis of the eye muscles impairing eye movement and causing drooping eyelids (ptosis); KSS may also manifest with muscle weakness in the limbs, deafness, renal pathology, and dementia
Pearson syndrome: PS	mtDNA deletions	Infantile onset, exocrine pancreatic insufficiency, sideroblastic anemia and bone marrow failure, tubular and liver dysfunction, encephalopathy; children who survive will develop classic Kearns-Sayre syndrome

MULTIFACTORIAL INHERITANCE

Many common diseases, such as cancer or congenital birth defects, cluster within the relatives of affected individuals more frequently than in the general population. Inheritance of these conditions generally does not follow one of the typical mendelian patterns of single-gene disorders because they are the result of the complex interactions among a number of genetic variants as well as certain environmental exposures. These types of disorders are **multifactorial** in origin.

Multifactorial disorders with complex inheritance can be classified by the use of the terms **qualitative traits** or **quantitative traits**. Qualitative traits are discrete types of traits that can most easily be understood from the fact that an individual either has the trait or does not have the trait. An example of a qualitative trait is the Rh blood type: an individual is either Rh-positive or Rh-negative. Quantitative traits are continuous traits such as measurable physical or biochemical quantities. Typical quantitative traits are blood pressure, height, or body mass index (BMI), each of which cannot be specified by a discrete category.

HIGH-YIELD CONCEPT

Many multifactorial disorders demonstrate a sex bias, appearing more frequently in one sex over the other (Table 35–3). The recurrence risk for multifactorial disorders is increased in the children of an individual if that individual is of the less commonly affected sex.

TABLE 35–3 Multifactorial conditions reported with a significant sex bias.

Increased in Males	
Condition	Increase (M:F)
Pyloric stenosis	5.0
Legg-Perthes	5.2
Hirschprung	3.7
Talipes equinovarus	2.0
Cleft lip + palate	1.6
Increased in Females	
Condition	Increase (F:M)
Idiopathic scoliosis	6.6
Cong. hip dysplasia	3.3
Anencephaly	1.6
Spina bifida	1.2
Cleft palate	1.4

HIGH-YIELD CONCEPT

In general, the recurrence risk for first-degree relatives of an individual affected by a multifactorial disorder is the square root of the incidence of that disorder in the general population.

Methods to determine the relative contributions of genetics and the environment to multifactorial disorders have involved the use of twin studies. Monozygotic twins (identical twins) share the same genotype and generally the same developmental environment. Dizygotic twins generally share the same developmental environment but differ genotypically as would any other typical non-twin sibling pair. When twins have the same disease, they are said to be **concordant** for that disease. Conversely, when one twin is affected, and the other is not, they are said to be **discordant**. By measuring the degree of concordance from twin studies, it is possible to get an estimate of the influence of genetics on multifactorial traits.

POPULATION GENETICS

Population genetics refers to the quantitative analysis of the distribution of genetic variation in populations. Population genetics is concerned not only with genetics but also with environmental and societal factors that, in combination, contribute to the distribution of alleles and genotypes in families and larger populations such as communities. A central concept of population genetics is that if a population meets certain assumptions a simple mathematical formula allows for the calculation of the frequency of alleles in a population and the genotypes in a population. This equation is known as the **Hardy-Weinberg law**.

HIGH-YIELD CONCEPT

For a population to be in Hardy-Weinberg equilibrium a set of assumptions must be met. A population under study must be large and matings must be random with respect to the gene (locus) being analyzed. The frequencies of alleles are assumed to remain constant over time. There is no appreciable rate of the appearance of new mutations. There is no selection such that all individuals are capable of mating and passing on their genes. There is no appreciable immigration of individuals, whose allele frequencies are very different, into the population under study.

In a population in Hardy-Weinberg equilibrium, the proportion of genotypes will remain constant from generation to generation if the allele frequencies remain constant. Using the typical "p" and "q" designations for the two alleles of a given gene,

TABLE 35–4 Genotype frequencies.

Genotype	Number of Individuals	Genotype Frequency
p-p	49	0.49 (49%)
p-q	42	0.42 (42%)
q-q	9	0.09 (9%)
Total	100	1.0 (100%)

where generally p represents the wild-type allele and q the mutant allele, the proportion of the different genotypes will be $p^2{:}2pq{:}q^2$ where p^2 is the homozygous wild-type frequency (A/A), $2pq$ is the heterozygous frequency (A/a), and q^2 is the homozygous mutant frequency (a/a). Since allele frequencies, as well as genotype frequencies, must sum to 100% (ie, be equal to 1), the Hardy-Weinberg equilibrium equation is $p^2 + 2pq + q^2 = 1$.

A simple example (Table 35–4) of the analysis of the frequencies of the genotypes for a single gene in a population of 100 people demonstrates the utility of the Hardy-Weinberg equilibrium equation. Given the frequencies of these three genotypes one can determine the frequencies of the two alleles (p and q) in this population. There are always two alleles for single genes and so there are a total of 200 alleles of the gene being studied in this population of 100 individuals.

There are 49 individuals with two copies of the p allele (homozygous wild-type), 42 individuals with one copy of each allele (heterozygous), and 9 individuals with two copies of the q allele (homozygous mutant). The frequency of the p allele is, therefore, $[(49 \times 2) + 42]/200 = 0.75$ (70%). Since the frequency of the two alleles must add up to 1 the frequency of the q allele is simply $1 - 0.7 = 0.3$ (30%). However, one can also calculate the frequency of the q allele: $[(9 \times 2) + 42]/200 = 0.3$.

Using these allele frequencies in the Hardy-Weinberg equation ($p^2 + 2pq + q^2 = 1$) would yield $(0.7)^2 + 2(0.7)(0.3) + (0.3)^2 = 1$ which results in $0.49 + 0.42 + 0.09 = 1$. What this demonstrates is that knowing the allele frequencies for a single gene allows for the calculation of genotype frequencies and conversely, knowing the genotype frequencies allows for the calculation of allele frequencies.

HIGH-YIELD CONCEPT

For autosomal recessive diseases q^2 (a/a) represents the incidence rate of the disease in a population. Using the Hardy-Weinberg law, and knowing the incidence rate, it is possible to calculate the frequency of carriers ($2pq$: A/a) of the mutant allele in the population. Conversely, knowing the rate of carriers in a population allows for the calculation of the incidence rate of the disease in that population.

When considering allele frequencies, it is useful to understand that the wild-type allele is much more prevalent than the mutant allele such that the value of p can always be assumed to be 1. Using this assumption allows for certain approximations to be made for the various forms of autosomal and sex-linked inheritance (Table 35–5).

TABLE 35–5 Applications/approximations from Hardy-Weinberg equation.

Inheritance	Assumption	Approximation
Autosomal recessive	Carriers = 2q	Number of carriers is twice the disease allele (q) frequency
Autosomal dominant	Number of affected individuals ~2q	Disease frequency is twice disease allele (q) frequency
X-linked recessive	Affected males = q: affected females = q^2	Female carriers are twice the frequency of affected males
X-linked dominant	Affected males = q: affected females ~2q	Twice as many affected females as males

HARDY-WEINBERG LAW AND AUTOSOMAL RECESSIVE DISEASES

The prevalent use of the Hardy-Weinberg law in clinical practice is in the genetic counseling for autosomal recessive diseases. Most autosomal recessive diseases are the result of many different mutations in the same gene (**allelic heterogeneity**) such that some individuals may be homozygous for the same mutation but, more often than not, they are compound heterozygotes harboring different mutant alleles of the gene. However, for convenience all disease-causing alleles (q) are treated as a single-mutant allele.

Using the pedigree shown in Figure 35–10, how would one calculate the likelihood of the child of II-1 and II-2 having a

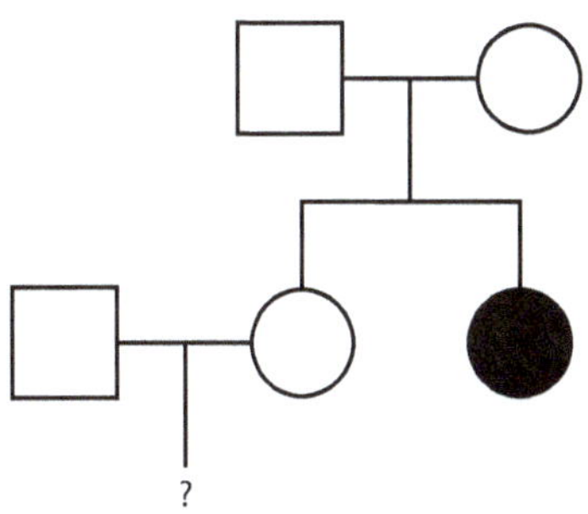

FIGURE 35–10 Practical application of the Hardy-Weinberg law. Using the Hardy-Weinberg law one can calculate the expected carrier frequency for individual II-1 and thus, the likelihood (recurrence rate) that the unborn child of II-1 and II-2 will inherit an autosomal recessive disease. (Reproduced with permission from themedicalbiochemistrypage, LLC.)

child with cystic fibrosis (CF). It is most useful to account for all the independent variables in calculating recurrence risks. In this pedigree each parent (II-1 and II-2) has a risk of being a carrier and a ½ chance of donating the mutant allele to their offspring. Therefore, the overall recurrence risk is the product of the four independent variables.

Since the pedigree most likely represents an autosomal recessive disease, and we know that CF is indeed an autosomal recessive disease, the likelihood that II-2 is a carrier is 2/3 since she is unaffected and she has a sibling with the disease. The four independent variables needed to calculate the risk of their unborn child having CF are the father's risk of being a carrier (calculate from Hardy-Weinberg law), the father's chance of donating mutant allele (1/2), the mother's risk of being a carrier (2/3), and the mother's chance of donating mutant allele (1/2). Since any individual always has a ½ chance of donating either of the two alleles for a single gene, many discussions of these calculations reduce the two independent variables of donating the mutant allele to their obvious product, 1/4, such that there are only three numbers in the calculation. However, always accounting for all the independent variables significantly reduces the risk of making errors in the calculations. This is particularly important in problems that introduce the likelihood of having a child of a particular sex AND the child having the disease. In this latter situation there is a fifth independent variable, the chance of having a male or a female child, which is ½.

Assume that the incidence rate of CF in a given population is 1 in 2000. Using the Hardy-Weinberg law it is possible to calculate the risk that individual II-1 is a carrier for CF. The incidence rate is q^2 so $q^2 = 1/2{,}000$ therefore, $q \sim 1/45$. Since we can assume $p = 1$ the carrier frequency for CF is $\sim 2q$ thus, $q = 1/22.5$. The father's likelihood of being a carrier is, therefore, 1/22.5 and that of the mother is 2/3. Each of them has a ½ chance of donating the mutant allele. Using each of the four independent variables the overall recurrence risk for their unborn child is $1/22.5 \times 1/2$ (father's two variables) $\times\ 2/3 \times 1/2$ (mother's two variables) = 1/135.

To demonstrate that it is acceptable to assign the value of 1 to p, remember that $p + q = 1$. The frequency for q (1/45) in this example was determined from the incidence rate. Therefore, the frequency for p must be 44/45 such that $p + q = 1$ which means that the actual frequency for p is 0.98 or essentially 1.

HARDY-WEINBERG LAW AND AUTOSOMAL DOMINANT DISEASES

Very rarely are individuals affected by an autosomal dominant disease homozygous for the mutant allele. This means that the incidence rate for autosomal dominant diseases is represented by the $2pq$ value of the Hardy-Weinberg law. As for autosomal recessive diseases it is possible to assign the frequency of the wild-type allele (p) the value of 1. This means that the number of individuals in a population that can be expected to have an autosomal dominant disease is very nearly twice the frequency of the mutant allele (q) in that population (as indicated in Table 35–5).

HARDY-WEINBERG LAW AND X-LINKED RECESSIVE DISEASES

Given that males are hemizygous for the X chromosome the Hardy-Weinberg law does not directly apply as there is no q^2 (x/x) value. However, because the presence of the mutant allele results in disease in males, the incidence rate in males is equal to the frequency of the mutant allele (x). Females have two X chromosomes so there is a q^2 value which represents the incidence rate in females. If the incidence rate of an X-linked recessive disease is 1/10,000 males (q) the incidence rate in females is q^2 which is $1/10^8$. Thus, using the Hardy-Weinberg law for females it is apparent that the frequency of X-linked recessive diseases is four orders of magnitude less in females than in males.

From the Hardy-Weinberg law the frequency of carrier females for an X-linked recessive is the same as for the frequency of autosomal recessive diseases, $2pq$. Since we can assign the value of 1 to p, the frequency of female carriers of mutant X alleles is $2q$ or as stated in Table 35–5 it is twice the incidence rate of the disease in males.

HARDY-WEINBERG LAW AND X-LINKED DOMINANT DISEASES

As for any X-linked disorder, males only have only one allele and thus, the incidence rate of X-linked dominant diseases in males is the frequency of the mutant allele. Also, as for autosomal dominant diseases, it is very rare to find homozygous females for X-linked dominant diseases. Thus, the incidence rate of these diseases in females is defined by $2pq$. However, since $p \sim 1$ the incidence rate in females is twice the frequency of the mutant allele (q). Since the incidence rate in males is equal to the frequency of the mutant allele, the incidence rate of X-linked dominant diseases in females is twice that in males. This is a useful approximation, however, due to X chromosome inactivation and epigenetic effects on the X chromosome this incidence rate assumption for females is not always that found in a population.

EXCEPTIONS TO HARDY-WEINBERG EQUILIBRIUM

A number of real-world factors violate the assumptions of the Hardy-Weinberg law that relate to a population being in equilibrium. In some diseases, such as Duchene muscular dystrophy, the rate of new mutations contributing to disease can be as high as 30%. Many populations have subgroups who choose to marry within their own subgroup and not the larger population, a phenomenon that is referred to as **stratification**. Individuals choose their mates based on many factors such as looks, intelligence, height, etc. such that matings in a given population are not random, a phenomenon referred to as **assortative mating**.

Consanguinity and inbreeding also result in increasing the frequency of mutant alleles in a population. For example, in the ethnic Ashkenazi Jewish population the frequency of carriers of mutant alleles of the gene encoding the α-subunit (*HEXA*) of β-hexosaminidase that result in Tay-Sachs disease is nearly 100 times higher than the frequency in the general population.

Due to a number of political and socio-economic factors, individuals emigrate all over the world such that the alleles from one location become mixed with those of another location. This process of population allele mixing is referred to as **genetic flow**.

Genetic drift refers to changes in allele frequency that are not related to natural selection but is the result of the random selection of certain genes. Genetic drift involves two related mechanisms, the **bottleneck effect** and the **founder effect**. A simple example of the bottleneck effect can be demonstrated using the near extinction of the America bison in the late 1800s. The small population of bison that remained, when they became protected, harbored a set of alleles that was dramatically less diverse than the pool of alleles in the vast herds that roamed North America prior to their near extinction. It is this small population of alleles that is resident in the genomes of the now much larger herd of American bison.

The simplest way to describe the founder effect is using a family into which a new member has been assimilated. If the new member harbors a dominant mutant allele, that was not originally in the family, and mates with someone in the family, the family will now demonstrate the characteristic inheritance of autosomal dominant diseases in each subsequent generation.

At the population level, the difference between bottleneck effect and founder effect is that in the former the change in the allele pool in the population occurs when the population size is reduced for at least one generation and in the latter the allele pool is derived from a small number of individuals that leave a large population to start a new colony.

CYTOGENETICS

Cytogenetics is the study of microscopically observable changes in the number or structure of the chromosomes. The diagnostic utility of cytogenetics relates to the fact that chromosomal abnormalities are the cause of numerous disorders and represent a major category of genetic disease. Chromosomal abnormalities account for half of all first trimester spontaneous abortions, are the cause of a large percentage of congenital malformations, and are the root cause of numerous cancers. Collectively chromosomal abnormalities are more common than all single-gene disorders combined.

Chromosome analysis involves the culture of dividing cells and arresting them in metaphase. Following treatment of the cells to release the metaphase chromosomes the chromosomes are fixed, stained, and spread onto slides (see Figure 35–1 for a stylized depiction). These metaphase spreads produce a **karyotype**, which is simply a picture of an individual's chromosomes. Classic cytogenetic techniques utilize chromosomal staining methods to generate specific patterns of banding for each chromosome. Molecular cytogenetics utilizes hybridization of fluorescently labelled probes to identify specific chromosomes as well as specific loci in chromosomes.

Abnormalities in chromosome structure and number can occur during mitosis and meiosis. Mitosis is the process by which homologous chromosomes of somatic cells are duplicated and one of each pair of sister chromatids is divided into each of the two resulting diploid daughter cells. Meiosis is of DNA replication and cell division that results in the formation of the gametes (eggs and sperm). Although mitosis and meiosis both involve DNA replication, meiosis is a reductive division that through two cycles (referred to as meiosis I and meiosis II) results in one copy of each type of chromosome being passed to each haploid gamete.

MEIOSIS

The various stages of meiosis, both during meiosis I and meiosis II, are similar to those occurring during mitosis: prophase, metaphase, anaphase, and telophase (Figure 35–11). The process of meiosis reduces the total chromosome number in the final cells (the gametes) by half. Meiosis is divided into two distinct events. In the first event, referred to as meiosis I, the DNA in the progenitor cell is duplicated and then the cell divides to produce two identical diploid cells. Since the duplicated chromosomes are separated in the final stages of meiosis I, this stage is referred to as **reductional cell division**.

In the second event, referred to as meiosis II, the two diploid cells divide without first undergoing DNA replication such that the final results are the generation of haploid gametes (four sperm and one egg) from the originating diploid germ cell progenitor (Figure 35–12). Since the sister chromatids are separated in meiosis II, without prior DNA replication, this is referred to as **equational cell division**. Each diploid nucleus that enters meiosis produces four haploid nuclei, each of which contains either the maternal or paternal copy of each chromosome, but not both. The gamete progenitor cells are called oogonia in females and spermatogonia in males.

The DNA of meiotic cells is replicated during interphase to produce chromosomes that are composed of two sister chromatids. Even though there is twice as much DNA content in the meiotic cells at the end of DNA replication (referred to as 4C) the sister chromatids are still considered a single chromosome so that the chromosome number (referred to as 2N) is not changed at the end of meiotic DNA replication and the cell is, therefore, still technically a diploid cell.

During prophase of meiosis I (prophase I) the chromosomes condense, the nuclear membrane is degraded, and the homologous chromosomes form structures that are referred to as bivalents. The term bivalent chromosome refers to the tetrad structure that is formed as a result of the interaction of homologous regions of DNA between sister chromatids. The interaction of homologous DNA regions results in DNA double-strand breaks that are subsequently repaired via the process referred to as **homology-directed repair**. The exchange of DNA segments between the sister chromatids occurs at sites in the chromosomes that are termed chiasma.

Meiosis II is the second meiotic division and is designed to result in the separation of sister chromatids, a process referred to

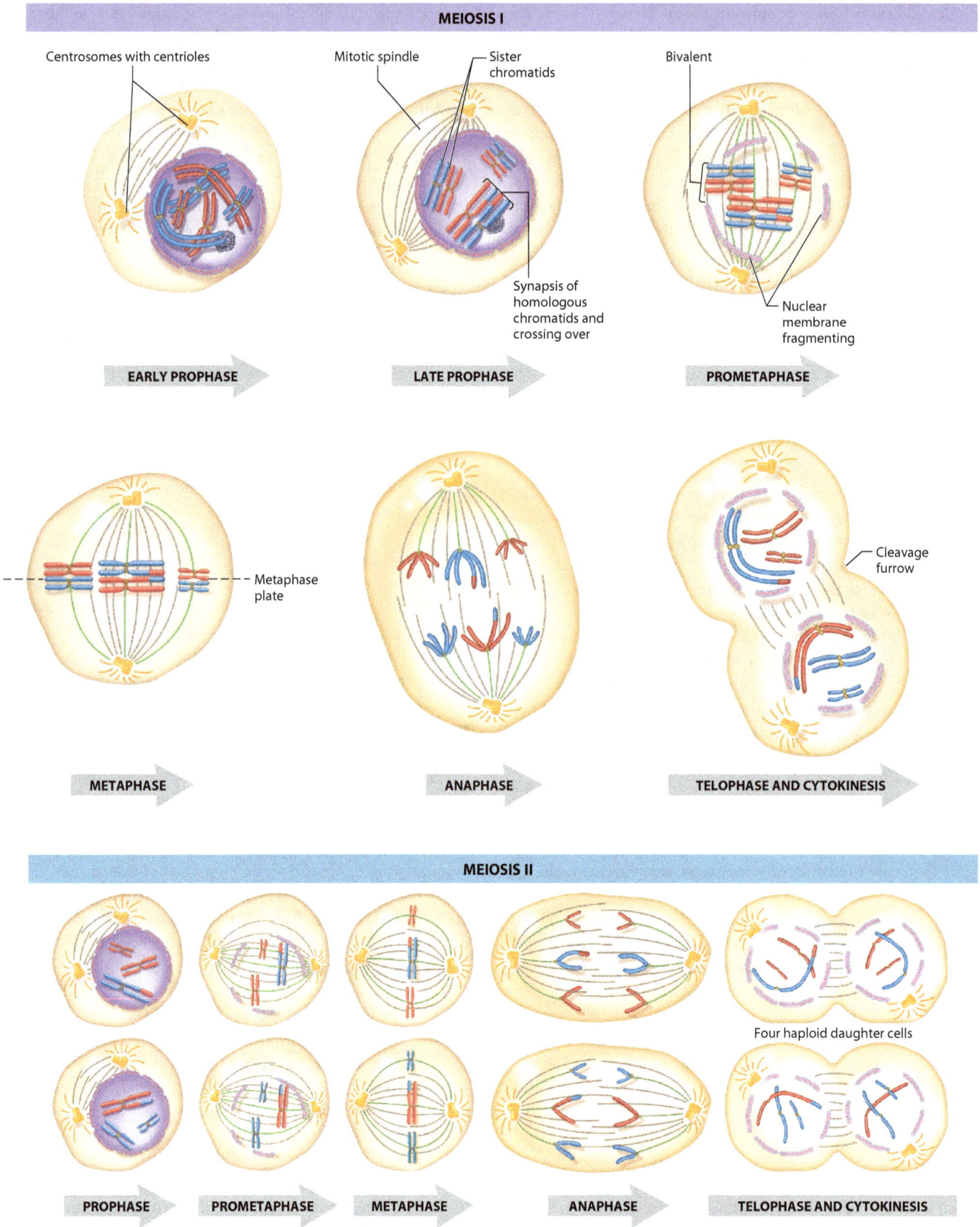

FIGURE 35–11 Meiosis involves two rounds of division and yields four haploid nuclei, each carrying one copy of each type of chromosome. Key events occur in prophase I of the first cycle including synapsis, or pairing, of homologous chromosome copies and recombination between them. (Reproduced with permission from Brooker RJ: *Genetics: Analysis & Principles*, 7th ed. New York, NY: McGraw Hill, 2021.)

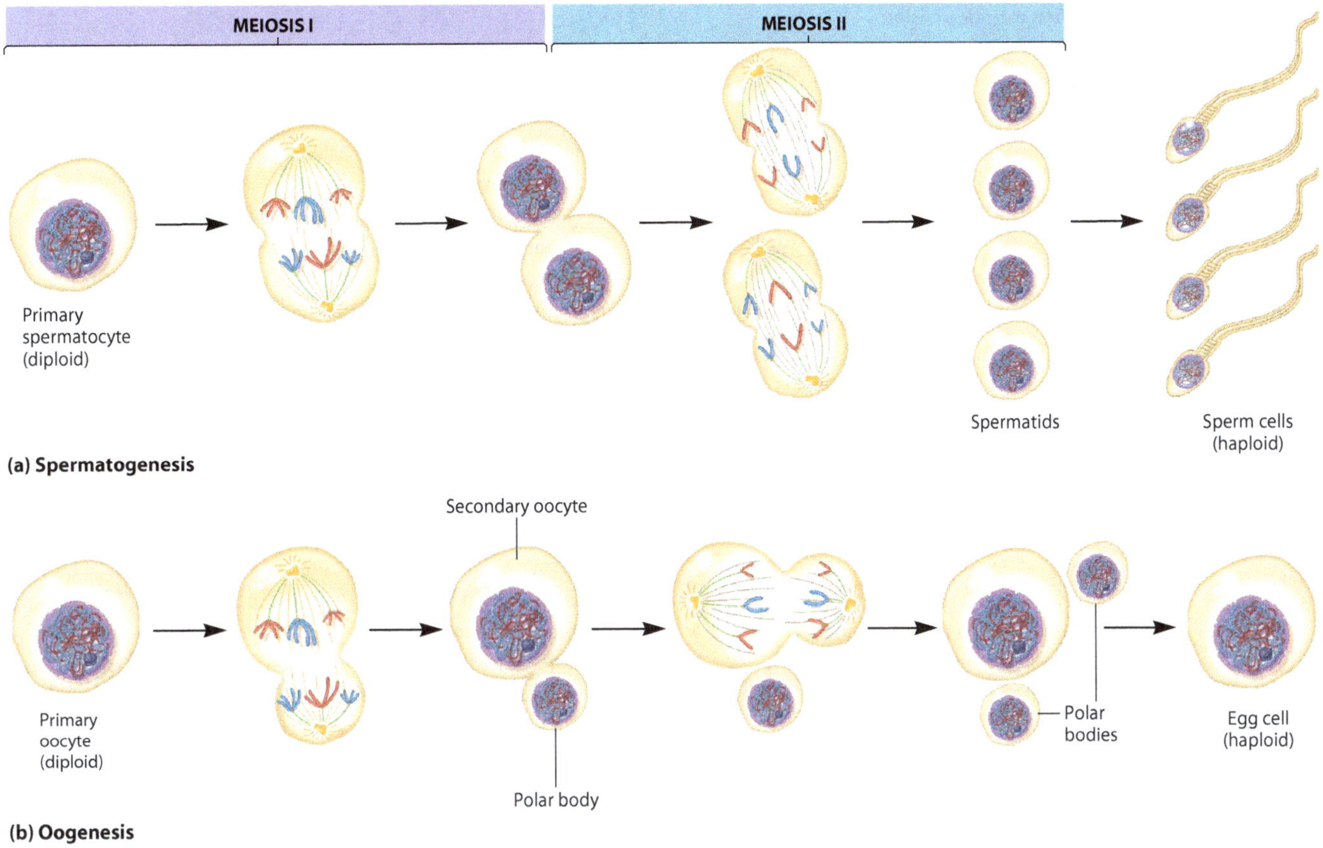

FIGURE 35–12 Comparison of: (a) spermatogenesis, which can yield four haploid sperm, and (b) oogenesis, which yields one haploid egg cell and up to three haploid polar bodies, which degenerate. (Reproduced with permission from Brooker RJ: *Genetics: Analysis & Principles*, 7th ed. New York, NY: McGraw-Hill, 2021.)

as equational segregation. Like mitosis, meiosis II occurs in four ordered steps identified, in order, as prophase II, metaphase II, anaphase II, and telophase II. The end result of meiosis II is production of haploid gametes.

During male spermatogenesis the spermatogonia yield four functional haploid gametes (sperm). In females the oogonia yield three polar bodies which are not functional gametes, and one functional gamete (ovum). When oogonia undergo meiosis, one of the two cells at the end of meiosis I represents the diploid cell that enters meiosis II, and one of the resultant cells is referred to as a polar body. The polar body then divides to become two polar bodies. Female eggs are arrested at the diplotene stage of prophase in meiosis I until puberty when ovulation is stimulated. This means that female eggs have the potential to be in this arrested stage of meiosis for many years. Only eggs that undergo ovulation complete meiosis I prior to their release from the ovary. When the egg is fertilized, only then does it complete meiosis II.

MEIOTIC NONDISJUNCTION

The proper sorting of the chromosomes during meiosis must be highly precise such that at the end of the process one complete set of chromosomes is distributed to each of the four resulting haploid gametes. In order to properly sort the original 92 chromatids, that result from the duplication of each of the 46 chromosomes in the original diploid progenitor cells, there needs to be accurate separation, first of the sister chromatids and then of the sister chromosomes. This process of separation is termed **disjunction**. Improper disjunction, termed **nondisjunction**, can occur either during meiosis I or during meiosis II (Figure 35–13).

When nondisjunction occurs some of the resulting haploid gametes will lack a particular chromosome while others will end up with more than one copy. Nondisjunction is especially common in human female meiosis as a result of the many years the eggs remain arrested in meiosis I. Indeed, nondisjunction in meiosis I increases dramatically as female age advances. Chromosomal nondisjunction during egg development represents the most common cause of both spontaneous abortion and intellectual impairment in humans.

When nondisjunction occurs during meiosis I the result will be two **disomic** (containing two copies of a chromosome) gametes and two **nullisomic** (lacking a particular chromosome) gametes. Because monosomy for any autosome is non-viable the two nullisomic gametes, if used for fertilization, will not lead to any viable fetus. The gametes that contain the extra chromosome will lead to aneuploidy and only a small set of aneuploid chromosomes result in viable embryos (trisomy 13, 18, or 21). Nondisjunction of chromosome 21 during female meiosis I represents the leading cause (75–80%) of Down syndrome. Because all autosomal

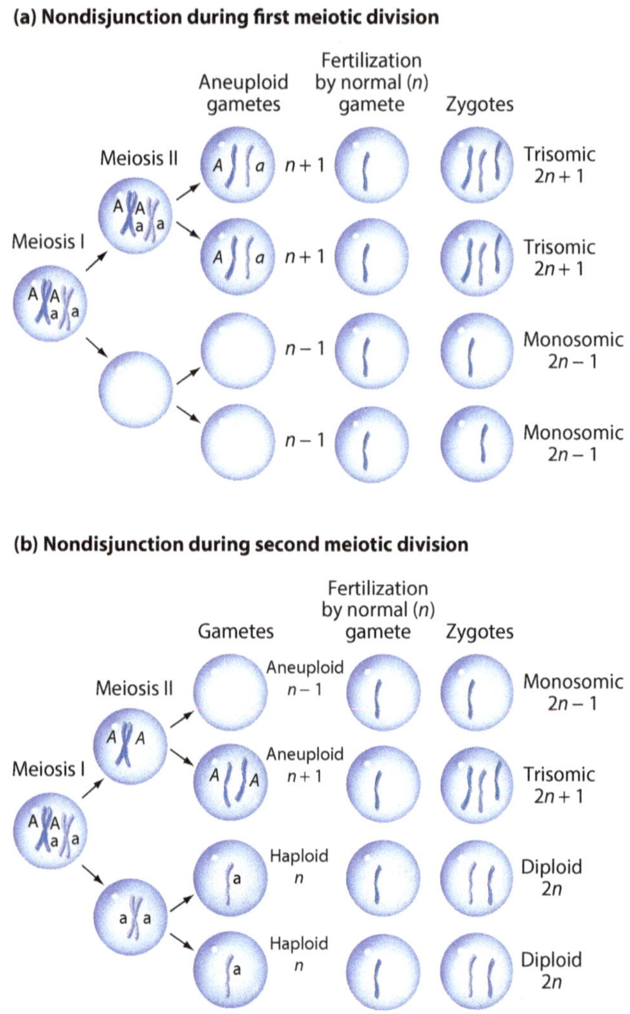

FIGURE 35–13 Results of non-disjunction during meiosis I or meiosis II. Non-disjunction during meiosis I yield two disomic and two nullisomic gametes. When these gametes are used during fertilization with normal gametes the outcomes are incompatible with viability except in the case of the resulting trisomies of chromosomes 13, 18, or 21. Non-disjunction during meiosis II will lead to at least 50% normal conceptuses, and so is a less detrimental result of non-disjunction. (Reproduced with permission from Goldberg ML, Fischer JA, Hood L, et al: Genetics: From Genes to Genomes, 7th ed. New York, NY: McGraw Hill; 2021.)

monosomies, and the vast majority of autosomal aneuploidies, are not compatible with life, the results of nondisjunction during meiosis I are almost always lethal.

When nondisjunction occurs during meiosis II the result will be two normal haploid gametes, one disomic gamete, and one nullisomic gamete. Because there are two normal haploid gametes, 50% of the outcomes from nondisjunction during meiosis II are viable embryos. If nondisjunction of chromosome 21 occurs during meiosis II the one disomic gamete would lead to a Down syndrome offspring. Indeed, nondisjunction of chromosome 21 during meiosis II represents approximately 20% of Down syndrome patients.

UNIPARENTAL DISOMY (UPD)

The most common consequence of chromosomal nondisjunction is trisomy or monosomy for the chromosome involved in the segregation error. However, nondisjunction can result in a disomic state for a given chromosome such that both copies of that chromosome derive from a single parent, referred to as uniparental disomy, UPD. When this phenomenon is associated with two copies of one of the maternal chromosomes it is referred to as maternal UPD, and if it is associated with two copies of a given paternal chromosome it is referred to as paternal UPD. If both chromosomes are derived from identical sister chromatids the situation is referred to as isodisomy, whereas if both homologs from one parent represent the two chromosomes the situation is referred to as heterodisomy.

The frequency of UPD is unknown but in some disorders, particularly in disorders involving imprinted regions of particular chromosomes, the presence of two copies of an imprinted region from one parent results from the process of UPD. Whereas the most common cause (65%–75%) of Prader-Willi syndrome (PWS) is deletion of the imprinted locus present in the q arm of the paternal chromosome 15 (see Clinical Box 22–5), it has been found that in 20%–30% of PWS patients the disorder is the result of maternal UPD. Angelman syndrome, AS (see Clinical Box 22–6), is another disease resulting from defects in the imprinted region of chromosome 15, and a small percentage, approximately 2%, of AS cases involve paternal UPD.

CHROMOSOME NUMBER ABNORMALITIES

Numerical chromosomal number abnormalities can be **euploid** (any exact multiple of the haploid chromosome content) or **aneuploid** (any chromosome number that is not 46 or a multiple of an exact haploid number). All autosomal monosomies are incompatible with life.

HIGH-YIELD CONCEPT

Aside from trisomy of chromosomes 13, 18, or 21 no other autosomal aneuploidy is compatible with life. Trisomy 13 is the cause of Patau syndrome, trisomy 18 is the cause of Edward syndrome, and trisomy 21 is the cause of Down syndrome. These three chromosomes harbor the lowest number of genes which likely explains why trisomy for any one of them is compatible with live birth.

Sex chromosome aneuploidies also occur. Turner syndrome, which afflicts females, results from the loss of one of the two X chromosomes such that their karyotype is 45,X. The loss of the X chromosome in Turner females is the result of a nondisjunction event during spermatogenesis. Turner syndrome is the only chromosomal monosomy that results in viable offspring. Other high-yield sex chromosome aneuploidies include triple X females (47,XXX), Kleinfelter males (47,XXY), and XYY males (47,XYY). The majority of triple X females result from nondisjunction during meiosis I of oogenesis. The XYY male genotype is due exclusively to nondisjunction during meiosis II of spermatogenesis.

Chromosomal triploidy (69,XX or 69,XY) is one of most common chromosome abnormalities in humans, found in 1–2% of all conceptions. Triploidy accounts for 10% of all miscarriages. Triploidy is termed **digyny**, when the extra set of chromosomes is of maternal origin, or **diandry**, when the extra set of chromosomes is of paternal origin. Diandry accounts for 2/3 of triploidy and is principally due to a failure in the normal block to polyspermy. Digyny most often results due to meiosis I failure.

The diandry phenotype is characterized by a normally sized or mildly symmetrically growth retarded fetus with normal adrenal glands, and is associated with an abnormally large, cystic placenta with histological features known as **partial hydatidiform mole** (PHM). The digyny phenotype is characterized by marked asymmetric intrauterine growth restriction, marked adrenal hypoplasia, and a very small, non-molar placenta.

CHROMOSOME STRUCTURE ABNORMALITIES

Chromosomal structural abnormalities are numerous and can result from a variety of different causes. Chromosomal structural abnormalities include translocations, insertions, deletions, inversions, duplications, isochromosomes, and ring chromosomes (Figure 35–14). Most chromosomal abnormalities occur during gametogenesis and are thus inherited. Somatic chromosomal abnormalities, particularly translocations, are commonly associated with the development of cancers, with lymphoid and hematopoietic cancers being very often caused by translocations.

Chromosomal structural rearrangements are termed **balanced** or **unbalanced**. Balanced alterations result in no gain or loss of genetic material although the function of some genes can be affected. Balanced alterations account for around 90% of the cases of chromosomal structural rearrangements that have been identified. Unbalanced alterations are those associated with the gain or loss of genetic material. Monosomies and trisomies, as

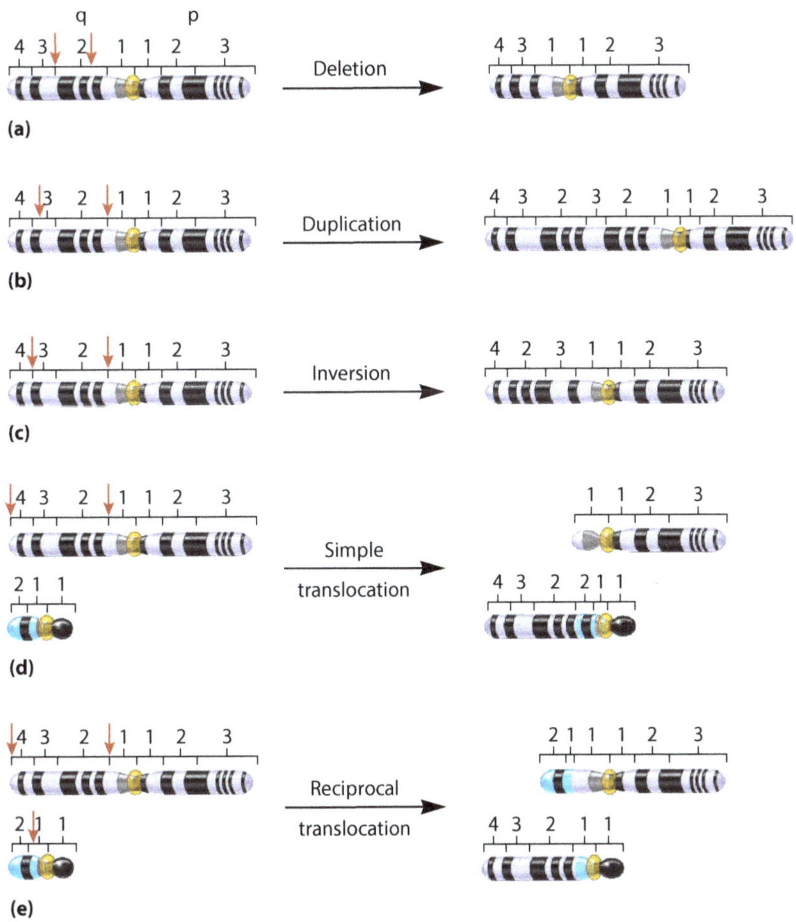

FIGURE 35–14 Chromosome aberrations are changes in chromosome structure. (a) Deletion is the loss of a segment of chromosome. (b) Duplication is the insertion of a section of chromosome so that two copies of each affected gene are present. (c) Inversions can occur when two breakpoints are reattached at alternate ends. (d) Simple translocation is the movement of a section of one chromosome to a different linkage group. (e) Reciprocal translocation involves the exchange of sections between nonhomologous chromosomes. (Reproduced with permission from Brooker RJ: *Genetics: Analysis & Principles*, 7th ed. New York, NY: McGraw Hill, 2021.)

well as partial monosomy or trisomy, represent the most obvious examples of unbalanced chromosomal rearrangements.

TRANSLOCATIONS

Translocations represent the major chromosomal structural abnormalities. Many translocations are balanced rearrangements since they are reciprocal, meaning a fragment of one chromosome becomes attached to another and vice versa. A special type of balanced translocation is termed the **Robertsonian translocation**. Robertsonian translocations involve the acrocentric chromosomes (13, 14, 15, 21, 22) where the two different chromosomes become fused at their centromeres with both chromosomes losing their p arms. Human ribosomal gene repeats are distributed among nucleolar organizer regions (NOR) on the p arms of the five acrocentric chromosomes and thus, loss of two p arms, as a result of a Robertsonian translocation, does not result in an overall loss of genetic material.

SEGREGATION OUTCOMES WITH TRANSLOCATED CHROMOSOMES

The consequences of germline translocations can be profound due to the process of segregation during meiosis. The regions of homology in the translocated chromosomes can pair up during meiosis leading to distinct types of segregation (Figure 35–15) termed **alternate** and **adjacent** segregation.

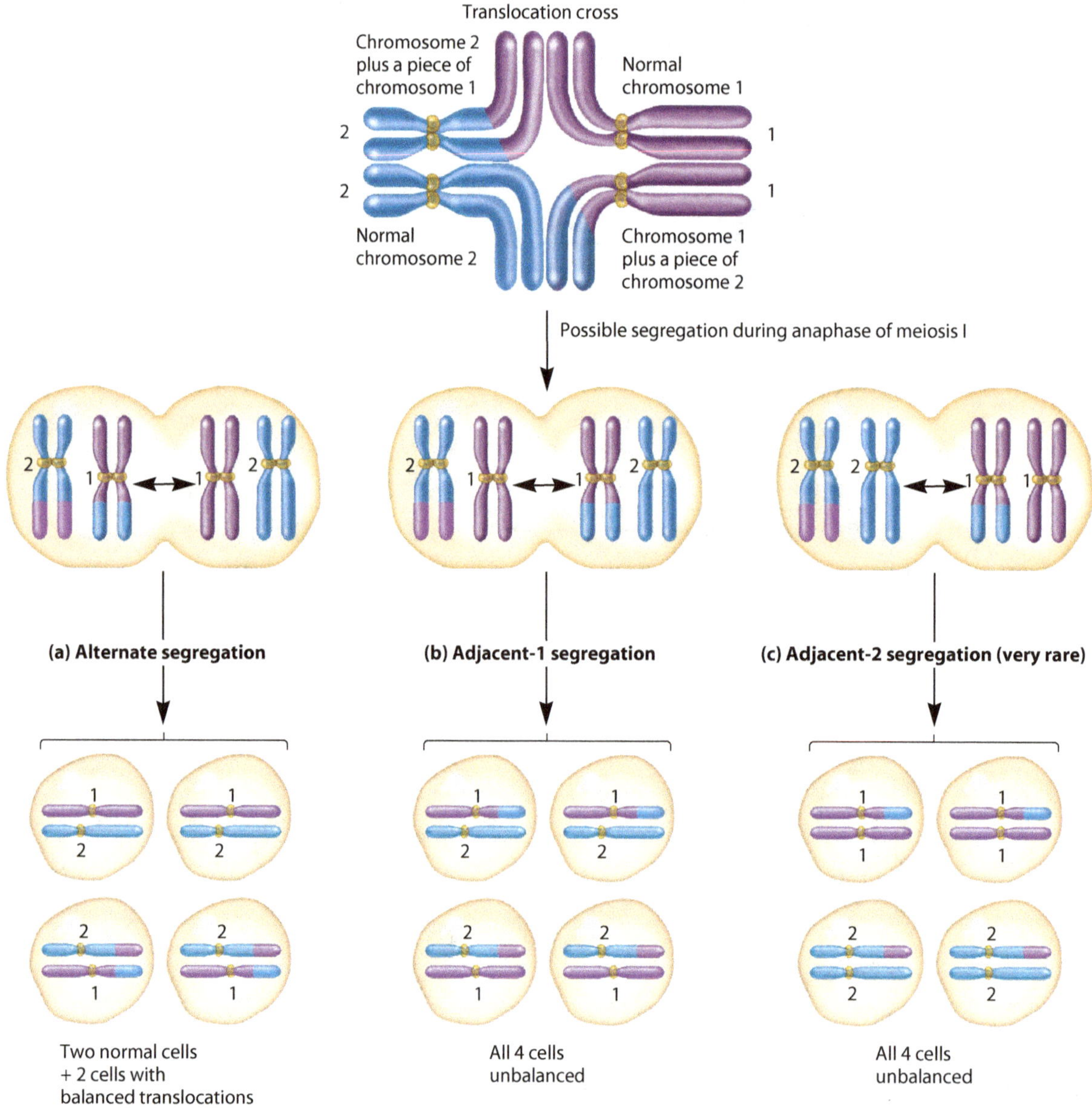

FIGURE 35–15 Translocation products depend on how the homologous centromeres attach to the spindle during meiosis. (Reproduced with permission from Brooker RJ: *Genetics: Analysis & Principles*, 7th ed. New York, NY: McGraw Hill, 2021.)

With alternate segregation the translocation chromosomes segregate (disjoin) to one spindle pole and the normal chromosomes segregate to the other spindle pole. The gametes that result are two normal haploid gametes and two gametes that harbor the same balanced translocations. The outcomes from the use of these gametes for fertilization will be viable. Adjacent segregation can be of two types identified as adjacent-1 and adjacent-2, with the latter being an extremely rare occurrence. With adjacent-1 the nonhomologous centromeres segregate to the same pole such that one normal and one translocated chromosome, of each type, segregate together. With adjacent-2 segregation the adjacent homologous centromeres segregate to the same pole. The outcomes from adjacent segregation will be four gametes harboring unbalanced translocations and therefore no viable conceptions will be possible.

A special circumstance resulting from Robertsonian translocations and meiotic segregation relates to the fact that the translocated chromosomes, whose q arms are attached at the single centromere, act like a single chromosome. If these chromosomes undergo alternate segregation, the resulting gametes are similar to the case for translocations that do not involve the acrocentric chromosomes, that is, normal gametes and translocation carrier gametes. However, if the Robertsonian translocation undergoes adjacent-1 segregation the outcomes will be two disomic and two nullisomic gametes. If the Robertsonian translocation involves chromosome 13 or 21 with another acrocentric chromosome one of the disomic gametes will harbor two copies of chromosome 13 or 21 resulting in a potentially viable trisomy. Indeed, approximately 3–5% of Down syndrome infants are the result of the gametes in the translocation carrier parent undergoing adjacent-1 segregation.

HIGH-YIELD CONCEPT

It is easy to appreciate the outcomes of translocation carrier gametes following segregation. With ***AL***ternate segregation **AL**L outcomes are viable. With ***AD***jacent segregation all outcomes are **AD**verse.

DELETIONS

As the term implies, deletions involve the loss of genetic material. Chromosomal deletions are broadly categorized as **interstitial** and terminal (Figure 35–16). Interstitial deletions are those that result from loss of chromosomal material in either the p or the q arm. Terminal deletions result in loss of chromosomal material from the tips of the p or q arms. High-yield diseases resulting from interstitial deletions in the q arm of chromosome 11 are Prader-Willi syndrome (see Clinical Box 22–5) and Angelman syndrome (see Clinical Box 22–6).

Terminal or interstitial deletions in the p arm of chromosome 5 result in the disorder termed cri du chat. Cri du chat (also written cri-du-chat; meaning "cry of the cat"), also known as 5p-syndrome, is a rare disorder where afflicted infants manifest with a high-pitched cat-like cry. The characteristic features of cri du chat are intellectual impairment, microcephaly (small head), hypotonia, and developmental delay. There are also characteristic facial features of cri du chat that include hypertelorism (wide-set eyes), a small jaw, low-set ears, and a rounded face.

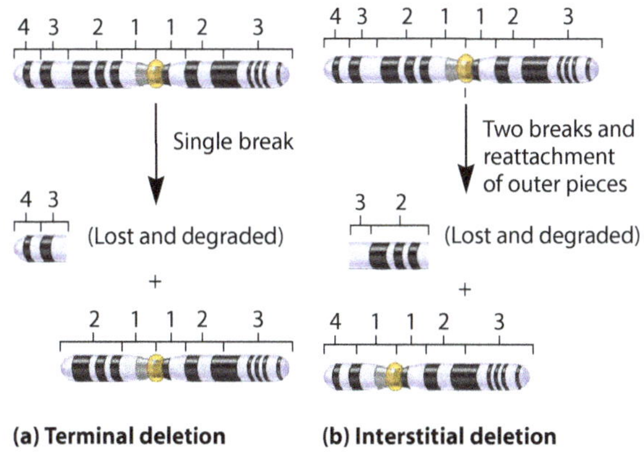

FIGURE 35–16 Loss of genetic material can occur from (a) terminal deletions in which the broken end of a chromosome is lost, or (b) interstitial deletions involving two breaks and the loss of the intervening section of the chromosome. (Reproduced with permission from Brooker RJ: *Genetics: Analysis & Principles*, 7th ed. New York, NY: McGraw Hill, 2021.)

The most common microdeletion syndrome is most often referred to as DiGeorge syndrome. This disorder results from a small deletion in the q arm of chromosome 22 (specifically 22q11.2) encompassing 30–40 genes and is, therefore, also known as 22q11.2 deletion syndrome. Individuals suffering from DiGeorge syndrome have increased susceptibility to infections as a consequence of decreased production of T cells. Although the full spectrum of the manifestations of DiGeorge syndrome is widely variable, in addition to immune deficit, patients frequently have a submucosal cleft palate, heart abnormalities, developmental delay, and distinctive facial features.

INVERSIONS

If two different strand breaks occur on the same chromosome simultaneously and the order of the broken ends are mismatched the result will be an inversion. Inversions are of two types, **pericentric** and **paracentric** (Figure 35–17). Pericentric inversions occur when the two breaks occur on either side of the centromere. Paracentric inversions occur when the breaks occur within the same arm (p or q) of a chromosome.

The consequences of inversion chromosomes during meiotic prophase I, the period of meiosis where homologous recombination occurs, can be profound (Figure 35–18). Paracentric inversion loops lead to one normal chromosome, one chromosome harboring the original paracentric inversion, one acentric (lack of centromere) chromosome that is lost, and one dicentric (two centromeres) chromosome that is broken randomly resulting in terminal deletions. The outcomes following meiosis II will be a normal gamete, an inversion gamete, and two deletion gametes. Pericentric inversion loops lead to one normal chromosome, one chromosome

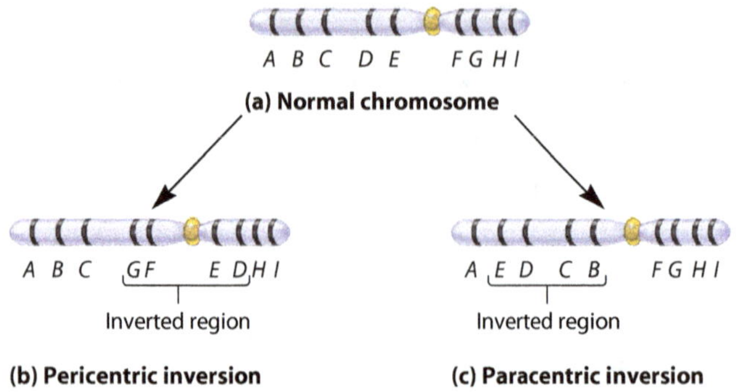

FIGURE 35–17 Inversions occur when the ends of chromosome segments are reattached incorrectly. The products can be classified as (a) pericentric or (b) paracentric, depending on whether the centromere is included in the inversion. (Reproduced with permission from Brooker RJ: *Genetics: Analysis & Principles*, 7th ed. New York, NY: McGraw Hill, 2021.)

harboring the original pericentric inversion, one chromosome with a duplication, and one chromosome with a deletion. The outcomes following meiosis II will be a normal gamete, an inversion gamete, and two different duplication gametes

GENETIC LINKAGE AND GENETIC ASSOCIATION

Genetic linkage analysis refers to the study of family pedigrees as a means to identify the chromosomal location of disease-causing genes and the inheritance of a disease in a family. A related technique, referred to as association analysis, is a population-based approach to look for increased or decreased frequency of various disease-causing alleles in affected individuals within the population when compared to unaffected individuals from the same

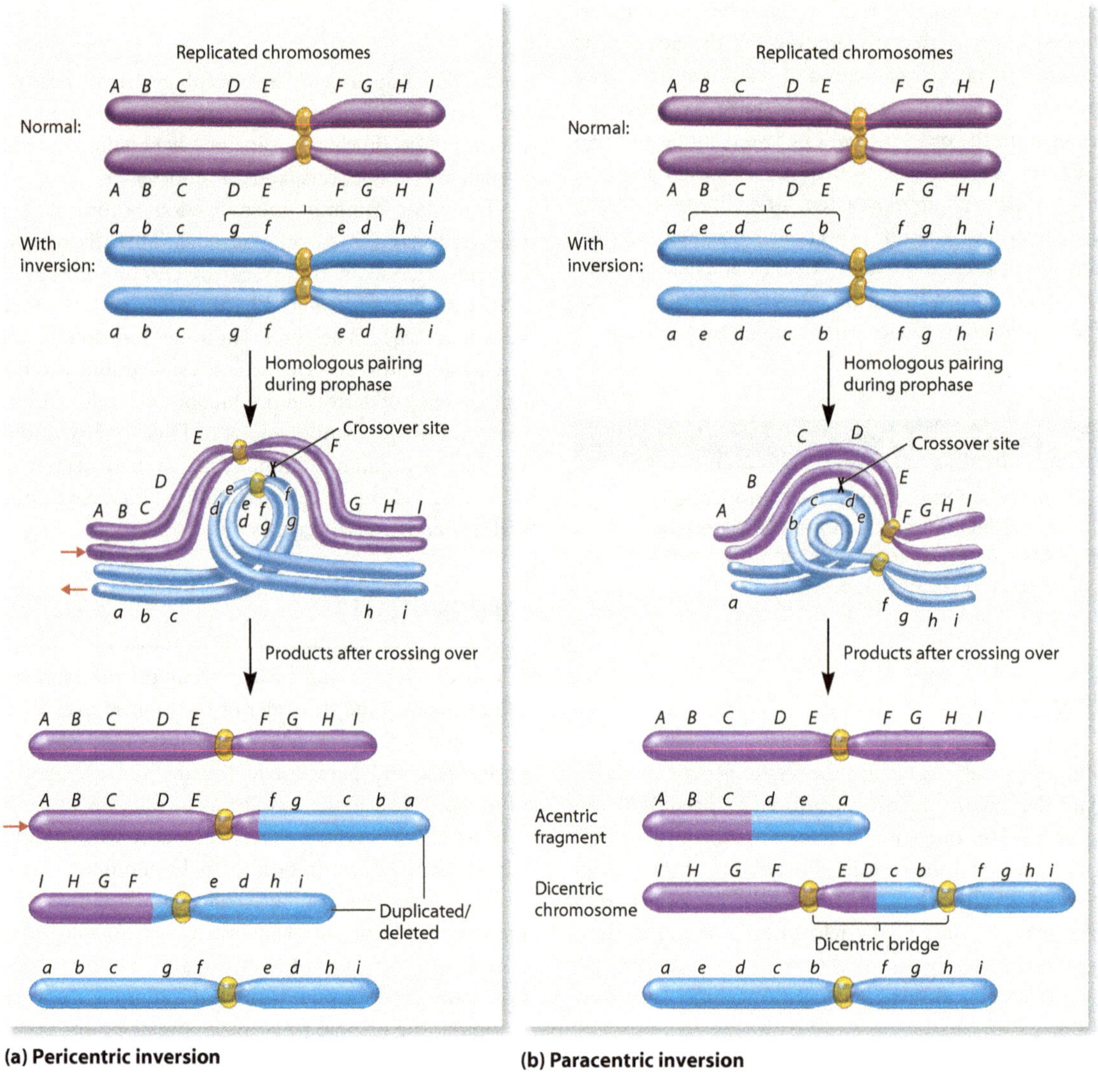

FIGURE 35–18 Crossing over in an inversion heterozygote yields deletions and duplications in half the haploid products of meiosis. In a paracentric inversion heterozygote, the centromere will be included in the segment that is either duplicated or deleted. This will result in dicentric bridges or acentric fragments, respectively. (Reproduced with permission from Brooker RJ: *Genetics: Analysis & Principles*, 7th ed. New York, NY: McGraw Hill, 2021.)

population. The modern approach to the identification of disease-causing alleles is the use of high throughput genome sequencing. The major advantage to genome sequencing, for the identification of disease gene linkage, is that rare disorders or family-specific disease alleles cannot be easily identified by the more traditional methods of genetic linkage analysis.

INDEPENDENT ASSORTMENT

During Gregor Mendel's studies of monohybrid crosses in pea plants he found that different genes were inherited independently of each other. He defined this observation as the Law of Independent Assortment.

During meiosis I the paternal and maternal chromosomes exchange homologous regions of DNA resulting in rearrangements that create new chromosomes that represent a mixture of the DNA from the grandmother's and grandfather's chromosomes. Any combination of alleles that results from recombination is as likely as any other combination which is the basis of independent assortment. An important exception to the law of independent assortment exists for genes that are located very close to one another on the same chromosome and thus, tend to be inherited together. This latter effect is the basis of genetic linkage.

The net effect of homologous recombination occurring during meiosis is chromosomes that look identical under a microscope but that differ substantially at the level of the DNA sequence. These DNA sequence differences represent polymorphisms.

Genes that reside on the same chromosome are termed **syntenic**. However, syntenic genes are not always genetically linked as can be appreciated when considering genes on different arms of the same chromosome. These genes are separated from one another such that they will always independently assort during meiotic homologous recombination.

Two genes, or a gene and a polymorphic marker, that are very close to one another on the same chromosome will tend to be inherited together. This genetic linkage can be used to identify the inheritance of a disease allele in a family as outlined in Figure 35–19. When ascertaining the genotype of individuals who are heterozygous at two syntenic loci, for example A/a and B/b, the designations are referred to as linkage phase. When two dominant or two recessive alleles are linked the linkage phase is termed **coupling**. Whereas, when a dominant and recessive allele are linked the linkage phase is termed **repulsion**.

RECOMBINATION FREQUENCY

Using the analysis of highly polymorphic loci, it is possible to detect the frequency with which closely linked DNA sequences rearrange during meiotic homologous recombination. Recombination frequency is, therefore, a measure of the distance between two loci. Because the possibilities are no recombination or some level of recombination, recombination frequency will fall between 0% and 50%. The closer two loci are to one another the smaller will be the likelihood of recombination and thus smaller the recombination frequency.

Recombination frequency can be theoretically equated to physical distance. This concept was first recognized by Thomas Hunt Morgan and so the distance measure is defined by the units termed **centimorgans, cM**. A centimorgan is defined as the genetic distance over which an average crossover occurs in 1% of the recombination events taking place in meiosis. The map distance of 1 cM is equivalent to the physical distance between approximately 1 million base pairs of DNA. The utility of this relationship between recombination frequency and physical chromosome map distance is that it allows for an approximation of how many bases of DNA need to be sequenced to reach a disease allele starting from a polymorphic marker that is linked to the disease allele.

Knowledge of recombination frequency is important to the risk assessment of disease in families. Using the disease described by the pedigree in Figure 35–19, it is possible to determine recombination frequency and thus, the contribution to disease risk. The pedigree describes an autosomal recessive disease allele (A) that is linked to the 1 allele of a polymorphic marker. Therefore, all children of II-4 and II-5 that inherit the 1 allele of the marker will most likely also inherit the disease allele. However, the child (III-6) is disease free yet has inherited two copies of the 1 allele of the marker, one from his mother and one from his father. This result could only occur if a recombination event occurred in his mother's gametes such that the wild-type allele of the disease gene recombined with the 1 allele of the marker as diagrammed in Figure 35–19.

Using the outcomes described in the pedigree in Figure 35–19 is it possible to calculate recombination frequency. The pedigree shows that, as a result of recombination, one individual that should have the disease does not and seven individuals have the disease. Therefore, the recombination frequency is the one recombinant individual divided by the total number of individuals that have the disease or should have the disease which is eight (1/8 = 12.5%). The overall risk of disease to the offspring of a mating pair, where one has the disease, is always 50% (1/2). However, because there is a 1/8 chance for recombination to occur, the future risk to any additional children of II-4 and II-5 is reduced by the recombination rate occurring in the mother's (II-4) gametes.

LINKAGE DISEQUILIBRIUM

When the alleles at two locations are linked, yet at a distance from one another of 0.1 cM to 1.0 cM, they will generally not show any preferred linkage phase in a population. Consider the situation where there are two genes or loci (eg, X and Y) both of which have two alleles where those for gene X are designated *A* and *a* and those for gene Y are designated *B* and *b*. Suppose for gene X the alleles *A* and *a* are found equally (50%) in the chromosomes of a given population and for gene Y the alleles *B* and *b* are found in 80% and 20% of the chromosomes in the same population, respectively.

The possible haplotypes for these alleles are *A*/*B*, *A*/*b*, *a*/*B*, and *a*/*b*. The frequency of any of these haplotypes is simply the product of the frequencies of the alleles in the haplotype. For example, the frequency of the *a*/*B* haplotype would be $0.5 \times 0.8 = 0.4$.

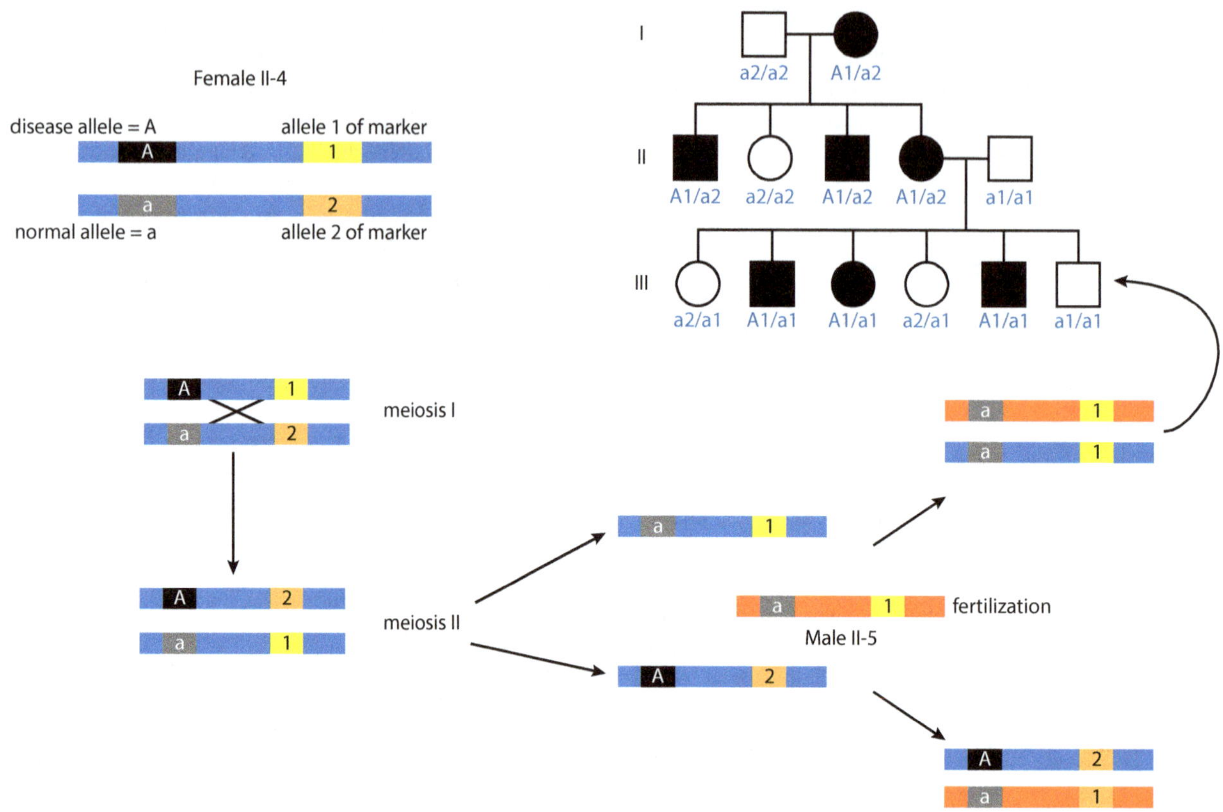

FIGURE 35–19 Recombination and linkage. Recombination occurring during prophase I of meiosis can result in the rearrangement of linked genes or markers. The pedigree shows the linkage of a particular marker allele with an autosomal dominant allele of a gene. The two different alleles of the linked marker are designated 1 and 2 and the two different alleles of the autosomal gene are designated A (dominant mutant) and a (wild-type). The genotypes represent the phase of the alleles in the individual family members. Analysis of the pedigree shows that the disease-causing allele is linked with the 1 allele of the marker in all individuals except III-6. Below each individual is shown their genotype with respect to the marker allele and the gene. All the sperm from male II-5 will have the wild-type allele of the gene and the 1 allele of the marker. The recombination event in a gamete from female II-4 is diagrammed showing how individual III-6 inherited the 1 allele of the marker from his mother but did not also inherit the disease allele of the gene and thus, is disease free. (Reproduced with permission from themedicalbiochemistrypage, LLC.)

All the possible allele frequencies cannot exceed 100%. Therefore, if the haplotype frequencies in a population are found to be as expected then the alleles are said to be in **linkage equilibrium**. However, when two loci are very close together the allele frequencies for these loci do not allow for an accurate prediction of the haplotype frequencies. If the frequency of an observed haplotype does not equal the product of the frequency of the two alleles generating that haplotype, then the alleles are said to be in **linkage disequilibrium**.

As a population expands the process of meiotic recombination can lead to the movement of a particular allele (e.g., a disease allele) onto a new haplotype such that the frequency of this new haplotype does not equal the product of the two alleles in a population. This example of linkage disequilibrium demonstrates that the number of possible recombination events (ie, the number of generations) will eventually lead to linkage disequilibrium for a disease allele in a population.

The process of natural selection can enhance or reduce a particular haplotype in a population. This will lead to either overrepresentation or underrepresentation of a particular haplotype in a population which is another example of linkage disequilibrium.

CHECKLIST

- ☑ Human somatic cell nuclei possess two copies each of 22 autosomes and 2 sex chromosomes, an X and a Y chromosome in males and two X chromosomes in females. The autosomes are numbered based on size with the largest being chromosome 1 and the smallest being chromosome 22.
- ☑ Chromosomes are divided on either side of the centromere into p arms and q arm, where the p arms are generally shorter than the q arms. Chromosomes with nearly equal p and q arms are termed metacentric, those where the p arm is demonstrably shorter than the q arm are termed submetacentric, and those with negligible p arms are termed acrocentric.
- ☑ All chromosomes undergo recombination during prophase of meiosis I which results in the DNA sequence composition of one's grandparental chromosomes being very different than that they inherit from their parents.
- ☑ Single-gene inheritance patterns are recessive (requiring two mutant alleles to manifest disease) or dominant (requiring a single mutant allele to manifest disease). Sex-linked disease inheritance is near exclusively associated with the X chromosome due to the small number of genes on the Y chromosome.
- ☑ Diseases of mitochondrial function can be due to nuclear or mitochondrial genome mutations. Disorders resulting from mutations in mitochondrial genes are inherited exclusively from females.
- ☑ Population genetics encompasses the assessment of genetic variation within populations that can be the small population of a given family or a large population of a region or country. One highly useful outcome from population genetics is the ability to determine the recurrence risk of a disease in the offspring of a mating pair in a family.
- ☑ The foundational work of Hardy and Weinberg, referred to as the Hardy-Weinberg law, determined the mathematical relationship between the frequencies of various alleles and the frequencies of the genotypes that result from various alleles.
- ☑ Chromosomal segregation during meiosis is termed disjunction and if this process fails, either in meiosis I or meiosis II, it is termed nondisjunction. The outcomes from nondisjunction during meiosis I include gametes that are disomic (contain two copies of a given chromosome) and are nullisomic (missing one chromosome). Nondisjunction in meiosis II will result in at least two normal gametes and is, therefore, a less severe event than that occurring during meiosis I.
- ☑ Translocation of chromosomal segments between different chromosomes represents the major contributor chromosomal rearrangements. Robertsonian translocation is the term used to denote translocations that occur between any two of the five acrocentric chromosomes.
- ☑ Meiotic segregations, occurring in the gametes of an individual who harbors a translocation, are of two types termed alternate and adjacent. The outcomes from alternate segregation are generally favorable while those from adjacent segregation are always lethal except in the case of Robertsonian translocations involving chromosomes 13 or 21.
- ☑ The principle of independent assortment is the basis for genetic linkage analysis. During meiosis the pairs of chromosomes share DNA through the process of homologous recombination and the new chromosomes randomly separate during the formation of the haploid gametes. Genes that are very close together tend to be inherited together and thus, "violate" the principle of independent assortment.
- ☑ The frequency of any given haplotype is determined from the product of the frequencies of the alleles in the haplotype. If the observed haplotype frequency is the same as expected the alleles are said to be in linkage equilibrium. Closely linked alleles tend to be inherited together such that the expected random distribution is not found and these alleles are said to be in linkage disequilibrium.

REVIEW QUESTIONS

1. A 37-year-old woman is being evaluated by a neurologist for clumsiness, stiffness in her legs, and a decline in cognitive function. At age 32, her father was noted to have symptoms of depression, choreiform movements, and cognitive decline. Her paternal grandfather committed suicide at age 53. Given the signs observed in this patient and the relevant family history, which of the following is most likely to be associated with genetic transmission of this disease?

(A) Allelic heterogeneity
(B) Anticipation
(C) Germline mosaicism
(D) Locus heterogeneity
(E) Pleiotropy

2. In a population of Native Americans, it is found that 26 individuals out of a total of 6000 have albinism. The form of albinism is recessive to normal skin color. The disease is manifest as a result of a single gene that is known to have two alleles. Assuming the population is in Hardy-Weinberg equilibrium, approximately how many of the individuals in the population would be predicted to be carriers for the recessive albino allele?

(A) 26
(B) 52
(C) 737
(D) 5238
(E) 5974

3. A 4-year-old girl is undergoing an evaluation for the cause of her ataxic jerking movements of her arms and legs and episodes of inappropriate laughter. Physical examination shows mild microcephaly and severe intellectual impairment. Karyotype analysis indicates the presence of deletion in the q arm of chromosome 15. Which of the following is the most disorder manifesting in this patient?
   (A) Angelman syndrome
   (B) Beckwith-Wiedemann syndrome
   (C) Down syndrome
   (D) Fragile X syndrome
   (E) Myotonic dystrophy type 1
   (F) Prader-Willi syndrome

4. Which of the following phenomena best explains the unaffected children of the parents affected by the autosomal recessive trait shown in the pedigree below?

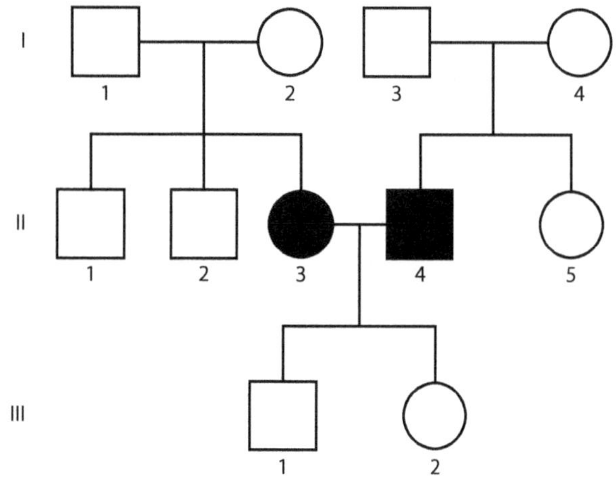

   (A) Allelic heterogeneity
   (B) Anticipation
   (C) Genomic imprinting
   (D) Locus heterogeneity
   (E) Pleiotropy

5. Homocystinuria is a metabolic disorder in which the toxic compound homocysteine accumulates in the blood and it's oxidized form, homocystine, is elevated in the urine. Mutations in at least three different enzymes can cause this disorder. With respect to the inheritance of homocystinuria, which of the following is most representative?
   (A) Allelic heterogeneity
   (B) Compound heterozygosity
   (C) Locus heterogeneity
   (D) Multifactorial inheritance
   (E) Variable expressivity

6. The disorder known as ectrodactyly (split hand-foot malformation) is an autosomal dominant disorder. In one family where this disorder is found, the grandfather and his grandson both exhibit the signs of this disease. However, the grandson's father does not have any signs of this disorder and is otherwise completely healthy. Which of the following is the most reasonable explanation for these observations?
   (A) Allelic heterogeneity
   (B) Anticipation
   (C) Germline mosaicism
   (D) Incomplete penetrance
   (E) New mutation
   (F) Variable expressivity

7. Two children, and their 31-year-old mother are being examined by their family physician following genetic testing identifying that they harbor mutations in the *NF1* gene. Mutations in this gene are responsible for type 1 neurofibromatosis. Physical examination of the mother shows multiple neurofibromas and the presence of Lisch nodules. Her 13-year-old daughter has a large plexiform neurofibroma and her 10-year-old son has multiple café au lait spots. Which of the following is the best explanation for the observations in these three individuals?
   (A) Epistasis
   (B) Incomplete penetrance
   (C) Pleiotropy
   (D) Somatic mosaicism
   (E) Variable expressivity

8. A couple are expecting their first child. The expectant mother has a sister that has cystic fibrosis. The unrelated father belongs to the same ethnic population as the wife. The incidence rate of the disease in this population 1 in 3600. Based upon the information in the pedigree, what is the most likely chance that the unborn child will have the same disease as the mother's sister?

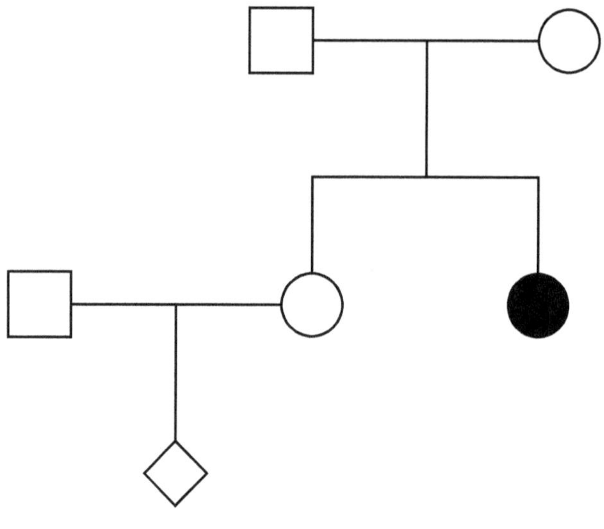

   (A) 1/720
   (B) 1/360
   (C) 1/180
   (D) 1/90
   (E) 1/45

9. A husband and wife seek genetic counseling when she is at 10-weeks gestation. The wife's brother has sickle cell anemia and the husband's sister also has the disease. The husband and wife do not have the disease, nor do any of their parents have the disease. The couple are concerned that their baby may be born with sickle cell anemia. What is the most likely recurrence risk for their unborn child?
   (A) 2%
   (B) 5%
   (C) 11%
   (D) 12.5%
   (E) 33.3%

10. A husband and wife seek genetic counseling when she is at 10-week gestation. The wife's brother was found to have alkaptonuria as a result of knee replacement surgery. The husband's aunt is a known carrier of a mutant allele for the disease. The couple are concerned that their baby may inherit the disease. What is the most likely risk that the wife is a carrier of a mutant allele?
(A) 0%
(B) 12%
(C) 25%
(D) 50%
(E) 67%

11. Physical examination of a 13-year-old boy shows myoclonic epilepsy, cerebellar ataxia, and progressive muscle weakness. His mother has had an unstable gait for the past 10 years. The mother's brother succumbed to a disorder of muscle function at the age of 37 years and his mother's sister suffers from progressive dementia and ataxia. Laboratory studies show elevated lactic acid in the blood and CSF of the patient. Which of the following is the most likely probability that this patient's female offspring will inherit the same disorder?
(A) 0%
(B) 12.5%
(C) 25%
(D) 50%
(E) 66.7%

12. A 32-year-old man who manifests the symptoms of an autosomal dominant disease has a brother who also has the syndrome, and his son is also affected. He has two daughters who show no signs of the disorder, and his wife is also not affected. The man and his wife are seeking counseling regarding risks to another child that they wish to have. Which of the following represents the recurrence risk for any of their additional children?
(A) 0%
(B) 25%
(C) 50%
(D) 67%
(E) 100%

13. A family with some members afflicted with retinitis pigmentosa is being studied. The pedigree for this family is shown. Individual III-3 plans to marry an unrelated and unaffected male. What is the recurrence risk to any future son?

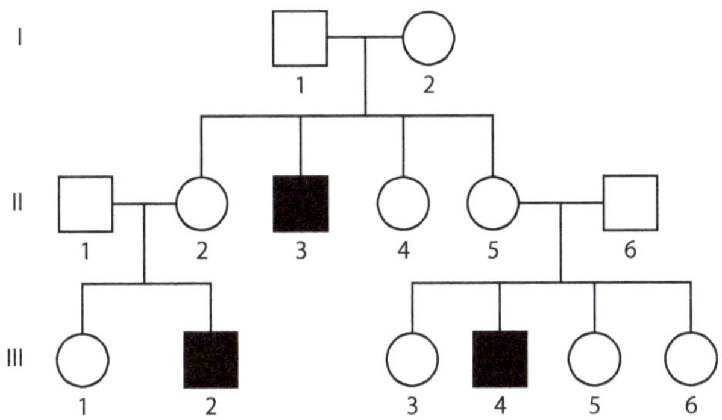

(A) 0%
(B) 25%
(C) 50%
(D) 67%
(E) 100%

14. A husband and wife have 3 children, two boys and one girl. The husband was diagnosed with Huntington disease at the age of 57. His father was also positive for the disease and died at the age of 68. The wife is 55 and has no symptoms nor family history of Huntington disease. Assuming the disease is 100% penetrant, what is the most likely probability that all three of their children will eventually develop Huntington disease?
(A) 1/8
(B) 1/4
(C) 1/2
(D) 3/4
(E) 1

15. The pedigree for a family in which a disorder has manifest in individual III-2 is shown. The affected female and her husband are concerned about the risks their unborn child might have for the same disease. Given the family pedigree shown, what is the most likely recurrence risk for the unborn child?

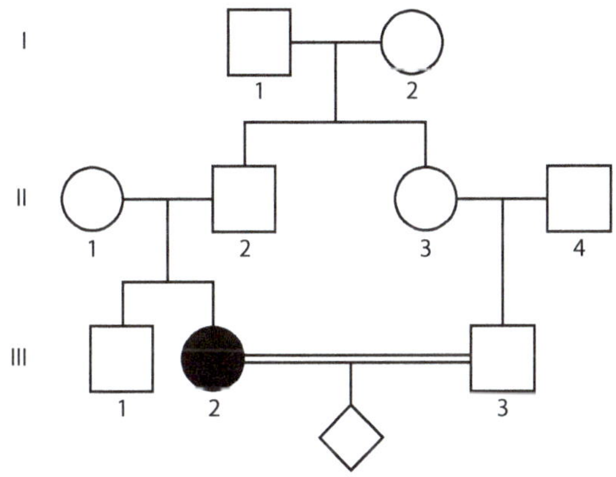

(A) 1/32
(B) 1/16
(C) 1/8
(D) 1/4
(E) 1/2

16. A family, that has several members afflicted with a form of degenerative muscle disease, is undergoing molecular studies of their disease. All members of the family represented by the pedigree shown have undergone PCR-based DNA testing (results presented below the pedigree). Based upon the results of the assay, which of the following is the most likely molecular cause of the disease in this family?

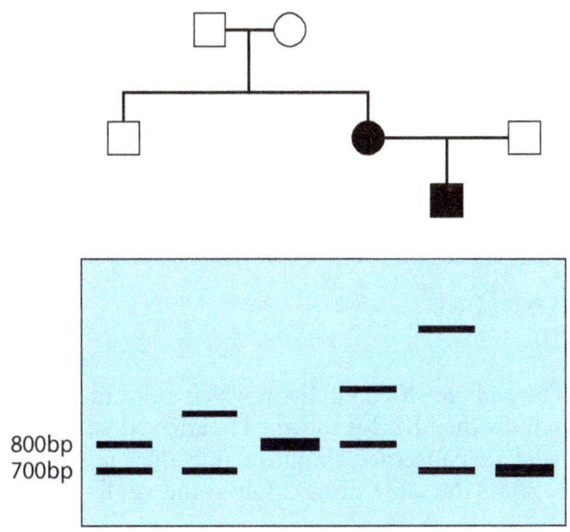

(A) Allelic heterogeneity
(B) Meiotic nondisjunction
(C) Microsatellite instability
(D) Trinucleotide repeat expansion
(E) Variable expressivity

17. The pedigree for a family in which some members are afflicted with a disorder associated with hyperuricemia and odd self-mutilation behavior is shown. Individual III-3 plans to marry an unrelated and unaffected male. What is the likelihood that she will have a son who is affected by the same disease?

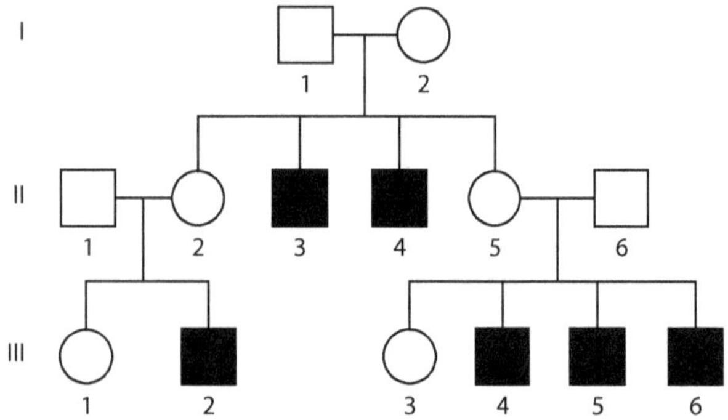

(A) 0
(B) 1/8
(C) 1/4
(D) 1/2
(E) 1

18. The pedigree for a family in which a disorder has manifest in individual III-1 is shown. The affected male exhibited a hemolytic crisis following the administration of Bactrim (sulfamethoxazole and trimethoprim) for the treatment of an ear infection. The sister of the affected individual has married her first cousin and she is pregnant with their first child. Given the family pedigree shown, what is the most likely chance that she will have a son with the same disease as her brother?

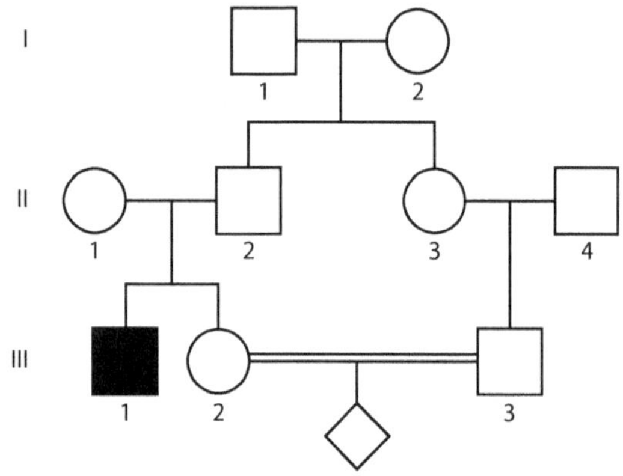

(A) 1/24
(B) 1/12
(C) 1/8
(D) 1/4
(E) 1/2

19. The pedigree for a family in which a disorder has manifested in individual III-2 is shown. The affected female and her husband are concerned about the risks their unborn child might have for the same disease. Given the family pedigree shown, what is the most likely chance that their unborn child will be a female with the same disease as her mother?

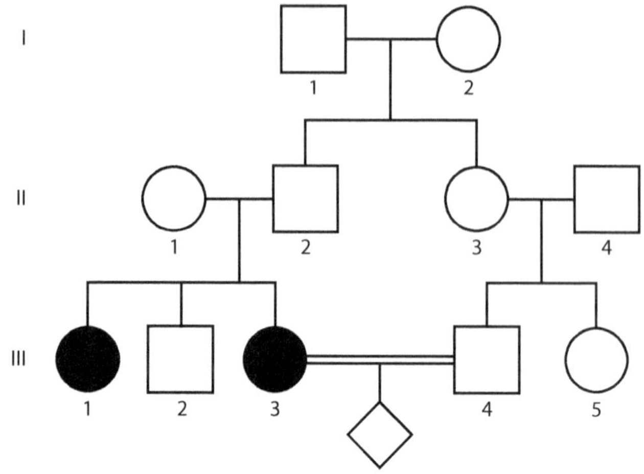

(A) 1/32
(B) 1/16
(C) 1/8
(D) 1/4
(E) 1/2

20. A 27-year-old woman has a brother with phenylketonuria, PKU. No one else in her family is affected. Given this limited information, which of the following most likely represents the risk that this woman is a carrier for the mutation present in her brother?
(A) 1/4
(B) 1/2
(C) 2/3
(D) 3/4
(E) Nearly 100%

21. In a given population, 4% of the individuals are affected with an autosomal recessive disease. Given this information, what is the most likely frequency of heterozygous carriers in the next generation?
(A) 0.1
(B) 0.25
(C) 0.4
(D) 0.67
(E) 0.75

22. In a small population of 93 individuals, the gene encoding an enzyme was analyzed. It was found that the gene has two alleles identified as A and A′. The genotype frequencies in this population were determined and shown to be:

A/A: 0.226
A/A′: 0.400
A′/A′: 0.374

Given the Hardy-Weinberg assumptions, which of the following represents the most likely predicted (not observed) frequency for the A/A genotype?
(A) 0.181
(B) 0.226
(C) 0.329
(D) 0.400
(E) 0.489

23. The following pedigree has been established for linkage analysis. Each family member in this pedigree has been typed for five highly polymorphic markers (A, B, C, D, E) all of which are known to be closely linked to a disease-causing gene in this family. As indicated in the red boxes, each marker has two alleles. Marker A is closest to the telomeric end of the chromosome, while marker E is closest to the centromere. From this information, which marker alleles are most likely inherited in phase with the disease-causing gene?

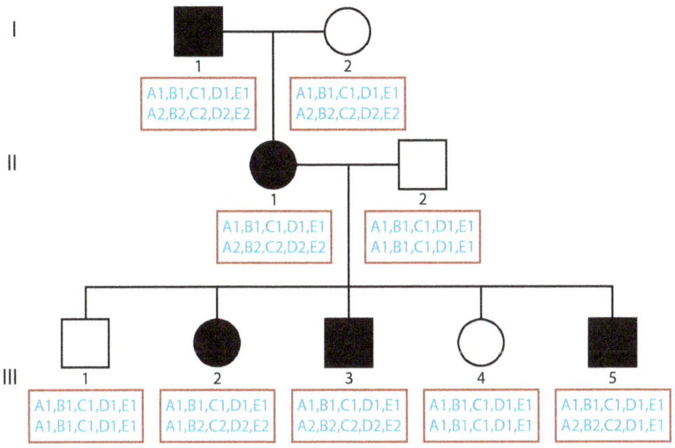

(A) The 1 allele of all of the markers
(B) The 2 allele of all of the markers
(C) The 1 allele of only the A marker
(D) The 2 allele of only the A marker
(E) The 1 allele of only the D marker
(F) The 2 allele of only the D marker

24. An autosomal recessive disease occurs with a frequency of 1/2500 in a particular population. A woman has a first cousin with this disease. She plans to marry an unrelated unaffected man. What is the most likely recurrence risk to any child of this woman and her husband?
(A) 1/400
(B) 1/200
(C) 1/100
(D) 1/50
(E) 1/25

25. The parents of a 1-year-old girl wish to know the likelihood that their daughter will be affected by the same disease present in her great-grandfather. The parents are first cousins. Assume that the disease is a rare autosomal recessive disorder with 100% penetration. What is the most likely probability that the child will be affected?
(A) 1/32
(B) 1/16
(C) 3/16
(D) 1/8
(E) 1/4

26. A divorced mother of a 4-year-old boy, who manifests an autosomal recessive disease, plans to re-marry an unrelated unaffected male. They plan to have another child and want to know the risk of having another affected child. The incidence of the disease in the general population is 1/9000. What is the most likely risk of this couple having an affected child?
(A) 1/190
(B) 1/90
(C) 1/45
(D) 1/9
(E) 1/4

27. Molecular diagnosis of a child manifesting an autosomal recessive disorder reveals that the child harbors a maternal uniparental disomic chromosome which carries the disease gene. This child's parents are phenotypically normal and not blood relatives. If the incidence of the disorder is 1/4000, what is the most likely risk that they would have another affected child?
(A) 1/250
(B) 1/125
(C) 1/50
(D) 1/25
(E) 1/4

28. What is the most likely frequency of affected males to affected females for Fragile X syndrome, assuming the disease is 100% penetrant?
(A) 1:0
(B) 1:1
(C) 1:2
(D) 2:1
(E) 4:1

29. The parents of a child with phenylketonuria (PKU) are divorced. The mother is planning to re-marry an unrelated unaffected male. The incidence of PKU is 1/8,100 in the ethnic population of the woman's future husband. What is the most likely recurrence risk for any children from this couple?
(A) 1/180
(B) 1/90
(C) 1/45
(D) 1/8
(E) 1/4

30. A man who has Marfan syndrome, and whose parents were phenotypically normal, is engaged to his phenotypically normal first cousin. What is the most likely chance that their first child will also have Marfan syndrome?
(A) 1/8
(B) 1/4
(C) 1/2
(D) 2/3
(E) 3/4

31. Hereditary hemochromatosis is a complex genetic disorder in which the majority of affected individuals are homozygous for mutations in the *HFE1* gene. From population studies, it has been determined that the frequency of carriers of mutant HFE1 alleles is approximately 10%. Assuming Hardy-Weinberg equilibrium, what is the most likely frequency of HFE1 mutant alleles in this population?
(A) 0.001
(B) 0.01
(C) 0.05
(D) 0.10
(E) 0.20

32. A young woman of northern European descent is the single parent of a child with cystic fibrosis. She marries her first cousin and becomes pregnant. What is the most likely probability that her child will have cystic fibrosis?
(A) 1/2500
(B) 1/100
(C) 1/32

(D) 1/16
(E) 1/8

33. A young woman is the single parent of a child who, in the neonatal period, experienced several episodes of severe hypoglycemia, lactic acidemia, hyperlipidemia, and hypoketonuria. She marries a healthy unrelated man, and they wish to have more children. The frequency of the disorder that afflicts the woman's first child in their population is 1/2,500. What is the most likely recurrence risk for the children of this couple?
(A) 1/250
(B) 1/100
(C) 1/50
(D) 1/25
(E) 1/4

34. If 1 out of every 250,000 people have a non-lethal autosomal recessive disorder, what is the most likely frequency of carriers of mutant alleles for this disorder?
(A) 1/1000
(B) 1/500
(C) 1/250
(D) 1/50
(E) 1/25

35. Assuming Hardy-Weinberg equilibrium for alleles of the phenylalanine hydroxylase gene, and given that the frequency of mutant alleles of this gene is 1/50, what is the most likely frequency of carriers in this population?
(A) $(1/50)^2$
(B) 1/100
(C) 1/50
(D) 1/25
(E) $(49/50)^2$

36. For a given autosomal recessive disease, the frequency of the mutant allele causing this disease is 1% in the population. Based upon this information what is the most likely percentage of individuals in this population that will harbor two wild-type copies of the gene?
(A) 2%
(B) 19%
(C) 90%
(D) 95%
(E) 98%

37. A karyotypically normal couple has a child with trisomy 21. DNA analysis of 21q polymorphic markers reveals the following results where the letters refer to polymorphic loci and the numbers refer to the various alleles at that locus. Given these results, which of the following is the most likely point where the meiotic nondisjunction occurred?

Marker Locus	Father's Alleles	Mother's Alleles	Child's Alleles
W	1,2	2,2	1,2,2
X	1,1	2,2	1,2,2
Y	1,1	1,1	1,1,1
Z	1,1	1,2	1,2,2

(A) Maternal meiosis I
(B) Maternal meiosis II
(C) Paternal meiosis I
(D) Paternal meiosis II
(E) Paternal meiosis I or II

38. A man and a woman, each with a normal karyotype, have a child with trisomy for chromosome 21. The haplotype, based on a polymorphic marker locus near the centromere of chromosome 21, is shown for the child, her mother, and her father. Based on this information, in which meiotic division did the non-disjunction event most likely occur?

Haplotype Mother:	C,D
Haplotype Father:	A,B
Haplotype affected child:	B,C,D

(A) Paternal meiosis I
(B) Paternal meiosis II
(C) Maternal meiosis I
(D) Maternal meiosis II
(E) Maternal meiosis I or paternal meiosis I

39. Of the following karyotypes, which would be most likely to be associated with a live birth?
(A) 46,XY,-11,+22
(B) 47,XX,+3
(C) 47,XX,+21
(D) 69,XXX
(E) 46,YY

40. A chromosomal analysis is obtained on a young woman with mild signs of Turner syndrome and reveals a 46,XX/45,X karyotype. This patient's karyotype is most likely indicative of nondisjunction occurring at which of the following steps of meiosis?
(A) Maternal meiosis I
(B) Maternal meiosis II
(C) Mitosis after fertilization
(D) Paternal meiosis I
(E) Paternal meiosis II

41. Examination of two genes on chromosome 12 shows that they are linked and that each gene has two different alleles. The frequency with which the two alleles of gene A appear in the general population is 0.3 for the A1 allele and 0.7 for the A2 allele. The frequency with which the two alleles of gene B appear in the general population is 0.8 for the B1 allele and 0.2 for the B2 allele. What is the most likely frequency with which the A2-B1 haplotype would be present in any given individual in this population?
(A) 0.16
(B) 0.21
(C) 0.24
(D) 0.56
(E) 1.00

42. A young couple is discussing having a first child. This couple belongs to a close-knit religious community where often times first cousins marry and have children. It is known that 1 in 30 individuals in this community is a carrier for the autosomal recessive disease gene. Given this knowledge, what is the most likely rate of prevalence of this disease within the community to which this couple belong?
(A) 1/7,200
(B) 1/3,600
(C) 1/1,500

(D) 1/200
(E) 1/30

43. Hemophilia A occurs in males in a particular population with a frequency of 1/10,000. Which of the following values represents the most likely rate of female carriers of this disease gene in this population?
(A) 1/100,000
(B) 1/15,000
(C) 1/10,000
(D) 1/5,000
(E) 1/2,500

44. A 10-year-old girl is admitted to the hospital because of a recurrent neurologic disorder. Her right arm and leg have become limp. Blood work demonstrates lactic acidosis. Two months earlier, the girl had a grand mal seizure followed by cortical blindness with slow resolution. Analysis of muscle biopsy tissue reveals abnormal mitochondria. Which of the following pedigrees is most likely related to her disease?

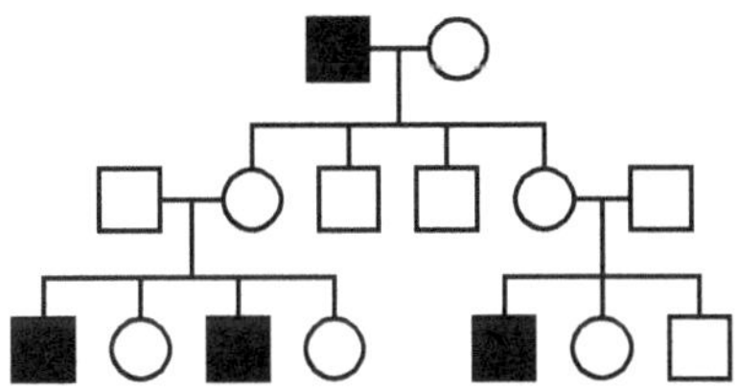

A

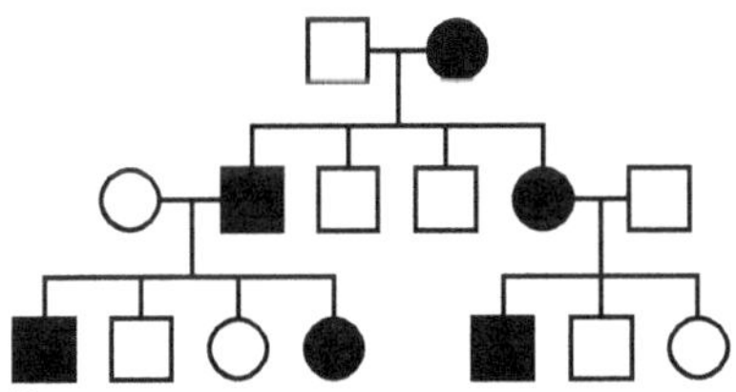

B

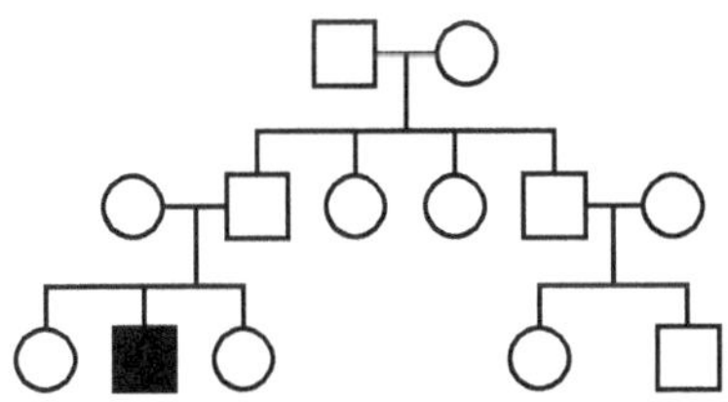

C

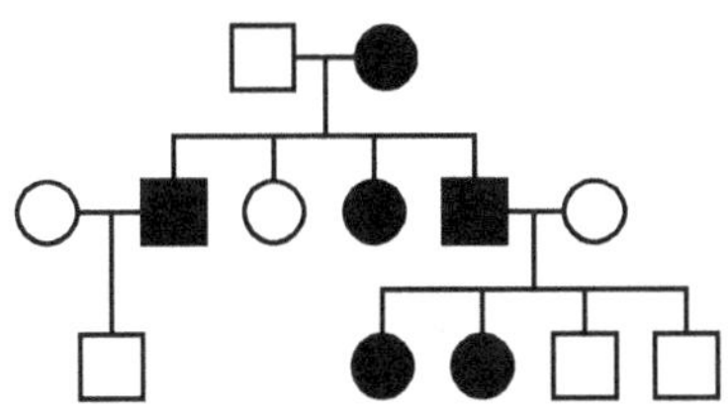

D

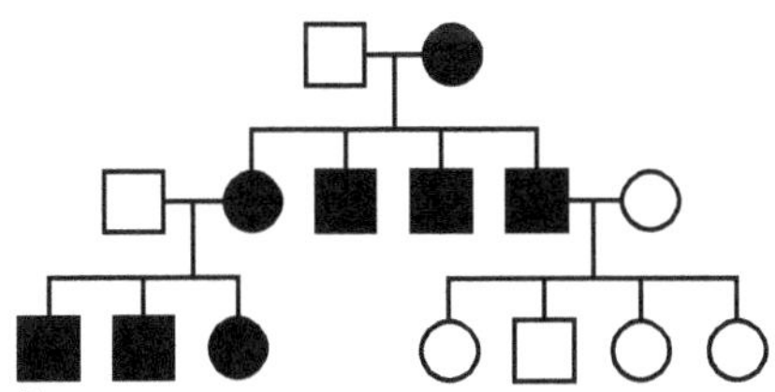

E

(A) A
(B) B
(C) C
(D) D
(E) E

45. A family in which a particular disease is found has been extensively studied. Based upon the phenotypic results from this study, the pedigree below was generated. Based upon this data, which of the following represents the most likely recurrence rate for unborn child of individuals IV-4 and IV-5?

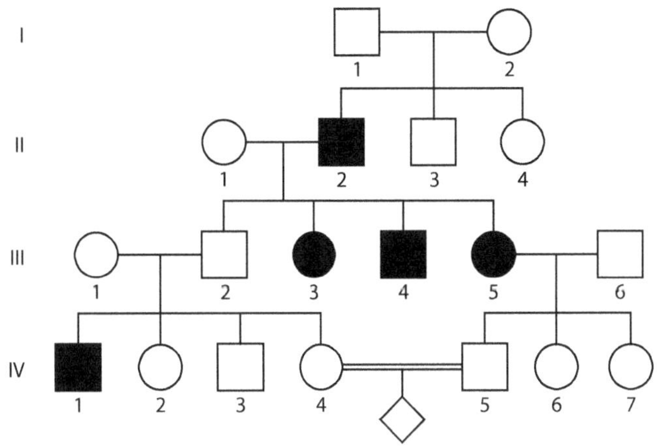

(A) 1/16
(B) 1/12
(C) 1/8
(D) 1/6
(E) 1.2

46. A 22-year-old woman has just given birth to her first child, a girl. The woman has phenylketonuria, but the father of the child does not have the disorder and there is no history of the disorder in the father's family. Physical examination of the neonate shows that she is smaller than predicted based upon the mother and father and has mild microcephaly. Blood analysis of the neonate finds elevated levels of phenylalanine. History reveals that the mother did not participate in regular prenatal examinations. Which of the following most likely explains the symptoms observed in the baby?
(A) A maternal translocation, involving the phenylalanine hydroxylase (*PAH*) gene, occurred with subsequent unbalanced segregation in meiosis I
(B) A spontaneous somatic mutation occurred in one of the father's *PAH* alleles
(C) The father is a carrier of a mutant phenylalanine hydroxylase (*PAH*) gene
(D) The mother did not adequately restrict phenylalanine from her diet during her pregnancy
(E) The neonate has two maternal copies of the mutant *PAH* gene due to maternal uniparental disomy

47. A 27-year-old man and his wide are getting genetic counseling before attempting to conceive a child. The man suffers from a particular condition and thus, they are concerned about the potential risks that their child will be born with the same condition. The accompanying pedigree demonstrates the mode of inheritance of the man's condition. Based on this information, the man is most likely afflicted with which of the following diseases?

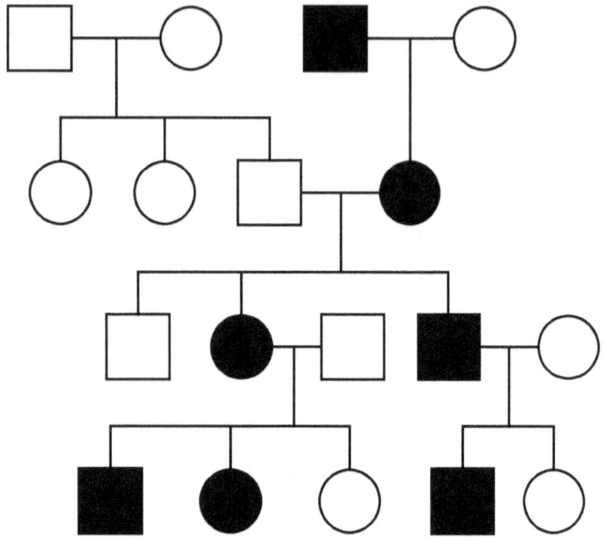

(A) Glucose-6-phosphate dehydrogenase deficiency
(B) Leber hereditary optic neuropathy
(C) Marfan syndrome
(D) Sickle cell anemia
(E) Tay-Sachs disease

48. A 12-year-old boy has just been diagnosed with myotonic dystrophy, type 1. Family history shows that the boy's father also has this same condition, as does his grandfather. The father began experiencing symptoms in his late twenties, while his grandfather was well into his forties before he began experiencing symptoms. Which of the following pedigrees is most closely associated with the family history of this disorder?

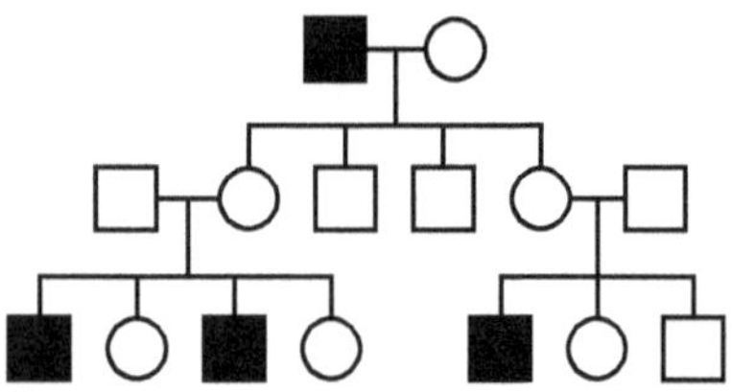

A

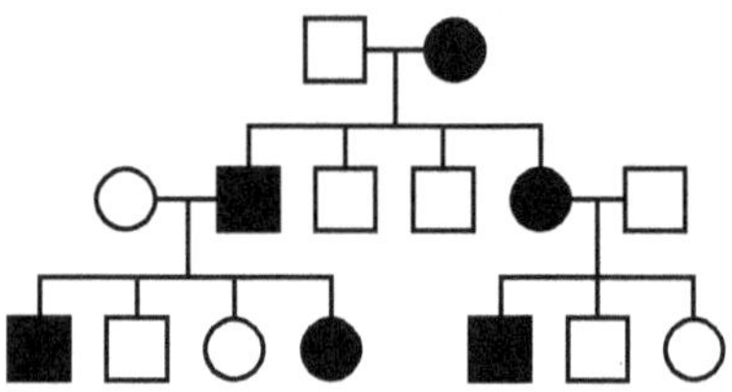

B

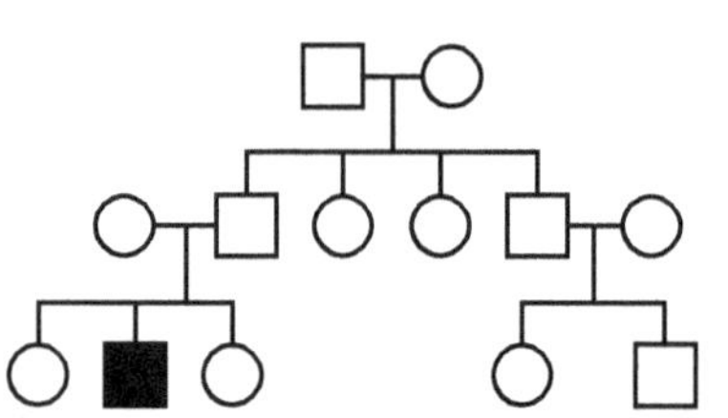

C

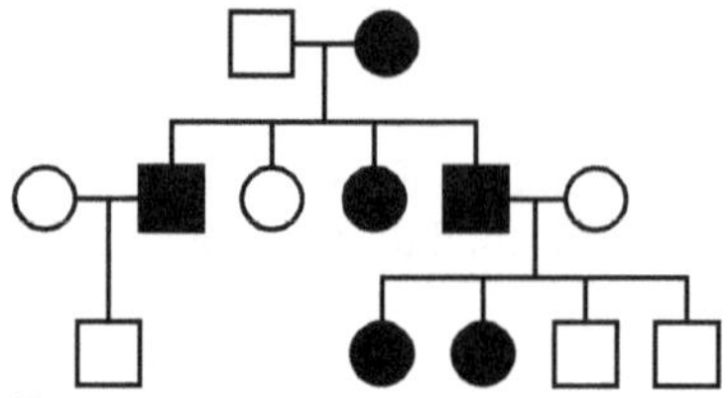

D

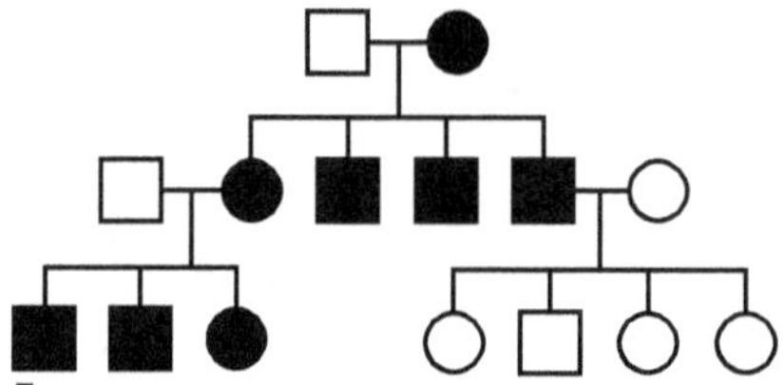

E

(A) A
(B) B
(C) C
(D) D
(E) E

49. An 18-month-old girl is undergoing an examination by her pediatrician due to concerns of her mother about her disproportionately looking limbs. The infant is at the 5th percentile for length. Physical examination shows distinctive rhizomelic limb shortening along with lordosis, macrocephaly, and midface hypoplasia. Which of the following represents the most likely mode of inheritance of the most likely disease manifesting in this patient?
(A) Autosomal dominant
(B) Autosomal recessive
(C) Mitochondrial
(D) X-linked dominant
(E) X-linked recessive

50. Medical geneticists are studying a family that has several members presenting with the distinctive symptoms of a particular disease. Based upon the pedigree that was generated following a detailed history, which of the following is the most likely disease affecting this family?

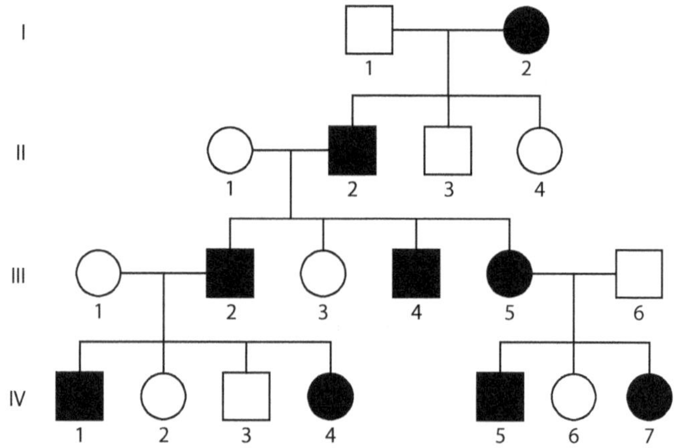

(A) Cystic fibrosis
(B) Fragile X syndrome
(C) Hemophilia A
(D) Marfan syndrome
(E) Myoclonic epilepsy with ragged red fibers, MERRF

51. A woman and her husband are seeking the advice of genetic counseling. Their first child was born prematurely and presented with dark sclera, a beaked nose, and frontal, parietal, and occipital bones that were extremely soft. History reveals that the woman's brother and father both had brittle bones that would break with minimal trauma. The woman's husband has no significant medical history, nor is there any family history on his side. Given the most likely disease presenting in their first child, what is the most likely chance that they have another child with similar symptoms?

(A) 0%
(B) 25% if the next child is male
(C) 25% regardless of sex
(D) 50%
(E) 100%

52. Physical examination of a male infant at birth shows a distinctive split on the left side of his upper lip extending into the nose. Examination of the inside of the infant's mouth also finds a small but distinctive opening in the front of the palate. Which of the following mechanisms is most likely to account for the physical manifestations discovered in this newborn?

(A) Autosomal recessive inheritance
(B) Imprinting error
(C) Mitochondrial inheritance
(D) Multifactorial inheritance
(E) Paternal uniparental disomy
(F) X-linked recessive

53. A husband and wife have come to a medical genetics' clinic for preconception counseling. Their primary concern is having a child with phenylketonuria because they were both born in countries where, they say, the incidence of this disease is high. Both individuals are healthy, and there are no siblings on either side with the disease. The wife's heritage is from a country where the frequency of carriers for the disease is 1/3500. The husband is from a bordering country where the carrier frequency for the disease is 1/2000. What is the most likely chance that this couple's first child will have phenylketonuria?

(A) 1/2000
(B) 1/3500
(C) 1/5,600,00
(D) 1/7,000,000
(E) 1/28,000,000
(F) 1/56,000,000

54. A newborn boy is undergoing an evaluation in the neonatal intensive care unit to ascertain the underlying circumstances for his subtle yet distinctive facial features that include a prominent nasal bridge, small ears, cleft palate, and hooded eyelids. The infant was born via spontaneous vaginal delivery following a full-term pregnancy. As a part of the examination, chest radiography finds a normal-sized heart silhouette with an upturned apex and a concave main pulmonary artery segment. Which of the following chromosomal abnormalities is most likely to account for the signs and symptoms found in this infant?

(A) Deletion of 5p15.2-p15.3
(B) Deletion of 15q11-q13
(C) Deletion of 22q11.2
(D) Trisomy 13
(E) Trisomy 18
(F) Trisomy 21

55. A family with several members who experience symptoms that include muscle weakness and pain, recurrent headaches, loss of appetite, vomiting, seizures, abdominal pain, extreme fatigue, muscle weakness, and difficulty breathing is being analyzed by the local medical genetics laboratory. Extensive history reveals that in some of the afflicted family members the symptoms are severe while in others they are mild. Also, the age of appearance is determined to be variable in the affected family members with some being affected in early childhood while others didn't experience significant symptoms until they were in their second decade of life. A detailed pedigree is generated from this family. Which of the following genetic principles best explains variable presentation of symptoms in this family?

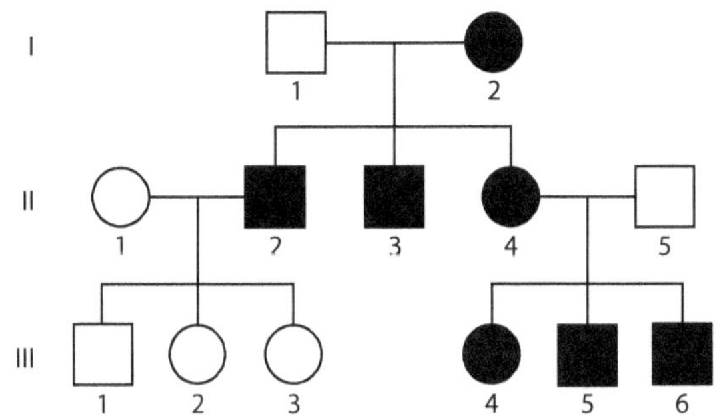

(A) Allelic heterogeneity
(B) Heteroplasmy
(C) Imprinting
(D) Locus heterogeneity
(E) Pleiotropy

56. A 46-year-old primigravida female is undergoing a routine ultrasound examination at 12 weeks in her pregnancy. The ultrasound technician notes an apparent anomaly and consults with the patient's obstetrician. They both concur that the ultrasound is detecting increased nuchal translucency. Based upon this observation, the obstetrician orders additional diagnostic testing to be performed. Which of the following processes is most likely to account for the most likely disorder manifesting in this fetus?

(A) Germline mosaicism
(B) Imprinting error
(C) Meiotic nondisjunction
(D) Unbalanced translocation
(E) Uniparental disomy

57. A husband and wife are visiting the genetics counseling center at the local University Medical School. The couple is concerned about the chances that they will have a child with Duchenne muscular dystrophy, DMD. Their concerns stem from the fact that the wife's brother has DMD. The husband states that there is no history of DMD in his family. Given that the carrier status of the wife is currently unknown, what is the most likely risk that this couple will have a child with DMD?

(A) 1/16
(B) 1/8
(C) 1/4
(D) 1/2
(E) 3/4

58. A man and woman are at the genetics clinic at the University Medical School seeking counseling regarding their potential risks for having a child with a disease that is present in several family members. The woman reports that she has a brother who experiences frequent episodes of fatigue, pain in his abdomen and limbs, and yellowing of his skin. The husband states that he has a brother who frequently experiences a similar constellation of symptoms. Based on this family history, which of the following represents the most likely probability that this couple will have a child who is affected by the same disease presenting in their siblings?
(A) 1/36
(B) 1/18
(C) 1/9
(D) 1/2
(E) 3/4

59. Medical geneticists are studying a family that has members presenting with what appears to be a novel disease. The following pedigree was generated following the examination of four generations of the family. Based upon the findings, which of the following is most likely associated with the inheritance of the disease in this family?

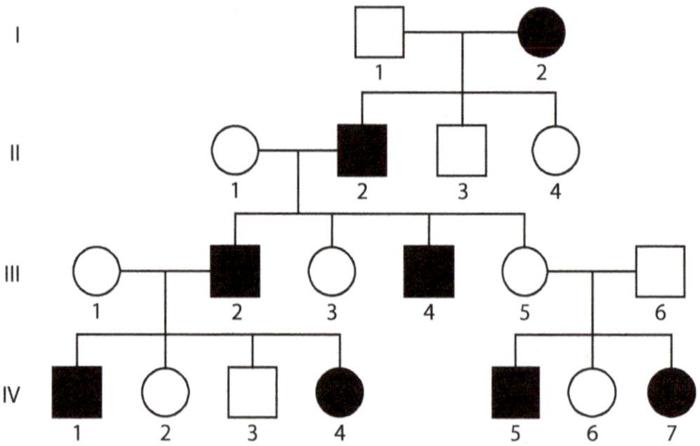

(A) Alellic heterogeneity
(B) Anticipation
(C) Codominance
(D) Imprinting
(E) Incomplete penetrance
(F) Variable expressivity

60. A 27-year-old man is being examined in the Emergency Department with a primary complaint of significant fatigue, dizziness, and shortness of breath. He reports that he was recently treated with tafenoquine as a prophylactic prior to a scheduled business trip to Mozambique. Physical examination finds diffuse abdominal pain on palpation with voluntary guarding, and the presence of scleral icterus is noted. Blood is drawn for analysis with the results of a peripheral blood smear shown. Given the most likely diagnosis in this patient, which of the following represents the most likely probability that any of his future sons will also have this disease?

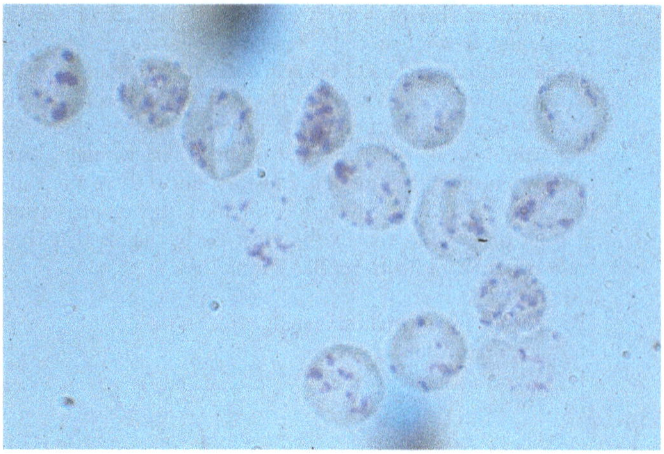

(A) 0%
(B) 25%
(C) 50%
(D) 67%
(E) 100%

61. Researchers are studying the occurrence of a progressive muscle weakness and degeneration that primarily affects the legs and is almost always observed in males. They discover that in some individuals, the symptoms begin around the age of 2 to 3 and ultimately result in death in the 3rd or 4th decade of life, most often from cardiomyopathy. In contrast, in some individuals, symptoms don't appear until the teens or 2nd decade of life and in these individuals their life expectancy can be into the 5th decade. Which of the following most closely reflects the genetics of the results identified by these researchers?
(A) Allelic heterogeneity
(B) Germline mosaicism
(C) Imprinting
(D) Locus heterogeneity
(E) Pleiotropy

62. A medical genetics researcher is studying a family in which several members harbor the same mutant allele that is associated with autosomal dominant inheritance. One of the affected members of this family is a 29-year-old man who has arachnodactyly, is at the 95th percentile for height, and has a late systolic murmur detectable with auscultation. This individual has a younger brother who is also very tall, but also has scoliosis and dural ectasia, as well as lens subluxation. Which of the following is the most likely explanation for the observations in this family?
(A) Anticipation
(B) Imprinting
(C) Incomplete penetrance
(D) Somatic mosaicism
(E) Variable expressivity

63. A medical geneticist is studying what appears to be a novel disorder in all three generations of a family. Individuals in the family who manifest the disease experience symptoms that first manifest with drooping eyelids (ptosis) progressing to weakness and paralysis (myopathy) of the muscles that move the eyes. The geneticist generates the following pedigree of the family based upon her examination of everyone in the family. Based upon these findings, which of the following is the most likely location for the genetic alteration responsible for the disease in this family?

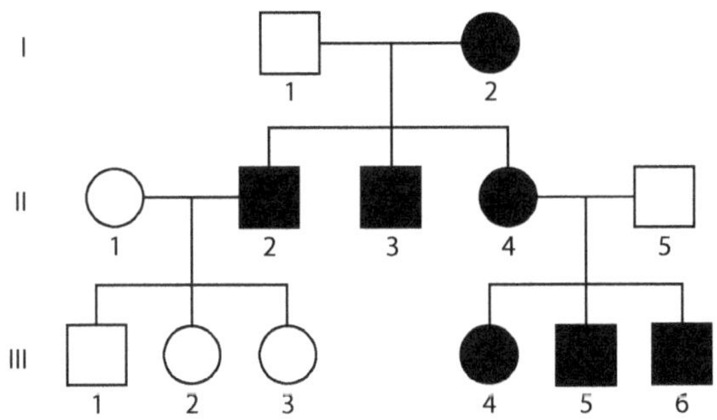

(A) Chromosome 5
(B) Chromosome 15
(C) Chromosome 21
(D) Mitochondrial DNA
(E) X chromosome
(F) Y chromosome

64. A 32-year-old man is taken to the Emergency Department by his wife because he is complaining of the acute onset of a squeezing pain in his chest that is radiating to left shoulder and arm. He reports that he has had high cholesterol for many years despite attempts to eat healthily and exercise. He is taking both ezetimibe and simvastatin to help lower his serum cholesterol. The results of an ECG show ST-segment elevation and hyperacute T waves. Blood work upon admission finds his total cholesterol is 485 mg/dL. In the absence of any additional family history, which of the following pedigrees most likely identifies the mode of inheritance of the most likely disorder manifesting in this patient?

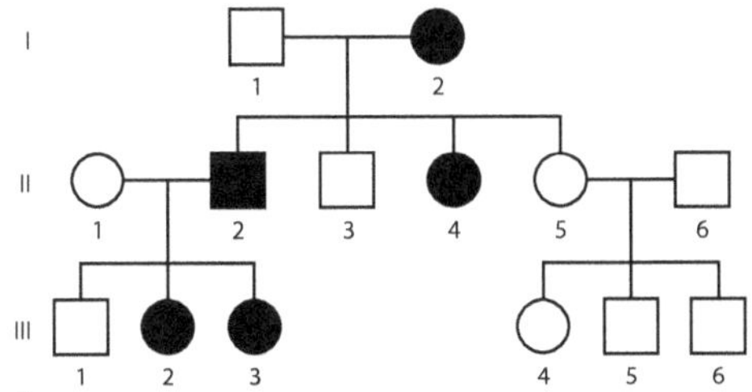

A

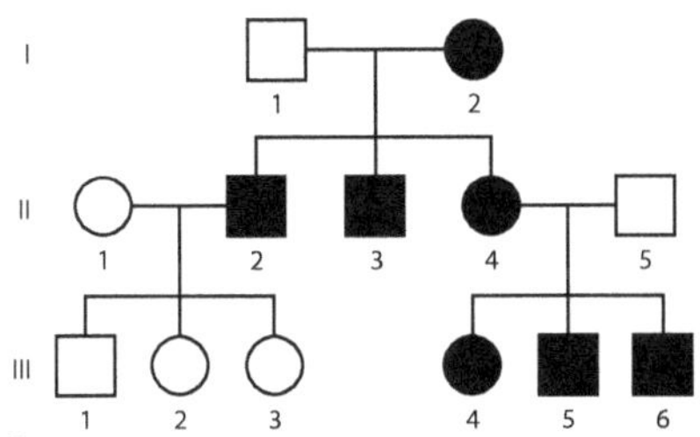

B

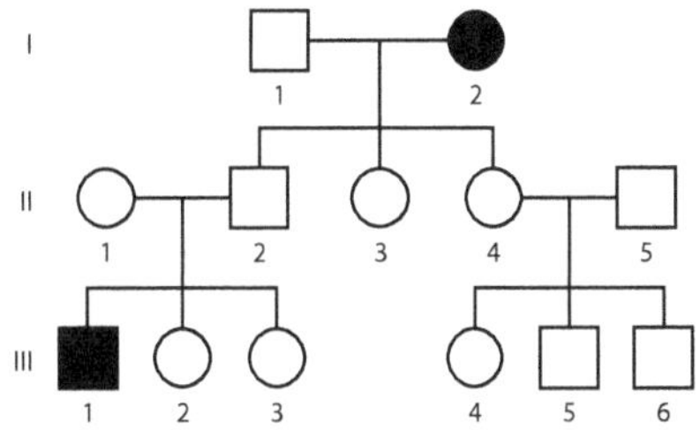

C

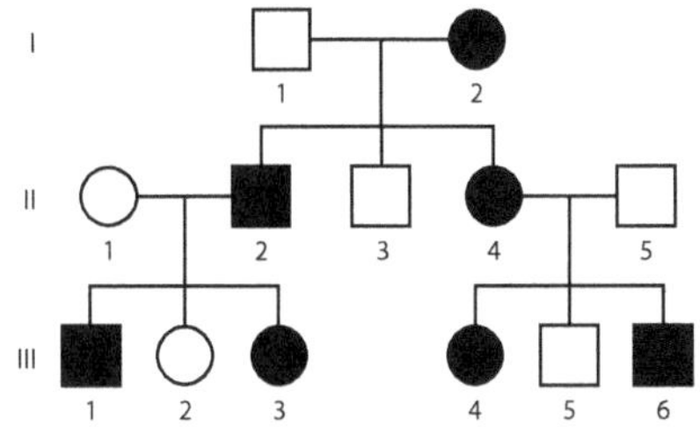

D

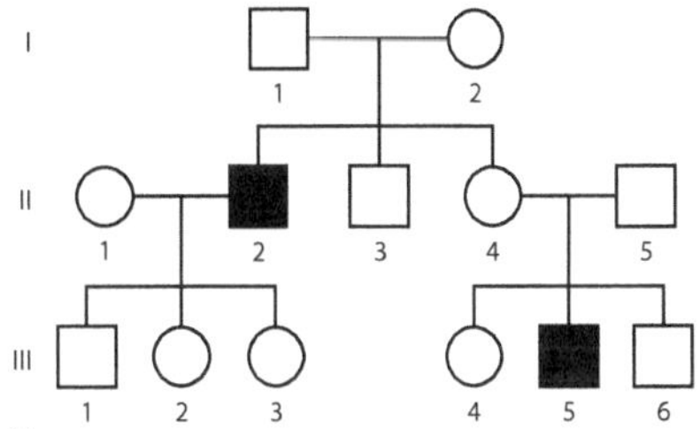

E

(A) A
(B) B
(C) C
(D) D
(E) E

65. A 26-year-old woman and her 30-year-old husband have come to the Medical Genetics clinic in their local hospital for counseling prior to conceiving a child. The husband states that he has a brother who has two children with a disorder that affects their joints and skin. The couple is concerned that their future children may inherit the same disorder. Both the wife and husband are currently healthy and have no known medical conditions. The genetics clinic is able to generate a pedigree from the husband's family. The husband and wife are indicated as individuals II-5 and II-6 in the generated pedigree shown below. Which of the following represents the most likely mode of inheritance of the disease in the husband's family?

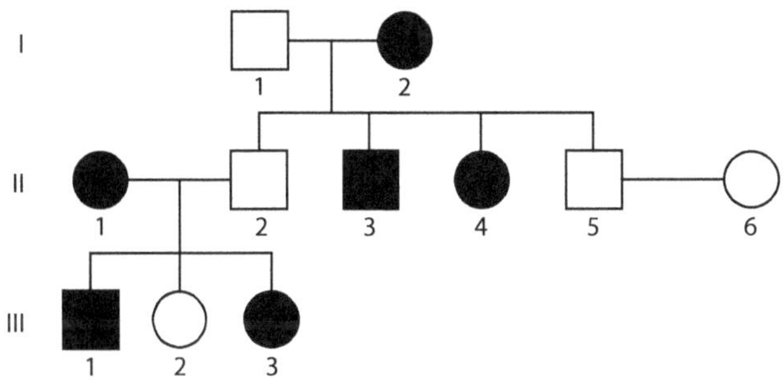

(A) Autosomal dominant
(B) Autosomal recessive
(C) Mitochondrial
(D) X-linked dominant
(E) X-linked recessive

66. A medical genetics research group has identified a novel locus associated with the inheritance of type 2 diabetes. They identify the gene associated with the inheritance and demonstrate that mutations in the gene exert a gain-of-function effect in the population under study. Data from the study demonstrates that the mutant allele responsible for diabetes in this population is present with a frequency of 20%. If the Hardy-Weinberg equilibrium assumptions are functioning in this population, what is the most likely percentage of individuals in the population harboring at least one allele for diabetes?
(A) 10%
(B) 18%
(C) 36%
(D) 72%
(E) 90%

67. A 4-year-old girl is being examined by her pediatrician because her parents are concerned about the rapid decline in her visual ability. Physical examination of the patient shows redness and swelling around her right eye. Closer examination of the patient's eyes shows strabismus and leukocoria. The pediatrician orders additional testing, the results of which demonstrate that there is a mutation in a gene on chromosome 11. Familial testing shows the same mutation in one of the two alleles of the gene in the mother. Given the most likely diagnosis, which of the following most correctly defines the genetic mechanism for the symptoms observed in this patient?
(A) Allelic heterogeneity
(B) Incomplete penetrance
(C) Imprinting
(D) Linkage disequilibrium
(E) Loss of heterozygosity

68. A husband and wife are at a genetics counseling center discussing their likelihood of having a child with cystic fibrosis. History reveals that both individuals are healthy, and neither is aware of any significant family histories. The counselor informs the couple that within their population, 75% of individuals do not have the disease. If Hardy-Weinberg equilibrium assumptions are operating in this population, what is the most likely frequency of the wild-type allele?
(A) 10%
(B) 35%
(C) 50%
(D) 67%
(E) 75%

69. A 15-year-old boy is being examined by an ophthalmologist to determine the cause of the gradual vision loss he is experiencing in both eyes. The patient reports that he has been experiencing blurriness and cloudiness in both eyes and that the intensity has gotten worse over the past 3 months prompting this most recent examination. Ophthalmoscopic examination finds optic disc hyperemia and peripapillary telangiectasias. Which of the following pedigrees most likely represents the mode of inheritance of the most likely disease in this patient?

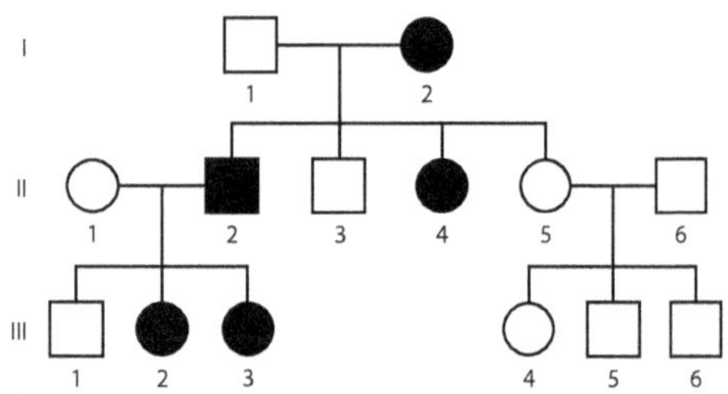
A

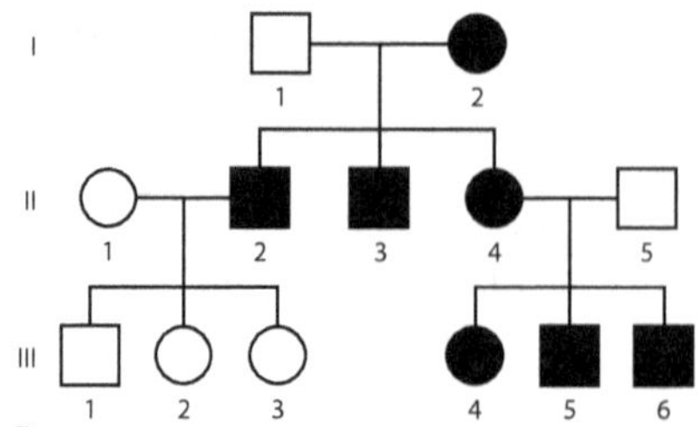
B

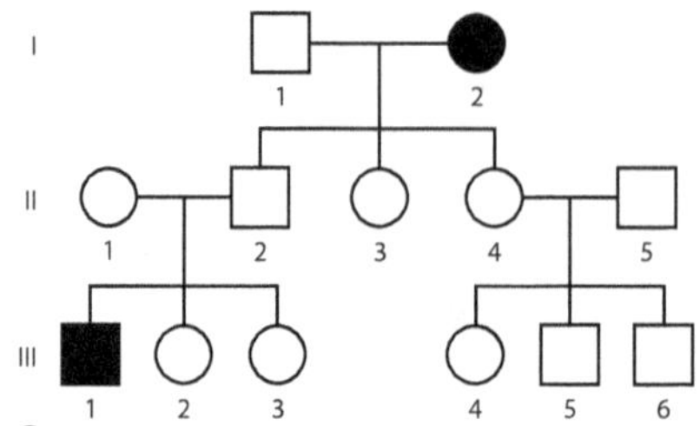
C

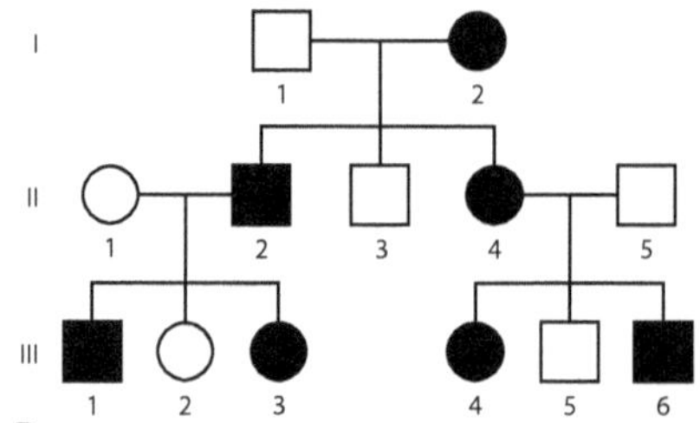
D

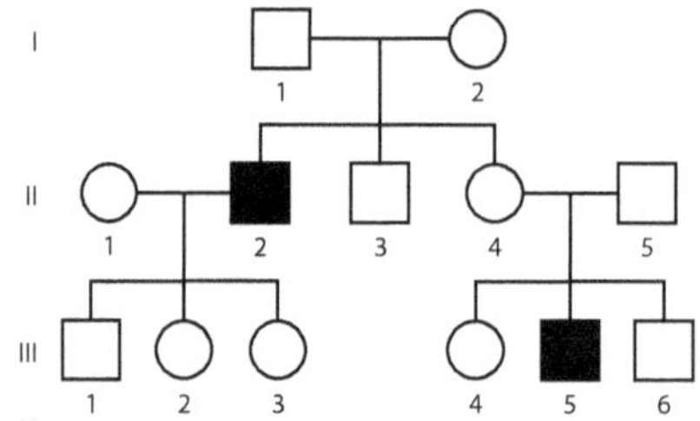
E

(A) A
(B) B
(C) C
(D) D
(E) E

70. A medical genetics group is studying the inheritance of phenylketonuria (PKU) in a population of 35,000 individuals that populate a remote region of Siberia. Their studies find that within this population, 96% of individuals do not have the disease. If Hardy-Weinberg equilibrium assumptions are operating in this population, what is the most likely frequency of the mutant allele responsible for PKU in this population?
(A) 4%
(B) 16%
(C) 20%
(D) 25%
(E) 50%

71. A 10-year-old boy is brought to the Emergency Department by his father following a seizure. The father reports that he is concerned that his son is experiencing the same disorder that resulted in the death of his mother 2 years ago from cardiomyopathy. He states that she also experienced a period of worsening seizures as well as muscle weakness. History reveals

that the patient's grandmother and maternal uncle both experienced seizures and muscle weakness beginning in their third decade of life. Which of the following inheritance patterns is most likely responsible for the most likely disease presenting in this patient?
(A) Autosomal dominant
(B) Autosoma recessive
(C) Mitochondrial
(D) Multifactorial
(E) X-linked recessive
(F) X-linked dominant

72. A husband and wife are discussing their likelihood of having a child with sickle cell anemia with a counselor at the local University's medical genetics clinic. History reveals that both individuals are healthy, and neither is aware of any significant family histories. The counselor informs the couple that the disease is present within the population, of which both individuals are members, at a frequency of 4%. If Hardy-Weinberg equilibrium assumptions are operating in this population, what is the most likely frequency of the disease-causing allele?
(A) 1%
(B) 5%
(C) 10%
(D) 20%
(E) 80%

73. A 24-year-old woman has come to the genetic counseling center of her local University Medical School to seek information on the likelihood that she and her husband will have the same disease that she has. The woman has a brother who is manifesting the same disease. Her husband does not have the disease, nor is there any history of the disease in his family. The medical geneticist constructs a pedigree of the woman's family and in this pedigree, she is designated as individual III-2. Given the constructed pedigree, which of the following most likely describes the mode of inheritance of the disease in this woman?

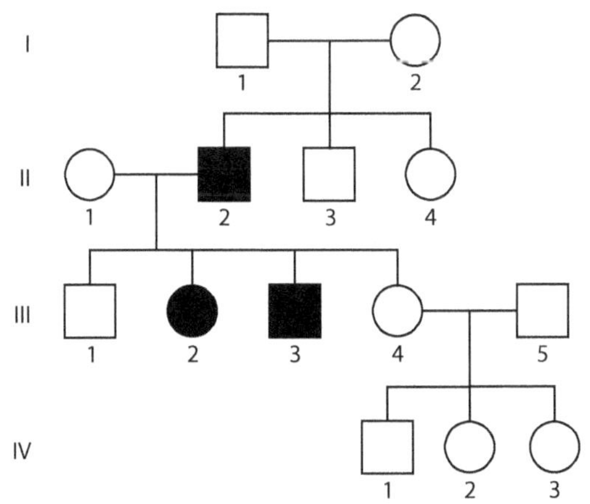

(A) Autosomal dominant
(B) Autosomal recessive
(C) Mitochondrial inheritance
(D) X-linked dominant
(E) X-linked recessive

74. An 8-year-old boy is undergoing an examination by a behavioral psychiatrist due to his extreme attention deficit and hyperactivity. The patient's history is significant for his large gestational size. Physical examination shows a boy with large ears, a prominent jaw, a long face, and flat feet. Which of the following genetic conditions is most likey to account for the signs and symptoms exhibited by this patient?
(A) Dominant negative inheritance
(B) Meiotic nondisjunction
(C) Somatic mutation
(D) Trinucleotide repeat expansion
(E) X-linked recessive inheritance

75. Studies are being conducted on a novel disease in an isolated population of 6000 individuals. Based on the results of this study it has been determined that the disease is transmitted in an autosomal recessive manner and that the disease has affected 15 individuals in this population. Further analysis finds that there has been no migration into or out of the studied population and that there is random mating among the members of the population. Evidence also points to the fact that no new novel mutations have been identified in the locus purportedly responsible for the disease. Given all the findings in this study, which of the following represents the most likely percentage of asymptomatic carriers of this disease within the population?
(A) 2.5%
(B) 5%
(C) 9.5%
(D) 18%
(E) 25.5%

76. A husband and wife are discussing their likelihood of having a child with sickle cell anemia with a counselor at the local University's medical genetics clinic. History reveals that both individuals are healthy, and neither is aware of any significant family histories. The counselor informs the couple that the disease is present within the population, of which both individuals are members, at a frequency of 4%. If Hardy-Weinberg equilibrium assumptions are operating in this population, what is the most likely frequency that either individual is an asymptomatic carrier of the sickle cell disease allele?
(A) 2%
(B) 4%
(C) 18%
(D) 32%
(E) 64%

77. A 9-year-old girl is undergoing a routine physical examination by her pediatrician. The patient is currently at the 25th percentile for height and the 40th percentile for weight. The patient's history includes the fact that she was born with swollen hands and feet and experienced feeding difficulties in infancy. The physical examination shows a female with short stature who has a short neck with a webbed appearance and low-set ears. Given the most likely diagnosis in this patient, an analysis of her Karyotype is most likely to find which of the following?
(A) 45, X
(B) 46, XY
(C) 46,XX,t(9;22)(q34;q11)
(D) 47, XXY
(E) Trisomy 21

78. A new disease is being studied in a population of 500 isolated individuals within whom the analysis finds there has been no evidence for natural selection nor migration into or out of the studied population. Genotyping of the population finds that the disease-causing allele is present at a frequency of 12%.

Given this finding, which of the following represents the most likely frequency of carriers for the disease in this isolated population?
(A) 5%
(B) 11%
(C) 21%
(D) 42%
(E) 88%

79. A husband and wife are discussing their likelihood of having a child with a particular disease with a counselor at the local University's medical genetics clinic. History reveals that both individuals are healthy, and neither is aware of any significant family histories. The geneticist determines that the husband is of a certain ethnicity within which the incidence rate of a particular autosomal recessive disorder is 1 in 3600. The incidence rate of this same disease is only 1 in 40,000 in the general population. Provided that the assumptions of the Hardy-Weinberg law are maintained within both the wife's and the husband's populations, what is the most likely probability that any of their offspring will be born with the disease?
(A) 1 in 400
(B) 1 in 3,000
(C) 1 in 6,000
(D) 1 in 12,000
(E) 1 in 24,000

80. A child born with cystic fibrosis will manifest with frequent respiratory issues that include coughing, shortness of breath, and infections. This child will also have digestive issues that can result in malabsorption of nutrients that, in turn, lead to slow growth. The manifestation of pathology with this disease is most likely the result of which of the following genetic phenomena?
(A) Allelic heterogeneity
(B) Locus heterogeneity
(C) Mosaicism
(D) Multifactorial inheritance
(E) Pleiotropy

ANSWERS

1. Correct answer is **B.** The disease most likely manifesting in this family is Huntington disease. Huntington disease is caused by expansion of a CAG trinucleotide repeat in the first exon of the huntingtin gene (*HTT*). The CAG repeat resides 17 codons downstream of the initiator AUG codon and its expansion results in a polyglutamine stretch in the amino terminus of the huntingtin protein that causes of defective function of the protein. Huntington disease is inherited as an autosomal dominant disorder that also exhibits a genetic phenomenon termed anticipation. Genetic anticipation means that the symptoms of the disease appear earlier and are more severe in subsequent generations. This phenomenon is explained by meiotic instability which increases the CAG repeat number and is greater in spermatogenesis than in oogenesis. Therefore, anticipation in Huntington disease is mainly observed when the mutation is inherited through the paternal line. Allelic heterogeneity (choice A) refers to the phenomenon of different mutations in the same gene being associated with the same disease. This phenomenon leads to the potential for variable phenotypic expression and is typical for most disease genes. As an example, there are over 1,500 identified mutations in the cystic fibrosis transmembrane conductance regulator (*CFTR*) gene all of which cause cystic fibrosis but not all mutations manifest with the same level of severity. Germline mosaicism (choice C) refers to mosaicism found exclusively in the gametes and not in any somatic cells. Genetic mosaicism occurs when an individual has two or more genetically different sets of cells in their body. Because the mutation is only present in gametes, and not somatic cells, the mutation will not be found during routine genetic testing which is accomplished using somatic cells. Germline mosaicism means an individual can have more than one affected offspring with an X-linked disorder (eg, Duchene muscular dystrophy) or an autosomal dominant disorder (eg, osteogenesis imperfecta) while they themselves do not manifest the disease. Locus heterogeneity (choice D) refers to the phenomenon whereby mutations in different genes are associated with the same disease. For example, osteogenesis imperfecta is a disorder that results from mutations in numerous genes, the most common forms being the result of mutations in collagen genes on chromosome 7 or 17. Pleiotropy (choice E) refers to the phenomenon whereby mutations in a single gene influence two or more seemingly unrelated phenotypic traits. For example, Marfan syndrome, which is caused by mutations in the gene (*FBN1*) encoding the connective tissue protein fibrillin, is associated with the skeletal anomaly known as arachnodactyly (long thin extremities) while in the cardiovascular system the disease leads to dilation of the aortic root.

2. Correct answer is **C.** Given the assumption that the population is in Hardy-Weinberg equilibrium, the frequency of individuals with the albino genotype is the square of the frequency of the albino allele. In other words, frequency of (a/a) = q^2. Thus, the frequency of (a/a) = 26/6000 = 0.0043333, and the square root of that is 0.0658, which is the value for q, the frequency of the albino allele. The frequency of the normal allele is p which is equal to 1 - q, so p = 0.934. The predicted frequency of individuals who are homozygous normal (genotype A/A) is p^2, which is 0.873. In other words, 87.3% of the population, or an estimated 5238 people, should be homozygous normal. The frequency of carriers would be predicted to be $2pq$, which is 0.123. Therefore, 12.3%, or 737 people, should be carriers of albinism, if the population is in Hardy-Weinberg equilibrium. The number of individuals in the population that are homozygous and therefore, manifest albinism is 26 (choice A). The number of individuals in the population that represents both the heterozygous carriers, and the homozygous normal individuals is 5974 (choice E). Neither choice B nor D reflects any pool of individuals from the total population of 6000 individuals.

3. Correct answer is **A.** The patient is most likely experiencing the symptoms associated with Angelman syndrome (AS). The characteristic clinical spectrum of AS include microcephaly, seizure disorder, ataxia, muscular hypotonia with hyperreflexia, and motor delay. The psychomotor delay in AS patients is evident by 6 months of age and is associated with hypotonia and feeding difficulties. The microcephaly is not apparent at birth but develops within the first 3 years. The seizure disorder associated with AS typically develops between the first and third years of life. AS results from loss of neuron-specific maternal expression of a ubiquitin ligase gene (*UBE3A*) in the chromosome 15q11.2-q13 region. Beckwith-Wiedemann syndrome (choice B) results from defects in genomic imprinting of genes present in chromosome 11p15.5. Down syndrome (choice C) is the result of trisomy of chromosome 21.

Fragile X syndrome (choice D) is the result of the amplification of a trinucleotide repeat in the *FMR1* gene located on the X chromosome. Myotonic dystrophy type 1 (choice E) is the result of the amplification of a trinucleotide repeat in the *DMPK* gene located on chromosome 19q13.32. Prader-Willi syndrome (choice F) is the result of the loss of expression of paternal specific genes in the same region of the p arm of chromosome 15 as in Angelman syndrome. Prader-Willi syndrome (PWS) is characterized by a failure to thrive in the neonatal period accompanied by muscular hypotonia. During early childhood PWS patients exhibit hyperphagia (excessive hunger and abnormally large intake of solid foods), obesity, hypogonadism, sleep apnea, behavior problems, and mild to moderate intellectual impairment. Hypogonadism is present in both males and females. A distinctive behavioral phenotype of PWS is temper tantrums, stubbornness, and manipulative and compulsive behaviors.

4. Correct answer is **D.** The disease defined by the pedigree is most likely autosomal recessive since it is distributed equally between males and females, and it is not found in all generations (not vertically penetrant). Given that individual II-3 and II-4 both manifest the disease their genotypes must both be a/a. If these mutant alleles were from the same gene in both parents all their children would inherit mutant alleles and be affected by the disease. Since neither child has the disease the most likely reason is that the disease can result from mutations in at least two different genes, the characteristic definition of locus heterogeneity. Allelic heterogeneity (choice A) refers to the phenomenon of different mutations in the same gene being associated with the same disease. This phenomenon leads to the potential for variable phenotypic expression and is typical for most disease genes. As an example, there are over 1,500 identified mutations in the cystic fibrosis transmembrane conductance regulator (*CFTR*) gene all of which cause cystic fibrosis but not all mutations manifest with the same level of severity. Anticipation (choice B) refers to the phenomenon with which the signs and symptoms of an inherited disorder tend to become more severe and/or appear at an earlier age as the disorder is passed from one generation to the next. Genomic imprinting (choice C) is an epigenetic phenomenon that is associated with parental specific gene expression. Genes can also be partially imprinted. Pleiotropy (choice E) refers to the phenomenon whereby mutations in a single gene influence two or more seemingly unrelated phenotypic traits. For example, Marfan syndrome, which is caused by mutations in the gene (*FBN1*) encoding the connective tissue protein fibrillin, is associated with the skeletal anomaly known as arachnodactyly (long thin extremities) while in the cardiovascular system the disease leads to dilation of the aortic root.

5. Correct answer is **C.** Locus heterogeneity refers to the phenomenon whereby mutations in different genes are associated with the same disease. In the case of homocystinura mutations in the genes (*CBS* and *MTR*) encoding cystathionine β-synthase and methionine synthase, respectively, both result in this disorder. Allelic heterogeneity (choice A) refers to the phenomenon of different mutations in the same gene being associated with the same disease. This phenomenon leads to the potential for variable phenotypic expression and is typical for most disease genes. As an example, there are over 1,500 identified mutations in the cystic fibrosis transmembrane conductance regulator (*CFTR*) gene all of which cause cystic fibrosis but not all mutations manifest with the same level of severity. Compound heterozygosity (choice B) defines the genotype in which two different mutant alleles of a gene are present as opposed to one wild-type allele and one mutant allele. For example, an individual that inherits a sickle cell anemia allele (HbS) from one parent and a hemoglobin C allele (HbC) from the other is an example of a compound heterozygote, defined as HbSC. Multifactorial inheritance (choice D) is commonly associated with many common diseases, such as cancer or congenital birth defects, and these diseases cluster within the relatives of affected individuals more frequently than in the general population. Inheritance of these conditions generally does not follow one of the typical Mendelian patterns of single gene disorders because they are the result of the complex interactions among a number of genetic variants as well as certain environmental exposures. Variable expressivity (choice E) refers to the extent or degree to which a genetic defect is expressed such as mild, severe, early, late, etc. Variable expressivity does not relate to penetrance.

6. Correct answer is **D.** Genetic penetrance refers to the proportion of people with a particular genetic variant, such as a dominant mutant allele, who exhibit signs and symptoms of a genetic disorder. In some individuals the presence of a mutant allele, which should manifest a clinical phenotype, does not actually result in the expected clinical phenotype and this circumstance is referred to as incomplete penetrance. Allelic heterogeneity (choice A) refers to the phenomenon of different mutations in the same gene being associated with the same disease. This phenomenon leads to the potential for variable phenotypic expression and is typical for most disease genes. As an example, there are over 1,500 identified mutations in the cystic fibrosis transmembrane conductance regulator (*CFTR*) gene all of which cause cystic fibrosis, but not all mutations manifest with the same level of severity. Anticipation (choice B) refers to the phenomenon with which the signs and symptoms of an inherited disorder tend to become more severe and/or appear at an earlier age as the disorder is passed from one generation to the next. Germline mosaicism (choice C) refers to mosaicism found exclusively in the gametes and not in any somatic cells. Genetic mosaicism occurs when an individual has two or more genetically different sets of cells in their body. Because the mutation is only present in gametes, and not somatic cells, the mutation will not be found during routine genetic testing which is accomplished using somatic cells. Germline mosaicism means an individual can have more than one affected offspring with an X-linked disorder (eg, Duchene muscular dystrophy) or an autosomal dominant disorder (eg, osteogenesis imperfecta) while they themselves do not manifest the disease. A dominant disease that manifests in a child of otherwise unaffected parents is most likely the result of a new mutation (choice E). Variable expressivity (choice F) refers to the extent or degree to which a genetic defect is expressed such as mild, severe, early, late, etc. Variable expressivity does not relate to penetrance.

7. Correct answer is **E.** Variable expressivity refers to the extent or degree to which a genetic defect is expressed such as mild, severe, early, late, etc., as evident in the variable levels of skin involvement in this family. Variable expressivity is probably caused by a combination of genetic, environmental, and lifestyle factors. Variable expressivity does not relate to penetrance. Epistasis (choice A) refers to the genetic phenomenon whereby the effect of a mutant allele is dependent on the presence or absence of mutations in one or more other genes. These other genes are referred to as modifier genes.

This means that the effect of a mutant allele is dependent on the genetic background in which it appears. Epistatic mutations will, therefore, have different effects on their own than when they occur together. Genetic penetrance refers to the proportion of people with a particular genetic variant, such as a dominant mutant allele, who exhibit signs and symptoms of a genetic disorder. In some individuals the presence of a mutant allele, which should manifest a clinical phenotype, does not actually result in the expected clinical phenotype and this circumstance is referred to as incomplete penetrance (choice B). Pleiotropy (choice C) refers to the phenomenon whereby mutations in a single gene influence two or more seemingly unrelated phenotypic traits. For example, Marfan syndrome, which is caused by mutations in the gene (*FBN1*) encoding the connective tissue protein fibrillin, is associated with the skeletal anomaly known as arachnodactyly (long thin extremities) while in the cardiovascular system the disease leads to dilation of the aortic root. Somatic mosaicism (choice D) refers to the occurrence of two, or more, genetically distinct populations of cells within an individual that are not the result of mutations in the germ cells from which the individual was generated. Somatic mosaicism is not generally inheritable and the likelihood of its occurrence in the same gene in multiple individuals in the same family is essentially zero.

8. Correct answer is **C.** The disease defined by the pedigree is most likely autosomal recessive. All siblings of affected individuals will have a 2/3 chance of themselves being carriers for the mutant allele. The father's chance of being a carrier for the mutant allele is determined from the $2pq$ value (carrier frequency) of the Hardy-Weinberg equation. The incidence rate is q^2 =1/3600 so q is 1/60. The frequency of the wild-type allele (p) is always assumed to be 1 since it is very close to this value. Therefore, the carrier frequency, $2pq$, is $2q$ [2(1/60)] = 1/30. What this result demonstrates is that for autosomal recessive diseases, the carrier frequency is always twice the frequency of the mutant allele in a given population. The overall risk for the unborn child is the product of the four independent variables (two for the father and two for the mother). Each parent has a 1/2 chance of donating the mutant allele. Most explanations of recurrence risk indicate the product of those two independent variables which is always 1/4. However, keeping track of all the independent variables during risk calculations (ie, two variables for each parent) prevents errors. The father's contributions (both independent variables) to the overall recurrence risk are 1/2 × 1/30 and the mother's contributions (both independent variables) to the overall recurrence risk are 1/2 × 2/3. Therefore, the overall recurrence risk is (1/2)(1/30)(1/2)(2/3) = 1/180. None of the other options (choices A, B, D, and E) represent the correct recurrence risk for the unborn child.

9. Correct answer is **C.** Sickle cell anemia is inherited as an autosomal recessive disease. Since the wife is unaffected and her brother is affected, her parents must both be carriers. Since the husband is unaffected and his sister is affected, his parents must also both be carriers. Because both the wife and husband are siblings of affected individuals, they both have a 2/3 chance of being a carrier of the mutant allele. The likelihood that the wife donates the mutant allele is 1/2 and the likelihood that the husband donates the mutant allele is also 1/2. The husband's contributions (both independent variables) to the overall recurrence risk are 1/2 × 2/3 and the wife's contributions (both independent variables) to the overall recurrence risk are also 1/2 × 2/3. Therefore, the overall recurrence risk is (1/2)(2/3)(1/2)(2/3) = 1/9 = 11%. None of the other options (choices A, B, D, and E) represent the correct recurrence risk for the unborn child.

10. Correct answer is **E.** Alkaptonuria is inherited as an autosomal recessive disease. If an individual has a sibling that is afflicted with an autosomal recessive disease, such as is the case for the wife, the risk of being a carrier is 2/3 (67%). None of the other options (choices A, B, C, and D) correspond to the correct percentage of likelihood of an individual with as sibling affected by an autosomal recessive disease being a carrier for the mutant allele.

11. Correct answer is **A.** The patient is most likely exhibiting the symptoms of the mitochondrial encephalomyopathy known as MERFF (myoclonic epilepsy with ragged red fibers). All of the gene mutations that have been identified as causing MERFF are in mitochondrial genome (mtDNA) encoded genes. The most common cause (80% of cases) of MERFF is inheritance of mutations in the *MT-TK* gene that encodes a Lys (K) tRNA. Symptoms of MERFF begin to appear in childhood or early adolescence and are characterized by myoclonus (muscle twitching), muscle weakness (myopathy), and progressive stiffness (spasticity). Additional common symptoms of MERFF are seizures, ataxia, peripheral neuropathy, optic neuropathy, hearing loss, and dementia. Mitochondrial encephalomyopathies, such as MERFF, are only transmitted by mothers never by fathers. This is due to the destruction of sperm mitochondria following fertilization. Therefore, if the patient ever decides to have children, they will not be able to inherit the disorder from him. None of the other options (choices B, C, D, and E) correctly reflect the likelihood of a male, with a strictly mtDNA-associated disorder, passing on the mutant allele.

12. Correct answer is **C.** Unless otherwise specified, the most likely genotype of an individual affected by an autosomal dominant disorder will be A/a and for individuals, such as the patient's wife, that are disease free the most likely genotype is a/a. From these two genotypes it can be easily determined from a Punnett square that the recurrence risk for an affected child will always be 50%. None of the other options (choices A, B, D, and E) correctly reflect the most likely recurrence risk for a child of parents, one of whom is afflicted with an autosomal dominant disorder.

13. Correct answer is **B.** The disease defined by the pedigree is most likely an X-linked recessive disease. Because neither individual in generation I have the disease it is not vertically penetrant, indicative of recessive inheritance. The presence, in the family, of only affected males strongly indicates an X-linked disorder and the absence of affected females makes autosomal dominance very unlikely. In X-linked recessive diseases all mothers of affected sons and all daughters of affected fathers are obligate carriers for the mutant X-linked gene. From the pedigree it is clear that individual II-4 is an obligate carrier. Since II-4 is obligate carrier, it is known that she has a 50% (1/2) chance of donating that mutant allele to any of her daughters. Therefore, the likelihood that individual III-3 is a carrier is 1/2 and she has a 1/2 chance of donating that mutant allele to any of her sons. Since males cannot transmit X-linked genes to their sons there is no need to consider the genetic status of any future mating partner that individual III-3 will have. Therefore, the recurrence risk for any of the sons of III-3 is (1/2) × (1/2) = 1/4 (25%). In questions such as this it is often worded in such a way that the sex of the child

is not a given. Since the likelihood of having a child that is a male is 50%, this would become an additional independent variable for calculation of recurrence risk. For example, if the actual question was worded. "What is the recurrence risk to any future children of individual III-3?" The most correct recurrence risk would need to include the 1/2 chance that individual III-3 has a son AND that he is affected making the overall risk (1/2) × (1/2) × (1/2) = 1/8. Another form of wording that would indicate the need to include the independent variable related to the likelihood of having a child of one sex for the other could be "What is the likelihood that she has a son affected by the disease?" None of the other options (choices A, C, D, and E) correctly define the recurrence risk for the son of a female who is an obligate carrier of an X-linked disease allele.

14. Correct answer is **A.** Huntington disease is inherited as an autosomal dominant disorder. The husband is most likely a heterozygote, A/a (mutant allele, A, from his father, normal allele, a, from his mother.) The wife is most likely homozygous normal, a/a. From the genotypes of the husband and wife it can be easily determined from a Punnett square that the recurrence risk for them to have an affected child will always be 50%. Thus, each child has a 50% (1/2) chance of the disease. Therefore, the probability that ALL three develop the disease is simply the product of the recurrence risk (1/2) for each child which is (1/2) × (1/2) × (1/2) = 1/8. None of the other options (choices B, C, D, and E) correctly define the overall recurrence risk for all three children to acquire Huntington disease.

15. Correct answer is **C.** The disease defined by the pedigree is most likely autosomal recessive. The genotype of individual III-2 is, therefore, denoted as a/a. Thus, this individual has a 100% (1) chance of harboring the mutant allele and has a 100% (1) chance of donating the mutant allele to any of her children. Individuals II-1 and II-2, the parents of III-1, must both be obligate carriers (heterozygotes: A/a) of the mutant allele. Individual II-2 must have acquired the mutant allele from one of his parents, either I-1 or I-2. This means that any children of I-1 and I-2 will have a 50% (1/2) chance of also acquiring the mutant allele. Therefore, individual II-3 has a 50% (1/2) chance of being a carrier of the mutant allele and a 50% (1/2) chance of donating the mutant allele to any of her children. This means that the first cousin (III-3) of individual III-2 has a (1/2) × (1/2) = 1/4 chance of being a carrier of the mutant allele. Therefore, the overall probability that any of their children will be born with the disorder (no different for 1st, 2nd, 3rd, etc.) is the product of the four independent variables, two for III-2 and two for III-3 which is (1) × (1) × (1/2) × (1/4) = 1/8. None of the other options (choices A, B, D, and E) correctly reflect the recurrence risk for any child of individuals III-2 and III-3.

16. Correct answer is **D.** The pedigree depicts a disease that is most likely inherited in an autosomal dominant manner, therefore only a single allele is necessary to manifest the disorder. In comparison of the PCR banding pattern, it is apparent that the three affected individuals all have one allele where the product of the PCR is larger than 800 bp. Additionally, it is apparent that in each subsequent generation the size of the disease allele is larger in the affected individuals. This molecular characteristic is typical of trinucleotide repeat disorders. Allelic heterogeneity (choice A) is the molecular feature where different mutations in the same gene result in very similar phenotypes, as is typical of most inherited diseases. Although it is remotely possible that allelic heterogeneity could result from different sized insertions in a gene it is much less likely to explain the results in this family than trinucleotide repeat expansion. Meiotic nondisjunction (choice B) would be evidenced molecularly as different numbers of alleles and very unlikely to be associated with different sized PCR products from a given allele. Microsatellite instability, MSI (choice C), refers to the molecular phenomenon where, most commonly, highly repetitive DNA elements are improperly replicated during S-phase of the cell cycle. Although the outcomes of MSI can be evidenced by increased size of PCR products and the inheritance of MSI-related disorders are autosomal dominant, the vast majority of MSI-associated disorders are cancers not degenerative muscle diseases. Variable expressivity (choice E) refers to the phenomenon of different presentation of symptoms in individuals harboring the same, or very similar alleles, and as such would not likely be associated with the molecular phenomena of different sized PCR products.

17. Correct answer is **B.** The disorder manifesting in the males in this family is most likely Lesch-Nyhan syndrome. Lesch-Nyhan syndrome is X-linked, and the pedigree confirms this pattern of inheritance. Female II-4 is an obligate carrier since all mothers of affected sons are obligate carriers. Since II-4 is an obligate carrier her daughter (III-3) has a 50% (1/2) chance of being a carrier as well. There will be no contribution from her unrelated unaffected mating partner since the recurrence risk relates to a son and only III-3 can give her sons a mutant X chromosome. The other independent variable in this question is that it is asking the likelihood of having a son (1/2) and that he is affected, therefore the overall likelihood is 1/2 chance of having a son times1/2 chance of being a carrier times 1/2 chance of donating the mutant X allele which is 1/2 × 1/2 × 1/2 = 1/8 (25%). None of the other options (choice A, C, D, and E) correctly reflect the likelihood that individual III-3 will have a son and that he will be afflicted with Lesch-Nyhan syndrome.

18. Correct answer is **C.** The pedigree depicts a disease that is most likely inherited in an X-linked recessive manner. The symptoms experienced by individual III-1 with Bactrim therapy strongly suggests that the disorder in the family is glucose-6-phosphate dehydrogenase deficiency, an X-linked disorder. Given that III-1 has the disease his mother, II-1 must be an obligate carrier (all mothers of affected sons are obligate carriers for X-linked disorders). Individual III-2, therefore, has a 50% (1/2) chance of also being a carrier. Individual III-3 cannot contribute an X chromosome to any son, so his genotype does not contribute to the overall recurrence risk. Individual III-2 has a 1/2 chance of being a carrier and has a 1/2 chance of donating the mutant allele to any of her children, and she also has a 1/2 chance of having a son. Therefore, the overall probability that she has a son with the disease is (1/2) × (1/2) × (1/2) = 1/8. None of the other options choice A, B, D, and E correctly reflect the likelihood that individual III-2 will have a son and that the son will have glucose-6-phosphate dehydrogenase deficiency.

19. Correct answer is **B.** The disease defined by the pedigree is most likely autosomal recessive. The genotype of individual III-2 is, therefore, denoted as a/a. Thus, this individual has a 100% (1) chance of harboring the mutant allele and has a 100% (1) chance of donating the mutant allele to any of her children. Individuals II-1 and II-2, the parents of III-1, must both be obligate carriers (heterozygotes) of the mutant allele. Individual II-2 must have acquired the mutant allele from one of his parents, either I-1 or I-2. This means that any children of I-1 and I-2 will have a 50% (1/2) chance of also acquiring the mutant allele. Therefore, individual II-3 has a 50% (1/2) chance of being a carrier of the mutant allele and a 50% (1/2) chance of donating the mutant allele to any of her children. This means that the first cousin (III-3) of individual III-2 has a (1/2) × (1/2) = 1/4 chance of being a carrier of the mutant allele. The likelihood that the unborn child of III-2 and III-3 is a female is 50% (1/2). Therefore, the overall probability that they have a girl and she has the disease is 1/2[(1) × (1) × (1/2) × (1/4)] = 1/16. None of the other options choice A, C, D, and E correctly reflect the likelihood that individuals III-2 and III-3 will have a daughter and that the daughter will have the disease.

20. Correct answer is **C.** Phenylketonuria (PKU) is an autosomal recessive disease. All siblings of affected individuals will have a 2/3 chance of themselves being carriers for the mutant allele. Since an unaffected individual cannot be homozygous for an autosomal recessive mutant allele (ie, cannot be genotype a/a) there are only three possible genotypes for this woman, A/A or two chances of being a carrier (A/a). Therefore, the woman has a 2/3 (66.7%) chance of being a carrier for the mutant allele causing PKU. None of the other options (choices A, B, D, and E) correctly reflect the most likely carrier frequency for individuals who have a sibling with an autosomal recessive disease.

21. Correct answer is **C.** Since 4% of the individuals in a population harbor an autosomal recessive disease, the incidence rate of the disease is 4%. From the Hardy-Weinberg equation this is the value of q^2 which would be 0.04 (or 1/25). Therefore, q = 0.2 (or 1/5). Carrier frequency in the next generation is the $2pq$ value from the Hardy-Weinberg equation. Given that the frequency of the mutant allele (q) for an autosomal recessive disease is always very low, the frequency of the wild-type allele (p) is always very nearly equal to 1. Therefore, the carrier frequency will be $2q = 2 \times (0.2) = 0.4$ or 1/2.5. Note that for autosomal recessive disorders the frequency of carriers of the mutant allele is always twice the frequency of the mutant allele (q). None of the other options (choices A, B, D, and E) is the correct frequency of carriers for an autosomal recessive disorder in which the incidence rate in a given population is 4%.

22. Correct answer is **A.** From the Hardy-Weinberg equation the predicted frequency for the A/A genotype can be assigned the value of p^2 and the predicted frequency for A′/A′ genotype can be assigned the value of q^2, while the predicted frequency for the heterozygote genotype (A/A′) is the value of $2pq$. Inserting the values of the determined genotype frequencies in the population gives the following results.

$$p^2 = (0.426)^2 = 0.181$$
$$2pq = 2(0.426)(0.574) = 0.489$$
$$q^2 = (0.574)^2 = 0.329$$

Therefore, according to the Hardy-Weinberg equation, the predicted homozygous (A/A) frequency would be 0.181 not the observed value of 0.226. Note that the sum of the predicted values for all three possible genotypes adds up to 1, as expected. The difference between the calculated and observed frequencies is most likely due to the fact that the size of the analyzed population is small and there could be a certain level of inbreeding in this small population. None of the other options (choices B, C, D, and E) correctly identify the predicted frequency of the A/A genotype from the Hardy-Weinberg equilibrium equation.

23. Correct answer is **B.** The 2 allele of all five markers is found in all individuals manifesting the disease. Therefore, this allele of the marker is most likely to be linked to, and in phase with, the disease allele. The findings for individual III-5 indicate that recombination has occurred at the D and E markers such that the result is this individual has inherited the 1 allele of both of these markers. None of the other options (choices A, C, D, E, and F) correctly identifies the allele of a given marker that is associated with the disease-causing gene

24. Correct answer is **A.** The determination of the likelihood that the future father is a carrier of a mutant allele for the autosomal recessive disease is accomplished using the Hardy-Weinberg equation. The incidence rate of the disease in the population to which the woman and her future husband belong is 1/2500 which is the q^2 value from the Hardy-Weinberg equation. Therefore q = 1/50 (0.02). The frequency of carriers is determined from the $2pq$ value of the Hardy-Weinberg equation. Given that the frequency of the mutant allele (q) for an autosomal recessive disease is always very low, the frequency of the wild-type allele (p) is always very nearly equal to 1. Therefore, the carrier frequency for any individual in this population will be $2q$ = [2(1/50)] = 1/25 (0.04). What this result demonstrates is that for autosomal recessive diseases, the carrier frequency is always twice the frequency of the mutant allele (q). The chance that a carrier donates the mutant allele to any child is 50% (1/2). The likelihood that the woman will be a carrier can be determined with the aid of a pedigree constructed from the information provided (shown in accompanying figure). One can make the assumption that her first cousin is the son of her mother's sister (the woman's aunt). Since her cousin has the autosomal recessive disease, both her aunt and uncle must be carriers. One of her maternal grandparents (her mother and aunt's parents) must harbor the mutant allele which means that all of their children, including the woman's mother, have a 50% (1/2) chance of acquiring the mutant allele. The woman's mother had a 50% (1/2) chance of donating the mutant allele to her such that her overall risk of being a carrier is (1/2) × (1/2) = 1/4. When carrying out these types of calculations, the consideration of the most likely probability that the woman's father (II-1) is also a carrier could be accomplished using the same $2q$ value used to determine the most likely probability that the potential father (III-1) is a carrier. However, this is not taken into consideration because it makes the overall risk of the woman being a carrier so small as to negate the predictive benefit. For this reason, individuals that are at least one generation removed are always assumed to be homozygous wild type (A/A) and, therefore, do not contribute to the recurrence risk calculation. The recurrence risk to any child of the woman and her future husband is determined from the product of the four independent variables (two for the mother and two for the father) which is (1/4) × (1/2) × (1/25) × (1/2) = 1/400 (0.0025). None of the other options (choice B, C, D, and E) correctly identifies the recurrence risk for any child of the woman and a man from this population.

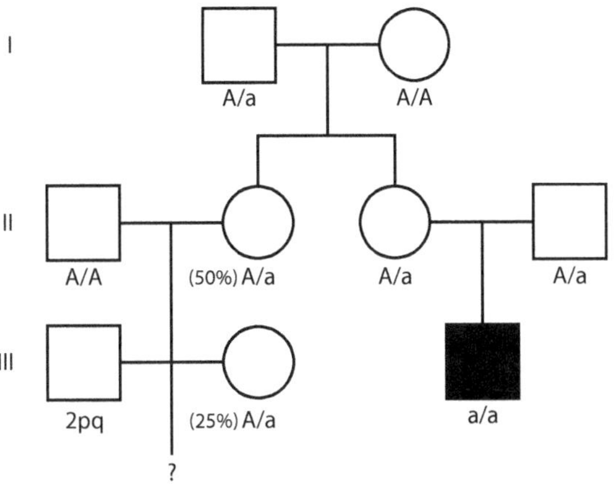

25. Correct answer is **B.** The great grandfather is stated to have had the autosomal recessive disease in question and must, therefore, have had the genotype, a/a. This means that all of his children, the maternal and paternal grandparents of the 1-year-old, would receive the mutant allele from him. The risk that the 1-year-old child's grandparents pass the mutant allele to the child's mother is 50% (1/2) as well as to the child's father is 50% (1/2). The two independent variables for the mother are that she is 50% likely to be a carrier and has a 50% chance of donating the mutant allele to her daughter. The two independent variables are identical for the father since they are first cousins. Therefore, the overall recurrence risk for the 1-year-old child is (1/2) × (1/2) × (1/2) × (1/2) = 1/16. None of the other options (choice A, C, D, and E) correctly identify the overall recurrence risk to the 1-year-old girl.

26. Correct answer is **A.** Since the woman's first child from her previous marriage has the autosomal recessive disease, the woman must be a carrier of the mutant allele. The two independent variables for the woman are 100% that she is a carrier and 50% (1/2) for the likelihood that she donates the mutant allele to any other children. The determination of the likelihood that the future husband is a carrier of a mutant allele for the autosomal recessive disease is accomplished using the Hardy-Weinberg equation. The incidence rate of the disease in the population to which the future husband belongs is 1/9000 which is the q^2 value from the Hardy-Weinberg equation. Therefore $q \approx 1/95$ (0.01). The frequency of carriers is determined from the $2pq$ value of the Hardy-Weinberg equation. Given that the frequency of the mutant allele (q) for an autosomal recessive disease is always very low, the frequency of the wild-type allele (p) is always very nearly equal to 1. Therefore, the carrier frequency for any individual in this population will be $2q$ = [2(1/95)] = 1/47.5 (0.021). The two independent variables for the future husband are 2.1% (1/47.5) that he is a carrier and 50% (1/2) for the likelihood that he donates the mutant allele to any of his children. Therefore, the overall recurrence risk for any child of this woman and her future husband is (1) × (1/2) × (1/47.5) × (1/2) = 1/190 (0.53%). None of the other options (choices B, C, D, and E) correctly identify the recurrence risk for any child of this woman and a man from the population in which the disease incidence rate is known.

27. Correct answer is **B.** Since the affected child acquired the disease as a consequence of non-Mendelian transmission, that is, the disease resulted from the inheritance of two copies of the mother's chromosome that harbors a mutant allele. Therefore, the phenotypically normal mother must be a carrier of the mutant allele. The two independent variables for the mother are 100% that she is a carrier and 50% (1/2) for the likelihood that she donates the mutant allele to any other children. The likelihood that non-Mendelian transmission of the mother's chromosome with the mutant allele occurs a second time is extremely rare and therefore not considered. The determination of the likelihood that the father is a carrier of a mutant allele for the autosomal recessive disease is accomplished using the Hardy-Weinberg equation. The incidence rate of the disease in the population to which the future husband belongs is 1/4000 which is the q^2 value from the Hardy-Weinberg equation. Therefore $q \approx 1/63$ (0.016). The frequency of carriers is determined from the $2pq$ value of the Hardy-Weinberg equation. Given that the frequency of the mutant allele (q) for an autosomal recessive disease is always very low, the frequency of the wild-type allele (p) is always very nearly equal to 1. Therefore, the carrier frequency for any individual in this population will be $2q \approx$ [2(1/63)] $\approx$ 1/31.5 (0.032). The two independent variables for the father are 1/31.5 that he is a carrier and 50% (1/2) for the likelihood that he donates the mutant allele to any of his children. Therefore, the overall recurrence risk for any child of this mother and father is (1) × (1/2) × (1/31.5) × (1/2) $\approx$ 1/125 (0.8%). None of the other options (choices A, C, D, and E) correctly identify the recurrence risk for any child of this woman and a man from the population in which the disease incidence rate is known.

28. Correct answer is **C.** Fragile X syndrome is identified as an X-linked dominant disorder. The frequency of X-linked dominant diseases in females is always twice that of males since females have two X chromosomes and thus, twice the chance for getting the dominant allele. None of the other options (choices A, B, D, and E) correctly identifies the frequency of males to females for any X-linked dominant disorder such as fragile X syndrome.

29. Correct answer is **A.** Phenylketonuria (PKU) is an autosomal recessive disorder. Since the mother's first child from her previous marriage has the autosomal recessive disease, the woman must be a carrier of the mutant allele. The two independent variables for the woman are 100% that she is a carrier and 50% (1/2) for the likelihood that she donates the mutant allele to any other children. The determination of the likelihood that the future husband is a carrier of a mutant allele for PKU is accomplished using the Hardy-Weinberg equation. The incidence rate of the disease in the population to which the future husband belongs is 1/8,100 which is the q^2 value from the Hardy-Weinberg equation. Therefore q = 1/90 (0.011). The frequency of carriers is determined from the $2pq$ value of the Hardy-Weinberg equation. Given that the frequency of the mutant allele (q) for an autosomal recessive disease is always very low, the frequency of the wild-type allele (p) is always very nearly equal to 1. Therefore, the carrier frequency for any individual in this population will be $2q$ = [2(1/90)] = 1/45 (0.022). The two independent variables for the future husband are 1/45 that he is a carrier and 50% (1/2) for the likelihood that he donates the mutant allele to any of his children. Therefore, the overall recurrence risk for any child of this woman and her future husband is (1) × (1/2) × (1/45) × (1/2) = 1/180 (0.56%). None of the other options (choices B, C, D, and E) correctly identify the recurrence risk for any child of this woman and a man from the population in which the disease incidence rate is known.

30. Correct answer is **C.** Marfan syndrome is inherited as an autosomal dominant disorder. Therefore, any children of the man will have a 50% (1/2) chance of acquiring Marfan syndrome. His future wife, his first cousin, is unlikely to harbor a mutant allele for Marfan syndrome since she is free of the symptoms of this autosomal dominant disorder. Although it is possible for the man's future wife to carry the mutant allele, but not penetrate the disease, there is insufficient evidence to calculate the potential penetration frequency for this disease in this family. None of the other options (choices A, B, D, and E) correctly identify the recurrence risk for autosomal dominant diseases, such as Marfan syndrome.

31. Correct answer is **C.** From the Hardy-Weinberg equilibrium equation it is known that the frequency of carriers for autosomal recessive disorders, such as primary hemochromatosis resulting from mutations in the *HFE1* gene, is the value of $2pq$. Given that the frequency of the mutant allele (q) for an autosomal recessive disease is always very low, the frequency of the wild-type allele (p) is always very nearly equal to 1. This means that the carrier frequency can be defined by $2q$ = 0.01. Therefore, the frequency of the mutant allele (q) in this population is 0.05. None of the other options (choices A, B, D, and E) correctly identifies the frequency of mutant HFE1 alleles in this population.

32. Correct answer is **C.** Cystic fibrosis (CF) is inherited as an autosomal recessive disorder. Since the woman's child has the autosomal recessive disease, the woman must be a carrier of the mutant allele. The two independent variables for the woman are 100% that she is a carrier and 50% (1/2) for the likelihood that she donates the mutant allele to any other children. The determination of the likelihood that her husband is a carrier of a mutant allele for CF is accomplished by knowing that he is her first cousin. Since the woman is a carrier, she must have gotten the mutant allele from one of her parents and it is 50% (1/2) likely that the mutant allele was carried by the parent who is a sibling of one the woman's first cousin's parents. This means that one of the common grandparents has a 50% (1/2) chance of being the carrier of the mutant allele that is now in the wife's genome. If one grandparent has a 50% (1/2) chance of being a carrier and a 50% (1/2) chance of donating the mutant allele to any of their children, one of the parents of the wife's first cousin (her spouse) has an overall chance of harboring the mutant allele of (1/2) × (1/2) = 1/4. This parent also has a 50% (1/2) chance of donating the mutant allele to any of their children (eg, the first cousin spouse) making the first cousin's risk of being a carrier of (1/4) × (1/2) = 1/8. The two independent variables for the husband are 1/8 that he is a carrier and 50% (1/2) for the likelihood that he donates the mutant allele to any of his children. Therefore, the overall recurrence risk for any child of this woman and her husband is (1) × (1/2) × (1/8) × (1/2) = 1/32 (3.12%). None of the other options (choices A, B, D, and E) correctly identify the recurrence risk for any child of this woman and her first cousin.

33. Correct answer is **B.** The child was most likely experiencing the symptoms of the glycogen storage disease identified as von Gierke disease. von Gierke disease is inherited as an autosomal recessive disorder. Since the woman's first child has the autosomal recessive disease, the woman must be a carrier of the mutant allele. The two independent variables for the woman are 100% that she is a carrier and 50% (1/2) for the likelihood that she donates the mutant allele to any other children. The determination of the likelihood that her husband is a carrier of a mutant allele for von Gierke disease is accomplished using the Hardy-Weinberg equation. The incidence rate of the disease in the population to which she and her husband belongs is 1/2,500 which is the q^2 value from the Hardy-Weinberg equation. Therefore q = 1/50 (0.02). The frequency of carriers is determined from the $2pq$ value of the Hardy-Weinberg equation. Given that the frequency of the mutant allele (q) for an autosomal recessive disease is always very low, the frequency of the wild-type allele (p) is always very nearly equal to 1. Therefore, the carrier frequency for any individual in this population will be $2q$ = [2(1/50)] = 1/25 (0.04). The two independent variables for the husband are 1/25 that he is a carrier and 50% (1/2) for the likelihood that he donates the mutant allele to any of his children. Therefore, the overall recurrence risk for any child of this woman and her future husband is (1) × (1/2) × (1/25) × (1/2) = 1/100 (1%). None of the other options (choices A, C, D, and E) correctly identify the recurrence risk for any child of this woman and a man from the population in which the disease incidence rate is known.

34. Correct answer is **C.** The determination of the carrier frequency for any mutant allele is accomplished using the Hardy-Weinberg equation. The incidence rate of the disease in the population is stated to be 1/250,000 which is the q^2 value from the Hardy-Weinberg equation. Therefore q = 1/500. The frequency of carriers is determined from the $2pq$ value of the Hardy-Weinberg equation. Given that the frequency of the mutant allele (q) for an autosomal recessive disease is always very low, the frequency of the wild-type allele (p) is always very nearly equal to 1. Therefore, the carrier frequency for any individual in this population will be $2q$ = [2(1/500)] = 1/250. None of the other options (choices A, B, D, and E) correctly identifies the carrier frequency of individuals from the population in which the disease incidence rate is known.

35. Correct answer is **D.** The determination of the carrier frequency for any mutant allele is accomplished using the Hardy-Weinberg equation. The mutant allele frequency is 1/50 and given that the sum of the frequencies of the mutant and wild-type alleles must be equal to 1 ($p + q = 1$), the frequency of the wild-type allele is 49/50. For a population in Hardy-Weinberg equilibrium, the heterozygote carrier frequency is $2pq = (2) \times (49/50) \times (1/50) = 98/2500 \approx 2/50 = 1/25$. None of the other options (choices A, B, C, and E) correctly identifies the carrier frequency of individuals from the population in which the frequency of the disease allele is 1/50.

36. Correct answer is **E.** The determination of the carrier frequency, homozygosity for the wild-type allele (p), and homozygosity for the mutant allele (q) can all be accomplished using the Hardy-Weinberg equation. Since the frequency of the mutant allele (q) is 0.01, and the sum of the frequencies of the mutant and wild-type alleles must equal 1 ($p + q = 1$), the frequency of the wild-type allele (p) is 1 – 0.01, or 0.99. Homozygous wild-type individuals are represented by the p^2 value from the Hardy-Weinberg equation, therefore, the percentage of homozygous wild-type individuals in this population is (0.99) × (0.99) = 0.98 = 98%. None of the other options (choices A, B, C, and D) correctly identifies the frequency of homozygous individuals in a population where the frequency of the disease allele is 1%.

37. Correct answer is **B.** Trisomy 21, Down syndrome, is the result of nondisjunction during maternal meiosis with a much greater frequency (93%) than paternal nondisjunction. The majority of Down syndrome cases result from maternal nondisjunction during meiosis I (86%). However, the results indicate that the child received a duplicate copy of only one of the maternal chromosomes (2,2,1,2). Therefore, nondisjunction most likely occurred at the second meiotic division (maternal meiosis II) after the grand paternally-derived and grand maternally-derived chromosomes separated. None of the other options (choices A, C, D, and E) can correctly explain the alleles of the marker genes present in the trisomy 21 child.

38. Correct answer is **C.** In meiosis I, each chromosome replicates into sister chromatids and then two homologous chromosomes separate to opposite poles of the cell, with each daughter cell retaining only one of the homologous pair. In meiosis II, the sister chromatids then separate resulting in haploid gametes. The affected child received both of the maternal alleles at this polymorphic locus (in addition to one paternal allele), so the nondisjunction event was most likely maternal. The child has both C and D alleles, so it must be maternal meiosis I. If the nondisjunction event occurred during maternal meiosis II (and assuming a B allele from the father), the child's haplotype would be either B,C,C or B,D,D. None of the other options (choices A, B, D, and E) correctly explains the mechanism that would generate the haplotype identified in this child.

39. Correct answer is **C.** The karyotype, 47,XX,+21, represents a female with trisomy of chromosome 21, Down syndrome. Down syndrome is the most common disorder resulting from chromosomal numerical abnormality. All autosomal monosomies such as 46,XY,−11,+21 (choice A) are incompatible with live birth. Most of the other trisomies, including 47,XX,+3 (choice B), rarely lead to live births except for trisomy 13 (Patau syndrome) and trisomy 18 (Edwards syndrome) which each occur in about 1/10,000 births. Triploidy, or 69,XXX (choice D), is seen in about 20% of spontaneously aborted fetuses but never in live births. The 46,YY karyotype (choice E) is not observed in live births as a result of the loss of critical X chromosome encoded gene functions.

40. Correct answer is **C.** The karyotype in this patient indicates that she is mosaic for monosomy of the X chromosome. A woman who is purely 45,X (Turner syndrome) most likely arose as the result of a paternal meiotic non-disjunction event (choice D and E) since more than 80% of these cases arise in this way. However, since the patient is mosaic, meaning she harbors cells that have a complete chromosome complement (46,XX) she must have received the appropriate amount of maternal and paternal genetic information at the time of fertilization. The cells in which the karyotype is 45,X would most likely have lost the second X chromosome post-fertilization. Therefore, the most likely mechanism to yield the mosaicism in this patient would be mitotic non-disjunction during development of the zygote. Maternal meiotic non-disjunction (choice A and B) is not possible for the same reason that paternal non-disjunction could not yield this particular mosaicism.

41. Correct answer is **D.** The frequency of any given haplotype is simply the product of the individual allele frequencies. Therefore, the most likely frequency of the A2-B1 haplotype is the product of the frequencies of the individual alleles which is $0.7 \times 0.8 = 0.56$. None of the other options (choices A, B, C, and E) correctly identifies the product of the frequencies of the two alleles constituting the A2-B1 haplotype.

42. Correct answer is **B.** The determination of the incidence rate of a given autosomal recessive disease can be determined using the Hardy-Weinberg equation. The carrier frequency ($2pq$) for this disease has been found to be 1/30. Given that the frequency of the mutant allele (q) for an autosomal recessive disease is always very low, the frequency of the wild-type allele (p) is always very nearly equal to 1. Therefore, the carrier frequency can be equated as $2q = 1/30$. Thus, q is equal to 1/60. The most likely incidence rate (q^2) in this close-knit community is $(1/60)^2$ or 1/3600. None of the other options (choice A, C, D, and E) correctly identifies the incidence rate for a disease in a population where the frequency of carriers of the mutant allele is 1/30.

43. Correct answer is **D.** Since males are hemizygous for the X chromosome the Hardy-Weinberg equilibrium equation cannot strictly be utilized. However, since males only have one X chromosome it can be stated that the frequency of the disease in males is equivalent to the frequency of the mutant allele (q) in males. Therefore, $q = 1/10,000$. Since females have two X chromosomes, the frequency of an X-linked recessive disease, such as hemophilia A, in females is $q^2 = 1/10^8$ which demonstrates the rarity of X-linked recessive disease manifestation in females. However, the carrier frequency for females is $2pq$ and since the frequency of the mutant allele (q) is always very low, the frequency of the wild-type allele (p) is always very nearly equal to 1. Therefore, the carrier frequency can be equated as $2q = (2) \times (1/10,000) = 1/5,000$. This demonstrates that the frequency of female carriers of recessive mutant X alleles is always twice the incidence rate of the disease in males. None of the other options (choices A, B, C, and E) correctly identifies the female carrier frequency for an X-linked recessive disease such as hemophilia A.

44. Correct answer is **E.** The patient is most likely experiencing the symptoms of a mitochondrial encephalomyopathy. The most common mitochondrial encephalomyopathies result from mutations in genes encoded by the mitochondrial genome, mtDNA. These diseases exhibit maternal specific inheritance because the mitochondria from the sperm are degraded at fertilization. All children of an affected mother will be affected with the disease regardless of their sex. None of the other pedigrees (choice A, B, C, and D) represent mitochondrially inherited diseases.

45. Correct answer is **D.** The disease represented by the pedigree is most likely autosomal recessive. Individual IV-4 is a sibling of an affected individual (IV-1) and, therefore, the most likely chance that she is a carrier of the mutant allele is 2/3. The two independent variables for individual IV-4 are 2/3 chance of being a carrier and 50% (1/2) chance of donating the mutant allele to her unborn child. Since individual IV-5 is the son of a woman with the disease (III-5) he has a 100% chance of having acquired the mutant allele. The two independent variables for individual IV-5 are 100% chance of being a carrier and 50% (1/2) chance of donating the mutant allele to his unborn child. The overall recurrence risk for their unborn child is $(2/3) \times (1/2) \times (1) \times (1/2) = 1/6$. None of the other options (choices A, B, C, and E) correctly identifies the recurrence risk for any child of individuals IV-4 and IV-5.

46. Correct answer is **D.** The child is affected at birth, indicating *in utero* exposure to high levels of maternally derived phenylalanine. Women with phenylketonuria (PKU) must strictly adhere to their special diet during pregnancy to avoid adversely affecting the fetus. Even if the father is a carrier of a mutant phenylalanine hydroxylase gene (choice C) and the child is homozygous for the mutant gene, there would have been no symptoms in the infant until 4-5 days after birth, providing the maternal blood phenylalanine level was in the normal range throughout pregnancy. Maternal translocation with unbalanced segregation in meiosis I (choice A) would likely have no effect on phenylalanine levels but might lead to trisomy. A spontaneous somatic mutation in one of the fathers *PAH* alleles (choice B) could not be passed on to the fetus and therefore, could not contribute to the symptoms observed in the neonate. Maternal uniparental disomy (choice E) simply means that two copies of a chromosome are derived from the mother and implies paternal nullisomy. Although there are rare occurrences of uniparental disomy, this mechanism is not known to be involved in any case of PKU. If maternal uniparental disomy had occurred, the child would be expected to have PKU, but symptoms would not occur until 4–5 days after birth.

47. Correct answer is **C.** The pedigree is demonstrating autosomal dominant inheritance. Marfan syndrome is autosomal dominant. Glucose-6-phosphate dehydrogenase (G6PD) deficiency (choice A) is an X-linked recessive disorder that affects the pentose phosphate pathway. The hallmark of X-linked recessive inheritance is an abundance of affected males and an absence of affected females. Males are hemizygous for the X chromosome, so the phenotype is expressed with only one dose of the gene. Females have two copies of the X chromosome, so they appear phenotypically normal although they may carry the recessive allele. Since a male inherits his X chromosome from his mother, if he is affected, she must carry the trait. Other common X-linked recessive disorders include Lesch-Nyhan syndrome, hemophilia A, and Duchenne muscular dystrophy. Leber hereditary optic neuropathy (choice B) is a relatively common cause of acute or subacute vision loss, especially in young men. It exhibits a mitochondrial inheritance pattern. The hallmark of this pattern is strict maternal inheritance. All the children of an affected woman will be affected since they receive mitochondrial genes only from the female parent. Affected males do not contribute mitochondria to progeny, so their children will not receive the trait. Sickle cell anemia (choice D) and Tay-Sachs disease (choice E) are both inherited in an autosomal recessive pattern. The distinguishing feature between autosomal dominant and recessive pedigrees is that with the former there is at least one affected individual in every generation, whereas in the latter there are skipped generation.

48. Correct answer is **B.** Myotonic dystrophy is an autosomal dominant disorder caused by the expansion of a trinucleotide repeat in the *DMPK* (dystrophia myotonica protein kinase) gene. Pedigree A represents a disease exhibiting an X-linked recessive inheritance. Pedigree C could equally be representative of an autosomal recessive or X-linked recessive mode of inheritance. Pedigree D represents a disease exhibiting X-linked dominant inheritance. Pedigree E represents a disease exhibiting mitochondrial inheritance.

49. Correct answer is **A.** The patient is most likely presenting the classic signs of achondroplasia, a disorder with autosomal dominant inheritance. Achondroplasia (ACH) is characterized by disproportionate short stature, where the limbs are shorter than the trunk, macrocephaly (excessive head size), midface hypoplasia, and lordosis (excessive inward curvature of the spine, particularly in the lumbar region). The limb shortening observed in ACH patients affects the proximal portion of the limbs such that they are shorter than the distal portions, clinically described as rhizomelic limb shortening. ACH is the result of mutations in the gene (*FGFR3*) encoding a member of the fibroblast growth factor receptor family. *FGFR3* is predominantly expressed in quiescent chondrocytes where it is responsible for restricting chondrocyte proliferation and differentiation. None of the other modes of inheritance (choices B, C, D, and E) are associated with the inheritance of ACH.

50. Correct answer is **D.** Based on the generated pedigree, the most likely mode of inheritance of the disease in the studied family is autosomal dominant. Of the diseases, only Marfan syndrome exhibits autosomal dominant inheritance. Cystic fibrosis (choice A) is inherited in an autosomal recessive manner. Fragile X syndrome is the most common form of inherited intellectual impairment and results from trinucleotide repeat expansion in the X-linked gene, *FMR1*. Hemophilia A (choice C) is a disorder of blood coagulation caused by mutations in the X-linked gene (*F8*) encoding factor VIII. Myoclonic epilepsy with ragged red fibers, MERFF (choice E) is a disorder of mitochondrial function resulting from mutations in any one of at least seven different genes encoded by the mitochondrial genome, mtDNA and as such exhibits maternal-specific mitochondrial inheritance.

51. Correct answer is **D.** The couple's first child is most likely manifesting the signs and symptoms of one of the four most common forms of osteogenesis imperfecta. The family history of the disease also strongly indicates autosomal dominant inheritance. Of the four forms of OI, type I and type II OI occur with a prevalence of 1 in 20,000 to 25,000 live births. Type II OI is a lethal form of the disorder. Infants with type II OI are usually born prematurely with a low birth weight. These infants have characteristic facial features that include dark sclera, a beaked nose and an extremely soft calvarium. Given that the infant is most likely manifesting the signs and symptoms of OI, none of the other modes of inheritance (choices A, B, C, and E) represent the most likely mode of inheritance of the disease in the infant.

52. Correct answer is **D.** The infant is most likely presenting with the classic signs of cleft lip and cleft palate. This congenital malformation syndrome is the result of multifactorial inheritance involving the impact of both one or more genes and environmental effects while *in utero*. The appearance of cleft lip and cleft palate in a newborn is not the result of any other mechanism or mode of inheritance (choices A, B, C, E, and F).

53. Correct answer is **E.** Phenylketonuria (PKU) is an autosomal recessive disease which would require a mutant allele from both parents to be passed on to any of their future children for the child to manifest this disease. The information for carrier frequency for the mother (1/3500) and the father (1/2000). In addition, they both have a 50% chance of donating the mutant allele if they are indeed carriers. Therfore, the overall likelihood that this couple having a child with phenylketonuria is $(1/3500) \times (1/2) \times (1/2000) \times (1/2) = 1/28,000,000$. Choice A represents the likelihood that the father is a carrier. Choice B represents the likelihood that the mother is a carrier. Choice D represents the most likey chance that this couple would have an affected child if the disease was transmitted in an autosomal dominant manner. Neither of the other options (choices C and F) correctly define the most likely chance of this couple having a child with PKU.

54. Correct answer is **C.** The infant is most likely exhibiting the typical congenital findings associated with DiGeorge syndrome. DiGeorge syndrome is also known as 22q11.2 deletion syndrome. The most common symptoms associated with DiGeorge syndrome are found in the newborn and include distinctive facial features such as a small chin, wide-set eyes, small low-set ears, and cleft palate. Most infants born with Digeorge syndrome also have varying degrees of heart defect ranging from mild to severe. Radiographic and echocardiographic findings in most DiGeorge syndrome infants show the characteristics of Tertralogy of Fallot, which reflects the upturned apex and concave main pulmonary artery observed in this infant. Deletion of 5p15.2-p15.3 (choice A) results in the disorder referred to as cri du chat. The characteristic features of cri du chat include a distinctive cat-like cry in infancy, low birth weight, macrocephaly, intellectual disability, and developmental delays. Deletion of 15q11-q13 (choice B) results in the imprinting disorders known as Prader Willi syndrome, PWS (associated with paternal chromosome deletion) or Angelman syndrome, AS (associated with maternal chromosome deletion). PWS patients exhibit excessive appetite and weight gain, hypotonia, developmental delay, intellectual disability, and behavioral problems. AS is also associated with developmental delay and intellectual disability, and is also associated with severe speech impairment, and hypotonia leading to movement and balance problems. Individuals with AS also often exhibit a happy demeanor with frequent laughter. Trisomy 13 (choice D) results in the disorder known as Patau syndrome, a disorder associated with heart defects, brain or spinal cord abnormalities, small or poorly developed eyes, extra fingers or toes, cleft lip, and hypotonia. Trisomy 18 (choice E) results in the disorder known as Edward syndrome that is associated with low birth weight, macrocephaly with an unusually shaped head, heart defects, and distinctive hand and foot malformations that includes clenched fists with overlapping fingers and "rocker-bottom" feet. Trisomy 21 (choice F) results in the disorder known as Down syndrome which is associated with some degree of intellectual disability and developmental delay along with a characteristic set of physical features that includes a flattened face, upward slanting eyes, and small ears.

55. Correct answer is **B.** The symptoms manifesting in this family are most likely reflective of mitochondrial encephalopathy, lactic acidosis, and stroke-like episodes (MELAS) which is a strictly mitochondrially inherited disorder. The pedigree generated from this family is also indicative of a mitochondrial disorder. Most disorders that are strictly mitochondrial, meaning they result solely from mutations in the mitochondrial genome (mtDNA), manifest with variable symptoms even within family members harboring the same mtDNA mutation. This phenomenon is a consequence of mitochondrial heteroplasmy which refers to the fact that a single cell in any given tissue, can contain several thousands of copies of mtDNA distributed within the several hundreds of individual mitochondria within that cell. Allelic heterogeneity (choice A) refers to the circumstance where the same disorder results from different mutations in the same gene, often presenting with variable levels of manifestation. Imprinting (choice C) involves the phenomenon of parental-specific manifestation of phenotype and is the result of differential DNA methylation status. Locus heterogeneity (choice D) refers to the circumstance where the same disorder results from mutations in different genes. Pleiotropy (choice E) refers to the phenomenon where mutations in a single gene influence multiple, seemingly unrelated phenotypic traits.

56. Correct answer is **C.** The increased nuchal translucency observed in the ultrasound is indictive, but not diagnostic, of Down syndrome, a syndrome resulting from chromosomal trisomy, specifically, trisomy 21. Down syndrome is highly correlated with maternal age as in the case for this woman. The identification of increased nuchal translucency with ultrasound would justify a more definitive diagnostic testing such as amniocentesis, chorionic villus sampling (CVS), and karyotype analysis of blood samples taken after birth. Although the use of noninvasive prenatal testing (NIPT) that analyzes fetal DNA in maternal blood can indicate a relative risk of a fetus having Down syndrome, like ultrasound, it is only indicative not diagnostic for the disorder. The majority of Down syndrome individuals acquired the trisomy 21 as a result of meiotic nondisjunction occurring during the completion of meiosis I in female eggs as a consequence of ovulation. Although Down syndrome can result from germline mosaicism (choice A) and from unbalanced translocations (choice D) involving chromosome 21 and another chromosome, these are not the most likely cause, being associated with less than 5% of Down syndrome patients. Neither of the other mechanisms (choices B and E) are associated with the cause of Down syndrome.

57. Correct answer is **B.** Duchenne muscular dystrophy is an X-linked recessive disorder so affected children are almost exclusively male. Since the wife's brother has DMD, her mother is an obligate carrier of the mutation in the dystrophin gene. All mothers of affected sons, and all daughters of affected fathers are obligate carriers for X-linked recessive alleles. Since the wife's mother is known to be an obligate carrier, the wife has a 50% chance of being a carrier herself and she has a 50% chance of donating the mutant allele to any of her children. However, since only males will manifest the symptoms of DMD, and there is a 50% chance that the couple will have a male child, the overall risk of them having a child with DMD is $(1/2) \times (1/2) \times (1/2) = 1/8$. Not taking into account the independent variable associated with one of two possible sexes would lead to ½ (choice D) being selected. None of the other options (choices A, C, and E) correctly identifies the most likely risk of this couple having a child with DMD.

58. Correct answer is **C.** The symptoms that the siblings of both the man and woman display most likely indicates that they have sickle cell anemia. Sickle cell anemia is an autosomal recessive disease which means that individuals who have siblings with the disease are themselves 2/3 likely to be carriers of the mutant allele. Both the man and the woman have a 50% chance of donating the mutant allele to any of their children so the most likely overall risk for this couple to have a child with the same disease manifesting in their siblings is $(2/3) \times (1/2) \times (2/3) \times (1/2) = 1/9$. None of the other options (choices A, B, D, and E) correctly identifies the most likely risk that this couple will have an affected child.

59. Correct answer is **E.** The pedigree generated from the family in question most likely demonstrates autosomal dominant inheritance associated with incomplete penetration. The incomplete penetration is evident in individual III-5 since she and her unrelated, unaffected male partner have three children, two of whom are affected with the disorder present in numerous individuals in the woman's family. In autosomal dominant inheritance, the likelihood affected individuals having affected children is 50% regardless of sex. The fact that individual III-5 had over 50% of her children affected by the disease is a strong indication of incomplete penetration. Allelic heterogeneity (choice A) refers to the circumstance where the same disorder results from different mutations in the same gene, often presenting with variable levels of manifestation. Anticipation (choice B) is a genetic phenomenon associated with disorders resulting, most commonly, from trinucleotide repeat expansion. These disorders exhibit increased severity and earlier onset with each successive generation. Codominance (choice C) refers to the phenotypes from two alleles for a trait being expressed equally in a heterozygote such that neither allele masks the other. Imprinting (choice D) involves the phenomenon of parental-specific manifestation of phenotype and is the result of differential DNA methylation status. Variable expressivity (choice F) refers to the phenomenon where two individuals harboring the same mutant allele exhibit different signs and symptoms.

60. Correct answer is **A.** The patient is most likely experiencing the signs and symptoms associated with glucose-6-phosphate dehydrogenase (G6PDH) deficiency (see Clinical Box 8–2). Many patients with G6PDH deficiency remain asymptomatic until an acute stimulus triggers a hemolytic attack, such as infections or drug interactions. Drugs used to treat and prevent malaria, such as primaquine and tafenoquine, are known to cause severe hemolytic anemia in G6PDH deficient individuals. The hemolytic anemia associated with G6PDH deficiency is a result of defective oxidant responses in red blood cells. The increased oxidation of hemoglobin results in its denaturation and cross-linking via cysteine sulfhydryl formation generating clumps of hemoglobin. These clumps can be visualized in a blood smear with the use of a supravital stain like new methylene blue as shown in the Figure with this question. The gene encoding glucose-6-phosphate dehydrogenase is located on the X chromosome and thus, G6PDH deficiency is an X-linked disorder. Therefore, this disorder cannot be transmitted from males to males. None of the other values (choices B, C, D, and E) correctly define the risk that this patient will have a male child with the same disease.

61. Correct answer is **A.** The researchers are most likely studying the related muscular dystrophies, identified as Duchenne muscular dystrophy (DMD) and Becker muscular dystrophy (BMD), that result from mutations in the gene encoding the intracellular protein, dystrophin. Given that the dystrophin gene is found on the X chromosome, both of these diseases are inherited in an X-linked manner. The primary clinical differences between DMD and BMD are due to the fact that the mutations in the *DMD* gene that cause Duchene muscular dystrophy result in virtually no functional dystrophin protein being made. With Becker muscular dystrophy the mutations result in some functional dystrophin protein ranging from 10% to 40% of the normal level of function. Allelic heterogeneity refers to the circumstance where the same, or similar, disorder results from different mutations in the same gene, often presenting with variable levels of manifestation. Germline mosaicism (choice B) refers to the condition where some of an individual's germ cells carry a mutation, while others do not. This means a parent harboring germline mosaicism may not show symptoms of a genetic condition themselves but can still pass the mutation on to their children, who may or may not exhibit the condition. Imprinting (choice C) involves the phenomenon of parental-specific manifestation of phenotype and is the result of differential DNA methylation status. Locus heterogeneity (choice D) refers to the circumstance where the same disorder results from mutations in different genes. Pleiotropy (choice E) refers to the phenomenon where mutations in a single gene influence multiple, seemingly unrelated phenotypic traits.

62. Correct answer is **E.** The disease that is most likely present in the family being studied is Marfan syndrome. Anticipation (choice A) is a genetic phenomenon associated with disorders resulting, most commonly, from trinucleotide repeat expansion. These disorders exhibit increased severity and earlier onset with each successive generation. Imprinting (choice B) involves the phenomenon of parental-specific manifestation of phenotype and is the result of differential DNA methylation status. Incomplete penetrance (choice C) refers to the circumstance where, in some individuals, the presence of a mutant allele, which should manifest a clinical phenotype, does not actually result in the expected clinical phenotype. Somatic mosaicism (choice D) refers to the circumstance where there is the presence of two or more cells, with different genetic or chromosomal compositions, within the same individual. This phenomenon results from post-zygotic mutation.

63. Correct answer is **D.** Based upon the pedigree generated by the medical geneticist, the most likely mode of inheritance in mitochondrial and thus, the genetic alteration responsible for the disease in this family is most likely associated with mitochondrial DNA, mtDNA. None of the other chromosomal locations (choices A, B, C, E, and F) can account for the pedigree generated from the individuals in the family studied by the medical geneticist.

64. Correct answer is **D.** The patient is most likely exhibiting the signs and symptoms of familial hypercholesterolemia, where the most common form (classic) of this disorder is the result of autosomal dominant inheritance of mutations in the gene encoding the LDL receptor. Classic familial hypercholesterolemia (FH) results in lifelong elevation of LDL-cholesterol (LDL-C) in the blood. The resultant hypercholesterolemia leads to premature coronary artery disease and atherosclerotic plaque formation in the coronary arteries and the aorta. None of the other pedigrees depict autosomal dominant inheritance. Pedigree A most likely represents an X-linked dominant disease since all the daughters of an affected male (II-2) have the disease and at least half of the children of an affected female (I-2) have the disease. Pedigree B most likely represents a mitochondrial disease since the transmission is found in individuals in each generation and, most telling, all the children, regardless of sex, of affected females (I-2 and II-4) have the disease. In addition, no children, regardless of sex, of an affected male (II-2) have the disease. Pedigree C most likely represents an autosomal recessive trait since there are very few affected individuals; there is very nearly always equal numbers of affected males and females, and the transmission is not vertically penetrant. Pedigree E most likely represents an X-linked recessive disorder since only males are affected, and the transmission is not fully vertically penetrant.

65. Correct answer is **A.** The pedigree generated from the husband's family most likely represents a disease that is transmitted as an autosomal dominant disorder. The disease is present in every generation and is nearly equally distributed between males and females, classical representation of an autosomal dominant form of inheritance. None of the other patterns of inheritance (choices B, C, D, and E) are represented by the generated pedigree.

66. Correct answer is **C.** Since mutations in the gene that was identified by the medical genetics research group exert effects in a gain-of-function manner, it is dominant and thus only one allele is required to confer the type 2 diabetes in this population. Given the Hardy-Weinberg assumptions, this means that individuals that harbor one mutant allele ($2pq$) and those that harbor 2 copies of the mutant allele (q^2) will harbor the disease. Since it has been determined that the frequency of the mutant allele (q) in this population is 20%, the frequency of the wild-type allele (p) must be 80%. If $q = 0.20$, then $q^2 = 0.04$. Therefore, the sum of $2pq + q^2$ is $(2) \times (0.8) \times (0.20) + 0.04 = 0.36$. In other words, 36% of individuals in this population must be harboring at least one mutant allele of the gene responsible for the inherited form of type 2 diabetes. None of the other values (choices A, B, D, and E) correctly define the most likely percentage of individuals harboring at least one disease allele.

67. Correct answer is **E.** The child is most likely exhibiting the signs associated with the childhood eye cancer, retinoblastoma. In the familial form of retinoblastoma individuals inherit a mutant, loss-of-function allele from an affected parent. A subsequent later somatic mutational event, referred to as loss of heterozygosity (LOH), inactivates the normal allele resulting in retinoblastoma development. This leads to an apparently dominant mode of inheritance. The requirement for an additional somatic mutational event at the unaffected allele means that penetration of the defect is not always complete. Indeed, the penetration frequency for retinoblastoma is not 100% but closer to 90%, meaning not all individuals who inherit what is supposed to be a genetically dominant disease-causing allele, actually develop retinoblastoma. Allelic heterogeneity (choice A) refers to the phenomenon of different mutations in the same gene being associated with the same disease. This phenomenon leads to the potential for variable phenotypic expression and is typical for most disease genes. Incomplete penetrance (choice B) refers to the circumstance where, in some individuals, the presence of a mutant allele, which should manifest a clinical phenotype, does not actually result in the expected clinical phenotype. This phenomenon is distinct from the LOH that is required for the development of retinoblastoma. Imprinting (choice C) involves the phenomenon of parental-specific manifestation of phenotype and is the result of differential DNA methylation status. Incomplete penetrance (choice C) refers to the circumstance where, in some individuals, the presence of a mutant allele, which should manifest a clinical phenotype, does not actually result in the expected clinical phenotype. Linkage disequilibrium (choice D) refers to the non-random association of alleles at different loci on a chromosome. What this means is that certain combinations of alleles tend to occur together more often than would be expected by chance.

68. Correct answer is **C.** Given that 75% of the population is free of the disease, and with Hardy-Weinberg assumptions, this value is represented by the sum of homozygous wild-type individuals (p^2) and carriers ($2pq$). From this it can be determined that the percentage of individuals with the disease (q^2) will be $q^2 = 1 - (p^2 + 2pq)$ which is $1 - 0.75 = 0.25$. Since the value of q^2 is 0.25, the disease allele (q) prevalence is 0.50. Given that the sum of p and q must be equal to 1, the prevalence of the wild-type allele (p) must also be 0.50. None of the other values (choices A, B, D, and E) correctly define the prevalence of the wild-type allele in the population preseting the husband and wife.

69. Correct answer is **B.** The patient is most likely manifesting the signs and symptoms of Leber hereditary optic neuropathy, LHON. Mutations in at least nine genes in the mitochondrial genome (mtDNA) have been identified as being responsible for the manifestation of the symptoms of LHON. The symptoms of LHON usually present in midlife (mean age of onset 27–35 years) and these symptoms are predominantly restricted to the visual system. The primary symptoms associated with LHON include acute or subacute central vision loss that initially manifests with blurring and clouding of vision ultimately leading to blindness. Typical ocular findings upon ophthalmoscopic examination of LHON patients optic disc hyperemia (redness and swelling) and peripapillary telangiectasias that are small, dilated vessels around the optic disc. The head of the optic nerve may also appear swollen. Males manifest symptoms of LHON more often than females. None of the other pedigrees depict mitochondrial inheritance. Pedigree A most likely represents an X-linked dominant disease since all the daughters of an affected male (II-2) have the disease and at least half of the children of an affected female (I-2) have the disease. Pedigree C most likely represents an autosomal recessive trait since there are very few affected individuals; there is very nearly always equal numbers of affected males and females, and the transmission is not vertically penetrant. Pedigree D most likely represents an autosomal dominant disorder since there is an affected individual in all generations, there are very nearly equal numbers of affected males and females, and there is male-to-male transmission, the latter eliminating X-linked inheritance. Pedigree E most likely represents an X-linked recessive disorder since only males are affected, and the transmission is not fully vertically penetrant.

70. Correct answer is **C.** Given that 96% of the population are free of the disease, and with Hardy-Weinberg assumptions, this value is represented by the sum of homozygous wild-type individuals (p^2) and carriers ($2pq$). From this it can be determined that the percentage of individuals with the disease (q^2) will be $q^2 = 1 - (p^2 + 2pq)$ which is $1 - 0.96 = 0.04$. Since the value of q^2 is 0.04, the disease allele (q) prevalence is 0.20 or 20%. None of the other values (choices A, B, D, and E) correctly define the prevalence of the mutant allele in the population being studied by the research group.

71. Correct answer is **C.** The patient is most likely manifesting the signs and symptoms of MELAS (mitochondrial encephalopathy, lactic acidosis, and stroke-like episodes), a disorder that results from mutations in any one of at least 10 genes located on the mitochondrial genome, mtDNA. Symptoms of MELAS usually appear in early childhood following a period of normal growth with more than 75% of patients experiencing symptoms before the age of 20. The earliest symptoms of MELAS include muscle weakness and pain, recurrent headaches, loss of appetite, vomiting, and seizures. Due to the involvement of mitochondria, skeletal muscle metabolism is greatly affected resulting in frequent and severe lactic acidosis. The lactic acidosis is a major contributor to the vomiting, abdominal pain, extreme fatigue, and muscle weakness experienced by MELAS patients. Most individuals with MELAS experience stroke-like episodes beginning before age 40. Since mtDNA mutations are very nearly exclusively transmitted by females, all children of affected females will manifest the disorder. The family history confirms the mitochondrial inheritance since the patient's mother most likely suffered from MELAS, leading to her death from cardiomyopathy, and similar symptoms were presented in his maternal grandmother and maternal uncle. The patient's disorder is most likey not transmitted by any of the other modes of inheritance (choices A, B, D, E, and F).

72. Correct answer is **D.** The incidence of sickle cell anemia in the population, of which the husband and wife are members, is 4% which is the value (0.04) for q^2. This means that the frequency of the disease allele (q) in this population is 20% or 0.2. None of the other values (choices A, B, C, and E) correctly represent the frequency of the disease-causing allele in the population to which the husband and wife belong.

73. Correct answer is **B.** The constructed pedigree most likely represents a disease whose mode of inheritance is autosomal recessive. There are three aspects of the pedigree that strongly indicate autosomal recessive inheritance. One is that the presence of the disease skips generations, that is, is not vertically penetrant, another is that the disease is found in nearly equal numbers of males and females, and lastly the disease is transmitted from males (II-2) to males (III-3) indicating that the transmission cannot be X-linked (choices D and E). Neither of the remaining two patterns of inheritance (choices A and C) are defined by the constructed pedigree.

74. Correct answer is **D.** The boy is most likely manifesting the signs and symptoms of Fragile X syndrome. Fragile X syndrome is an X-linked dominant disorder, not X-linked recessive (choice E), representing the most common form of inherited intellectual impairment. Fragile X syndrome results from the expansion of a CGG trinucleotide repeat in the *FMR1* (fragile X messenger ribonucleoprotein 1) gene which encodes the FMRP protein. The CGG repeat resides in the 5′-untranslated region (UTR) of the *FMR1* gene. The molecular consequences of the amplification of the CGG repeat are the presentation of CpG dinucleotide sites that can be methylated on the cytidine. Indeed, the trinucleotide repeat expansion leads to epigenetic transcriptional silencing due to hypermethylation of the promoter region of the *FMR1* gene. Dominant negative inheritance (choice A), also known as antimorph inheritance, refers to a genetic mechanism where a mutated gene product interferes with the normal function of the corresponding wild-type gene product, resulting in the manifestation of an abnormal phenotype even in the presence of the normal allele. Meiotic nondisjunction (choice B) refers to the abnormal process that occurs during meiosis resulting in the failure of the separation of sister chromatids (meiosis I) or sister chromosomes (meiosis II). Nondisjunction can occur either during meiosis I or during meiosis II. When nondisjunction occurs, some of the resulting haploid gametes will lack a particular chromosome while others will end up with more than one copy. Somatic mutation (choice C) refers to the generation of a mutation in a gene in post-zygotic (somatic) cells. These types of mutations are commonly observed in cancers but they cannot be transmitted to the affected individual's children.

75. Correct answer is **C.** The incidence of the disease in this population is 15 out of 6000 or 0.25%. This means that the value for $q^2 = 0.0025$ so $q = 0.05$. Since the value of the wild-type allele (p) frequency and the mutant allele frequency must be equal to 1, the value of $p = 0.95$. Since the disease is adherent to the assumptions of the Hardy-Weinberg law the value of carriers is equal to $2pq$. Therefore, the carrier frequency is $(2) \times (0.95) \times (0.05) = 0.095$ or 9.5%. None of the other values (choices A, B, D, and E) correctly represent the frequency of carriers in the population under study.

76. Correct answer is **D.** The incidence of sickle cell anemia in the population, of which the husband and wife are members, is 4% which is the value (0.04) for q^2. This means that the frequency of the disease allele (q) in this population is 20% or 0.2. Since the value of the wild-type allele (p) frequency and the mutant allele frequency must be equal to 1, the frequency of the wild-type allele (p) must be 80% or 0.8. From the Hardy-Weinberg equilibrium equation it is understood that the frequency of carriers is equal to $2pq$, or $(2) \times (0.8) \times (0.2) = 0.32$ or 32%. None of the other values (choices A, B, C, and E) correctly represent the likelihood that the husband or the wife are carriers of the sickle cell disease allele.

77. Correct answer is **A.** The patient is most likely manifesting the signs and symptoms of Turner syndrome. Turner syndrome is a female-specific disorder that results from the loss of part or all one of the two X chromosome, thus the karyotype of these individuals is designated 45,X, also sometimes designated as 45,X0. The karyotype 46,XY (choice B) designates a genetically normal male. The karyotype 46,XX,t(9;22)(q34;q11) (choice C) represents a female with the Philadelphia chromosome associated form of chronic myelogenous leukemia, CML. The karyotype 47,XXY (choice D) is associated with the disorder referred to as Kleinfelter syndrome. Kleinfelter syndrome is exclusive to males and thus cannot be representative of the patient in this question. An individual with trisomy 21 (choice E) will manifest the symptoms of Down syndrome which is associated with some degree of intellectual disability and developmental delay along with a characteristic set of physical features that includes a flattened face, upward slanting eyes, and small ears. These physical signs and symptoms do not reflect the observations in this patient.

78. Correct answer is **C.** Given that the sum of the frequency of the mutant allele (q) and the wild-type allele (p) must be equal to 100%, with a disease allele frequency of 12% the frequency of the wild-type allele must be 88%. From the Hardy-Weinberg equilibrium equation it is understood that the frequency of carriers is equal to $2pq$, or $(2) \times (.88) \times (.12) = 0.21$ or 21%. None of the other values (choices A, B, D, and E) correctly represent the frequency of disease allele carriers in the population being studied.

79. Correct answer is **D.** Given the incidence rate in the husband's population the value for q^2 is 1/3600, therefore the disease allele frequency is 1/60. Given the incidence rate in the general population, which presumes the wife's population, the value for q^2 is 1/40,000; therefore, the disease allele frequency is 1/200. Since carrier frequency for autosomal recessive diseases is $2pq$, and the value for the wild-type allele, p, is statistically very nearly equal to 1, the carrier frequency for the husband is $2q = 1/30$ and for the wife is $2q = 1/100$. To bear a child with the disease, the mutant allele must be transmitted from each parent, both of whom have a ½ chance of doing so. Therefore, the overall risk for this couple to have a child with the autosomal recessive disease is $(1/2) \times (1/30) \times (1/2) \times (1/100) = 1$ in 12,000. None of the other options (choices A, B, C, and E) correctly identify the most likely probability that any of the offspring of the couple being counseled will be affected by the disease.

80. Correct answer is **E.** Diseases, like cystic fibrosis, that are the result of mutations in a single gene, yet display multiple diverse phenotypes in different organ systems, exhibit the phenomenon of pleiotropy. Pleiotropy refers to the phenomenon whereby mutations in a single gene influence two or more seemingly unrelated phenotypic traits. For example, Marfan syndrome, which is caused by mutations in the gene (*FBN1*) encoding the connective tissue protein fibrillin, is associated with the skeletal anomaly known as arachnodactyly (long thin extremities), while in the cardiovascular system the disease leads to dilation of the aortic root. Allelic heterogeneity (choice A) refers to the phenomenon of different mutations in the same gene being associated with the same disease. This phenomenon leads to the potential for variable phenotypic expression and is typical for most disease genes. Locus heterogeneity (choice B) refers to the circumstance where the same disorder results from mutations in different genes. Mosaicism (choice C) can be either somatic or germline. Somatic mosaicism refers to the occurrence of two, or more, genetically distinct populations of cells within an individual that are not the result of mutations in the germ cells from which the individual was generated. Germline mosaicism refers to the condition where some of an individual's germ cells carry a mutation, while others do not. Multifactorial inheritance (choice D) refers to disorders that generally do not follow one of the typical Mendelian patterns inheritance of single gene disorders because they are the result of the complex interactions among a number of genetic variants as well as certain environmental exposures.

www.ingramcontent.com/pod-product-compliance
Lightning Source LLC
LaVergne TN
LVHW082003200926
848481LV00010B/2794